MEDICAL-SURGICAL NURSING

Patient-Centered Collaborative Care

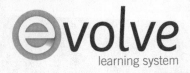
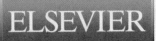

MEDICAL-SURGICAL NURSING

Patient-Centered Collaborative Care

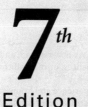

7th

Edition

Donna D. Ignatavicius, MS, RN, ANEF

Speaker and Curriculum Consultant for Academic Nursing Programs
Founder, Boot Camp for Nurse Educators®
President, DI Associates, Inc.
Placitas, New Mexico

M. Linda Workman, PhD, RN, FAAN

Senior Volunteer Faculty
College of Nursing
University of Cincinnati
Cincinnati, Ohio;
Formerly Gertrude Perkins Oliva Professor of Oncology
Frances Payne Bolton School of Nursing
Case Western Reserve University
Cleveland, Ohio

ELSEVIER

ELSEVIER
SAUNDERS

3251 Riverport Lane
St. Louis, Missouri 63043

MEDICAL-SURGICAL NURSING:
PATIENT-CENTERED COLLABORATIVE CARE-

ISBN (single volume): 978-1-4377-2801-9
ISBN (2-volume set): 978-1-4377-2799-9

International Standard Book Number (single volume): 978-1-4377-2801-9
International Standard Book Number (2-volume set): 978-1-4377-2799-9

Executive Content Strategist: Lee Henderson
Senior Content Development Specialist: Rae L. Robertson
Publishing Services Manager: Deborah L. Vogel
Senior Project Manager: Jodi M. Willard
Design Direction: Paula Catalano

Printed in United States of America

Last digit is the print number: 9 8 7 6 5 4 3

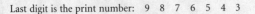

QSEN CONSULTANTS

Gail Armstrong, DNP, ACNS-BC, CNE
Assistant Professor
University of Colorado—Denver
College of Nursing
Denver, Colorado

Mary A Dolansky, PhD, RN
Veterans Administration Quality
  Scholarship Faculty
Assistant Professor
Frances Payne Bolton School of Nursing
Case Western Reserve University
Cleveland, Ohio

CONTRIBUTORS

Judy Laver Bierschbach, MSN, ARNP
Nurse Practitioner
Center for Perioperative Care, UC Health
Cincinnati, Ohio

Deanne A. Blach, MSN, RN
Nurse Educator;
President, DB Productions
Green Forest, Arkansas
Concept Maps

Katherine L. Byar, MSN, ANP-BC
Hematological Malignancy Nurse
  Practitioner
University of Nebraska Medical Center
Omaha, Nebraska

Robin Chard, PhD, RN, CNOR
Adjunct Faculty
College of Allied Health & Nursing
Nova Southeastern University
Fort Lauderdale, Florida

Tammy L. Coffee, MSN
Acute Care Nurse Practitioner
MetroHealth Medical Center
Cleveland, Ohio

Janice Cuzzell, RN, MA
Certified Wound Specialist and Clinical
  Consultant
Savannah, Georgia

Laura M. Dechant, APN, MSN, CCRN, CCNS, BC
Clinical Nurse Specialist
Christiana Care Health System
Newark, Delaware

Cheryl J. Dumont, PhD, RN
Director of Nursing Research and Vascular
  Access Team
Winchester Medical Center
Winchester, Virginia

Ronald L. Hickman, Jr., PhD, RN, ACNP-BC
Assistant Professor
Frances Payne Bolton School of Nursing
Case Western Reserve University
Cleveland, Ohio

Mary Justice, MSN, CNE
Associate Professor
University of Cincinnati—Raymond
  Walters College
Cincinnati, Ohio

Mary K. Kazanowski, APRN, PhD, CHPN
Palliative Care Nurse Practitioner
VNA Home Care and Hospice of
  Manchester and Southern New
  Hampshire
Manchester, New Hampshire;
Concord Hospital
Concord, New Hampshire

Linda A. LaCharity, PhD, RN
Accelerated Program Director
Assistant Professor
College of Nursing
University of Cincinnati
Cincinnati, Ohio

Linda Laskowski-Jones, RN, MS, ACNS-BC, CEN, FAWM
Vice President, Emergency, Trauma &
  Aeromedical Services
Christiana Care Health System
Wilmington, Delaware

Rona F. Levin, PhD, RN
Professor
Pace University
Pleasantville, New York

Richard Lintner, RT(R), (CV), (MR), (CT), ARRT
Program Director
School of Interventional Radiology;
Manager
Interventional Radiology
Kansas University Medical Center
Kansas City, Kansas
Interventional radiology content

Tami Kathleen Little, MS, RN
Nursing Faculty
School of Nursing
Brookline College
Phoenix, Arizona

Margaret Elaine McLeod, MSN, BC-ADM, ACNS-BC, CDE
Clinical Nurse Specialist
Veterans Administration Medical Center
Tennessee Valley Healthcare System
Nashville, Tennessee

Rachel L. Palmieri, MS, RN-C/ANP
Adult Nurse Practitioner
Armed Forces Services Corporation
Arlington, Virginia

Cherie R. Rebar, PhD, RN, MBA, FNP
Associate Director, Division of Nursing;
Chair, AS & BSN Nursing Programs
Kettering College
Kettering, Ohio

Harry C. Rees III, MSN, ACNP-BC
Acute Care Nurse Practitioner
Anesthesia Critical Care
Cleveland Clinic;
Anticoagulation Clinic
MetroHealth Medical Center
Cleveland, Ohio

James G. Sampson, DNP, ANP-C, AAHNS
Adult Nurse Practitioner, Clinical Supervisor
Infectious Disease/AIDS Clinic
Denver Health Medical Center
Denver, Colorado

Karen Toulson, MSN, RN, MBA, CEN, NE-BC
Nurse Manager, Emergency Department
Christiana Care Health System
Newark, Delaware

Shirley E. Van Zandt, MS, MPH, CRNP
Instructor and Nurse Practitioner, School of Nursing
Johns Hopkins University
Baltimore, Maryland

Chris Winkelman, PhD, RN, CCRN, ACNP
Associate Professor
Frances Payne Bolton School of Nursing
Case Western Reserve University;
Cleveland, Ohio

Fay Wright, RN, MS, ACNP-BC
Doctoral Student
College of Nursing
New York University
New York, New York

Pamela C. Zickafoose, EdD, MSN, RN, CNA-BC, CNE
Instructor of Nursing
Delaware Technical & Community College—Terry Campus
Dover, Delaware

CONTRIBUTORS TO TEACHING/LEARNING RESOURCES

Audience Response System Questions (in PowerPoint® Slides)

Mary Beth Flynn Makic, PhD, RN, CNS, CCNS, CCRN
Assistant Professor, Adjoint
College of Nursing
University of Colorado—Anschutz Medical Campus;
Research Nurse Scientist
University of Colorado Hospital
Aurora, Colorado

QSEN Content in TEACH® for Nurses Lesson Plans

Gail Armstrong, DNP, ACNS-BC, CNE
Assistant Professor
College of Nursing
University of Colorado
Denver, Colorado

Tammy Sue Spencer, RN, MS, CNE, ACNS-BC, CCNS
Senior Instructor
Department of Nursing
University of Colorado College of Nursing
Aurora, Colorado

PowerPoint® Slides

Katrina Allen, RN, MSN, CCRN
Nursing Instructor, Clinical Coordinator
Faulkner State Community College
Bay Minette, Alabama

Linda A. LaCharity, PhD, RN
Accelerated Program Director
Assistant Professor
College of Nursing
University of Cincinnati
Cincinnati, Ohio

Cherie R. Rebar, PhD, MBA, RN, FNP
Associate Director, Division of Nursing;
Chair, AS & BSN Nursing Programs
Kettering College
Kettering, Ohio

TEACH® for Nurses Lesson Plans

Carolyn Gersch, MSN, RN, CNE
Assistant Director; Associate Professor
Division of Nursing
Kettering College
Kettering, Ohio

Cherie R. Rebar, PhD, MBA, RN, FNP
Associate Director, Division of Nursing;
Chair, AS & BSN Nursing Programs
Kettering College
Kettering, Ohio

Teaching Tips

Rosalinda Alfaro-LeFevre, RN, MSN, ANEF
President
Teaching Smart/Learning Easy
Stuart, Florida

Gail Armstrong, DNP, ACNS-BC, CNE
Assistant Professor
College of Nursing
University of Colorado
Denver, Colorado

Amy J. Barton, PhD, RN, FAAN
Professor and Associate Dean, Clinical and Community Affairs
College of Nursing
University of Colorado—Anschutz Medical Campus
Aurora, Colorado

Tim Bristol, PhD, RN, CNE
Director
Nursing Education Consultants
Ingram, Texas

Test Bank

Meg Blair, PhD, MSN, RN, CEN
Associate Professor, Nursing
Nebraska Methodist College
Omaha, Nebraska

Linda Hughes, PhD, RN, CCRN
Director of Undergraduate Programs, Nursing
Nebraska Methodist College
Omaha, Nebraska

Tami Little, MS, RN
Nursing Faculty
School of Nursing
Brookline College
Phoenix, Arizona

Karen Montalto, PhD
BSN Chair and Associate Professor
School of Nursing and Allied Health Professions
Holy Family University
Philadelphia, Pennsylvania

Key Points (Expanded)

Peggy Slota, RN, DNP, FAAN
Associate Professor; Director
DNP and Graduate Nursing Leadership Programs
School of Nursing
Carlow University
Pittsburgh, Pennsylvania

NCLEX® Examination Challenge and Decision-Making Challenge Answers

Nancy Haugen, PhD, MN, RN
Associate Professor and ABSN Program Chair
Samuel Merritt University
Oakland, California

Tamara Kear, PhD, RN
Assistant Professor of Nursing
College of Nursing
Villanova University
Villanova, Pennsylvania

M. Linda Workman, PhD, RN, FAAN
Senior Volunteer Faculty
College of Nursing
University of Cincinnati
Cincinnati, Ohio;
Formerly Gertrude Perkins Oliva Professor
of Oncology
Frances Payne Bolton School of Nursing
Case Western Reserve University
Cleveland, Ohio

Review Questions for the NCLEX® Examination

Susan Nickell Behmke, MS, RN
Professor
College of Southern Maryland
La Plata, Maryland

Stephanie C. Butkus, MSN, APRN, CPNP
Associate Professor
Division of Nursing
Kettering College
Kettering, Ohio

Marilyn J. Herbert-Ashton, MS, RN, BC
Associate Professor
Virginia Western Community College
Roanoke, Virginia

Lisa A. Hollett, BSN, RN, MA, MICN
Trauma Program Manager
Department of Trauma Services
St. John Medical Center
Tulsa, Oklahoma

Andrea Rothman Mann, MSN, RN, CNE
Third Level Chair and Instructor
Aria Health School of Nursing
Philadelphia, Pennsylvania

Mitch Seal, EdD, Med-IT, RN-BC
Commander, Nurse Corps, U.S. Navy
Associate Director of Standards &
Evaluation
Medical Education & Training Campus
Fort Sam Houston, Texas

Diane K. Daddario, MSN, ACNS-BC, RN-BC, CMSRN
Nursing Instructor
Pennsylvania College of Technology
Williamsport, Pennsylvania;
Nurse Specialist
Geisinger Medical Center
Danville, Pennsylvania;
Staff Nurse
Evangelical Community Hospital
Lewisburg, Pennsylvania

Fernande E. Deno, MSN, RN
Anoka Ramsey Community College
Coon Rapids, Minnesota

Jennifer Duhon, RN, MS
Director of Health Services
Lutheran Hillside Village
Peoria, Illinois

Helen Freeman, MSN, RN, BC
Web Development Manager
Chamberlain College of Nursing
Columbus, Ohio

Bradley R. Harrell, DNP, ACNP-BC, CRN
Assistant Professor
School of Nursing
Union University
Germantown, Tennessee

Mimi Haskins, MS, RN, CMSRN
Roswell Park Cancer Institute
Buffalo, New York

Nancy Haugen, PhD, MN, RN
Associate Professor and ABSN Program
 Chair
Samuel Merritt University
Oakland, California

LaWanda Herron, PhD, RN, MSA, FNP-BC
Holmes Community College
Grenada, Mississippi

Paula Hopper, MSN, RN
Jackson Community College
Jackson, Mississippi

Jamie Lynn Jones, MSN, RN
University of Arkansas at Little Rock
Little Rock, Arkansas

Tamara Marie Kear, PhD, RN
Gwynedd-Mercy College
Gwynedd Valley, Pennsylvania

Mary Ann Kolis, MSN, RN, ANP-BC, APNP
Instructor
Gateway Technical College
Kenosha, Wisconsin

Charles Preston Molsbee, EdD, MSN, RN, CNE
University of Arkansas at Little Rock
Little Rock, Arkansas

Jason Mott, MSN, RN
Instructor of Nursing
School of Nursing
Bellin College
Green Bay, Wisconsin

Kristin E. Oneail, MSN, RN
Instructor
University of Detroit Mercy
Detroit, Michigan

Rebecca Lynn Purdy, MSN, RN
Assistant Professor of Nursing
Morehead State University
Morehead, Kentucky

Cherie R. Rebar, PhD, MBA, RN, FNP
Associate Director, Division of Nursing;
Chair, AS & BSN Nursing Programs
Kettering College
Kettering, Ohio

Mary Lou Robinson, PhD, RN
Professor and Assistant to the Chair
Lewis-Clark State College
Lewiston, Idaho

Mitchell J. Seal, EdD, Med-IT, RN-BC
Deputy Director of Standards & Evaluation
Medical Education & Training Campus;
Adjunct Faculty
Cerro Coso College
San Antonio, Texas

Susan M. Seiboldt, MSN, RN, CNE
Assistant Professor of Nursing
Carl Sandburg College
Galesburg, Illinois

Denise Sevigny, RN, MSN
Adjunct Faculty
School of Nursing
Old Dominion University
Norfolk, Virginia

Brenda K. Shelton, MS, RN, CCRN, AOCN
The Sidney Kimmel Comprehensive Cancer
 Center at Johns Hopkins
Baltimore, Maryland

Leah R. Shreves, MSN, RN
Assistant Professor of Nursing
Edison Community College
Piqua, Ohio

Karyn Skiathitis, MSN, RN, CPAN
Clinical Coordinator/Faculty
Department of Nursing
California State University—Northridge
Northridge, California

Jana Wiscaver Thompson, MSNc, RN
Assistant Professor
Department of Nursing
University of Arkansas at Little Rock
Little Rock, Arkansas

Cynthia W. Ward, MSN, RN-BC, CMSRN, ACNS-BC
RN IV
Centra—Lynchburg General Hospital
Lynchburg, Virginia

Julie M. Willenbrink, MSN, RN
Edison Community College
Piqua, Ohio

Lisa J. Wolf, MS, RN, CMSRN
Mount Carmel West Hospital
Columbus, Ohio

The first edition of this textbook, entitled *Medical-Surgical Nursing: A Nursing Process Approach,* received widespread acclaim in the early 1990s. The following five editions built on that achievement and further solidified the book's position as a major trendsetter for the practice of adult health nursing. Now in its seventh edition, "Iggy" charts an essential course for the future of adult nursing practice—a course reflected in its current title: *Medical-Surgical Nursing: Patient-Centered Collaborative Care.* The focus of this new edition continues to be to help students learn how to provide safe, quality care that is patient-centered, evidence-based, and collaborative.

The book's subtitle was carefully chosen to emphasize the nurse's role in providing patient care in collaboration with members of the interdisciplinary team in both acute care and community-based settings. The Institute of Medicine (IOM), The Joint Commission, the National Quality Forum, and other health care organizations have called for all health professionals to coordinate and deliver patient care as a collaborative care team. In addition, the 2010 IOM *Future of Nursing* report states that nurses need to have requisite competencies, including research and evidence-based practice, and teamwork and collaboration to deliver safe, high-quality care in specific content areas such as community health and geriatrics.

Patient safety is also emphasized in this edition with references to The Joint Commission's National Patient Safety Goals initiative (http://www.jointcommission.org/standards_information/npsgs.aspx). A new feature for the seventh edition, Nursing Safety Priority boxes, enables students to immediately identify the most important care needed for patients with specific health problems. These highlighted features are further classified as Action Alerts, Drug Alerts, or Critical Rescue boxes.

KEY THEMES FOR THE 7TH EDITION

The seventh edition continues to use the term "patient" instead of "client" throughout. Although the use of these terms remains a subject of discussion among nursing educators, we have not defined the patient as a dependent person. Rather, the patient can be an individual, a family, or a group, all of whom have rights that are respected in a mutually trusting nurse-patient relationship. Most health care agencies and professional organizations use "patient" in their practice and publications. In addition, many nursing organizations support the term.

As in the sixth edition, the seventh edition relates the focus of critical thinking to an emphasis on nursing judgment to make timely and appropriate clinical decisions. To help achieve that focus, all new case-based Decision-Making Challenges based on the Quality and Safety Education (QSEN) core competencies have been integrated throughout the text. These exercises provide clinical situations in which students can practice on-the-spot decision making to help prepare them for the fast-paced world of medical-surgical nursing and become competent nurses. Suggested answer guidelines

for these Decision-Making Challenges are provided on the book's Evolve website (http://evolve.elsevier.com/Iggy/).

In addition to this key theme of clinical decision-making, the seventh edition also emphasizes "readiness"—readiness for the NCLEX® Examination, readiness for major emergencies such as we saw in the aftermath of the events of 9/11 and recent natural disasters, readiness for safe drug administration, and readiness for the new world of genetics and genomics that is unfolding before us. An increased number of NCLEX® Examination Challenges, now including some with alternate-format items, are interspersed throughout the text to allow students the opportunity for practice in test-taking.

As the nursing shortage becomes more acute, it is more critical than ever that students be ready to pass the licensure exam on the first try. To help both students and faculty achieve that outcome, chapter-opening Learning Outcomes are consistent with the objectives outlined in the detailed NCLEX-RN® Test Plan. The seventh edition also continues to include an innovative end-of-chapter feature called "Get Ready for the NCLEX® Examination!" This unique and popular learning aid consists of a list of Key Points *organized by Client Needs Category* as found in the NCLEX-RN® Test Plan.

To further help students connect previously learned concepts with new information in the text, six Concept Overviews introduce groups of content units. These unique features review basic concepts learned in nursing fundamentals courses—such as oxygenation and protection—to help students make connections between fundamental concepts and patient care for medical-surgical conditions. At the end of each body system chapter, Nursing Concept Reviews apply these same concepts to the health problems presented in the chapter. Dr. Christine Tanner's clinical judgment framework is used to help students apply these concepts (Tanner, 2006). The components of this model include that clinical nurses use nursing judgment to provide quality care by:

- Noticing
- Interpreting
- Responding
- Reflecting

This seventh edition includes a new chapter—Chapter 7: Evidence-Based Practice in Medical-Surgical Nursing—written by evidence-based practice (EBP) experts Dr. Rona F. Levin and Fay Wright. This chapter discusses the importance of EBP and incorporating it into nursing care. This chapter, along with the Evidence-Based Practice boxes throughout the book, offers a solid foundation in this increasingly important aspect of nursing practice emphasized by the QSEN initiative.

Additional themes carried over from the previous edition are an emphasis on women's health issues, genetic/genomic considerations, cultural awareness, complementary and alternative therapies, and the special needs of older adults. In addition, concepts of case management and community-based care are interwoven throughout to help students identify the role of the nurse in providing continuing patient care.

CLINICAL CURRENCY AND ACCURACY

To ensure the book's currency and accuracy, we listened to students and faculty who have used the previous editions, focusing on their impressions of and experiences with the book. We reviewed documents crafted by a variety of health care organizations, including the Institute of Medicine (IOM), The Joint Commission (TJC), and the Institute for Healthcare Improvement (IHI). Recent nursing education publications were also examined, such as those authored by the National League for Nursing (NLN), the American Association of Colleges of Nursing (AACN), and Dr. Patricia Benner and her colleagues in their book *Educating Nurses: A Call for Radical Transformation* (2010). A thorough nursing education literature search of best current evidence helped us validate best practices and national health care trends to help shape the focus of the seventh edition.

We also commissioned in-depth reviews of every chapter by clinicians and instructors from across the United States and used their reviews to guide us in revising the chapters into their final form. A well-respected interventional radiologist ensured the accuracy of selected diagnostic testing procedures and associated patient care.

The results of these efforts are reflected in the seventh edition's:

- Strong, consistent focus on NCLEX-RN® Examination preparation, clinical decision making, patient-centered collaborative care, pathophysiology, drug therapy, evidence-based clinical practice, and community-based care
- Foundation of relevant research and best practice guidelines
- Emphasis on the critical "need to know" information that beginning nurses must master to provide safe patient care

Best Practice for Patient Safety & Quality Care charts help highlight the most important nursing care. Our Evidence-Based Practice boxes include a Commentary section, as well as a rating of the level of evidence based on a well-respected scale outlined in Chapter 7.

With today's knowledge explosion, it is easy for a book to become larger with each new edition. However, today's nursing students have a limited time to absorb and begin to apply the information essential for medical-surgical nursing care. Therefore in this seventh edition we eliminated some of the content found in previous foundation courses or other specialty textbooks. We limited our discussions to how these concepts are used in adult nursing and focused on content that was "need to know" for safe, quality nursing practice.

OUTSTANDING READABILITY

Today's students need to be able to read information once and understand it; they do not have time to repeatedly read the same information. To achieve this level of readability, the text has a more direct-address style (wherever appropriate) that speaks directly to the reader, and sentences are as short as possible without sacrificing essential content.

Reading level is highly influenced by the length of sentences and the length of words. Although we can control the length of the sentences, medical terms are often 4 to 5 syllables long and tend to skew a chapter's reading level.

Nevertheless, the result of our efforts is a med-surg text of consistently outstanding readability. The average reading level is 10th to 11th grade. It is important to note that reducing the reading level of this edition did not reduce the quality or depth of content that students need to know. Instead, the content is clear, focused, and accessible.

EASE OF ACCESS

To make the text as easy to use as possible, we have maintained the previous editions' approach of smaller chapters of more uniform length. Although we eliminated some of the foundational content in the first unit of the last edition and added one new chapter, the seventh edition remains 76 chapters long.

We also have maintained the unit structure of previous editions, with vital body systems (cardiovascular, respiratory, and neurologic) appearing earlier in the book. In these three units we continue to provide complex care content in separate chapters that discuss managing critically ill patients with coronary artery disease, respiratory health problems, and neurologic health problems.

To help break up long blocks of text and also to highlight key information, we continue to include numerous headings, bulleted lists, tables, charts, and in-text highlights. Key Terms are in boldface color type and are defined in the text to foster the learning of need-to-know vocabulary. A glossary is located in the back of the book. Chapter bibliographies have been moved to the back of the book to save space in chapters for need-to-know content. These current bibliographic resources include research articles, nationally accepted clinical guidelines, and other sources of evidence when available for each chapter. Classic sources from before 2008 are noted with an asterisk (*).

A PATIENT-CENTERED COLLABORATIVE CARE APPROACH

As in all previous editions, we take a collaborative care approach to patient care. We believe that in the real world of health care, nurses, patients, and other health care providers (including physicians, advanced-practice nurses, and physician's assistants) *share* responsibility for the management of patient problems. Thus we present patient care in a collaborative care framework. In this framework we make no *artificial* distinctions between medical treatment and nursing care. Instead, under each Patient-Centered Collaborative Care heading we discuss how the nurse coordinates care and interacts with members of the health care team as appropriate for the patient's health problems, including health promotion and illness prevention.

This edition includes newly redesigned patient-centered Concept Maps that underscore this collaborative care approach. Each Concept Map contains a case scenario. It then shows how a selected complex health problem is addressed. Each Concept Map spells out the steps of the nursing process and related concepts to illustrate the relationships among disease processes, priority patient problems, collaborative management, and more.

Although our approach is collaborative, the text is first and foremost a *nursing* text. We therefore use a nursing process approach as a tool to organize discussions of patient health problems and their management. Discussions of *major* health problems follow a full nursing process format using this structure:

[Health problem]
    Pathophysiology
        Etiology (and Genetic Risk when appropriate)
        Incidence/Prevalence
    Health Promotion and Maintenance (when appropriate)
    Patient-Centered Collaborative Care
        Assessment
        Analysis
        Planning and Implementation
            [Collaborative Intervention Statement (based on priority patient problems)]
            Planning: Expected Outcomes
            Interventions
        Community-Based Care
            Home Care Management
            Teaching for Self-Management
            Health Care Resources
        Evaluation: Outcomes

The Analysis sections list the priority patient problems (collaborative problems and nursing diagnoses) associated with major medical disorders. This seventh edition uses official NANDA-I nursing diagnosis language where it applies; however, most health care agencies prefer to identify collaborative patient problems or needs as the basis for the interdisciplinary plan of care rather than being restricted to NANDA-I language, which addresses primarily nursing-oriented patient problems. With its more flexible interweaving of NANDA-I diagnoses and collaborative patient problems or needs, the seventh edition more closely aligns with the language of actual clinical practice. The nursing diagnoses used in this edition are the 2012-2014 NANDA-I diagnoses—the most recently approved diagnoses at the time of publication of this edition. Health Promotion and Maintenance sections are found in selected discussions.

Discussions of less common or less complex disorders, although not given this complete subhead structure, nonetheless follow the same basic format: a discussion of the problem itself (including pertinent information on pathophysiology) followed by a section on collaborative care of patients with the disorder. To demonstrate our commitment to providing the content foundational to nursing education and consistent with the recommendations of Benner and colleagues through the Carnegie Foundation for the Future of Nursing Education, we highlight throughout this edition essential pathophysiologic concepts that are key to understanding the basis for collaborative management.

Integral to this collaborative care approach is a clear delineation of just who is responsible for what. When a responsibility is primarily the nurse's, the text says so. When a decision must be made jointly by the patient, nurse, physician, and physical therapist, for example, this is clearly stated. When different health care practitioners in different care settings might be involved in the patient's care, this is stated.

ORGANIZATION

The 76 chapters of *Medical-Surgical Nursing: Patient-Centered Collaborative Care* are grouped into 16 units. Unit 1, Foundations for Medical-Surgical Nursing, lays the foundation for the health care concepts incorporated throughout the text. Unit 2 consists of three chapters on concepts of emergency and trauma care and disaster preparedness.

Unit 3 consists of three chapters on the management of patients with fluid, electrolyte, and acid-base imbalances. Chapters 13 and 14 review key assessments and related patient care in a clear, concise discussion. The chapter on infusion therapy (Chapter 15) is supplemented with an online Fluids & Electrolytes Tutorial on the companion Evolve website.

Unit 4 presents the perioperative nursing content that medical-surgical nurses need to know. This content provides a solid foundation to help the student better understand the collaborative care required for the surgical patient.

Unit 5 provides core content on health problems related to immune system function. This content includes normal inflammation and the immune response, altered cell growth and cancer development, and interventions for patients with connective tissue disease, HIV infection, and other immunologic disorders, cancers, and infections.

The remaining 11 units, subdivided and introduced by the six Concept Overviews, cover medical-surgical content by body system. Each of these units begins with an Assessment chapter and continues with one or more Nursing Care chapters for patients with selected health problems in that body system. This framework is familiar to students who learn the body systems in preclinical foundational science courses such as anatomy and physiology.

MULTINATIONAL, MULTICULTURAL, MULTIGENERATIONAL FOCUS

To reflect the increasing diversity of our society, *Medical-Surgical Nursing: Patient-Centered Collaborative Care* takes a multinational, multicultural, and multigenerational focus. Addressing the needs of both U.S. and Canadian readers, we have included examples of trade names of drugs available in the United States and in Canada. Drugs that are available only in Canada are designated with a ✺ symbol. When appropriate, we identify specific Canadian health care resources, including their websites.

To help nurses provide quality care for patients whose cultural background may differ from their own, numerous Cultural Awareness boxes highlight important aspects of culturally competent care throughout the text. A revised and expanded cultural health chapter (Chapter 4) includes specific information about lesbian, gay, bisexual, and transgender (LGBT) health and health care, as well as special needs associated with homelessness and dwarfism. Located in an appendix is an innovative Communication Quick Reference for Spanish-Speaking Patients. This Quick Reference helps ensure clear communication between native English speakers and the rapidly growing population who speak Spanish as a first language.

Increases in life expectancy and the "graying" of the baby-boom generation add up to a steadily increasing older adult population. To help equip nurses for this challenge, the seventh edition continues to provide thorough coverage of the care of older adults. Chapter 3 offers content on the role of the nurse and health care team in promoting health for older adults in the community. It also provides coverage of common health problems that older adults may have in the health care setting, such as falls and inadequate nutrition. The text includes many Nursing Focus on the Older Adult charts. Laboratory values and drug dosages typical for older patients are also included throughout the book. Charts specifying normal physiologic changes to expect in the older population are found in each Assessment chapter. In addition, Considerations for Older Adults boxes are included throughout the text to emphasize key points to consider when caring for these patients.

Also appearing throughout the text are Women's Health Considerations boxes, which address topics of concern to women and their health care providers. These in-text highlights alert the reader to gender-related differences in assessment parameters and in the incidence, severity, and treatment of common health problems.

ADDITIONAL LEARNING AIDS

As in previous editions, the seventh edition continues to include a rich array of learning aids geared toward adult learners to help students quickly identify and understand key information and to serve as study aids.

- Written in "patient-friendly" language, Patient and Family Education: Preparing for Self-Management charts provide the types of instructions that nurses must learn to provide to patients and their families to help them cope with life changes caused by illness.
- Laboratory Profile charts summarize important information on laboratory tests commonly used to evaluate health problems. Information typically includes normal ranges of laboratory values (including differences for older adults, when appropriate) and the possible significance of abnormal findings.
- Common Examples of Drug Therapy charts summarize important information about commonly used drugs. Most charts include both U.S. and Canadian trade names for typically used drugs, usual dosages (including dosages for older patients, as appropriate), and nursing interventions with rationales.
- Key Features charts highlight the clinical manifestations of important health problems based on pathophysiologic concepts.
- Evidence-Based Practice boxes, provided in nearly every chapter, give synopses of recent nursing research articles and other scientific articles applicable to nursing. Each box provides a brief summary of the research, its level of evidence (LOE), and a brief commentary with implications for nursing practice and future research. The purpose of this feature is to help students identify the strengths and weaknesses of the research and to see how research guides nursing practice.
- As in the previous editions, Home Care Assessment charts serve as a convenient summary of essential assessment points for patients who need follow-up home health nursing care.
- Assessment Using Gordon's Functional Health Patterns charts provide a convenient one-stop list of questions to ask patients about the impact of health conditions on everyday function.
- New to this edition, subtypes of Decision-Making Challenges emphasize the six QSEN core competencies:

Patient-Centered Care, Teamwork and Collaboration, Evidence-Based Practice, Quality Improvement, Safety, and Informatics.

AN INTEGRATED MULTIMEDIA RESOURCE BASED ON PROVEN STRATEGIES FOR STUDENT ENGAGEMENT AND LEARNING

Medical-Surgical Nursing: Patient-Centered Collaborative Care, 7th edition, is the centerpiece of a comprehensive package of electronic and print learning resources that break new ground in the application of proven strategies for student engagement, learning, and evidence-based educational practice. This integrated multimedia resource actively engages the student in problem solving and practicing clinical decision-making skills.

Resources for Instructors

For the convenience of faculty, all Instructor Resources are available on a streamlined, secure instructor area of the Evolve website (http://evolve.elsevier.com/Iggy/). Included among these Instructor Resources are the exciting new *TEACH for Nurses* Lesson Plans. These Lesson Plans focus on the most important content from each chapter and provide innovative strategies for student engagement and learning. Lesson Plans are provided for each chapter and are categorized into several parts:

    Objectives
    Teaching Focus
    Key Terms
    Nursing Curriculum Standards
        QSEN
        Concepts
        BSN Essentials
    Student Chapter Resources
    Instructor Chapter Resources
    Teaching Strategies

Additional Instructor Resources provided on the Evolve website include:

- A completely revised, updated, high-quality Test Bank consisting of 2260 items, both traditional multiple-choice and NCLEX-RN® "alternate" item types. Each question is coded for correct answer, rationale, cognitive level, NCLEX Integrated Process, and NCLEX Client Needs Category. Page references are provided for Remembering (Knowledge)- and Understanding (Comprehension)-level questions. (Questions at the Applying [Application] and above cognitive level require the student to draw on understanding of multiple or broader concepts not limited to a single textbook page, so page cross references are not provided for these higher-level critical thinking questions.) The Test Bank is provided in ExamView, ParTest, and rich-text formats.
- An electronic Image Collection containing all images from the book (approximately 630 images), delivered in a format that makes incorporation into lectures, presentations, and online courses easier than ever.
- PowerPoint Presentations—a collection of over 2000 slides corresponding to each chapter in the text and highlighting key content with integrated images and

Unfolding Case Studies. Audience Response System Questions (three discussion-oriented questions per chapter for use with iClicker and other audience response systems) are folded into these slide presentations.

- Guest Lectures—Seven ready-to-use narrated Power-Point presentations by Dr. Workman covering topics with which both students and faculty tend to struggle.
- Faculty Development Videos—two videos by Donna Ignatavicius addressing (1) the implications of changes in the NCLEX-RN® Examination for faculty and (2) curriculum transformation.

Also available for adoption and separate purchase, Simulation Learning System (SLS) helps faculty make the best use of high-fidelity patient simulators.

Resources for Students

Resources for students include a revised and updated Clinical Decision-Making Study Guide, a Clinical Companion, a Virtual Clinical Excursions workbook/CD-ROM, and Evolve Learning Resources.

The *Clinical Decision-Making Study Guide* has been revised and updated and features a continued emphasis on clinical decision making, priorities of delegation, management of care, and pharmacology. The use of Case Studies is expanded in this edition, and documentation questions have been added to most chapters to provide practice with this important aspect of the evaluation step of the nursing process.

The pocket-sized *Clinical Companion* is a handy clinical resource that retains a popular alphabetical organization and streamlined format. It now includes new "Critical Rescue," "Drug Alert," and "Action Alert" highlights throughout based on the Nursing Safety Priority features in the textbook. National Patient Safety Goals highlights underscore the importance of observing vital patient safety standards. This "pocket-sized Iggy" has been tailored to the special needs of students preparing for clinicals and clinical practice.

The *Virtual Clinical Excursions 3.0* workbook/CD-ROM package, featuring an updated and easy-to-navigate "virtual" clinical setting, will once again be available for the seventh edition. This unique learning tool guides students through a virtual clinical environment and helps them "learn by doing" in the safety of a "virtual" hospital. The clinical simulations and workbook represent the next generation of research-based learning tools to promote critical thinking and meaningful learning.

Also available for students is a dynamic collection of Evolve Student Resources, available at http://evolve.elsevier.com/Iggy/. The Evolve Student Resources —*organized by student learning needs* —include the following:

- Review Questions for the NCLEX® Examination
- Answer Guidelines for NCLEX® Examination and Decision-Making Challenges
- Interactive Case Studies
- Concept Maps (digital versions of the 12 Concept Maps from the text)
- Concept Map Creator (a handy tool for creating customized Concept Maps)
- Fluid & Electrolyte Tutorial (a complete self-paced tutorial on this perennially difficult content)
- Chapter Reviews (downloadable expanded key points for each chapter)
- Health Assessment Image Collection (supplemental images of common assessment findings)
- Audio Glossary
- Audio Clips, Animations, and Video Clips
- Content Updates

For more information on any of these innovative companion resources, contact your Elsevier Educational Solutions Consultant, visit http://www.us.elsevierhealth.com/, or contact Elsevier Faculty Support at 1-800-222-9570 or sales.inquiry@elsevier.com.

In summary, *Medical-Surgical Nursing: Patient-Centered Collaborative Care*, 7th edition, together with its fully integrated multimedia ancillary package, provides the tools you will need to meet the challenge of nursing in the second decade of the 21st century and beyond. The only elements that remain to be added to this package are those that you alone can provide—your diligence, your commitment, your innovation, *your nursing expertise.*

Donna D. Ignatavicius
M. Linda Workman

To Charles and Stephanie
Thank you for your unending support, love, and understanding
during every edition; I could not do this without you!
Stephanie, I especially appreciate your editorial help.

To students and faculty
Thank you for your feedback, support, and guidance
during my journey as an author over many years.

Donna

To students everywhere, who inspire us to make each edition better.

To GBW: Your courage and integrity are limitless.

Linda

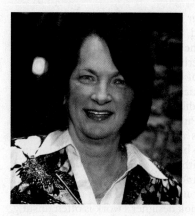

Donna D. Ignatavicius received her diploma in nursing from the Peninsula General School of Nursing in Salisbury, Maryland. After working as a charge nurse in medical-surgical nursing, she became an instructor in staff development at the University of Maryland Medical Center. She then received her BSN from the University of Maryland School of Nursing. For 5 years she taught in several schools of nursing while working toward her MS in Nursing, which she received in 1981. Donna then taught in the BSN program at the University of Maryland, after which she continued to pursue her interest in gerontology and accepted the position of Director of Nursing of a major skilled-nursing facility in her home state of Maryland. Since that time, she has served as an instructor in several associate degree nursing programs. Through her consulting activities and faculty development workshops, Donna has gained national recognition in nursing education. She is currently the President of DI Associates, Inc. (http://www.diassociates.com/), a company dedicated to improving health care through education and consultation for faculty. In recognition of her contributions to the field, she was inducted as a charter Fellow of the prestigious Academy of Nursing Education in 2007.

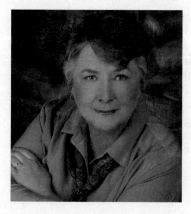

M. Linda Workman, a native of Canada, received her BSN from the University of Cincinnati College of Nursing and Health. After serving in the U.S. Army Nurse Corps and working as an Assistant Head Nurse and Head Nurse in civilian hospitals, Linda earned her MSN from the University of Cincinnati College of Nursing and a PhD in Developmental Biology from the University of Cincinnati College of Arts and Sciences. Linda's 30-plus years of academic experience include teaching at the diploma, associate degree, baccalaureate, and master's levels. Her areas of teaching expertise include medical-surgical nursing, physiology, pathophysiology, genetics, oncology, and immunology. Linda has been recognized nationally for her teaching expertise and was inducted as a Fellow into the American Academy of Nursing in 1992. She received Excellence in Teaching awards at the University of Cincinnati and at Case Western Reserve University. She is a former American Cancer Society Professor of Oncology Nursing and held an endowed chair in oncology for 5 years. In addition to authoring several textbooks and serving as a consult for major universities, she is Senior Volunteer Faculty at the College of Nursing, University of Cincinnati.

Publishing a textbook and ancillary package of this depth and breadth would not be possible without the combined efforts of many people. Stephanie M. Ignatavicius assisted with literature searches and the revision of Chapter 4 (Cultural Aspects of Health and Illness). Paul W. Elliott, Jr. helped develop the Concept Overview feature for Mobility, Sensation, and Cognition.

Our contributing authors once again provided consistently excellent manuscripts in a timely fashion. Special thanks to Deanne Blach, who redesigned our Concept Maps. Our reviewers—expert clinicians and instructors from around the United States and Canada—provided invaluable suggestions and encouragement throughout the book's development.

The staff of Elsevier/Saunders once again provided us with crucial guidance and support throughout the planning, writing, revision, and production of the seventh edition. In particular, Executive Content Strategist Lee Henderson worked closely with us from the early stages of this edition to help us hone and focus our revision plan, and Lee coordinated the project from start to finish. Senior Content Development Specialist Rae Robertson then worked with us step-by-step to bring the seventh edition from vision to publication. Rae, Julia Curcio, and Kelly McGowan held the reins of our complex ancillary package and worked with a gifted group of writers and content experts to provide an outstanding library of resources to complement and enhance the text. Special thanks to Content Coordinator Kelly McGowan, who not only managed the *Clinical Companion* but also handled the countless administrative details associated with a project of this size.

Senior Project Manager Jodi Willard was once again a joy to work with. If, as is said, the mark of a good editor is that her work is invisible to the reader, then Jodi is the consummate editor. Her unwavering attention to detail, flexibility, and conscientiousness not only helped to make this edition the most consistently readable ever, but also made the entire production process incredibly smooth.

Special thanks also to Publishing Services Manager Debbie Vogel. For three editions now, Debbie has worked quietly behind the scenes to help bring the book to publication precisely on schedule and with a very high level of quality.

Designer Paula Catalano is responsible for the beautiful cover and the completely new interior design of the seventh edition. The praise of a book designer's work is often unsung, but Paula's work on this edition has cast important features in exactly the right light, with neither too much nor too little emphasis, making this edition not only practical and easy to read, but also beautiful.

Our acknowledgments would not be complete without recognizing our dedicated team of Educational Solutions Consultants and other key members of the Sales and Marketing staff who helped to put this book into your hands.

Finally, we wish to thank Sally Schrefer (Managing Director, Nursing and Health Professions), Loren Wilson (Vice President and Publisher, Nursing), Tom Wilhelm (Vice President, eSolutions, Nursing), and Robin Carter (Director, eContent Solutions, Nursing) for their ongoing vision, direction, and support for state-of-the-art educational resources for nurses.

Donna D. Ignatavicius
M. Linda Workman

CONTENTS

UNIT VI	PROBLEMS OF PROTECTION: MANAGEMENT OF PATIENTS WITH PROBLEMS OF THE SKIN, HAIR, AND NAILS

CONCEPT OVERVIEW: OXYGENATION AND TISSUE PERFUSION

UNIT VII   PROBLEMS OF OXYGENATION: MANAGEMENT OF PATIENTS WITH PROBLEMS OF THE RESPIRATORY TRACT

UNIT VIII   PROBLEMS OF CARDIAC OUTPUT AND TISSUE PERFUSION: MANAGEMENT OF PATIENTS WITH PROBLEMS OF THE CARDIOVASCULAR SYSTEM

UNIT XII   **PROBLEMS OF MOBILITY: MANAGEMENT OF PATIENTS WITH PROBLEMS OF THE MUSCULOSKELETAL SYSTEM**

CONCEPT OVERVIEW: NUTRITION, METABOLISM, AND BOWEL ELIMINATION

UNIT XIII   **PROBLEMS OF DIGESTION, NUTRITION, AND ELIMINATION: MANAGEMENT OF PATIENTS WITH PROBLEMS OF THE GASTROINTESTINAL SYSTEM**

UNIT XIV   PROBLEMS OF REGULATION AND METABOLISM: MANAGEMENT OF PATIENTS WITH PROBLEMS OF THE ENDOCRINE SYSTEM

GUIDE TO SPECIAL FEATURES

COMMON EXAMPLES OF DRUG THERAPY

CONCEPT MAP

EVIDENCE-BASED PRACTICE

FOCUSED ASSESSMENT

HOME CARE ASSESSMENT

KEY FEATURES

LABORATORY PROFILE

NURSING FOCUS ON THE OLDER ADULT

PATIENT AND FAMILY EDUCATION: PREPARING FOR SELF-MANAGEMENT

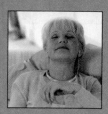

CHAPTER

48

Assessment of the Eye and Vision

M. Linda Workman

evolve WEBSITE

http://evolve.elsevier.com/Iggy/

Answer Key for NCLEX Examination Challenges and
    Decision-Making Challenges
Audio Glossary
Key Points

Review Questions for the NCLEX® Examination
Video Clip: Central Vision
Video Clip: External Eye
Video Clip: Pupil Responses

LEARNING OUTCOMES

Safe and Effective Care Environment

1. Use aseptic technique when touching the eyelids or external eye structures.
2. Use appropriate technique when instilling eyedrops or eye ointments.
3. Verify that informed consent has been obtained before invasive tests of the eye or vision are performed.

Health Promotion and Maintenance

4. Teach all people about the use of eye protection equipment and strategies.
5. Perform health history and risk assessment for eye and vision problems.
6. Teach patients who have systemic health problems that may affect eye health and vision to adhere to prescribed therapies and to have yearly eye examinations by an ophthalmologist.

Psychosocial Integrity

7. Teach patients and family members about what to expect during tests and procedures to assess vision and eye problems.
8. Provide the opportunity for the patient and family to express their concerns about a possible change in vision.

Physiological Integrity

9. Explain the concept of refraction in relation to how the cornea, lens, aqueous humor, and vitreous humor contribute to vision.
10. Explain the relationship between intraocular pressure and eye health.
11. Use knowledge of anatomy and psychomotor skills when assessing the eye and vision.
12. Explain the eye changes associated with aging and their impact on vision.
13. Interpret the findings of visual acuity by the Snellen chart.

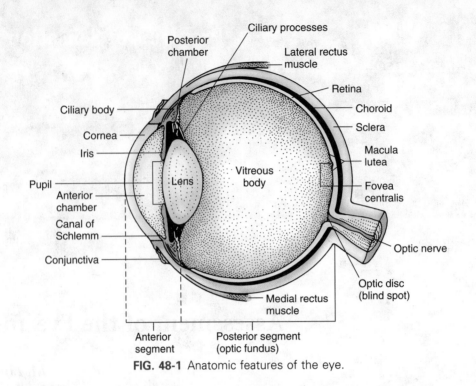

FIG. 48-1 Anatomic features of the eye.

The eye works with the brain to cause vision. Many people consider vision to be the most important sense for sensation and cognition. It is used to assess surroundings, allow independence, warn of danger, appreciate beauty, work, play, and interact with other people.

Vision begins with the eye, where light is changed into nerve impulses. These impulses are sent to the brain, where images are fully perceived. Many systemic conditions, as well as eye problems, affect the eye and change vision temporarily or permanently. Changes in the eye and vision can provide information about the patient's general health status and problems that might occur in self-care.

ANATOMY AND PHYSIOLOGY REVIEW

Structure

The eyeball, a round, ball-shaped organ, is located in the front part of the eye orbit. The orbit is the bony socket of the skull that surrounds and protects the eye along with the attached muscles, nerves, vessels, and tear-producing glands.

Layers of the Eyeball

The eye has three layers, or coats (Fig. 48-1). The external layer is the sclera (the opaque tissue making up the "white" of the eye) and the transparent cornea on the front of the eye.

The middle layer, or uvea, is heavily pigmented and consists of the choroid, the ciliary body, and the iris. The choroid, a dark brown membrane between the sclera and the retina, lines most of the sclera. It has many blood vessels that supply nutrients to the retina.

The ciliary body connects the choroid with the iris and secretes aqueous humor. The iris is the colored portion of the external eye; its center opening is the pupil. The muscles of the iris contract and relax to control pupil size and the amount of light entering the eye.

The innermost layer is the retina, a thin, delicate structure made up of sensory photoreceptors that begin the transmission of impulses to the optic nerve. The retina contains blood vessels and two types of photoreceptors called *rods* and *cones*. The rods work at low light levels and provide peripheral vision. The cones are active at bright light levels and provide color and central vision.

The optic fundus is the area at the inside back of the eye that can be seen with an ophthalmoscope. This area contains the optic disc, a creamy pink or white depressed area where the fine nerve fibers that synapse with the photoreceptors join together to form the optic nerve and exit the eyeball. The optic disc is sometimes called the "blind spot" because it contains only nerve fibers and no photoreceptor cells. To one side of the optic disc is a small, yellowish pink area called the *macula lutea.* The center of the macula is the *fovea centralis,* where vision is the most acute.

Refractive Structures and Media

Light waves pass through these structures on the way to the retina: cornea, aqueous humor, lens, and vitreous humor. Each structure has a different density, which causes the light waves to bend (refract) and focus images on the retina. Together, these structures are the eye's *refracting media.*

The cornea is the clear layer that forms the external bump on the front of the eye (see Fig. 48-1). The aqueous humor is a clear, watery fluid that fills the anterior and posterior chambers of the eye. Aqueous humor is continually produced by the ciliary processes and passes from the posterior chamber, through the pupil, and into the anterior chamber. This fluid drains through the canal of Schlemm into the blood to maintain a balanced intraocular pressure (IOP), the pressure within the eye (Fig. 48-2).

The lens is a circular, convex structure that lies behind the iris and in front of the vitreous body. It is normally transparent and bends the rays of light entering through the pupil so

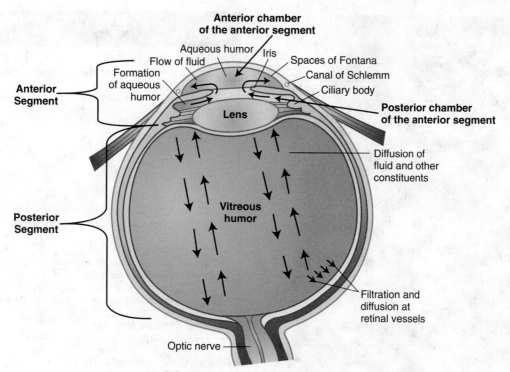

FIG. 48-2 Flow of aqueous humor.

that they focus properly on the retina. The curve of the lens changes to focus on near or distant objects. A *cataract* is a lens that has lost its transparency.

The vitreous body is a clear, thick gel that fills the *vitreous chamber* (the space between the lens and the retina). This gel transmits light and maintains eye shape.

The eye is a hollow organ and must be kept in the shape of a ball for vision to occur. To maintain this shape, the gel in the posterior segment *(vitreous humor)* and the fluid in the anterior segment *(aqueous humor)* must be present in set amounts that apply pressure inside the eye to keep it inflated (McCance et al., 2010). This pressure is known as intraocular pressure or IOP. IOP has to be just right. If the pressure is too low, the eyeball is soft and collapses, preventing light from getting to the light-sensitive photoreceptors in the back of the eye on the retina. If the pressure becomes too high, the extra pressure compresses capillaries and nerve fibers in the eye. Pressure on retinal blood vessels prevents blood from flowing through them, and as a result the photoreceptors and nerve fibers become hypoxic. Compression of the fine nerve fibers prevents intracellular fluid flow, which also reduces nourishment to the distal portions of these thin nerve fibers. The increased intraocular pressure and resulting hypoxia of the photoreceptors and their synapsing nerve fibers is a condition called *glaucoma*. Continued hypoxia inside the eye result in photoreceptor necrosis and death and permanent nerve fiber damage. With extensive photoreceptor loss and nerve fiber damage, vision is lost and the person is permanently blind.

External Structures

The eyelids are thin, movable skinfolds that protect the eyes, shut out light during sleep, and keep the cornea moist. The upper eyelid is larger than the lower one. The canthus is the place where the two eyelids meet at the corner of the eye.

The conjunctivae are the mucous membranes of the eye. The palpebral conjunctiva is a thick membrane with many blood vessels that lines the undersurface of each eyelid. The thin, transparent bulbar conjunctiva covers the entire front of the eye.

Tears are produced by a small lacrimal gland, which is located in the upper outer part of each orbit (Fig. 48-3). Tears flow across the front of the eye, toward the nose, and into the inner canthus. They drain through the punctum (an opening at the nasal side of the lid edges), into the lacrimal duct and sac, and then into the nose through the nasolacrimal duct.

Muscles, Nerves, and Blood Vessels

Six voluntary muscles rotate the eye and coordinate eye movements (Fig. 48-4 and Table 48-1). Coordinated eye movements ensure that the retina of each eye receives an image at the same time so only a single image is seen.

The muscles around the eye are innervated by cranial nerves (CNs) III (oculomotor), IV (trochlear), and VI (abducens). The optic nerve (CN II) is the nerve of sight, connecting the optic disc to the brain. Part of the trigeminal nerve (CN V) stimulates the blink reflex when the cornea is touched. The facial nerve (CN VII) innervates the lacrimal glands and muscles controlling lid closure.

The ophthalmic artery brings oxygenated blood to the eye and structures in the orbit. This artery branches to supply blood to the retina. The ciliary arteries supply the sclera, choroid, ciliary body, and iris. Venous drainage occurs through the two ophthalmic veins.

Function

The four eye functions that provide clear images and vision are refraction, pupillary constriction, accommodation, and convergence.

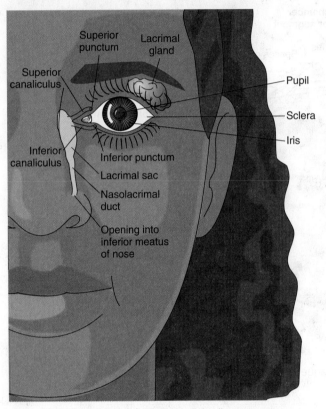

FIG. 48-3 Front view of the eye and adjacent structures.

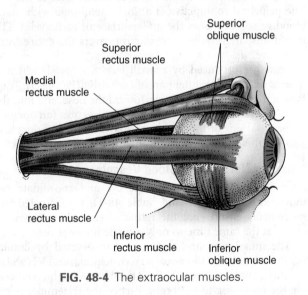

FIG. 48-4 The extraocular muscles.

Refraction involves bending light rays from the outside world into the eye. The different curved surfaces and refractive media of the eye allow light to pass through to the retina. Each surface and media bends (refracts) light differently to focus an image on the retina. Emmetropia is the perfect refraction of the eye: with the lens at rest, light rays from a distant source (20 feet [6 m] or more) are focused into a sharp image on the retina. Fig. 48-5 shows the normal refraction of light within the eye. Images fall on the retina inverted and reversed left to right. For example, an object in the lower nasal visual field strikes the upper outer area of the retina.

TABLE 48-1	FUNCTIONS OF OCULAR MUSCLES

Superior Rectus Muscle
- Together with the lateral rectus, this muscle moves the eye diagonally upward toward the side of the head.
- Together with the medial rectus, this muscle moves the eye diagonally upward toward the middle of the head.

Lateral Rectus Muscle
- Together with the medial rectus, contraction of this muscle holds the eye in a straight position.
- Contracting alone, this muscle turns the eye toward the side of the head.

Medial Rectus Muscle
- Contracting alone, this muscle turns the eye toward the nose.

Inferior Rectus Muscle
- Together with the lateral rectus, this muscle moves the eye diagonally downward toward the side of the head.
- Together with the medial rectus, this muscle moves the eye diagonally downward toward the middle of the head.

Superior Oblique Muscle
- Contracting alone, this muscle pulls the eye downward.

Inferior Oblique Muscle
- Contracting alone, this muscle pulls the eye upward.

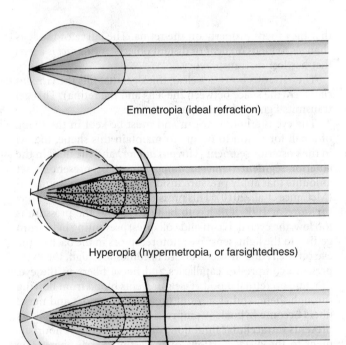

FIG. 48-5 Refraction and correction in emmetropia, hyperopia, and myopia.

Errors of refraction are common. Hyperopia (farsightedness or *hypermetropia*) occurs when the eye does not refract light enough. As a result, images actually fall *(converge)* behind the retina (see Fig. 48-5). Vision beyond 20 feet is normal, but near vision is poor. Hyperopia is corrected with a convex lens in eyeglasses or contact lenses.

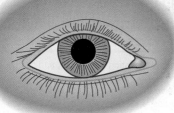
Normal pupil slightly dilated for moderate light

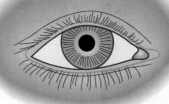
Miosis—pupil constricted when exposed to increased light or close work, such as reading

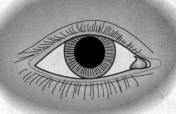
Mydriasis—pupil dilated when exposed to reduced light or when looking at a distance

FIG. 48-6 Miosis and mydriasis.

CHART 48-1   NURSING FOCUS ON THE OLDER ADULT

Changes in the Eye and Vision Related to Aging

STRUCTURE/ FUNCTION	CHANGE	IMPLICATION
Appearance	Eyes appear "sunken." Arcus senilis forms. Sclera yellows or appears blue.	Do not use eye appearance as an indicator for hydration status. Reassure patient that this change does not affect vision. Do not use sclera to assess for jaundice.
Cornea	Cornea flattens, which blurs vision.	Encourage older adults to have regular eye examinations and wear prescribed corrective lenses for best vision.
Ocular muscles	Muscle strength is reduced, making it more difficult to maintain an upward gaze or maintain a single image.	Reassure patient that this is a normal happening and to re-focus gaze frequently to maintain a single image.
Lens	Elasticity is lost, increasing the near point of vision (making the near point of best vision farther away). Lens hardens, compacts, and forms a cataract.	Encourage patient to wear corrective lenses for reading. Stress the importance of yearly vision checks and monitoring for when intervention is needed.
Iris	Decrease in ability to dilate results in small pupil size and poor adaptation to darkness.	Teach older adults the need for good lighting for best vision to avoid tripping and bumping into objects.
Pupil	Pupil size is smaller, reducing the ability to see in dim light.	Teach older adults the need for good lighting for best vision to avoid tripping and bumping into objects.
Color vision	Discrimination among greens, blues, and violets decreases.	The patient may not be able to use "dipstick" or other color-indicator monitors of health status.
Tears	Tear production is reduced, resulting in dry eyes, discomfort, and increased risk for corneal damage or eye infections.	Teach patient to use saline eyedrops on a schedule to reduce dryness. Teach patient to increase humidity in the home.

Myopia (nearsightedness) occurs when the eye overbends the light and images converge in front of the retina (see Fig. 48-5). Near vision is normal, but distance vision is poor. Myopia is corrected with a biconcave lens in eyeglasses or contact lenses.

Astigmatism is a refractive error caused by unevenly curved surfaces on or in the eye, especially of the cornea. These uneven surfaces distort vision.

Pupillary constriction and dilation control the amount of light that enters the eye. If the level of light to one or both eyes is increased, both pupils constrict (become smaller). The amount of constriction depends on how much light is available and how well the retina can adapt to light changes. Pupillary constriction is called miosis, and pupillary dilation is called mydriasis (Fig. 48-6). Drugs can alter pupillary constriction.

Accommodation allows the healthy eye to focus images sharply on the retina whether the image is close to the eye or distant. The process of maintaining a clear visual image when the gaze is shifted from a distant to a near object is known as accommodation. The eye can adjust its focus by changing the curve of the lens.

Convergence is the ability to turn both eyes inward toward the nose at the same time. This action helps ensure that only a single image of close objects is seen.

Eye Changes Associated with Aging

Changes inside the eye cause visual acuity to decrease with age (Touhy & Jett, 2010). Age-related changes of the nervous system and in the eye support structures also reduce visual function (Chart 48-1).

Structural changes occur with aging, including decreased eye muscle tone that reduces the ability to keep gaze focused on a single object. The lower eyelid may relax and fall away from the eye (*ectropion*), leading to dry-eye symptoms.

Arcus senilis, an opaque, bluish white ring within the outer edge of the cornea, is caused by fat deposits (Fig. 48-7). Although very common, this change does not affect vision.

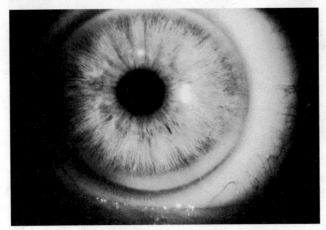

FIG. 48-7 Arcus senilis of the iris.

The clarity and shape of the cornea change with age. After age 65 years, the cornea flattens and the curve of its surface becomes irregular. This change causes or worsens astigmatism and blurs vision.

Fatty deposits cause the sclera to develop a yellowish tinge. A bluish color may be seen as the sclera thins. With age, the iris has less ability to dilate, which leads to difficulty in adapting to dark environments. Older adults may need additional light for reading and other "close up" work and to avoid tripping over objects.

Functional changes also occur with aging. The lens yellows with aging, reducing the ability of the eye to transmit and focus light. The aging lens hardens, shrinks, and loses elasticity. As the lens loses elasticity, the eye reduces accommodation. The near point of vision (the closest distance at which the eye can see an object clearly) increases. Near objects, especially reading material, must be placed farther from the eye to be seen clearly. This age-related change is called presbyopia. The far point (farthest point at which an object can be distinguished) decreases. Together these changes narrow the visual field of an older adult.

As a person ages, general color perception decreases, especially for green, blue, and violet. More light is needed to stimulate the photoreceptors. Intraocular pressure (IOP) is slightly higher in older adults.

Health Promotion and Maintenance

Vision is important to everyday function and quality of life. Many vision and eye problems can be avoided, and others can be corrected or managed if discovered early. Teach all people about eye protection methods, adequate nutrition, and the importance of regular eye examinations.

The risks for cataract formation and for cancer of the eye (ocular melanoma) increase with exposure to ultraviolet (UV) light. Teach people to protect the eyes by using sunglasses that filter UV light whenever they are outdoors. Also explain that UV protection should be used in tanning salons and in work environments that have UV exposure.

Vision can be affected by injury, and eye injury also increases the risk for both cataract formation and glaucoma. Urge all people to wear eye and head protection during work in occupations that involve particulate matter, fluid or blood spatter, high temperatures, or sparks. Eye and head protection should be worn during participation in sports, such as

---

baseball, or any activity that increases the risk for the eye being hit by objects in motion. Teach people to avoid rubbing the eyes because excessive eye rubbing can traumatize the delicate outer eye surfaces.

Eye infections can lead to vision loss. Although the eye surface is not sterile, the sclera and cornea have no separate blood supply and thus are at risk for infection because the immunities in the blood do not reach these structures. Teach everyone to wash their hands before touching the eye or eyelid. Teach people who use eyedrops about the proper technique to use these drugs (Chart 48-2) and to not share eyedrops with others. If an eye has a discharge, teach the patient to use a separate eyedrop bottle for this eye and to wash the unaffected eye before washing the affected eye.

Other health problems, especially diabetes mellitus and hypertension, can have serious adverse effects on vision. Teach patients who have these health problems about the importance of controlling blood glucose levels and managing blood pressure to reduce the risk for vision loss. Explain that yearly consultation with an ophthalmologist is needed to ensure coordination with their regular health care provider to slow or prevent eye complications.

Teach all people who have a refractive error to have an eye examination yearly. Young adults who do not have vision problems may need an eye examination only every 3 to 5 years unless a problem develops. Adults older than 40 years should have an eye examination yearly that includes assessment of intraocular pressure and visual fields, because the risk for both glaucoma and cataract formation increases with age.

CHART 48-3   EYE AND VISION ASSESSMENT

Using Gordon's Functional Health Patterns

Cognitive-Perceptual Pattern
- Do you have any difficulty seeing objects at a distance?
- Do you have any difficulty reading fine print or doing close work?
- Do you wear eyeglasses or contact lenses?
- What type of light do you use for reading?
- Do you wear sunglasses or a hat when outdoors?
- Do you have frequent headaches?
- Have you noticed any change in your ability to see things at night?
- When did you last have your eyes examined?
- Do you go to an ophthalmologist or an optometrist?
- When were you last tested for glaucoma?

Based on Gordon, M. (2011). *Manual of nursing diagnosis* (12th ed.). New York: Jones & Bartlett.

! NURSING SAFETY PRIORITY

Action Alert

Teach people to see a health care provider *immediately* when an eye injury occurs or an eye infection is suspected.

? NCLEX EXAMINATION CHALLENGE

Psychosocial Integrity

The older adult client asks whether the white ring in the iris of both eyes is a cataract that can be removed to improve her vision. What is the nurse's best response?
A. "A cataract forms inside the eye, not on the surface. This growth should be assessed for cancer."
B. "This type of ring in the eye gets worse as intraocular pressure increases, leading to glaucoma."
C. "The ring is a cataract, and it cannot be removed until it reaches and covers over the pupil."
D. "The ring is just a buildup of deposits, not a cataract, and never interferes with vision."

ASSESSMENT METHODS

Patient History

Collect information to determine whether problems with the eye or vision have an impact on ADLs or other daily functions. Chart 48-3 lists questions to ask when assessing the eye and vision.

Age is an important factor to consider when assessing the visual processes and eye structure. The incidence of glaucoma and cataract formation increases with aging. Presbyopia commonly begins in the 40s.

Gender also may be important. For example, retinal detachments are more common in men and dry-eye syndromes are more common in women.

Occupation and leisure activities can affect vision. Ask patients about work and specifically how the eyes are used. In some occupations, such as computer programming, constant exposure to monitor screens may lead to eyestrain. Machine operators are at risk for eye injury because of the high speeds at which particles can be thrown at the eye. Ask the patient who works in industrial settings about the use of protective eyewear, such as goggles. Chronic exposure to infrared or ultraviolet light may cause photophobia and

TABLE 48-2   SYSTEMIC CONDITIONS AND COMMON DRUGS AFFECTING THE EYE AND VISION

Systemic Conditions and Disorders
- Diabetes mellitus
- Hypertension
- Lupus erythematosus
- Sarcoidosis
- Thyroid dysfunction
- Acquired immune deficiency syndrome
- Cardiac disease
- Multiple sclerosis
- Pregnancy

Drugs
- Antihistamines
- Decongestants
- Antibiotics
- Opioids
- Anticholinergics
- Cholinergic agonists
- Sympathomimetics
- Oral contraceptives
- Chemotherapy agents
- Corticosteroids
- Carbonic anhydrase inhibitors
- Beta blockers

cataract formation. Teach the patient about the use of eye protection during work.

Ask whether the patient plays sports, the type of sport played, and whether eye protection is used. Even a blow to the head near the eye, such as with a baseball, can damage external eye structures, the eye, the connections with the brain, or the area of the brain where vision is perceived.

Systemic health problems can affect vision. Check whether the patient has any condition listed in Table 48-2. Ask about past accidents, injuries, surgeries, or blows to the head that may have led to the present problem. Specifically ask about previous laser surgeries because patients often do not classify laser treatment as surgery.

Drugs, even systemic drugs, can affect vision and the eye (see Table 48-2). Ask about the use of any prescription or over-the-counter drugs, especially decongestants and antihistamines, which tend to dry the eye and may increase intraocular pressure (IOP). Many patients do not consider over-the-counter eyedrops to be drugs. Record the name, strength, dose, and scheduling for all drugs the patient uses. Ocular effects from drugs include pruritus (itching), foreign body sensation, redness, tearing, photophobia (sensitivity to light), and the development of cataracts or glaucoma.

Nutrition History

Because some ocular problems are caused by or made worse with vitamin deficiencies, ask the patient about his or her food choices. For example, vitamin A deficiency can cause eye dryness, keratomalacia, and blindness. However, nutrients and antioxidants such as lutein and beta carotene may help maintain retinal function. A diet rich in fruit and red, orange, and dark green vegetables is important to eye health. Teach all people to eat five to ten servings of these foods daily.

Family History and Genetic Risk

Ask about a family history of eye problems. Some conditions, such as a refractive error, show a familial tendency. Some genetic problems lead to visual impairment in adulthood (Nussbaum et al., 2007). When a patient tells you that other relatives, especially first-degree relatives (parents, siblings, and children), have eye problems, record the gender of the affected person, his or her relationship to the patient, the exact nature of the problem, and the age that the problem was first noted.

Current Health Problems

Ask the patient about the onset of visual changes. Did the change occur rapidly or slowly? Determine whether the symptoms are present to the same degree in both eyes.

Ask these questions if ocular injury or eye trauma is involved:

- How long ago did the injury occur?
- What was the patient doing when it happened?
- If a foreign body was involved, what was its source?
- Was any first aid administered at the scene? If so, what actions were taken?

! NURSING SAFETY PRIORITY

Critical Rescue

Notify the ophthalmologist immediately for any patient who has a sudden or persistent loss of vision within the past 48 hours, eye trauma, a foreign body in the eye, or sudden ocular pain.

Physical Assessment
Inspection

Look for head tilting, squinting, or other noticeable actions that indicate the patient is compensating to try to attain clear vision. For example, patients with double vision may cock the head to the side to focus the two images into one or they may close one eye to see more clearly.

Assess for symmetry in the appearance of the eyes. Check the eyes to determine whether they are equal distance from the nose, are the same size, and have the same degree of prominence. Assess the eyes for their placement in the orbits and for symmetry of movement. Exophthalmos (proptosis) is protrusion of the eye. Enophthalmos is the sunken appearance of the eye.

Examine the eyebrows and eyelashes for hair distribution, and determine the direction of the eyelashes. Eyelashes normally point outward and away from the eyelid. Assess the eyelids for ptosis (drooping), redness, lesions, or swelling. The lids normally close completely, with the upper and lower lid edges touching. When the eyes are open, the upper lid covers a small portion of the iris. The edge of the lower lid lies below the line between the cornea and sclera. No sclera should be visible between the eyelid and the iris.

Scleral and corneal assessment requires a penlight. Examine the sclera for color; it is usually white. A yellow color may indicate jaundice or systemic problems. In dark-skinned people, the normal sclera may appear yellow and small, pigmented dots may be visible (Jarvis, 2012).

The cornea is best observed by directing a light at it from the side using several angles. The cornea should be transparent, smooth, shiny, and bright. Any cloudy areas or specks may be the result of accidents or injuries.

Assess the blink reflex by bringing a fist quickly toward the patient's face; patients with vision will blink. This reflex can also be assessed by expelling a syringe full of air toward the eyes. The patient blinks if the reflex is intact.

Pupillary assessment involves examining each pupil separately and comparing the results. This examination is also part of a rapid neurologic assessment. The pupils are usually round and of equal size. About 5% of people normally have a noticeable difference in the size of their pupils, which is known as anisocoria (Jarvis, 2012). Pupil size varies in people exposed to the same amount of light. Pupils are smaller in older adults. People with myopia have larger pupils. People with hyperopia have smaller pupils. The normal pupil diameter is between 3 and 5 mm. Smaller pupils reduce vision in low light conditions.

Observe the pupils for their response to light. Increasing light causes constriction, whereas decreasing light causes dilation. Constriction of both pupils is the normal response to direct light and to accommodation. Assess pupillary reaction to light by asking the patient to look straight ahead while you quickly bring the beam of a penlight in from the side and direct it at the right pupil. Constriction of the right pupil is a direct response to shining the penlight into that eye. Constriction of the left pupil when light is shined at the right pupil is known as a consensual response. Assess the responses for each eye. (You may see the abbreviation "PERRLA" in a patient's medical record, which stands for *p*upils *e*qual, *r*ound, *r*eactive to *l*ight, and *a*ccommodative.)

Evaluate each pupil for speed of reaction. The pupil should immediately constrict when a light is directed at it. This rapid response is termed *brisk*. If the pupil takes more than 1 second to constrict, the response is termed *sluggish*. Pupils that fail to react are termed *nonreactive* or *fixed*. Compare the reactivity speed of right and left pupils, and document any difference.

To assess for accommodation, hold your finger about 18 cm from the patient's nose and move it toward the nose. The patient's eyes normally converge during this movement, and the pupils constrict equally. When accommodation stops, the pupils first enlarge and then return to their normal size.

Vision Testing

Vision is measured by various tests. First test each eye separately, and then test both eyes together. Patients who wear corrective lenses are tested both without and with their lenses.

Visual acuity tests measure both distance and near vision. The Snellen chart, or "eye chart," is a simple tool to measure distance vision. This chart has letters, numbers, pictures, or a single letter presented in various positions (Fig. 48-8). The chart with one letter in different positions is used for patients who cannot read, who do not speak the language used at the facility, or who cannot speak but do have adequate cognition. Have the patient stand 20 feet from the chart, cover one eye, and use the other eye to read the line that appears most clear. If the patient can do this accurately, ask him or her to read the next lower line. Repeat this sequence to the last line on which the patient can correctly identify most characters. Repeat the procedure with the other eye. Record findings as a comparison between what the patient can read at 20 feet and the distance at which a person with normal vision can read the same line. For example, 20/50 means that the patient can see at 20 feet from the chart what a "healthy eye" can see at 50 feet.

LETTER CHART FOR 20 FEET
Snellen Scale

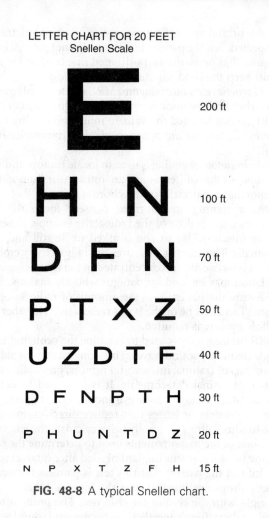

E	200 ft
H N	100 ft
D F N	70 ft
P T X Z	50 ft
U Z D T F	40 ft
D F N P T H	30 ft
P H U N T D Z	20 ft
N P X T Z F H	15 ft

FIG. 48-8 A typical Snellen chart.

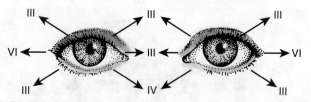

FIG. 48-9 Checking extraocular movements in the six cardinal positions indicates the functioning of cranial nerves III, IV, and VI.

For patients who are in a confined space that does not permit a 20-foot distance to the eye chart or who cannot see the 20/400 character, assess visual acuity by holding fingers in front of their eyes and asking them to count the number of fingers. Acuity is recorded as "count fingers vision at 5 feet," or the farthest distance at which fingers are counted correctly.

Patients who cannot count fingers are tested for hand motion (HM) acuity. Stand about 2 to 3 feet in front of the patient. Ask him or her to cover the eye not being tested. Direct a light onto your hand from behind the patient. Demonstrate the three possible directions in which the hand can move during the test (stationary, left-right, or up-down). Move your hand slowly (1 second per motion), and ask the patient, "What is my hand doing now?" Repeat this procedure five times. Visual acuity is recorded as HM at the farthest distance at which most of the hand motions are identified correctly.

If the patient cannot detect hand movement, test acuity by measuring light perception (LP). Ask the patient first to cover the left eye. In a darkened room, direct the beam of a penlight at the patient's right eye from a distance of 2 to 3 feet for 1 to 2 seconds. Instruct the patient to say "on" when the beam of light is perceived and "off" when it is no longer detected. If the patient identifies the presence or absence of light three times correctly, acuity is recorded as LP.

Near vision is tested for patients who have difficulty reading without using glasses or other means of vision correction. Use a small, handheld miniature chart called a *Rosenbaum Pocket Vision Screener* or a *Jaeger card*. Ask the patient to hold the card 14 inches away from his or her eyes and read the characters. Test each eye separately and then together. Record the value of the lowest line on which the patient can identify more than half the characters.

Visual field testing is used to determine the degree of peripheral vision. It can be performed formally with a computerized machine or informally with a "confrontation test" for a crude but rapid check of peripheral vision. During the confrontation test, sit facing the patient and ask him or her to look directly into your eyes while you look into the patient's eyes. Cover your right eye and have the patient cover his or her left eye so that you both have the same visual field. Then move a finger or an object from a nonvisible area into the patient's line of vision. The patient with normal peripheral vision should notice the object at about the same time you do. Repeat this examination by covering your left eye and the patient covering his or her right eye. Note any areas in which you can see but the patient cannot.

Extraocular muscle function is assessed using the corneal light reflex and the six cardinal positions of gaze. These tests not only assess smoothness of eye movements but also test the function of cranial nerves III, IV, and VI.

The corneal light reflex determines alignment of the eyes. After asking the patient to stare straight ahead, shine a penlight at both corneas from a distance of 12 to 15 inches. The bright dot of light reflected from the shiny surface of the cornea should be in a symmetric position (e.g., at the 1 o'clock position in the right eye and at the 11 o'clock position in the left eye). An asymmetric reflex indicates a deviating eye and possible muscle weakness.

Use the six cardinal positions of gaze to assess muscle function (Fig. 48-9). The eye will not turn to a particular position if the muscle is weak or if the controlling nerve is affected. Ask the patient to hold his or her head still and to move only the eyes to follow a small object. Move the object to the patient's right (lateral), upward and right (temporal), down and right, left (lateral), upward and left (temporal), and down and left (see Fig. 48-9). While the patient moves the eyes to these positions, note whether both eyes move in a parallel manner and any deviation of movement. Nystagmus, an involuntary and rapid twitching of the eyeball, is a normal finding for the far lateral gaze. It may also be caused by abnormal nerve function.

Color vision is usually tested using the *Ishihara chart*, which shows numbers composed of dots of one color within a circle of dots of a different color (Fig. 48-10). Test each eye separately by asking the patient what numbers he or she sees on the chart. Reading the numbers correctly indicates normal color vision.

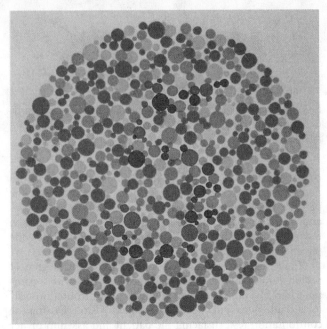

FIG. 48-10 An Ishihara chart for testing color vision.

❓ NCLEX EXAMINATION CHALLENGE

Safe and Effective Care Environment

Which client assessment finding does the nurse report to the health care provider immediately?

A. The left pupil is slightly smaller than the right pupil.

B. Both eyes twitch when the client looks to the far lateral gaze position.

C. The right pupil does not change size when a light is shined directly at it.

D. The lowest line the client can read clearly at 20 feet on the Snellen chart is marked 50 feet.

Psychosocial Assessment

A patient with changes in visual perception may be anxious about possible vision loss. Patients with severe visual defects may be unable to perform ADLs or engage in some leisure activities. Dependency resulting from reduced vision can affect self-esteem. Ask the patient how he or she feels about the vision changes, and assess the effectiveness of coping techniques. Discuss these concerns with the family to determine available support. Also assess the patient's knowledge and use of services for the visually impaired. Provide information about local resources and services for reduced vision.

Diagnostic Assessment

Laboratory Assessment

Cultures of corneal or conjunctival swabs and scrapings help diagnose infections. Obtain a sample of the exudate for culture before antibiotics or topical anesthetics are instilled. Take swabs from the conjunctivae and any ulcerated or inflamed areas.

Imaging Assessment

Computed tomography (CT) is a useful diagnostic tool for looking at the eyes, the bony structures around the eyes, and the extraocular muscles. It is also used for detecting tumors in the orbital space. Contrast dye is used unless trauma is suspected. Tell the patient that this test is not painful but does require that he or she be positioned in a confined space and must keep the head still during the procedure.

Magnetic resonance imaging (MRI) is often used to examine the orbits and the optic nerves and to evaluate ocular tumors. MRI cannot be used to evaluate injuries involving metal in the eyes. *Metal in the eye is an absolute contraindication for MRI.*

Radioisotope scanning is used to locate tumors and lesions. Isotope studies differentiate an intraocular tumor from a hemorrhage, especially in the choroid layer.

After signing an informed consent form, the patient receives a tracer dose of the radioactive isotope, either orally or by injection. He or she is asked to lie still and breathe normally. The scanner measures the radioactivity emitted by the radioactive atoms concentrated in the area being studied. Sedation may be used for patients who are anxious.

Assure the patient that the amount of radioisotope used is small and that he or she is not radioactive. No other special follow-up care is required.

Ultrasonography is used to examine the orbit and eye with high-frequency sound waves. This noninvasive test aids in the diagnosis of trauma, intraorbital tumors, proptosis, and choroidal or retinal detachments. It is also used to determine gross outline changes in the eye and the orbit in patients with cloudy corneas or lenses that reduce direct examination of the fundus. Ultrasonography helps calculate the length of the eye, one of the measurements used to determine the strength of the intraocular lens implant needed after cataract removal.

Inform the patient that this test is painless because anesthetic drops are instilled into the lower lid. He or she sits upright with the chin in the chin rest. The probe is touched against the patient's anesthetized cornea, and sound waves are bounced through the eye. The sound waves create a reflective pattern on a computer screen that can be examined for abnormalities. No special follow-up care is needed. Remind the patient not to rub or touch the eye until the effects of the anesthetic drops have worn off.

Other Diagnostic Assessment

Many tests are used to examine specific eye structures but are not needed for routine vision assessment. Such tests may be indicated for those with special risks, symptoms, or exposures. These tests are performed only by physicians, optometrists, or advanced practice nurses.

Slit-lamp examination magnifies the anterior eye structures (Fig. 48-11). The patient leans on a chin rest to stabilize the head. A narrow beam (slit) of light is aimed so that only a narrow segment of the eye is brightly lighted. The examiner can then locate the position of any abnormality in the cornea, lens, or anterior vitreous humor.

Corneal staining consists of placing fluorescein or other topical dye into the conjunctival sac. The dye outlines irregularities of the corneal surface that are not easily visible. This test is used for corneal trauma, problems caused by a contact lens, or the presence of foreign bodies, abrasions, ulcers, or other corneal disorders.

This procedure is noninvasive and is performed under aseptic conditions. The dye is applied topically to the eye, and the eye is then viewed through a blue filter. Nonintact areas of the cornea stain a bright green color.

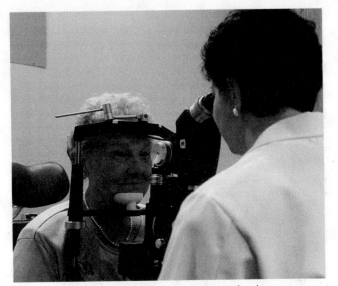

FIG. 48-11 Slit-lamp ocular examination.

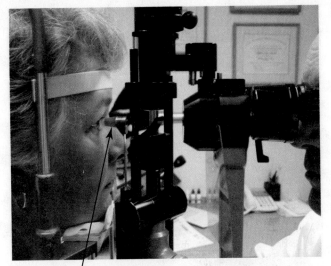

Goldman's applanation tonometer

FIG. 48-12 Use of Goldman's applanation tonometer and a slit lamp to measure intraocular pressure (IOP).

Tonometry measures intraocular pressure (IOP) using a tonometer. This instrument applies pressure to the outside of the eye until it equals the pressure inside the eye as indicated when the cornea begins to indent. Normal IOP readings have always been considered to range from 10 to 21 mm Hg; however, this number is not absolute and must be considered along with corneal thickness. The thickness of the cornea affects how much pressure must be applied before indentation occurs. For example, a person with a thicker cornea will have a higher tonometer reading that may falsely indicate increased IOP. A person with a thinner-than-normal cornea may have a low tonometer reading even when higher IOP is present.

About 5% of patients with healthy eyes have a slightly higher pressure. Tonometer readings are indicated for all patients older than 40 years. Adults with a family history of glaucoma should have their IOP measured once or twice a year. The most common method to measure IOP by an ophthalmologist is the Goldman's applanation tonometer used with a slit lamp (Fig. 48-12). This method involves direct eye contact. Another instrument, the Tono-Pen (Fig. 48-13), is designed for use by patients in the home to measure IOP daily.

Intraocular pressure varies throughout the day. It is often higher in the morning but may peak at any time of the day. Therefore always document the time of IOP measurement and teach patients who are measuring IOP at home to perform the measurement at the same time or times each day.

Ophthalmoscopy allows viewing of the eye's external and interior structures with an instrument called an *ophthalmoscope*. This examination can be performed by any nurse but usually is performed by a physician, advanced practice nurse, or physician assistant. It is easiest to examine the fundus when the room is dark, because the pupil will dilate. Stand on the same side as the eye being examined. Tell the patient to look straight ahead at an object on the wall behind you. Placing your thumb on the patient's eyebrow can help you know the distance from the ophthalmoscope to the patient. Hold the ophthalmoscope firmly against your face, and align it so that your eye sees through the sight hole (Fig. 48-14).

When using the ophthalmoscope, move toward the patient's eye from about 12 to 15 inches away and to the side

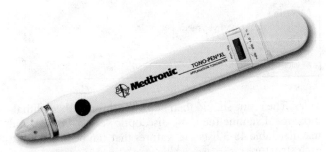

FIG. 48-13 The Tono-Pen.

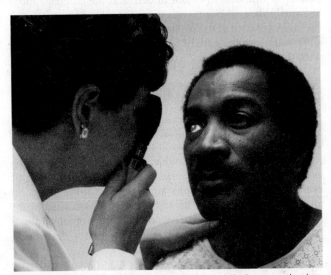

FIG. 48-14 Proper technique for direct ophthalmoscopic visualization of the retina.

of his or her line of vision. As you direct the ophthalmoscope at the pupil, a red glare (red reflex) should be seen in the pupil as a reflection of the light on the retina. An absent red reflex may indicate a lens opacity or cloudiness of the vitreous. Move toward the patient's pupil while following the red

TABLE 48-3 STRUCTURES ASSESSED BY DIRECT OPHTHALMOSCOPY

Red Reflex
- Presence or absence

Optic Disc
- Color
- Margins (sharp or blurred)
- Cup size
- Presence of rings or crescents

Optic Blood Vessels
- Size
- Color
- Kinks or tangles
- Light reflection
- Narrowing
- Nicking at arteriovenous crossings

Fundus
- Color
- Tears or holes
- Lesions
- Bleeding

Macula
- Presence of blood vessels
- Color
- Lesions
- Bleeding

CHART 48-4 BEST PRACTICE FOR PATIENT SAFETY & QUALITY CARE

Instillation of Eyedrops

- Check the name, strength, expiration date, color, and clarity of the eyedrops to be instilled.
- Check to see whether only one eye is to have the drug or if both eyes are to receive the drug.
- If both eyes are to receive the same drug and one eye is infected, use two separate bottles and carefully label each bottle with "right" or "left" for the correct eye.
- Wash your hands.
- Put on gloves if secretions are present in or around the eye.
- Explain the procedure to the patient.
- Have the patient sit in a chair, and you stand behind the patient.
- Ask the patient to tilt the head backward, with the back of the head resting against your body and looking up at the ceiling.
- Gently pull the lower lid down against the patient's cheek, forming a small pocket.
- Hold the eyedrop bottle (with the cap off) like a pencil, with the tip pointing down.
- Rest the wrist holding the bottle against the patient's check.
- Without touching any part of the eye or lid with the tip of the bottle, gently squeeze the bottle and release the prescribed number of drops into the pocket you have made with the patient's lower lid.
- Gently release the lower lid.
- Tell the patient to close the eye gently (without squeezing the lids tightly).
- Gently press and hold the corner of the eye nearest the nose to close off the punctum and prevent the drug from being absorbed systemically.
- Without pressing on the lid, gently blot away any excess drug or tears with a tissue.
- Remove your gloves, and place the cap back on the bottle.
- Ask the patient to keep the eye closed for about 1 minute.
- Wash your hands again.

reflex. The retina should then be visible through the ophthalmoscope. Examine the optic disc, optic vessels, fundus, and macula. Table 48-3 lists the features that can be observed in each structure.

The use of an ophthalmoscope may make a confused patient or one who does not understand the language more anxious. When working with a patient who does not speak the language used at the facility, use an interpreter, when possible, to ensure the patient's understanding and cooperation with the examination.

! NURSING SAFETY PRIORITY

Action Alert

Avoid using an ophthalmoscope with a confused patient.

Fluorescein angiography, which is performed by a physician or advanced practice nurse, provides a detailed image of eye circulation. Photographs are taken in rapid succession after the dye is given IV. This test is useful for assessing problems of retinal circulation (e.g., diabetic retinopathy, retinal hemorrhage, and macular degeneration) or for diagnosing intraocular tumors.

Explain the procedure to the patient, and instill mydriatic eyedrops (cause pupil dilation) 1 hour before the test. Chart 48-4 lists the best practice for correct eyedrop instillation. Check that the informed consent has been signed by the patient or responsible person. Warn that the dye may cause the skin to appear yellow for several hours after the test. The stain is eliminated through the urine, which also changes color.

Intravenous access must be obtained. After the needle is in the vein, 5 mL of a 10% solution of fluorescein is injected.

A digital camera is set up with equipment to photograph retinal and choroidal blood vessels as the dye passes through them. The results can be viewed immediately on a computer screen. The procedure takes only a few minutes because the vessels fill quickly.

? DECISION-MAKING CHALLENGE

Patient-Centered Care; Safety; Teamwork and Collaboration

The patient is a 75-year-old woman from Mexico who was brought to the clinic by her daughter. The patient speaks no English, and the daughter serves as her interpreter. The daughter explains that even though her mother wears nonprescription glasses that she bought at the drugstore to do close work, she says that everything is always blurry. A complete eye examination is planned with an eye chart, an ophthalmoscope, a slit lamp, and tonometry.

1. What type of Snellen chart would be most appropriate for this patient? Explain your choice.
2. Should the daughter be allowed to stay with her? Why or why not? After an explanation by her daughter of what is expected of her, the patient participates in the Snellen chart test and "reads" the 70-foot line correctly but is incorrect on the 50-foot line. She then sits quietly and cooperates during the examination with the ophthalmoscope. However, when a slit-lamp examination is attempted, the patient keeps moving her head to the side and shouts "no, no, no," and tells her daughter that she is afraid of this big machine.
3. Is a slit-lamp examination important to perform for this patient? Why or why not?
4. What technique or techniques could be used to allay her fears?

Encourage patients to drink fluids to help eliminate the dye. Remind them that any yellow or green staining of the skin will disappear in a few hours. After the test, the urine will be bright green until the dye is excreted. Teach the patient to wear dark glasses and avoid direct sunlight until pupil dilation returns to normal, because the bright light will cause eye pain.

Electroretinography is the process of graphing the retina's response to light stimulation. This test is helpful in detecting and evaluating blood vessel changes from disease or drugs. The graph is obtained by placing a contact lens electrode on an anesthetized cornea. Lights at varying speeds and intensities are flashed, and the neural response is graphed. The measurement from the cornea is identical to the response that would be obtained if electrodes were placed directly on the retina.

Perimetry is a commonly used test to screen the visual fields. During this computerized test, the patient is asked to look straight ahead and then indicate, by pressing a control button, when a moving light enters the peripheral vision. This process draws a "map" of the person's peripheral vision and any deficits.

Gonioscopy is a test performed when a high IOP is found and determines whether open angle or closed angle glaucoma is present. It uses a special lens that eliminates the corneal curve, is painless, and allows visualization of the angle where the iris meets the cornea.

Laser imaging of the retina and optic nerve creates a three-dimensional view of the back of the eye. It is commonly used for those people with ocular hypertension or who are at risk for glaucoma from other problems. This type of computerized examination assesses the thickness and contours of the optic nerve and retina for changes that indicate damage as a result of high IOP. This type of test can be used serially for a person at risk for glaucoma to detect early changes and indicate when intervention is needed.

NURSING CONCEPT REVIEW

What should you expect to NOTICE in a patient with adequate sensation related to the eye and vision?

Physical Assessment
- Eyes are symmetric on the face on a line just about even with the tops of the ears.
- Eyes are clear with no drainage or open areas.
- Patient does not squint or tilt the head.
- Patient does not close one eye to read or see at a distance.
- Patient startles when a sudden move is made at the face.
- Patient blinks 5 to 10 times per minute.
- Pupils are the same size in each eye.
- Both pupils constrict when a light is shined at only one eye.
- Appearance is neat with buttons properly buttoned and hair combed or brushed.
- Patient comments on the presence of art or unusual visual objects in the immediate environment.
- Patient walks without hesitation into a room without bumping into objects in his or her path.

Psychological Assessment
- Patient is oriented and not confused.
- Patient makes eye contact when speaking.

GET READY FOR THE NCLEX® EXAMINATION!

KEY POINTS

Review these Key Points for each NCLEX Examination Client Needs Category.

Safe and Effective Care Environment
- Wash your hands before moving a patient's eyelids.
- If a patient has discharge from one eye, examine the eye without the discharge first.
- Wear gloves when examining an eye with drainage.
- Avoid using an ophthalmoscope on a confused patient.

Health Promotion and Maintenance
- Teach patients not to rub their eyes.
- Identify patients at risk for eye injury as a result of work environment or leisure activities.
- Urge all patients to wear eye protection when they are performing yard work, working in a woodshop or metal shop, using chemicals, or are in any environment in which drops or particulate matter is airborne.

Psychosocial Integrity
- Provide opportunities for the patient and family to express their concerns about a possible change in vision status.
- Explain all diagnostic procedures, restrictions, and follow-up care to the patient scheduled for tests.

Physiological Integrity
- Ask the patient about vision problems in any other members of the family, because some vision problems have a genetic component.
- Test the visual acuity of both eyes immediately of any person who experiences an eye injury or any sudden change in vision.

49

Care of Patients with Eye and Vision Problems

M. Linda Workman

LEARNING OUTCOMES

Safe and Effective Care Environment

1. Use aseptic technique when performing an eye examination or instilling drugs into the eye.
2. Apply the principles of infection control when caring for a patient with an eye infection.
3. Orient the patient with reduced vision to his or her immediate environment.
4. Ensure that all members of the health care team are aware of a patient's visual limitations and need for assistance.

Health Promotion and Maintenance

5. Teach all people, especially those older than 40 years, to have an annual eye examination including measurement of intraocular pressure.
6. Teach patients and family members how to correctly instill ophthalmic drops and ointment into the eye.
7. Teach the patient and family how to alter the home environment for patient safety.

Psychosocial Integrity

8. Teach patients and family members about what to expect during procedures to correct vision and eye problems.

9. Provide opportunities for the patient and family to express concerns about a change in vision.
10. Refer the patient with reduced vision to local services for the blind.
11. Teach the patient with reduced vision about techniques for performing ADLs and self-care independently.

Physiological Integrity

12. Explain the consequences of increased intraocular pressure (IOP).
13. Identify common actions, conditions, and positions that increase IOP.
14. Prioritize educational needs for the patient after cataract surgery with lens replacement.
15. Prioritize educational needs for patients with primary open-angle glaucoma.
16. Describe the mechanisms of action and nursing implications of drug therapy for glaucoma.

Vision is affected by many factors and problems. Some problems occur gradually, such as cataracts, and others can result from an acute insult or illness. Even when reduced vision is temporary, the patient must make some changes in function or lifestyle.

EYELID DISORDERS

The eyelid is composed of thin skin attached to small muscles. It protects the eye surface and spreads tears. Problems can occur with changes in the structure, function, or position of the eyelid. Lid structure may also be altered by age.

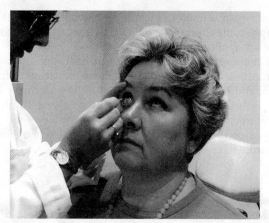

FIG. 49-1 Application of ophthalmic ointment.

Blepharitis

Blepharitis, an inflammation of the eyelid edges, occurs most often in the older adult and those with dry eye syndrome (see the Keratoconjunctivitis Sicca section, p. 1056). Reduced tear production often leads to bacterial infection of the eye, because tears inhibit bacterial growth.

Patients usually have itchy, red, and burning eyes. Seborrhea (greasy, itchy scaling) of the eyebrows and eyelids is often present. Greasy scales and mattering may be seen where the eyelashes exit the eyelid.

Blepharitis is controlled with eyelid care using warm, moist compresses followed by gentle scrubbing with dilute baby shampoo. Instruct the patient to avoid rubbing the eyes, because if infection is present, this action can spread the infection to other eye structures.

Entropion and Ectropion

An entropion is the turning inward of the eyelid causing the lashes to rub against the eye. Entropion can be caused by eyelid muscle spasms or by scarring and deformity of the eyelid after trauma. It occurs often among older adults because of age-related loss of tissue support.

The patient usually reports "feeling something in my eye." Pain and tears may also be present. The eyelid is turned inward, and the conjunctiva is red. Corneal abrasion may result from constant irritation.

Surgery corrects eyelid position by either tightening the orbicular muscles and moving the eyelid to a normal position or by preventing inward rotation of the eyelid. After surgery, the eye is covered with a patch and the patient is discharged a few hours later.

Demonstrate instillation of eyedrops, and evaluate the patient's ability to instill the drops. Instruct the patient to leave the patch in place until he or she is seen by the ophthalmologist and to report any pain or drainage under the patch. Teach the patient or family member how to clean the suture line with a cotton swab and the prescribed solution. A small amount of antibiotic ointment may be applied (Fig. 49-1). Chart 49-1 describes how to apply ophthalmic ointment. Chart 49-2 lists information on common ophthalmic drugs for eye inflammation and infection.

An ectropion is the turning outward and sagging of the eyelid, which often occurs with aging, caused by muscle

---

CHART 49-1 BEST PRACTICE FOR PATIENT SAFETY & QUALITY CARE

Instillation of Ophthalmic Ointment

- Check the name, strength, and expiration date of the ointment to be instilled. Be sure it is an ophthalmic (eye) preparation and not a general topical ointment.
- Check to see whether only one eye is to receive the drug or if both eyes are to receive the drug.
- If both eyes are to receive the same drug and one eye is infected, use two separate tubes and carefully label each tube with "right" or "left" for the correct eye.
- Wash your hands and put on gloves.
- Explain the procedure to the patient.
- Have the patient sit in a chair, and you stand behind the patient.
- Ask the patient to tilt the head backward, with the back of the head resting against your body and looking up at the ceiling.
- Gently pull the lower lid down against the patient's cheek, forming a small pocket.
- Hold the tube (with the cap off) like a pencil, with the tip pointing down.
- Rest the wrist holding the tube against the patient's cheek.
- Without touching any part of the eye or lid with the tip of the tube, gently squeeze the tube and release about a ¼- to ½-inch thin strip of ointment into the pocket you have made with the patient's lower lid. Start at the nose side of the pocket, and move toward the outer edge of the pocket.
- Gently release the lower lid.
- Tell the patient to close the eye gently (without squeezing the lids tightly).
- With the patient's eye closed, gently wipe away any excess ointment with a tissue.
- Tell the patient that sight in that eye will be blurred while the ointment is present in the eye and that he or she should not drive or operate heavy machinery until the ointment is removed.
- Remove your gloves, and place the cap back on the tube.
- Ask the patient to keep the eye closed for about 1 minute.
- Wash your hands again.
- To remove ointment from the eye, wear gloves if drainage is present.
- Then ask the patient to close the eye; wipe the closed lids with a clean tissue from the corner of the eye nearest the nose outward. If you are wiping the same eye twice, use a different area of the tissue or use a new one.

! NURSING SAFETY PRIORITY

Drug Alert

Check the route of administration for ophthalmic drugs. Most are administered as eye instillation route, not the oral route. Administering these drugs orally can cause systemic side effects in addition to not having a therapeutic effect on the eye.

---

relaxation or weakness. This lid position reduces the washing action of tears, leading to corneal drying and ulceration.

Patients often have constant tears and a sagging lower eyelid. Surgery can restore lid alignment. After surgery, the eye is covered with a patch and the patient is discharged. Nursing care is the same as for an entropion.

Hordeolum

A hordeolum, or *stye,* is an infection of the sweat glands in the eyelid (external hordeolum) or of the eyelid sebaceous gland (internal hordeolum). A red, swollen, tender area occurs on the skin surface side of the eyelid. The most common causative organisms are *Staphylococcus aureus*, *Staphylococcus epidermidis*, and *Streptococcus*. The hordeolum usually affects only one eyelid at a time. Vision is not affected.

Small, beady, swollen areas may be on the skin side of the eyelid or on the conjunctival side of the eyelid. Pain occurs as the hordeolum fills with purulent material.

Management includes applying warm compresses four times a day and an antibacterial ointment. When the lesion opens, the pus drains and the pain subsides.

Nursing interventions include instructing the patient how to apply compresses. Chart 49-3 describes the proper technique for application of an eye compress.

After compresses have been applied, instill antibiotic ointment. Advise the patient that ointments may cause blurred vision, and teach him or her to remove the ointment from the eyes before driving or operating machinery. To remove the ointment, teach the patient to close the eye and then gently wipe the closed eyelid from the nasal side of the eye outward.

CHART 49-2 COMMON EXAMPLES OF DRUG THERAPY

Eye Inflammation and Infection

DRUG	NURSING INTERVENTIONS*†	RATIONALES
Topical Anesthetics		
Proparacaine HCl, or proxymetacaine (AK-Taine, Alcaine, Ocu-Caine, Ophthetic)	Remind the patient not to rub or touch the eye while it is anesthetized.	Touching may injure the eye.
Tetracaine HCl, cocaine HCl (Pontocaine)	Patch the eye if the patient leaves the facility before the anesthetic wears off.	The use of a patch prevents injury, such as corneal abrasion.
	Instruct the patient not to use discolored solution.	Discoloration is a sign of altered drug composition.
	Teach the patient to store the bottle tightly closed.	Air may cause drug contamination and oxidation.
Topical Steroids		
Prednisolone acetate (Ocu-Pred, Ophtho-Tate ♣)	Tell the patient to shake the bottle vigorously before use.	Drug is a suspension; shaking is required to distribute the drug evenly in the solution.
Prednisolone phosphate (Inflamase)	Teach the patient to check for corneal ulceration (pain, reduced vision, secretions).	Steroid use predisposes the patient to local infection.
Dexamethasone (Dexair, Dexotic, Maxidex)		
Betamethasone (Betnesol)	Warn the patient not to share eyedrops with others.	Disease transmission is possible when sharing eyedrops.
Fluorometholone (Fluor-Op, Liquifilm)		
Anti-Infective Agents		
Gentamicin (Genoptic, Gentak Alcomicin ♣)	Teach the patient the importance of using the drug exactly as prescribed, even if he or she needs to use it hourly.	Bacterial and fungal eye infections worsen rapidly and can lead to blindness if not treated adequately.
Tobramycin (Tobrex)		
Ciprofloxacin (Ciloxan)		
Erythromycin (Ilotycin)	Teach the patient how to clean exudate from the eyes before using drops.	Cleansing decreases the risk for contaminating the drug and increases contact of the conjunctiva with the drug.
Chlortetracycline (Aureomycin)		
Sulfisoxazole (Gantrisin)	Reinforce the importance of completing the prescribed drug regimen.	Adherence is critical to maintain a therapeutic level of drug.
Ofloxacin (Ocuflox)		
Levofloxacin (Quixin)		
Antibiotic-Steroid Combinations		
Tobramycin with dexamethasone (TobraDex)	This is the same as for the general anti-infective agents alone and for the steroids alone.	This is the same as for the general anti-infective agents alone and for the steroids alone.
Neomycin sulfate with polymyxin B sulfate and dexamethasone (Maxitrol)		
Topical Antiviral Agents		
Trifluridine (Viroptic)	Teach the patient to refrigerate the drug and protect it from light.	Drug stability is affected by warm temperatures and light.
Vidarabine (Vira-A)	Teach the patient to assess for itching lids and burning eyes.	Sensitivity to these drugs is common.
Antifungal Agents		
Amphotericin B	Teach the patient to assess for itching lids and burning eyes.	Sensitivity to these drugs is common.
Natamycin (Natacyn)		
Nonsteroidal Anti-Inflammatory Agents		
Flurbiprofen (Ocufen)	Teach the patient to check for bleeding in the eye.	These drugs disrupt platelet aggregation.
Diclofenac (Voltaren)		
Bromfenac (Xibrom)	Teach the patient not to wear soft contact lenses during therapy with these drugs.	These drugs interact with contact lens materials and increase the risk for infection.
Ketorolac (Acular)		

*When instilling eyedrops, teach patients to use nasal punctal occlusion to reduce the risk for systemic absorption and side effects.
†When more than one topical ophthalmic drug is prescribed, teach patients to separate the instillation of each drug by 10-15 minutes (or package recommendations).

CHART 49-3   PATIENT AND FAMILY EDUCATION: PREPARING FOR SELF-MANAGEMENT

Application of an Ocular Compress

- Wash your hands.
- Fold a clean washcloth into fourths.
- Soak the washcloth with running tap water that is warm to your inner wrist. (If cool compresses are needed, follow the same steps using cold running tap water.)
- Place the cloth over your closed eye.
- Keep the cloth in place with minimal pressure until the cloth cools (or warms, if cool compresses are prescribed).
- Refold the washcloth so that a different "fourth" will be held against the eye.
- Resoak the cloth with running tap water.
- Repeat applications three times for as many times each day as prescribed by your health care provider.

Chalazion

A *chalazion* is an inflammation of a sebaceous gland in the eyelid. It begins with redness and tenderness, followed by a gradual *painless* swelling. Later, redness and tenderness are not present. Most chalazia protrude on the inside of the eyelid. The patient has eye fatigue, light sensitivity, and excessive tears.

Management includes applying warm compresses four times a day, followed by instillation of ophthalmic ointment. If the chalazion is large enough to affect vision or is cosmetically displeasing, it may be removed surgically.

After surgery, antibiotic ointment is instilled and the eye is covered with a patch. Best practices for application of a nonpressure eye patch are described in Chart 49-4.

Instruct the patient to leave the eye patch in place for about 6 hours and then remove the patch and apply warm, wet compresses. Antibiotic eyedrops are instilled after use of

CHART 49-4   BEST PRACTICE FOR PATIENT SAFETY & QUALITY CARE

Application of an Eye Patch

Nonpressure Eye Patch

1. Assemble the equipment:
   - Eye patch
   - Skin preparation pad
   - Nonallergenic paper tape
2. Explain the procedure to the patient.
3. Wash your hands.
4. Apply a skin preparation to the patient's forehead and cheek.
5. Instruct the patient to close both eyes gently.
6. Place a patch over the closed eyelid.

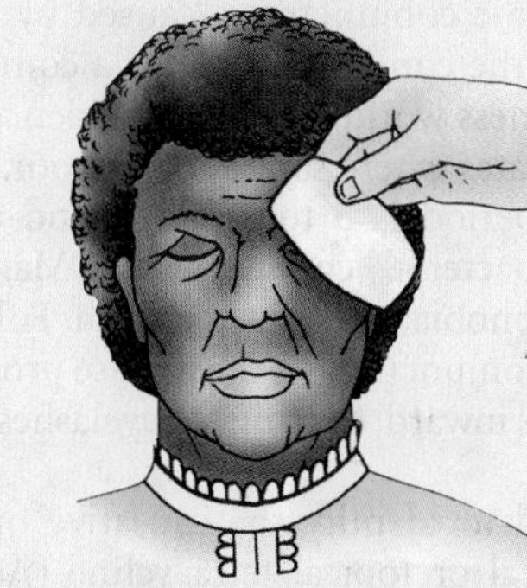

7. Apply tape from the cheek to the middle of the forehead in a diagonal line.

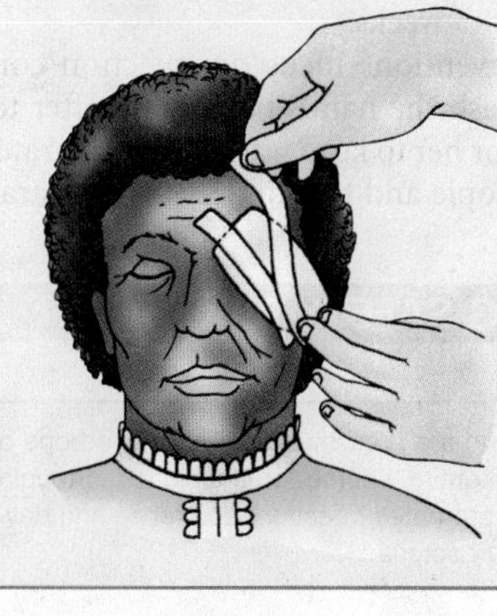

8. Cover the patch with overlapping pieces of tape.

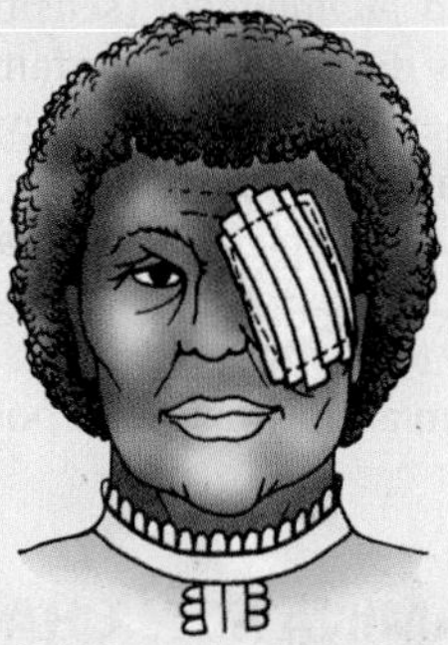

Pressure Eye Patch

1. Assemble the equipment:
   - Two eye patches for each eye requiring treatment
   - Skin preparation pad
   - Nonallergenic paper tape
2-5. Follow corresponding steps under Nonpressure Eye Patch.
6. Fold one eye patch in half, place it over the closed eyelid, and apply a second eye patch (unfolded) over the folded one.

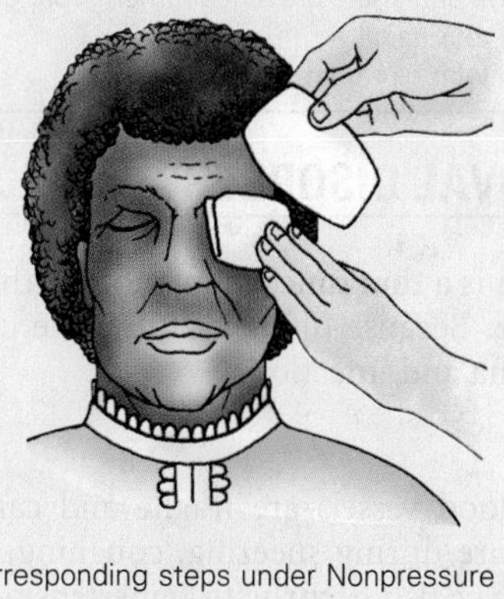

7, 8. Follow corresponding steps under Nonpressure Eye Patch.

the compresses. Teach him or her to immediately report increasing redness, purulent drainage, or reduced vision to the ophthalmologist.

KERATOCONJUNCTIVITIS SICCA

Pathophysiology

The lacrimal system moistens the eye surface with tears and removes tears from the eye. Problems arise from reduced tear production, infection, or inflammation in the lacrimal system.

Keratoconjunctivitis sicca, or dry eye syndrome, results from changes in tear production, tear composition, or tear distribution. Drugs (e.g., antihistamines, beta-adrenergic blocking agents, anticholinergic drugs) also can reduce tear production. Diseases associated with decreased tear production include rheumatoid arthritis, leukemia, sarcoidosis, and Sjögren's syndrome. Radiation or chemical burns to the eye also decrease tear production. Injury to cranial nerve VII inhibits tears. Eye dryness may follow vision-enhancing surgery. Dry eye syndromes are much more common in women than in men (Pullen & Hall, 2010).

PATIENT-CENTERED COLLABORATIVE CARE

The patient has a foreign body sensation in the eye, burning and itching eyes, and *photophobia* (sensitivity to light). The corneal light reflex is dulled. Tears contain mucus strands.

Management depends on symptom severity. Cyclosporine (Restasis) eyedrops may be prescribed to increase tear production. Artificial tears (HypoTears, Refresh) also can be used to reduce daytime dryness. A lubricating ointment (Lacri-Lube SOP, Refresh P.M.) is used at night. If the dry eye syndrome is caused by an abnormal eyelid position, surgery may be needed.

? NCLEX EXAMINATION CHALLENGE

Health Promotion and Maintenance

Which precaution is most important for the nurse to teach a client who is prescribed to use an ophthalmic ointment?

A. "Keep the tube in the refrigerator to make the ointment easier to control when you squeeze the tube."

B. "Wear gloves when you apply the ointment to prevent absorbing the drug through your skin."

C. "Patch your eye at night to prevent ointment from getting on your bedding or in your hair."

D. "Do not drive with ointment in your eyes."

CONJUNCTIVAL DISORDERS

The conjunctiva is a thin mucous membrane that covers and protects the eye. Because of its location, the conjunctiva is subject to trauma and infection.

Hemorrhage

Conjunctival blood vessels are fragile and can break with increased pressure during sneezing, coughing, or vomiting. Hemorrhages may also occur with hypertension, trauma, or blood clotting problems.

The small, well-defined area of hemorrhage is bright red under the conjunctiva. The patient is usually concerned about its appearance although no pain or visual impairment occurs with the hemorrhage. It resolves within 14 days without treatment.

Conjunctivitis

Conjunctivitis is an inflammation or infection of the conjunctiva. Inflammation occurs from exposure to allergens or irritants. Infectious conjunctivitis occurs with bacterial or viral infection and is readily transmitted from person to person (Saligan & Yeh, 2008).

Allergic conjunctivitis manifestations are edema, a sensation of burning, a "bloodshot" eye appearance, excessive tears, and itching. Management includes vasoconstrictor and corticosteroid eyedrops (see Chart 49-2). Teach women to avoid using makeup near the eye until all symptoms have subsided.

Bacterial conjunctivitis, or "pink eye," is usually caused by *Staphylococcus aureus* or *Haemophilus influenzae.* Manifestations are blood vessel dilation, mild edema, tears, and discharge. The discharge is watery at first and then becomes thicker, with shreds of mucus.

Cultures of the drainage are obtained to identify the organism. Drug therapy with topical antibiotics is prescribed to eliminate the infection. Nursing interventions focus on preventing infection spread to the other eye or to other people. Document the amount, color, and type of drainage. Remind the patient to wash his or her hands after touching the eye and before using eyedrops. Warn him or her not to touch the unaffected eye without first washing the hands and to avoid sharing washcloths and towels with others. Instruct women to discard eye makeup and applicators used at the time the infection developed to avoid the possibility of recontamination.

Trachoma

Trachoma is a chronic conjunctivitis caused by *Chlamydia trachomatis.* It scars the conjunctiva and is a common cause of preventable blindness worldwide. The incidence is highest in warm, moist climates where sanitation is poor.

The incubation period is 5 to 14 days, and at first the disease resembles bacterial conjunctivitis. Manifestations include tears, photophobia, and eyelid edema. Follicles form on the upper eyelid conjunctiva. As the disease progresses, the eyelid scars and turns inward, causing the eyelashes to damage the cornea.

Cultures are used to identify the causative organism. A 4-week course of oral or topical tetracycline (Achromycin, Apo-Tetra ✿) or erythromycin (Apo-Erythro-EC ✿, E-Mycin, E.E.S.) is given. Azithromycin (Zithromax) can be used once per week for 1 to 3 weeks.

Nursing interventions focus on infection control. Teach the patient to wash the hands before and after touching the eyes. Teach him or her to keep washcloths separate from those of unaffected people and to launder them separately.

! NURSING SAFETY PRIORITY

Action Alert

Teach patients who are prescribed antibiotic eyedrops or ointments to complete the entire course of antibiotics. Stopping antibiotic therapy too soon promotes infection recurrence and development of antibiotic-resistant bacteria.

CORNEAL DISORDERS

For a sharp image to be focused on the retina, the cornea must be transparent and intact. Corneal problems may be caused by irritation or infection (keratitis) with ulceration of the corneal surface, degeneration of the cornea (keratoconus), or deposits in the cornea. All corneal problems reduce the refracting power of the cornea, and some can lead to blindness.

CORNEAL ABRASION, ULCERATION, AND INFECTION

Pathophysiology

A corneal abrasion is a scrape or scratch of the cornea that disrupts its integrity. This painful condition can be caused by a small foreign body, trauma, or, most commonly, contact lens use. Other conditions that promote loss of corneal integrity include malnutrition, dry eye syndromes, and some cancer therapies. The abrasion allows organisms to enter, leading to corneal infection. Bacterial, protozoal, and fungal infections can lead to corneal ulceration, which is a deeper disruption of the epithelium. *This problem is an emergency because the cornea has no separate blood supply and infections that can permanently impair vision develop rapidly.* Use of homemade contact lens solutions and the use of large-volume solution containers that can easily become contaminated have led to a sharp rise in the incidence of corneal ulcers infected with *Pseudomonas aeruginosa* and fungi.

PATIENT-CENTERED COLLABORATIVE CARE

The patient with a corneal disorder has pain, reduced vision, photophobia, and eye secretions. Cloudy or purulent fluid may be present on the eyelids or lashes. Wear gloves when examining the eye.

The entire cornea may look hazy or cloudy with a patchy area of ulceration. When fluorescein stain is used, the patchy areas appear green. Microbial culture and corneal scrapings can help determine the causative organism. Anti-infective therapy is started before the organism is identified because of the high risk for vision loss. For culture, obtain swabs from the ulcer and its edges. For corneal scrapings, the cornea is anesthetized with a topical agent and a physician or advanced practice nurse remove samples from the center and edge of the ulcer.

Antibiotics, antifungals, and antivirals are prescribed to reduce or eliminate the organisms. Usually, a broad-spectrum antibiotic is prescribed first and may be changed when culture results are known. Steroids may be used with antibiotics to reduce the inflammatory response in the eye. Drugs can be given topically as eyedrops, injected subconjunctivally, or injected IV. Chart 48-4 in Chapter 48 lists best practices for instilling eyedrops. The nursing priorities are to begin the drug therapy, to ensure patient understanding of the drug therapy regimen, and to prevent infection spread.

Often, the anti-infective therapy involves instilling eyedrops *every hour* for the first 24 hours. Teach the patient how to apply the eyedrops correctly. (See Chart 48-2 in Chapter 48.) Use sterile saline eyedrops to demonstrate the technique, and obtain a return demonstration. If the patient cannot safely self-apply the drugs, teach a family member how to do it.

If the eye infection occurs from a corneal abrasion or ulcer, only one eye is affected. Teach the patient not to use the drug in the unaffected eye. In addition, teach him or her to wash hands after touching the affected eye and before touching or doing anything to the healthy eye. If both eyes are infected, separate bottles of drugs are needed for each eye. Teach the patient to clearly label the bottles "right eye" and "left eye" and not to switch the drugs from eye to eye. Also teach him or her to completely care for one eye, then wash the hands, and using the drugs for the remaining eye, care for that eye. Teach the patient not to wear contact lenses during the entire time that these drugs are being used because the eye then has fewer protections against infection or injury. In addition, the drugs can cloud or damage the contact lenses.

Stress the importance of applying the drug as often as prescribed, even at night. Stopping the infection at this stage can save the vision in the infected eye. Also instruct the patient to make and keep all follow-up appointments; usually the patient is seen again in 24 hours or less.

The type of anti-infective used and the frequency of application may change when the organism is identified and the infection is responding to the therapy. Drug therapy may continue for 3 or more weeks to ensure eradication of the infection. Warn women to avoid using makeup around the eye until the infection has cleared to prevent spread of infection. Instruct patients to discard all open containers of contact lens solutions and bottles of eyedrops because these may be contaminated. Patients should not wear contact lenses for weeks to months until the infection is gone and the ulcer is healed.

KERATOCONUS AND CORNEAL OPACITIES

Pathophysiology

The cornea can permanently lose it shape, become scarred or cloudy, or become thinner. When these conditions occur, refraction is reduced and images are not focused sufficiently for useful vision. Keratoconus, the degeneration of the corneal tissue resulting in abnormal corneal shape, can occur with trauma or may be an inherited disorder (Fig. 49-2). Inadequately treated corneal infections and severe trauma

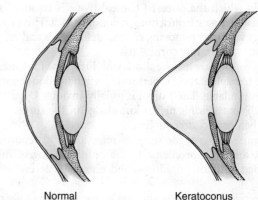

Normal   Keratoconus

FIG. 49-2 Profile of a normal cornea and one with keratoconus.

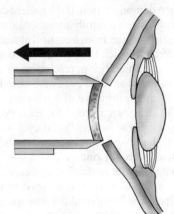
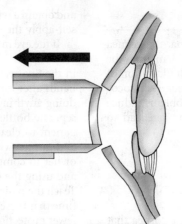
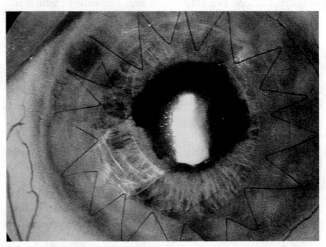

The diseased cornea is removed with a trephine.

A button, or graft, of donor cornea is removed with the same trephine so the cuts are identical.

The donor cornea is placed on the eye and stitched into place with suture material that is finer than a human hair.

FIG. 49-3 The steps involved in corneal transplantation (penetrating keratoplasty).

can damage and scar the cornea and lead to severe visual impairment that can be improved only by surgical interventions.

PATIENT-CENTERED COLLABORATIVE CARE

For a misshaped cornea that is still clear, surgical management involves a corneal implant that adjusts the shape of the cornea. The device approved for this procedure is the Intacs corneal ring. With this procedure, the shape of the cornea is changed by placing a flexible ring in the outer edges of the cornea (outside of the optical zone).

The procedure is performed on both eyes during one surgery under local anesthesia. Improvement to best vision is immediate. Overcorrection or undercorrection of refraction is possible. However, removal, replacement, or adjustment of ring tightness can enhance satisfaction. In addition, replacements can be made if the patient's vision changes further as a result of aging. Because the ring is applied to the cornea outside of the optical zone, the risk for corneal clouding or scarring is lower than with other surgical eye procedures.

Surgery to improve clarity for a permanent corneal disorder that obscures vision is a **keratoplasty** (corneal transplant), in which the diseased corneal tissue is removed and replaced with tissue from a human donor cornea. This process improves vision by removing corneal deformities and replacing them with healthy corneal tissue.

Preoperative care may be short, with little time for teaching because transplantation is performed when the donor cornea becomes available. The patient is usually anxious. Use a calm approach to assess his or her knowledge of the surgery and of care before and after surgery.

Examine the eyes for signs of infection, and report any redness, drainage, or edema to the ophthalmologist. Instill prescribed antibiotic eyedrops, and obtain IV access before surgery.

Operative procedures are *keratoplasties* and are usually performed with local anesthesia in an ambulatory surgical setting. The transplant may involve the entire depth of corneal

FIG. 49-4 The appearance of the eye with sutures in place after corneal transplantation.

tissue (penetrating keratoplasty) or only certain layers of the corneal tissue (lamellar keratoplasty). The nerves around and behind the eye are numbed so that the patient cannot move or see out of the eye. The center 7 to 8 mm of the diseased cornea is removed (Fig. 49-3) with an instrument that works like a cookie cutter. The same instrument is used to cut the tissue graft from the donor cornea so that the graft will be a perfect fit. The donor corneal graft is sutured into place on the eye. Fig. 49-4 shows the eye after transplantation. The procedure usually takes about an hour, and the patient is discharged to home 1 to 2 hours after the procedure.

Postoperative care involves extensive patient teaching. After the procedure, an antibiotic is injected under the conjunctiva and an antibiotic ointment instilled. The eye is covered with a pressure patch and a protective shield until the next day, when the patient returns to the surgeon.

Notify the ophthalmologist of changes in vital signs or of drainage on the dressing. Instruct the patient to lie on the nonoperative side to reduce intraocular pressure (IOP).

TABLE 49-1	ACTIVITIES THAT INCREASE INTRAOCULAR PRESSURE
• Bending from the waist • Lifting objects weighing more than 10 lbs • Sneezing, coughing • Blowing the nose • Straining to have a bowel movement	• Vomiting • Having sexual intercourse • Keeping the head in a dependent position • Wearing tight shirt collars

Show the patient or family member how to apply a patch, and obtain a return demonstration. The patch may need to be worn during the day for the first 3 to 5 days. Teach the patient to wear the shield at night for the first month after surgery and whenever he or she is around small children or pets. Instruct him or her *not* to use an ice pack on the eye. Complications after surgery include bleeding, wound leakage, infection, and graft rejection. Teach the patient how to instill eyedrops, and obtain a return demonstration. Show pictures of what the eye and sutures should look like. Teach him or her to examine the eye (or have a family member do the examination) daily for the presence of infection or graft rejection. The presence of purulent discharge, a continuous leak of clear fluid from around the graft site (not tears), or excessive bleeding should be reported immediately to the surgeon. Other complications include decreased vision, increased reddening of the eye, pain, increased sensitivity to light, and the presence of light flashes or "floaters" in the field of vision. Teach the patient to report any of these manifestations to the surgeon if they develop after the first 48 hours and persist for more than 6 hours.

The eye should be protected from any activity that can increase the pressure on, around, or inside the eye. Teach the patient to avoid jogging, running, dancing, and any other activity that promotes rapid or jerky head motions for several weeks after surgery. Other activities that may raise intraocular pressure (IOP) and should be avoided are listed in Table 49-1. Returning to work depends on the type of work. Patients who have sedentary jobs, such as secretaries, may return to work in 1 week, whereas those who perform heavy lifting or manual labor may need to be off work for 6 to 8 weeks.

Graft rejection can occur. Inflammation starts in the donor cornea near the graft edge and moves toward the center. Vision is reduced, and the cornea becomes cloudy. Topical corticosteroids and other immunosuppressants are used to stop the rejection process. If rejection continues, the graft becomes opaque and blood vessels branch into the opaque tissue.

Eye donation is a common procedure and needed for corneal transplantation. Corneal tissue is obtained from a local eye or tissue bank. An eye bank obtains its supply of corneal tissue from volunteer donors. These donors must be free of infectious disease or cancer at the time of death. If a deceased patient is a potential eye donor, follow these steps:

- Raise the head of the bed 30 degrees.
- Instill prescribed antibiotic eyedrops, such as Neosporin or tobramycin.
- Close the eyes, and apply a *small* ice pack to the closed eyes.
- Contact the family and physician to discuss eye donation.

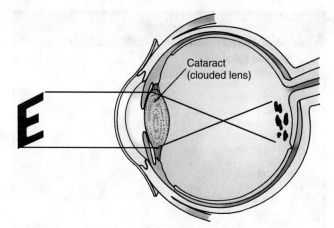

FIG. 49-5 The visual impairment produced by the presence of a cataract.

CATARACT

Pathophysiology

The lens is a transparent, refractive elastic structure suspended behind the iris. A cataract is a lens opacity that distorts the image projected onto the retina (Fig. 49-5). With aging, the lens gradually loses water and increases in density (Touhy & Jett, 2010). This increased density occurs as older lens fibers are compressed and new fibers are produced in the outer layers. Lens proteins dry out and form crystals. As the density of the lens increases, it becomes opaque with a painless loss of transparency. Both eyes may have cataracts; however, the rate of progression in each eye is usually different.

Etiology and Genetic Risk

Cataracts are classified by nature or by onset. They may be present at birth or develop at any time. Cataracts may be age-related or caused by trauma or exposure to toxic agents. They also occur with other diseases and eye disorders (Table 49-2).

Incidence/Prevalence

About 20 to 22 million people in North America have cataracts (National Eye Institute, 2010; Statistics Canada, 2010). The age-related cataract is the most common type. Some degree of cataract formation is expected in all people older than 70 years.

TABLE 49-2	COMMON CAUSES OF CATARACTS

Age-Related Cataracts
• Lens water loss and fiber compaction

Traumatic Cataracts
• Blunt injury to eye or head
• Penetrating eye injury
• Intraocular foreign bodies
• Radiation exposure, therapy

Toxic Cataracts
• Corticosteroids
• Phenothiazine derivatives
• Miotic agents

Associated Cataracts
• Diabetes mellitus
• Hypoparathyroidism
• Down syndrome
• Chronic sunlight exposure

Complicated Cataracts
• Retinitis pigmentosa
• Glaucoma
• Retinal detachment

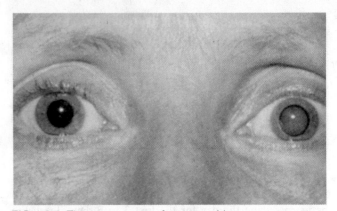

FIG. 49-6 The appearance of an eye with a mature cataract.

Health Promotion and Maintenance

Although most cases of cataracts in North America are age-related, the onset of cataract formation occurs earlier with heavy sun exposure or exposure to other sources of ultraviolet (UV) light. Teach people to reduce the risk for cataract by wearing sunglasses that limit exposure to UV light whenever they are out in bright sunlight. Cataracts also may result from direct eye injury. Urge all people to wear eye and head protection during sports, such as baseball, or any activity that increases the risk for the eye being hit by objects in motion.

PATIENT-CENTERED COLLABORATIVE CARE

ASSESSMENT

History

Age is important because cataracts are most prevalent in the older adult. Ask about these predisposing factors:
• Recent or past trauma to the eye
• Exposure to radioactive materials, x-rays, or UV light
• Systemic disease (e.g., diabetes mellitus, hypoparathyroidism, Down syndrome)
• Prolonged use of corticosteroids, chlorpromazine, beta blockers, or miotic drugs
• Intraocular disease (e.g., recurrent uveitis)

Ask the patient to describe his or her vision. For example, you might say, "Tell me what you can see well and what you have difficulty seeing."

Physical Assessment/Clinical Manifestations

Early manifestations of cataracts are slightly blurred vision and decreased color perception. At first, the patient may think his or her glasses or contact lenses are smudged. As lens cloudiness continues, blurred and double vision occur and the patient may have difficulty with ADLs. Without surgical intervention, visual impairment progresses to blindness. *No pain or eye redness is associated with age-related cataract formation.*

Vision is tested using a Snellen chart and brightness acuity testing (see Chapter 48). Examine the lens with an ophthalmoscope, and describe any observed densities by size, shape, and location. As the cataract matures, the opacity makes it difficult to see the retina and the red reflex may be absent. When this occurs, the pupil is white (Fig. 49-6).

Psychosocial Assessment

Loss of vision is gradual, and the patient may not be aware of it until reading or driving is affected. Fear of blindness can be overwhelming, and the patient has anxiety about loss of independence. Encourage the patient and family to express concerns about reduced vision.

PLANNING AND IMPLEMENTATION

The priority problem for the patient with cataracts is reduced vision, which is a safety risk. Patients often live with reduced vision for years before the cataract is removed. Interventions for safety and independence before surgery are on pp. 1073-1075 in Patient-Centered Collaborative Care in the Reduced Vision section.

Improving Vision

Planning: Expected Outcomes. The patient with cataracts is expected to recognize when he or she is no longer able to perform ADLs safely and independently and then is expected to have cataract surgery. This procedure is covered by Medicare for patients who are 65 years or older.

Interventions. Surgery is the only "cure" for cataracts. After vision is reduced to the extent that ADLs are affected, the surgery should be performed as soon as possible.

Preoperative Care. The health care provider has the responsibility of (1) giving the patient accurate information so that he or she can make informed decisions about treatment and (2) obtaining informed consent. Reinforce this information, and teach about the nature of cataracts, their progression, and their treatment.

Because cataract surgery is usually an ambulatory procedure and most patients are older, preoperative teaching is challenging. Assess how the patient's vision affects ADLs, especially dressing, eating, and ambulating. Stress that care

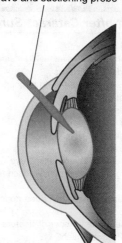

Sound wave and suctioning probe

Sound waves break up the lens, pieces are sucked out, and the capsule remains largely intact

FIG. 49-7 Cataract removal by phacoemulsification.

after surgery requires the instillation of different types of eyedrops several times a day for 2 to 4 weeks. Careful assessment of eye appearance is also needed. If the patient is unable to perform these tasks, help him or her make arrangements for this care.

Ask the patient whether he or she takes any drugs that affect blood clotting, such as aspirin, warfarin (Coumadin), clopidogrel (Plavix), and dabigatran (Pradaxa). Ensure that this information is communicated to the surgeon because some of these drugs may need to be discontinued before cataract surgery.

An IV infusion may or may not be started in the operating room. A sedative is given before surgery, and a series of ophthalmic drugs are instilled just before surgery to dilate the pupils and cause vasoconstriction. Other eyedrops are instilled to induce paralysis to prevent lens movement. When the patient is in the surgical area, a local anesthetic is injected into the muscle cone behind the eye for anesthesia and eye paralysis.

Operative Procedures. Extraction of the lens is most commonly performed by *phacoemulsification* (Fig. 49-7). A probe is inserted through the capsule, and high-frequency sound waves break the lens into small pieces, which are then removed by suction. The capsule remains intact, and the replacement intraocular lens (IOL) is placed inside it to focus light rays in the retina. The IOL is a small, clear, plastic lens. Different types are available, and one is selected by the surgeon and patient to allow correction of a specific refractive error. Some patients have distant vision restored to 20/20 and may need glasses only for reading or close work. Some replacement lenses have multiple focal planes and may correct all vision for a patient to the extent that glasses or contact lenses may not be needed. Lens replacement surgery is now performed for people who do not have cataracts but who want corrected vision.

Postoperative Care. Immediately after surgery, antibiotics are given subconjunctivally. Usually antibiotic and steroid

ointments also are instilled. The eye is left unpatched, and the patient is discharged within an hour after surgery. Instruct him or her to wear dark glasses outdoors or in brightly lit environments until the pupil responds to light. Teach the patient and family members how to instill the prescribed eyedrops. (See Chart 48-2 in Chapter 48.) Work with them in creating a written schedule for the timing and the order of eyedrops administration. Stress the importance of keeping all follow-up appointments.

Remind the patient that mild eye itching is normal, as is a "bloodshot appearance." The eyelid may be slightly swollen. However, significant swelling or bruising is abnormal. Cool compresses may be beneficial. Discomfort at the site is controlled by a mild analgesic such as acetaminophen (Abenol ✦, Tylenol) or acetaminophen with oxycodone (Endocet ✦, Percocet, Tylox). Remind him or her to avoid aspirin because of its effects on blood clotting.

Pain early after surgery may indicate increased intraocular pressure (IOP) or hemorrhage. Teach patients to contact the surgeon if pain occurs with nausea or vomiting.

To reduce increases in IOP, teach the patient and family about activity restrictions. Activities that can cause a sudden rise in IOP are listed in Table 49-1.

Another major complication is infection. Teach the patient and family to observe for increasing redness of the eye, a change in visual acuity, tears, and photophobia. Creamy white, dry, crusty drainage on the eyelids and lashes is normal. However, yellow or green drainage indicates infection and must be reported.

Patients experience a dramatic improvement in vision on the day of surgery. Remind them that final best vision will not be present until 4 to 6 weeks after surgery. However, vision is not expected to become worse after the procedure.

> **! NURSING SAFETY PRIORITY**
> ***Action Alert***
> Instruct the patient who has had cataract surgery to immediately report any reduction of vision after surgery in the eye that had the cataract removed.

Community-Based Care

The patient is usually discharged within an hour after cataract surgery. Nursing interventions focus on helping the patient and family with plans for return to the home, assisted-living, or extended-care setting.

Home Care Management

If the patient has difficulty instilling eyedrops, a supportive neighbor, friend, or family member can be taught the procedure. Adaptive equipment that positions the bottle of eyedrops directly over the eye can also be purchased (Fig. 49-8). Eyedrops are often prescribed for 2 to 6 weeks after cataract surgery.

Teaching for Self-Management

The best outcome of cataract removal requires close adherence to the drug regimen after surgery. Providing the patient or family with accurate information and demonstration of needed skills are nursing priorities for this patient population (Lockey, 2009). Review these indications of complications

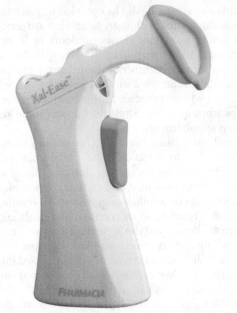

FIG. 49-8 The Xal-Ease adaptive device for self-administering eyedrops.

after cataract surgery with the patient and family before discharge:

- Sharp, sudden pain in the eye
- Bleeding or increased discharge
- Green or yellow, thick drainage
- Lid swelling
- Reappearance of a bloodshot sclera after the initial appearance has cleared
- Decreased vision
- Flashes of light or floating shapes

Remind the patient to avoid activities that might increase IOP (see Table 49-1). Hair may be washed a day or two after surgery but only with the head tilted back, such as in a beauty salon or barber shop, to avoid getting water in the eye. Teach the patient to stand in the shower with the face away from the showerhead for the first week after surgery.

Teach the patient about activity restrictions. Cooking and light housekeeping are permitted, but vacuuming should be avoided for several weeks because of the forward flexion involved and the rapid, jerky movements required. Advise him or her to refrain from driving, operating machinery, and participating in sports until given specific permission from the ophthalmologist. Chart 49-5 lists items to cover in the focused assessment of a patient in the home environment after cataract surgery.

Health Care Resources

If the patient lives alone and has no support, arrange for a home care nurse to assess him or her and the home situation. If the patient is unable to instill eyedrops independently, a friend, neighbor, or family member can be taught this technique.

EVALUATION: OUTCOMES

Evaluate the care of the patient with cataracts on the basis of improving vision. The expected outcomes include that the patient after cataract surgery will:

CHART 49-5   HOME CARE ASSESSMENT

The Patient after Cataract Surgery

Assess the eye and vision:
- Visual acuity in both eyes using a Jaeger card
- Visual fields of both eyes
- Compare operative eye with nonoperative eye for presence or absence of:
    Redness
    Tearing
    Drainage

Ask the patient about:
- Pain in or around the operative eye
- Any change in visual acuity (decreased or improved) in the operative eye
- Whether any of these has been noticed in the operative eye:
    Dark spots
    Increase in the number of floaters
    Bright flashes of light

Assess the home environment for:
- Safety hazards (especially tripping and falling hazards)
- Kitchen hazards
- Level of room lighting

Assess patient adherence with and understanding of treatment and limitations, such as:
- Signs and symptoms to report
- Drug regimen
- Activity restrictions

Assess functional ability:
- Activities of daily living
- Adherence to drug regimen

- Have improved sensory function (vision)
- Recognize manifestations of complications

Specific indicators for these outcomes are listed under the Planning and Implementation section (see earlier).

❓ NCLEX EXAMINATION CHALLENGE

Safe and Effective Care Environment

A client who had cataract removal with placement of an intraocular implant 1 week ago now calls in and reports that her eye is more bloodshot than it was yesterday and that a small amount of greenish drainage is present. What is the priority nursing action?
- A. Reassure the client that these symptoms are normal for this stage of recovery after cataract surgery.
- B. Explain how to apply a wet compress to the affected eye for 15 minutes four times daily.
- C. Instruct the client to come to the office immediately to be seen by the ophthalmologist.
- D. Instruct the client to use the antibiotic eyedrops four times daily instead of twice daily.

GLAUCOMA

Pathophysiology

Glaucoma is a group of eye disorders resulting in increased IOP. Intraocular pressure (IOP) is the fluid pressure within the eye. As described in Chapter 48, the eye is a hollow organ. For proper eye function, the gel in the posterior segment (vitreous humor) and the fluid in the anterior segment (aqueous humor) must be present in set amounts that apply pressure inside the eye to keep it ball-shaped.

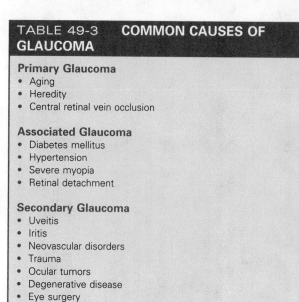

TABLE 49-3   COMMON CAUSES OF GLAUCOMA

Primary Glaucoma
- Aging
- Heredity
- Central retinal vein occlusion

Associated Glaucoma
- Diabetes mellitus
- Hypertension
- Severe myopia
- Retinal detachment

Secondary Glaucoma
- Uveitis
- Iritis
- Neovascular disorders
- Trauma
- Ocular tumors
- Degenerative disease
- Eye surgery

The gel-like vitreous humor is made as the eyes form and grow. Once eye growth is complete, this volume does not change. The aqueous humor, however, is continuously made from blood plasma. The ciliary bodies located behind the iris and just in front of the lens make and secrete this fluid (see Fig. 48-2 in Chapter 48). The fluid flows through the pupil into the bulging area in front of the iris. At the outer edges of the iris beneath the cornea, blood vessels collect fluid and return it to the blood. Usually about 1 mL of aqueous humor is present at all times, but it is continuously made and reabsorbed at a rate of about 5 mL daily. *A normal IOP requires a balance between production and outflow of aqueous humor. If the IOP becomes too high, the extra pressure compresses retinal blood vessels and photoreceptors and their synapsing nerve fibers. This compression results in poorly oxygenated photoreceptors and nerve fibers. These sensitive nerve tissues become ischemic and die. When too many have died, sight is lost and the person is permanently blind.* Tissue damage usually starts in the periphery and moves inward toward the fovea centralis. Left untreated, glaucoma can result in blindness. Glaucoma is usually painless, and the patient may be unaware of a gradual reduction in vision.

There are several causes and types of glaucoma (Table 49-3). It is classified as primary, secondary, or associated. In primary glaucoma, the most common form, the structures involved in circulation and reabsorption of the aqueous humor undergo direct pathologic change.

Primary open-angle glaucoma (POAG), the most common form of primary glaucoma, usually affects both eyes and has no symptoms in the early stages. Outflow of aqueous humor through the chamber angle is reduced. Because the fluid cannot leave the eye at the same rate it is produced, IOP gradually increases. Primary angle-closure glaucoma (also called *PACG* or *acute glaucoma*) is less common, has a sudden onset, and is an emergency. The basic problems are a narrowed angle and forward displacement of the iris. The iris pressing against the cornea closes the chamber angle, obstructing the outflow of aqueous humor. This can happen suddenly and without warning. It is more common in women and Asian patients (Kock & Sikes, 2009).

Glaucoma is a common cause of blindness in affluent countries. It is age-related, occurring in about 10% of people older than 80 years (McCance et al., 2010).

PATIENT-CENTERED COLLABORATIVE CARE

Primary open-angle glaucoma (POAG) develops slowly, with gradual loss of visual fields that may go unnoticed because central vision is unaffected. At times, the patient may have foggy vision, reduced accommodation, mild aching in the eyes, or headaches and may require frequent changes in eyeglass prescriptions. Late manifestations occur after irreversible damage to optic nerve function and include seeing halos around lights, losing peripheral vision, and having decreased vision that does not improve with eyeglasses. The Concept Map on p. 1066 addresses collaborative care issues for patients who have glaucoma.

ASSESSMENT

Physical Assessment/Clinical Manifestations

Ophthalmoscopic examination of the patient with glaucoma shows cupping and atrophy of the optic disc. It becomes wider and deeper and turns white or gray. Visual fields are measured to determine the extent of peripheral vision loss. In POAG, the visual fields first show a small defect that gradually progresses to a larger field defect.

Manifestations of acute angle-closure glaucoma differ from those of POAG. The onset is acute, and the patient has sudden, severe pain around the eyes that radiates over the face. Headache or brow pain, nausea, and vomiting may occur. Other manifestations include seeing colored halos around lights and sudden blurred vision with decreased light perception. The sclera may appear reddened and the cornea foggy. Ophthalmoscopic examination reveals a shallow anterior chamber, cloudy aqueous humor, and a moderately dilated, nonreactive pupil.

Diagnostic Assessment

An elevated intraocular pressure (IOP) is measured by tonometry. In open-angle glaucoma, the tonometry reading is between 22 and 32 mm Hg (normal is 10 to 21 mm Hg). In angle-closure glaucoma, the tonometry reading may be 30 mm Hg or higher. Visual field testing by perimetry is performed, as is visualization by gonioscopy to determine whether the angle is open or closed (Sharts-Hopko & Glynn-Milley, 2009). Usually, the optic nerve is imaged to determine to what degree nerve damage is present. All of these diagnostic assessment techniques are described in Chapter 48.

INTERVENTIONS

Nonsurgical Management

Blindness from glaucoma can be prevented by early detection, lifelong treatment, and close monitoring with follow-up care. Some degree of vision loss occurs, although use of topical agents that reduce IOP has been found to delay or prevent damage. Chart 49-6 lists ways to assist the person with impaired vision to remain as independent as possible.

Concept Map: Primary Open-Angle Glaucoma (POAG)

Concept Map by Deanne A. Blach, MSN, RN

HISTORY

80-year-old Donald Vincent has just been diagnosed with POAG. He states he has been having a gradual loss of vision, including foggy vision with occasional eye aches. He has recently had the prescription changed on his eyeglasses but still has vision issues.

OBJECTIVE DATA
- PERRL with reduced accommodation
- Tonometry reading — 28 mm Hg (N = 10-21 mm Hg)
- Cupping and atrophy of the optic disc noted
- Peripheral vision decreased
- Patient instills 1 drop of Travatan (travoprost ophthalmic solution) 0.004% to the left eye daily

SUBJECTIVE DATA

"Everything is a little bit deteriorated. I have a little double vision sometimes. I can't read very much, that's why I like to watch the news on TV. I can't see far away, I can just see a figure walking...not their facial features. I have to use a magnifying glass to read the label on the eyedrop bottle."

Perform and Interpret Physical Assessment

Planning

EXPECTED OUTCOMES

Prevent blindness by early detection, lifelong treatment, and close monitoring with follow-up care.

INTERVENTIONS

1 **Physical Assessment/Clinical Manifestions**

Perform eye exam; glaucoma will show cupping and atrophy of the optic disc. *Measures visual fields to determine the extent of peripheral vision loss.*

2 **Priority Nursing Intervention**

Provide written instructions about the prescribed medication schedule. When more than one drug is given, instruct to wait 10-15 minutes between drops. *Prevents one drug from "washing out" or diluting the other.*

3 **Nursing Safety Priority: Drug Alert**

Teach the correct technique to instill eyedrops (punctual occlusion). *Prevents drugs for glaucoma from being systemically absorbed and causing serious side effects.*

4 **Safe & Effective Care Environment**

Teach principles of infection control (e.g., hand hygiene), and teach the patient not to touch the tip of the eyedrop container or dropper to any part of the eye. *Protects the patient from infection transmission.*

5 **Patient Education**

Educate the patient about what to expect when instilling eyedrops. *Informs the patient that most eye medications cause tearing, mild burning, and blurred vision for a few minutes after instillation. The sclera may also become red and itchy.*

6 **Blindness Prevention Strategy**

Encourage the patient to keep follow-up appointments to check IOP. *Monitors IOP. If it becomes too high, the extra pressure can cause sensitive nerve tissues to become ischemic and die, leading to permanent blindness.*

7 **Travaprost (Travatan) Side Effects**

Teach the patient to report emergent signs of allergy—hives, difficulty breathing, angioedema. Stop using drops and call the provider for serious side effects: redness, swelling, itching, eye pain, discharge, increased light sensitivity, visual changes, or chest pain. *Educates the patient and prevents medication complications.*

8 **Psychosocial Aspects**

Encourage the patient and family to express concerns about reduced vision. *Helps patient and family to cope with fear of blindness and anxiety about loss of independence.*

CHART 49-6   NURSING FOCUS ON THE OLDER ADULT

Promote Independent Living in Patients with Impaired Vision

Drugs
- Having a neighbor, relative, friend, or visiting nurse visit once a week to measure the proper drugs for each day may be helpful.
  - If the patient is to take drugs more than once each day, it is helpful to use a container of a different shape (with a lid) each time. For example, if the patient is to take drugs at 9 AM, 1 PM, and 9 PM, the 9 AM drugs would be placed in a round container, the 1 PM drugs in a square container, and the 9 PM drugs in a triangular container.
  - It is helpful to place each day's drug containers in a separate box with raised letters on the side of the box spelling out the day.
- "Talking clocks" are available for the patient with low vision.
- Some drug boxes have alarms that can be set for different times.

Communication
- Telephones with large, raised block numbers may be helpful. The best models are those with black numbers on a white phone or white numbers on a black phone.
- Telephones that have a programmable, automatic dialing feature are very helpful. Programmed numbers should include those for the fire department, police, relatives, friends, neighbors, and 911.

Safety
- It is best to leave furniture the way the patient wants it and not move it.
- Throw rugs are best eliminated.
- Appliance cords should be short and kept out of walkways.
- Lounge-style chairs with built-in footrests are preferable to footstools.
- Nonbreakable dishes, cups, and glasses are preferable to breakable ones.
- Cleansers and other toxic agents should be labeled with large, raised letters.
- Hook-and-loop (Velcro) strips at hand level may help mark the locations of switches and electrical outlets.

Food Preparation
- Meals on Wheels is a service that many older adults find helpful. This service brings meals at mealtime, cooked and ready to eat.

The cost of this service varies, depending on the patient's ability to pay.
- Many grocery stores offer a "shop by telephone" service. The patient can either complete a computer booklet indicating types, amounts, and brands of items desired, or the store will complete this booklet over the telephone by asking the patient specific information. The store then delivers groceries to the patient's door (many stores also offer a "put away" service) and charges the patient's bank card.
- A microwave oven is a safer means of cooking than a standard stove, although many older patients are afraid of microwave ovens. If the patient has and will use a microwave oven, others can prepare meals ahead of time, label them, and freeze them for later use. Also, many microwavable complete frozen dinners that comply with a variety of dietary restrictions are available.
- Friends or relatives may be able to help with food preparation. Often relatives do not know what to give an older person for birthdays or other gift-giving occasions. One suggestion is a homemade prepackaged frozen dinner that the patient enjoys.

Personal Care
- Handgrips should be installed in bathrooms.
- The tub floor should have a nonskid surface.
- Male patients should use an electric shaver rather than a razor.
- Choosing a hairstyle that is becoming but easy to care for (avoiding parts) helps in independent living.
- Home hair care services may be available.

Diversional Activity
- Some patients can read large-print books, newspapers, and magazines (available through local libraries and vision services).
- Books, magazines, and some newspapers are available on audiotapes or discs.
- Patients experienced in knitting or crocheting may be able to create items fashioned from straight pieces, such as afghans.
- Card games, dominoes, and some board games that are available in large, high-contrast print may be helpful for patients with low vision.

Drug therapy for glaucoma focuses on reducing IOP through these mechanisms:
- Constricting the pupil so that the ciliary muscle is contracted, allowing better circulation of the aqueous humor to the site of absorption
- Reducing the production or increasing the absorption of aqueous humor

Eyedrop drugs are the mainstay of control for glaucoma. They do not improve lost vision but prevent more damage by decreasing IOP. The classes of drugs to manage glaucoma are the prostaglandins agonists, adrenergic agonists, beta-adrenergic blockers, cholinergic agonists, and carbonic anhydrase inhibitors. Most eyedrops cause tearing, mild burning, and blurred vision for a few minutes after instilling the drug. The sclera may also become red and itchy. Specific drug actions and nursing interventions are listed in Chart 49-7.

The priority nursing intervention for the patient on drug therapy for glaucoma is teaching. Provide written instructions similar to those in Chart 48-2 in Chapter 48. The benefit of drug therapy is achieved only when the drugs are used on the prescribed schedule, usually every 12 hours. Teach patients

the importance of instilling the drops on time and not skipping doses. When more than one drug is prescribed, teach him or her to wait 10 to 15 minutes between drug instillations to prevent one drug from "washing out" or diluting another drug. Stress the need for good handwashing, keeping the eyedrop container tip clean, and avoiding touching the tip to any part of the eye. Also teach the technique of punctal occlusion (placing pressure on the corner of the eye near the nose) immediately after eyedrop instillation to prevent systemic absorption of the drug. Fig. 49-9 demonstrates this technique.

! NURSING SAFETY PRIORITY

Drug Alert

Most eyedrops used for glaucoma therapy can be absorbed systemically and cause serious systemic problems. Although punctal occlusion should be used after instilling any type of eyedrop, it is critical to teach patients to use the technique with eyedrops for glaucoma.

Systemic osmotic drugs may be given for angle-closure glaucoma as part of emergency management to rapidly

CHART 49-7 COMMON EXAMPLES OF DRUG THERAPY (EYEDROPS)

Categories for Management of Glaucoma

CATEGORY AND DRUG	PURPOSE/ACTIONS	NURSING IMPLICATIONS	RATIONALES
Prostaglandin Agonists Bimatoprost (Lumigan) Latanoprost (Xalatan) Travoprost (Travatan)	Drugs lower IOP by dilating the blood vessels in the trabecular mesh of the eye, where the aqueous humor is reabsorbed, collecting more aqueous humor and allowing more fluid to leave the eye.	Teach the patient to check the cornea for abrasions or other signs of trauma. Remind the patient that, over time, the eye color darkens and eyelashes elongate in the eye receiving the drug. If only one eye is to be treated, teach the patient *not* to place drops in the other eye to try to make the eye colors similar. Warn the patient that using higher doses than are prescribed can reduce the effectiveness of the drug in controlling the glaucoma.	Drugs should not be used when the cornea is not intact. Knowing the side effects in advance reassures the patient that their presence is expected and normal. Using the drug in an eye with normal IOP can cause a *lower-than-normal* IOP, which reduces vision. Drug action is based on blocking receptors, which can increase in number when the drug is overused.
Adrenergic Agonists Apraclonidine (Iopidine) Brimonidine tartrate (Alphagan) Dipivefrin hydrochloride (Propine)	These drugs bind to receptors in the eye, reducing the amount of aqueous humor produced by the ciliary bodies. In addition, the pupil of the eye is dilated and flow of the fluid through the pupil is improved. Both these actions reduce the amount of fluid present in the eye at any one time, lowering the intraocular pressure.	Ask whether the patient is taking any antidepressants from the MAO inhibitor class, such as phenelzine (Nardil) or tranylcypromine (Parnate). Teach the patient to wear dark glasses outdoors and also indoors when lighting is bright. Teach the patient not to use the eyedrops with contact lenses in place and to wait 15 minutes after using the drug to put in the lenses.	These enzyme inhibitors increase blood pressure as do the adrenergic agonists. When taken together, the patient may experience hypertensive crisis. The pupil dilates (mydriasis) and remains dilated, even when there is plenty of light, causing discomfort. These drugs are absorbed by the contact lens, which can become discolored or cloudy.
Beta-Adrenergic Blockers Betaxolol hydrochloride (Betopic) Carteolol (Cartrol, Ocupress) Levobunolol (Betagan) Timolol (Betimol, Istalol, Timoptic) Timoptic GFS (gel-forming solution) (Timoptic-XE, Timolol-GFS)	By selectively blocking beta-adrenergic receptors in the eye, less aqueous humor is produced by the ciliary bodies. The fluid also appears to be absorbed slightly faster as a result of this drug therapy. Both actions reduce IOP.	Ask whether the patient has moderate to severe asthma or COPD. Warn diabetic patients to check their blood glucose levels more often when taking these drugs. Teach patients who also take oral beta blockers to check their pulse at least twice per day and to notify the health care provider if the pulse is consistently below 58 beats per minute.	If these drugs are absorbed systemically, they constrict pulmonary smooth muscle and narrow airways. These drugs induce hypoglycemia and also mask the hypoglycemic symptoms. These drugs potentiate the effects of systemic beta blockers and can cause an unsafe drop in heart rate and blood pressure.
Cholinergic Agonists Carbachol (Carboptic, Isopto Carbachol, Miostat) Echothiophate (Phospholine Iodide) Pilocarpine (Adsorbocarpine, Akarpine, Isopto Carpine, Ocu-Carpine, Ocusert, Piloptic, Pilostat)	These drugs lower IOP by decreasing the amount of aqueous humor produced and by improving flow of the fluid. They make the pupil smaller (miosis) but, at the same time, make more room between the iris and the lens, allowing the fluid to flow through the pupil better even though it is smaller.	Teach the patient not to use more eyedrops than are prescribed and to report increased salivation or drooling to the health care provider. Teach the patient to use good light when reading and to take care in darker rooms.	These drugs are readily absorbed by conjunctival mucous membranes and can cause systemic side effects of headache, flushing, increased saliva, and sweating. The pupil of the eye will not open more to let in more light, and it may be harder to see objects in dim light. This problem can increase the risk for falls.

COPD, Chronic obstructive pulmonary disease; *IOP,* intraocular pressure; *MAO,* monamine oxidase.

CHART 49-7	**COMMON EXAMPLES OF DRUG THERAPY (EYEDROPS)**		

Categories for Management of Glaucoma—cont'd

CATEGORY AND DRUG	PURPOSE/ACTIONS	NURSING IMPLICATIONS	RATIONALES
Carbonic Anhydrase Inhibitors			
Brinzolamide (Azopt) Dorzolamide (Trusopt)	Drugs reduce IOP by directly inhibiting production of aqueous humor from the zonules of the ciliary bodies. They do not affect the flow or absorption of the fluid.	Ask whether the patient has an allergy to sulfonamide antibacterial drugs.	Drugs are similar to the sulfonamides, and if a patient is allergic to the sulfonamides, an allergy is likely with these drugs, even as eyedrops.
		Teach the patient to shake the drug before applying.	Drug separates on standing.
		Teach the patient not to use the eyedrops with contact lenses in place and to wait 15 minutes after using the drug to put in the lenses.	These drugs are absorbed by the contact lens, which can become discolored or cloudy.
Combination Drugs			
Brimonidine tartrate and timolol maleate (Combigan)	Same as for each drug alone.	Same as for each drug alone.	Same as for each drug alone.

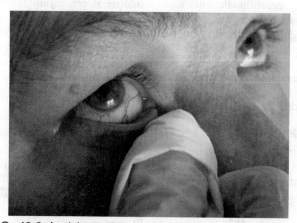

FIG. 49-9 Applying punctal occlusion to prevent systemic absorption of eyedrops.

reduce IOP. These agents include oral glycerin and IV mannitol (Osmitrol).

Surgical Management

Surgery is used when drugs for the patient with open-angle glaucoma are not effective at controlling IOP. Two common procedures are laser trabeculoplasty and filtering microsurgery. A *laser trabeculoplasty* burns the trabecular meshwork, scarring it and causing the meshwork fibers to tighten. Tight fibers increase the size of the spaces between the fibers, improving outflow of aqueous humor and reducing IOP. *Filtering microsurgery* creates a drainage hole in the iris between the posterior and anterior chambers. Both are ambulatory surgery procedures.

If glaucoma fails to respond to common approaches or if the drainage hole does not remain open, other more invasive procedures may be used. These include deep sclerectomy, viscocanalostomy, or an implanted shunt (Sharts-Hopko & Glynn-Milley, 2009).

A *sclerectomy* for glaucoma involves removing a section of sclera and trabecular meshwork along with a section of the canal of Schlemm to allow more direct drainage of aqueous humor. A *viscocanalostomy* requires removal of a section of

sclera but the main focus is artificially widening the canal of Schlemm to improve drainage. The *implanted shunt* has a small tube or filament connected to a flat plate positioned on the outside of the eye in the eye orbit. (The plate is not visible on the front part of the eye.) The open part of the fine tube is placed into the front chamber of the eye, just in front of the iris. The fluid then drains through the tube (or along the outside of the tube) into the area around the flat plate where it collects and is reabsorbed into the bloodstream.

A serious complication after glaucoma surgery is choroidal hemorrhage. If IOP is too low, fluid may enter the suprachoroid space and cause a choroidal detachment. Extra fluid in this space may break blood vessels located there. Manifestations of choroidal hemorrhage include:

- Acute pain deep in the eye
- Decreased vision
- Vital sign changes

? NCLEX EXAMINATION CHALLENGE

Safe and Effective Care Environment

Which assessment question is most important for the nurse to ask a client with glaucoma who has just been prescribed the drug apraclonidine (Iopidine)?
A. "Are you allergic to sulfa drugs?"
B. "What other drugs do you currently take?"
C. "Do you have any difficulty passing urine?"
D. "Do you have asthma or any other respiratory problem?"

VITREOUS HEMORRHAGE

The vitreous is the gel that fills the posterior two thirds of the eye and maintains the eye's shape. Vitreous hemorrhage (bleeding into the vitreous cavity) may result from aging, systemic diseases, or trauma. With aging, the vitreous may spontaneously detach from the retina. Torn blood vessels allow bleeding into the vitreous. Diabetes and hypertension damage retinal blood vessels and cause vitreal hemorrhage.

Reduced visual acuity is the main manifestation of vitreous hemorrhage. A mild hemorrhage may cause the patient to see a red haze or "floaters." A moderate hemorrhage may cause the patient to see "black streaks" or "tiny black dots." Severe hemorrhage may reduce visual acuity to hand motion. The eye has a reduced red reflex because light rays do not reach the retina. The location and extent of the hemorrhage are determined by ultrasonography.

The hemorrhage may absorb slowly with no treatment. Leaking blood vessels can be sealed with laser therapy. If the hemorrhage is still present several weeks to months later, a vitrectomy (surgical removal of the vitreous) may be needed.

UVEITIS

The eye's uveal tract has three related parts: the iris, the ciliary body, and the choroid. Any of these anterior or posterior structures can become inflamed (uveitis).

Anterior uveitis is inflammation of the iris or of the ciliary body, or both. The cause is unknown but uveitis often follows exposure to allergens, infectious agents, trauma, or systemic disease (rheumatoid arthritis, herpes simplex, herpes zoster). It can follow any local or systemic bacterial infection. Manifestations include aching around the eye; tearing; blurred vision; photophobia; a small, irregular, nonreactive pupil; and a "bloodshot" appearance of the sclera.

Posterior uveitis is another term for retinitis (inflammation of the retina) and chorioretinitis (inflammation of the choroid and the retina). It occurs with tuberculosis, syphilis, and toxoplasmosis.

The onset of symptoms is slow and painless. Reduced vision in the affected eye results from fluid, fibrin, and cells leaking into the vitreous cavity. The pupil is small, nonreactive, and irregularly shaped. Black dots are visible against the red background of the fundus. Lesions appear as grayish yellow patches on the retinal surface.

Management of uveitis includes resting the ciliary body with a cycloplegic drug to paralyze the ciliary muscles and dilate the pupil. This action prevents adhesions from forming between the iris and the lens. Steroid drops are given hourly to reduce the inflammation and to prevent adhesion of the iris to the cornea and lens. Ocular injections of steroids are used in posterior uveitis or when topical steroids have been ineffective. Analgesics that contain neither aspirin nor opioids are prescribed for pain. Systemic antibiotic therapy may be started for posterior uveitis or when infection is present with anterior uveitis.

Cool or warm compresses are applied for ocular pain. Darkening the room and wearing sunglasses reduce the discomfort of photophobia. Because of blurred vision from the cycloplegic drops, instruct the patient not to drive or operate machinery. Review the manifestations of bacterial and fungal ulcers and those of increased intraocular pressure (IOP).

RETINAL DISORDERS

MACULAR DEGENERATION

Pathophysiology

Macular degeneration is the deterioration of the macula (the area of central vision) and can be age-related or exudative. Age-related macular degeneration (AMD) has two types. The most common type is *dry* AMD, caused by gradual blockage of retinal capillaries, allowing retinal cells in the macula to become ischemic and necrotic. Rod and cone photoreceptors die. Central vision declines, and patients describe mild blurring and distortion at first. Eventually, the person loses all central vision (National Eye Institute, 2010). About 2 million older adults in the United States and Canada have dry AMD (National Eye Institute, 2010; Statistics Canada, 2010). This vision loss affects independence, well-being, and quality of life, as well as health care costs. It is often the impetus for an older adult leaving his or her independent living environment and moving into assisted living (Touhy & Jett, 2010).

Dry AMD is more common and progresses at a faster rate among smokers than among nonsmokers (Noble & Chaudhary, 2010). Other risk factors include hypertension, female gender, short stature, family history, and a long-term diet poor in carotene and vitamin E (National Eye Institute, 2010).

Another cause of AMD is the growth of new blood vessels in the macula, which have thin walls and leak blood and fluid (*wet* AMD). Exudative macular degeneration is also a type of wet macular degeneration but can occur at any age. The condition can occur in only one eye or in both eyes. In addition, the person with AMD can also develop exudative macular degeneration. Patients with exudative degeneration have a sudden decrease in vision after a serous detachment of pigment epithelium in the macula. Newly formed blood vessels invade this injured area and cause fluid and blood to collect under the macula (like a blister), resulting in scar formation and visual distortion.

PATIENT-CENTERED COLLABORATIVE CARE

Dry AMD has no cure. Management of dry AMD is focused on slowing the progression of the vision loss and helping the patient maximize remaining vision (Watkinson, 2010). Current research findings suggest that the risk for dry macular degeneration can be reduced by increasing long-term dietary intake of antioxidants, vitamin B_{12}, and the carotenoids *lutein* and *zeaxanthin*. The same dietary treatments appear to slow the progression of macular degeneration.

The loss of central vision reduces the ability to read, write, recognize safety hazards, and drive. Suggest alternative strategies (e.g., large-print books, public transportation) and referrals to community organizations that provide a wide range of adaptive equipment. See pp. 1073-1075 of Patient-Centered Collaborative Care in the Reduced Vision section for a complete discussion of patient care needs.

Management of patients with exudative or wet macular degeneration is geared toward slowing the process and identifying further changes in visual perception. Fluid and blood may resorb in some patients with exudative degeneration. Laser therapy to seal the leaking blood vessels in or near the macula can limit the extent of the damage. Recent clinical trials with agents that slow or prevent new blood vessel formation, the vascular endothelial growth factor inhibitors (VEGFIs), have shown success in the management of wet macular degeneration. This therapy uses either bevacizumab (Avastin), which is a drug used as targeted therapy for cancer, or ranibizumab (Lucentis), which is a VEGFI approved specifically for ocular problems. Management involves monthly injections of the drug into the vitreal chamber. The results were a reduction of vitreal fluids and an increase in visual acuity (Tao et al., 2010).

RETINAL HOLES, TEARS, AND DETACHMENTS

Pathophysiology

A retinal hole is a break in the retina. These holes can be caused by trauma or can occur with aging. A retinal tear is a more jagged and irregularly shaped break in the retina. It can result from traction on the retina. A retinal detachment is the separation of the retina from the epithelium. Detachments are classified by the nature of their development.

Rhegmatogenous detachments occur following a hole or tear in the retina caused by mechanical force, creating an opening for the vitreous to move under the retina. When sufficient fluid collects in this space, the retina detaches. *Traction* detachments occur when the retina is pulled away from the support tissue by bands of fibrous tissue in the vitreous. *Exudative* detachments are caused by fluid collecting under the retina. These often occur with a systemic disease or with ocular tumors. No retinal break occurs.

PATIENT-CENTERED COLLABORATIVE CARE

The onset of a retinal detachment is usually sudden and painless because no pain fibers are located in the retina. Patients may suddenly see bright flashes of light (photopsia) or floating dark spots in the affected eye. During the initial phase of the detachment or if the detachment is partial, the patient may describe the sensation of a curtain being pulled over part of the visual field. The visual field loss corresponds to the area of detachment.

On ophthalmoscopic examination, detachments are seen as gray bulges or folds in the retina that quiver. Depending on the cause of the detachment, a hole or tear also may be seen at the edge of the detachment.

If a retinal hole or tear is discovered before it causes a detachment, the defect may be closed or sealed. Closure prevents fluid from collecting under the retina and reduces the risk for a detachment. Treatment involves creating an inflammatory response that will bind the retina and choroid together around the break. The inflammatory response can be created using cryotherapy (a freezing probe), photocoagulation (laser), or diathermy (high-frequency current).

Spontaneous reattachment of the retina is rare. Surgical repair is needed to place the retina in contact with the underlying structures. A common repair procedure is scleral buckling.

Preoperative Care

The patient is usually anxious and fearful about a possible permanent loss of vision. *Nursing priorities include providing information and reassurance to allay fears.*

Instruct the patient to restrict activity and head movement before surgery to prevent further tearing or detachment and to promote drainage of any fluid under the retina. An eye patch is placed over the affected eye to reduce eye movement. Topical drugs are given before surgery to inhibit pupil constriction and accommodation.

Operative Procedures

The surgery is performed with the patient under general anesthesia. In scleral buckling, the ophthalmologist repairs wrinkles or folds in the retina so that the retina can assume its normal smooth position. To promote reattachment, a small piece of silicone is placed against the sclera and held in place by an encircling band (which is the actual "buckle"). This device keeps the retina in contact with the choroid and sclera to promote attachment. Any fluid under the retina is drained.

A gas or silicone oil placed inside the eye can be used to promote retinal reattachment. These agents float up against the retina to hold it in place until healing occurs.

Postoperative Care

After surgery, an eye patch and shield usually are applied. Monitor the patient's vital signs, and check the eye patch and shield for any drainage.

Activity after surgery varies. If gas or oil has been placed in the eye, position the patient on his or her abdomen. Instruct the patient to lie with the head turned so that the affected eye is facing up, for several days or until the gas has been absorbed. As an alternative, he or she can sit on the side of the bed and place the head on an over-the-bed table.

Give drugs as prescribed for pain and nausea. Teach the patient to report any sudden increase in pain or pain occurring with nausea. Report these symptoms to the surgeon immediately because they may indicate the development of complications. Remind the patient to avoid activities that increase intraocular pressure (IOP) (see Table 49-1).

Teach the patient to avoid reading, writing, and close work, such as sewing, in the first week after surgery because these activities cause rapid eye movements and promote detachment. Teach him or her the manifestations of infection and detachment (sudden reduced visual acuity, eye pain, pupil that does not respond to light by constricting). Instruct the patient to notify the surgeon immediately if these manifestations occur.

RETINITIS PIGMENTOSA

Several types of retinal disorders can cause progressive degeneration of the retina and lead to blindness. Retinitis pigmentosa (RP) is a condition in which retinal nerve cells degenerate and the pigmented cells of the retina grow and move into the sensory areas of the retina, causing further degeneration.

The earliest manifestation of RP is night blindness, often occurring in childhood. Over time, decreased visual acuity progresses to total blindness. Examination of the retina shows heavy pigmentation in a lacy pattern. Cataracts may accompany this disorder.

No current therapy is effective in preventing the degenerative process. Current management strategies focus on protecting active retinal cells and slowing the progression of disease. Teach patients with RP to avoid drugs that are known to adversely affect retinal cells, such as isotretinoin (Accutane) and drugs for erectile dysfunction (e.g., sildenafil [Viagra]). Also remind them to wear eyeglasses that provide ultraviolet protection. The ingestion of 15,000 international units of vitamin A daily is recommended to slow the progression of the disorder, as is the daily ingestion of docosahexaenoic acid (DHA), an omega-3 fatty acid and antioxidant (Foundation Fighting Blindness, 2010). Additional supplements that appear to slow the progression of RP include beta carotene, lutein, and zeaxanthin. When macular edema is present, oral acetazolamide (Diamox) can reduce the edema. Cataract surgery and lens replacement is recommended when cataracts further reduce vision. Other treatments under investigation include retinal microchip implantation, retinal tissue transplantation, and stem cell therapy.

❓ NCLEX EXAMINATION CHALLENGE

Psychosocial Integrity

A client whose sister was just diagnosed with autosomal recessive retinitis pigmentosa is pregnant with a male fetus. The client's husband has no relatives with the disorder. She asks what the chances are that her son could be affected. What is the nurse's best response?

A. "Because it is likely that you are a carrier and your husband does not have any affected relatives, only your daughters can develop the disease."

B. "Because it is likely that you are a carrier and your husband does not have any affected relatives, none of your children will have the disease but each child will have a 50% risk for being a carrier."

C. "Because your sister actually has retinitis pigmentosa, the risk for your children having the disorder is 50% with each pregnancy."

D. "Because you are a woman, your daughters will each have a 50% risk for having the disease, and all of your sons will be carriers."

REFRACTIVE ERRORS

Pathophysiology

The ability of the eye to focus images on the retina depends on the length of the eye from front to back and the refractive power of the lens system. Refraction is the bending of light rays. Problems in either eye length or refraction can result in refractive errors.

Myopia is nearsightedness, in which the eye over-refracts the light and the bent images fall in front of, not on, the retina. Hyperopia, also called *hypermetropia,* is farsightedness, in which refraction is too weak, causing images to be focused behind the retina. Presbyopia is the age-related problem in which the lens loses its elasticity and is less able to change shape to focus the eye for close work. As a result, images fall behind the retina. This problem usually begins in people in their 30s and 40s. Astigmatism occurs when the curve of the cornea is uneven. Because light rays are not refracted equally in all directions, the image does not focus on the retina.

PATIENT-CENTERED COLLABORATIVE CARE

Refractive errors are diagnosed through a process known as refraction. The patient is asked to view an eye chart while lenses of different strengths are systematically placed in front of the eye. With each lens strength, he or she is asked whether the lenses sharpen or worsen vision. The strength of the lens needed to focus the image on the retina is expressed in measurements called *diopters.*

Nonsurgical Management

Refractive errors are corrected with a lens that focuses light rays on the retina (see Fig. 48-5 in Chapter 48). Hyperopic vision is corrected with a convex lens that moves the image forward. Myopic vision is corrected with a biconcave lens to move the focused image back to the retina.

Eyeglasses are used to correct refractive errors. They are easy to use, durable, and relatively low cost. Disadvantages are a change in appearance, the weight of the frame on the nose, and reduced peripheral vision (only central vision is corrected with eyeglasses).

Contact lenses also correct refractive errors. Round plastic disks rest against the cornea and fit under the eyelid. Hard contact lenses correct errors in two ways—by changing the shape of the cornea and by providing direct refraction. Changing corneal shape increases its refracting ability. Direct refraction from the contact lens places the specific refractive power and shape needed in front of the eye so that light rays are correctly focused onto the retina.

Complications of hard contact lens wear include corneal edema, which occurs when the lenses are worn for an extended period. Corneal abrasion can result from overwear, which dries the cornea and causes small breaks, or from the irritation of the contact lens against the cornea.

Soft contact lenses are better tolerated than hard contact lenses. They are about the thickness of plastic wrap and can be worn for longer periods because they allow greater corneal access to moisture and oxygen. Problems with soft lenses are related to lens deterioration, deposits in the lens, and failure to follow correct lens care practices.

There are two types of soft contact lenses: daily-wear lenses (worn only during waking hours) and extended-wear lenses. Extended-wear contact lenses are worn continuously for days to several weeks, depending on the patient's environment, activities, and tolerance of the lenses.

Surgical Management

Surgery is a popular alternative for the treatment of refractive errors. The most common vision-enhancing surgery is laser in-situ keratomileusis (LASIK). This procedure is much more expensive than eyeglasses or any type of contact lens, and it is rarely covered by insurance.

LASIK can correct nearsightedness, farsightedness, and astigmatism using the excimer laser. The superficial layers of the cornea are lifted temporarily as a flap, and brief but powerful laser pulses reshape the deeper corneal layers. After reshaping is complete, the corneal flap is placed back into its original position.

Usually both eyes are treated at the same time, which is most convenient for the patient, although this practice has some risks. If the laser malfunctions or if instruments are contaminated, the vision in both eyes could be adversely affected (Ayers, 2010). Many patients have improved vision within an hour after surgery, although complete healing to best vision may take up to 4 weeks. The outer corneal layer is not damaged, and pain is minimal.

After LASIK correction of refractive errors, many patients no longer require eyeglasses or contact lenses. Overcorrection or undercorrection is possible, however, and some patients may need a mild prescription for a continued refractive error.

Complications include corneal clouding, chronic dry eyes, and refractive errors. Some patients have developed blurred vision and other refractive errors months to years after this surgery as a result of keratectasia. This problem is related to the formation of the corneal flap during surgery and laser-thinning of the cornea. The cornea then becomes unstable and does not refract appropriately.

Although it is a relatively safe procedure, not everyone should have LASIK. People for whom risks may outweigh benefits of LASIK surgery include anyone who has a disorder or is taking drugs that delay wound healing (e.g., human immune deficiency virus [HIV] disease, rheumatoid arthritis, other autoimmune diseases, diabetes), those whose refractive errors are unstable and require yearly changes in prescriptive correction, those who routinely engage in contact sports, those who have thin corneas, and those who have any type of dry eye syndrome (Ayers, 2010).

Another procedure, Intacs corneal ring placement, can enhance vision for nearsightedness. However, this procedure is most often performed for keratoconus. For more information about the procedure, see surgical intervention for keratoconus on p. 1058.

TRAUMA

Trauma to the eye or orbital area can result from almost any activity. Care varies depending on the area of the eye affected and whether the globe of the eye has been penetrated.

Hyphema

A hyphema is a hemorrhage in the anterior chamber occurring when a force is applied to the eye and breaks the blood vessels. If the hyphema is large, it may block the pupil and reduce vision, possibly causing pain and photophobia. Hemolysis of the blood occurs, and the blood is filtered out of the eye through the trabecular meshwork. If the blood particles obstruct the meshwork, increased intraocular pressure (IOP) results.

Management includes bedrest in semi-Fowler's position to use gravity as an aid in keeping the hyphema away from the optical center of the cornea. Minimal or no sudden eye movements are permitted for 3 to 5 days to decrease the risk for rebleeding. Cycloplegic (paralyzing) eyedrops may be prescribed, and the eye is protected by a patch and shield. Television and reading are restricted. A hyphema usually resolves in 5 to 7 days.

Contusion

A contusion of the eyeball and surrounding tissue is caused by traumatic contact with a blunt object. The force of the blow pushes the eye back in the socket. The globe is compressed, and stretching of the ocular soft tissues occurs, which can damage and possibly rupture the globe. Results of the injury may not be immediate and include edema of the eyelids, subconjunctival hemorrhage, corneal edema, and hyphema.

Periorbital ecchymosis, or "black eye," a common contusion injury, is usually caused by blunt trauma. Bleeding into the soft tissue occurs, creating the bruise. The color fades gradually and disappears in 10 to 14 days. Visual acuity is usually not affected, although orbital pain, photophobia, eyelid edema, and diplopia may be present.

Treatment begins at the time of injury. Ice is applied immediately. The patient should have a thorough eye examination to rule out any other eye injuries.

Foreign Bodies

Eyelashes, dust, fingernails, dirt, and airborne particles can come in contact with the conjunctiva or cornea and irritate or abrade the surface. If nothing is seen on the cornea or conjunctiva, the eyelid is everted to examine the conjunctivae. The patient usually has a feeling of something being in the eye and may have blurred vision. Pain occurs if the corneal surface is injured. Tearing and photophobia may be present.

Evaluation of vision is done before treatment. The eye of any patient with a suspected corneal abrasion is examined with fluorescein, followed by irrigation with normal saline (0.9%) to gently remove the particles. Best practices for ocular irrigation are listed in Chart 49-8.

If an eye patch is applied after the foreign body is removed, tell the patient how long the patch must be left in place. Follow-up with the ophthalmologist is needed.

Lacerations

Lacerations are wounds caused by sharp objects and projectiles. The injury can occur to any part of the eye, but the most commonly injured areas are the eyelids and the cornea.

Initially, close the eye and apply a small ice pack to decrease bleeding. The patient should receive medical attention as soon as possible. If the patient can open the eye, check visual acuity and clean the eyelids. Minor lacerations of the eyelid can be sutured in an emergency department, an urgent care center, or an ophthalmologist's office. A microscope is needed in the operating room if the patient has a laceration that involves the eyelid margin, affects the lacrimal system, involves a large area, or has jagged edges.

Corneal lacerations are an emergency because eye contents may prolapse through the laceration. Manifestations include severe eye pain, photophobia, tearing, decreased visual acuity, and inability to open the eyelid. If the laceration is the result of a penetrating injury, an object may be seen protruding from the eye. *The object is removed only by the ophthalmologist, because it may be holding eye structures in place.*

CHART 49-8   BEST PRACTICE FOR PATIENT SAFETY & QUALITY CARE

Ocular Irrigation

1. Assemble equipment:
   - Normal saline IV (1000-mL bag)
   - Macrodrip IV tubing
   - IV pole
   - Eyelid speculum
   - Topical anesthetic (proparacaine hydrochloride)
   - Gloves
   - Collection receptacle (emesis basin works well)
   - Towels
   - pH paper
2. Quickly obtain a history from the patient while flushing the tubing with normal saline:
   - Nature and time of the injury
   - Type of irritant or chemical (if known)
   - Type of first aid administered at the scene
   - Any allergies to the "caine" family of medications
3. Evaluate the patient's visual acuity *before* treatment:
   - Ask the patient to read your name tag with the affected eye while covering the good eye.
   - Ask the patient to "count fingers" with the affected eye while covering the good eye.
4. Put on gloves.
5. Place a strip of pH paper in the cul-de-sac of the patient's affected eye to test the pH of the agent splashed into the eye and to know when it has been washed out.
6. Instill proparacaine hydrochloride eyedrops as prescribed.
7. Place the patient in a supine position with the head turned slightly toward the affected eye.
8. Have the patient hold the affected eye open, or position an eyelid speculum.
9. Direct the flow of normal saline across the affected eye from the nasal corner of the eye toward the outer corner of the eye.
10. Assess the patient's comfort during the procedure.
11. If both eyes are affected, irrigate them simultaneously using separate personnel and equipment.

Antibiotics are given to reduce the risk for infection. Depending on the depth of the laceration, scarring may develop. If the scar alters vision, a corneal transplant may be needed later. If the eye contents have prolapsed through the laceration or if the injury is severe, enucleation (surgical eye removal) may be indicated.

Penetrating Injuries

Patients with penetrating eye injuries have the poorest chance of retaining vision in the injured eye. Glass, high-speed metal or wood particles, BB pellets, and bullets are common causes of penetrating injuries. The particles can enter the eye and lodge in or behind the eyeball.

The patient has eye pain and reports "I suddenly felt something hit my eye." An entrance wound may be visible. Depending on where the object enters and rests within the eye, vision may be affected.

X-rays and computed tomography (CT) scans of the orbit are usually performed. Computer-generated reconstructions of the CT images are created to study this complex area to ensure the orbit is intact and to look for fractures that might entrap orbital muscles. *Magnetic resonance imaging (MRI) is contraindicated because the procedure may move any metal-containing projectile and cause more injury.*

Surgery is usually needed to remove the foreign object. In some cases, foreign bodies need to be removed by a vitrectomy. IV antibiotics are started before surgery to reduce the risk for infection. A tetanus booster is given if necessary.

Assess and document visual acuity. If the patient cannot see print, determine whether he or she can count fingers or see hand motions. If the patient cannot see movement, assess his or her ability to see light.

OCULAR MELANOMA

Pathophysiology

Melanoma is the most common malignant eye tumor in adults (American Cancer Society, 2011; Simar, 2009). This tumor occurs most often in the uveal tract among people in their 30s and 40s and is associated with exposure to ultraviolet (UV) light. Because of its rich blood supply, a melanoma can spread by extension through the sclera or invasion into nearby tissue and the brain.

PATIENT-CENTERED COLLABORATIVE CARE

Manifestations of melanoma may not be readily apparent; the tumor may be discovered during a routine examination. Blurred vision may occur if the macular area is invaded. Visual acuity is reduced if the tumor grows inward toward the center of the eye from the choroid and alters the visual pathway. Increased intraocular pressure (IOP) can result if the tumor obstructs flow of aqueous humor. Iris color changes when the tumor infiltrates the iris. Sudden loss of a visual field may result from tumor invasion that causes retinal detachment.

Diagnostic tests for a melanoma depend on the size and tumor growth rate. Ultrasonography or MRI is performed to determine the tumor's location and size. Treatment depends on the tumor's size and growth rate, as well as the condition of the other eye. Small iris lesions are monitored until growth is observed. Tumors of the choroid are treated by surgical enucleation or by radiation therapy with a radioactive plaque (Simar, 2009).

Enucleation (surgical removal of the entire eyeball) is the most common surgery for ocular melanoma and is performed under general anesthesia. After the eye is removed, a ball implant is inserted as a base for the socket prosthesis.

The implant is covered with surrounding tissue, muscles, and conjunctiva. A plastic conformer is placed over the conjunctiva to maintain the shape of the eyelids until a prosthesis can be fitted. After the dressing is removed, a pressure patch is placed over the eye for 24 hours.

Until the prosthesis is fitted (after about 1 month), an antibiotic-steroid ointment is inserted into the cul-de-sac once daily. Best practices for prosthesis care are listed in Chart 49-9.

Radiation therapy is an "eye-sparing" procedure that can reduce the size and thickness of melanomas but rarely eliminates the tumors completely. The radioactive plaque—a round, flat disk about the size of a dime and containing a radioactive material—is sutured to the sclera overlying the tumor site. The length of time the plaque remains sutured to the sclera depends on the size of the tumor and the dose of radiation to be delivered.

Insertion and Removal of an Ocular Prosthesis

Insertion

1. Assemble equipment:
   - Prosthesis
   - Gloves
   - Towel
2. Explain the procedure to the patient.
3. Wash your hands.
4. Cover the work area with a cloth or towel.
5. Don gloves.
6. Remove the prosthesis from its container, and rinse it with warm water.
7. Lift the patient's upper lid using your nondominant hand.

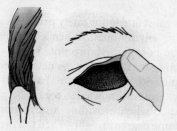

8. Place the prosthesis between the thumb and forefinger of your dominant hand. The notched end of the prosthesis should be closest to the patient's nose.

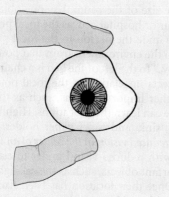

9. Insert the prosthesis with the top edge slipping under the upper lid. Continue until most of the iris is covered by the upper lid.

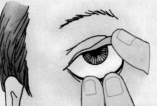

10. Gently release the upper eyelid.
11. Retract the lower lid slightly until the bottom edge of the prosthesis slips behind it.

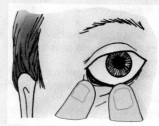

12. Release your hands slowly.

Removal

1. Assemble equipment:
   - Normal saline–filled, labeled container
   - Gloves
2. Explain the procedure to the patient.
3. Wash your hands.
4. Don gloves.
5. Instruct the patient to sit up and tilt the head slightly downward.
6. Place your hand against the patient's cheek, palm side up.
7. Pull the lower lid slightly down and laterally.
8. Allow the prosthesis to slide out onto your hand, or pull gently if necessary.
9. Place the prosthesis in a container filled with normal saline labeled with the patient's name. Cover the container.

Complications of radiation therapy include vascular changes, retinopathy, glaucoma, necrosis of the sclera, and cataract formation. Vitreous hemorrhage may develop as the tumor becomes smaller and pulls or breaks blood vessels.

While the plaque is in place, an eye patch may or may not be used. Cycloplegic eyedrops and an antibiotic-steroid combination are given. Teach the patient how to instill eyedrops.

REDUCED VISION

Pathophysiology

Different forms of reduced vision may affect any or all aspects of vision, including color, light, image, movement, and acuity. Reduced vision may be temporary, such as when cataracts obscure vision but surgery has not yet been planned or performed. Patients are legally blind if their best visual acuity with corrective lenses is 20/200 or less in the better eye or if the widest diameter of the visual field in that eye is no greater than 20 degrees.

Blindness can occur in one or both eyes. When one eye is affected, the field of vision is narrowed and depth perception is impaired. Central vision can be impaired by diseases involving the macula, such as macular edema or macular degeneration. Loss of peripheral vision occurs with glaucoma. The loss of side vision affects the patient's ability to drive and awareness of hazards in the periphery.

PATIENT-CENTERED COLLABORATIVE CARE

Priorities for nursing involve teaching the patient techniques to make better use of existing vision (Watkinson, 2009). Moving the head slightly up and down can enhance a three-dimensional effect. When shaking hands or pouring water, the patient can line up the object and move toward it. He or she should choose a position that favors the eye with better vision. For example, people with vision in the right eye should position people and items on their right.

CHART 49-10 BEST PRACTICE FOR PATIENT SAFETY & QUALITY CARE

Providing Care to the Patient with Reduced Vision

- Always knock or announce your entrance into the patient's room or area and introduce yourself.
- Ensure that all members of the health care team also use this courtesy of announcement and introduction.
- Ensure that the patient's reduced vision is noted in the medical record, is communicated to all staff, is marked on the call board, and is identified on the door of the patient's room.
- Determine to what degree the patient can see anything.
- Orient the patient to the environment, counting steps with him or her to the bathroom.
- Assist the patient in placing objects on the bedside table or in the bed and around the bed and room, and do not move them without the patient's permission.
- Remove all objects and clutter between the patient's bed and the bathroom.
- Ask the patient what type of assistance he or she prefers for grooming, toileting, eating, and ambulating, and communicate these preferences with the staff.
- Describe food placement on a plate in terms of a clock face.
- Open milk cartons; open salt, pepper, and condiment packages; and remove lids from cups and bowls.
- Unless the patient also has a hearing problem, use a normal tone of voice when speaking.
- When walking with the patient, offer him or her your arm and walk a step ahead.
- Using tape and a heavy black marker, mark the 350-degree temperature setting on the oven and mark the 70-degree temperature setting on the heating or cooling thermostat.
- Paint or mark light switches in a deep color that contrasts with the surrounding wall.
- Label canned goods with large, bold, black letters on white tape.
- Teach the patient to feel for the crease in paper milk cartons that indicates the place to open the spout.
- Help the patient differentiate different drugs by altering the shape or contours of a bottle. Rubber bands can be wound around a bottle to change its texture. Raised symbols can be glued to caps to make identification easier.

Nursing interventions for the patient with reduced sight focus on communication, safety, ambulation, self-care, and support (Watkinson, 2009). Chart 49-10 lists ways to help patients with reduced vision to function as independently as possible.

Communication is important in helping the patient remain independent and connected to the world. Reduced vision is a common occurrence, and many adaptive devices are available to help the person maintain independence. Many towns and cities have auditory traffic signals so that persons with reduced vision can know when it is safe to cross a street. Curbs in these areas may have high-contrast color paint to let the person know when to step up or down. Libraries have large-print books and books on tape. "Talking" clocks, watches, and timers are available. Playing cards, games, restaurant menus, calendars, and instruction booklets are available in large print sizes. Computer keyboards with high contrast and larger letters in the keys are available, as are large screens. Direct the patient with reduced vision to the local resources to obtain adaptive items and to learn how to use them (Watkinson, 2009).

Safety is a major issue for the person with reduced vision. For patients at home with reduced vision, the home is the place where they feel most safe. They are familiar with room and item location. For example, they may have counted the number of footsteps needed to move from one area to another within the home. It is important to stress to family and friends that changes in item location should not be made without input from the person with reduced vision.

Even people who have experienced gradually reduced vision over time and who have had time to adjust may benefit from having a person with vision assist in making adaptations in the home. Adaptations may include the following:

The patient is most at risk for safety problems in an unfamiliar or changing environment. When a person with reduced vision must be hospitalized, promote safety and independence by orienting him or her to the new environment.

Most people with reduced vision had sight at some time and have background knowledge regarding size and shape that can be used when providing information. Many blind people have some degree of sight. When talking with a person who has limited sight or is blind, always use a normal tone of voice unless he or she is has a hearing problem.

First orient the patient to the immediate environment, including the size of the room. Use one object in the room, such as a chair or hospital bed, as the focal point during your description. Guide the person to the focal point, and orient him or her to the environment from that point. For example, you might say, "To the left of the bed is a chair." Then describe all other objects in relation to the focal point. Go with the patient to other important areas, such as the bathroom, so that he or she can learn their locations. Highlight the location of the toilet, sink, and toilet paper holder. *Never leave the patient with reduced vision in the center of an unfamiliar room.*

Patients with reduced vision prefer to establish the location of important objects, such as the call light, water pitcher, and clock. Once their location has been fixed, do not move these items without the patient's consent. Do not move the location of chairs, stools, and wastebaskets without consulting the patient.

At mealtime, set up food on the tray using clock placement. For example, "There is sliced ham at the 6 o'clock position; peas are located at the 3 o'clock position; to the right of the plate is coffee; salt and pepper are next to the coffee."

Ambulation with a patient who has reduced vision involves allowing him or her to grasp your arm at the elbow. Keep the arm close to your body so that he or she can detect your direction of movement. Alert the patient when obstacles are in the path ahead.

Patients may use a cane to detect obstacles, such as furniture, walls, or curbs. The cane is held in the dominant hand several inches off the floor and sweeps the ground where his or her foot will be placed next. The laser cane sends out signals to help detect obstacles.

Self-care and the ability to control the environment are important. Knock on the door before entering the hospital room or any other environment of a patient with reduced vision. State your name and the reason for visiting when entering the room. Coordinate with other members of the health care team to ensure this etiquette is used consistently.

Mark the door to the room to indicate it is occupied by a person with reduced vision.

Support is needed, especially when the reduced vision is of sudden onset and may be permanent. Patients' reactions to the loss of sight are similar to the reaction to loss of a body part. Allow the newly blind person a period of grieving for the "dead" (nonseeing) eye. He or she may feel hopeless and angry. With time, anger usually gives way to acceptance. The ability to cope may begin within days, but some patients mourn for months or years.

Patients benefit from the honest support that you can provide. They need to hear that it is normal to mourn, to cry, and to feel the loss. Help them move toward acceptance by encouraging the mastery of one task at a time and by providing positive reinforcement for each success.

❓ NCLEX EXAMINATION CHALLENGE
Psychosocial Integrity

A client with reduced vision who is 1 day postoperative for a non-vision problem expresses concern to the nurse that he is afraid if a hospital fire occurred he would not be able to get out in time. Which nurse response or action is most likely to allay his fears?
A. Demonstrating how to close the door and place wet towels at the bottom edge of the door.
B. Reminding him that the hospital meets all current fire codes and has never experienced a major fire.
C. Helping him count the steps to the stairway exit and reminding him that he is on the second floor.
D. Reassuring him that even if a fire broke out, the nurses and other personnel would stay on the unit with him.

NURSING CONCEPT REVIEW

What might you NOTICE if the patient is experiencing reduced sensation as a result of vision problems?

Perform and interpret focused physical assessment findings, including:
- Patient squints or tilts the head when viewing objects or print at a distance.
- Patient closes one eye to read or see at a distance.
- Patient moves reading materials either very close to his or her face or as far away from the face as he or she can reach.
- Patient may not startle when a sudden move is made at the face.
- Pupils are unequal and may not react to light.
- Eyes do not focus on a distant object and track it as it is moved closer to the face.
- Red reflex may be absent or present in only one eye.
- Appearance is disheveled with buttons not properly buttoned and clothing colors or patterns not complementary.
- Patient does not make eye contact and turns head toward sounds rather than sights.
- Patient walks with hesitation into a room or bumps into objects in his or her path.
- Patient may seem confused about time and place.

What should you INTERPRET and how should you RESPOND to a patient experiencing reduced sensation as a result of vision problems?

Interpret by:
- Assessing visual acuity with a Snellen chart, counting fingers, hand motion, or light perception.
- Asking the patient to describe the objects in the room and their colors.
- Asking the patient what he or she can see well and what is more difficult to see.

Respond by:
- Orienting the patient to the immediate surroundings.
- Offering your arm for the patient to hold when he or she is moving to a different location.
- Not leaving the patient alone in the center of a strange room.
- Asking him or her what assistance is needed for independent activity.
- Assessing the immediate environment for safety hazards and removing the hazard.

On what should you REFLECT?
- Consider what environmental changes could make the unit safer or more manageable for a person with reduced vision.

GET READY FOR THE NCLEX® EXAMINATION!

KEY POINTS

Review these Key Points for each NCLEX Examination Client Needs Category

Safe and Effective Care Environment
- Use gloves when examining an eye with drainage from the eye or tear duct.
- Avoid performing an ophthalmoscopic examination on a confused patient.
- Orient the patient with reduced vision to his or her immediate surroundings, including how to call for help and where the bathroom is located.

- Identify the room of a patient with reduced vision (without identifying the patient).

Health Promotion and Maintenance

- Identify people at risk for vision problems as a result of work environment or leisure activities, and teach them specific ways to protect the eyes.
- Encourage all patients to wear eye protection when they are performing yard work, are working in a woodshop or metal shop, are using chemicals, or are in any environment in which drops or particulate matter is airborne.
- Encourage all adult patients older than 40 years to have an eye examination with measurement of intraocular pressure every year.
- Encourage everyone to use polarizing sunglasses whenever outdoors in bright sunlight.
- Teach all patients to wash their hands before and after touching the eyes.

Psychosocial Integrity

- Use a normal tone of voice to talk with a patient who has a vision problem and normal hearing.

- Knock on the door before entering the room of a patient with reduced vision, and introduce yourself.
- Allow the patient and family the opportunity to express concerns about a vision change.
- Refer patients newly diagnosed with visual impairment to appropriate local resources and support groups.

Physiological Integrity

- Ask the patient about vision problems in any other members of the family, because many vision problems have a genetic component.
- Teach patients the proper techniques for self-instillation of eyedrops and eye ointment.
- Stress the importance of completing an antibiotic regimen for an eye infection.
- Teach patients who are at risk for increased intraocular pressure what activities to avoid (see Table 49-1).
- Teach patients with an infection of the eye or eyelid not to rub the eye (to avoid infecting the other eye).
- Never attempt to remove any object protruding from the eye.

Assessment of the Ear and Hearing

Judith Laver Bierschbach

evolve WEBSITE

http://evolve.elsevier.com/Iggy/

Animation: Ears: Weber Test
Answer Key for NCLEX Examination Challenges and
   Decision-Making Challenges
Audio Glossary

Key Points
Review Questions for the NCLEX® Examination
Video Clip: Ear Canal
Video Clip: External Ear

LEARNING OUTCOMES

Safe and Effective Care Environment

1. Apply principles of infection control when examining an ear with drainage.

Health Promotion and Maintenance

2. Teach all people how to perform ear hygiene safely.
3. Teach all people to use ear protection equipment and strategies.

Psychosocial Integrity

4. Teach patients and family members about what to expect during tests and procedures to assess ear and hearing problems.
5. Provide opportunities for the patient and family to express feelings and concerns about a possible change in hearing.

Physiological Integrity

6. Identify people at risk for hearing problems as a result of drug therapy, genetic predisposition, or exposure to environmental hazards.
7. Perform a clinical ear and hearing assessment, including health history and psychosocial assessment.
8. Describe adaptations needed when caring for patients who have age-related changes in the structure of the ear and hearing.
9. Identify 10 common drugs that affect hearing.
10. Demonstrate the correct use of an otoscope.

The ear and the brain together allow hearing. Hearing is one of the five senses important for communicating with the world. Functional hearing assists in the concepts of sensation and cognition. It is used to assess surroundings, allow independence, warn of danger, appreciate music, work, play, and interact with other people.

Ear and hearing problems are common among adults of all ages. Assessment of the ear and hearing is an important skill for nurses in any care environment. Therefore an understanding of the anatomy and physiology of the ear is essential. Many ear and hearing problems develop over long periods and may be affected by drugs or systemic health problems.

ANATOMY AND PHYSIOLOGY REVIEW

Structure

The ear has three divisions: the external ear, the middle ear, and the inner ear. Each part is important to hearing.

External Ear

The external ear develops in the embryo at the same time as the kidneys and urinary tract. Thus any person with a defect of the external ear should be examined for possible problems of the kidney and urinary systems.

The pinna is the part of the external ear that is composed of cartilage covered by skin and attached to the head at about a 10-degree angle. It is embedded in the temporal bone on both sides of the head at the level of the eyes. The external ear also includes the mastoid process, which is the bony ridge located over the temporal bone behind the pinna. The external ear extends from the pinna through the external ear canal to the tympanic membrane (eardrum) (Fig. 50-1). The ear canal is slightly S-shaped and lined with cerumen (wax)-producing glands, sebaceous glands, and hair follicles. Cerumen helps protect and lubricate the ear canal. The hair follicles and cerumen protect the eardrum and the middle ear. The distance from the opening of the ear canal to the eardrum in an adult is 1 to 1½ inches (2.5 to 3.75 cm).

Middle Ear

The middle ear begins at the medial or inner side of the eardrum. The eardrum separates the external ear and the middle ear.

The middle ear consists of a compartment called the epitympanum. Located in the epitympanum are the top opening of the eustachian tube and three small bones known as the bony ossicles, which are the malleus (hammer), the incus (anvil), and the stapes (stirrup) (Fig. 50-2). The bony ossicles are joined loosely, thereby moving with vibrations created when sound waves hit the eardrum.

The eardrum, a thick sheet of tissue, is transparent, opaque, or pearly gray and moves when air is injected into the external canal. The landmarks on the eardrum include the *annulus*, the *pars flaccida*, and the *pars tensa*. These correspond to the parts of the malleus that can be seen through the transparent eardrum. The eardrum is attached to the first bony ossicle, the malleus, at the umbo (Fig. 50-3). The umbo is seen

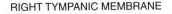

RIGHT TYMPANIC MEMBRANE

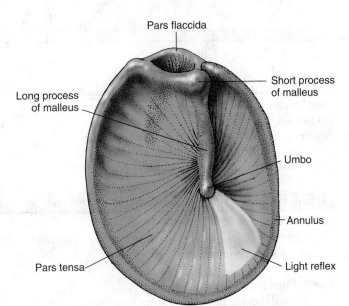

FIG. 50-3 Landmarks on the tympanic membrane.

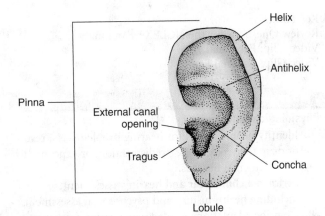

FIG. 50-1 Anatomic features of the external ear.

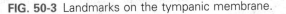

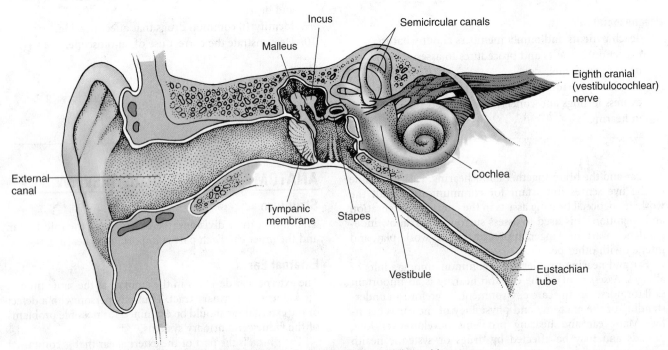

FIG. 50-2 Anatomic features of the middle and inner ear.

through the eardrum membrane as a white dot and is one end of the long process of the malleus. The pars flaccida is that portion of the eardrum above the short process of the malleus. The pars tensa is that portion surrounding the long process of the malleus.

The middle ear is separated from the inner ear by the round window and the oval window. The eustachian tube begins at the floor of the middle ear and extends to the throat. The tube opening in the throat is surrounded by adenoid lymphatic tissue (Fig. 50-4). The eustachian tube allows the pressure on both sides of the eardrum to equalize. Secretions from the middle ear drain through the tube into the throat.

Inner Ear

The inner ear is on the other side of the oval window and contains the semicircular canals, the cochlea, the vestibule, and the distal end of the eighth cranial nerve (see Fig. 50-2). The semicircular canals are tubes made of cartilage and contain fluid and hair cells. These canals are connected to the sensory nerve fibers of the vestibular portion of the eighth cranial nerve. The fluid and hair cells within the canals help maintain the sense of balance.

The cochlea, the spiral organ of hearing, is divided into the scala tympani and the scala vestibuli. The scala media is filled with *endolymph,* and the scala tympani and scala vestibuli are filled with *perilymph.* These fluids protect the cochlea and the semicircular canals by allowing these structures to "float" in the fluids and be cushioned against abrupt head movements.

The organ of Corti is the receptor of hearing located on the basilar membrane of the cochlea. The cochlea contains hair cells that detect vibration from sound and stimulate the eighth cranial nerve.

The vestibule is a small, oval-shaped, bony chamber between the semicircular canals and the cochlea. It contains the utricle and the saccule, organs that are important for balance.

Function

Hearing is the main function of the ear and occurs when sound is delivered through the air to the external ear canal and the temporal bone covering the mastoid air cells. The sound waves strike the mastoid and the movable eardrum, creating vibrations. The eardrum is connected to the first bony ossicle, which allows the sound wave vibrations to be transferred from the eardrum to the malleus, the incus, and the stapes. From the stapes, the vibrations are transmitted to the cochlea. Receptors at the cochlea transduce (change) the vibrations into action potentials. The action potentials are conducted to the brain as nerve impulses by the cochlear portion of the eighth cranial (auditory) nerve. The nerve impulses are processed and interpreted as sound by the brain in the auditory cortex of the temporal lobe.

Ear and Hearing Changes Associated with Aging

Ear and hearing changes related to aging are listed in Chart 50-1, along with implications for care of older patients who have these changes. Some of the ear changes, such as an increase in ear size, are harmless. Other changes to ear structures may pose threats to the hearing ability of older adults.

All older adults should be screened for hearing acuity. Many scales or tools are available to assess hearing loss. However, asking "Do you have a hearing problem now?" may be just as helpful as these scales. Family members may have noticed behaviors that suggest changes in a patient's hearing.

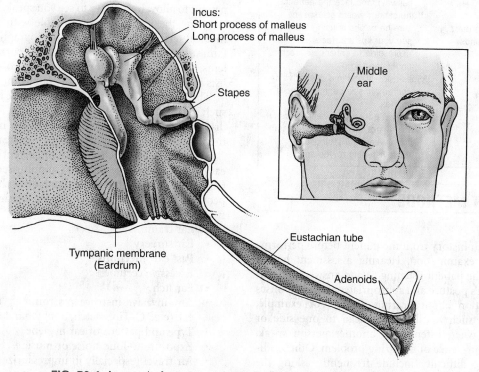

FIG. 50-4 Anatomic features and attached structures of the middle ear.

CHART 50-1 NURSING FOCUS ON THE OLDER ADULT

Age-Related Changes in the Ear and Hearing

EAR OR HEARING CHANGE	NURSING ADAPTATIONS AND ACTIONS
Pinna becomes elongated because of loss of subcutaneous tissues and decreased elasticity.	Reassure the patient that this is normal and does not indicate a problem. When positioning a patient on his or her side, take care not to "fold" the ear under the head.
Hair in the canal becomes coarser and longer, especially in men.	Reassure the patient that this is normal. The patient may require more frequent ear irrigation to keep cerumen from clumping in the hair.
Cerumen is drier and impacts more easily, reducing hearing function.	Teach the patient to irrigate the ear canal weekly or whenever he or she notices a change in hearing.
Tympanic membrane loses elasticity and may appear dull and retracted.	Do not use this finding as the only indication of otitis media.
Hearing acuity decreases (in some people).	Establish that a hearing deficiency exists, using simple, noninvasive tests such as the voice test and the watch test. If a deficit is present, refer the patient to an ear, nose, and throat specialist to determine what type of hearing loss is present and what can be done to improve hearing. Do not assume all older adults have a hearing loss!!
The ability to hear high-frequency sounds is lost first. Older adults may have particular problems hearing the *f*, *s*, *sh*, and *pa* sounds.	Provide a quiet environment when speaking (close the door to the hallway), and face the patient. If the patient wears glasses, be sure he or she is using them to see your lips and facial expression to enhance speech understanding. Speak slowly and in a deeper voice, and emphasize beginning word sounds. Some patients with a hearing loss that is not corrected may benefit from wearing a stethoscope while listening to you speak.

ASSESSMENT METHODS

Patient History

Obtain a thorough history from the patient before performing the physical examination. Hearing assessment begins while observing the patient listening to and answering questions. The patient's posture and appropriateness of responses provide information about hearing acuity. For example, posture changes, such as tilting the head to one side or leaning forward when listening to another person speak, may indicate the presence of a hearing problem. Other indicators of hearing difficulty include frequently asking the speaker to repeat statements or frequently saying "What?" or

CHART 50-2 EAR AND HEARING ASSESSMENT

Using Gordon's Functional Health Patterns

Cognitive-Perceptual Pattern
- Do you have any hearing difficulty?
- Do you use any type of hearing aid?
- Do you notice that you have the volume of the television or radio set at an increased level?
- Are you sitting closer to the television or radio to hear more clearly?
- Do you have difficulty in your ability to hear or follow conversations in a noisy environment, such as a restaurant?
- Do you have difficulty hearing high-pitched sounds like the doorbell?

Health Perception–Health Management Pattern
- Have you had your hearing checked?
- If you are or were exposed to environmental noise, have you consistently used appropriate hearing protection?
- Do you avoid cleaning your ear canals with foreign objects such as toothpicks or paper clips?
- Have you discussed with your health care provider the side effects of any drugs you may be taking that might affect your ear and hearing?

Based on Gordon, M. (2011). *Manual of nursing diagnosis* (12th ed.). New York: Jones & Bartlett.

"Huh?" Notice whether the patient responds to whispered questions and conversations and startles when an unexpected sound occurs in the environment. Also assess whether the patient's responses match the question asked. For example, when you ask the patient "How old are you?" does the patient respond with an age or does he or she say "No, I don't have a cold."

During the interview, sit in adequate light and face the patient to allow him or her to see you speak. Use short, simple language the patient is comfortable with rather than long medical terms. Obtain data on demographics, personal and family history, socioeconomic status, current health problems, and the use of remedies for ear problems. Chart 50-2 lists important questions to ask about functional hearing.

The patient's gender is important. Some hearing disorders, such as otosclerosis, are more common in women. Other disorders, such as Ménière's disease, are more common in men. Age is also an important factor in hearing loss.

Personal history includes past or current manifestations of ear pain, ear discharge, vertigo (spinning sensation), tinnitus (ringing), decreased hearing, and difficulty understanding people when they talk or difficulty hearing environmental noise. Ask the patient about:
- Ear trauma
- Ear surgery
- Past ear infections
- Excessive cerumen
- Ear itch
- Any invasive instruments routinely used to clean the ear (e.g., Q-Tip, match, bobby pin, key)
- Type and pattern of ear hygiene
- Exposure to loud noise or music
- Air travel (especially in unpressurized aircraft)
- Swimming and whether ear protection is used

- History of hereditary factors that can cause progressive hearing loss
- History of health problems that can decrease the blood supply to the ear such as heart disease, hypertension, or diabetes
- History of vitiligo (a pigment disorder in which there may be a loss of melanin-containing cells in the inner ear, resulting in hearing loss)
- History of smoking (reduces oxygenation of the cochlea)
- History of vitamin B$_{12}$ and folate deficiency (associated with age-related hearing loss)

If the patient uses foreign objects to clean the ear canal (e.g., bobby-pins, Q-tips, toothpicks, keys), explain the danger in using these objects. They can scrape the skin of the canal, push cerumen up against the eardrum, and even puncture the eardrum. If the patient says that cerumen buildup is a problem, teach him or her to use an ear irrigation syringe and proper solutions to remove it. Chart 50-3 describes techniques to teach patients how to remove cerumen safely.

! NURSING SAFETY PRIORITY

Action Alert

Teach patients the safe way to clean their ears, stressing that nothing smaller than his or her own fingertip should be inserted into the canal.

If the patient uses a hearing aid, assess whether hearing is improved with its use. Obtain the date of the last hearing test, the type of test given, and the results. Ask about problems that may impair hearing such as allergies, upper respiratory infections, hypothyroidism, arteriosclerosis, head trauma, and recent head, facial, or dental surgery. A thorough drug history is important because many drugs are *ototoxic* (damaging to the ear) (Table 50-1).

Ask about the patient's occupation and hobbies that involve exposure to loud noise or music. Assess whether protective ear devices are used. Also ask whether any devices are consistently inserted into the ear, such as ear plugs or earpiece headsets, and for how long each day they are used. Use this opportunity to teach the patient about protecting his or her ears from loud noises by wearing protective ear devices, such as over-the-ear headsets or foam ear inserts, when persistent loud noises are in the environment. Also suggest the use of earplugs when engaging in water sports to prevent ear infections.

Assess the patient's socioeconomic status to determine the availability and affordability of health care. Some people might hesitate to have their hearing loss diagnosed because of the fear of needing to wear a hearing aid and the cost associated with these devices.

Family History and Genetic Risk

Family history, as well as personal history, is important in determining genetic risk for hearing loss. Although most genetic hearing loss is seen in childhood, some genetic problems can lead to progressive hearing loss in adults (Nussbaum et al., 2007). For example, most people with Down syndrome develop hearing loss as adults. People with osteogenesis imperfecta have bilateral and progressive hearing loss by their 30s.

CHART 50-3   PATIENT AND FAMILY EDUCATION: PREPARING FOR SELF-MANAGEMENT

Self–Ear Irrigation for Cerumen Removal

- *Do not attempt to remove ear wax or irrigate the ears if you have ear tubes or if you have blood, pus, or other drainage from the ear.*
- Use an ear syringe designed for the purpose of wax removal. These are inexpensive, available at most drug stores, reusable, and can be used by more than one person when cleaned properly between uses.
- The safest type of ear syringe to use is one that has a right-angle or "elbow" in the tip.
- Irrigating your ears in the shower is an easy method.
- Always use tap water that feels just barely warm to you. If you are using a thermometer, keep the water temperature as close as possible to 98° or 99° F. Water that is warmer or colder can make you feel dizzy and nauseated.
- If your ear wax is thick and sticky, you may need to place a few drops of a warm ceruminolytic (commercial eardrops that soften ear wax) into the ear an hour or so before you irrigate the ear. Other substances that can be used for this purpose include baby oil or mineral oil.
- Fill the syringe with the lukewarm tap water.
- If you are using a syringe with an elbow tip, place only the last part of the tip into your ear and aim it toward the roof of your ear canal.
- If you are using a straight-tipped syringe, insert the tip only about ½- to ¾-inch into your ear canal, aiming toward the roof of the canal.
- Hold your head at a 30-degree angle to the side you are irrigating.
- Use one hand to hold the syringe and the other to push the plunger or squeeze the bulb.
- Apply gentle but firm continuous pressure, allowing the water to flow against the top of the canal.
- *Do not use blasts or bursts of sudden pressure.*
- The ear canal should fill, and water will begin to flow out, bringing ear wax and debris with it.
- If a dental water-pressure irrigator is used, put it on the lowest possible setting.
- This process should not be painful! If pain occurs, decrease the pressure. If pain persists, stop the irrigation.
- Continue the irrigation until at least a cup of solution has washed into and out from your ear canal. (You may have to refill the syringe.)
- Tilting your head at a 90-degree angle to the side should allow most, if not all, of the water to drain out of your ear.
- Repeat the procedure on the other ear.
- If you feel that water is still in the canal, hold a hair dyer on a low setting near the ear.
- Irrigate your ears anytime from weekly to monthly, depending on how fast your ear wax collects.

GENETIC/GENOMIC CONSIDERATIONS

Mutations in several different genes are associated with hearing loss. One type of hearing loss among adults has a genetic basis with a mutation in gene *GJB2* on chromosome 1. This mutation causes poor production of the protein *connexin-26*, which has a role in the function of cochlear hair cells. Other genetic problems slow the metabolism and excretion of drugs, including ototoxic drugs. This allows ototoxic drugs to remain in the body longer, thus increasing the risk for hearing loss.

TABLE 50-1   OTOTOXIC DRUGS

DRUG TYPE	DRUG	DRUG TYPE	DRUG
Antibiotics	Amikacin	Nonsteroidal anti-inflammatory agents	Ibuprofen (Advil, Nuprin, Motrin)
	Capreomycin		Indomethacin (Indocin)
	Chloramphenicol		Naproxen (Aleve, Naprosyn, Anaprox)
	Dihydrostreptomycin		Piroxicam (Feldene), diflunisal (Dolobid), diclofene
	Erythromycin		(Voltaren), etodolac (Lodine), nabumetone
	Gentamicin (Garamycin, Cidomycin)		(Relafen), ketorolac (Toradol)
	Kanamycin		Salicylates (aspirin, Disalcid, Bufferin, Ecotrin,
	Metronidazole (vestibulotoxicity rarely)		Trilisate, Ascriptin, Empirin, Excedrin, Fiorinal)
	Neomycin		
	Netilmicin		
	Streptomycin		
	Tobramycin		
Diuretics	Acetazolamide (Apo-Acetazolamide 🍁, Diamox)	Chemotherapy agents	Actinomycin
			Bleomycin
	Ethacrynic acid (Edecrin)		Cisplatin (Abiplatin, Platinol)
	Bumetanide		Carboplatin
	Furosemide (Lasix, Apo-Furosemide 🍁,		Nitrogen mustard (Mustargen)
	Furoside 🍁)		Vincristine
		Miscellaneous	Carbamazepine
			Hydroxychloroquine (Plaquenil)
			Quinine (Legatrin, Novo-Quinine 🍁, Quinamm)
			Quinidine (Apo-Quinidine 🍁, Cardioquin, Quinidex)

Ask the patient:
- Who in your family has hearing problems?
- Are the problems present in men and women equally or are they present more in one gender?
- At what age was hearing loss diagnosed in your relative(s)?
- Are both ears affected?

Current Health Problems

Assess current ear-related problems by asking the patient about any ear "trouble," ear pain, or discharge, including earwax. Ask about any change in hearing, such as hyperacusis (the intolerance for sound levels that do not bother other people) or tinnitus (ringing in the ears). If a change in hearing is reported, ask whether one or both ears are involved and if the change was sudden or gradual. Also ask about problems with dizziness, sensations of being "off-balance," or vertigo (sensation of spinning movement).

? NCLEX EXAMINATION CHALLENGE
Physiological Integrity

The client is a 28-year-old woman who reports to the nurse that she has experienced reduced hearing in both ears during the past 2 years. Which health issue or personal factor is most likely to be associated with the reduced hearing?

A. Use of cotton-tipped applicators to clean the ears for her entire adult life.
B. Use of oral contraceptives as the method of birth control for the past 3 years.
C. Participation in a vegetarian diet that permits milk and eggs for the past 5 years.
D. Management of chronic joint pain with daily naproxen (Aleve) for the past 3 years.

Physical Assessment

Inspection and palpation are used to assess the ear. Begin the examination by placing the patient in a sitting or supine position. Remove any hearing aids before the examination. Inspect the hearing aid for cracks, debris, and a proper fit. A complete ear examination is usually performed by a physician, advanced practice nurse, or physician assistant. The brief assessment of the ear and hearing usually performed by a medical-surgical nurse is described next.

External Ear and Mastoid Assessment

Inspect the entire external ear for shape, location of attachment to the head, and condition, including the condition of the visible external canal. The normal pinna is uniformly shaped without skin tags or deformity. The pinna should be attached to the side of the head at a posterior angle of 10 degrees or less. The normal external canal is dry, clean, free from lesions, and not reddened.

Abnormalities of the pinna include swelling, nodules, and lesions. In chronic gout, collections of uric acid crystals result in hard, irregular, painless nodules called tophi on the pinna. Other nodules on the pinna might also be from basal cell carcinoma or rheumatoid arthritis. Small, crusted, ulcerated, or indurated lesions on the pinna that fail to heal could be squamous cell carcinoma.

Inspect the mastoid process for redness and swelling, which indicate inflammation. To assess for tenderness, gently tap with one finger over the mastoid process, compress the tragus with one finger, and gently move the pinna forward and backward. Any tenderness suggests an inflammatory process in either the external ear or the mastoid.

Assess for and record these problems:
- Furuncles
- Large amounts of cerumen
- Scaliness

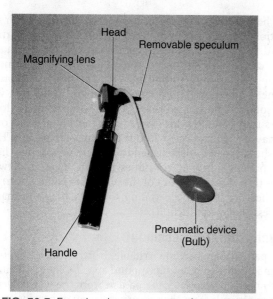

FIG. 50-5 Functional components of an otoscope.

Labels: Head, Magnifying lens, Removable speculum, Handle, Pneumatic device (Bulb)

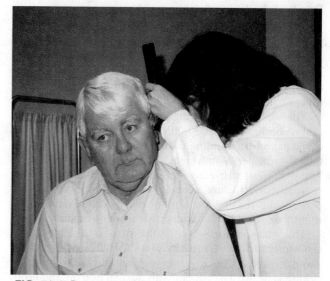

FIG. 50-6 Proper technique for an otoscopic examination.

- Redness
- Swelling of or drainage from the ear associated with a foreign object (insects or other substances), trauma, or infection
- Drainage such as blood, cerebrospinal fluid, pus, or serous fluid, and its character

Otoscopic Assessment

The purpose of a brief otoscopic examination is to assess the patency of the external canal, identify lesions or excessive cerumen in the canal, and assess whether the eardrum is intact or inflamed. An instrument called an otoscope is used to examine the ear. Many types are available. It consists of a light, a handle, a magnifying lens, and a pressure bulb for injecting air into the external canal to test mobility of the eardrum (Fig. 50-5). Specula of various diameters attach to the head of the otoscope. Select the largest speculum that most comfortably fits the patient's external canal.

> ### ! NURSING SAFETY PRIORITY
> **Action Alert**
>
> Do not use an otoscope to examine the ears of any patient who is unable to hold his or her head still during the examination.

If the patient has pain during the external ear examination, cautiously attempt an otoscopic examination. The speculum will cause extreme pain if it comes in contact with inflamed tissue in the external canal.

When performing an otoscopic examination, tilt the patient's head slightly away and hold the otoscope upside down, like a large pen (Fig. 50-6). This position permits your hand to lie against the patient's head for support. If the patient moves, both your hand and the otoscope also move, preventing damage to the external canal or eardrum. Hold the otoscope in your dominant hand, and gently pull the pinna up and back with your nondominant hand to straighten the canal. View the ear canal while you slowly insert the speculum. Use caution to avoid the pain associated with

touching the speculum on the walls of the external canal. More experienced clinicians may use the down position during the otoscopic examination, with fingers placed on the patient's cheek for safety.

> ### ! NURSING SAFETY PRIORITY
> **Action Alert**
>
> Observe the ear canal through the otoscope as you insert the speculum into the external canal to avoid the risk for perforating the eardrum.

After the otoscope is comfortably introduced in the external canal, assess for lesions and the amount, consistency, and color of cerumen and hair. The normal external canal is skin colored, intact, and without lesions. It contains various amounts of soft cerumen and small, fine hairs.

Assess the eardrum for intactness and color. *The normal eardrum is always intact.* The eardrum is shiny, transparent, and opaque or pearly gray and without lesions. Redness is seen in otitis media. Reflection of the otoscope's light from the normal eardrum is the light reflex, and it appears as a clearly outlined triangle of light. The base of the triangle is on the annulus, and the point of the triangle is on the umbo. On the right eardrum, the light reflex appears in the right lower quadrant. On the left eardrum, the light reflex appears in the left lower quadrant. The light reflex is termed diffuse when the light reflex is spotty or multiple because of a changed eardrum shape from retraction or bulging.

> ### ⊕ CULTURAL AWARENESS
>
> Cerumen is generally moist and tan or brown in Euro-Americans and African Americans. It is dry and light brown to gray in Asians and American Indians. The distinction of dry or moist ear wax is a genetically inherited trait. The color of the lining of the external ear canal varies with the patient's skin tone. Variations should not be mistaken for indications of problems. Patients with more moist earwax may form cerumen impactions more easily than patients with drier, flaky earwax and require more frequent ear irrigations.

General Auditory Assessment

After assessing the external ear and the canals of both ears, briefly assess the patient's hearing acuity. Several rapid and simple tests for hearing can be performed at the patient's bedside. Although these tests do not determine the true extent or type of hearing loss, they can indicate a patient's functional hearing ability.

The *voice test* for hearing is a simple hearing acuity test that is conducted by asking the patient to block one external ear canal while standing 1 to 2 feet (30 to 60 cm) away. Quietly whisper a statement, and then ask the patient to repeat it. Test each ear separately. If the patient does not respond correctly, use a louder whisper. If you suspect the patient is lip-reading, use your hand to block the view of your mouth, or stand behind him or her while whispering.

The *watch test* for hearing is the use of a ticking watch to test acuity for high-frequency sounds. Hold a ticking watch about 5 inches (12.7 cm) from each ear and ask whether the ticking is heard. The patient with normal hearing should be able to hear it. If a watch that ticks cannot be found, test hearing by clicking the fingernails of your thumb and fore-finger together about 12 inches from the patient's ear or just behind his or her head. More complex assessments of hearing, performed by audiologists, physicians, advanced practice nurses, specialty nurses, and physician assistants, can determine the type and extent of hearing loss.

Sound is transmitted by air conduction and bone conduction. Air conduction of sound is normally more sensitive than bone conduction. If hearing acuity is decreased, the hearing loss is categorized as:

- **Conductive hearing loss,** which results from physical obstruction of sound wave transmission such as a foreign body in the external canal, a retracted or bulging tympanic membrane, or fused bony ossicles.
- **Sensorineural hearing loss,** which results from a defect in the cochlea, the eighth cranial nerve, or the brain itself. Exposure to loud noise and music may cause this type of hearing loss as a result of damage to the cochlear hair cells.
- **Mixed conductive-sensorineural hearing loss,** which is a profound hearing loss resulting from both conductive and sensorineural hearing loss.

Each auditory function test determines the degree of hearing loss and differentiates the type of loss.

Audioscopy testing involves the use of a handheld device to generate tones of varying intensities to test hearing. Hearing can be measured at a 40-decibel (dB) intensity at frequencies of 500, 1000, 2000, and 4000 cycles per second (cps), or hertz (Hz). The audioscope is larger than a standard otoscope and is easily used to assess hearing.

Tuning fork tests for hearing acuity are the Weber and Rinne tests. These tests are useful, although limited, in distinguishing between conductive and sensorineural hearing losses. The frequency range of the tuning fork used for these tests corresponds to that of normal speech.

The Weber tuning fork test is performed by placing a vibrating tuning fork on the middle of the patient's head and asking him or her to indicate in which ear the sound is louder. The normal test result is sound heard equally in both ears. The term *lateralization* is used if the sound is louder in one ear. For example, lateralization to the right means that the sound is heard loudest in the right ear.

The Rinne tuning fork test compares hearing by air conduction with hearing by bone conduction. Sound is normally heard two to three times longer by air conduction than by bone conduction. The Rinne tuning fork test is performed by placing the vibrating tuning fork stem on the mastoid process (bone conduction) and asking the patient to indicate when the sound is no longer heard. When the patient no longer hears the sound, the fork is brought quickly in front of the pinna (air conduction) without touching the patient. He or she should then indicate when this sound is no longer heard. The patient normally continues to hear the sound two to three times longer in front of the pinna (air conduction) after not hearing it with the tuning fork touching the mastoid process (bone conduction).

Psychosocial Assessment

The patient may become irritable, frustrated, and depressed by an inability to hear and respond appropriately. The inability to hear often isolates the patient from the world. Depression may result from the sensory isolation of hearing loss. Be sensitive to the patient, and conduct the interview at a pace appropriate for that person.

Ask about social and work relationships to determine whether the patient is isolated because of hearing problems. In addition, encourage the patient to express feelings related to hearing loss and discuss any changes in daily living activities that have been made as a result of a change in hearing. Also obtain information from family members, especially if the patient does not acknowledge having a hearing problem.

> **? DECISION-MAKING CHALLENGE**
>
> ### Safety
>
> You are admitting a 78-year-old man to a rehabilitation and long-term care facility on discharge from the hospital after a transurethral resection prostatectomy. He is not very steady on his feet and is still dribbling urine. The hand-off report indicates that he did not seem to understand his care instructions although his family states he has no cognitive, vision, or hearing problems. When you tell the patient your name (Terry), he repeats it as "Mary." When you repeat your name a little louder, he says "Just quit mumbling and shouting. I have perfect hearing."
> 1. Should you apologize for this misunderstanding? Why or why not?
> 2. You plan to make a hearing assessment as part of your admission assessment. How should you introduce this assessment to the patient after his statement of having perfect hearing?
> 3. What types of issues could be affecting his hearing?

Diagnostic Assessment
Laboratory Assessment

Laboratory tests generally are not of value in determining hearing acuity. For an external ear infection, the typical causative organisms are known and this infection is treated without obtaining cultures. If the usual antibiotic therapy is not successful at clearing the infection, microbial culture and antibiotic sensitivity tests may be performed.

Imaging Assessment

Computed tomography (CT), with or without contrast enhancement, shows the structures of the ear in great detail by multiple x-ray scans of the head. These scans are then averaged by a computer. CT is especially helpful in diagnosing acoustic tumors.

Magnetic resonance imaging (MRI) is a noninvasive, non-radioactive diagnostic tool that uses a computer to generate images. Because of its superior contrast resolution, bones do not obscure the tissue image, so the MRI most accurately reflects soft-tissue changes. Patients with older internal metal vascular clips cannot have MRI. Newer clips are made from titanium and are not a contraindication for MRI.

Specific Auditory Assessment

Audiometry. Audiometry is the measurement of hearing acuity. It is performed by audiologists, audiology technicians, or nurses with special training. Frequency is the highness or lowness of tones (expressed in hertz). The greater the number of vibrations per second, the higher the frequency (pitch) of the sound. The fewer the number of vibrations per second, the lower the frequency (pitch).

Intensity of sound is expressed in decibels (dB). Threshold is the lowest level of intensity at which pure tones and speech are heard by a patient about 50% of the time.

The lowest intensity at which a young, normal ear can detect sound about 50% of the time is 0 dB. Sound at 110 dB is so intense (loud) that it is painful for most people with normal hearing. Conversational speech is around 60 dB, and a soft whisper is around 20 dB (Table 50-2). A hearing loss of 45 to 50 dB renders the person unable to hear speech without a hearing aid. A person with a hearing loss of 90 dB may not be able to hear speech even with a hearing aid.

Pure tones are generated by an audiometer to determine hearing acuity. The two types of audiometry are pure-tone audiometry and speech audiometry.

Pure-Tone Audiometry. Pure-tone audiometry generates tones with an audiometer that are presented to the patient at frequencies for hearing speech, music, and other common sounds. It can be performed by air-conduction testing or bone-conduction testing. The results of pure-tone audiometry are graphed on an audiogram. The hearing of one ear may be masked while the hearing of the other ear is tested.

Pure-tone air-conduction testing determines whether a patient hears normally or has a hearing loss. It is designed to test air-conduction hearing sensitivity (through earphones) at frequencies ranging from 125 to 8000 Hz. Thresholds are usually confined to the frequencies of 250, 500, 1000, 2000, 4000, and 8000 Hz. The intensities for pure tones generally range from 10 to 110 dB.

The patient sits in a sound-isolated room to reduce background noise. Earphones are placed over the ears, and tones of varying frequencies and intensities are delivered through the earphones, testing one ear at a time. The patient presses a button or raises a hand to indicate when he or she hears a tone. No special follow-up care is needed.

Pure-tone bone-conduction testing determines whether the hearing loss detected by air-conduction testing is due to conductive or sensorineural factors or to a combination of the two. It is used only when the results of air-conduction testing are abnormal. Testing is similar to air-conduction testing except that a bone-conduction vibrator, placed firmly behind the pinna on the mastoid process, is used instead of earphones. No special follow-up care is needed.

Interpretation of audiometric evaluation determines whether the patient's hearing is within normal limits or, with a hearing impairment, whether the hearing loss is conductive, sensorineural, or mixed. The type of loss can be determined by an experienced clinician who examines the shape of the audiogram after completion of pure-tone air- and bone-conduction audiometry.

Speech Audiometry. In speech audiometry, the patient's ability to hear spoken words is measured through a microphone connected to an audiometer. The two components of speech audiometry are the speech reception threshold and speech discrimination.

Speech reception threshold is the minimum loudness at which a patient can repeat simple words. This test determines how loud a simple speech stimulus must be before the patient can hear it well enough to repeat it correctly. In one common test, lists of two-syllable words called spondee are used (i.e., words in which there is generally equal stress on each syllable, such as *airplane, railroad,* and *cowboy*).

The speech reception threshold measured by the audiometer is the hearing level at which the patient can repeat simple words correctly 50% of the time. The test is conducted in a manner similar to the pure-tone tests.

Speech discrimination testing determines the patient's ability to discriminate among similar sounds or among words that contain similar sounds. The ability to understand speech is the most important measurable aspect of human hearing. Speech discrimination testing assesses *understanding* of speech. A hearing loss may decrease sensitivity to sound and impair understanding of what is being said.

A standard format contains lists of 25 to 50 monosyllabic (one-syllable) words, such as *carve, day, toe,* and *ran,* and phonemically balanced words, with equal word difficulty between lists. The lists are presented to the patient through earphones at a selected loudness level, generally about 30 to 40 dB above the speech reception threshold, or at the patient's most comfortable listening level. A percentage score is derived from the number of words repeated correctly.

Tympanometry. Tympanometry assesses mobility of the eardrum and structures of the middle ear by systematically changing air pressure in the external auditory canal. The progression or resolution of serous otitis and otitis media can be accurately monitored with this procedure.

TABLE 50-2 DECIBEL INTENSITY AND SAFE EXPOSURE TIME FOR COMMON SOUNDS

SOUND	DECIBEL INTENSITY (DB)	SAFE EXPOSURE TIME*
Threshold of hearing	0	
Whispering	20	
Average residence or office	40	
Conversational speech	60	
Car traffic	70	>8 hr
Motorcycle	90	8 hr
Chain saw	100	2 hr
Rock concert, front row	120	3 min
Jet engine	140	Immediate danger
Rocket launching pad	180	Immediate danger

*For every 5-dB increase in intensity, the safe exposure time is cut in half.

This test is helpful in distinguishing middle ear pathologic conditions, such as otosclerosis, ossicular disarticulation, otitis media, and perforation of the eardrum. It is also useful for assessing patency of the eustachian tube and for checking recovery of middle ear function after surgery.

Auditory Brainstem-Evoked Response. Auditory brainstem-evoked response (ABR) assesses hearing in patients who are unable to indicate their recognition of sound stimuli during standard hearing tests. This test helps diagnose both conductive and sensorineural hearing losses. Electrodes are placed on the scalp during the test. After the test, clean the patient's hair to remove the electrode gel.

To prepare the patient for ABR:
- Tell the patient that no fasting or sedation is needed
- Carefully explain the procedure and its purpose
- Inform the patient that the procedure usually takes about 30 minutes

Assessment of Balance

Electronystagmography (ENG) is a test that is sensitive in detecting both central and peripheral disease of the vestibular system in the ear. The ENG detects and records nystagmus (involuntary eye movements) because the eyes and ears depend on each other for balance. Electrodes are taped to the skin near the eyes, and one or more procedures (caloric testing, changing gaze position, or changing head position) are performed to stimulate nystagmus. Failure of nystagmus to occur with cerebral stimulation suggests an abnormality in the vestibulocochlear apparatus, the cerebral cortex, the auditory nerve, or the brainstem.

To prepare the patient for ENG:
- Carefully explain the procedure and its purpose. The examiners will be asking the patient to name names or do simple math problems during the test to ensure he or she stays alert.
- Tell the patient to fast for several hours before the test and to avoid caffeine-containing beverages for 24 to 48 hours before the test.
- Tell patients with pacemakers that they should not have the test because pacemaker signals interfere with the sensitivity of ENG.

- Carefully introduce oral fluids after the test to prevent nausea and vomiting.

Caloric testing evaluates the vestibular (inner ear) portion of the auditory nerve. Warm water or warm air is infused into the ear. A normal response is the onset of vertigo and nystagmus within 20 to 30 seconds. Prepare the patient for caloric testing by:
- Carefully explaining the procedure and its purpose.
- Telling the patient to fast for several hours before the test.
- Telling the patient that the affected side will be tested first.
- Explaining that he or she will be on bedrest after the procedure with careful introduction of oral fluids to prevent nausea and vomiting.

Dix-Hallpike testing for vertigo is performed by assisting the patient to a sitting position on an examination table. Stand to the side of the patient, and quickly reposition him or her from sitting to supine with the head extending beyond the end of the table. This change of position is done first to one side and then to the other side. A patient with benign positional vertigo will have a burst of nystagmus after a delay of 5 to 10 seconds.

To prepare the patient for the Dix-Hallpike test:
- Carefully explain the procedure and its purpose.
- Tell him or her to keep the eyes open and try not to blink.
- Explain that double vision may occur during the test.

? NCLEX EXAMINATION CHALLENGE
Health Promotion and Maintenance

Which precaution or action is the priority for the nurse to teach the client who is scheduled to undergo tympanometry, pure-tone audiometry, and caloric testing?

A. Avoid aspirin and aspirin-containing products for 1 week before testing.
B. Shower and wash your hair the night before testing.
C. Do not eat or drink within 4 hours before testing.
D. Do not smoke for 24 hours before the testing.

NURSING CONCEPT REVIEW

What should you expect to NOTICE in a patient with adequate sensation related to the ear and hearing?

- Ears are symmetric on the face on a line about even with the corners of the eyes and with the tops of the ears rotated slightly toward back.
- Outer ear (pinna) has no open areas, scales, or bumps.
- No drainage occurs from the ear canal.
- Does not tilt one side of the head or lean forward when listening to another person speak.
- Startles when a loud or unexpected sound occurs in the environment.

- Responds appropriately to questions.
- Does not consistently ask a speaker to repeat himself or herself; does not say "What?" or "Huh?" frequently.
- Responds appropriately to greetings with other people in the immediate environment.
- Responds appropriately to whispered questions and conversations, even when the speaker is not facing the patient.

GET READY FOR THE NCLEX® EXAMINATION!

KEY POINTS

Review these Key Points for each NCLEX Examination Client Needs Category.

Safe and Effective Care Environment
- Use a separate speculum cover for each ear when conducting an otoscopic examination.
- Slowly and gently introduce the otoscopic speculum into the external ear canal during assessment.
- Use Standard Precautions with any patient who has drainage from the ear canal.
- Do not perform an otoscopic examination on a confused patient.
- Use the suggestions presented in the Patient History section to enhance communication with a patient who has a hearing impairment.

Health Promotion and Maintenance
- Teach patients the proper way to clean the pinna and external ear canal.
- Identify patients at risk for hearing impairment as a result of work environment or leisure activities.
- Encourage all patients, even if they already have a hearing impairment, to use ear protection in loud environments.
- Inform all patients who smoke that smoking increases the risk for development of hearing problems.

Psychosocial Integrity
- Allow the patient the opportunity to express fear or anxiety about a change in hearing status.
- Explain all diagnostic procedures, restrictions, and follow-up care to the patient scheduled for tests.

Physiological Integrity
- Ask the patient about hearing problems in any other members of the family, because many hearing problems have a genetic component.
- Ask the patient whether he or she has ever used any ototoxic drugs (see Table 50-1).

Care of Patients with Ear and Hearing Problems

Judith Laver Bierschbach

⊖volve WEBSITE

http://evolve.elsevier.com/Iggy/

Answer Key for NCLEX Examination Challenges and
   Decision-Making Challenges
Audio Glossary

Concept Map Creator
Key Points
Review Questions for the NCLEX® Examination

LEARNING OUTCOMES

Safe and Effective Care Environment

1. Apply principles of infection control when examining an ear with drainage.
2. Implement precautions to prevent falls in patients experiencing vertigo or dizziness.
3. Correctly instill eardrops.

Health Promotion and Maintenance

4. Teach patients using hearing aids how to use and care for them properly.

Psychosocial Integrity

5. Teach patients and family members about what to expect during tests, procedures, and follow-up to manage ear and hearing problems.
6. Provide opportunities for the patient and family to express feelings and concerns about a change in hearing.

7. Refer hearing-impaired patients and families to local and Internet-based support services.

Physiological Integrity

8. Compare the clinical manifestations and interventions for external otitis with those of otitis media.
9. Safely remove impacted cerumen from the ear canal of an older patient.
10. Coordinate the care of the patient with Ménière's disease.
11. Prioritize nursing care needs for the patient after tympanoplasty.
12. Prioritize educational needs for the patient after stapedectomy.
13. Identify an appropriate method for communicating with a patient who has recently become hearing impaired.

The ears are important for hearing and balance. Ear disorders may lead to hearing difficulty, balance problems, and impaired general function. Hearing problems reduce the ability of patients to fully communicate with the world around them. They can lead to confusion, mistrust, social isolation, and the inability to give and receive accurate information. Although ear and hearing disorders are often easily managed, early recognition and intervention are necessary to prevent additional damage and to promote a maximum level of wellness.

CONDITIONS AFFECTING THE EXTERNAL EAR

The external ear is the outermost part of the ear structures and is subject to outside factors that can cause problems. Disorders of the external ear include congenital malformation (birth defects), trauma, and infectious or noninfectious lesions of the pinna, auricle, or auditory canal. The presence of birth defects in one area does not necessarily mean that other areas of the ear also will be affected. Abnormalities of the external ear range from crumpling or falling forward of the pinna to complete absence (atresia) of the auditory canal. Trauma can damage or destroy the auricle and external canal. Surgical reconstruction can re-form the pinna with skin grafts and plastic prostheses. Trauma to the auricle resulting in a hematoma requires the removal of blood via needle aspiration to prevent calcification and hardening, which is often referred to as a cauliflower or boxer's ear.

Benign cysts or polyps of the auricle or external canal are surgically removed if they block the canal and affect hearing. Cancer cells, usually basal cell carcinoma, can occur on the pinna. Usually, treatment consists of simple excision. When the lesion becomes larger, its location near the skull and facial nerve makes treatment more difficult.

EXTERNAL OTITIS

Pathophysiology

External otitis is a painful condition caused when irritating or infective agents come into contact with the skin of the external ear. The result is either an allergic response or inflammation with or without infection. Affected skin becomes red, swollen, and tender to touch or movement. Swelling of the ear canal can lead to temporary hearing loss due to obstruction. Allergic external otitis is often caused by contact with cosmetics, hair sprays, earphones, earrings, or hearing aids. The most common infectious organisms are *Pseudomonas aeruginosa, Streptococcus, Staphylococcus,* and *Aspergillus.*

External otitis occurs more often in hot, humid environments, especially in the summer, and is known as swimmer's ear because it occurs most often in people involved in water sports. Patients who have traumatized their external ear canal with sharp or small objects (e.g., hairpins, cotton-tipped applicators) or with headphones also are more susceptible to external otitis.

Necrotizing or *malignant otitis* is the most virulent form of external otitis. Organisms spread beyond the external ear canal into the ear and skull. The high mortality rate seen with malignant external otitis results from complications such as meningitis, brain abscess, and destruction of cranial nerve VII.

PATIENT-CENTERED COLLABORATIVE CARE

Manifestations of external otitis range from mild itching to pain with movement of the pinna or tragus, particularly when upward pressure is applied to the external canal. Patients report feeling as if the ear is plugged and hearing is reduced.

Use caution during otoscopic examination to avoid pressing on the walls of the external canal, which causes pain. Drainage from the ear is often greenish white. To prevent cross-contamination, examine the unaffected ear first. Hearing loss in the affected ear can be severe when inflammation obstructs the ear canal and prevents sounds from reaching the eardrum (tympanic membrane).

Management focuses on reducing inflammation, edema, and pain. Nursing priorities include comfort measures, such as applying heat to the ear for 20 minutes three times a day. This can be accomplished by using towels warmed with water and then wrapped in a plastic bag or by using a heating pad placed on a low setting. Teach the patient that minimizing head movements reduces pain.

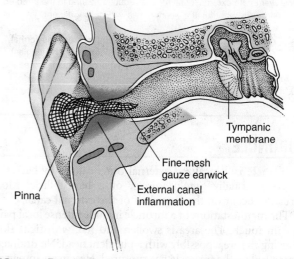

FIG. 51-1 Earwick for instillation of antibiotics into the external canal. When edema occludes the external auditory canal, it is difficult for antibiotic solutions to enter the canal adequately. An earwick is placed through the meatus. Solutions placed on the external portion of the earwick are absorbed through the canal.

Topical antibiotic and steroid therapies are most effective in decreasing inflammation and pain. Review best practices for instilling eardrops with the patient, as shown in Chart 51-1. Observe the patient self-administer the eardrops to make sure that proper technique is used. If edema obstructs the external canal, an earwick is inserted past the blockage, with drugs applied to the outside end (Fig. 51-1). A long piece of gauze dressing serves as an earwick, which the health care provider inserts using forceps to push carefully through the blocked external auditory canal to the eardrum. The earwick may be removed when eardrops can flow freely into the canal. Use handwashing whenever the infected ear is touched. Oral or IV antibiotics are used in severe cases, especially when infection spreads to surrounding tissue or area lymph nodes are enlarged.

Analgesics, including opioids, may be needed for pain relief during the initial days of treatment. NSAIDs, such as acetylsalicylic acid (aspirin, Entrophen ✦) and ibuprofen (Advil), or acetaminophen (Tylenol, Abenol ✦) may relieve less-severe pain.

After the inflammation has subsided, a solution of 50% rubbing alcohol, 25% white vinegar, and 25% distilled water may be dropped into the ear to keep it clean and dry and to prevent recurrence. Teach the patient not to use cotton-tipped applicators to dry the ears, because this use could damage the canal and increase the risk for infection or inflammation. Teach him or her to use preventive measures for minimizing ear canal moisture, trauma, or exposure to materials that lead to local irritation or contact dermatitis. Recommend the use of earplugs when engaging in water sports to those patients with recurrent episodes of external otitis.

FURUNCLE

A furuncle is a localized external otitis caused by bacterial infection, usually *Staphylococcus*, of a hair follicle. Most furuncles occur on the outer half of the external canal.

The manifestations of a furuncle include intense local pain to light touch. The area is swollen and red, with tight skin covering the area, possibly with a purulent head. No drainage is seen unless the furuncle has ruptured. Hearing is impaired if the lesion blocks the canal.

Treatment consists of local and systemic antibiotics and local heat application. An earwick may be used with one-half strength Burow's solution to relieve pain. The furuncle may need to be incised and drained if it does not resolve with antibiotic therapy.

PERICHONDRITIS

Perichondritis is an infection of the perichondrium, a tough, fibrous tissue layer that surrounds the cartilage and shapes the pinna. This tissue supplies blood to the ear cartilage. Infection can be caused by opening an area of pus or localized infection, insect bites, trauma, postoperative complication of tympanoplasty, and cartilage ear piercing. When infection occurs between the perichondrium and the cartilage, blood flow to the cartilage can be reduced to the point that necrosis occurs and the pinna may become deformed. This can occur as a complication of high helical ear piercing and may require removal of necrotic tissue.

The purposes of management are to eliminate the infection and ensure that the perichondrium stays in direct contact

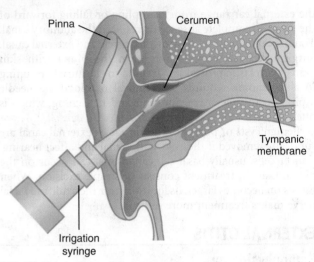

FIG. 51-2 Irrigation of the external canal. Cerumen and debris can be removed from the ear by irrigation with warm water. The stream of water is aimed above or below the impaction to allow back-pressure to push it out rather than further down the canal.

with the cartilage. In addition to systemic antibiotic therapy, a wide incision is made and suction drainage is used to remove pus and other fluid.

CERUMEN OR FOREIGN BODIES

Pathophysiology

Cerumen (wax) is the most common cause of an impacted canal. A canal can also become impacted as a result of foreign bodies that can enter or be placed in the external ear canal, such as vegetables, beads, pencil erasers, and insects. Although uncomfortable, cerumen or foreign bodies are rarely true emergencies and can be carefully removed by a health care professional. Cerumen impaction in the older adult is common, and removal of the cerumen from older adults often improves hearing (Holcomb, 2009).

▌PATIENT-CENTERED COLLABORATIVE CARE

Patients with a cerumen impaction or a foreign body in the ear may experience a sensation of fullness in the ear, with or without hearing loss, and may have ear pain, itching, dizziness, or bleeding from the ear. The object may be visible with direct inspection.

When the occluding material is cerumen, management options include watchful waiting, manual removal, and the use of ceruminolytic agents followed by either manual irrigation or the use of a low-pressure, electronic, oral irrigation device (Holcomb, 2009). The canal can be irrigated with a mixture of water and hydrogen peroxide at body temperature (Fig. 51-2), following best practices for proper irrigation (Chart 51-2). Removal of a cerumen obstruction by irrigation is a slow process and may take more than one sitting. When it is the cause of hearing loss, cerumen removal may improve hearing. Between 50 and 70 mL of solution is the maximum

CHART 51-2 BEST PRACTICE FOR PATIENT SAFETY & QUALITY CARE

Ear Irrigation

- Wash your hands.
- Use an otoscope to check the location of the impacted cerumen; ascertain that the eardrum is intact and that the patient does not have otitis media.
- Gather the proper equipment: basin, syringe (without needle), otoscope, towel.
- Warm tap water (or other prescribed solution) to body temperature.
- Fill a syringe with the warmed irrigating solution.
- Place a towel around the patient's neck.
- Place a basin under the ear to be irrigated.
- Place the tip of the syringe at an angle so that the fluid pushes on one side of and not directly on the impaction (this helps loosen the impaction instead of forcing it further into the canal).
- Apply gentle but firm continuous pressure, allowing the water to flow against the top of the canal.
- Do not use blasts or bursts of sudden pressure.
- If pain occurs, decrease the pressure. If pain persists, stop the irrigation.
- Watch the fluid return for signs of cerumen plug removal.
- Continue to irrigate the ear with about 70 mL of fluid.
- If the cerumen does not drain out, wait 10 minutes and repeat the irrigation procedure.
- Monitor the patient for signs of nausea.
- If the patient becomes nauseated, stop the procedure.
- If the cerumen cannot be removed by irrigation, place (or the patient may place) mineral oil into the ear three times a day for 2 days to soften dry, impacted cerumen, after which irrigation may be repeated.
- After completion of the irrigation, have the patient turn his or her head to the side just irrigated to drain any remaining irrigation fluid.
- Wash your hands.

CHART 51-3 NURSING FOCUS ON THE OLDER ADULT

Cerumen Impaction

- Assess the hearing of all older patients using simple voice tests (see Chapter 50).
- Perform a gentle otoscopic inspection of the external canal and eardrum of any older patient who has a problem with hearing acuity, especially the patient who wears a hearing aid.
- Use ear irrigation to remove any impacted cerumen.
- Make certain that the irrigating fluid is about 98.6° F (37° C) to reduce the chance for stimulating the vestibular sense.
- Use no more than 5 to 10 mL of irrigating fluid at a time.
- If nausea, vomiting, or dizziness develops, stop the irrigation immediately.
- Teach the patient how to irrigate his or her own ears.
- Obtain a return demonstration of ear irrigation from the patient, observing for specific areas in which the patient may need assistance.
- Encourage the patient to wash the external ears daily using a soapy, wet washcloth over the index finger (best done in the shower or while washing the hair).

the far end) to clean the ears or remove cerumen. Chart 50-3 in Chapter 50 describes steps to teach patients regarding ear hygiene and self–ear irrigation. Refer to Chart 51-3 for nursing care considerations of older adult patients with cerumen impaction.

Insects are killed before removal unless they can be coaxed out by a flashlight or a humming noise. Lidocaine, a numbing agent, can be placed in the ear canal for pain relief. Mineral oil or diluted alcohol instilled into the ear can suffocate the insect, which is then removed with ear forceps.

If the patient has local irritation, an antibiotic or steroid ointment may be applied to prevent infection and reduce local irritation. Hearing acuity is tested if hearing loss is not resolved by removal of the object.

Surgical removal of the foreign object may be required. The object is removed through the ear canal (transcanal route) using a wire bent at a 90-degree angle. The wire is looped around the object, and the object is pulled out.

amount that the patient with an impaction usually can tolerate at one sitting.

! NURSING SAFETY PRIORITY

Action Alert

Do not irrigate an ear with an eardrum perforation or otitis media because this may spread the infection to the inner ear. Also, do not irrigate the ear when the foreign object is vegetable matter, because this material expands when wet, making the impaction worse. For vegetable matter, the object needs to be physically removed by an experienced health care professional.

If the cerumen is thick and dry or cannot be removed easily, suggest an over-the-counter ceruminolytic product such as Cerumenex to soften the wax before trying to remove it. Another way to soften cerumen is to add 3 drops of glycerin or mineral oil to the ear at bedtime and 3 drops of hydrogen peroxide twice a day. After several days of this treatment, the cerumen is more easily removed by irrigation. In some cases, a small curette or cerumen spoon may be used by a health care professional to scoop out the wax. Care is taken with this method because damage to the canal or the eardrum can occur with improper technique.

Discourage the use of cotton swabs and ear candles (hollow tubes coated in wax inserted into the ear and then lighted at

? DECISION-MAKING CHALLENGE

Safety; Patient-Centered Care

A 78-year-old woman who is an assisted-living resident reports pain in and drainage from her right ear. She also reports decreased hearing in the affected ear. When you examine her, she asks if she can just have some medicine without an examination of the ear. You reassure her that you will be gentle and not cause more pain. She reluctantly agrees to be examined.

1. Describe exactly how you would proceed with this ear assessment.
2. What other vital signs should you take and why?

As you prepare to perform an otoscopic examination of the right ear, the patient tells you that last week her ear itched and that she used a pencil to scratch the ear canal. When she removed the pencil, the eraser was missing. Her ear pain and discharge began about 3 days later.

3. Should you proceed with an otoscopic examination now? Why or why not?
4. What type of problem do you suspect with this situation?

Because this procedure is painful, general anesthesia is needed.

CONDITIONS AFFECTING THE MIDDLE EAR

OTITIS MEDIA

Pathophysiology

The three common forms of otitis media are acute otitis media, chronic otitis media, and serous otitis media. Each type affects the middle ear but has different causes and pathologic changes. If otitis progresses or is untreated, permanent conductive hearing loss may occur.

Acute otitis media and chronic otitis media, also known as *suppurant* or *purulent* otitis media, are similar. An infecting agent in the middle ear causes inflammation of the mucosa, leading to swelling and irritation of the small bones *(ossicles)* within the middle ear, followed by purulent inflammatory exudate. Acute disease has a sudden onset and lasts 3 weeks or less. Chronic otitis media often follows repeated acute episodes, has a longer duration, and causes greater middle ear injury. It may be a result of the continuing presence of a biofilm in the middle ear. A biofilm is a community of bacteria working together to overcome host defense mechanisms to continue to survive and proliferate (Lee et al., 2009). (See Chapter 25 for more information about biofilms.) Therapy for complications associated with chronic otitis media, unlike that of acute otitis media, usually involves surgical intervention.

The eustachian tube and mastoid, connected to the middle ear by a sheet of cells, are also affected by the infection. If the eardrum membrane perforates and infective materials spill into the external ear, external otitis develops that thickens and scars the middle ear if left untreated. Necrosis of the ossicles destroys middle ear structures and causes hearing loss.

PATIENT-CENTERED COLLABORATIVE CARE

ASSESSMENT

The patient with acute or chronic otitis media has ear pain with and without movement of the external ear. Acute otitis media causes more intense pain. As the pressure in the middle ear increases, there is a sensation of fullness in the ear. Hearing is reduced and distorted. The patient may notice a sticking or cracking sound in the ear upon yawning or swallowing or may have tinnitus in the form of a low hum or a low-pitched sound. Conductive hearing loss may occur as sound wave transmission is obstructed. Headaches and systemic symptoms such as malaise, fever, nausea, and vomiting can occur. As the pressure on the middle ear pushes against the inner ear, the patient may have dizziness or vertigo.

Otoscopic examination findings vary, depending on the stage of the condition. The eardrum is initially retracted, which allows landmarks of the ear to be seen clearly. At this early stage, the patient has only vague ear discomfort. As the condition progresses, the eardrum's blood vessels dilate and appear red (Fig. 51-3). In the third stage, the eardrum becomes red, thickened, and bulging, with loss of landmarks. Decreased eardrum mobility is evident on inspection with a pneumatic otoscope. Pus may be seen behind the membrane.

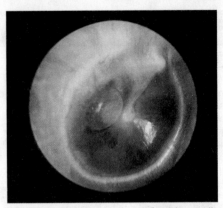

FIG. 51-3 Otoscopic view of otitis media.

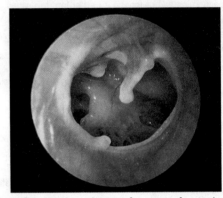

FIG. 51-4 Otoscopic view of a perforated tympanic membrane.

If the condition progresses, the eardrum spontaneously **perforates** (ruptures) and pus or blood drains from the ear (Fig. 51-4). When the membrane ruptures, the patient notices a marked decrease in pain as the pressure on middle ear structures is relieved (Fig. 51-5). Eardrum perforations from any cause may heal if the underlying problem is controlled. Initially, the eardrum membrane is thinner over the healed perforation. A simple central perforation does not interfere with hearing unless the small bones of the middle ear are damaged or the perforation is large. Repeated perforations with extensive scarring can cause hearing loss.

Cultures of drainage after a perforation from uncontrolled otitis media may reveal the infecting agent. Cultures are taken only when previous treatment is ineffective. When the eardrum is not perforated, a needle aspiration or myringotomy may be performed by a physician or nurse practitioner to withdraw fluid for culture.

INTERVENTIONS

Nonsurgical Management

Management can be as simple as putting the patient in a quiet environment. Bedrest limits head movements that intensify the pain. Heat may be applied by using a heating pad adjusted to a low setting. Application of cold also may relieve pain.

Topical antibiotics are not used to treat otitis media. Systemic antibiotic therapy decreases pain by reducing inflammation. Teach the patient to complete the antibiotic therapy as prescribed and to not stop taking the drug when manifestations are no longer present. Stopping the drug early may

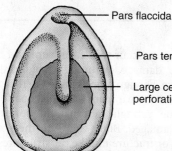

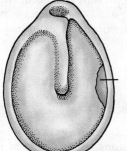

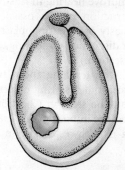

With a **large central perforation,**
patients report significant hearing loss.

With a **marginal perforation,**
patients may report significant hearing loss.

With a **small inferior pars tensa perforation,**
patients do not report much interference with hearing.

FIG. 51-5 Perforations of the tympanic membrane. Central perforations heal more quickly than marginal perforations. Marginal perforations that do not heal allow cholesteatoma formation.

result in infection recurrence and contributes to antibiotic resistance. Analgesics such as aspirin, ibuprofen (Advil), and acetaminophen (Tylenol, Abenol ♣) relieve pain and reduce fever, helping the patient feel better. When pain is severe, opioid analgesics such as codeine also may be prescribed.

Antihistamines and decongestants are prescribed to decrease fluid in the middle ear. The body can then reabsorb the fluid, reducing pressure and pain.

Surgical Management

If pain persists after antibiotic therapy and the eardrum continues to bulge, a *myringotomy* (surgical opening of the pars tensa of the eardrum) is performed. This procedure drains middle ear fluids and immediately relieves pain.

Preoperative care includes reassuring the patient that the myringotomy will relieve pain and is usually performed

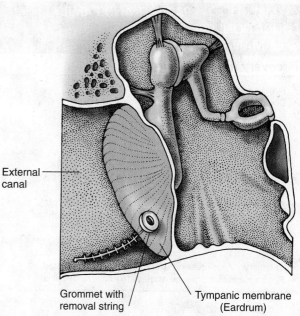

FIG. 51-6 Grommet through the tympanic membrane. A small grommet is placed through the tympanic membrane away from the margins, which allows prolonged drainage of fluids from the middle ear. The grommet can be removed later and the tympanic membrane allowed to heal naturally or patched with a small piece of homogenous tissue.

without anesthesia. Many people are concerned about a perforation and its effect on hearing. To relieve some of this anxiety, discuss the reasons for the procedure and encourage the patient to use techniques such as deep breathing before and during the procedure. Systemic antibiotic therapy continues before and after this procedure. Clean the external canal with a bacteriostatic solution such as povidone-iodine (Betadine) before the myringotomy.

The operative procedure is a small surgical incision often performed in an office or clinic setting and heals rapidly. Another approach is the removal of fluid from the middle ear with a needle. For relief of pressure caused by serous otitis media and for those patients who have repeated episodes of otitis media, a small grommet (polyethylene tube) may be surgically placed through the eardrum to allow continuous drainage of middle ear fluids (Fig. 51-6).

Postoperative care priorities include teaching the patient to keep the external ear and canal free of other substances while the incision is healing. Instruct him or her to keep the head dry by not washing the hair or showering for several days. Other instructions after surgery are listed in Chart 51-4.

MASTOIDITIS

Pathophysiology

The lining of the middle ear is continuous with the lining of the mastoid air cells, which are embedded in the temporal bone. Mastoiditis is an infection of the mastoid air cells caused by untreated or inadequately treated otitis media. This infection can be acute or chronic. Antibiotic therapy is used to treat the middle ear infection before it progresses to mastoiditis.

PATIENT-CENTERED COLLABORATIVE CARE

The manifestations of mastoiditis include swelling behind the ear and pain with minimal movement of the tragus, the pinna, or the head. Pain is *not* relieved by myringotomy. Cellulitis (infection spreading sideways through the tissues of the skin) develops on the skin or external scalp over the mastoid process. The ear is pushed sideways and down. Otoscopic examination shows a red, dull, thick, immobile eardrum with or without perforation. Lymph nodes behind the ear are tender and enlarged. Patients may have low-grade fever, malaise, ear drainage, and loss of appetite. Hearing loss occurs, and computed tomography (CT) scans show fluid in the air cells of the mastoid process.

Interventions focus on halting the infection before it spreads to other structures. IV antibiotics are used to prevent the spread of infection. These drugs have limited use in actual mastoiditis treatment because they do not easily penetrate the infected bony structure of the mastoid. Cultures of the ear drainage determine which antibiotics should be most effective. Surgical removal of the infected tissue is needed if the infection does not respond to antibiotic therapy within a few days. A simple or modified radical mastoidectomy with tympanoplasty is the most common treatment. All infected tissue must be removed so that the infection does not spread to other structures. A tympanoplasty is then performed to reconstruct the ossicles and the eardrum to restore hearing. Patient preparation, the operative procedure, and follow-up care for tympanoplasty are discussed on pp. 1101 and 1102.

Complications occur when infective material is not removed completely or when other structures are contaminated. Complications include damage to cranial nerves VI and VII, decreasing the patient's ability to look sideways (cranial nerve VI) and causing a drooping of the mouth on the affected side (cranial nerve VII). Other complications include vertigo, meningitis, brain abscess, chronic purulent otitis media, and wound infection.

TRAUMA

Pathophysiology

Trauma and damage may occur to the eardrum and ossicles by infection, by direct damage, or through rapid changes in the middle ear pressure. Foreign objects placed in the external canal exert pressure on the eardrum and cause perforation. If the objects continue through the canal, the bones of the middle ear may be damaged. Blunt injury to the skull and ears can also damage or fracture middle ear structures. Slapping the external ear increases the pressure in the ear canal and can tear the eardrum. The eardrum has a limited stretching ability and gives way under high pressure. Excessive nose blowing and rapid changes of pressure that occur with nonpressurized air flight (barotrauma) can increase pressure within the middle ear. High pressure damages the ossicles and can perforate the eardrum.

PATIENT-CENTERED COLLABORATIVE CARE

Most eardrum perforations heal within a week or two without treatment. Repeated perforations, especially from chronic otitis media, heal more slowly, with scarring. Depending on the amount of damage to the ossicles, hearing may or may not return. Hearing aids can improve hearing in this type of hearing loss. Surgical reconstruction of the ossicles and eardrum through a tympanoplasty or a myringoplasty may also improve hearing. (See later discussion of nursing care on p. 1102 in the Tympanoplasty section.)

Nursing care priorities focus on teaching about trauma prevention. Caution patients to avoid inserting objects into the external canal and to follow the steps in Chart 50-3 in Chapter 50 for ear hygiene. Stress the importance of using ear protectors when blunt trauma is likely, especially in sports such as boxing and wrestling.

NEOPLASMS

Tumors of the middle ear are rare, and the most common type is the *glomus jugulare*, a benign lesion arising from the jugular vein. Malignant ear tumors also can occur. The growth of any lesion within the middle ear area disrupts conductive hearing, erodes the ossicles, and may spread to the inner ear and nearby cranial nerves.

Patients have progressive hearing loss and tinnitus. Infection and pain rarely occur with *glomus jugulare* tumors. Otoscopic examination shows a bulging eardrum or a mass extending to the external ear canal. The many blood vessels of the *glomus jugulare* tumor give it a reddish color and a visible pulsation when seen through the eardrum.

Diagnosis is made by physical examination, tomography, and angiography. Tumors are removed by surgery, which often destroys hearing in the affected ear. If all of the edges of the tumor can be seen clearly through the eardrum, surgery is performed through the ear canal to remove the tumor. When the tumor edges extend past the eardrum, more testing is needed to determine the extent of involvement. Radiation therapy is used to decrease the blood supply of the *glomus jugulare* tumor but is not the preferred method of treatment.

TABLE 51-1 RESOURCE AGENCIES FOR EAR AND HEARING IMPAIRMENT

House Research Institute
2100 West Third Street, Fifth Floor
Los Angeles, CA 90057
Voice: (800) 388-8612
Fax: (213) 483-8789
www.hei.org
E-mail: info@hei.org

American Speech-Language-Hearing Association
2200 Research Boulevard
Rockville, MD 20850-3289
Voice: (800) 638-8255
Fax: (301) 296-8580
www.asha.org

Laurent Clerc National Deaf Education Center
Gallaudet University
800 Florida Avenue NE
Washington, DC 20002
Voice/TTY: (202) 651-5051

Hearing Loss Association of America
7910 Woodmont Avenue, Suite 1200
Bethesda, MD 20814
Voice/TTY: (301) 657-2248
Fax: (301) 657-2248
www.shhh.org

American Academy of Otolaryngology/Head and Neck Surgery
One Prince Street
Alexandria, VA 22314-3357
Voice/TTY: (703) 836-4444
www.entnet.org

American Tinnitus Association
P.O. Box 5
Portland, OR 97207-0005
Voice: (800) 634-8978
www.ata.org

Benign tumors are removed because, with continued growth, other structures can be affected, further damaging the facial or trigeminal nerve. When possible, reconstruction of the middle ear structures is performed later to restore conductive hearing.

CONDITIONS AFFECTING THE INNER EAR

TINNITUS

Tinnitus (continuous ringing or noise perception in the ear) is a common hearing problem. Diagnostic testing cannot confirm tinnitus, nor can the disorder be observed. Testing is performed, however, to assess hearing and rule out other disorders.

Manifestation of tinnitus range from mild ringing, which can go unnoticed during the day, to a loud roaring in the ear, which can interfere with thinking and attention span. Some patients feel as if the constant ringing could drive them mad. When patients report tinnitus, consider the many factors that cause tinnitus: presbycusis, otosclerosis (irregular bone growth around ossicles), Ménière's disease, certain drugs, exposure to loud noise, and other inner ear problems (Bauer & Brozoski, 2008).

The problem and its management vary with the underlying cause (Newman et al., 2008). When no cause can be found or the disorder is untreatable, therapy focuses on ways to mask the tinnitus with background sound, noise-makers, and music during sleeping hours. Ear mold hearing aids can amplify sounds to drown out the tinnitus during the day. The American Tinnitus Association assists patients in coping with tinnitus. Refer patients with tinnitus to local and online support groups to help cope with this problem (Table 51-1).

VERTIGO AND DIZZINESS

Vertigo and dizziness are common manifestations of many ear disorders. Dizziness is a disturbed sense of a person's relationship to space. Patients vary greatly in defining dizziness. Vertigo is often used interchangeably with dizziness, but the definition and cause are somewhat different (Warren, 2008). True vertigo is a real sense of whirling or turning in space.

The visual system, the vestibular system (cochlea, semicircular canals), and the proprioceptive system (muscles and nerve endings) combine to give input to the brain about balance. Problems in any of these areas lead to a disturbed sense of balance and motion. Problems that cause vertigo include Ménière's disease, labyrinthitis, acoustic neuromas, motion sickness, and drug or alcohol ingestion.

Manifestations of vertigo include nausea, vomiting, falling, nystagmus, hearing loss, and tinnitus. Until the cause of the vertigo can be identified, each manifestation is treated. Teach patients these strategies to reduce manifestations:

- Restrict head motion and change position slowly.
- Maintain adequate hydration, especially after vomiting.
- Take drugs that reduce the vertigo effects such as over-the-counter dimenhydrinate (Dramamine, Gravol ✿) or prescription drugs such as diazepam (Valium, Apo-Diazepam ✿), meclizine (Antivert, Bonamine ✿), and scopolamine (Transderm Scop, Transderm-V ✿).

Many patients are dissatisfied with drug side effects, especially drowsiness, which can be worse than the vertigo. Teach patients to maintain a safe, uncluttered environment to prevent accidents during periods of vertigo and to use a cane or walker to maintain balance. Also instruct them to not drive or operate machinery when taking these drugs.

LABYRINTHITIS

Labyrinthitis is an infection of the labyrinth, which may occur as a complication of acute or chronic otitis media. Infection results from an erosion of the bony capsule, allowing organisms to invade the inner ear. Labyrinthitis often results from the growth of a cholesteatoma (benign overgrowth of squamous cell epithelium) from the middle ear into the semicircular canal. It may follow middle ear or inner ear surgery when infection is present. Labyrinthitis is often viral in origin and may occur with an upper respiratory infection or mononucleosis.

Manifestations include hearing loss, tinnitus, nystagmus to the affected side, and vertigo with nausea and vomiting. Meningitis (infection of the brain covering) is a common complication of labyrinthitis.

Labyrinthitis is usually a self-limiting condition. If it does not resolve with supportive therapy, management includes systemic antibiotics. Teach the patient to complete the antibiotic therapy as prescribed and to not stop taking the drug when manifestations are no longer present. Stopping the drug early can lead to infection recurrence and antibiotic resistance. Advise patients to stay in bed in a darkened room until manifestations are reduced. Antiemetics and antivertiginous drugs, such as dimenhydrinate (Dramamine, Gravol ✿) and meclizine (Antivert, Bonamine ✿), relieve symptoms.

The patient also needs psychosocial support. Hearing loss on the affected side may be permanent, although vertigo subsides as the inflammation resolves. Persistent balance problems may improve with gait training and physical therapy.

? NCLEX EXAMINATION CHALLENGE

Safe and Effective Care Environment

Which problem is most important for the nurse to prevent with a client who has any degree of dizziness from an ear disorder?
A. Pain
B. Falls
C. Dehydration
D. Hearing loss

MÉNIÈRE'S DISEASE

Pathophysiology

Ménière's disease has three features: tinnitus, one-sided sensorineural hearing loss, and vertigo, occurring in attacks that can last for several days. (Some patients have continuous manifestations of varying intensity rather than intermittent attacks.) Patients are almost totally incapacitated during an attack, and full recovery often takes several days. The pathology of Ménière's disease is an excess of endolymphatic fluid that distorts the entire inner-canal system. This distortion decreases hearing by dilating the cochlear duct, causes vertigo because of damage to the vestibular system, and stimulates tinnitus (Peate, 2009). At first, hearing loss is reversible, but repeated damage to the cochlea from increased fluid pressure leads to permanent hearing loss.

The exact cause of Ménière's disease is unknown, but it often occurs with infections, allergic reactions, and fluid imbalances. Long-term stress may also have a role in the disease.

PATIENT-CENTERED COLLABORATIVE CARE

ASSESSMENT

Ménière's disease usually first occurs in people between the ages of 20 and 50 years. The disease is more common in men and in white people. Severe, debilitating attacks alternate with symptom-free periods. Patients often have certain manifestations before an attack of vertigo, such as headaches, increasing tinnitus, and a feeling of fullness in the affected ear.

Patients describe the tinnitus as a continuous, low-pitched roar or a humming sound, which worsens just before and during an attack. Hearing loss occurs first with the low-frequency tones but worsens to include all levels after repeated episodes. In the early stages of Ménière's disease, hearing is normal or nearly normal between episodes, but permanent hearing loss develops as the attacks increase.

Patients describe the vertigo as periods of whirling, which might even cause them to fall. The vertigo is so intense that even while lying down, the patient often holds the bed or ground to keep from falling. Severe vertigo usually lasts 3 to 4 hours, but he or she may feel dizzy long after the attack. Nausea and vomiting are common. Other manifestations include rapid eye movements (nystagmus) and severe headaches.

INTERVENTIONS

Nonsurgical Management

Teach patients to move the head slowly to prevent worsening of the vertigo. Nutrition and lifestyle changes can reduce the amount of endolymphatic fluid. Encourage patients to stop smoking because of the blood vessel–constricting effects.

Nutrition therapy with a hydrops diet may stabilize body fluid levels to prevent excess endolymph accumulation. The basic structure of this diet involves:

- Distributing food and fluid intake evenly throughout the day and from day to day
- Avoiding foods or fluids that have a high salt content
- Drinking adequate amounts of fluids (low in sugar) daily
- Avoiding caffeine-containing fluids and foods
- Limiting alcohol intake to one glass of beer or wine each day
- Avoiding foods containing monosodium glutamate (MSG)

Coordinate with a dietitian for more detailed information about hydrops diet therapy for reduction of Ménière's manifestations.

Drug therapy may reduce the vertigo and vomiting and restore normal balance. Mild diuretics are prescribed to decrease endolymph volume, which reduces vertigo, hearing loss, tinnitus, and aural fullness. Nicotinic acid has been found to be useful because of its vasodilatory effect. Antihistamines such as diphenhydramine hydrochloride (Benadryl, Allerdryl ✦) and dimenhydrinate (Dramamine, Gravol ✦), and antivertiginous drugs such as meclizine (Antivert, Bonamine ✦), help reduce the severity of or stop an acute attack. Antiemetics such as chlorpromazine hydrochloride (Thorazine, Novo-Chlorpromazine ✦), droperidol (Inapsine), promethazine (Phenergan), and ondansetron (Zofran) help reduce the nausea and vomiting. Diazepam (Valium, Apo-Diazepam ✦) calms the patient; reduces vertigo, nausea, and vomiting; and allows the patient to rest quietly during an attack. Intratympanic therapy with gentamicin and steroids is another method for preventing manifestations; however, some or all hearing is lost in the ear receiving this drug combination.

Another nonsurgical treatment is the Meniett device, which applies low-pressure micropulses to the inner ear for 5 minutes three times daily. This action displaces inner ear fluid and relieves manifestations. Placement of a tympanostomy tube in the eardrum of the affected ear is needed to use this therapy. Long-term success in control of vertigo is over 80%. Although hearing loss is not improved, Meniett device usage does not adversely affect balance, as do most forms of surgical therapy for Ménière's disease.

Surgical Management

For years, surgical treatment of Ménière's disease was a last resort because the hearing in the affected ear was often lost with the more radical procedures. When medical therapy is ineffective and the patient's general function is decreased significantly, surgery may be performed. The choice of the surgical procedure depends on the degree of usable hearing, the severity of the spells, and the condition of the opposite ear.

The most radical procedure involves resection of the vestibular nerve or total removal of the labyrinth (labyrinthectomy), performed through the ear canal. The footplate of the stapes is moved aside, and the labyrinth is removed through the oval window.

Another procedure performed early in the course of the disease is endolymphatic decompression with drainage and a shunt (Lee & Pensak, 2008). The effectiveness of this procedure varies. The endolymphatic sac is drained, and a small tube is inserted to improve fluid drainage. Some patients report relief of vertigo with retention of their hearing. If an endolymphatic decompression has been performed, movement of the vestibular structures of the inner ear causes vertigo early after surgery. Reassure the patient that the vertigo is a temporary result of the surgical procedure, not the disease.

❓ NCLEX EXAMINATION CHALLENGE

Safe and Effective Care Environment

Which new symptom in a 68-year-old man taking diphenhydramine (Benadryl) for vertigo from Ménière's disease will the nurse report to the prescriber?
A. Decreased urination
B. Drowsiness
C. Dry mouth
D. Cough

ACOUSTIC NEUROMA

An acoustic neuroma is a benign tumor of cranial nerve VIII that often damages other structures as it grows. Depending on the size and exact location of the tumor, damage to hearing, facial movements, and sensation can occur (McCance et al., 2010). An acoustic neuroma can cause many neurologic manifestations as the tumor enlarges in the brain.

Manifestations begin with tinnitus and progress to gradual sensorineural hearing loss in most patients. Later, patients have constant mild to moderate vertigo. As the tumor enlarges, nearby cranial nerves are damaged.

Acoustic neuromas are diagnosed with computed tomography (CT) scanning and magnetic resonance imaging (MRI). Audiograms show sensorineural hearing loss. Cerebrospinal fluid assays show increased pressure and protein.

Surgical removal through a craniotomy is performed, and the remaining hearing is lost. Care is taken to preserve the function of the facial nerve (cranial nerve VII). Care after craniotomy is discussed in Chapter 47. Acoustic neuromas rarely recur after surgical removal.

HEARING LOSS

Pathophysiology

Hearing loss is a common handicap worldwide. It may be conductive, sensorineural, or a combination of the two (Fig. 51-7). Conductive hearing loss occurs when sound waves are blocked from contact with inner ear nerve fibers because of external ear or middle ear disorders. If the inner ear sensory nerve fibers that lead to the cerebral cortex are damaged, the hearing loss is *sensorineural*. Combined hearing loss is *mixed conductive-sensorineural.*

The differences in conductive and sensorineural hearing loss are listed in Table 51-2. Disorders that cause conductive hearing loss are often corrected with minimal or no permanent damage. Sensorineural hearing loss is often permanent, and measures must be taken to prevent further damage or to amplify sounds as a means to improve hearing.

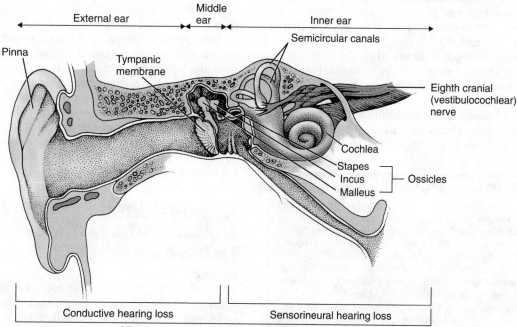

FIG. 51-7 Anatomy of hearing loss. Hearing loss can be divided into three types: (1) conductive (difficulty in the external or the middle ear); (2) sensorineural (difficulty in the inner ear or the acoustic nerve); and (3) mixed conductive-sensorineural (a combination of the two).

TABLE 51-2 DIFFERENTIAL FEATURES OF CONDUCTIVE AND SENSORINEURAL HEARING LOSS

CONDUCTIVE HEARING LOSS	SENSORINEURAL HEARING LOSS
Causes	
Cerumen	Prolonged exposure to noise
Foreign body	Presbycusis
Perforation of the tympanic membrane	Ototoxic substance
	Ménière's disease
Edema	Acoustic neuroma
Infection of the external ear or middle ear	Diabetes mellitus
	Labyrinthitis
Tumor	Infection
Otosclerosis	Myxedema
Assessment Findings	
Evidence of obstruction with otoscope	Normal appearance of external canal and tympanic membrane
Abnormality in tympanic membrane	Tinnitus common
	Occasional dizziness
Speaking softly	Speaking loudly
Hearing best in a noisy environment	Hearing poorly in loud environment
Rinne test: air conduction greater than bone conduction	Rinne test: air conduction less than bone conduction
Weber test: lateralization to affected ear	Weber test: lateralization to unaffected ear

Etiology and Genetic Risk

Conductive hearing loss can be caused by any inflammation or obstruction of the external or middle ear by cerumen or foreign objects. Changes in the eardrum such as bulging, retraction, and perforations may indicate damage to middle ear structures, which leads to conductive hearing loss. Tumors, scar tissue, and overgrowth of soft bony tissue (otosclerosis) on the ossicles from previous middle ear surgery also lead to conductive hearing loss.

Sensorineural hearing loss occurs when the inner ear or auditory nerve (cranial nerve VIII) is damaged. Prolonged exposure to loud noise can damage the hair cells of the cochlea. Many drugs are toxic to the inner ear structures, and their effects on hearing can be transient or permanent, dose related or non–dose related, and affect one or both ears. When ototoxic drugs (e.g., those listed in Table 50-1 in

GENETIC/GENOMIC CONSIDERATIONS

Some types of hearing loss in adults can have a genetic origin. Some syndromes in which a single gene mutation results in many abnormal manifestations also increase the risk for progressive hearing loss in adults. Two such syndromes are Usher's syndrome and Alport's syndrome (Nussbaum et al., 2007). Usher's syndrome, in addition to hearing loss, occurs with blindness as a result of retinitis pigmentosa. This syndrome has an autosomal recessive pattern of inheritance. Alport's syndrome, which causes abnormal kidney function in addition to hearing loss, has many forms and many patterns of inheritance. One type of adult-onset hearing loss that does not have any other physical problems is associated with a mutation in the *GJB2* gene on chromosome 1 (Online Mendelian Inheritance in Man [OMIM], 2010). This problem has an autosomal dominant pattern of inheritance.

Chapter 50) are given to patients with reduced kidney function, increased ototoxicity can result because drug elimination is slower. Older patients are especially at risk for ototoxicity because of reduced kidney function.

Presbycusis is a sensorineural hearing loss that occurs as a result of aging (Ko, 2010). It is caused by breakdown or atrophy of cochlear nerve cells, loss of elasticity of the basilar membrane, or a decreased blood supply to the inner ear. Deficiencies of vitamin B_{12} and folic acid may play a role in presbycusis. Other causes include atherosclerosis, hypertension, infections, fever, Ménière's disease, diabetes, and ear surgery. Each disorder accelerates degenerative changes of the cochlea (Touhy & Jett, 2010). Trauma to the ear also contributes to sensorineural hearing loss (Laubach, 2010).

Incidence/Prevalence

Because hearing loss may be gradual and affect only some aspects of hearing, many adults are unaware that their hearing is impaired. The actual incidence of hearing loss is not known, but hearing loss dramatically increases among people in their 70s and 80s (Pratt et al., 2009) (see the Evidence-Based Practice box on p. 1099).

Health Promotion and Maintenance

For most people, hearing is an important factor in social interactions and to gain knowledge. With special care to the ears, hearing can be preserved at maximum levels. Address barriers to the use of hearing protection, exposure to loud music, and other modifiable risk factors that lead to hearing loss (Stephenson, 2009). Encourage everyone to have simple hearing testing performed as part of their annual health assessment.

Teach everyone the danger in using foreign objects (e.g., bobby-pins, Q-tips, toothpicks, keys) to clean the ear canal. These objects can scrape the skin of the canal, push cerumen up against the eardrum, and even puncture the eardrum. Explain that nothing smaller than a person's own fingertip should be inserted into the canal. If cerumen buildup is a problem, teach the person to use an ear irrigation syringe and proper solutions to remove it. (Chart 50-3 in Chapter 50 describes techniques to remove cerumen safely.)

Teach all people about protecting their ears from loud noises by wearing protective ear devices, such as over-the-ear headsets or foam ear inserts, when exposed to persistent loud noises. Suggest the use of earplugs when engaging in water sports to prevent ear infections, as well as using an over-the-counter product such as Swim-Ear to assist with drying the ear after swimming.

PATIENT-CENTERED COLLABORATIVE CARE

ASSESSMENT

History

Ask patients how long they have noticed a difference in their hearing and whether the changes occurred suddenly or gradually. Age is an important factor, because some ear and hearing changes occur with advancing age. Chronic otitis media occurs more often in the older adult. Ask about occupational exposure to loud or continuous noises, as well as current or previous use of ototoxic drugs. Also ask about any

EVIDENCE-BASED PRACTICE

What Is the Incidence of Hearing Loss Among Older Adults?

Pratt, S.R., Kuller, L., Talbott, E.O., McHugh-Pemu, K., Buhari, A.M., & Xu, X. (2009). Prevalence of hearing loss in black and white elders: Results of the cardiovascular health study. *Journal of Speech, Language, and Hearing Research, 52*(4), 973-989.

Hearing loss is more common among older adults; however, the actual incidence and the personal characteristics more closely associated with hearing loss are not known. The purpose of this study was to determine the influence of age, gender, and race on both the incidence and severity of hearing loss. The subjects were 548 persons who were part of a cohort of participants in a large cardiovascular health cohort study sponsored by the National Heart, Lung, and Blood Institute of the National Institutes of Health; they represented a cross-section of the original 5201 members of the original cohort. Subjects ranged in age from 72 to 96 years and consisted of 48 black men, 74 black women, 179 white men, and 247 white women. Hearing was assessed after otoscopic examination determined no impediment to conduction through the ear canal existed. Hearing tests were performed by audiologists using pure-tone air-conduction testing measuring standard and extended high-frequency thresholds. In addition to descriptive statistics, multiple linear regression analyses were performed to examine relationships between hearing and variables of age, gender, race, smoking, and cardiovascular disease.

Age was the most significant contributor to hearing loss, with subjects in their 80s experiencing greater and more severe hearing loss than those in their 70s. Overall, men had more hearing loss than women and hearing loss was greater among whites than among blacks. A surprising outcome of the study was that neither smoking history nor cardiovascular disease had a negative effect on hearing.

Level of Evidence: 4
Although very large, the study was descriptive in nature without randomization of subject selection or assignment. The methods of statistical analysis were appropriate for the research questions posed.

Commentary: Implications for Practice and Research
The results of this study indicated that more than 50% of adults older than 80 years experienced significant hearing loss, especially men. Nurses must consider this when communicating with older adults, especially during assessment and teaching sessions when miscommunication could result in serious problems. Although nurses should not assume that all older adults have a hearing loss, it is important to use communication techniques that improve information transfer in all situations. These include:
- Facing the patient during any communication
- Ensuring that your mouth is visible to the patient when you speak
- Making the environment as quiet as possible (turning radios and televisions off or down, closing the door to the hall, moving to a treatment room or conference room if the noise in the room is too loud and cannot be managed)
- Speaking clearly and at a pace that is slightly slower (such as that you would use for public speaking)
- Asking the patient to repeat the main points of what has been said in his or her own words
- Observing the patient's face and body language for cues that communication is effective or ineffective

---

CHART 51-5   **FOCUSED ASSESSMENT**

The Patient with Suspected Hearing Loss

Assess whether the patient has any of these ear problems:
- Pain
- Feeling of fullness or congestion
- Dizziness or vertigo
- Tinnitus
- Difficulty understanding conversations, especially in a noisy room
- Difficulty hearing sounds
- The need to strain to hear
- The need to turn the head to favor one ear or the need to lean forward to hear

Assess visible ear structures, particularly the external canal and tympanic membrane:
- Position and size of the pinna
- Patency of the external canal; presence of cerumen or foreign bodies, edema, or inflammation
- Condition of the tympanic membrane: intact, edema, fluid, inflammation

Assess functional ability, including:
- Frequency of asking people to repeat statements
- Withdrawal from social interactions or large groups
- Shouting in conversation
- Failing to respond when not looking in the direction of the sound
- Answering questions incorrectly

---

ask about recent upper respiratory infection and allergies affecting the nose and sinuses.

Physical Assessment/Clinical Manifestations

Chart 51-5 lists focused assessment techniques for patients with suspected hearing loss. Hearing loss may be sudden or gradual and often affects both ears. The ability to hear high-frequency soft consonants—especially *s, sh, f, th,* and *ch* sounds—is lost first. Patients often state that they have no problem with hearing but cannot understand specific words. They might think that the speaker is mumbling. They often have continuous tinnitus in both ears. Vertigo may be present, depending on the extent of inner ear involvement.

Tuning fork tests help diagnose hearing loss (see Chapter 50). With the Weber test, the patient can usually hear sounds well in the ear with a conductive hearing loss because of bone conduction. With the Rinne test, the patient reports that sound transmitted by bone conduction is louder and more sustained than that transmitted by air conduction.

Otoscopic examination is performed to assess the external ear canal, the eardrum, and structures of the middle ear that can be seen through the eardrum (see Chapter 50). Findings from examination vary, depending on the cause of the hearing loss.

External ear canal obstruction can result in hearing loss. Inspect the canal, looking for:
- Whether the canal is open
- The amount and character of cerumen present
- The integrity of the skin lining the canal
- The presence of redness, exudates, lesions, or foreign objects

Middle ear infections can also reduce hearing. In infection or inflammation, the eardrum appears red, thickened, and bulging, with a loss of landmarks. Loss of eardrum mobility

---

history of external ear or middle ear infection and whether eardrum perforation occurred. Ask patients about any direct trauma to the ears. Because some types of hearing loss have a genetic basis, ask whether any family members are hearing impaired. When pain occurs with acute-onset hearing loss,

is seen with inspection through a pneumatic otoscope. Document the presence of scars or perforations on the eardrum.

Psychosocial Assessment

For people with a hearing loss, communication can become a struggle and they may isolate themselves because of the difficulty in talking and listening. Social isolation can lead to depression, fear, and despair. Be sensitive to emotional changes that may be related to reduced hearing and a decline in conversational skills. Encourage the patient and family to express their feelings and concerns about an actual or potential hearing loss.

Laboratory Assessment

No laboratory test diagnoses hearing loss. However, some laboratory findings can indicate problems that affect hearing.

White blood cell counts are elevated in the patient with acute or chronic otitis media. Microbial culture and antibiotic sensitivity tests can determine the causative organism and appropriate drug therapy when infection causes hearing loss.

The patient with hearing loss from peripheral neuropathy may have other systemic diseases, including human immune deficiency virus (HIV) disease or diabetes. Patients undergoing cancer chemotherapy or interferon therapy are at risk for neuropathic hearing loss.

Imaging Assessment

Imaging assessment can determine non-auditory problems affecting hearing ability. Skull x-rays are used to determine bony involvement in otitis media and the location of otosclerotic lesions, and CT and MRI are used to determine soft-tissue involvement and the presence and location of tumors.

Other Diagnostic Assessment

Audiometry can help determine the extent and type of hearing loss. An audiogram shows whether hearing loss is only conductive or whether it has a sensorineural component. This is important in determining possible causes of the hearing loss and in planning interventions.

ANALYSIS

The priority problems for the patient with any degree of hearing impairment are:

1. Difficulty hearing related to obstruction, infection, damage to the middle ear, or damage to the auditory nerve
2. Potential for reduced communication related to difficulty hearing

PLANNING AND IMPLEMENTATION

Increasing Hearing

Planning: Expected Outcomes. The patient with hearing impairment is expected to either have an increase in functional hearing or maintain existing hearing levels. Indicators include:

- No or minimal loss of high pitch tones
- No or minimal loss of ability to distinguish conversation from background environmental noise
- Turning toward sound
- Identifying discrete sounds

Interventions. Interventions are expected to identify the problem, halt the pathologic processes, and increase usable hearing. Nursing care priorities focus on teaching the patient about the use and care of an appropriate assistive device, providing support to the patient and family who are working to maintain or increase communication, and assisting patients to find local and Internet-based support services.

Nonsurgical Management. Interventions include early detection of hearing impairment, use of drug therapy and comfort measures, and use of assistive devices to amplify or augment the patient's usable hearing.

Early detection helps correct the problem causing the hearing loss. Assess for indications of hearing loss, as listed in Chart 51-5.

Drug therapy is focused on either correcting the underlying pathologic change or reducing the side effects of problems occurring with hearing loss. Topical antibiotics are given to patients with external otitis. Systemic antibiotics are needed when patients have other ear infections. Teach the patient receiving antibiotic therapy the importance of taking the drug or drugs exactly as prescribed and completing the entire course. Caution him or her to not stop the drug just because manifestations have improved. By treating the infection, antibiotics reduce local edema and improve hearing. When pain occurs with hearing disorders, analgesics are used, depending on the location and type of pain. Many ear disorders disturb equilibrium, causing vertigo and dizziness with nausea and vomiting. Antiemetic, antihistamine, antivertiginous, and benzodiazepine drugs can help correct nausea, vertigo, and dizziness.

Assistive devices are useful for patients with permanent, progressive hearing loss. Portable amplifiers can be used while watching television to avoid increasing the volume and disturbing others. Telephone amplifiers increase telephone volume, allowing the caller to speak in a normal voice. Flashing lights activated by the ringing telephone or a doorbell alert patients visually. In some cases, patients may have a specially trained dog to help them be aware of sounds (ringing telephones or doorbells, cries of other people, and potential dangers), in much the same way that a seeing-eye dog assists a blind person. Provide information about agencies that can assist the hearing-impaired person.

Small, portable audio amplifiers can assist in communicating with patients with hearing loss but who have chosen not to use a hearing aid. The use of audio amplifiers or allowing patients to use a stethoscope for listening helps you communicate with anyone who requires additional volume to hear speech.

A hearing aid is a miniature electronic amplifier that is usually used for patients with conductive hearing loss. Hearing aids are less effective for sensorineural hearing loss and may make hearing worse by amplifying background noise. The amplifier can be worn in one or both ears. Some hearing-impaired patients refuse to use hearing aids, believing that other people will think they are old. Most common hearing aids are small. Some are attached to a person's glasses and are visible to other people. Another type fits into the ear and is less noticeable. Newer devices fit completely in the canal with only a fine, clear filament visible. The cost of smaller hearing aids is greater than the cost of larger ones. Local agencies offer special classes for the hearing impaired that help the users benefit from this device.

Offer some special tips to help the patient adjust to the hearing aid. Hearing with a hearing aid is different from natural hearing. Teach the patient to start using the hearing aid slowly, at first wearing it only at home and only during part of the day. Listening to television and the radio and reading aloud can help the patient get used to new sounds. The tone or volume of the hearing aid can be adjusted. A difficult aspect of a hearing aid is the amplification of background noise. The patient must learn to concentrate and filter out background noises.

Teach the patient how to care for the hearing aid (Chart 51-6). Hearing aids are delicate devices that should be handled only by people who know how to care for them properly. The cost of the aids varies greatly but is a significant investment.

Cochlear implantation may help patients with sensorineural hearing loss. Although a superficial surgical procedure is needed to implant the device, the procedure does not enter the inner ear and thus is not considered a surgical correction for hearing impairment. A small computer converts sound waves into electronic impulses. Electrodes are placed near the internal ear, with the computer attached to the external ear. The electronic impulses then directly stimulate nerve fibers. Some patients have a 50% return of their hearing with this method (Bassim & Fayad, 2010).

Surgical Management. Many surgical interventions are available for patients with specific disorders leading to hearing loss.

Tympanoplasty. Tympanoplasty reconstructs the middle ear to improve conductive hearing loss. The procedures vary from simple reconstruction of the eardrum (myringoplasty) to replacement of the ossicles within the middle ear (ossiculoplasty). A type I tympanoplasty is used for a myringoplasty; a type II tympanoplasty is used in cases of greater damage, and it provides more extensive reconstruction (Fig. 51-8).

Preoperative Care. The patient requires specific instructions before surgery. Systemic antibiotics reduce the risk for infection. Before surgery, irrigate the ear with a solution of equal parts of vinegar and sterile water to restore normal ear pH. Teach the patient to follow other measures to decrease the risks for infection, such as avoiding people with upper respiratory infections, getting adequate rest, eating a balanced diet, and drinking adequate amounts of fluid.

Assure the patient that hearing loss immediately after surgery is normal because of canal packing and that hearing will improve when it is removed. Teach about deep breathing and coughing after surgery, but stress that forceful coughing increases middle ear pressure and must be avoided.

Operative Procedures. Surgery is performed only when the middle ear is free of infection. If an infection is present, the graft is more likely to become infected and not heal. Surgery

---

CHART 51-6 PATIENT AND FAMILY EDUCATION: PREPARING FOR SELF-MANAGEMENT

Hearing Aid Care

- Keep the hearing aid dry.
- Clean the ear mold with mild soap and water while avoiding excessive wetting.
- Clean debris from the hole in the middle of the part that goes into your ear with a toothpick.
- Turn off the hearing aid and remove the battery when not in use.
- Check and replace the battery frequently.
- Keep extra batteries on hand.
- Keep the hearing aid in a safe place.
- Avoid dropping the hearing aid or exposing it to temperature extremes.
- Adjust the volume to the lowest setting that allows you to hear, to prevent feedback squeaking.
- Avoid using hair spray, cosmetics, oils, or other hair and face products that might come into contact with the receiver.
- If the hearing aid does not work:
  - Change the battery.
  - Check the connection between the ear mold and the receiver.
  - Check the on/off switch.
  - Clean the sound hole.
  - Adjust the volume.
  - Take the hearing aid to an authorized service center for repair.

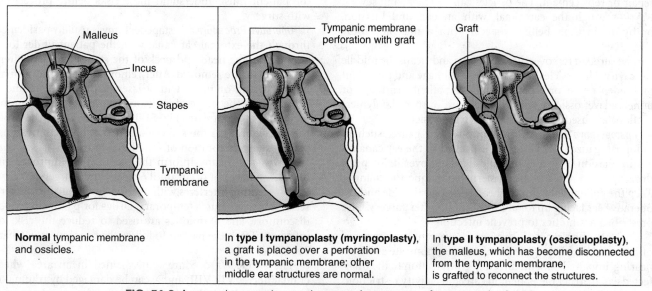

Normal tympanic membrane and ossicles.

In **type I tympanoplasty (myringoplasty)**, a graft is placed over a perforation in the tympanic membrane; other middle ear structures are normal.

In **type II tympanoplasty (ossiculoplasty)**, the malleus, which has become disconnected from the tympanic membrane, is grafted to reconnect the structures.

FIG. 51-8 A normal tympanic membrane and two types of tympanoplasties.

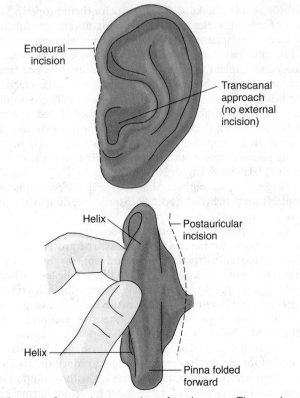

FIG. 51-9 Surgical approaches for the ear. The endaural approach is used when the external canal is too small to use for a transcanal approach. The postauricular approach is used for more extensive repair of the middle ear and inner ear structures.

of the eardrum and ossicles requires the use of a microscope and is a delicate procedure. Local anesthesia can be used, although general anesthesia is often used to prevent the patient from moving.

The surgeon can repair the eardrum with many materials, including muscle fascia, a skin graft, and venous tissue. If the ossicles are damaged, more extensive surgery is needed for repair or replacement. The ossicles can be reached in several ways—through the ear canal, with an endaural incision, or by an incision behind the ear with a mastoidectomy (Fig. 51-9).

The surgeon removes diseased tissue and cleans the middle ear cavity. The ossicles are assessed for damage and the extent of needed repair or replacement. The patient's cartilage or bone, cadaver ossicles, stainless steel wire, or special polymers (Teflon) are used to repair or replace the ossicles.

Postoperative Care. An antiseptic-soaked gauze, such as iodoform gauze (NU GAUZE), is packed in the ear canal. If a skin incision is used, a dressing is placed over it. Keep the dressing clean and dry, using sterile technique for changes. Keep the patient flat, with the head turned to the side and the operative ear facing up for at least 12 hours after surgery. Give prescribed antibiotics to prevent infection.

Patients often report hearing improvement after removal of the canal packing. Until that time, communicate as with a hearing-impaired patient, directing conversation to the unaffected ear. Instruct the patient in care and activity restrictions (see Chart 51-4).

Stapedectomy. A partial or complete stapedectomy with a prosthesis corrects some types of hearing loss. This procedure is most effective for patients with hearing loss related to otosclerosis. The average age for patients undergoing primary stapes surgery is increasing. Regardless of age, hearing usually improves after primary stapes surgery; however, some patients redevelop conductive hearing loss after surgery and revision surgery is needed.

Preoperative Care. To prevent infection, the patient must be free from external otitis at surgery. Teach the patient to follow measures that prevent middle ear or external ear infections (Chart 51-7).

Review with the patient the expected outcomes and possible complications of the surgery. Hearing is initially worse after a stapedectomy. The success rate of this procedure is high. However, there is always a risk for failure that might lead to total deafness on the affected side. Possible complications include vertigo, infection, and facial nerve damage, and the patient must understand these risks before proceeding with surgery.

Operative Procedures. A stapedectomy is usually performed through the external ear canal with the patient under local anesthesia. The head and neck of the stapes and, less often, the footplate are removed. After removal of the bone, a small hole is drilled or made with a laser in the footplate and a prosthesis in the shape of a piston is connected between the incus and the footplate (Fig. 51-10). Sounds cause the prosthesis to vibrate as the stapes did. After stapedectomy, most patients have restoration of functional hearing.

Postoperative Care. Inform the patient that improvement in hearing may not occur until 6 weeks after surgery. At first, the ear packing interferes with hearing. Swelling after surgery reduces hearing but is temporary. Drugs for pain help reduce discomfort, and antibiotics are used to reduce the risk for infection. Teach the patient to follow the procedures in Chart 51-4.

The surgical procedure is performed in an area where cranial nerves VII, VIII, and X can be damaged by trauma or by swelling after surgery. *Assess for facial nerve damage or*

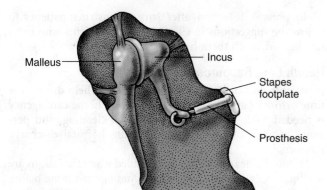

FIG. 51-10 Prosthesis used with stapedectomy. The stapes is removed, leaving the footplate. After a hole is made in the footplate, a metal or plastic prosthesis is connected to the incus and inserted through the hole to act as a vibration device, much as the stapes worked before the development of otosclerosis.

muscle weakness. Indications include an asymmetric appearance or drooping of features on the affected side of the face. Ask the patient about changes in facial perception of touch and in taste. Vertigo, nausea, and vomiting are common after surgery because of the nearness to inner ear structures.

Antivertiginous drugs, such as meclizine (Antivert, Bonamine ✦), and antiemetic drugs, such as droperidol (Inapsine), are given. Take care to prevent injury, especially during times of increased vertigo.

! NURSING SAFETY PRIORITY

Action Alert

Prevent injury by assisting the patient with ambulation during the first 1 to 2 days after stapedectomy. In addition, keep top bed siderails up, and remind the patient to move his or her head slowly when changing position to avoid vertigo.

Totally Implanted Devices. A newly approved device to treat bilateral moderate to severe sensorineural hearing loss is the Esteem system. It is designed to improve hearing to the same or better level as a high quality hearing aid but without any visible part. The device has three components that are totally implanted: a sound processor, a sensor, and a computer driver. Vibrations of the eardrum and ossicles are picked up by the sensor and converted to electric signals that are processed by the sound processor. Each processor is specifically programmed to the patient's specific hearing pathology. The processor filters out some background noise and amplifies the desired sound signal, which is then transferred to the driver. The driver then converts the processed signal into vibrations that are transmitted to the inner ear for sound perception (U.S. Food and Drug Administration, 2010). Patient criteria for this new device include:

- Bilateral stable sensorineural hearing loss determined by pure-tone audiometry
- Speech discrimination score of 40% or higher (see Chapter 50)
- Healthy tympanic membrane, eustachian tube, and ossicles of the middle ear

- Large enough space in the ear cavity to accommodate the parts of the device
- Minimum of 30 days of experience with an appropriately fitted hearing aid
- Absence of acute or chronic middle ear, inner ear, or mastoid infection
- Absence of Ménière's disease or recurring vertigo that requires treatment
- Absence of excessive sensitivity to silicone rubber, polyurethane, stainless steel, titanium, or gold

Possible complications of the device and the surgery required to implant it include:

- Temporary facial paralysis
- Changes in taste sensation
- Ongoing or new-onset tinnitus

Unlike more standard cochlear implants, the middle ear is entered and it is considered a surgical procedure. Care before and after surgery is similar to that required with stapedectomy. A distinct disadvantage is the cost of the implant and procedure, which exceeds $30,000 and is not currently covered by insurance.

Maximizing Communication

Planning: Expected Outcomes. The patient with hearing loss or impairment is expected to become proficient in hearing compensation behaviors to maintain or improve communication. Indicators include that the patient consistently demonstrates these behaviors:

- Uses hearing assistive devices
- Cares for external hearing assistive devices
- Uses sign language, lip-reading, or closed captioning (for television viewing)
- Accurately interprets messages
- Uses nonverbal language
- Exchanges messages accurately with others

Interventions. Nursing priorities focus on facilitating communication and reducing anxiety.

Use best practices that are listed in Chart 51-8 for communicating with a hearing-impaired patient. Do not shout at the patient because the sound may be projected at a higher frequency, making him or her less able to understand. The most obvious means of communicating is by the written word (if he or she is able to see, read, and write) or with pictures of familiar phrases and objects. Many television programs are now closed captioned (subtitled).

Assistive devices, described on p. 1100, can greatly increase communication for the patient with a hearing impairment.

Lip-reading and *sign language* can also increase communication. In lip-reading classes, patients are taught the special cues to look for when lip-reading and how to understand body language. However, the best lip-reader still misses more than half of what is being said. Because hearing is assisted by even minimal lip-reading, urge patients to wear their eyeglasses when talking with someone to see lip movement.

Sign languages, such as American Sign Language (ASL), combine speech with hand movements that signify letters, words, and phrases. These languages take time and effort to learn, and many people cannot learn them, just as many people cannot learn foreign languages.

Managing anxiety can increase the effectiveness of communication efforts. One source of anxiety is the possibility of permanent hearing loss. Provide accurate information about the likelihood of hearing returning. When the hearing impairment is likely to be permanent or become more profound, reassure patients that communication and social interaction can be maintained.

To reduce anxiety and prevent social isolation, assist patients to use resources and communication to make social contact satisfying. Ask about past or present diversional activities to identify the patient's most satisfying activities and social interactions, and determine the effort necessary to continue them. Activities can be altered to improve patient satisfaction. Someone accustomed to large gatherings might choose smaller groups instead. A quiet evening meal at home with friends might substitute for dinner in a noisy restaurant.

Community-Based Care

Lengthy hospitalization is rare for most patients with ear and hearing disorders. If surgical repair is needed and the procedure is completed without complications, the procedure may be completed in an ambulatory setting or the hospital stay is usually only 1 day.

Home Care Management

Patients who have persistent vertigo, either with the disorder or as a side effect of surgery, remain in danger of falling. Assess the home for potential hazards and to determine whether family members or significant others are available to assist with meal preparation and other ADLs. A nurse case manager can coordinate with the home care nurse to assist patients and their families in determining the best ways to maintain adequate self-care abilities, maintain a safe environment, decide about assistance needs, and provide needed care.

Teaching for Self-Management

Give patients written instructions about how to take drugs and when to return for follow-up care. If the patient cannot read, give these instructions to a family member who may assist with care. Teach patients how to instill eardrops (see Chart 51-1) and irrigate the ears (see Chart 51-2), and obtain a return demonstration.

To prevent infection after surgery, instruct patients to follow the suggestions in Chart 51-7. For patients who use a hearing aid, teach them how to use it effectively.

Health Care Resources

If patients do not have family or friends to help during the time before or after surgery, a referral to a home care agency is needed. Help with meal preparation, cleaning, and personal hygiene can be arranged by the hospital discharge planners.

Follow-up hearing tests are scheduled when the lesions are well healed, in about 6 to 8 weeks. Audiograms done before and after treatment are compared, and evaluation for further intervention to improve hearing begins. A complication of surgery is continued disability or complete loss of hearing in the affected ear. Surgery is performed on the ear with the greatest hearing loss. If the surgery does not improve hearing, patients must decide to either attempt surgical correction of the other ear or continue to use an amplification device. When the underlying disorder causing the hearing impairment is progressive, this decision is difficult. Support patients by listening to their concerns and giving additional information when needed.

Costs to the person with a hearing impairment can be extensive. Information and support can come from several organizations that publish informative articles to help patients reduce hearing loss (see Table 51-1). Many public and private agencies offer hearing evaluations, as well as supply information and counseling for patients with hearing disorders.

EVALUATION: OUTCOMES

Evaluate the care of the patient with hearing loss or hearing impairment based on the identified priority patient problems. The expected outcomes include that the patient will:

- Have at least partial improvement of hearing
- Have minimal anxiety
- Use appropriate hearing compensation behaviors
- Be able to communicate effectively with family, friends, co-workers, and health care professionals

Specific indicators for these outcomes are listed for each priority problem under the Planning and Implementation section (see earlier).

❓ DECISION-MAKING CHALLENGE

Patient-Centered Care

The patient is a 48-year-old man who is an advertising executive in a large agency. He has recently been diagnosed with bilateral sensorineural hearing loss. His other health issues include hypertension (which he manages with losartan [Cozaar]) and gastroesophageal reflux disease (which he manages with esomeprazole [Nexium]). He also has completed chemotherapy for Hodgkin's lymphoma within the past 6 months. He is surprised by his diagnosis because he works at keeping himself physically fit. He is distraught and very concerned that his co-workers will consider him "over the hill" with an "old man's" disease. He says that using a hearing aid is out of the question.

1. Is there any possibility that his hearing loss is related to current or past health problems? If so, which one(s) and why?
2. What additional personal and family information should you obtain from this patient?
3. How would you approach his concern about being considered old?
4. What options are available to improve his hearing?

NURSING CONCEPT REVIEW

What might you NOTICE if the patient is experiencing hearing problems?

- Person tilts one side of the head or leans forward to listen when another person speaks.
- Person watches the lips of a speaker closely.
- Person does not startle when a loud or unexpected sound occurs in the environment.
- Person frequently asks the speaker to repeat statements or questions.
- Person does not verbally interact with those around him or her.
- When a sentence is whispered to the person, he or she does not accurately repeat it back to the speaker.
- Person responds inappropriately to questions. For example, if asked "Is the room too cold?" the patient may respond "No, I don't feel old."

How should you RESPOND to a patient experiencing hearing problems?

- Reduce the background sound when speaking to the person (close the door to the hall, use a private area, turn off televisions and radios).
- Speak slowly, distinctly, and with a deeper tone.
- Face the patient while speaking.
- Ensure that all members of the health care team are aware of the patient's impairment and use an appropriate method to communicate with the patient.
- Determine whether the patient can communicate by sign language.
- Identify safety issues specific for the patient with a hearing impairment.
- Use a certified medical interpreter when taking a history from, explaining procedures to, or teaching the patient who has a hearing impairment.

GET READY FOR THE NCLEX® EXAMINATION!

KEY POINTS

Review these Key Points for each NCLEX Examination Client Needs Category.

Safe and Effective Care Environment

- Use Contact Precautions with any patient who has drainage from the ear canal.
- Avoid performing an otoscopic examination on a confused or uncooperative patient.
- Use the suggestions presented under History in the Hearing Loss section to enhance communication with a patient who has a hearing impairment.
- Protect the patient with vertigo or dizziness from injury, and assist with ambulation.

Health Promotion and Maintenance

- Teach patients the proper way to clean the pinna and external ear canal.
- Encourage all patients, even if they already have a hearing impairment, to use ear protection in a loud environment.
- Teach patients how to properly care for their hearing aids.
- Instruct patients to avoid closing off one naris when blowing the nose.
- Remind patients who engage in water sports and who are at risk for external otitis to wear earplugs when in the water.
- Teach proper ear hygiene for cleaning cerumen from the external canal.

- Urge everyone to avoid exposure to loud noises for extended periods without proper OSHA-approved ear protection.

Psychosocial Integrity

- Encourage the patient and family to express feelings and concerns about a change in hearing status.
- Refer patients newly diagnosed with hearing impairment or any chronic ear problem to appropriate local resources and support groups.
- Explain therapeutic procedures, restrictions, and follow-up care to the patient and family.
- Teach family members ways to communicate with a hearing-impaired patient with and without a hearing aid.

Physiological Integrity

- Ask the patient about hearing problems in any other members of the family, because many hearing problems have a genetic component.
- Check the hearing of any patient receiving an ototoxic drug (Table 50-1 in Chapter 50) for more than 5 days.
- Teach patients the proper techniques for self-instillation of eardrops and ear irrigation.
- Stress the importance of completing an antibiotic regimen for an ear infection.
- Follow the guidelines in Chart 51-2 when irrigating the ear canal.
- Avoid ear canal irrigation if the eardrum is perforated or if the canal contains vegetative matter.

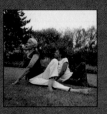

CHAPTER 52

Assessment of the Musculoskeletal System

Donna D. Ignatavicius

℮volve WEBSITE

http://evolve.elsevier.com/Iggy/

Animation: Classification of Joints: Condyloid Joint
Animation: Classification of Joints: Gliding Joint (Hand)
Animation: Classification of Joints: Hinge Joint
Answer Key for NCLEX Examination Challenges
Audio Glossary

Key Points
Review Questions for the NCLEX® Examination
Video Clip: Gait
Video Clip: Muscular Development and Strength

LEARNING OUTCOMES

Safe and Effective Care Environment

1. Collaborate with the physical and occupational therapists to perform a complete musculoskeletal assessment, including functional status, as needed.

Health Promotion and Maintenance

2. Explain how physiologic aging changes of the musculoskeletal system affect care of older adults.

Psychosocial Integrity

3. Assess the patient's and family's reaction to change in body image caused by a major musculoskeletal health problem.
4. Recognize the importance of support systems and effective strategies for the patient with unexpected altered body image caused by a musculoskeletal health problem.

Physiological Integrity

5. Recall the anatomy and physiology of the musculoskeletal system.
6. Conduct a musculoskeletal history using Gordon's Functional Health Patterns.
7. Assess patients for mobility, gait, motor skills, pain, and the use of assistive devices.
8. Interpret assessment findings in a patient with a musculoskeletal health problem.
9. Assess patients regarding iodine allergy before imaging assessments.
10. Explain the use of laboratory testing for a patient with a musculoskeletal health problem.
11. Develop a teaching plan to educate the patient and family about diagnostic procedures.

The musculoskeletal system is the second largest body system. It includes the bones, joints, and skeletal muscles, as well as the supporting structures needed to move them. *Mobility* (movement) is a basic human need that is essential for performing ADLs. When a patient cannot move to perform ADLs or other daily routines, self-esteem and a sense of self-worth can be diminished.

Disease, surgery, and trauma can affect one or more parts of the musculoskeletal system, often leading to decreased mobility. When mobility is impaired for a long time, other body systems can be affected. For example, prolonged immobility can lead to skin breakdown, constipation, and thrombus formation. If nerves are damaged by trauma or disease, patients may also have problems with *sensation*.

ANATOMY AND PHYSIOLOGY REVIEW

Skeletal System

The skeletal system consists of 206 bones and multiple joints. The growth and development of these structures occur during childhood and adolescence and are not discussed in this text. Common physical skeletal differences among ethnic groups are listed in Table 52-1.

Bones

Types and Structure. Bone can be classified in two ways—by shape and by structure. Long bones, such as the femur, are cylindric with rounded ends and often bear weight. Short bones, such as the phalanges, are small and bear little or no weight. Flat bones, such as the scapula, protect vital organs and often contain blood-forming cells. Bones that have unique shapes are known as irregular bones. The carpal bones in the wrist and the small bones in the inner ear are examples of irregular bones. The sesamoid bone is the least common type and develops within a tendon; the patella is a typical example.

The second way bone is classified is by *structure* or composition. As shown in Fig. 52-1, the outer layer of bone, or cortex, is composed of dense, compact bone tissue. The inner layer, in the medulla, contains spongy, cancellous tissue. Almost every bone has both tissue types but in varying quantities. The long bone typically has a shaft, or diaphysis, and two knoblike ends, or epiphyses.

The structural unit of the cortical compact bone is the haversian system, which is detailed in Fig. 52-1. The haversian system is a complex canal network containing microscopic blood vessels that supply nutrients and oxygen to bone, as well as lacunae, which are small cavities that house osteocytes (bone cells). The canals run vertically within the hard cortical bone tissue.

The softer cancellous tissue contains large spaces, or trabeculae, which are filled with red and yellow marrow. Hematopoiesis (production of blood cells) occurs in the red marrow. The yellow marrow contains fat cells, which can be dislodged and enter the bloodstream to cause fat embolism syndrome (FES), a life-threatening complication. Volkmann's canals connect bone marrow vessels with the haversian system and periosteum, the outermost covering of the bone. In the deepest layer of the periosteum are osteogenic cells, which later differentiate into osteoblasts (bone-forming cells) and osteoclasts (bone-destroying cells).

Bone also contains a matrix, or *osteoid*, consisting chiefly of collagen, mucopolysaccharides, and lipids. Deposits of inorganic calcium salts (carbonate and phosphate) in the matrix provide the hardness of bone.

TABLE 52-1	MUSCULOSKELETAL DIFFERENCES IN SELECTED GROUPS
GROUP	**MUSCULOSKELETAL DIFFERENCES**
African Americans	Greater bone density than Europeans, Asians, and Hispanics. Accounts for decreased incidence of osteoporosis.
Amish	Greater incidence of dwarfism than in other populations.
Chinese Americans	Bones are shorter and smaller with less bone density. Increased incidence of osteoporosis.
Egyptian Americans	Shorter in stature than Euro-Americans and African Americans.
Filipino/Vietnamese	Short in stature; adult height about 5 feet.
Irish Americans	Taller and broader than other Euro-Americans. Less bone density than African Americans.
Navajo American Indians	Taller and thinner than other American Indians.

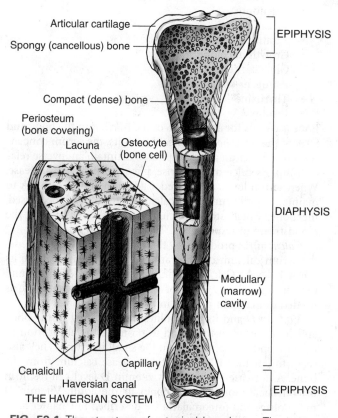

FIG. 52-1 The structure of a typical long bone. The cortex, or outer layer, is composed of dense, compact tissue. The microscopic structure of this compact cortical tissue is the haversian system.

Bone is a very vascular tissue. Its estimated total blood flow is between 200 and 400 mL/min. Each bone has a main nutrient artery, which enters near the middle of the shaft and branches into ascending and descending vessels. These vessels supply the cortex, the marrow, and the haversian system. Very few nerve fibers are connected to bone. Sympathetic nerve fibers control dilation of blood vessels. Sensory nerve fibers transmit pain signals experienced by patients who have primary lesions of the bone, like bone tumors.

Function. The skeletal system:

- Provides a framework for the body and allows the body to be weight bearing, or upright
- Supports the surrounding tissues (e.g., muscle and tendons)
- Assists in movement through muscle attachment and joint formation
- Protects vital organs, such as the heart and lungs
- Manufactures blood cells in red bone marrow
- Provides storage for mineral salts (e.g., calcium and phosphorus)

After puberty, bone reaches its maturity and maximum growth. Bone is a dynamic tissue. It undergoes a continuous process of formation and resorption, or destruction, at equal rates until the age of 35 years. In later years, bone resorption increases, decreasing bone mass and predisposing patients to injury, especially older women.

Numerous minerals and hormones affect bone growth and metabolism, including:

- Calcium
- Phosphorus
- Calcitonin
- Vitamin D
- Parathyroid hormone (PTH)
- Growth hormone
- Glucocorticoids
- Estrogens and androgens
- Thyroxine
- Insulin

Bone accounts for about 99% of the *calcium* in the body and 90% of the *phosphorus.* In healthy adults, the serum concentrations of calcium and phosphorus maintain an inverse relationship. As calcium levels rise, phosphorus levels decrease. When serum levels are altered, calcitonin and PTH work to maintain equilibrium. If the calcium in the blood is decreased, the bone, which stores calcium, releases calcium into the bloodstream in response to PTH stimulation.

Calcitonin is produced by the thyroid gland and *decreases* the serum calcium concentration if it is increased above its normal level. Calcitonin inhibits bone resorption and increases renal excretion of calcium and phosphorus as needed to maintain balance in the body.

Vitamin D and its metabolites are produced in the body and transported in the blood to promote the absorption of calcium and phosphorus from the small intestine. They also seem to enhance PTH activity to release calcium from the bone. A decrease in the body's vitamin D level can result in osteomalacia (softening of bone) in the adult. Vitamin D metabolism and osteomalacia are described in Chapter 53.

When serum calcium levels are lowered, *parathyroid hormone* (PTH, or parathormone) secretion increases and stimulates bone to promote osteoclastic activity and *release* calcium to the blood. PTH reduces the renal excretion of calcium and facilitates its absorption from the intestine. If serum calcium levels increase, PTH secretion diminishes to preserve the bone calcium supply. This process is an example of the feedback loop system of the endocrine system.

Growth hormone secreted by the anterior lobe of the pituitary gland is responsible for increasing bone length and determining the amount of bone matrix formed before puberty. During childhood, an increased secretion results in gigantism and a decreased secretion results in dwarfism. In the adult, an increase causes acromegaly, which is characterized by bone and soft-tissue deformities (see Chapter 65).

Adrenal glucocorticoids regulate protein metabolism, either increasing or decreasing catabolism to reduce or intensify the organic matrix of bone. They also aid in regulating intestinal calcium and phosphorus absorption.

Estrogens stimulate osteoblastic (bone-building) activity and inhibit PTH. When estrogen levels decline at menopause, women are susceptible to low serum calcium levels with increased bone loss (osteoporosis). *Androgens,* such as testosterone in men, promote anabolism (body tissue building) and increase bone mass.

Thyroxine is one of the principal hormones secreted by the thyroid gland. Its primary function is to increase the rate of protein synthesis in all types of tissue, including bone. *Insulin* works together with growth hormone to build and maintain healthy bone tissue.

Joints

A joint is a space in which two or more bones come together. This is also referred to as *articulation* of the joint. The major function of a joint is to provide movement and flexibility in the body.

There are three types of joints in the body:

- Synarthrodial, or completely immovable, joints (e.g., in the cranium)
- Amphiarthrodial, or slightly movable, joints (e.g., in the pelvis)
- Diarthrodial (synovial), or freely movable, joints (e.g., the elbow and knee)

Although any of these joints can be affected by disease or injury, the synovial joints are most commonly involved.

The diarthrodial, or synovial, joint is the most common type of joint in the body. Synovial joints are the only type lined with synovium, a membrane that secretes synovial fluid for lubrication and shock absorption. As shown in Fig. 52-2, the synovium lines the internal portion of the joint capsule but does not normally extend onto the surface of the cartilage at the spongy bone ends. Articular cartilage consists of a collagen fiber matrix impregnated with a complex ground substance. Patients with inflammatory types of arthritis often have synovitis (synovial inflammation) and breakdown of the cartilage. Bursae, small sacs lined with synovial membrane, are located at joints and bony prominences to prevent friction between bone and structures adjacent to bone. These structures can also become inflamed, causing bursitis.

Synovial joints are described by their anatomic structures. *Ball-and-socket* joints (shoulder, hip) permit movement in any direction. *Hinge* joints (elbow) allow motion in one plane—flexion and extension. The knee is often classified as a hinge joint, but it rotates slightly, as well as flexes and extends. It is best described as a *condylar* type of synovial

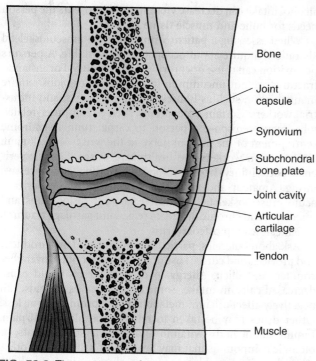

FIG. 52-2 The structure of a synovial joint. Synovium lines the joint capsule but does not extend into the articular cartilage.

joint. The gliding movement of the wrist is characteristic of the *biaxial* joint. *Pivot* joints permit rotation only, as in the radioulnar area.

Muscular System

There are three types of muscle in the body: smooth muscle, cardiac muscle, and skeletal muscle. Smooth, or non-striated, involuntary muscle is responsible for contractions of organs and blood vessels and is controlled by the autonomic nervous system. Cardiac muscle, or striated, involuntary muscle, is also controlled by the autonomic nervous system. The smooth and cardiac muscles are discussed with the body systems to which they belong in the assessment chapters.

In contrast to smooth and cardiac muscle, skeletal muscle is striated, voluntary muscle controlled by the central and peripheral nervous systems. The junction of a peripheral motor nerve and the muscle cells that it supplies is sometimes referred to as a motor end plate. Muscle fibers are held in place by connective tissue in bundles, or fasciculi. The entire muscle is surrounded by dense fibrous tissue, or fascia, which contains the muscle's blood, lymph, and nerve supply.

The main function of skeletal muscle is *movement* of the body and its parts. When bones, joints, and supporting structures are adversely affected by injury or disease, the adjacent muscle tissue is often involved, limiting mobility. During the aging process, muscle fibers decrease in size and number, even in well-conditioned adults. Atrophy results when muscles are not regularly exercised and they deteriorate from disuse.

Supporting structures for the muscular system are very susceptible to injury. They include tendons (bands of tough, fibrous tissue that attach muscles to bones) and ligaments, which attach bones to other bones at joints.

Changes in the Musculoskeletal System Related to Aging

PHYSIOLOGIC CHANGE	NURSING INTERVENTIONS	RATIONALES
Decreased bone density	Teach safety tips to prevent falls.	Porous bones are more likely to fracture.
	Reinforce need to exercise, especially weight-bearing exercise.	Exercise slows bone loss.
Increased bone prominence	Prevent pressure on bone prominences.	There is less soft tissue to prevent skin breakdown.
Kyphotic posture: widened gait, shift in the center of gravity	Teach proper body mechanics; instruct the patient to sit in supportive chairs with arms.	Correction of posture problems prevents further deformity; the patient should have support for bony structures.
Cartilage degeneration	Provide moist heat, such as a shower or warm, moist compresses.	Moist heat increases blood flow to the area.
Decreased range of motion (ROM)	Assess the patient's ability to perform ADLs and mobility.	The patient may need assistance with self-care skills.
Muscle atrophy, decreased strength	Teach isometric exercises.	Exercises increase muscle strength.
Slowed movement	Do not rush the patient; be patient.	The patient may become frustrated if hurried.

MUSCULOSKELETAL CHANGES ASSOCIATED WITH AGING

Osteopenia, or decreased bone density (bone loss), occurs as one ages. Many older adults, especially white, thin women, have severe osteopenia, a disease called *osteoporosis*. This condition causes postural and gait changes and predisposes the person to fractures. Chapter 53 discusses this health problem in detail.

Synovial joint cartilage can become less elastic and compressible as a person ages. As a result of these cartilage changes and continued use of joints, the joint cartilage becomes damaged, leading to osteoarthritis (OA). Genetic defects in cartilage may also contribute to joint disease. The most common joints affected are the weight-bearing joints of the hip, knee, and cervical and lumbar spine, but joints in the shoulder and upper extremity, feet, and hands can be affected. Refer to Chapter 20 for a complete discussion of OA.

As one ages, muscle tissue atrophies. Increased activity and exercise can slow the progression of atrophy and restore muscle strength. Musculoskeletal changes cause decreased coordination, loss of muscle strength, gait changes, and a risk for falls with injury. (See Chapter 3 for discussion on fall prevention.) Chart 52-1 lists the major anatomic and physiologic changes and implications for nursing care.

Based on Gordon, M. (2011). *Manual of nursing diagnosis* (12th ed.). New York: Jones & Bartlett.

CHART 52-2   MUSCULOSKELETAL ASSESSMENT

Using Gordon's Functional Health Patterns

Activity-Exercise Pattern
- Do you have sufficient energy for desired/required activities?
- What is your exercise pattern? Type of exercise? Regularity?
- What spare time (leisure) activities do you engage in?
- What is your perceived ability for (code for level according to key below):

Feeding?	Level 0: Full self-care
Bathing?	Level I: Requires use of equipment or
Toileting?	device
Bed mobility?	Level II: Requires assistance of or
Dressing?	supervision by another person
Grooming?	Level III: Requires assistance of or
General mobility?	supervision by another person and
Cooking?	equipment or device
Home maintenance?	Level IV: Is dependent and does not
Shopping?	participate

Cognitive-Perceptual Pattern
- Do you experience any discomfort?
- Do you have pain? If so, how do you manage it?
- What is the easiest way for you to learn things?
- Do you have any difficulty learning?

ASSESSMENT METHODS

Patient History

In the assessment of a patient with an actual or potential musculoskeletal problem, a detailed and accurate history is helpful in identifying priority problems and nursing interventions (Chart 52-2). The history reveals information about the patient that can direct the physical assessment.

Accidents, illnesses, lifestyle, and drugs may contribute to a patient's current problem. Young men are at the greatest risk for trauma related to motor vehicle crashes. Older adults are at the greatest risk for falls that result in fractures and soft-tissue injury. When taking a personal health history, question the patient about any traumatic injuries and sports activities, no matter when they occurred. An injury to the lumbar spine 30 years ago may have caused a patient's current low back pain. A motor vehicle crash or sports injury can cause osteoarthritis years after the event.

Previous or current illness or disease may affect musculoskeletal status. For example, a patient with diabetes who is treated for a foot ulcer is at high risk for acute or chronic osteomyelitis (bone infection). In addition, diabetes slows the healing process. Ask the patient about any previous hospitalizations and illnesses or complications. Inquire about his or her ability to perform ADLs independently or if assistive/adaptive devices are used.

Current lifestyle also contributes to musculoskeletal health. Weight-bearing activities such as walking can reduce risk factors for osteoporosis and maintain muscle strength. High-impact sports, such as excessive jogging or running, can cause musculoskeletal injury to soft tissues and bone. Tobacco use slows the healing of musculoskeletal injuries. Excessive alcohol intake can decrease vitamins and nutrients the person needs for bone and muscle tissue growth.

When assessing a patient with a possible musculoskeletal alteration, inquire about occupation or work life. A person's occupation can cause or contribute to an injury. For instance, fractures are not uncommon in patients whose jobs require manual labor, such as housekeepers, mechanics, and industrial workers. Certain occupations, such as computer-related jobs, may predispose a person to carpal tunnel syndrome (entrapment of the median nerve in the wrist) or neck pain. Construction workers and health care workers may experience back injury from prolonged standing and excessive lifting. Amateur and professional athletes often experience acute musculoskeletal injuries (e.g., joint dislocations and fractures) and chronic disorders (e.g., joint cartilage trauma), which can lead to osteoarthritis.

Ask about allergies, particularly allergy to dairy products, and previous and current use of drugs—prescribed, over-the-counter, and illicit. Allergy to dairy products could cause decreased calcium intake. Some drugs, such as steroids, can negatively affect calcium metabolism and promote bone loss. Other drugs may be taken to relieve musculoskeletal pain. Inquire about herbs, vitamin and mineral supplements, or biologic compounds that may be used for arthritis and other musculoskeletal problems, such as glucosamine and chondroitin. Complementary and alternative therapies are commonly used by patients with various types of arthritis and arthralgias (joint aching).

Nutrition History

A brief review of the patient's nutrition history helps determine any risks for inadequate nutrient intake. For example, most people, especially women, do not get enough calcium in their diet. Determine if the patient has had a significant weight gain or loss.

Ask the patient to recall a typical day of food intake to help identify deficiencies and excesses in the diet. Lactose intolerance is a common problem that can cause inadequate calcium intake. People who cannot afford to buy food are especially at risk for undernutrition. Some older adults and others are not financially able to buy the proper foods for adequate nutrition.

Inadequate protein or insufficient vitamin C or D in the diet slows bone and tissue healing. Obesity places excess stress and strain on bones and joints, with resulting fractures and trauma to joint cartilage. In addition, obesity inhibits mobility in patients with musculoskeletal problems, which predisposes them to complications such as respiratory and circulatory problems. People with eating disorders such as anorexia nervosa and bulimia nervosa are also at risk for osteoporosis related to decreased intake of calcium and vitamin D.

Family History and Genetic Risk

Obtaining a family history assists in identifying disorders that have a familial or genetic tendency. Osteoporosis (age-related bone loss) and gout, for instance, often occur in several generations of a family. Osteogenic sarcoma, a type of bone cancer, may be genetically influenced by *Tp53* gene mutation (Nussbaum et al., 2007). Positive family history of these types of disorders can increase risks to the patient. Chapters 20 and

53 provide a more complete description of musculoskeletal problems that have strong genetic links.

Current Health Problems

The most common reports of persons with a musculoskeletal problem are pain and weakness, either of which can impair mobility. Collect data pertinent to the patient's presenting health problem as follows:

- Date and time of onset
- Factors that cause or exacerbate (worsen) the problem
- Course of the problem (e.g., intermittent or continuous)
- Clinical manifestations (as expressed by the patient) and the pattern of their occurrence
- Measures that improve clinical manifestations (e.g., heat, ice)

Assessment of pain can present many challenges. Pain can be related to bone, muscle, or joint problems. *Pain* may be described as acute or chronic, depending on the onset and duration. Pain with movement could indicate a fracture and/or muscle or joint injury. Assess the intensity of pain by using a pain scale and asking the patient to rate the level of pain he or she is experiencing. Quality of pain may be described as dull, burning, aching, or stabbing. Determine the location of pain and areas to which the pain may radiate. With any pain assessment, it is always best if the patient describes the pain in his or her own words and points to its location, if possible.

Weakness may be related to individual muscles or muscle groups. Determine if weakness occurs in proximal or distal muscles or muscle groups. Proximal weakness may indicate myopathy (a problem in muscle tissue), whereas distal weakness may indicate neuropathy (a problem in nerve tissue). Muscle weakness in the lower extremities may increase the risk for falls and injury. Weakness in the upper extremities may interfere with ADLs.

Assessment of the Skeletal System

Although bones, joints, and muscles are usually assessed simultaneously in a head-to-toe approach, each subsystem is described separately for emphasis and understanding. For physical assessment of the musculoskeletal system, use inspection, palpation, and range of motion (ROM). A general assessment is described in this chapter. More specific assessment techniques are discussed in the musculoskeletal problem chapters in this unit.

General Inspection

Observe the patient's posture, gait, and general mobility for gross deformities and impairment. Note unusual findings, and coordinate with the physical or occupational therapist for an in-depth physical assessment.

Posture and Gait. Posture includes the person's body build and alignment when standing and walking. Assess the curvature of the spine and the length, shape, and symmetry of extremities. Fig. 52-3 illustrates several common spinal deformities. Inspect muscle mass for size and symmetry.

Most patients with musculoskeletal problems eventually have a problem with *gait*. The nurse or therapist evaluates the patient's balance, steadiness, and ease and length of stride. Any limp or other asymmetric leg movement or deformity is

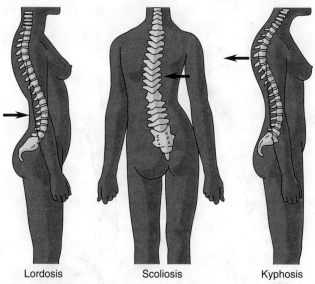

Lordosis   Scoliosis   Kyphosis

FIG. 52-3 Common spinal deformities.

noted. An abnormality in the stance phase of gait is called an antalgic gait. When part of one leg is painful, the patient shortens the stance phase on the affected side. An abnormality in the swing phase is called a lurch. This abnormal gait occurs when the muscles in the buttocks and/or legs are too weak to allow the person to change weight from one foot to the other. In this case, the shoulders are moved either side-to-side or front-to-back for help in shifting the weight from one leg to the other. Some patients, such as those with chronic hip pain and muscle atrophy from arthritic disorders, have a combination of an antalgic gait and lurch.

Mobility and Functional Assessment. In collaboration with the physical or occupational therapist, assess the patient's need for ambulatory devices, such as canes and walkers, during transfer from bed to chair and while walking and climbing stairs. Observe his or her ability to perform ADLs, such as dressing and bathing (see Chart 52-2). Pain and deformity may limit physical mobility and function. Coordinate with the physical and occupational therapists to assess the patient's functional status. A complete discussion of functional assessment is found in Chapter 8.

Assess major bones, joints, and muscles by inspection, palpation, and determination of ROM. Pay special attention to areas that are affected or may be affected, according to the patient's history or current problem.

A goniometer is a tool that may be used by rehabilitation therapists or nurses to provide an exact measurement of flexion and extension or joint ROM. Active range of motion (AROM) can be evaluated by asking the patient to move each joint through the ROM himself or herself. If the patient cannot actively move a joint through range of motion, ask him or her to relax the muscles in the extremity. Hold the part with one hand above and one hand below the joint to be evaluated and allow passive range of motion (PROM) to evaluate joint mobility. Movements shown in Fig. 52-4 may be used to evaluate active and passive ROM. Circumduction is a movement that can also be evaluated in the shoulder by having the patient move the arm in circles from the shoulder joint. As long as the patient can function to meet personal

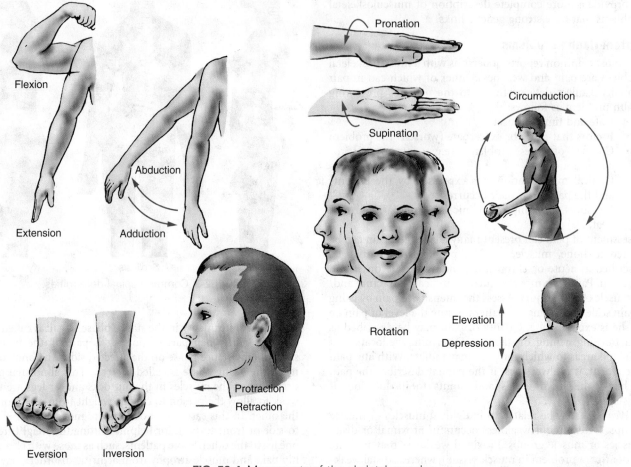

FIG. 52-4 Movements of the skeletal muscles.

needs, a limitation in ROM may not be significant. For each anatomic location, observe the skin for color, elasticity, and lesions that may relate to musculoskeletal dysfunction. For instance, redness or warmth may indicate an inflammatory process and/or pressure injury to skin.

❓ NCLEX EXAMINATION CHALLENGE
Health Promotion and Maintenance

A nurse is performing a musculoskeletal assessment on an older adult. What physiologic changes of aging will the nurse expect? **Select all that apply.**
A. Scoliosis
B. Muscle atrophy
C. Slowed movement
D. Rheumatoid arthritis
E. Antalgic gait

Specific Assessments

If the patient has pain or weakness in the *face* or *neck*, inspect and palpate this area for tenderness and masses. Ask the patient to open his or her mouth while palpating the temporomandibular joints (TMJs). Common abnormal findings are tenderness or pain, crepitus (a grating sound), and a spongy swelling caused by excess synovium and fluid.

Inspect and palpate each vertebra of the spine in the neck. Proceed cautiously and gently if pain is present. Clinical findings may include malalignment; tenderness; or inability to flex, extend, and rotate the neck as expected. Muscle and nerve pain often accompany neck pain if spinal nerves are involved.

The thoracic *spine*, lumbar spine, and sacral spine are evaluated in the same manner as the neck. Spinal alignment problems are common (see Fig. 52-3). Place both hands over the posterior iliac crests with the thumbs over the lumbosacral area. Apply pressure with the thumbs along the lumbosacral spine to elicit tenderness. Many patients do not have discomfort until the area is palpated. Lordosis is a common finding in adults who have abdominal obesity. During screening for scoliosis, ask the patient to flex forward from the hips and inspect for a lateral curve in the spine.

If the extremities are affected by a musculoskeletal problem, assess arms or legs at the same time for side-to-side comparisons. For example, inspect and palpate both shoulders for size, swelling, deformity, poor alignment, tenderness or pain, and mobility. A shoulder injury may prevent the patient from combing his or her hair with the affected arm, but severe arthritis may inhibit movement in both arms. Assess the elbows and wrists in a similar way.

Because the hand has multiple joints in a single digit, assessment of hand function is perhaps the most critical part of the examination. If the hands are affected, inspect and palpate the metacarpophalangeal (MCP), proximal interphalangeal (PIP), and distal interphalangeal (DIP) joints. The

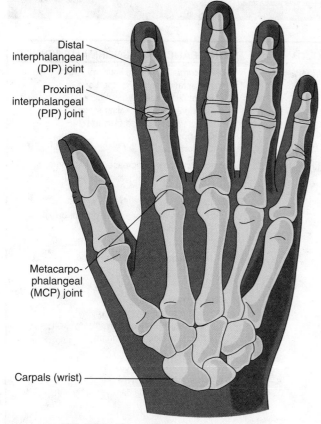

Distal
interphalangeal
(DIP) joint

Proximal
interphalangeal
(PIP) joint

Metacarpo-
phalangeal
(MCP) joint

Carpals (wrist)

FIG. 52-5 The small joints of the hand.

TABLE 52-2	LOVETT'S SCALE FOR GRADING MUSCLE STRENGTH
RATING	**DESCRIPTION**
5	Normal: ROM unimpaired against gravity with full resistance
4	Good: can complete ROM against gravity with some resistance
3	Fair: can complete ROM against gravity
2	Poor: can complete ROM with gravity eliminated
1	Trace: no joint motion and slight evidence of muscle contractility
0	Zero: no evidence of muscle contractility

ROM, Range of motion.

NURSING SAFETY PRIORITY

Action Alert

Perform a complete neurovascular assessment (also called a "circ" check), which includes *palpation of pulses in the extremities below the level of injury and assessment of sensation, movement, color, temperature, and pain in the injured part.* If pulses are not palpable, use a Doppler to find pulses in the extremities. See Chart 54-3 in Chapter 54 for more details about neurovascular assessment.

---

same digits are compared on the right and left hands (Fig. 52-5). Determine the range of motion (ROM) for each joint by observing active movement. If movement is not possible, evaluate passive motion. For a quick and easy assessment of ROM, ask the patient to make a fist and then appose each finger to the thumb. If he or she can perform these maneuvers, ROM of the hand is not seriously restricted.

Evaluation of the hip joint relies primarily on determination of its degree of mobility, because the joint is deep and difficult to inspect or palpate. The patient with hip pain usually experiences it in the *groin* or has pain that radiates to the knee. The knee is readily accessible for physical assessment, particularly when the patient is sitting and the knee is flexed. Fluid accumulation, or effusion, is easily detected in the knee joint. Limitations in movement with accompanying pain are common findings. The knees may be poorly aligned, as in genu valgum ("knock-knee") or genu varum ("bow-legged") deformities.

The ankles and feet are often neglected in the physical examination. However, they contain multiple bones and joints that can be affected by disease and injury. Observe and palpate each joint and test for ROM if feet are affected by musculoskeletal problems.

Neurovascular Assessment

While completing a physical assessment of the musculoskeletal system, perform an assessment of peripheral vascular and nerve integrity. Beginning with the injured side, always compare one extremity with the other.

Assessment of the Muscular System

During the skeletal assessment, notice the size, shape, tone, and strength of major skeletal muscles. The circumference of each muscle may be measured and compared symmetrically for an estimation of muscle mass if abnormalities are observed.

Ask the patient to demonstrate muscle strength. Apply resistance by holding the extremity and asking the patient to move against resistance. As an option, place your hands on the patient's upper arms and ask the patient to try to raise the arms. Although movement against resistance is not easily quantified, several scales used by nurses and therapists are available for grading the patient's strength. A commonly used scale is shown in Table 52-2.

Psychosocial Assessment

The data from the history and physical assessment provide clues for anticipating psychosocial problems. For instance, prolonged absence from employment or permanent disability may cause job or career loss. Further stress may be experienced if chronic pain continues and the patient cannot cope with numerous stressors. Anxiety and depression are common when patients have chronic pain. Deformities resulting from musculoskeletal disease or injury, such as an amputation, can affect a person's body image and self-concept. Help the patient identify support systems and coping mechanisms that may be useful if he or she has long-term musculoskeletal health problems. Encourage him or her to verbalize feelings related to loss and body image changes. Refer the patient for psychological or spiritual counseling if needed and if it is culturally appropriate.

Diagnostic Assessment
Laboratory Assessment

Chart 52-3 lists the common laboratory tests used in assessing patients with musculoskeletal disorders. There is no special patient preparation or follow-up care for any of these

CHART 52-3   **LABORATORY PROFILE**

Musculoskeletal Assessment

TEST	NORMAL RANGE FOR ADULTS	SIGNIFICANCE OF ABNORMAL FINDINGS
Serum calcium	9.0-10.5 mg/dL (2.25-2.75 mmol/L) *Older adults:* decreased	*Hypercalcemia* (increased calcium) • Metastatic cancers of the bone • Paget's disease • Bone fractures in healing stage *Hypocalcemia* (decreased calcium) • Osteoporosis • Osteomalacia
Serum phosphorus	3.0-4.5 mg/dL (0.97-1.45 mmol/L) *Older adults:* decreased	*Hyperphosphatemia* (increased phosphorus) • Bone fractures in healing stage • Bone tumors • Acromegaly *Hypophosphatemia* (decreased phosphorus) • Osteomalacia
Alkaline phosphatase (ALP)	30-120 units/L *Older adults:* slightly increased	*Elevations* may indicate: • Metastatic cancers of the bone • Paget's disease • Osteomalacia
Serum muscle enzymes Creatine kinase (CK-MM)	Total CK: *Men:* 55-170 units/L *Women:* 30-135 units/L	*Elevations* may indicate: • Muscle trauma • Progressive muscular dystrophy • Effects of electromyography
Lactic dehydrogenase (LDH)	Total LDH: 100-190 units/L LDH_1: 17%-27% LDH_2: 27%-37% LDH_3: 18%-25% LDH_4: 3%-8% LDH_5: 0% to 5%	*Elevations* may indicate: • Skeletal muscle necrosis • Extensive cancer • Progressive muscular dystrophy
Aspartate aminotransferase (AST)	0-35 units/L *Older adults:* increased	*Elevations* may indicate: • Skeletal muscle trauma • Progressive muscular dystrophy
Aldolase (ALD)	3.0-8.2 units/dL	*Elevations* may indicate: • Polymyositis and dermatomyositis • Muscular dystrophy

tests. Teach the patient about the purpose of the test and the procedure that can be expected. Additional tests performed for patients with connective tissue diseases, such as rheumatoid arthritis, are described in Chapter 20.

Disorders of bone and the parathyroid gland are often reflected in an alteration of the serum calcium or phosphorus level. Therefore these electrolytes, especially calcium, are monitored.

Alkaline phosphatase (ALP) is an enzyme normally present in blood. The concentration of ALP increases with bone or liver damage. In metabolic bone disease and bone cancer, the enzyme concentration rises in proportion to the osteoblastic activity, which indicates bone formation. The level of ALP is normally slightly increased in older adults.

The major *muscle enzymes* affected in skeletal muscle disease or injuries are:

• Creatine kinase (CK-MM)
• Aspartate aminotransferase (AST)
• Aldolase (ALD)
• Lactic dehydrogenase (LDH)

As a result of damage, the muscle tissue releases additional amounts of these enzymes, which increases serum levels.

The serum CK level begins to rise 2 to 4 hours after muscle injury and is elevated early in muscle disease, such as muscular dystrophy. The CK molecule has two subunits: M (muscle) and B (brain). Three isoenzymes have been identified. Skeletal muscle CK (CK-MM, or CK_3) is the only isoenzyme that rises in concentration with damage to skeletal muscle, such as trauma, surgery, and neuromuscular disease. This test is 90% accurate because it is affected by exercise and certain drugs, such as anticoagulants, furosemide, and statins (Kress et al., 2008).

AST is moderately elevated (three to five times normal) in certain muscle diseases, such as muscular dystrophy. The levels of the isoenzymes aldolase A (ALD-A) and LDH_5 also increase in patients with these disorders.

Imaging Assessment

The skeleton is very visible on *standard x-rays.* Anteroposterior and lateral projections are the initial screening views used most often. Other approaches, such as oblique or stress views, depend on the part of the skeleton to be evaluated and the necessity of the x-ray.

Bone density, alignment, swelling, and intactness can be seen on x-ray. The conditions of joints can be determined, including the size of the joint space, the smoothness of articular cartilage, and synovial swelling. Soft-tissue involvement may be evident but not clearly differentiated.

Inform the patient that the x-ray table is hard and cold, and instruct him or her to remain still during the filming process. Coordinate with the radiology department or clinic to keep older adults and those at risk for hypothermia as warm as possible (e.g., by using blankets).

Whereas standard x-rays superimpose one structure on another, tomography produces planes, or slices, for focus and blurs the images of other structures. This procedure is helpful in detailing the musculoskeletal system, because the many close structures make visualization difficult.

Xeroradiography highlights the contrast between structures. Margins and edges can be clearly seen (edge enhancement). Disadvantages of xeroradiography are the higher radiation dose to the patient and inability of the test to determine tissue densities.

Myelography involves the injection of contrast medium into the subarachnoid space of the spine, usually by spinal puncture. The vertebral column, intervertebral disks, spinal nerve roots, and blood vessels can be visualized. Although this test is still performed, it is far less popular. Computed tomography (CT) and magnetic resonance imaging (MRI) have often replaced such invasive and potentially painful and risky diagnostic techniques. The post-test care is similar to that for lumbar puncture, except that the patient is usually placed with the head of the bed elevated 30 to 50 degrees to prevent the contrast medium from getting into the brain (see Chapter 43).

An arthrogram is an x-ray study of a joint after contrast medium (air or solution) has been injected to enhance its visualization. Double-contrast arthrography, which uses both air and contrast, may be performed when a traumatic injury is suspected. The physician can often determine bone chips, torn ligaments, or other loose bodies within the joint. This test is not used commonly because of newer advances in diagnostic imaging. Most joints are now studied by MRI.

Computed tomography (CT) has gained wide acceptance for detecting musculoskeletal problems, particularly those of the vertebral column and joints. The scanned images can be used to create additional images from other angles or to create three-dimensional images and view complex structures from any position. The nurse or radiology technologist should ask the patient about iodine-based contrast allergies.

Nuclear Scans. The bone scan is a radionuclide test in which radioactive material is injected for viewing the entire skeleton. It may be used primarily to detect tumors, arthritis, osteomyelitis, osteoporosis, vertebral compression fractures, and unexplained bone pain. Bone scans are used less commonly today as more sophisticated MRI equipment becomes more available. However, it may be very useful for detecting hairline fractures in patients with unexplained bone pain and diffuse metastatic bone disease.

The gallium and thallium scans are similar to the bone scan but are more specific and sensitive in detecting bone problems. Gallium citrate (^{67}Ga) is the radioisotope most commonly used. This substance also migrates to brain, liver, and breast tissue and therefore is used in examination of these structures when disease is suspected.

For patients with osteosarcoma, thallium (^{201}Tl) is better than gallium or technetium for diagnosing the extent of the disease. Thallium has traditionally been used for the diagnosis of myocardial infarctions but can be used for additional evaluation of cancers of the bone.

Because bone takes up gallium slowly, the nuclear medicine physician or technician administers the isotope 4 to 6 hours before scanning. Other tests that require contrast media or other isotopes cannot be given during this time.

Instruct the patient that the radioactive material poses no threat because it readily deteriorates in the body. Because gallium is excreted through the intestinal tract, it tends to collect in feces after the scanning procedure.

Depending on the tissue to be examined, the patient is taken to the nuclear medicine department 4 to 6 hours after injection. The procedure takes 30 to 60 minutes, during which time the patient must lie still for accurate test results to be achieved. The scan may be repeated at 24, 48, and/or 72 hours. Mild sedation may be necessary to facilitate relaxation and cooperation during the procedure for confused older adults or those in severe pain.

No special care is required after the test. The radioisotope is excreted in stool and urine, but no precautions are taken in handling the excreta. Remind the patient to push fluids to facilitate urinary excretion.

Magnetic Resonance Imaging. Magnetic resonance imaging (MRI), with or without the use of contrast media, is commonly used to diagnose musculoskeletal disorders. It is more accurate than computed tomography (CT) and myelography for many spinal and knee problems. MRI is most appropriate for joints, soft tissue, and bony tumors that involve soft tissue. CT is still the test of choice for injuries or pathology that involves only bone.

The image is produced through the interaction of magnetic fields, radio waves, and atomic nuclei showing hydrogen density. Simply put, the radio waves "bounce" off the body tissues being examined. Because each tissue has its own density, the computer image clearly distinguishes normal and abnormal tissues. For some tissues, the cross-sectional image is better than that produced by radiography or CT. The lack of hydrogen ions in cortical bone makes it easily distinguishable from soft tissues. The test is particularly useful in identifying problems with muscles, tendons, and ligaments.

Ensure that the patient removes all metal objects and checks for clothing zippers and metal fasteners. Although joint implants made of titanium or stainless steel are usually safe, depending on the age of the MRI equipment, pacemakers, stents, and surgical clips usually are not. Chart 52-4 lists questions that the nurse or technician should consider in preparing the patient for MRI. Open MRIs prevent the claustrophobia that occurs with the older, encased machines.

Ultrasonography. Sound waves produce an image of the tissue in ultrasonography. An ultrasound procedure may be used to view:

- Soft-tissue disorders, such as masses and fluid accumulation
- Traumatic joint injuries
- Osteomyelitis
- Surgical hardware placement

A jelly-like substance applied to the skin over the site to be examined promotes the movement of a metal probe. No special preparation or post-test care is necessary. A quantitative ultrasound (QUS) may be done for determining fractures or bone density.

Preparing the Patient for Magnetic Resonance Imaging

- Is the patient pregnant?
- Does the patient have ferromagnetic fragments or implants, such as an older-style aneurysm clip?
- Does the patient have a pacemaker, stent, or electronic implant?
- Does the patient have chronic kidney disease? (Gadolinium contrast agents may cause severe systemic complications if the kidneys do not function.)
- Can the patient lie still in the supine position for 45 to 60 minutes? (May require sedation.)
- Does the patient need life-support equipment available?
- Can the patient communicate clearly and understand verbal communication?
- Did the patient get any tattoo *more than* 20 years ago? (If so, metal particles *may* be in the ink.)
- Is the patient claustrophobic? (Ask this question for closed MRI scanners; open MRIs do not cause claustrophobia.)

Other Diagnostic Assessment

Biopsies. In a bone biopsy, the physician extracts a specimen of the bone tissue for microscopic examination. This invasive test may confirm the presence of infection or neoplasm, but it is not commonly done today. One of two techniques may be used to retrieve the specimen: needle (closed) biopsy or incisional (open) biopsy. It is important to watch for bleeding from the puncture site and for tenderness, redness, or warmth that could indicate infection. Mild analgesics may be used.

Muscle biopsy is done for the diagnosis of atrophy (as in muscular dystrophy) and inflammation (as in polymyositis). The procedure and care for patients undergoing muscle biopsy are the same as those for patients undergoing bone biopsy.

Electromyography. Electromyography (EMG) is used to evaluate diffuse or localized muscle weakness. EMG is usually accompanied by nerve conduction studies for determining the electrical potential generated in an individual muscle. EMG helps in the diagnosis of neuromuscular, lower motor neuron, and peripheral nerve disorders. This test is contraindicated for patients undergoing anticoagulant therapy.

Inform the patient that EMG may cause temporary discomfort, especially when the patient is subjected to episodes of electrical current. For selected patients, mild sedation is prescribed. The physician may also prescribe a temporary discontinuation of skeletal muscle relaxants several days before the procedure to prevent drugs from affecting the test results.

The test may be performed at the bedside or in an EMG laboratory. When both EMG and nerve conduction studies are done, nerve conduction is usually tested first. Flat electrodes are placed along the nerve to be evaluated, and low electrical currents are passed through the electrodes to the nerve and muscle innervated. If nerve conduction occurs, the muscle contracts.

For testing muscle potential, multiple small needle electrodes are inserted. The patient is asked to perform activities for measurement of muscle potential during minimal and maximal contraction. The degree of nerve and muscle activity is recorded for later interpretation.

A few medical complications are associated with EMG. The nurse provides comfort measures and inspects the needle sites for hematoma formation. The application of ice can prevent this complication. The patient may also report increased pain and anxiety after the test.

Arthroscopy. The arthroscopy may be used as a diagnostic test or a surgical procedure. An arthroscope is a fiberoptic tube inserted into a joint for direct visualization of the ligaments, menisci, and articular surfaces of the joint. The knee and shoulder are most commonly evaluated. In addition, synovial biopsy and surgery to repair traumatic injury can be done through the arthroscope as an ambulatory care procedure.

Patient Preparation. Because the knee is most commonly "scoped," the care described for the patient undergoing arthroscopy relates to that joint. Arthroscopy is performed on an ambulatory basis or as same-day surgery. The patient must be able to flex the knee. Those who cannot flex the knee at least 40 degrees or who have an infected knee are not candidates for the procedure. If the patient cannot flex the knee, the arthroscope cannot be inserted into the joint space to allow visualization. Joint infection may worsen from the mechanical trauma of arthroscope insertion.

If the procedure is done for surgical repair, the patient may have a physical therapy consultation before arthroscopy to learn the leg exercises that are necessary after the test. Straight-leg raises (SLRs) and quadriceps setting exercises (isometrics with the leg extended) are practiced in sets of 10 each. ROM exercises are also taught but may not be allowed immediately after arthroscopic surgery. The nurse in the surgeon's office or at the surgical center can teach these exercises or reinforce the information provided by the physical therapist. The nurse also reinforces the explanation of the procedure and post-test care and ensures that the patient has signed an informed consent.

Procedure. The patient is usually given local, light general, or epidural anesthesia, depending on the purpose of the procedure. In some settings, a large pneumatic tourniquet is used around the thigh to minimize bleeding during the procedure. Drugs that promote vasoconstriction for control of bleeding may be used alone or in conjunction with the tourniquet.

The knee is flexed to at least 40 degrees and is irrigated. As shown in Fig. 52-6, the arthroscope is inserted through a small incision less than $\frac{1}{4}$-inch (0.6 cm) long. Multiple incisions may be required to allow inspection at a variety of angles. After the procedure, a dressing may be applied, depending on the amount of manipulation during the test or surgery.

Postprocedure Care. The immediate care after an arthroscopy is the same for patients having the procedure for diagnostic purposes and those having an arthroscopy for surgical intervention.

> **! NURSING SAFETY PRIORITY**
> **Action Alert**
>
> The priority for postprocedure care after arthroscopy is to assess the neurovascular status of the patient's affected limb every hour or according to agency or surgeon protocol. Monitor and document distal pulses, warmth, color, capillary refill, pain, movement, and sensation of the affected extremity.

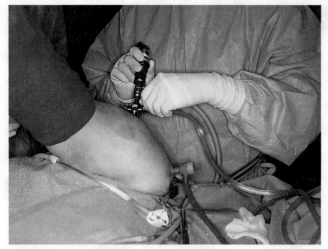

FIG. 52-6 An arthroscope is used in the diagnosis of pathologic changes in the joints. This patient is undergoing arthroscopy of the shoulder.

Encourage the patient to perform exercises as taught before the procedure, if appropriate. For the mild discomfort experienced after the diagnostic arthroscopy, the physician prescribes a mild analgesic, such as acetaminophen (Tylenol, Ace-Tabs ✦). If postoperative, the patient may have short-term activity restrictions, depending on the musculoskeletal problem. Ice is often used for 24 hours, and the extremity should be elevated for 12 to 24 hours. When arthroscopic surgery is performed, the health care provider usually prescribes an opioid-analgesic combination, such as oxycodone and acetaminophen (Percocet, Tylox).

Although complications are not common, monitor and teach the patient to observe for:
- Swelling
- Increased joint pain attributable to mechanical injury
- Thrombophlebitis
- Infection

Severe joint or limb pain after discharge may indicate a possible complication. Teach the patient to contact the physician immediately. The surgeon usually sees the patient about 1 week after the procedure to check for complications.

> **❓ NCLEX EXAMINATION CHALLENGE**
> ### Safe and Effective Care Environment
>
> A client returns to PACU after an arthroscopy to repair several knee ligaments. What is the nurse's priority when caring for this client?
> A. Take vital signs every hour.
> B. Check for swelling and bleeding.
> C. Perform frequent neurovascular assessments.
> D. Ensure that the surgical dressing is intact.

NURSING CONCEPT REVIEW

What should you NOTICE in a patient with adequate mobility and sensation related to the musculoskeletal system?

Physical Assessment
- No gross deformities or impairments in posture or gait
- Adequate size, strength, and symmetry of muscle for age
- Can perform ADLs independently
- Can perform other routine daily activities independently
- Can ambulate with or without assistive devices
- No pain or tenderness on palpation or passive range-of-motion (ROM) of joints
- Active ROM of joints within normal limits for age
- No crepitus when moving joints
- No swelling of joints or extremities
- Equal size and alignment of extremities
- Equal sensation in extremities

Diagnostic Assessment
- Muscle enzymes (e.g., CK-MM, ALD) within normal limits for age
- Bone density adequate for age and gender
- Joint changes within normal limits for age

GET READY FOR THE NCLEX® EXAMINATION!

KEY POINTS

Review these Key Points for each NCLEX Examination Client Needs Category.

Safe and Effective Care Environment
- Collaborate with the physical and/or occupational therapist to perform a complete musculoskeletal assessment if indicated.

Health Promotion and Maintenance
- Be aware that older adults have physiologic changes that affect their musculoskeletal system (see Chart 52-1).

Psychosocial Integrity
- Assess the patient's support systems and coping mechanisms when musculoskeletal trauma or disease affects his or her body image.

GET READY FOR THE NCLEX® EXAMINATION!—cont'd

- Ask about the patient's occupation, because heavy manual labor may cause back injury and other musculoskeletal trauma.

Physiological Integrity

- Assess the patient's pain intensity, quality, duration, and location.
- Assess the patient's mobility, including gait, posture, and muscle strength.
- Assess for musculoskeletal changes associated with aging (see Chart 52-1).
- Interpret the patient's laboratory values that are related to musculoskeletal disease (see Chart 52-3).

- Teach the patient that mild discomfort can be expected during electromyography, a test to assess the electrical potential of muscles and their innervation.
- Instruct the patient to report swelling, infection, and increased pain after an arthroscopy.
- Ask the patient questions to ensure safety before an MRI (see Chart 52-4).
- Ask the patient about allergy to contrast media before diagnostic testing such as CT scans.
- Evaluate the neurovascular status of the patient's affected extremity after an arthroscopic procedure as the *priority for care.*

Care of Patients with Musculoskeletal Problems

Donna D. Ignatavicius

℮volve WEBSITE

http://evolve.elsevier.com/Iggy/

Answer Key for NCLEX Examination Challenges and
  Decision-Making Challenges
Audio Glossary

Concept Map Creator
Key Points
Review Questions for the NCLEX® Examination

LEARNING OUTCOMES

Safe and Effective Care Environment

1. Coordinate with health care team members when planning and providing care for patients with musculoskeletal problems.
2. Teach the patient and family about home safety when the patient has a metabolic bone problem such as osteoporosis.
3. Identify community resources for patients with musculoskeletal problems that impair mobility.
4. Apply principles of infection control for patients with osteomyelitis, including Contact Precautions if needed.

Health Promotion and Maintenance

5. Develop a teaching plan for all age-groups about ways to decrease the risk for osteoporosis.
6. Perform health risk assessments for people at risk for osteoporosis and osteomalacia.
7. Assess the genetic risk for patients who have parents with muscular dystrophy.
8. Refer patients with genetic-associated diseases for genetic counseling and testing.

Psychosocial Integrity

9. Assess the patient's and family's responses to a bone cancer diagnosis and treatment options.
10. Evaluate patient's and family's coping strategies and fears related to grief and loss before and after bone cancer surgery.

Physiological Integrity

11. Educate the patient and family about common drugs used for bone diseases, such as calcium supplements and bisphosphonates.
12. Compare and contrast osteoporosis and osteomalacia.
13. Identify key features of Paget's disease of the bone.
14. Differentiate acute and chronic osteomyelitis.
15. Prioritize care for patients with osteomyelitis.
16. Identify collaborative management options for treating patients with primary and metastatic bone cancer.
17. Describe common disorders of the foot, including hallux valgus and plantar fasciitis, that can affect mobility.
18. Explain the role of the nurse when caring for an adult patient with muscular dystrophy.

Musculoskeletal disorders include metabolic bone diseases, such as osteoporosis and Paget's disease, bone tumors, and a variety of deformities and syndromes. Older adults are at the greatest risk for most of these problems, although primary bone cancer is most often found in adolescents and young adults. As technologic advances occur and patients survive longer with primary cancers, metastatic lesions have become more prevalent among older adults. Almost all musculoskeletal health problems can cause the patient to have difficulty meeting the human need of *mobility*. This chapter focuses on selected disorders not covered in Chapter 20 on arthritis and other connective tissue diseases.

METABOLIC BONE DISEASES

OSTEOPOROSIS

Pathophysiology

Osteoporosis is a chronic metabolic disease in which bone loss causes decreased density and possible fracture. It is often referred to as a "silent disease" because the first sign of osteoporosis in most people follows some kind of a fracture. The spine, hip, and wrist are most often at risk, although any bone can fracture (National Osteoporosis Foundation, 2010).

Osteoporosis is a major health problem in the world. The estimated cost for osteoporosis-related health care alone in the United States is more than $18 billion each year with continual cost increases each year. By 2040, that number is expected to double or triple (National Osteoporosis Foundation, 2010).

Bone is a dynamic tissue that is constantly undergoing changes in a process referred to as bone remodeling. Osteoporosis and osteopenia (low bone mass) occur when osteoclastic (bone resorption) activity is greater than osteoblastic (bone building) activity. The result is a decreased bone mineral density (BMD). BMD determines bone strength and peaks between 25 and 30 years of age. Before and during the peak years, osteoclastic activity and osteoblastic activity work at the same rate. After the peak years, bone resorption activity exceeds bone-building activity, and bone density decreases. BMD decreases most rapidly in postmenopausal women as serum estrogen levels diminish. Although estrogen does not build bone, it helps prevent bone loss. Trabecular, or cancellous (spongy), bone is lost first, followed by loss of cortical (compact) bone. This results in thin, fragile bone tissue that is at risk for fracture.

Standards for the diagnosis of osteoporosis are based on BMD testing that provides a T-score for the patient. A T-score represents the number of standard deviations above or below the average BMD for young, healthy adults. *Osteopenia is present when the T-score is at −1 and above −2.5. Osteoporosis is diagnosed in a person who has a T-score at or lower than −2.5.* Medicare reimburses for BMD testing every 2 years in people ages 65 years and older who (National Osteoporosis Foundation, 2010):

- Are estrogen deficient
- Have vertebral abnormalities
- Receive long-term steroid therapy
- Have primary hyperparathyroidism
- Are being monitored while on osteoporosis drug therapy

Osteoporosis can be classified as generalized or regional. *Generalized* osteoporosis involves many structures in the skeleton and is further divided into two categories, primary and secondary. *Primary* osteoporosis is more common and occurs in postmenopausal women and in men in their seventh or eighth decade of life. Even though men do not experience the rapid bone loss that postmenopausal women have, they do have decreasing levels of testosterone (which builds bone) and altered ability to absorb calcium. This results in a slower loss of bone mass in men, especially those older than 75 years. *Secondary* osteoporosis may result from other medical conditions, such as hyperparathyroidism; long-term drug therapy, such as with corticosteroids; or prolonged immobility, such as that seen with spinal cord injury (Table 53-1). Treatment

TABLE 53-1	CAUSES OF SECONDARY OSTEOPOROSIS
Diseases/Conditions	**Drugs (Chronic Use)**
• Diabetes mellitus • Hyperthyroidism • Hyperparathyroidism • Cushing's syndrome • Growth hormone deficiency • Metabolic acidosis • Female hypogonadism • Paget's disease • Osteogenesis imperfecta • Rheumatoid arthritis • Prolonged immobilization • Bone cancer • Cirrhosis • HIV/AIDS • Chronic airway limitation	• Corticosteroids • Heparin • Anticonvulsants (phenobarbital, phenytoin) • Ethanol (alcohol) • Drugs that induce hypogonadism (decreased levels of sex hormones) • High levels of thyroid hormone • Cytotoxic agents • Immunosuppressants • Loop diuretics • Aluminum-based antacids

AIDS, Acquired immune deficiency syndrome; *HIV,* human immune deficiency virus.

CHART 53-1	BEST PRACTICE FOR PATIENT SAFETY & QUALITY CARE

Assessing Risk Factors for Primary Osteoporosis

Assess for:
- Older age in both genders and all races
- Parental history of osteoporosis, especially mother
- History of low-trauma fracture after age 50 years
- Low body weight, thin build
- Chronic low calcium and/or vitamin D intake
- Estrogen or androgen deficiency
- Current smoking (active or passive)
- High alcohol intake (3 or more drinks a day)
- Lack of physical exercise or prolonged immobility

of the secondary type is directed toward the cause of the osteoporosis when possible.

Regional osteoporosis, an example of secondary disease, occurs when a limb is immobilized related to a fracture, injury, or paralysis. Immobility for longer than 8 to 12 weeks can result in this type of osteoporosis. Bone loss also occurs when people spend prolonged time in a gravity-free or weightless environment (e.g., astronauts).

Etiology and Genetic Risk

Primary osteoporosis is caused by a combination of genetic, lifestyle, and environmental factors. Chart 53-1 lists the major factors that contribute to the development of this disease.

Primary osteoporosis most often occurs in women after menopause as a result of decreased estrogen levels. Women lose about 2% of their bone mass every year in the first 5 years after natural or surgical (ovary removal) menopause. For women of any age who do not take estrogen replacement, the risk for osteoporosis increases.

Men also develop osteoporosis after the age of 50 because their testosterone levels decrease. Testosterone is the major sex hormone that builds bone tissue. Men are often underdiagnosed, even when they become older adults. A recent study of almost 1200 men in a VA rehabilitation center showed that screening for osteoporosis had not been conducted. As a result of bone mineral density screening, the researchers found 33 study patients who had osteoporosis and were at

GENETIC/GENOMIC CONSIDERATIONS

The genetic and immune factors that cause osteoporosis are very complex. Strong evidence demonstrates that genetics is a significant factor, with a heritability of 50% to 90% (Chang et al., 2010). Many genetic changes have been identified as possible causative factors, but there is no agreement about which ones are most important or constant in all patients. For example, changes in the vitamin D receptor *(VDR)* gene and calcitonin receptor *(CTR)* gene have been found in some patients with the disease. Receptors are essential for the uptake and use of these substances by the cells.

The bone morphogenetic protein-2 *(BMP-2)* gene has a key role in bone formation and maintenance. Some osteoporotic patients who have had fractures have changes in their *BMP-2* gene. Alterations in growth hormone-1 (GH-1) have been discovered in petite Asian-American women, those who are predisposed to developing osteoporosis.

Hormones, tumor necrosis factor (TNF), interleukins, and other substances in the body help control osteoclasts in a very complex pathway. The recent identification of the importance of the cytokine receptor activator of nuclear factor kappa-B ligand *(RANKL)*, its receptor *RANK*, and its decoy receptor osteoprotegerin *(OPG)* has helped researchers understand more about the activity of osteoclasts in metabolic bone disease. Disruptions in the *RANKL, RANK,* and *OPG* system can lead to increased osteoclast activity in which bone is rapidly broken down (McCance et al., 2010).

high risk for fractures, especially of the hip. Those who were diagnosed with the disease were the oldest patients who had a lower body mass index and weight (Swislocki et al., 2010).

Body build and weight seems to influence who gets the disease. Osteoporosis occurs most often in older, lean-built Euro-American and Asian women, particularly those who do not exercise regularly. However, African Americans are at risk for decreased vitamin D, which is needed for adequate calcium absorption in the small intestines. Obese women can store estrogen in their tissues for use as necessary to maintain a normal level of serum calcium. Weight-bearing exercise reduces bone resorption (loss) and stimulates bone formation. Prolonged immobility produces rapid bone loss.

The relationship of osteoporosis to nutrition is well established. For example, excessive caffeine in the diet can cause calcium loss in the urine. A diet lacking enough calcium and vitamin D stimulates the parathyroid gland to produce parathyroid hormone (PTH). PTH triggers the release of calcium from the bony matrix. Activated vitamin D is needed for calcium uptake in the body. Malabsorption of nutrients in the GI tract also contributes to low serum calcium levels. Institutionalized or homebound patients who are not exposed to sunlight may be at a higher risk because they do not receive adequate vitamin D for the metabolism of calcium.

Calcium loss occurs at a more rapid rate when phosphorus intake is high. (Chapter 13 describes the usual relationship between calcium and phosphorus in the body.) People who drink large amounts of carbonated beverages each day (over 40 ounces) are at high risk for calcium loss and subsequent osteoporosis, regardless of age or gender.

Protein deficiency may also reduce bone density. Because 50% of serum calcium is protein bound, protein is needed to use calcium. However, excessive protein intake may increase calcium loss in the urine. For instance, people who are on high-protein, low-carbohydrate diets, like the Atkins diet, may consume too much protein to replace other food not allowed. Dietary protein intake in healthy adults is

recommended at 0.8 grams per kilogram of body weight. Protein is needed for bone healing when a fracture occurs.

Excessive alcohol and tobacco use are other risk factors for osteoporosis. Although the exact mechanisms are not known, these substances promote acidosis, which in turn increases bone loss. Alcohol also has a direct toxic effect on bone tissue, resulting in decreased bone formation and increased bone resorption. For those people who have excessive alcohol intake, alcohol calories decrease hunger and the need to take in adequate amounts of nutrients.

Osteoporosis also occurs in young adults who participate in excessive exercise or weight-loss dieting or in those who have eating disorders, such as anorexia nervosa or bulimia nervosa. Young females with these risk factors have a low body weight and absent menstruation, which contribute to the development of osteoporosis. Dancers, gymnasts, and other athletes may overtrain without sufficient caloric intake, which also results in severe weight loss. Young girls and women may have an obsession with being slim. Particular attention must be paid to bone health for these groups.

Incidence/Prevalence

Osteoporosis is a potential health problem for more than 44 million Americans. About 10 million people in the United States have the disease, and about 34 million people 50 years of age and older have osteopenia and are at risk for development of osteoporosis. Women remain the largest group affected by osteoporosis, although men, especially those older than 75 years, also have the disease. After the age of 50, men are at increased risk for osteoporosis and osteoporotic-related fractures (Voda, 2009b).

People of all ethnic and racial backgrounds are at some degree of risk, but white, thin women are likely to get primary osteoporosis at an earlier age (National Osteoporosis Foundation, 2010).

CULTURAL AWARENESS

Although there is some advantage of increased bone density in dark-skinned women, lifestyle and health beliefs about prevention may put all women at an equal risk for osteoporosis. Dietary preferences or the ability to afford high-nutrient food may influence the woman's rate of bone loss. For example, many blacks have lactose intolerance and cannot drink milk or eat other dairy-based foods. Milk and cheese are good sources of protein, a nutrient needed to bind calcium for use by the body.

Osteoporosis results in more than 1.5 million fractures each year. A woman who experiences a hip fracture has a four times greater risk for a second fracture. Fractures as a result of osteoporosis and falling can decrease a patient's *mobility* and quality of life. The mortality rate for older patients with hip fractures is very high, especially within the first 6 months, and the debilitating effects can be devastating.

Nursing home residents fall 11 times more often than their community-dwelling counterparts (Parikh et al., 2009). Yet, skilled nursing facilities (SNFs) do not routinely screen residents for osteoporosis. A national study by Gloth and Simonson (2008) reported the results of osteoporosis screening for more than 34,000 SNF residents in 26 states. Over 42% of residents were categorized as having a high risk for osteoporosis and associated fractures (see the Evidence-Based Practice box on p. 1122).

EVIDENCE-BASED PRACTICE

Is Osteoporosis Underdiagnosed in Residents Admitted to Skilled Nursing Facilities?

Gloth, F.M., 3rd, & Simonson, W. (2008). Osteoporosis is underdiagnosed in skilled nursing facilities: A large-scale heel BMD screening study. *Journal of the American Medical Directors Association, 9*(3), 190-193.

The purpose of this nationwide study in the United States was to investigate the belief that osteoporosis is underdiagnosed in the skilled nursing facility (SNF) setting. Local consultant pharmacists screened 34,486 SNF residents in 26 states using the peripheral dual-energy x-ray absorptiometry (DXA) scan to determine bone mineral density (BMD) of the heel. Residents ranged in age from younger than 59 years to older than 80 years. Of the total screened residents, 22.4% were categorized as low risk, 35.1% as moderate risk, and 42.5% as high risk for osteoporosis and related fractures. The researchers concluded that osteoporosis is grossly underdiagnosed and BMD screening should be a part of the resident's admission assessment.

Level of Evidence: 4

Although the sample was very large and the study answered the research question, no experimental or quasi-experimental design was used. However, it would be inappropriate to use these designs to answer the research question.

Commentary: Implications for Practice and Research

Nurses working with older adults in any setting need to be aware of the prevalence of osteoporosis among this population. They can be instrumental in developing screening programs that can identify the most at-risk older adults so they can be treated and monitored more carefully for fractures. Those at risk need to have health teaching about drug therapy and lifestyle changes that could slow or improve the disease process.

Health Promotion and Maintenance

Peak bone mass is achieved by about 30 years of age in most women. *Building strong bone as a young person may be the best defense against osteoporosis in later adulthood. Young women need to be aware of appropriate health and lifestyle practices that can prevent this potentially disabling disease.*

Nurses can play a vital role in patient education to prevent and manage osteoporosis. *Teaching should begin with young women because they begin to lose bone after 30 years of age.*

The focus of osteoporosis prevention is to decrease modifiable risk factors. For example, teach patients who do not include enough dietary calcium which foods should be included, such as dairy products and dark green, leafy vegetables. Teach them to read food labels for sources of calcium content. Explain the importance of sun exposure (but not so much as to get sunburned) and adequate vitamin D in the diet. In 2010, the Institute of Medicine published recommendations for healthy people younger than 71 years to take 600 international units of activated vitamin D each day; 800 to 1000 international units each day is recommended for people older than 71 years. The National Osteoporosis Foundation recommends higher doses for healthy people. Patients being treated for osteoporosis or osteomalacia (vitamin D deficiency) are prescribed much higher therapeutic doses.

Teach the need to limit the amount of carbonated beverages consumed each day. Remind patients who have sedentary lifestyles about the importance of exercise and what types of exercise builds bone tissue. Weight-bearing exercises, such as regularly scheduled walking, are preferred. Teach people to avoid activities that cause jarring, such as horseback riding, to prevent potential vertebral compression fractures.

PATIENT-CENTERED COLLABORATIVE CARE

ASSESSMENT

A complete health history with assessment of risk factors is important in the prevention, early detection, and treatment of osteoporosis. Patients who have risk factors for osteoporosis are at increased risk for fractures when falls occur. Include a fall risk assessment in the health history, especially for older adults. Assess for fall risk factors, including:

- Delirium
- Dementia
- Immobility
- Muscular weakness
- History of falls
- Visual or hearing deficits
- Current drugs

The Joint Commission's National Patient Safety Goals (NPSG) specify the need to reduce risk for harm to patients resulting from falls. *People with osteoporosis are at an increased risk for fracture if a fall occurs. The World Health Organization (WHO) Fracture Risk Algorithm (FRAX) is often used to determine the patient's risk for fractures associated with bone loss.* Chapter 3 discusses falls in older adults in more detail.

Physical Assessment/Clinical Manifestations

When performing a musculoskeletal assessment, inspect and palpate the vertebral column. The classic "dowager's hump," or kyphosis of the dorsal spine, is often present (Fig. 53-1). The patient may state that he or she has gotten shorter, perhaps as much as 2 to 3 inches (5 to 7.5 cm) within the previous 20 years. Take or delegate height and weight measurements, and compare with previous measurements if they are available.

The patient may have back pain, which often occurs after lifting, bending, or stooping. The pain may be sharp and acute in onset. Pain is worse with activity and is relieved by rest. Palpation of the vertebrae, particularly the lower thoracic and lumbar vertebrae, can increase the patient's discomfort. Therefore palpation should be gentle.

Back pain accompanied by tenderness and voluntary restriction of spinal movement suggests one or more compression vertebral fractures, the most common type of osteoporotic fracture. Movement restriction and spinal deformity may result in constipation, abdominal distention, reflux esophagitis, and respiratory compromise in severe cases. The most likely area for spinal fracture is between T8 and L3. This problem is discussed in more detail in Chapter 54.

Fractures are also common in the distal end of the radius (wrist) and the upper third of the femur (hip). Ask the patient to locate all areas that are painful, and observe for signs and symptoms of fractures, such as swelling and malalignment.

Psychosocial Assessment

Women associate osteoporosis with menopause, getting older, and becoming less independent. The disease can result in suffering, deformity, and disability that can affect the patient's well-being and life satisfaction. The quality of life

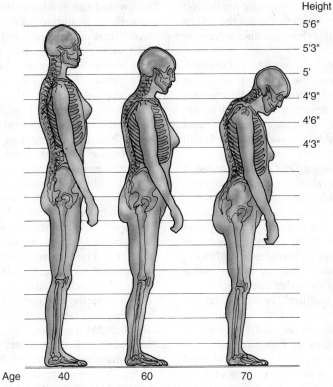

Height
5'6"
5'3"
5'
4'9"
4'6"
4'3"

Age   40   60   70

FIG. 53-1 A normal spine at age 40 years and osteoporotic changes at ages 60 and 70 years. These changes can cause a loss of as much as 6 inches in height and can result in the so-called *dowager's hump (far right)* in the upper thoracic vertebrae.

may be further impacted by pain, insomnia, depression, and **fallophobia** (fear of falling).

Assess the patient's concept of body image, especially if he or she is severely kyphotic. For example, the patient may have difficulty finding clothes that fit properly. Social interactions may be avoided because of a change in appearance or the physical limitations of being unable to sit in chairs in restaurants, movie theaters, and other places. Changes in sexuality may occur as a result of poor self-esteem or the discomfort caused by positioning during intercourse.

Because osteoporosis poses a risk for fractures, teach the patient to be extremely cautious about activities. As a result, the threat of fracture can create anxiety and fear and result in further limitation of social or physical activities. Assess for these feelings to assist in treatment decisions and health teaching. For example, the patient may not exercise as prescribed for fear that a fracture will occur.

Laboratory Assessment

There are no definitive laboratory tests that confirm a diagnosis of primary osteoporosis, although a number of *biochemical markers* can provide information about bone resorption and formation activity. These biochemical markers are sensitive to bone changes and can be used to monitor effectiveness of treatment for osteoporosis. *Bone-specific alkaline phosphatase (BSAP)* is found in the cell membrane of the osteoblast and indicates bone formation status. *Osteocalcin* is a protein substance in bone and increases during bone resorption activity. Pyridinium (PYD) cross-links are released into circulation during bone resorption. *N-teleopeptide (NTX)* and *C-teleopeptide (CTX)* are proteins released when bone is

broken down. Some laboratories require a 24-hour urine collection for testing, whereas others use a double-voided specimen. Some markers, like NTX and CTX, can also be measured in the blood using immunoassay techniques. Increased levels of any of these markers indicate a risk for osteoporosis. Increased levels are found in patients with osteoporosis, Paget's disease, and bone tumors (Pagana & Pagana, 2010).

A battery of tests can be performed to rule out secondary osteoporosis or other metabolic bone diseases, such as osteomalacia and Paget's disease. These include measurements of serum calcium, vitamin D, and phosphorus. Urinary calcium levels may also be assessed. Serum protein measurements and thyroid function tests are done to check for hyperthyroidism.

Imaging Assessment

Conventional x-rays of the spine and long bones show decreased bone density but only after a 25% to 40% bone loss has occurred. Fractures can also be seen on x-ray.

The most commonly used screening and diagnostic tool for measuring bone mineral density (BMD) is **dual x-ray absorptiometry (DXA).** The spine and hip are most often assessed when central DXA (cDXA) scan is performed. Many physicians recommend that women in their 40s have a baseline screening DXA scan so that later bone changes can be detected and compared. DXA is a painless scan that emits less radiation than a chest x-ray. *It is the best tool currently available for a definite diagnosis of osteoporosis.* The patient stays dressed but is asked to remove any metallic objects such as belt buckles, coins, keys, or jewelry that might interfere with the test. The results are displayed on a computer graph, and a T-score is calculated. No special follow-up care for the test is required. However, the patient needs to discuss the results with the physician for any decisions about possible preventive or management interventions.

A peripheral DXA (pDXA) scan assesses BMD of the heel, forearm, or finger. It is often used for large-scale screening purposes. For example, Gloth and Simonson (2008) reported a large-scale heel BMD study for screening over 34,000 skilled nursing facility residents. The pDXA is also commonly used for screening at community health fairs and women's health centers.

Quantitative computed tomography (QCT) can also measure bone density, using either a central or peripheral technique. This procedure analyzes trabecular and cortical bone separately and is especially sensitive to changes in the vertebral column. The test is more expensive than the DXA scan and exposes the patient to more radiation; however, it is a safe screening test (National Osteoporosis Foundation, 2010).

Peripheral quantitative ultrasound (pQUS) is an effective and low-cost peripheral screening tool that can detect osteoporosis and predict risk for hip fracture. The heel, tibia, and patella are most commonly tested. The procedure requires no special preparation, is quick, and has no radiation exposure or specific follow-up care (Pagana & Pagana, 2010). The National Osteoporosis Foundation recommends that men older than 70 years have the pQUS as a screening tool for the disease.

ANALYSIS

The most common problem for patients with osteoporosis or osteopenia is potential for fractures related to weak, porous bone tissue.

PLANNING AND IMPLEMENTATION

Planning: Expected Outcomes

The expected outcome is that the patient avoids fractures by preventing falls, managing risk factors, and adhering to preventive or treatment measures for bone loss.

Interventions

Because the patient is predisposed to fractures, nutritional therapy, exercise, lifestyle changes, and drug therapy are used to slow bone resorption and form new bone tissue. Patient education can help prevent osteoporosis or slow the progress. These measures help reduce the chance of fractures and their complications. The role of drug therapy has increased over the past decade and helps prevent fractures related to osteoporosis. Drug therapy should begin when the BMD T-score for the hip is below −2.0 with no other risk factors or when the T-score is below −1.5 with one or more risk factors or previous fracture.

Nutrition Therapy. The nutritional considerations for the treatment of a patient with a diagnosis of osteoporosis are the same as those for preventing the disease. Teach patients about the adequate amounts of protein, magnesium, vitamin K, and trace minerals that are needed for bone formation. Calcium and vitamin D intake should be increased. Teach patients to avoid excessive alcohol and caffeine consumption. For the patient who has sustained a fracture, adequate intake of protein, vitamin C, and iron is important to promote bone healing. People who are lactose intolerant can choose a variety

of soy and rice products that are fortified with calcium and vitamin D. In addition, calcium and vitamin D are added to many fruit juices, bread, and cereal products.

A variety of nutrients are needed to maintain bone health. *The promotion of a single nutrient will not prevent or treat osteoporosis.* Help the patient develop a nutritional plan that is most beneficial in maintaining bone health; the plan should emphasize fruits and vegetables, low-fat dairy and protein sources, increased fiber, and moderation in alcohol and caffeine (National Osteoporosis Foundation, 2010).

Lifestyle Changes. Exercise is important in the prevention and management of osteoporosis. It also plays a vital role in pain management, cardiovascular function, and an improved sense of well-being.

In collaboration with the health care provider, the physical therapist may prescribe exercises for strengthening the abdominal and back muscles for those at risk for vertebral fractures. These exercises improve posture and support for the spine. Abdominal muscle tightening, deep breathing, and pectoral stretching are stressed to increase lung capacity. Exercises for the extremity muscles include muscle-tightening, resistive, and range-of-motion (ROM) exercises. Encourage active ROM exercises, which improve joint mobility and increase muscle tone, as well as prescribed exercise activities. Swimming provides overall muscle exercise.

In addition to exercises for muscle strengthening, a general weight-bearing exercise program should be implemented. Teach patients that *walking for 30 minutes three to five times a week is the single most effective exercise for osteoporosis prevention.* Teach the patient that certain high-impact recreational activities, such as running, bowling, and horseback riding, may cause vertebral compression fractures and should be avoided.

In addition to nutrition and exercise, other lifestyle changes may be needed. Teach the patient to avoid tobacco in any form, especially cigarette smoking. The patient must be careful to prevent falls and other activities that can cause a fracture. Teach the patient about the importance of having a hazard-free environment, including avoiding scatter rugs, cluttered rooms, and wet floor areas.

Hospitals and long-term care facilities have risk management programs to assess for the risk for falls. For those patients at high risk, communicate this information to other members of the health care team, using colored armbands or other easy-to-recognize methods (National Patient Safety Goals). Chapter 3 discusses fall prevention in health care agencies and at home in more detail.

❓ NCLEX EXAMINATION CHALLENGE

Health Promotion and Maintenance

Which statement by the client regarding lifestyle changes to prevent osteoporosis indicates a need for further teaching by the nurse?
A. "I need to eat more green, leafy vegetables and dairy products."
B. "I will cut down the amount of wine I drink each night."
C. "I plan to begin smoking cessation classes at the hospital."
D. "I am going to want to work out 3 days a week at the gym."

Drug Therapy. The health care provider may prescribe calcium and vitamin D supplements, bisphosphonates, or estrogen agonist/antagonists (formerly called *selective estrogen receptor modulators*), or a combination of several drugs to treat or prevent osteoporosis (Chart 53-2). Estrogen and combination hormone therapy are not used solely for osteoporosis prevention or management because they can increase other health risks such as breast cancer and myocardial infarction (Woman's Health Initiative, 2005).

Calcium and Vitamin D. Intake of *calcium* alone is not a treatment for osteoporosis, but calcium is an important part of a *prevention* program to promote bone health. Most people cannot or do not have enough calcium in their diet, and therefore calcium supplements are needed. Calcium carbonate, found in over-the-counter (OTC) drugs such as Os-Cal, is one of the most cost-effective supplement formulas. Calcium citrate, available OTC as Citracal, is often recommended for those who have gastric upset when taking a calcium supplement. Teach patients to take calcium supplements with food and 6 to 8 ounces of water, although Citracal can be taken anytime. It is best to divide the daily dose, with at least one third of the daily dose being taken in the evening. Teach women to start taking supplements in young adulthood to assist in maintaining peak bone mass. Instruct patients of any age to take calcium supplements that also contain activated vitamin D, such as Os-Cal Ultra.

Remind patients to take these supplements under the supervision of a health care provider. Hypercalcemia (excess serum calcium) can cause serious damage to the urinary system and other body systems. Teach patients to drink plenty of fluids to prevent urinary or renal calculi (stones). Chapter 13 describes the clinical manifestations of hypercalcemia.

Bisphosphonates. Bisphosphonates (BPs) slow bone resorption by binding with crystal elements in bone, especially spongy, trabecular bone tissue. They are the most common drugs used for osteoporosis, but some are also approved for Paget's disease and hypercalcemia related to cancer. Three FDA-approved BPs—alendronate (Fosamax), ibandronate (Boniva), and risedronate (Actonel)—are commonly used for the *prevention and treatment* of osteoporosis (National Osteoporosis Foundation, 2010). These drugs are available as oral preparations, with ibandronate (Boniva) also available as an IV preparation.

> ### ! NURSING SAFETY PRIORITY
> **Drug Alert**
>
> Do not confuse Fosamax with Flomax, a selective alpha-adrenergic blocker used for benign prostatic hyperplasia (BPH).

Oral BPs are commonly associated with a serious problem called esophagitis (inflammation of the esophagus). Esophageal ulcers have also been reported with the use of BPs, especially when the tablet is not completely swallowed.

> ### ! NURSING SAFETY PRIORITY
> **Drug Alert**
>
> Teach patients to take bisphosphonates (BPs) early in the morning with 8 ounces of water and wait 30 to 60 minutes in an upright position before eating. If chest discomfort occurs, a symptom of esophageal irritation, instruct patients to discontinue the drug and contact their health care provider. Patients with poor renal function, hypocalcemia, or gastroesophageal reflux disease (GERD) should not take BPs.

The most recent additions to the bisphosphonates are IV zoledronic acid (Reclast) and IV pamidronate (Aredia). For management of osteoporosis, Reclast is needed only once a year and Aredia is given every 3 to 6 months. Both drugs have been linked to a complication called jaw osteonecrosis (jaw bone death) in which infection and necrosis of the mandible or maxilla occur (Lee, 2009). The incidence of this serious problem is low but can be a complication of this infusion therapy.

> ### ! NURSING SAFETY PRIORITY
> **Drug Alert**
>
> Teach the patient to have an oral assessment and preventive dentistry before beginning any bisphosphonate therapy. Instruct the patient to inform any dentist who is planning invasive treatment, such as a tooth extraction or implant, that he or she is taking a BP (Cohen, 2010).

Estrogen Agonist/Antagonists. Formerly called the *selective estrogen receptor modulators (SERMs)*, estrogen agonist/antagonists are a class of drugs designed to mimic estrogen in some parts of the body while blocking its effect elsewhere. Raloxifene (Evista) is currently the only approved drug in this class and is used for *prevention and treatment* of osteoporosis in postmenopausal women. Raloxifene increases bone mineral density (BMD), reduces bone resorption, and reduces the incidence of osteoporotic vertebral fractures. The drug should not be given to women who have a history of thromboembolism.

Other Agents. Parathyroid hormone is prepared as *teriparatide* under the brand name *Forteo* and is a bone-building agent approved for *treatment* of osteoporosis in postmenopausal women with high risk for fracture. Teach patients to self-administer Forteo as a daily subcutaneous injection. This drug stimulates new bone formation, thus increasing BMD. Reduced risk for fracture in the spine, hip, and wrist has been reported in women, and reduced risk for hip fracture has been reported in men. Patients may experience dizziness or leg cramping as side effects of Forteo (National Osteoporosis Foundation, 2010). Teach the patient to lie down if these problems occur and notify the health care provider as soon as possible.

Calcitonin is a thyroid hormone that inhibits osteoclastic activity, thus decreasing bone loss. It is used for the *treatment* of osteoporosis, Paget's disease, and hypercalcemia associated with cancer. The drug also has an analgesic effect after vertebral fracture, thereby promoting early recovery.

Calcitonin can be given subcutaneously or intranasally. The nasal route is preferred because it improves drug adherence, decreases side effects, and is convenient. However, the effect of calcitonin may decrease after use for 2 or more years. Patients may require a holiday from this treatment to maintain effectiveness. Teach the patient to alternate nares to prevent mucosal irritation, a common side effect. The drug must be refrigerated.

Community-Based Care

Patients with osteoporosis are usually managed at home. Osteoporosis disease-management programs managed by nurse practitioners have helped diagnose and treat the disease. Greene and Dell (2010) reported that over a 6-year period, a

CHART 53-2 **COMMON EXAMPLES OF DRUG THERAPY**

Osteoporosis

DRUG AND USUAL DOSAGE	PURPOSE OF DRUG	NURSING INTERVENTIONS	RATIONALES
Supplements			
Calcium (with vitamin D if needed) (e.g., Os-Cal, Citracal) 1-1.5 g in divided doses orally daily	Increases calcium intake (and vitamin D if needed)	Give a third of daily dose at bedtime. Push fluids.	Calcium is most readily utilized by the body when the patient is fasting and immobile. Increased fluid intake aids in preventing the formation of calcium-based urinary stones.
		Assess for a history of urinary stones.	Calcium supplements are not given to patients who are susceptible to urinary stone formation.
		Monitor serum calcium level.	Hypercalcemia, or calcium excess, is a side effect of calcium supplementation.
		Monitor urinary calcium level (no more than 4 mg/kg in 24 hr).	The kidneys attempt to excrete excess calcium.
		Observe for signs of hypercalcemia.	Hypercalcemia can result in urinary stones, cardiac dysrhythmias, and an increase or decrease in skeletal muscle tone.
Bisphosphonates			
Alendronate (Fosamax) or (Fosamax plus D) **For Prevention:** 5 mg orally daily or 35 mg orally weekly (available as tablet or liquid) **For Treatment:** 10 mg orally daily or 70 mg orally weekly with 2800-5600 international units of vitamin D	Prevents bone loss and increases bone density	Take on an empty stomach, first thing in the morning with a full glass of water. Take 30 minutes before food, drink, or other drugs. Remain upright, sitting or standing, for 30 minutes after administration. Take liquid (75 mL) and follow with 2 ounces of water.	Difficulty swallowing, esophagitis, esophageal ulcers, and gastric ulcers can result from alendronate therapy. Any of these should be reported to a health care provider as soon as possible.
Risedronate (Actonel) or (Actonel with Calcium) 5 mg orally daily, 35 mg orally every week, or 150 mg monthly	Same as for alendronate	Follow interventions for alendronate. Observe for CNS side/adverse effects, such as drowsiness, anxiety, agitation.	Same as for alendronate. Drug can also cause CNS effects that may not be tolerated.
Ibandronate (Boniva) 150 mg orally once every month or 3.375 mg IV every 3 months	Same as for alendronate	Take on the same day each month. Take on an empty stomach, first thing in the morning with a full glass of water. Take 60 minutes before food, drink, or other drugs. Remain upright for 1 hour after administration.	Same as for alendronate.
Zoledronic acid (Reclast, Zometa) **For Prevention:** 5 mg IV once every 2 years **For Treatment:** 5 mg IV once a year	Same as for other bisphosphonates	Infuse over 15-30 minutes.	The drug should not be infused too quickly to prevent rare complications such as atrial fibrillation.
		Make sure the patient has a dental examination before starting the drug.	The drug can cause jaw or maxillary osteonecrosis, particularly if oral hygiene is poor.
		Do not give to patients who are sensitive to aspirin.	The patient may experience bronchoconstriction.
		Check serum creatinine before and after administering the drug.	The drug can cause renal insufficiency or kidney failure.
Estrogen Agonist/Antagonists*			
Raloxifene (Evista) 60 mg orally daily	Prevents bone loss and increases bone density	Teach patient signs and symptoms of VTE.	Raloxifene can cause increased risk for VTE, especially in the first 4 months of therapy.
		Monitor liver function tests (LFTs) in collaboration with health care provider.	Raloxifene can cause increased LFT values or worsen hepatic disease (should not be given to patient who has liver disease).

CNS, Central nervous system; *VTE*, venous thromboembolism.
*Formerly Selective Estrogen Receptor Modulators (SERMs).

❓ DECISION-MAKING CHALLENGE

Patient-Centered Care; Evidence-Based Practice

A 62-year-old patient visits the physician's office to receive her first treatment for osteoporosis. She has a recent history of a badly fractured ankle and osteopenia (for which she has been taking Actonel). Her mother and grandmother had osteoporosis and osteoarthritis. The patient does not smoke but enjoys an occasional glass of wine when she and her husband go out for dinner. She drinks only 1 or 2 cups of caffeinated beverages a day. Although she realizes the importance of regular exercise, she has no time to fit that into her schedule because she travels throughout the country for her job. As her office nurse, you will be monitoring her as she has her first dose of Reclast.

1. What risk factors does this patient have for osteopenia and osteoporosis?
2. What health teaching might this patient need? How can you help her plan time for increasing her physical activity level? What does current evidence show that supports your answer?
3. What actions will you take before starting her Reclast?
4. How fast will you administer the drug, and what method will you use?

large osteoporosis disease-management program resulted in a 263% increase in the number of DXA scans done each year, a 153% increase in the number of patients treated with drug therapy, and a 38.1% decrease in the expected hip fracture rate.

Some patients have fractures that may require hospitalization or medical management in an emergency department (ED) or urgent care setting. In any setting, assess for risk factors for osteoporosis and provide health teaching as appropriate.

The patient with osteoporosis who has one or more fractures may be discharged to the home setting. In some instances, though, the patient is transferred to a long-term care facility for rehabilitation or permanent residence when support systems are not available. Collaborate with case managers or discharge planners to assist in preparing patients and their families for placement in long-term care facilities. Chapter 54 discusses continuing care for patients who have fractures.

Refer patients to the National Osteoporosis Foundation (www.nof.org) in the United States to provide information to patients and health care professionals regarding the disease and its treatment. The Osteoporosis Society of Canada (www.osteoporosis.ca) has similar services. Large hospitals often have osteoporosis specialty clinics and support groups for patients with osteoporosis.

OSTEOMALACIA

Pathophysiology

Osteomalacia is loss of bone related to a vitamin D deficiency. It causes softening of the bone resulting from inadequate deposits of calcium and phosphorus in the bone matrix. Normal remodeling of the bone is disrupted, and calcification does not occur. Osteomalacia is the adult equivalent of rickets, or vitamin D deficiency, in children.

Vitamin D deficiency is the most important factor in development of osteomalacia. In its natural form, vitamin D is activated by the ultraviolet radiation of the sun and obtained from certain foods as a nutritional supplement. In combination with calcium and phosphorus, the vitamin is necessary for bone formation.

TABLE 53-2	DIFFERENTIAL FEATURES OF OSTEOPOROSIS AND OSTEOMALACIA	
CHARACTERISTIC	**OSTEOPOROSIS**	**OSTEOMALACIA**
Definition	Decreased bone mass	Demineralized bone
Pathophysiology	Lack of calcium	Lack of vitamin D
Radiographic findings	Osteopenia, fractures	Pseudofractures, Looser's zones, fractures
Calcium level	Low or normal	Low or normal
Phosphate level	Normal	Low or normal
Parathyroid hormone	Normal	High or normal
Alkaline phosphatase	Normal	High

TABLE 53-3	CAUSES OF OSTEOMALACIA

Vitamin D Disturbance
- Inadequate production
- Lack of sunlight exposure
- Dietary deficiency
- Abnormal metabolism
- Drug therapy
  - Phenytoin (Dilantin)
  - Fluoride
  - Barbiturates
- Liver disease
- Renal disease

- Inadequate absorption
  - Postgastrectomy
  - Malabsorption syndrome
- Inflammatory bowel disease

Kidney Disease
- Chronic kidney disease
- Acute tubular disorders
  - Acidosis
  - Hypophosphatemia

Familial Metabolic Error
- Hypophosphatemia

Osteomalacia is frequently confused with osteoporosis because of similar characteristics shared by the two disease processes. Table 53-2 compares and contrasts osteoporosis and osteomalacia.

In addition to primary disease related to lack of sunlight exposure or dietary intake, vitamin D deficiency caused by various health problems may result in osteomalacia (Table 53-3). Malabsorption of vitamin D from the small bowel is a common complication of partial or total gastrectomy and bypass or resection surgery of the small intestine. Disease of the small bowel, such as Crohn's disease, may cause decreased vitamin and mineral absorption.

Liver and pancreatic disorders disrupt vitamin D metabolism and decrease its production. Chronic kidney disease (CKD) interferes with the synthesis of calcitriol, the most active vitamin metabolite. Osteomalacia can also be caused by bone tumors (oncogenic or tumor-induced osteomalacia).

Conditions that contribute to phosphate depletion (hypophosphatemia) lead to osteomalacia because they stimulate movement from bone and prevent calcium uptake in the bone. Osteomalacia is also an adverse effect of certain drugs, particularly anticonvulsants, barbiturates, and fluoride. The exact mechanism for the drug effects is not known. Genetic deviations in vitamin D or phosphate metabolism may contribute to bone changes seen in osteomalacia.

Osteomalacia is not common in the United States and Western Europe. However, it is more common in less affluent nations and in countries where famine is common.

Newcomers from these countries may seek health care in the United States. Older adults are most at risk. This group may have inadequate exposure to sunlight or intake of vitamin D–fortified foods. People who adhere to very restrictive vegan diets without adequate supplement of vitamin D can also be at risk. Assess for the risk for osteomalacia in anyone who has poor nutritional intake related to homelessness, who severely abuses drugs or alcohol, or who is very poor.

Health Promotion and Maintenance

To prevent or help treat osteomalacia, teach patients to increase vitamin D through dietary intake, sun exposure, and drug supplements. Instruct the at-risk patient about foods high in vitamin D, such as milk and food that has had it added. Remind patients that cheese and yogurt rarely contain vitamin D although they are rich in calcium. Instruct them to read food labels for nutrient content. Remind patients, especially those who are homebound, about the importance of daily sun exposure (at least 5 minutes each day) for the most important source of vitamin D.

Some people are lactose intolerant or do not use dairy products because of their vegan diets. However, many products are available for people who avoid dairy products. Soy and rice milk, tofu, and soy products are substitutes, but they are expensive. Teach patients to choose those products that are fortified with vitamin D. Other foods rich in the vitamin are eggs, swordfish, chicken, and liver, as well as enriched cereals and bread products. The at-risk patient should also take vitamin D supplements as prescribed by his or her health care provider.

PATIENT-CENTERED COLLABORATIVE CARE

ASSESSMENT

Collect important data for the patient with osteomalacia or suspected osteomalacia, including age, ability to be exposed to sunlight, and skin pigmentation. The older adult who has been homebound or chronically institutionalized is at the greatest risk. People who have dark skin and who may consume minimal protein are more at risk than light-skinned people with the same dietary habits. Dark-skinned people tend to avoid the sun and need protein for calcium binding. Take a thorough nutritional history to determine the intake of foods containing vitamin D and calcium. Coordinate the assessment with the dietitian.

Assessment includes any history of chronic disease processes of the GI tract including inflammatory bowel disease, gastric or intestinal bypass surgery, or any problem that interferes with absorption from the GI tract. A history of renal or liver dysfunction may lead to ineffective metabolism of vitamin D. Drugs such as phenytoin (Dilantin) or fluoride preparations may also interfere with metabolism of vitamin D.

Osteomalacia is easily confused with osteoporosis, and both disorders may occur at the same time (see Table 53-2). In the early stages of osteomalacia, the manifestations are nonspecific. Muscle weakness and bone pain may be misdiagnosed as arthritis or other connective tissue disorder. In some cases, proximal muscle weakness in the shoulder and pelvic girdle area is the only presenting symptom.

Muscle weakness in the lower extremities may cause a waddling and unsteady gait, which contributes to falls and subsequent fractures. Hypophosphatemia leads to an inadequate production of muscle cell adenosine triphosphate, thus resulting in a decrease in muscle cell energy. If hypocalcemia is present, muscle cramping may occur with weakness.

In collaboration with the physical therapist, assess muscle strength and observe the patient's gait. Document concerns about muscle cramps and bone pain. Skeletal discomfort is often vague and generalized. The spine, ribs, pelvis, and lower extremities are most often affected. The patient usually describes the pain as aggravated by activity and worse at night.

Palpate the affected bones for tenderness. Bone tenderness may occur when pressure is applied to the tibia or rib cage. Skeletal malalignment, like long-bone bowing or spinal deformity, may be similar to that seen in osteoporosis. In extreme cases, the pelvis narrows, so vaginal childbirth is difficult. If osteomalacia is untreated, vertebral, rib, and long-bone fractures may occur. The patient may be misdiagnosed as having bone cancer or osteoporosis.

X-rays of bone in patients with osteomalacia reveal a decrease in the cancellous bone and lack of osteoid sharpness. The classic diagnostic finding specific to the disease, however, is the presence of radiolucent bands (Looser's lines or zones). Looser's zones represent stress fractures that have not mineralized. They often appear symmetrically in the medial area of the femoral neck, ribs, and pelvis and may progress to complete fractures with minimal trauma. Bone biopsy of these areas may be needed for complete diagnosis. DXA scan may assist in diagnosis of osteomalacia.

INTERVENTIONS

The major treatment for osteomalacia is vitamin D in an active form, such as ergocalciferol. Studies indicate that large doses over a short period can correct low vitamin D status. For example, Przybelski et al. (2008) measured the serum vitamin D levels of 63 nursing home residents. Twenty-five residents had low serum levels and were given ergocalciferol 50,000 international units three times a week. After the treatment period, the mean total vitamin D serum concentration in the treated residents increased from 17.3 to 63.8 ng/mL. The researchers concluded that nursing home residents should be routinely screened to identify and treat those with low vitamin D levels to decrease the risk for fractures from osteomalacia and osteoporosis. Vitamin D is needed to adequately absorb and utilize calcium in the body.

Nurses play a vital role in educating other health care professionals about the need to screen patients for low vitamin D levels. For all at-risk patients, teach them about which high calcium and vitamin D foods to eat and the important of adequate daily sunlight. Additional health teaching is discussed above in the Health Promotion and Maintenance section.

PAGET'S DISEASE OF THE BONE

Pathophysiology

Paget's disease, or osteitis deformans, is a chronic metabolic disorder in which bone is excessively broken down (osteoclastic activity) and re-formed (osteoblastic activity). The result is bone that is structurally disorganized, causing bones to be weak with increased risk for bowing of long bones and fractures. Two types of Paget's disease can occur—familial and sporadic.

Three pathophysiologic phases of the disorder have been described: active, mixed, and inactive. In the first phase (the active phase), a rapid increase in osteoclasts (cells that break down bone) causes massive bone destruction and deformity. The osteoclasts of pagetic bone are large and multinuclear, unlike the osteoclasts of normal bone tissue.

In the mixed phase, the osteoblasts (bone-forming cells) react to compensate in forming new bone. The result is bone that is vascular, structurally weak, and deformed. Paget's disease occurs in one bone or in multiple sites. The most common areas of involvement are the vertebrae, femur, skull, clavicle, humerus, and pelvis.

When the osteoblastic activity exceeds the osteoclastic activity, the inactive phase occurs. The newly formed bone becomes sclerotic and very hard.

GENETIC/GENOMIC CONSIDERATIONS

Because Paget's disease is often present in identical twins, an autosomal dominant pattern has been suggested. The disease has been noted in up to 30% of people with a positive family history for Paget's disease. Several complex genetic factors have been identified in families with the disease, including mutations in the:

- *RANKL/RANK/OPG* system, which is needed for osteoclast development and activity (see p. 1121 in the Osteoporosis section)
- Valosin-containing gene of complement binding protein *(VCP)*, an important inflammatory factor
- Sequestosome 1 *(SQSTM1)* or *p62*, an expressed adaptor protein that can bind to ubiquitin and the atypical protein kinase C (Najat et al., 2009).

Teach patients the importance of genetics in familial Paget's disease, and refer them to the appropriate genetic counseling resource. Ask the patient if genetic testing is desired.

Paget's disease is second only to osteoporosis as one of the most common bone diseases in the United States, affecting about one million people. The disease is seen more frequently in people ages 50 years and older and in those of European heritage. The risk for developing Paget's disease increases as a person ages, particularly in those 80 years old and older. Men are affected twice as often as women (National Institute of Arthritis and Musculoskeletal and Skin Diseases, 2010).

PATIENT-CENTERED COLLABORATIVE CARE

ASSESSMENT

Physical Assessment/Clinical Manifestations

Most patients are asymptomatic, and the disease may be confined to one bone. It may be accidentally discovered during a routine laboratory or x-ray examination. In more severe disease, the manifestations are diverse and potentially fatal (Chart 53-3).

Ask the patient about a history of fracture and current bone pain. Bone pain, usually described as mild to moderate, may cause the patient to seek medical attention. The most common sites for pain are the hip and pelvis, but even the bones in the ear may be affected, causing hearing loss. The pain is usually described as aching, poorly defined, deep, and worsened by pressure. It is most noticeable at night or when

---

CHART 53-3   **KEY FEATURES**

Paget's Disease of the Bone

Musculoskeletal Manifestations
- Bone and joint pain (may be in a single bone) that is aching, poorly described, and aggravated by walking
- Low back and sciatic nerve pain
- Bowing of long bones
- Loss of normal spinal curvature
- Enlarged, thick skull
- Pathologic fractures
- Osteogenic sarcoma (bone cancer)

Skin Manifestations
- Flushed, warm skin

Other Manifestations
- Apathy, lethargy, fatigue
- Hyperparathyroidism
- Gout
- Urinary or renal stones
- Heart failure from fluid overload

---

the patient is resting. Patients may report redness and warmth at affected sites. These manifestations may be related to increased vascularity and blood flow.

The pain associated with the disorder may result from metabolic bone activity, secondary arthritis, impending fracture, or nerve impingement. Arthritis often occurs at the joints (cartilage) of the affected bones, resulting from bowing in the long bones of the leg. Some patients have joint replacements as a result of very painful weight-bearing joints. Nerve impingement is particularly common in the lumbosacral area of the vertebral column, presenting as back pain that radiates along one or both legs.

Observe posture, stance, and gait to identify gross bony deformities. Because of the enlargement of the vertebrae, loss of normal spinal curvature, and lower extremity malalignment, the patient may have decreased height. Assess for kyphosis or scoliosis of the spinal column. Note any long-bone bowing in the legs with subsequent varus (bow-leg) deformity. Long bones of the arms may also develop bowing. Flexion contracture in the hip joint is often present. Any of these deformities may be asymmetric. This weakened bone is at risk for fracture from even a minor injury. All of these problems interfere with the patient's need for independent mobility.

When performing a musculoskeletal assessment in a patient with Paget's disease, pay particular attention to the size and shape of the skull, which is typically soft, thick, and enlarged. Pressure from an enlarged temporal bone may lead to deafness and vertigo (dizziness). Basilar (in the occipital area) complications can compress any of the cranial nerves and result in neurologic problems. Assess the patient for changes in vision, swallowing, hearing, and speech. Platybasia, or basilar invagination, causes brainstem (vital sign center) damage that threatens life. In some cases, the bony enlargement of the skull blocks cerebrospinal fluid (CSF), resulting in hydrocephalus.

Pathologic fractures may be the presenting clinical manifestation of the disorder. The femur and the tibia are most often affected, and fracture of these bones can result from minimal trauma. The fracture line is usually perpendicular to the long axis of the bone, and healing is unpredictable because of abnormal metabolic activity within the bone.

Although rare, bones affected by Paget's disease may develop malignant changes. The most dreaded complication of Paget's disease is cancer, most commonly osteogenic sarcoma. Increased incidence of sarcoma occurs in men in the 70- to 80-year-old group. It affects the femur, humerus, and old fracture sites and has a grave prognosis because of early metastasis to the lung or extensive local invasion. When severe bone pain is present in a patient with Paget's disease, bone cancer is suspected.

Assess the skin for its color and temperature. In people with Paget's disease, the skin is typically flushed and warm because of increased blood flow. In addition, assess the patient's energy level because apathy, lethargy, and fatigue are common.

Other less common manifestations of Paget's disease include hyperparathyroidism and gout. Secondary hyperparathyroidism leads to an increase in serum and urinary calcium levels. In severe cases, serum calcium excess results from prolonged immobilization. Calcium deposits occur in joint spaces or as stones in the urinary tract. **Hyperuricemia** (serum uric acid excess) and gout occur because the increased metabolic activity of bone creates an increase in nucleic acid catabolism. Therefore kidney stones are more common in people with Paget's disease.

In a few cases, increased blood flow causes the heart to work harder to increase cardiac output, resulting in heart failure if not treated. Cardiac complications tend to occur only when more than a third of the skeleton is involved.

Diagnostic Assessment

Increases in *serum alkaline phosphatase (ALP)* and urinary hydroxyproline levels are the primary laboratory findings indicating possible Paget's disease. Overactive osteoblasts cause an altered ALP level. ALP can be further evaluated by alkaline phosphatase isoenzymes. The isoenzyme testing can further break ALP into three fractions—liver, bone, and intestinal. Elevated bone isoenzymes can help in a more definitive diagnosis of Paget's disease. Serum isoenzyme levels of bone ALP are used to monitor effectiveness of treatment (Pagana & Pagana, 2010).

The 24-hour *urinary hydroxyproline* level reflects bone collagen turnover and indicates the degree of disease severity. The higher the hydroxyproline, the more severe is the disease.

The *calcium* levels in blood and urine may be low, normal, or elevated. The immobilized patient is more likely to have an increase in calcium levels as a result of calcium moving from bone into the blood.

Paget's disease often causes an elevated *uric acid* because nucleic acid from overactive bone metabolism increases. This finding may be misinterpreted as primary gout.

X-rays are also used to diagnose Paget's disease. They reveal characteristic changes including the presence of osteolytic lesions and enlarged bones with radiolucent, or punched-out, appearance. Decrease in joint space may be seen with arthritic changes in joints. Malalignment deformities, fractures, and secondary arthritic changes may be present.

Radionuclide bone scan may be most sensitive in detecting Paget's disease. A radiolabeled bisphosphonate is injected IV and shows pagetic bone in areas of high bone turnover activity. This test can determine the extent of Paget's disease in the skeleton. Computed tomography (CT) is useful in the detection of cancerous tumors, changes in the skull, and spinal cord or nerve compression. Magnetic resonance imaging (MRI) may also be used for the same purpose as the CT scan.

▌INTERVENTIONS

Nonsurgical or surgical management may be necessary to reduce pain and promote *mobility*. Nonsurgical interventions are used first.

Drug Therapy

The primary intervention for Paget's disease is drug therapy. Potent prescription drugs are used to treat Paget's disease. In addition, simple analgesics such as OTC NSAIDs can be used to control pain.

The purpose of *drug therapy* in Paget's disease is to relieve pain and to decrease bone resorption. Management of mild to moderate pain may include the use of aspirin or NSAIDs such as ibuprofen (Motrin, Apo-Ibuprofen ✦). When the calcium level is more than twice the normal value and the disease is widespread, the health care provider usually prescribes more potent drugs, such as selected bisphosphonates. Treatment with these agents for Paget's disease requires dosages and duration of therapy different from those for osteoporosis. Chart 53-2 includes information about some of these commonly used drugs.

Oral bisphosphonates are a first-line treatment choice for Paget's disease when alkaline phosphatase levels are at least twice the normal serum level. Alendronate (Fosamax), risedronate (Actonel), etidronate (Didronel), and tiludronate (Skelid) are given in tablet form. When oral agents are not effective, pamidronate (Aredia) and zoledronic acid (Reclast, Zometa) are administered IV. Aredia is given once every 3 months, and Reclast is given once a year as a single IV dose. These drugs are usually highly effective. To reduce the risk for hypocalcemia, patients should receive 1500 mg of calcium daily in divided doses and 800 international units of vitamin D daily for at least 2 weeks after zoledronic acid infusion unless they are prone to kidney stones. Chart 53-2 provides additional information about caring for patients receiving bisphosphonates.

Calcitonin is a hormone that seems to reduce bone resorption and, subsequently, relieve pain. The drug often causes a dramatic decrease in the alkaline phosphatase level in a few weeks. Calcitonin is approved for subcutaneous administration in treating Paget's disease because the nasal spray has shown to be ineffective. It binds to osteoclast receptors, therefore slowing bone breakdown. The drug may be used for those patients who do not tolerate bisphosphonates. Side effects of calcitonin include nausea, flushing, and skin rash. Skin testing may be done before administration of the first dose.

Other Interventions

In addition to administering drugs, implement physical measures to reduce pain and increase *mobility*. These measures may include application of heat and gentle massage. An exercise program may be started with the help of a physical therapist. Exercise may be difficult because of pain and danger of fracture. Non-impact exercise should be used, but the patient may benefit from strengthening and weight-bearing exercises. In collaboration with the physical therapist, teach the patient about ROM and gentle stretching. Additional interventions for pain relief, such as relaxation techniques, are discussed in Chapter 5.

Measures to promote bone health are also important and include a diet rich in calcium and vitamin D. Nutrition therapy for bone health is described on p. 1124 in the discussion of Interventions in the Osteoporosis section.

Provide the patient with information to contact the U.S. local chapter of The Paget Foundation (www.paget.org) and the Arthritis Foundation (www.arthritis.org). The Arthritis

Society in Canada (www.arthritis.ca) is also an excellent service. These resources provide information and support for the patient and family or significant others. Nutritional instruction should be similar to information given to the patient with osteoporosis.

💡 NCLEX EXAMINATION CHALLENGE

Physiological Integrity

A client is starting on alendronate (Fosamax) for prevention of osteoporosis. What precaution will the nurse include in the client's health teaching about this drug?
A. "Take with food or milk to prevent stomach upset."
B. "Monitor the drug injection site for redness or itching."
C. "Take the drug at night before you go to bed."
D. "Do not lie down for at least 30 minutes after taking the drug."

OSTEOMYELITIS

Infection in bony tissue can be a severe and difficult-to-treat problem. Bone infection can result in chronic recurrence of infection, loss of function and mobility, amputation, and even death.

Pathophysiology

Bacteria, viruses, or fungi can cause infection in bone known as osteomyelitis. Invasion by one or more pathogenic microorganisms stimulates the inflammatory response in bone tissue. The inflammation produces an increased vascular leak and edema, often involving the surrounding soft tissues. Once inflammation is established, the vessels in the area become thrombosed and release exudate (pus) into bony tissue. Ischemia of bone tissue follows and results in necrotic bone. This area of necrotic bone separates from surrounding bone tissue, and sequestrum is formed. The presence of sequestrum prevents bone healing and causes superimposed infection, often in the form of bone abscess. As shown in Fig. 53-2, the cycle repeats itself as the new infection leads to further inflammation, vessel thromboses, and necrosis.

Osteomyelitis is categorized as exogenous, in which infectious organisms enter from outside the body as in an open fracture, or endogenous, in which organisms are carried by the bloodstream from other areas of infection in the body.

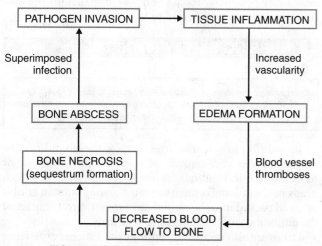

FIG. 53-2 Infection cycle of osteomyelitis.

Endogenous osteomyelitis may also be referred to as hematogenous osteomyelitis. A third category is contiguous, in which bone infection results from skin infection of adjacent tissues. Osteomyelitis can be further divided into two major types: acute osteomyelitis and chronic osteomyelitis.

Etiology

Each type of bone infection has its own causative factors. Pathogenic microbes favor bone that has a rich blood supply and a marrow cavity. Acute hematogenous infection results from bacteremia, underlying disease, or nonpenetrating trauma. Urinary tract infections, particularly in older men, tend to spread to the lower vertebrae. Long-term IV catheters (e.g., Hickman catheters) can be primary sources of infection. Patients undergoing long-term hemodialysis and IV drug abusers are also at risk for osteomyelitis. *Salmonella* infections of the GI tract may spread to bone. Patients with sickle cell disease and other hemoglobinopathies often have multiple episodes of salmonellosis, which can cause bone infection.

Poor dental hygiene and periodontal (gum) infection can be a causative factor in contiguous osteomyelitis in facial bones. Minimal nonpenetrating trauma can cause hemorrhages or small-vessel occlusions, leading to bone necrosis. Regardless of the source of infection, many infections are caused by *Staphylococcus aureus*. Treatment of infection may be complicated further by the presence of methicillin-resistant *Staphylococcus aureus* (MRSA) or other drug-resistant microorganism, which is very common in hospitalized and other institutionalized patients. One of the major desired outcomes in health care settings today is to reduce the number of MRSA infections from any source.

CONSIDERATIONS FOR OLDER ADULTS

Malignant external otitis media involving the base of the skull is sometimes seen in older adults with diabetes. The most common cause of contiguous spread in older adults, however, is found in those who have slow-healing foot ulcers. Multiple organisms tend to be responsible for the resulting osteomyelitis.

Penetrating trauma leads to acute osteomyelitis by direct inoculation. A soft-tissue infection may be present as well. Animal bites, puncture wounds, and bone surgery can result in bone infection. The most common offending organism is *Pseudomonas aeruginosa*, but other gram-negative bacteria may be found.

If bone infection is misdiagnosed or inadequately treated, chronic osteomyelitis may develop. Inadequate care management results when the treatment period is too short or when the treatment is delayed or inappropriate. About half of cases of chronic osteomyelitis are caused by gram-negative bacteria. Although bacteria are the most common causes of osteomyelitis, viruses and fungal organisms also may cause infection.

Incidence/Prevalence

Hematogenous osteomyelitis is the most common type of osteomyelitis. It occurs more often in children but is becoming increasingly common in adults, particularly older adults. Acute infection is more common in children. Chronic infection is more common in adults. Men have osteomyelitis more often than women, related to a higher incidence of blunt or penetrating trauma. Conditions such as malnutrition, alcoholism, diabetes, kidney or liver disease, and immune-suppressing disorders increase the risk and complicate effective treatment. Bone tissues in the vertebrae and long bones are common sites of infection. The adult with a compromised blood supply is at greatest risk for chronic infection. Advanced age and concurrent disease may prolong the course of the infection for as long as a year or more.

PATIENT-CENTERED COLLABORATIVE CARE

ASSESSMENT

Bone pain, with or without other manifestations, is a common concern of patients with bone infection. The pain is described as a constant, localized, pulsating sensation that worsens with movement.

The patient with *acute* osteomyelitis has fever, usually with temperature greater than 101° F (38.3° C). *Older adults may not have an extreme temperature elevation because of lower core body temperature and compromised immune system that occur with normal aging.* The area around the infected bone swells and is tender when palpated. Erythema (redness) and heat may also be present. When vascular compromise is severe, patients may not feel discomfort because of nerve damage from lack of blood supply.

When vascular insufficiency is suspected, assess circulation in the distal extremities. Ulcerations may be present on the feet or hands, indicating inadequate healing ability as a result of poor circulation.

Fever, swelling, and erythema are less common in those with *chronic* osteomyelitis. Ulceration resulting in sinus tract formation, localized pain, and drainage is more characteristic of chronic infection (Chart 53-4).

The patient with acute osteomyelitis usually has an elevated white blood cell (leukocyte) count, which may be double the normal value. In chronic infection, normal values or slight elevations may be seen.

The erythrocyte sedimentation rate (ESR) may be normal early in the course of the disease but rises as the condition progresses. It may remain elevated for as long as 3 months after drug therapy is discontinued.

If bacteremia is present, a potentially life-threatening complication that could lead to septic shock, a blood culture identifies the offending organisms to determine which antibiotics should be used in treatment. Both aerobic and anaerobic blood cultures should be collected before therapy is started.

Although bone changes cannot be detected early with standard x-rays, changes in blood flow can be seen early in the course of the disease by radionuclide scanning. A bone scan, using technetium or gallium, is extremely helpful in the diagnosis of osteomyelitis and identifies most cases. In some cases, MRI may be more sensitive than traditional bone scanning in the diagnosis of osteomyelitis.

INTERVENTIONS

The specific treatment protocol depends on the type and number of microbes present in the infected tissue. If other measures fail to resolve the infectious process, surgical management may be needed.

Nonsurgical Management

To reverse *acute* osteomyelitis, the health care provider starts antimicrobial (e.g., antibiotic) therapy as soon as possible. In the presence of copious wound drainage, Contact Precautions are used to prevent the spread of the offending organism to other patients and health care personnel. Teach patients, visitors, and staff members how to use these precautions. (See Chapter 25 for a discussion of Contact Precautions.)

IV antimicrobial therapy is usually prescribed for several weeks for acute osteomyelitis. More than one agent may be needed to combat multiple types of organisms. The hospital or home care nurse gives the drugs at specifically prescribed times so that therapeutic serum levels are achieved. Observe for the actions, side effects, and toxicity of these drugs. *Teach family members or other caregivers in the home setting how to administer antimicrobials if they are continued after hospital discharge or are used only at home.*

The optimal drug regimen for patients with chronic osteomyelitis is not well established. Prolonged therapy for more than 3 months may be needed to eliminate the infection. Because of the cost of lengthy hospital stays, patients are typically cared for in the home setting with long-term vascular access catheters, such as the peripherally inserted central catheter (PICC), for drug administration. After discontinuation of IV drugs, oral therapy may be needed for weeks or months. Patients and families must understand the complications of inadequate treatment or failure to follow up with health care providers. Teach them that drug therapy must be continued over a long period to be effective.

! NURSING SAFETY PRIORITY

Drug Alert

Even when symptoms of osteomyelitis appear to be improved, teach the patient and family that the full course of IV and oral antimicrobials must be completed to ensure that the infection is resolved.

In addition to systemic drug therapy, the wound may be irrigated, either continuously or intermittently, with one or more antibiotic solutions. A medical technique in which beads made of bone cement are impregnated with an antibiotic and packed into the wound can provide direct contact of the antibiotic with the offending organism.

Drugs are also needed to control pain. Patients experience acute and chronic pain and must receive a regimen of drug

---

CHART 53-4   KEY FEATURES

Acute and Chronic Osteomyelitis

Acute Osteomyelitis	Chronic Osteomyelitis
• Fever; temperature usually above 101° F (38.3° C)	• Ulceration of the skin
• Swelling around the affected area	• Sinus tract formation
• Erythema of the affected area	• Localized pain
• Tenderness of the affected area	• Drainage from the affected area
• Bone pain that is constant, localized, and pulsating; intensifies with movement	

therapy for control. Chapter 5 describes pharmacologic and nonpharmacologic interventions for both acute and chronic pain.

If an open wound or ulcer is present in the hospital or long-term care setting, the patient's treatment usually includes Standard Precautions for limited infections in which the wound is not draining but is covered. This practice may vary according to health care agency policy. Contact Precautions are reserved for more severe infections, particularly when the purulent material cannot be adequately contained by a dressing. Cover the open area and use clean technique when dressings are changed to prevent further contamination. The previous clinical practice was to use strict aseptic technique, but most agencies are now using clean technique for contaminated ("dirty") wounds. Wounds may be managed through the window of a cast, which must remain dry during dressing or irrigation procedures. Teach patients and families how to continue clean dressing procedures at home.

A treatment to increase tissue perfusion for patients with chronic, unremitting osteomyelitis is the use of a hyperbaric chamber or portable device to administer hyperbaric oxygen (HBO) therapy. These devices are usually available in large tertiary care centers and may not be accessible to all patients who might benefit from them. With HBO therapy, the affected area is exposed to a high concentration of oxygen that diffuses into the tissues to promote healing. In conjunction with high-dose drug therapy and surgical débridement, HBO has proven very useful in treating a number of anaerobic infections. Other wound-management therapies are described in Chapter 27.

Surgical Management

Antimicrobial therapy alone may not meet the desired outcome of treatment. Surgical techniques may be used to minimize the disfigurement that can be a devastating result of severe osteomyelitis. Surgery is reserved for patients with chronic osteomyelitis.

Because bone cannot heal in the presence of necrotic tissue, a *sequestrectomy* may be performed to débride the necrotic bone and allow revascularization of tissue. The excision of dead and infected bone often results in a sizable cavity, or bone defect. The use of bone *grafts* to repair bone defects is also widely used.

When infected bone is extensively resected, reconstruction with *microvascular bone transfers* may be done. This procedure is reserved for larger skeletal defects. The most common donor sites are the patient's fibula and iliac crest. The bone graft may have an attached muscle or skin flap, if necessary. The steps of the procedure are similar to those of bone grafting in that débridement of dead or necrotic bone is done before bone transfer.

Nursing care of the patient after surgery is similar to that for any postoperative patient (see Chapter 18). However, the important difference is that neurovascular (NV) assessments must be done frequently because the patient experiences increased swelling after the surgical procedure. Elevate the affected extremity to increase venous return and thus control swelling. Assess and document the patient's NV status, including:

- Pain
- Movement
- Sensation
- Warmth
- Temperature
- Distal pulses
- Capillary refill (not as reliable as the above indicators)

> **⚠ NURSING SAFETY PRIORITY**
> *Critical Rescue*
>
> *After surgery to treat osteomyelitis, frequently check for signs of neurovascular compromise, including **p**ain that cannot be controlled, **p**aresis or **p**aralysis (weakness or inability to move), **p**aresthesia (abnormal, tingling sensation), **p**allor, and **p**ulselessness. If any of these findings occur, report them immediately to the surgeon.*

If the bony defect is small, a *muscle flap* may be the only surgery required. Local muscle flaps are used in the treatment of chronic osteomyelitis when soft tissue does not fill the dead space, or cavity, resulting from bone débridement. The flap provides wound coverage and enhances blood flow to promote healing. A split-thickness skin graft is often applied several days after the muscle flap.

When the previously described surgical procedures are not appropriate or successful and as a last resort, the affected limb may need to be amputated. The physical and psychological care for a patient who has undergone an amputation is discussed in Chapter 54.

For all of the surgical procedures and their recovery phases, long-term antimicrobial treatment is necessary. The preoperative and postoperative nursing care is similar to that for repair of musculoskeletal trauma and is also discussed in Chapter 54.

BENIGN BONE TUMORS

Pathophysiology

Benign (noncancerous) bone tumors are often asymptomatic and may be discovered on routine x-ray examination or as the cause of pathologic fractures. The cause of benign bone tumors is not known. Tumors may arise from several types of tissue. The major classifications include chondrogenic tumors (from cartilage), osteogenic tumors (from bone), and fibrogenic tumors (from fibrous tissue and found most often in children). Although many specific benign tumors have been identified, only the common ones are described here.

The most common benign bone tumor is the *osteochondroma*. Although its onset is usually in childhood, the tumor grows until skeletal maturity and may not be diagnosed until adulthood. The tumor may be a single growth or multiple growths and can occur in any bone. The femur and the tibia are most often involved.

The *chondroma*, or endochondroma, is a lesion of mature hyaline cartilage affecting primarily the hands and the feet. The ribs, sternum, spine, and long bones may also be involved. Chondromas are slow growing and often cause pathologic fractures after minor injury. They are found in people of all ages, occur in both men and women, and can affect any bone.

The origin of the *giant cell tumor* remains uncertain. This lesion is aggressive and can be extensive and may involve surrounding soft tissue. Although classified as benign, giant cell tumors can metastasize (spread) to the lung. Unlike most other benign bone tumors, giant cell tumors affect women older than 20 years. The peak incidence occurs in patients in their 30s.

PATIENT-CENTERED COLLABORATIVE CARE

Assess for pain, the most common manifestation of benign bone tumors. Pain can range from mild to moderate. It can be caused by direct tumor invasion into soft tissue, compressing peripheral nerves, or by a resulting pathologic fracture.

In addition to assessing the patient's pain, observe and palpate the suspected involved area. When the tumor affects the lower extremities or the small bones of the hands and feet, local swelling may be detected as the tumor enlarges. In some cases, muscle atrophy or muscle spasm may be present. Carefully palpate the bone and muscle to detect these changes and elicit tenderness.

Routine x-rays and tomography are used to find bone tumors. Tumors are characterized by sharp margins, intact cortices, and smooth, uniform periosteal bone.

CT is less useful except in complex anatomic areas, such as the spinal column and sacrum. The test is helpful in evaluating the extent of soft-tissue involvement. MRI may be especially helpful in viewing problems of the spinal column.

The health care provider uses drug therapy and surgery in combination when possible. Non-drug pain relief measures are also used. Depending on the patient's preference and tolerance, measures such as heat or cold may help relieve pain.

In addition to prescribing analgesics to reduce pain, the health care provider usually prescribes one or more NSAIDs to inhibit prostaglandin synthesis that increases pain and inflammation. Give these drugs after meals or with food to reduce GI side effects.

The most common surgical procedure used for benign bone tumors is removal. If the tumor is small, surgery may not be needed. When the tumor is very extensive, as in a giant cell tumor, it is removed with care to restore or maintain the function of the adjacent joint, most often the knee. In some cases, the knee is replaced with a prosthetic device and, less often, is fused (arthrodesis). Bone grafting may be needed. The collaborative care for patients undergoing these surgical procedures is discussed in Chapter 20.

BONE CANCER

Cancerous bone tumors may be primary or secondary (those that originate in other tissues and metastasize to bone). *Primary tumors* occur most often in people between 10 and 30 years of age and make up a small percentage of bone cancers. As for other forms of cancer, the exact cause of bone cancer is unknown. *Metastatic lesions* most often occur in the older age-group and account for most bone cancers.

Previous radiation therapy in the anatomic area is a big risk factor. For example, bone cancer of the ribs in the path of radiation for breast cancer is fairly common.

Pathophysiology

Osteosarcoma, or osteogenic sarcoma, is the most common type of *primary* malignant bone tumor. More than 50% of cases occur in the distal femur, followed in decreasing order of occurrence by the proximal tibia and humerus.

The tumor is relatively large, causing acute pain and swelling. The involved area is usually warm because the blood flow to the site increases. The center of the tumor is sclerotic from increased osteoblastic activity. The periphery is soft, extending through the bone cortex in the classic sunburst appearance associated with the neoplasm. An inward spread into the medullary canal is also common.

Osteosarcoma typically metastasizes (spreads) to the periphery of the lung within 2 years of treatment. Metastasis usually results in death.

Osteosarcoma occurs twice as often in males as in females between ages 10 and 30 years and in older patients with Paget's disease. Patients who have received radiation for other forms of cancer or who have benign lesions are also at high risk.

Although *Ewing's sarcoma* is not as common as other tumors, it is the most malignant. Like other primary tumors, it causes pain and swelling. In addition, systemic manifestations, particularly low-grade fever, leukocytosis, and anemia, characterize the lesions. The pelvis and the lower extremity are most often affected. Pelvic involvement is a poor prognostic sign. It often extends into soft tissue. Death results from metastasis to the lungs and other bones. Although the tumor can be seen in patients of any age, it usually occurs in children and young adults in their 20s. Men are affected more often than women.

In contrast to the patient with osteosarcoma, the patient with *chondrosarcoma* experiences dull pain and swelling for a long period. The tumor typically affects the pelvis and proximal femur near the diaphysis. Arising from cartilaginous tissue, it destroys bone and often calcifies. The patient with this type of tumor has a better prognosis than one with osteogenic sarcoma. Chondrosarcoma occurs in middle-aged and older people, with a slight predominance in men.

Arising from fibrous tissue, *fibrosarcomas* can be divided into subtypes, of which malignant fibrous histiocytoma (MFH) is the most malignant. Usually, the clinical presentation of MFH is gradual, without specific symptoms. Local tenderness, with or without a palpable mass, occurs in the long bones of the lower extremity. As with other bone cancers, the lesion can metastasize to the lungs. Although MFH affects people of all ages, it typically occurs in middle-aged men but is not common.

Primary tumors of the prostate, breast, kidney, thyroid, and lung are called *bone-seeking* cancers because they spread to the bone more often than other primary tumors. The vertebrae, pelvis, femur, and ribs are the bone sites commonly affected. Simply stated, primary tumor cells, or seeds, are carried to bone through the bloodstream. *Pathologic fractures caused by metastatic bone are a major concern in patient care management.* The most commonly affected areas for fracture are the acetabulum and the proximal femur.

Metastatic bone tumors greatly outnumber primary bone tumors. They affect primarily people older than 40 years. In patients with a history of cancer and local pain, bone metastasis is suspected.

PATIENT-CENTERED COLLABORATIVE CARE

ASSESSMENT

The data collected for the patient suspected of having a malignant bone tumor are similar to the data needed for the patient with a benign growth. In addition, ask whether the patient has had previous radiation therapy for cancer and determine the status of the patient's general health.

The clinical manifestations seen in the patient with primary bone cancer or metastatic disease vary, depending on the specific type of lesion. Usually, the patient has a group of nonspecific concerns, including pain, local swelling, and a tender, palpable mass. Marked disability and impaired mobility may occur in those with advanced metastatic bone disease.

In a patient with Ewing's sarcoma, a low-grade fever may occur because of the systemic features of the neoplasm. For this reason, it is often confused with osteomyelitis. Fatigue and pallor resulting from anemia are also common.

In performing a musculoskeletal assessment, inspect the involved area and palpate the mass for size and tenderness. In collaboration with the physical and occupational therapists, assess the patient's ability to perform mobility tasks and ADLs.

Patients with malignant bone tumors may be young adults whose productive lives are just beginning. They need strong support systems to help cope with the diagnosis and its treatment. Family, significant others, and health care professionals are major components of the needed support. Determine what systems or resources are available.

Patients often experience a loss of control over their lives when a diagnosis of cancer is made. As a result, they become anxious and fearful about the outcome of their illness. Coping with the diagnosis becomes a challenge. As patients progress through the grieving process, there may be initial denial. Identify the anxiety level, and assess the stage or stages of the grieving process. Explore any maladaptive behavior, indicating ineffective coping mechanisms. Chapter 24 further describes the psychosocial assessment for patients with cancer.

The patient with a malignant bone tumor typically shows elevated serum alkaline phosphatase (ALP) levels, indicating the body's attempt to form new bone by increasing osteoblastic activity. The patient with Ewing's sarcoma or metastatic bone cancer often has anemia. In addition, leukocytosis is common with Ewing's sarcoma. The progression of Ewing's sarcoma may be evaluated by elevated serum lactic dehydrogenase (LDH) levels.

In some patients with bone metastasis from the breast, kidney, or lung, the serum calcium level is elevated. Massive bone destruction stimulates release of the mineral into the bloodstream. In patients with Ewing's sarcoma and bone metastasis, the erythrocyte sedimentation rate (ESR) may be elevated because of secondary tissue inflammation.

As with benign bone tumors, routine x-rays and CT reveal malignant lesions. Although each tumor type has its own characteristic radiographic pattern, certain findings are common to all. Cancerous tumors typically show poor demonstration of bone margins, bone destruction, irregular periosteal new bone, and breakthrough of the cortical layer.

Metastatic lesions may increase or decrease bone density, depending on the amount of osteoblastic and osteoclastic activity. CT is helpful in determining the extent of soft-tissue damage. The patient may have an MRI for difficult-to-visualize areas such as the vertebrae.

In some cases, a needle bone biopsy may be performed, usually under fluoroscopy to guide the surgeon. Needle biopsy is an outpatient procedure with rare complications. After biopsy, the cancer is staged for size and degree of spread. One popular method is the TNM staging system, based on tumor size and number (T), the presence of cancer cells in lymph nodes (N), and metastasis (spread) to distant sites (M).

Another staging method is to correlate the tumor grade (high or low), tumor site (intracompartmental or extracompartmental), and presence of metastatic disease (positive or negative). Staging guides the health care team in their decision regarding patient-centered collaborative care.

INTERVENTIONS

Because the pain is often due to direct primary tumor invasion, treatment is aimed at reducing the size of or removing the tumor. The expected outcome of treating metastatic bone tumors is palliative rather than curative. Palliative therapies may prevent further bone destruction and improve patient function. A combination of nonsurgical and surgical management is used. Members of the interdisciplinary health care team collaborate to plan the best approach for positive patient outcomes.

Nonsurgical Management

In addition to analgesics for local pain relief, chemotherapeutic agents and radiation therapy are often administered to shrink the tumor. In patients with spinal involvement, bracing and immobilization with cervical traction may reduce back pain. Interventional radiology techniques are used to decrease vertebral pain and treat compression fractures.

Drug Therapy. The physician may prescribe *chemotherapy* to be given alone or in combination with radiation or surgery. Certain proliferating tumors, such as Ewing's sarcoma, are sensitive to cytotoxic drugs. Others, such as chondrosarcomas, are often totally drug resistant. Chemotherapy seems to work best for small, metastatic tumors and may be administered before or after surgery. In most cases, the physician prescribes a combination of agents. At present, there is no universally accepted protocol of chemotherapeutic agents. The drugs selected are determined in part by the primary source of the cancer in metastatic disease. For example, when metastasis occurs from breast cancer, estrogen and progesterone blockers may be used. Chapter 24 describes the general nursing care of patients who receive chemotherapy. Remember that all chemotherapeutic agents are categorized as high-alert medications (Institute for Safe Medication Practices, 2008).

Other drugs are given for specific metastatic cancers, depending on the location of the primary site. For example, biologic agents, such as cytokines, are given to stimulate the immune system to recognize and destroy cancer cells, especially in patients with renal cancer. Zoledronic acid (Zometa) and pamidronate (Aredia) are two IV bisphosphonates that are approved for bone metastasis from the breast, lung, and prostate. These drugs help protect bones and prevent fractures. Inform patients that osteonecrosis of the jaw may also occur, especially in those who have invasive dental procedures. Monitor associated laboratory tests, such as serum creatinine and electrolytes, because these drugs can be toxic to the kidneys.

Radiation Therapy. Radiation, either brachytherapy or external radiation, is used for selected types of malignant tumors. For patients with Ewing's sarcoma and early osteosarcoma, radiation may be the treatment of choice in reducing tumor size and thus pain.

For patients with metastatic disease, radiation is given primarily for palliation. The therapy is directed toward the painful sites to provide a more comfortable life span. One or more treatments are given, depending on the extent of disease. With precise planning, radiation therapy can be used with minimal complications. The general nursing care for patients receiving radiation therapy is described in Chapter 24.

Interventional Radiology. Interventional radiologists can perform several noninvasive procedures to help relieve pain in the patient with metastasis to the spinal column. Two types of *thermal ablation techniques, radiofrequency ablation (RFA)* and cryoablation, can be done under moderate sedation or general anesthesia. RFA kills the targeted tissue with heat using a small needle inserted into the tumor. Most patients have pain relief or control after this ambulatory care procedure. *Cryoablation* is similar to RFA, but the radiologist uses an extremely cold gas through a probe into the tumor. Although this procedure has been available for years, newer surgical equipment allows a small incision and the patient can return to usual daily activities in a day or two.

The radiologist may also perform a *vertebroplasty* if the patient with spinal metastasis has pathologic compression fractures. After making a small incision, bone cement is injected through a needle into the fractured area. The cement hardens within 15 minutes. Like thermal ablation, this procedure is done in an ambulatory care setting and the patient is placed under moderate sedation.

Surgical Management

Primary bone tumors are usually reduced or removed with surgery and often combined with radiation or chemotherapy.

Preoperative Care. In addition to the nature, progression, and extent of the tumor, the patient's age and general health state are considered. Chemotherapy may be administered preoperatively.

As for any patient preparing for cancer surgery, the patient with bone cancer needs psychological support from the nurse and other members of the health care team. Assess the level of the patient's and family's understanding about the surgery and related treatments. As an advocate, encourage the patient and family to discuss concerns and questions and provide information regarding hospital routines and procedures. Spiritual support is important to some patients. They may prefer to contact a member of the clergy or a spiritual leader or talk with a clergy member affiliated with the hospital. Assist in arranging for spiritual assistance if requested.

Anticipate postoperative needs as much as possible before the patient undergoes surgery. Remind the patient what to expect postoperatively and how to help ensure adequate recovery.

Operative Procedures. Wide or radical resection procedures are used for patients with bone sarcomas to salvage the affected limb. Wide excision is removal of the lesion surrounded by an intact cuff of normal tissue and leads to cure of low-grade tumors only. A radical resection includes removal of the lesion, the entire muscle, bone, and other tissues directly involved. It is the procedure used for high-grade tumors.

Large bone defects that result from tumor removal may require either:

- Total joint replacements with prosthetic implants, either whole or partial
- Custom metallic implants
- Allografts from the iliac crest, rib, or fibula

As an alternative to total replacement, an allograft may be implanted with internal fixation for those patients who do not have metastases. This is a common procedure for sarcomas of the proximal femur. Allograft procedures for the knee are also performed, particularly in young adults. Preoperative chemotherapy is given to enhance the likelihood of success. Allografts with adjacent tendons and ligaments are harvested from cadavers and can be frozen or freeze-dried for a prolonged period. The graft is fixed with a series of bolts, screws, or plates.

Although not commonly done, patients with metastatic disease intractable (not reversible) pain can be surgically treated with percutaneous cordotomy (cutting of the spinal nerve roots). Cryosurgery (cold application) may reduce pain and tumor size.

Postoperative Care. The surgical incision for a limb salvage procedure is often extensive. A pressure dressing with wound suction is typically maintained for several days. The patient who has undergone a limb salvage procedure has some degree of impaired physical mobility and a self-care deficit. The nature and extent of the alterations depend on the location and extent of the surgery.

> ### ! NURSING SAFETY PRIORITY
> #### Action Alert
>
> *For patients who have allografts, observe for signs of hemorrhage, infection, or fracture. Report these changes to the surgeon immediately.*

Muscle strengthening and range-of-motion (ROM) exercises begin immediately postoperatively and continue for at least a year. After upper extremity surgery, the patient can engage in active-assistive exercises by using the opposite hand to help achieve motions such as forward flexion and abduction of the shoulder. Continuous passive motion (CPM) using a CPM machine may be initiated as early as the first postoperative day for either upper extremity or lower extremity procedures.

After lower extremity surgery, the emphasis is on strengthening the quadriceps muscles by using passive and active motion when possible. Maintaining muscle tone is an important prerequisite to weight bearing, which progresses from toe touch or partial weight bearing to full weight bearing by 3 months postoperatively. Coordinate the patient's plan of care for ambulation and muscle strengthening with the physical therapist.

The patient who has had a bone graft may have a cast or other supportive device for several months. Weight bearing is prohibited until there is evidence that the graft is incorporated into the adjacent bone tissue.

During the recovery phase, the patient may also need assistance with ADLs, particularly if the surgery involves the upper extremity. Assist if needed, but at the same time encourage the patient to do as much as possible unaided. Some patients need assistive/adaptive devices for a short period while they are healing. Coordinate the patient's plan of care for promoting independence in ADLs with the occupational therapist.

Surrounding tissues, including nerves and blood vessels, may be removed during surgery. Vascular grafting is common, but the lost nerve(s) is (are) usually not replaced. Assess the neurovascular status of the affected extremity and hand or foot every 1 to 2 hours immediately after surgery. Splinting or casting of the limb may also cause neurovascular (NV) compromise and needs to be checked for proper placement. Assess for NV compromise as described on p. 1133 under Surgical Management in the Osteomyelitis section.

Pelvic lesions, although not common, may also be surgically removed. Reconstruction generally entails bone fusion with muscle and nerve preservation. A hip spica cast or other device may be necessary until the graft has been incorporated. The patient may need a cane, crutches, or walker for ambulation.

The major complications of reconstructive surgery, such as a joint replacement, are superficial and deep wound infection, dislocation or loosening of the implants, and rapid neurovascular compromise. Report an increase in pain or temperature or a rapid deterioration in circulation to the surgeon promptly. Chapter 20 discusses postoperative care of patients having total joint replacements.

In addition to needing emotional support to cope with physical disabilities, the patient may need help coping with the surgery and its effects. Help identify available support systems as soon as possible.

As a result of most of the surgical procedures, the patient experiences an altered body image. Suggest ways to minimize cosmetic changes. For example, a lowered shoulder can be covered by a custom-made pad worn under clothing. The patient can cover lower extremity defects with pants.

The nurse's most important role is to be an active listener and to encourage the patient and family or significant others to verbalize their feelings. Counselors and members of the clergy or spiritual leaders may provide additional assistance in promoting acceptance of the diagnosis, treatment, or, possibly, impending death. Chapter 9 provides information about loss, death, and dying.

Regardless of the prognosis, a diagnosis of bone cancer is a major stressor that causes the patient and family or significant others to grieve. Help the patient and others cope with the loss and resolve the grief. Although patients are asked on admission to a health care agency if they want advance directives, they may have chosen not to have them. If a patient has terminal metastatic bone cancer, though, ask if he or she would like to complete advance directives, like a living will. If the patient already has written advance directives, be sure that a copy is on the medical record and has been given to the health care provider.

Advocate for the patient and the family to promote the physician-patient relationship. For instance, the patient may not completely understand the medical or surgical treatment plan but may hesitate to question the physician. The nurse's intervention can increase communication, which is essential in successful management of the patient with cancer.

Community-Based Care

After medical treatment for a primary malignant tumor, the patient is usually managed at home with follow-up care. The patient with metastatic disease may remain in the home or, when home support is not available, may be admitted to a long-term care facility for extended or hospice care. Coordinate the patient's discharge plan and continuity of care with

? DECISION-MAKING CHALLENGE

Patient-Centered Care; Teamwork and Collaboration; Safety

A 75-year-old widow reports pain in her right rib cage area. She had a right simple mastectomy 8 years ago and was thought to be cancer-free until this time. A chest x-ray revealed bone metastasis in several ribs. On additional testing, the patient was found to also have multiple bone lesions in her right femur and pelvis. The patient is admitted to the cancer center for intensive treatment. Her only daughter is with her.

1. The patient states that she is very angry that her cancer has returned because she thought it was cured. She wonders if she should not have had a double mastectomy 8 years ago and perhaps the bone cancer could have been prevented. How will you respond to her feelings?
2. What treatment options does this patient have to manage her bone cancer? What is the purpose of treating the cancer at this time?
3. For what major complications is this patient most at risk and how will you plan to help prevent them? (Hint: See Chapter 24.)
4. With what health care team members will you collaborate and why?
5. What will you tell the daughter about her condition?
6. What are the major considerations for discharge planning?

the case manager and other health care team members, depending on the patient's needs.

Home Care Management

In collaboration with the occupational therapist, evaluate the patient's home environment for structural barriers that may hinder mobility. The patient may be discharged with a cast, walker, crutches, or a wheelchair.

Accessibility to eating and toileting facilities is essential to promote ADL independence. Because the patient with metastatic disease is susceptible to pathologic fractures, potential hazards that may contribute to falls or injury should be removed.

Teaching for Self-Management

For the patient receiving intermittent chemotherapy or radiation on an ambulatory basis, emphasize the importance of keeping appointments. Review the expected side and toxic effects of the drugs with the patient and family. Teach how to treat less serious side effects and when to contact the health care provider. If the drugs are administered at home via long-term IV catheter, explain and demonstrate the care involved with daily dressing changes and potential catheter complications. Chapter 15 describes the health teaching required for a patient receiving infusion therapy at home.

If the patient has undergone surgery, he or she has a wound and limited *mobility*. Teach the patient, family, and/or significant others how to care for the wound. Help the patient learn how to perform ADLs and mobility activities independently for self-management. Coordinate with the physical and occupational therapists to assist in ADL teaching, and provide or recommend assistive and adaptive devices, if necessary. The physical therapist also teaches the proper use of ambulatory aids, such as crutches, and exercises.

Pain management can be a major problem, particularly for the patient with metastatic bone disease. Discuss the various options for pain relief, including relaxation and music therapy. Emphasize the importance of those techniques that worked during hospitalization.

The patient with bone cancer may fear that the malignancy will return. Acknowledge this fear, but reinforce confidence in the health care team and medical treatment chosen.

Mutually establish realistic outcomes regarding returning to work and participating in recreational activities. Encourage the patient to resume a functional lifestyle, but caution that it should be gradual. Certain activities, such as participating in sports, may be prohibited.

Help the patient with advanced metastatic bone disease prepare for death. The nurse and other support personnel assist the patient through the stages of death and dying. Identify resources that can help the patient write a will, visit with distant family members, or do whatever he or she thinks is needed for a peaceful death. In the later stages of the disease, hospice care may be an option (see Chapter 9). Nurses working in this area of care can be most helpful in managing end-of-life care.

Health Care Resources

In addition to family and significant others, cancer support groups are helpful to the patient with bone cancer. Some organizations, such as *I Can Cope*, provide information and emotional support. Others, such as *CanSurmount*, are geared more toward patient and family education. The American Cancer Society (www.cancer.org) and the Canadian Cancer Society (www.cancer.ca) can also provide education and resources for patients and families.

The hospital staff nurse, discharge planner, or case manager also ensures that follow-up care, including nursing care and physical or occupational therapy, is available in the home. The patient with terminal cancer may choose to become part of a hospice program.

DISORDERS OF THE HAND

Dupuytren's Contracture

Dupuytren's contracture, or deformity, is a slowly progressive thickening of the palmar fascia, resulting in flexion contracture of the fourth (ring) and fifth (little) fingers of the hand. The third or middle finger is occasionally affected. Although Dupuytren's contracture is a common problem, the cause is unknown. It usually occurs in older Euro-American men, tends to occur in families, and can be bilateral.

When function becomes impaired, surgical release is required. A partial or selective fasciectomy (cutting of fascia) is performed. After removal of the surgical dressing, a splint may be used. Nursing care is similar to that for the patient with carpal tunnel repair (see Chapter 54).

Ganglion

A ganglion is a round, benign cyst, often found on a wrist or foot joint or tendon. The synovium surrounding the tendon degenerates, allowing the tendon sheath tissue to become weak and distended. Ganglia are painless on palpation, but they can cause joint discomfort after prolonged joint use or minor trauma or strain. The lesion can rapidly disappear and then recur. Ganglia are most likely to develop in people between 15 and 50 years of age. With local or regional anesthesia in a physician's office or clinic, the fluid within the cyst can be aspirated through a small needle. A cortisone injection

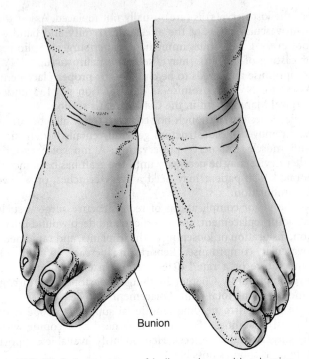

FIG. 53-3 Appearance of hallux valgus with a bunion.

may follow. If the cyst is very large, it is removed using a small incision. Patients should avoid strenuous activity for 48 hours after surgery and report any signs of inflammation to their physician.

DISORDERS OF THE FOOT

Foot Deformities

The hallux valgus deformity is a common foot problem in which the great toe drifts laterally at the first metatarsophalangeal (MTP) joint (Fig. 53-3). The first metatarsal head becomes enlarged, resulting in a bunion. As the deviation worsens, the bony enlargement causes pain, particularly when shoes are worn. Women are affected more often than men. Hallux valgus often occurs as a result of poorly fitted shoes—in particular, those with narrow toes and high heels. Other causes include osteoarthritis, rheumatoid arthritis, and family history.

The surgical procedure, a simple bunionectomy, involves removal of the bony overgrowth and bursa and realignment. When other toe deformities accompany the condition or if the bony overgrowth is large, several osteotomies, or bone resections, may be performed. Fusions may also be performed. Screws or wires are often inserted to stabilize the bones in the great toe and first metatarsal during the healing process. If both feet are affected, one foot is usually treated at a time. Surgery usually is performed as a same-day procedure.

Most patients are allowed partial weight bearing while wearing an orthopedic boot or shoe. Walking is difficult because the feet bear body weight. The healing time after surgery may be more than 6 to 12 weeks because the feet receive less blood flow than other parts of the body because of their distance from the heart.

Often patients have hammertoes and hallux valgus deformities at the same time. As shown in Fig. 53-4, a hammertoe

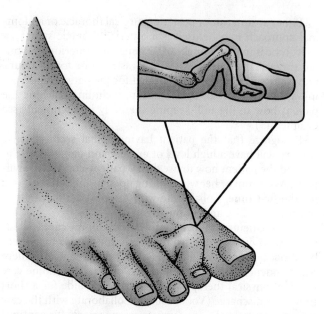

FIG. 53-4 Hammertoe of the second metatarsophalangeal joint.

TABLE 53-4	TREATMENT OF COMMON FOOT PROBLEMS
DESCRIPTION/CAUSE	**TREATMENT**
Corn Induration and thickening of the skin caused by friction and pressure; painful conical mass	Surgical removal by podiatrist
Callus Flat, poorly defined mass on the sole over a bony prominence caused by pressure	Padding and lanolin creams; overall good skin hygiene
Ingrown Nail Nail sliver penetration of the skin, causing inflammation	Removal of sliver by podiatrist; warm soaks; antibiotic ointment
Hypertrophic Ungual Labium Chronic hypertrophy of nail lip caused by improper nail trimming; results from untreated ingrown nail	Surgical removal of necrotic nail and skin; treatment of secondary infection

is the dorsiflexion of any MTP joint with plantar flexion of the proximal interphalangeal (PIP) joint next to it. The second toe is most often affected. As the deformity worsens, uncomfortable corns may develop on the dorsal side of the toe and calluses may appear on the plantar surface. Patients are uncomfortable when wearing shoes and walking.

Hammertoe may be treated by surgical correction of the deformity with osteotomies (bone resections) and the insertion of wires or screws for fixation. The postoperative course is similar to that for the patient with hallux valgus repair. The patient uses crutches until full weight bearing is allowed several weeks after surgery.

Morton's Neuroma

In the patient with Morton's neuroma, or plantar digital neuritis, a small tumor grows in a digital nerve of the foot. The patient usually describes the pain as an acute, burning sensation in the web space. The pain involves the entire surface of the third and fourth toes. Management involves surgical removal of the neuroma and application of a pressure dressing. Ambulation is usually permitted immediately after surgery.

Plantar Fasciitis

Plantar fasciitis is an inflammation of the plantar fascia, which is located in the area of the arch of the foot. It is often seen in middle-aged and older adults, as well as in athletes, especially runners. In ambulatory care settings, plantar fasciitis accounts for 10% of running injuries. Obesity is also a contributing factor.

Patients report severe pain in the arch of the foot, especially when getting out of bed. The pain is worsened with weight bearing. Although most patients have unilateral plantar fasciitis, the problem can affect both feet.

Most patients respond to conservative management, which includes rest, ice, stretching exercises, strapping of the foot to maintain the arch, shoes with good support, and orthotics. NSAIDs or steroids may be needed to control pain and

inflammation. If conservative measures are unsuccessful, endoscopic surgery to remove the inflamed tissue may be required.

Teach the patient about the importance of adhering to the treatment plan and coordinating care with the physical therapist for instruction in exercise.

Other Problems of the Foot

Table 53-4 lists other common foot problems and how they are managed. Although patients are usually not hospitalized for these conditions, the nurse may recognize a foot disorder and alert the physician. Even small deformities or other foot deformities can be very annoying and painful for the patient and may hinder ambulation, as well as interfere with ADLs.

SCOLIOSIS

Pathophysiology

Scoliosis occurs when the vertebrae rotate and begin to compress. The spinal column begins to move into a lateral curve, most commonly in the right lateral thoracic area (see Fig. 52-3 in Chapter 52). As the degree of curvature increases, damage to the vertebral bodies results. The degree of the curvature increases during periods of growth, such as in adolescence. Curvature of greater than 50 degrees results in an unstable spine, and curvature of greater than 60 degrees in the thoracic spine results in compromise of cardiopulmonary function.

The exact cause of scoliosis is not well understood, yet it affects about 6 million people in the United States. The process may result from some problem in the balance mechanism located in the central nervous system. Females are affected more often than males, and onset is often in adolescence. School health nurses screen children for scoliosis during the middle school years. Information about caring for children with scoliosis is found in most pediatric nursing textbooks. Scoliosis that occurs in childhood or early adolescence may persist into adulthood.

Three types of scoliosis can be described: congenital, neuromuscular, and idiopathic; the most common curve pattern in adults is idiopathic scoliosis and the cause is unknown (Voda, 2009a). Congenital scoliosis occurs during embryonic development. Neuromuscular scoliosis can result from a neuromuscular condition in childhood or adulthood, such as cerebral palsy or spinal cord tumors. Untreated scoliosis can lead to back pain, deformity, and cardiopulmonary complications.

PATIENT-CENTERED COLLABORATIVE CARE

ASSESSMENT

A complete history of the patient with spinal deformity should include onset of problem, in adolescence or adulthood, and what treatments may have been used in the past. Patients who had surgery for scoliosis during adolescence are returning with progressive, debilitating back pain from degenerative disk disease below the level of vertebral fusion. A loss of lumbar curvature, or lordosis, described as "flat back" syndrome, may also be present. Complete a thorough pain assessment for patients reporting back pain.

Observe the patient from the front and back, while standing and during forward flexion from the hips. Physical examination usually reveals asymmetry of hip and shoulder height, prominence of the thoracic ribs and scapula on one side, and visible curve in the spinal column. Observation from the side may reveal kyphosis of the thoracic spine. Assess for leg length differences as well.

Methods of managing adult scoliosis differ from those used for children. The adult spinal column is less flexible and therefore less likely to respond to exercises, weight reduction, bracing, and casting for correction of the deformity. In the adult, the disorder is progressive and can result in an additional one degree of deviation each year.

INTERVENTIONS

Adults with less than 50 degrees of curvature of the spine may be treated conservatively with moist heat, pain medication, and exercise. Those with greater than 50 degrees of curvature may require surgical intervention to prevent shortness of breath and fatigue, osteoarthritis, and severe back pain.

The *surgical* reconstructive procedure consists of surgical fusion and insertion of instrumentation, including plates, screws, or rods to stabilize the spine. The surgeon performs spinal fusion by packing cancellous bone chips, usually from the iliac crest, between the affected vertebrae for support and stabilization. Both an anterior and a posterior approach may be needed. If so, the surgeon may perform both procedures during the same operative day or may stage them 7 to 10 days apart. The metal instrumentation supports the spine and immobilizes the fused area during healing.

! NURSING SAFETY PRIORITY

Action Alert

The priority for nursing care after spinal reconstructive surgery is to assess the patient's respiratory status and encourage deep breathing. Teach the patient how to use the incentive spirometer to prevent atelectasis.

Either an anterior or posterior surgical thoracic or abdominal approach may be used. For anterior thoracic surgery, a chest tube is in place for about 72 hours; for anterior abdominal surgery, the patient has a nasogastric tube for 24 hours. Other nursing care is similar to that for the patient undergoing a laminectomy or spinal fusion, including teaching the patient how to log roll, keeping the body in alignment (see Chapter 45).

Recognize that the patient having spinal reconstructive surgery will have a high level of anxiety and pain. Be sure to remind the patient how to use the IV patient-controlled analgesia. Assist him or her when sitting up, standing, and walking for the first time. Collaborate with the physical therapist to improve mobility and ambulation.

Teach patients and their families about home care, including how to care for the wound; body mechanics to prevent bending, twisting, and lifting; and how to adapt to achieve ADLs independently. Some patients may require home care nursing, physical therapy, or a home health aide for a short time after discharge (Voda, 2009a). Collaborate with the case manager to make the appropriate arrangements for continuity of care to meet the patient's needs.

For some patients, a return to work in about 3 to 6 weeks is realistic. Other surgical procedures may prevent the patient from performing these activities until 3 to 6 months postoperatively. Refer patients and their families to the National Scoliosis Foundation (www.scoliosis.org) for information and support services.

PROGRESSIVE MUSCULAR DYSTROPHIES

Many types of muscular dystrophy (MD) have been categorized as slowly progressive or rapidly progressive. The slowly progressive types are most commonly seen in adults. Most pediatric nursing books describe the care for patients with MD in detail. Four forms of MD are often seen in adults. Each type has its own distinct characteristics and causes, but all are progressive (Table 53-5).

The exact pathophysiologic mechanisms are unknown, but several causes are possible. These include:

GENETIC/GENOMIC CONSIDERATIONS

The major pathologic change that occurs in most types of MD is the production or faulty action of a muscle protein called dystrophin. The purpose of this protein is to maintain muscle integrity by sending signals to coordinate smooth, synchronous muscle fiber contraction. The coding of this protein is by a large gene that has many parts located on the X chromosome. Different mutations of the gene where dystrophin is located determine the degree of muscle weakness. Because this protein connects with other substances for final muscle action, genetic mutations of these other substances can make dystrophin fail to work properly.

The most common forms of MD are Duchenne MD (DMD) and Becker MD (BMD). Both are X-linked recessive disorders. Women who are *carriers* (able to pass on the gene without having the disorder) have a 50% chance of passing the MD gene to their daughters, who are then carriers, and to their sons, who then have the disease. These types of MD, then, affect only males. In DMD, most patients die very young and therefore do not have children. In BMD, the patient lives longer and may have children. None of these men's sons will have the disease, but their daughters will be carriers (Nussbaum et al., 2007). Refer carriers for genetic testing and counseling.

TABLE 53-5	DIFFERENTIAL FEATURES OF COMMON MUSCULAR DYSTROPHIES SEEN IN ADULTS		
ONSET	GENETIC LINK	CLINICAL MANIFESTATIONS	PROGRESSION
Becker (Benign X-Linked) Dystrophy			
5-25 yr	Sex-linked recessive; expression in males	Wasting of pelvic and shoulder muscles; normal cardiac and mental function	Gradual progression; inability to walk 25 yr after onset; usually normal life span
Limb-Girdle Dystrophy			
Usually 20s or 30s	Usually autosomal dominant; expression in either gender	Upper extremity and neck muscles and lower extremity and hip muscle weakness	Extremely variable; severe disability within 10-20 yr after onset; life span shortened by 10-20 yr
Facioscapulohumeral (Landouzy-Dejerine) Dystrophy			
Usually in 20s	Autosomal dominant; expression in either gender	Facial and shoulder girdle muscle involvement	Usually benign; normal life span
Myotonic (Steinert) Dystrophy			
Birth to 40s	Autosomal dominant; expression in either gender	Muscle atrophy with multiple organ involvement (e.g., heart, lungs, smooth muscle, and endocrine system)	Usually gradual if onset in adulthood

- Poor blood flow to muscle resulting in reduced tissue oxygenation
- Disturbance in nerve-muscle interaction
- Loss of cell membrane integrity as a result of increased enzyme activity

Regardless of the type of MD, the primary problem is progressive muscle weakness. The major cause of death is respiratory failure caused by profound respiratory muscle weakness. Cardiac failure also occurs because dystrophin activity is needed for cardiac muscle contraction and maintenance.

Diagnosis of MD is often difficult because the clinical manifestations are similar to those of other muscular disorders. Muscle biopsy often confirms the diagnosis. Muscle weakness and trophic changes are characteristic of all types of MD. Serum muscle enzyme values, such as aldolase and creatine kinase, may be elevated, and electromyographic (EMG) findings are often abnormal.

Collaborative care of the patient with MD is supportive and involves the entire health care team. Physical and occupational therapy help the patient maintain as much function, *mobility*, and independence as possible. Refer the patient and family to the local chapter of the Muscular Dystrophy Association (www.mda.org) for support services and information.

Major organ or body system involvement is medically managed, but the life span is often shortened from these manifestations of the disease. With the exception of steroids, no drug has been found to slow the progression of the disorder, although immunosuppressive agents, anabolic steroids, and growth factors have been tried.

An experimental treatment, myoblast transfer therapy (MTT), has been supported by the Food and Drug Administration (FDA). MTT involves injections of healthy muscle cells (myoblasts) taken from a donor and multiplied in a laboratory. The cells are then given to the patient with MD, where they theoretically fuse with each other and the recipient's unhealthy muscle cells. Gene therapy may also be an option for curing MD in the future.

Nursing interventions focus on making the patient as comfortable as possible and reinforcing techniques and exercises taught in the physical therapy program. The nurse's role in caring for a patient with cardiac or other organ involvement is the same as for any patient with dysfunction of these systems.

NURSING CONCEPT REVIEW

What might you NOTICE if the patient has impaired mobility as a result of chronic musculoskeletal disorders?

- Spinal deformity (e.g., kyphosis, lateral deviation)
- Bone malalignment (e.g., leg bowing)
- Muscle weakness
- Bone swelling or deformity
- Fracture
- Joint inflammation
- Flushed skin (Paget's disease)
- Fever (bone infection)
- Report of pain
- Report of weight loss

What should you INTERPRET and how should you RESPOND to a patient with impaired mobility as a result of chronic musculoskeletal disorders?

Perform and interpret focused physical assessment findings, including:

- Ability to ambulate (with or without assistive device)
- ADLs ability
- Body weight
- Pain intensity and quality
- Neurovascular assessment findings
- Ability to cope with decreased mobility

NURSING CONCEPT REVIEW—cont'd

Respond:

- Provide pain control interventions, including drugs and nonpharmacologic measures.
- Collaborate with members of the health care team, including PT, OT, dietitian, as needed.
- Teach about drugs that may be needed for long-term use, including side and toxic effects.
- Explain about the need for adequate calcium and vitamin D for healthy bones and bone healing.
- Assist with ADLs and ambulation as needed, but encourage independence when possible.
- Implement measures to prevent patient falls in the inpatient and home setting.
- Encourage the patient to discuss feelings related to disorders causing impaired mobility.

- Refer patients to appropriate community resources, such as the National Osteoporosis Foundation and Paget Disease Foundation.

On what should you REFLECT?

- Monitor the patient's response to pain control interventions.
- Prevent and monitor the patient for falls.
- Evaluate the patient's knowledge of nutrition and drug therapy.
- Evaluate the patient's coping ability related to disease diagnosis and treatment.
- Think about what else you might do to promote mobility.
- Decide whether you need to provide alternative interventions or additional health teaching.

GET READY FOR THE NCLEX® EXAMINATION!

KEY POINTS

Review these Key Points for each NCLEX Examination Client Needs Category.

Safe and Effective Care Environment

- Coordinate with health care team members when assessing patients with osteoporosis for risk for falls.
- In coordination with the physical and occupational therapists, educate the patient and family on home safety when the patient has a metabolic bone disease, such as osteoporosis.
- Refer to The Joint Commission for information about National Patient Safety Goals related to fall injury prevention.

Health Promotion and Maintenance

- Teach patients at risk for osteoporosis to minimize risk factors, such as stopping smoking, decreasing alcohol intake, exercising regularly, and increasing dietary calcium.
- Remind patients at risk for osteoporosis to have regular screening tests, such as the DXA scan.
- Instruct older adults to have at least 5 minutes of sun per day and to eat vitamin D–fortified foods to prevent osteomalacia.
- Refer patients with genetic-associated diseases for genetic testing and counseling.
- Assess the genetic risk for patients who have parents with muscular dystrophy.
- Refer patients with musculoskeletal problems to appropriate community resources, such as the Paget Disease Foundation and the National Osteoporosis Foundation.

Psychosocial Integrity

- Assist patients with osteoporosis to overcome fear of falling, or fallophobia, which prevents them from socializing or going outside their homes. Collaborate with the physical therapist to determine whether ambulatory devices such as canes are indicated.

Physiological Integrity

- Remind patients taking bisphosphonates (BPs) to take them early in the morning, at least 30 to 60 minutes before breakfast, with a full glass of water and to remain sitting upright during that time to prevent esophagitis, a common complication of BP therapy.
- Most patients are unaware that they have osteoporosis until they experience a fracture, the most common complication of the disease.
- Osteomalacia, the result of a deficiency in vitamin D, can be caused by the factors listed in Table 53-3.
- Remember that severe chronic pain is a priority for patients with metastatic bone disease.
- Use appropriate infection control practices when caring for patients with an open wound associated with osteomyelitis.
- For patients who have surgery for bone cancer, report postoperative manifestations of infection, dislocation, or neurovascular compromise to the surgeon promptly.
- Assess for key features of Paget's disease as summarized in Chart 53-3.
- Remember that bone tumors can be benign or malignant.
- Be aware that even minor hand and foot problems can be very painful. Common foot problems are described in Table 53-4.
- In collaboration with the health care team, provide supportive care for the patient with muscular dystrophy.
- Recognize that most major types of muscular dystrophy are genetic and manifest usually in childhood. Care is supportive.

Care of Patients with Musculoskeletal Trauma

Donna D. Ignatavicius

evolve WEBSITE

http://evolve.elsevier.com/Iggy/

Answer Key to NCLEX Examination Challenges and
  Decision-Making Challenges
Audio Glossary

Concept Map Creator
Key Points
Review Questions for the NCLEX® Examination

LEARNING OUTCOMES

Safe and Effective Care Environment

1. Explain the importance of collaborating with the health care team when providing care for patients with fractures and amputations.
2. Apply principles of infection control when caring for a patient with a compound fracture.

Health Promotion and Maintenance

3. Identify community resources about amputations for patients and their families.
4. Recognize the importance of teaching the public about ways to prevent fractures and other musculoskeletal injuries.
5. Plan discharge teaching for patients with fractures or amputations.
6. Plan care that meets the special needs of older adults with hip fractures, including interventions to increase mobility.

Psychosocial Integrity

7. Describe how to assess the patient's and family's reaction to changes in body image resulting from amputation.
8. Explain how to assist patients in coping with loss of a body part.

Physiological Integrity

9. Compare and contrast common types of fractures.
10. Describe the usual healing process for bone.

11. Assess patients with musculoskeletal trauma to prioritize interventions for their care.
12. Explain the typical clinical manifestations that are seen in patients with fractures.
13. Delineate nursing care needed to maintain casts for patients with fractures.
14. Delineate nursing care needed to maintain traction and external fixation for patients with fractures.
15. Plan pain management for patients with musculoskeletal trauma.
16. Identify the risk for complications from fractures, and take measures to help prevent them.
17. Describe how to perform focused musculoskeletal and neurovascular assessment for patients with musculoskeletal trauma.
18. Develop a postoperative plan of care, including health teaching, for a patient after fracture repair.
19. Describe emergency care for people who have a traumatic amputation.
20. Plan postoperative care, including health teaching, after an elective amputation.
21. Identify common causes of amputations.
22. Identify appropriate complementary and alternative therapies for patients with phantom limb pain.
23. Describe the patient-centered collaborative care needed to manage complex regional pain syndrome.
24. Plan care for patients with common types of sports-related injuries.

Musculoskeletal trauma accounts for about two thirds of all injuries and is one of the primary causes of disability in the United States. It ranges from simple muscle strain to multiple bone fractures with severe soft-tissue damage.

Fractures and other musculoskeletal trauma impair a patient's *mobility* in varying degrees, depending on the severity and extent of the injury. These injuries also affect *sensation* because of pressure on nerve endings from edema. In some cases, peripheral nerves are directly damaged as a result of musculoskeletal injury.

FRACTURES

Pathophysiology

A fracture is a break or disruption in the continuity of a bone that often affects *mobility and sensation*. It can occur anywhere in the body and at any age. All fractures have the same basic pathophysiologic mechanism and require similar patient-centered collaborative care, regardless of fracture type or location.

Classification of Fractures

A fracture is classified by the extent of the break:
- *Complete fracture.* The break is across the entire width of the bone in such a way that the bone is divided into two distinct sections.
- *Incomplete fracture.* The fracture does not divide the bone into two portions because the break is through only part of the bone.

A fracture is described by the extent of associated soft-tissue damage as open (or compound) or closed (or simple). The skin surface over the broken bone is disrupted in a *compound* fracture, which causes an external wound. These fractures are often graded to define the extent of tissue damage. A *simple* fracture does not extend through the skin and therefore has no visible wound.

Fig. 54-1 shows common types of fractures. In addition to being identified by type, fractures are described by their cause. A pathologic (spontaneous) fracture occurs after minimal trauma to a bone that has been weakened by disease. For example, a patient with bone cancer or osteoporosis can

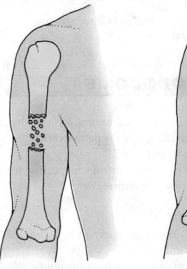

Closed, nondisplaced

Open (compound)

Comminuted (fragmented)

Displaced

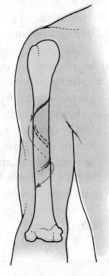

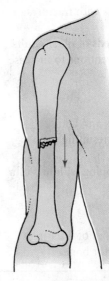

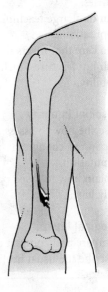

Oblique

Spiral

Impacted

Greenstick

FIG. 54-1 Common types of fractures.

easily have a pathologic fracture. A fatigue (stress) fracture results from excessive strain and stress on the bone. This problem is commonly seen in recreational and professional athletes. Compression fractures are produced by a loading force applied to the long axis of cancellous bone. They commonly occur in the vertebrae of older patients with osteoporosis and are extremely painful.

Stages of Bone Healing

When a bone is fractured, the body immediately begins the healing process to repair the injury and restore the body's equilibrium. Fractures heal in five stages that are a continuous process and not single stages. In stage one, within 24 to 72 hours after the injury, a hematoma forms at the site of the fracture because bone is extremely vascular. Stage two occurs in 3 days to 2 weeks when granulation tissue begins to invade the hematoma. This then prompts the formation of fibrocartilage, providing the foundation for bone healing. Stage three of bone healing occurs as a result of vascular and cellular proliferation. The fracture site is surrounded by new vascular tissue known as a *callus* (within 3 to 6 weeks). Callus formation is the beginning of a nonbony union. As healing continues in stage four, the callus is gradually resorbed and transformed into bone. This stage usually takes 3 to 8 weeks. During the fifth and final stage of healing, consolidation and remodeling of bone continue to meet mechanical demands. This process may start as early as 4 to 6 weeks after fracture and can continue for up to 1 year, depending on the severity of the injury and the age and health of the patient. Fig. 54-2 summarizes the stages of bone healing.

In young, healthy adult bone, healing takes about 4 to 6 weeks. In the older person who has reduced bone mass, healing time is lengthened. Complete healing often takes 3 to 6 months or longer in people who are older than 70 years. Other factors also affect healing. Examples include the severity of the trauma, the type of bone injured, how the fracture is managed, infections at the fracture site, and ischemic or avascular necrosis (AVN).

CONSIDERATIONS FOR OLDER ADULTS

Bone healing is often affected by the aging process. Bone formation and strength rely on adequate nutrition. Calcium, phosphorus, vitamin D, and protein are necessary for the production of new bone (see Chapter 53). For women, the loss of estrogen after menopause decreases the body's ability to form new bone tissue. Chronic diseases can also affect the rate at which bone heals. For instance, peripheral vascular diseases, such as arteriosclerosis, reduce arterial circulation to bone. Thus the bone receives less oxygen and fewer nutrients, both of which are needed for repair.

Complications of Fractures

Regardless of the type or location of the fracture, several limb- and life-threatening acute and chronic complications can result from the injury. Clinical manifestations of beginning complications must be treated early to prevent serious consequences. In some cases, careful monitoring and assessment can prevent these complications:

- Acute compartment syndrome
- Crush syndrome
- Hypovolemic shock
- Fat embolism syndrome
- Venous thromboembolism
- Infection
- Chronic complications, such as ischemic necrosis and delayed union

Acute Compartment Syndrome. Compartments are areas in the body in which muscles, blood vessels, and nerves are contained within fascia. Most compartments are located in the extremities. Fascia is an inelastic tissue that surrounds groups of muscles, blood vessels, and nerves in the body. Acute compartment syndrome (ACS) is a serious condition in which increased pressure within one or more compartments reduces circulation to the area. The most common sites for this problem in patients with musculoskeletal trauma are the compartments in the lower leg and forearm.

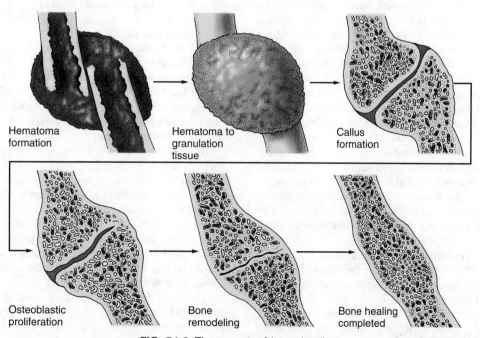

Hematoma formation

Hematoma to granulation tissue

Callus formation

Osteoblastic proliferation

Bone remodeling

Bone healing completed

FIG. 54-2 The stages of bone healing.

CHART 54-1   KEY FEATURES

Compartment Syndrome

PHYSIOLOGIC CHANGE	CLINICAL FINDINGS
Increased compartment pressure	No change
Increased capillary permeability	Edema
Release of histamine	Increased edema
Increased blood flow to area	Pulses present Pink tissue
Pressure on nerve endings	Pain
Increased tissue pressure	Referred pain to compartment
Decreased tissue perfusion	Increased edema
Decreased oxygen to tissues	Pallor
Increased production of lactic acid	Unequal pulses Flexed posture
Anaerobic metabolism	Cyanosis
Vasodilation	Increased edema
Increased blood flow	Tense muscle swelling
Increased tissue pressure	Tingling Numbness
Increased edema	Paresthesia
Muscle ischemia	Severe pain unrelieved by drugs
Tissue necrosis	Paresis/paralysis

The pathophysiologic changes of increased compartment pressure are sometimes referred to as the *ischemia-edema cycle.* Capillaries within the muscle dilate, which raises capillary pressure. Capillaries then become more permeable because of the release of histamine by the ischemic muscle tissue. As a result, plasma proteins leak into the interstitial fluid space and edema occurs. Edema increases pressure on nerve endings and causes pain. Blood flow to the area is reduced, and further ischemia results. Sensory deficits or paresthesia generally appears before changes in vascular or motor signs. The color of the tissue pales, and pulses begin to weaken but rarely disappear. The affected area is usually palpably tense, and pain occurs with passive motion of the extremity. If the condition is not treated, cyanosis, tingling, numbness, paresis, necrosis, and severe pain can occur. Chart 54-1 summarizes the sequence of pathophysiologic events in compartment syndrome and the associated clinical assessment findings.

The pressure to the compartment can be from an external or internal source. Tight, bulky dressings and casts are examples of *external* pressure. Blood or fluid accumulation in the compartment is a common source of *internal* pressure. The injury or trauma causing the problem is above the compartment involved, which decreases blood flow to the more distal area of injury. ACS is not limited to patients with musculoskeletal problems. It can also occur in those with severe burns, extensive insect bites or snakebites, or massive infiltration of IV fluids. In these situations, edema increases internal pressure in one or more compartments.

Problems resulting from compartment syndrome include infection, persistent motor weakness in the affected extremity, contracture, and myoglobinuric renal failure. In extreme cases, amputation becomes necessary.

Infection from necrosis may become severe enough that amputation of the limb is needed. *Motor weakness* from

injured nerves is not reversible, and the patient may require an orthotic device for assistance in mobility. Volkmann's *contractures* of the forearm, which can begin within 12 hours of the pressure increase, result from shortening of the ischemic muscle and from nerve involvement.

Myoglobinuric renal failure from muscle breakdown is a potentially fatal complication of compartment syndrome. It occurs when large or multiple compartments are involved. Injured muscle tissues release myoglobulin (muscle protein) into the circulation, where it can clog the renal tubules and cause acute renal failure. Although the exact pathophysiologic mechanisms are unknown, it is suspected that myoglobulin has a direct toxic effect on the kidney. Damaged muscle cells also release potassium, which cannot be excreted because of the renal failure. The resulting hyperkalemia may cause dysrhythmias and cardiac arrest.

Crush Syndrome. Crush syndrome (CS) occurs from an external crush injury that compresses one or more compartments in the leg, arm, or pelvis. It is a potentially life-threatening, systemic complication that results from hemorrhage and edema after a severe fracture injury. As muscle becomes ischemic and necrotic from pressure within the compartment, myoglobin is released into circulation, where it can occlude the distal renal tubules and result in kidney failure.

Specific causes of CS include:
- Twisting-type injuries
- Natural disasters, such as earthquakes
- Work-related injuries, such as being trapped under heavy equipment such as a car
- Drug or alcohol overdose, when one or more limbs may be compressed by body weight for a prolonged time
- Older adults who fall, are unable to get up, and lie for a prolonged time

Regardless of the cause, CS is indicated by:
- Acute compartment syndrome
- Hypovolemia (decreased circulating blood volume)
- Hyperkalemia (increased serum potassium)
- Rhabdomyolysis (myoglobulin release from skeletal muscle into the bloodstream)
- Acute tubular necrosis (ATN) resulting from hypovolemia and rhabdomyolysis
- Dark brown urine
- Muscle weakness and pain

Management focuses on preventing (1) ATN from myoglobin release and (2) cardiac dysrhythmias related to hyperkalemia. Kayexalate may reduce serum potassium adequately, but hemodialysis may be required if potassium levels remain high or kidney failure occurs.

Hypovolemic Shock. Bone is very vascular. Therefore there is a risk for bleeding with bone injury. In addition, trauma can cut nearby arteries and cause hemorrhage, resulting in rapidly developing hypovolemic shock. (The pathophysiology of hypovolemic shock is described in Chapter 39.)

Fat Embolism Syndrome. Fat embolism syndrome (FES) is another serious complication in which fat globules are released from the yellow bone marrow into the bloodstream within 12 to 48 hours after an injury or other illness. These globules clog small blood vessels that supply vital organs, most commonly the lungs, and impair organ perfusion. FES usually results from long bone fractures or fracture repair but occasionally is seen in patients who have a total

Pulmonary Emboli: Fat Embolism Versus Blood Clot Embolism

FAT EMBOLISM	BLOOD CLOT EMBOLISM
Definition	
Obstruction of the pulmonary vascular bed by fat globules	Obstruction of the pulmonary artery by a blood clot or clots
Origin	
95% from fractures of the long bones; occurs usually within 48 hr of injury	85% from deep vein thrombosis in the legs or pelvis; can occur anytime
Assessment Findings	
Altered mental status (earliest sign)	Same as for fat embolism, except no petechiae
Increased respirations, pulse, temperature	
Chest pain	
Dyspnea	
Crackles	
Decreased SaO₂	
Petechiae (50%-60%)	
Retinal hemorrhage (not common)	
Mild thrombocytopenia	
Treatment	
Bedrest	Preventive measures (e.g., leg exercises, antiembolism stockings, SCDs)
Gentle handling	
Oxygen	
Hydration (IV fluids)	Bedrest
Possibly steroid therapy	Oxygen
Fracture immobilization	Possibly mechanical ventilation
	Anticoagulants
	Thrombolytics
	Possible surgery: pulmonary embolectomy, vena cava umbrella

SaO_2, Arterial oxygen saturation; *SCD,* sequential compression device.

joint replacement. It may also occur, although less often, in those with pancreatitis, osteomyelitis, blunt trauma, or sickle cell disease.

The problem can occur at any age or in either gender, but young men between ages 20 and 40 years and older adults between ages 70 and 80 years are at the greatest risk. Patients with fractured hips have the highest risk, but FES is also common in those with fractures of the pelvis.

The earliest manifestation of FES is altered mental status, which is caused by a low arterial oxygen level. Dyspnea and chest pain may follow. Petechiae, a macular, measles-like rash, may appear over the neck, upper arms, or chest and abdomen. This rash is a classic manifestation but can be a late sign.

Abnormal laboratory findings include:
- Increased erythrocyte sedimentation rate (ESR)
- Decreased serum calcium levels
- Decreased red blood cell and platelet counts
- Increased serum lipase level

These changes in blood values are poorly understood, but they aid in diagnosis of the condition.

FES can result in respiratory failure or death, often from pulmonary edema. When the lungs are affected, the complication may be misdiagnosed as a pulmonary embolism from a blood clot (Chart 54-2).

Venous Thromboembolism. Venous thromboembolism (VTE) includes deep vein thrombosis (DVT) and its major complication, pulmonary embolism (PE). It is the most common complication of lower extremity surgery or trauma and the most often fatal complication of musculoskeletal surgery. Factors that make patients with fractures most likely to develop VTE include:
- Cancer or chemotherapy
- Surgical procedure longer than 30 minutes
- History of smoking
- Obesity
- Heart disease
- Prolonged immobility
- Oral contraceptives or hormones
- History of VTE complications
- Older adults (especially with hip fractures)

The pathophysiology and management of VTE is described in Chapter 38.

Infection. Whenever there is trauma to tissues, the body's defense system is disrupted. Wound infections are the most common type of infection resulting from orthopedic trauma. They range from superficial skin infections to deep wound abscesses. Infection can also be caused by implanted hardware used to repair a fracture surgically, such as pins, plates, or rods. Clostridial infections can result in gas gangrene or tetanus and can prevent the bone from healing properly.

Bone infection, or osteomyelitis, is most common with open fractures in which skin integrity is lost and after surgical repair of a fracture. For patients experiencing this type of trauma, the risk for hospital-acquired infections is increased. These infections are common, and many are from multidrug-resistant organisms, such as methicillin-resistant *Staphylococcus aureus* (MRSA). Reducing MRSA infections is a primary desired outcome for all health care agencies.

Chronic Complications. Ischemic necrosis and delayed bone healing are later complications of musculoskeletal trauma. Ischemic necrosis is sometimes referred to as aseptic or avascular necrosis (AVN) or osteonecrosis. Blood supply to the bone is disrupted, leading to the death of bone tissue. This problem is most often a complication of hip fractures or any fracture in which there is displacement of bone. Surgical repair of fractures also can cause necrosis because the hardware can interfere with circulation. Patients on long-term corticosteroid therapy, such as prednisone, are also at high risk for ischemic necrosis.

Delayed union is a fracture that has not healed within 6 months of injury. Some fractures never achieve union; that is, they never completely heal (nonunion). Others heal incorrectly (malunion). These problems are most common in patients with tibial fractures, fractures that involve many treatment techniques (e.g., cast, traction), and pathologic fractures. Union may also be delayed or not achieved in the older patient. If bone does not heal, he or she typically has chronic pain and immobility from deformity.

Etiology and Genetic Risk

The primary cause of a fracture is trauma from a motor vehicle crash or fall, especially in older adults. The trauma may be a direct blow to the bone or an indirect force from muscle contractions or pulling forces on the bone. Sports, vigorous exercise, and malnutrition are contributing factors. Bone diseases, such as osteoporosis, increase the risk for a fracture in older adults (see Chapter 53). Genetic factors that increase risk for fracture are discussed with these specific health problems throughout this text.

Incidence/Prevalence

The incidence of fractures depends on the location of the injury. Rib fractures are the most common type in the adult population. Femoral shaft fractures occur most often in young and middle-aged adults. The incidence of proximal femur (hip) fractures is highest in older adults. Humeral fractures are common in adults; the older the person, usually the more proximal is the fracture. Wrist (Colles') fractures are typically seen in middle and late adulthood and usually result from a fall.

Health Promotion and Maintenance

Airbags and seat belts have decreased the number of severe injuries and deaths, but they have increased the number of leg and ankle fractures, especially in older adults. Encourage people to use seat belts, and support legislation for improved vehicle design and re-evaluation of the federal standards for motor vehicle safety. Health teaching should also focus on other risks for musculoskeletal injury, including:

- Osteoporosis screening and education
- Fall prevention
- Home safety assessment and modification, if needed
- Dangers of drinking and driving
- Drug safety (prescribed, over-the-counter, and illicit)
- Older adults and driving
- Helmet use when riding bicycles, motorcycles, all-terrain vehicles (ATVs), and skateboards

These educational interventions are discussed throughout this book and in other texts. Fall prevention is discussed in detail in Chapter 3 as part of care for older adults.

PATIENT-CENTERED COLLABORATIVE CARE

ASSESSMENT

History

If the patient is in severe pain, delay the interview until he or she is more comfortable. Then, ask about the cause of the fracture, which helps in developing an individualized plan of care. Some type of force, such as incisional, crush, acceleration or deceleration, and shearing and friction, leads to most musculoskeletal injuries. As a result, several body systems are often affected.

Incisional injuries, as from a knife wound, and *crush* injuries cause hemorrhage and decrease blood flow to major organs. *Acceleration or deceleration* injuries cause direct trauma to the spleen, brain, and kidneys when these organs are moved from their fixed locations in the body. *Shearing and friction* damage the skin and cause a high level of wound contamination.

Asking about the events leading to the injury helps identify which forces have been experienced and therefore which body systems or parts of the body to assess. For example, a forward fall often results in Colles' fracture of the wrist because the person tries to catch himself or herself with an outstretched hand. Knowing the mechanism of injury also

helps determine whether other types of injury, such as head and spinal cord injury, might be present.

A drug history, including substance abuse, is important regardless of the patient's age. For example, a young adult may have had an excessive amount of alcohol, which contributed to a motor vehicle crash or to a fall at the work site. Many older adults also consume alcohol and an assortment of prescribed and over-the-counter drugs, which can cause dizziness and loss of balance.

A medical history may identify possible causes of the fracture and gives clues as to how long it will take for the bone to heal. Certain diseases such as bone cancer and Paget's disease cause pathologic fractures that often do not achieve total healing or union.

Ask about the patient's occupation and recreational activities. Some occupations are more hazardous than others. For instance, construction work is potentially more physically dangerous than office work. Certain hobbies and recreational activities are also extremely hazardous, such as skiing. Contact sports, such as football and ice hockey, often result in musculoskeletal injuries, including fractures. Other activities do not have such an obvious potential for injury but can cause fractures nonetheless. For instance, daily jogging or running can lead to fatigue fractures.

Physical Assessment/Clinical Manifestations

The patient with a fracture often has trauma to other body systems. Therefore assess all major body systems *first* for life-threatening complications, including head, chest, and abdominal trauma. For example, some fractures can cause internal organ damage resulting in hemorrhage. When a pelvic fracture is suspected, assess vital signs, skin color, and level of consciousness for indications of possible hypovolemic shock. Check the urine for blood, which indicates possible damage to the urinary system, often the bladder. If the patient cannot void, suspect that the bladder or urethra has been damaged. Complete assessment of these areas is described elsewhere in this text.

❗ NURSING SAFETY PRIORITY

Action Alert

> The most common manifestation of fractures is moderate to often severe pain. Patients with severe or multiple fractures of the arms, legs, or pelvis have severe pain. Vertebral compression factures are also extremely painful. Patients *with a fractured hip may have groin pain or pain referred to the back of the knee or lower back*. Pain is usually due to muscle spasm and edema, which result from the fracture. Patients with one or more fractured ribs have severe pain when they take deep breaths. Monitor respiratory status, which may be severely compromised from pain or pneumothorax (air in the pleural cavity). Assess the patient's pain level and manage pain *before* continuing the physical assessment.

For fractures of the shoulder and upper arm, the physical assessment is best done with the patient in a sitting or standing position, if possible, so that shoulder drooping or other abnormal positioning can be seen. Support the affected arm and flex the elbow to promote comfort during the assessment. For more distal areas of the arm, perform the assessment with the patient in a supine position so that the extremity can be elevated to reduce swelling.

Place the patient in a supine position for assessment of the legs and pelvis. A patient with an impacted hip fracture may be able to walk for a short time after injury, although this is not recommended.

When inspecting the site of a possible fracture, look for a change in bone alignment. The bone may appear deformed, a limb may be internally or externally rotated, and/or one or more bones may also be dislocated (out of their joint capsules). Observe for extremity shortening or a change in bone shape.

If the skin is intact (closed fracture), the area over the fracture may be ecchymotic (bruised) from bleeding into the underlying soft tissues. Subcutaneous emphysema, the appearance of bubbles under the skin because of air trapping, may be present but is usually seen later.

Swelling at the fracture site is rapid and can result in marked neurovascular compromise. *Gently perform a thorough neurovascular assessment, and compare extremities. Assess skin color and temperature, sensation, mobility, pain, and pulses distal to the fracture site. If the fracture involves an extremity and the patient is not in severe pain, check the nails for capillary refill by applying pressure to the nail and observing for the speed of blood return. If nails are brittle or thick, assess the skin next to the nail. Checking for capillary refill is not as reliable as other indicators of perfusion.* Chart 54-3 describes the procedure for a neurovascular assessment, which evaluates circulation, movement, and sensation (CMS function).

DECISION-MAKING CHALLENGE

Patient-Centered Care; Evidence-Based Practice

A 68-year-old woman slipped on ice on her walkway to her driveway. Her neighbor, an RN, was awakened by her scream for help and rushed to find the woman holding her deformed and swollen ankle. The nurse called 911, performed a rapid head-to-toe assessment, and stayed with her, trying to make her as comfortable as possible. The woman is alert and has no other apparent injury or problem. Upon arrival at the emergency department (ED), another nurse and you greet the patient and help her transfer into a room reserved for her.

1. What are your priority assessments for the patient when coming into the ED? What sources of evidence would you seek to answer this clinical question?
2. The patient has a dislocated ankle (distal tibia and fibula) and reports that she is still in pain even though the EMT gave her IV fentanyl. How will you respond to this patient, and what action will you take?
3. The patient's daughter comes to the ED and asks you if her mother's history of osteopenia may have caused the fracture. How will you answer her?
4. What factors may have contributed to this patient's "slip and fall?"

Psychosocial Assessment

The psychosocial status of a patient with a fracture depends on the extent of the injury, possible complications, coping ability, and the availability of support systems. Hospitalization is not required for a single, uncomplicated fracture, and the patient returns to usual daily activities within a few days. Examples include a single fracture of a finger, wrist, foot, or toe.

In contrast, a patient suffering severe or multiple traumas may be hospitalized for weeks and may undergo many surgical procedures, treatments, and prolonged rehabilitation. These disruptions in lifestyle can create a high level of stress.

The stresses that result from a long-term condition affect relationships between the patient and family members or

CHART 54-3 BEST PRACTICE FOR PATIENT SAFETY & QUALITY CARE

Assessment of Neurovascular Status in Patients with Musculoskeletal Injury

ASSESSMENT METHOD	NORMAL FINDINGS
Skin Color Inspect the area distal to the injury.	No change in pigmentation compared with other parts of the body.
Skin Temperature Palpate the area distal to the injury (the dorsum of the hands is most sensitive to temperature).	The skin is warm.
Movement Ask the patient to move the affected area or the area distal to the injury (active motion).	The patient can move without discomfort.
Move the area distal to the injury (passive motion).	No difference in comfort compared with active movement.
Sensation Ask the patient if numbness or tingling is present (paresthesia).	No numbness or tingling.
Palpate with a paper clip (especially the web space between the first and second toes or the web space between the thumb and forefinger).	No difference in sensation in the affected and unaffected extremities. (Loss of sensation in these areas indicates peroneal nerve or median nerve damage.)
Pulses Palpate the pulses distal to the injury.	Pulses are strong and easily palpated; no difference in the affected and unaffected extremities.
Capillary Refill (Least Reliable) Press the nail beds distal to the injury until blanching occurs (or the skin near the nail if nails are thick and brittle).	Blood returns (return to usual color) within 3 sec (5 sec for older patients).
Pain Ask the patient about the location, nature, and frequency of the pain.	Pain is usually localized and is often described as stabbing or throbbing. (Pain out of proportion to the injury and unrelieved by analgesics might indicate compartment syndrome.)

friends. Assess the patient's feelings, and ask how he or she coped with previously experienced stressful events. Body image and sexuality may be altered by deformity, treatment modalities for fracture repair, or long-term immobilization. Assess the availability of support systems, such as family, church, or community groups who can help patients during the acute and rehabilitation phases needed when multiple or severe fractures occur. Active patients of any age or those who are older and live alone may become depressed during the healing process. Acute and chronic pain can decrease energy levels and may also cause sadness or depression.

Laboratory Assessment

No special laboratory tests are available for assessment of fractures. Hemoglobin and hematocrit levels may often be low because of bleeding caused by the injury. If extensive soft-tissue damage is present, the erythrocyte sedimentation rate (ESR) may be elevated, which indicates the expected inflammatory response. If this value increases during fracture healing, the patient may have a bone infection. During the healing stages, serum calcium and phosphorus levels are often increased as the bone releases these elements into the blood.

Imaging Assessment

The health care provider requests standard x-rays and tomograms to confirm a diagnosis of fracture. These reveal the bone disruption, malalignment, or deformity. If the x-ray does not show a fracture but the patient is symptomatic, the x-ray is usually repeated with additional views.

The computed tomography (CT) scan is useful in detecting fractures of complex structures, such as the hip and pelvis. It also identifies compression fractures of the spine. Magnetic resonance imaging (MRI) is useful in determining the amount of soft-tissue damage that may have occurred with the fracture.

ANALYSIS

The most common problems for patients with fractures are:

1. Acute Pain related to one or more fractures, soft-tissue damage, muscle spasm, and edema
2. Potential for neurovascular compromise related to tissue edema and/or bleeding
3. Potential for infection related to a wound caused by an open fracture
4. Impaired Physical Mobility related to acute or chronic pain

PLANNING AND IMPLEMENTATION

Managing Acute Pain

Planning: Expected Outcomes. The patient with a fracture is expected to state that he or she has adequate pain control after fracture reduction and immobilization.

Interventions. A fracture can happen anywhere and may be accompanied by multiple injuries to vital organs. Patient-centered collaborative care depends on the severity and extent of the injury and the number of fractures the patient has.

Emergency Care: Fracture. For any patient who experiences trauma in the community, first call 911 and assess for **a**irway, **b**reathing, and **c**irculation (ABCs, or primary survey). Then provide lifesaving care if needed before being concerned about the fracture (Chart 54-4). If CPR is needed, ensure circulation first, followed by airway and breathing (see Chapter 36).

If the person is clothed, cut away clothing from the fracture site, and remove any jewelry from the affected extremity. Control any bleeding by direct pressure on the area and digital pressure over the artery above the fracture. To prevent shock, place the patient in a supine position and keep him or her warm.

After a head-to-toe assessment (secondary survey) and patient stabilization by the prehospital team, pain is managed with IV opioids such as fentanyl. Cardiac monitoring for patients who are older than 50 years is established before drug administration. To prevent further tissue damage, reduce

---

CHART 54-4   BEST PRACTICE FOR PATIENT SAFETY & QUALITY CARE

Emergency Care of the Patient with an Extremity Fracture

1. Assess the patient's airway, breathing, and circulation, and perform a quick head-to-toe assessment.
2. Remove the patient's clothing (cut if necessary) to inspect the affected area while supporting the area above and below the injury. Do not remove shoes because this can cause increased trauma.
3. Remove jewelry on the affected extremity in case of swelling.
4. Apply direct pressure on the area if there is bleeding and pressure over the proximal artery nearest the fracture.
5. Keep the patient warm and in a supine position.
6. Check the neurovascular status of the area distal to the fracture, including temperature, color, sensation, movement, and capillary refill. Compare affected and unaffected limbs.
7. Immobilize the extremity by splinting; include joints above and below the fracture site. Recheck circulation after splinting.
8. Cover any open areas with a dressing (preferably sterile).

---

pain, and increase circulation, the prehospital or emergency team immobilizes the fracture by splinting. An air splint or any object or device that extends to the joints above and below the fracture to immobilize it can be used as a splint. Sterile gauze is placed loosely over open areas to prevent further contamination of the wound.

In the emergency department (ED), physician's office, or urgent care center, fracture management begins with reduction and immobilization of the fracture, while attending to continued pain assessment and management.

Reduction, or realignment of the bone ends for proper healing, is accomplished by a closed method or an open (surgical) procedure. In some cases, dislocated bones are also reduced, such as when the distal tibia and fibula are dislocated with a fractured ankle. Immobilization is achieved by the use of bandages, casts, traction, internal fixation, or external fixation.

The health care provider selects the treatment method based on the type, location, and extent of the fracture. These interventions prevent further injury and reduce pain.

Nonsurgical Management. Nonsurgical management includes closed reduction and immobilization with a bandage, splint, cast, or traction. For some small, closed bone fractures in the hand or foot, reduction is not required. Immobilization with an orthotic device or special orthopedic shoe or boot may be the only management during the healing process.

For each modality, the primary nursing concern is assessment and prevention of neurovascular dysfunction or compromise. Assess the patient's neurovascular status every hour for the first 24 hours and every 1 to 4 hours thereafter, depending on the injury (see Chart 54-3). The patient usually reports discomfort that is unrelieved by analgesics if the bandage, splint, or cast is too tight. Elevate the fractured extremity higher than the heart, and apply ice for the first 24 to 48 hours as needed to reduce edema.

Closed Reduction and Immobilization. Closed reduction is the most common nonsurgical method for managing a simple fracture. While applying a manual pull, or traction, on the bone, the health care provider moves the bone ends so that they realign. Moderate sedation and/or analgesia is often

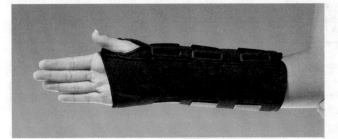

FIG. 54-3 A universal wrist and forearm splint used for immobilization.

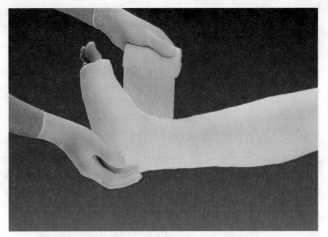

FIG. 54-4 Application of fiberglass synthetic cast.

used during this procedure to decrease pain. An x-ray shows that the bone ends are approximated (aligned) before the bone is immobilized.

Bandages and Splints. For certain areas of the body, such as the scapula (shoulder) and clavicle (collarbone), an elastic bandage or commercial immobilizer may be used to keep the bone in place during healing. Because upper extremity bones do not bear weight, splints may be sufficient to keep bone fragments in place for a closed fracture. Fig. 54-3 shows a wrist splint for fracture immobilization. Thermoplastic, a durable, flexible material for splinting, allows custom fitting to the patient's body part. Splints for lower extremities are also custom-fitted using flexible materials and held in place with elastic bandages (e.g., ace wrap).

Casts. For more complex fractures or fractures of the lower extremity, the physician or orthopedic technician applies a cast to hold bone fragments in place after reduction. A cast is a rigid device that immobilizes the affected body part while allowing other body parts to move. It also allows early mobility and reduces pain. Although its most common use is for fractures, a cast may be applied for correction of deformities (e.g., clubfoot) or for prevention of deformities (e.g., those seen in some patients with rheumatoid arthritis).

Several types of materials are used to make casts. The traditional plaster-of-Paris cast is no longer commonly used for management of most fractures. It requires application of a well-fitted stockinette under the material. If the stockinette is too tight, it may impair circulation. If it is too loose, wrinkles can lead to the development of pressure ulcers. Padding is applied over the stockinette, followed by wet plaster rolls wrapped around the extremity or other body part. The cast feels hot because an immediate chemical reaction occurs, but it soon becomes damp and cool. This type of cast takes 24 to 72 hours to dry, depending on the size and location of the cast. A wet cast feels cold, smells musty, and is grayish. The cast is dry when it feels hard and firm, is odorless, and has a shiny white appearance.

If the skin under the cast is open, the health care provider, orthopedic technician, or specially trained nurse cuts a window in the cast so that the wound can be observed and cared for. The piece of cast removed to make the window must be retained and replaced after wound care to prevent localized edema in the area. This is most important when a window is cut from a cast on an extremity. Tape or elastic bandage wrap may be used to keep the "window" in place. A window is also an access for taking pulses, removing wound drains, or preventing abdominal distention when the patient is in a body or spica cast.

If the cast is too tight, it may be cut with a cast cutter to relieve pressure or allow tissue swelling. The health care provider may choose to bivalve the cast (i.e., cut it lengthwise into two equal pieces) if bone healing is almost complete. Either half of the cast can be removed for inspection or for provision of care. The two halves are then held in place by an elastic bandage wrap.

Synthetic materials for casts are much more common and include fiberglass and polyester-cotton knit (Fig. 54-4). These materials are lighter than plaster and require minimal drying time. Fiberglass casts are dry in 10 to 15 minutes and can bear weight 30 minutes after application. Polyester-cotton knit casts take 7 minutes to dry and can withstand weight bearing in about 20 minutes. Some health care providers may use synthetic casts for upper extremities and plaster-of-Paris casts for lower extremities because plaster casts can bear more weight for a longer time. However, newer synthetic materials are stronger than earlier ones. Synthetic casts can be bivalved as needed.

Casts can be generally divided into four main groups: arm casts, leg casts, cast braces, and body or spica casts. Table 54-1 describes specific casts that are used for various parts of the body.

When a patient is in bed with an *arm cast,* teach him or her to elevate the arm above the heart to reduce swelling. The hand should be higher than the heart. Ice may be prescribed for the first 24 to 48 hours. When the patient is out of bed, the arm is supported with a sling placed around the neck to alleviate fatigue caused by the weight of the cast. The sling should distribute the weight over a large area of the shoulders and trunk, not just the neck. Some health care providers prefer that the patient not use a sling after the first few days in an arm cast, particularly a short-arm cast. This encourages normal movement of the mobile joints and enhances bone healing.

A *leg cast* allows mobility and requires the patient to use ambulatory aids such as crutches. A cast shoe, sandal, or boot that attaches to the foot or a rubber walking pad attached to the sole of the cast assists in ambulation (if weight bearing is allowed) and helps prevent damage to the cast. Teach the patient to elevate the affected leg on several pillows to reduce swelling and to apply ice for the first 24 hours or as prescribed.

TABLE 54-1	TYPES OF CASTS USED FOR MUSCULOSKELETAL TRAUMA
TYPE AND CHARACTERISTICS OF CAST	**USE**
Upper Extremity Casts	
Short-arm cast (SAC) (extends from below the elbow to and including part of the hand)	Stable fractures of the wrist (metacarpals, carpals, or distal radius)
Long-arm cast (LAC) (includes the upper arm to and including part of the hand)	Unstable fractures of the wrist, distal humerus, radius, or ulna
Hanging-arm cast (same as LAC but heavier, with added loop at the mid-forearm)	Fractures of the humerus that cannot be aligned by LAC (light traction is possible while the patient is in bed or by an attached strap that extends around the neck)
Thumb spica (gauntlet) cast (similar to SAC with the thumb casted in abduction)	Fractures of the thumb
Shoulder spica cast (the shoulder is casted in abduction with the elbow flexed)	Unstable fractures of the shoulder girdle or humerus; dislocations of the shoulder
Lower Extremity Casts	
Short-leg cast (SLC) (from below the knee to the base of the toes)	Fractures of the ankle, metatarsals, or foot
Long-leg cast (LLC) (from the mid-upper thigh to the base of the toes)	Unstable fractures of the tibia, fibula, or ankle
Walking cast (a walking device on the bottom of SLC or LLC)	Same as for SLC or LLC
Leg cylinder (similar to SLC, but the ankle and foot are not casted)	Stable fractures of the tibia, fibula, or knee
Long-leg cylinder (similar to LLC, but the ankle and foot are not casted)	Stable fractures of the distal femur, proximal tibia, or knee
Cast Braces (or Brace Casts) (Not As Common)	
Patellar weight-bearing cast (similar to SLC or leg cylinder)	Mid-shaft or distal shaft fractures of the femur
External polycentric knee hinge cast (a hinge connects the lower and upper leg and allows 90 degrees of knee flexion)	Same as for the patellar weight-bearing cast
Body Casts (Not As Common)	
Hip spica (extends from below the nipple line down the affected leg [single], down the leg and half of the unaffected leg [1½], or down both legs [double])	Dislocation of the hip; pelvic or hip injuries
Risser cast (the body jacket extends from the shoulders to beyond the iliac crests and hips, with a large opening over the anterior chest)	Scoliosis; thoracic spinal fractures
Halo cast (the body jacket contains a halo brace)	Fractures of the cervical spine

A *body cast* encircles the trunk of the body and is not commonly used for adults. A spica cast encases a portion of the trunk and one or two extremities. A patient with either of these casts presents a special challenge for nursing care. Potential complications related to severe impairment in mobility include:

- Skin breakdown
- Respiratory dysfunction, such as pneumonia and atelectasis
- Constipation
- Joint contractures

Cast syndrome (superior mesenteric artery syndrome), an uncommon but serious complication, may be seen in orthopedic patients who have been placed in a hip spica or body cast. Partial or complete upper intestinal obstruction results in classic symptoms: abdominal distention, epigastric pain, nausea, and vomiting. The vomiting often occurs after meals, and patients may have normal bowel sounds. Partial obstruction occurs initially from compression of the third portion of the duodenum between the superior mesenteric artery and the aorta. This can progress to complete obstruction from duodenal edema caused by continued vomiting and distention. Placing a window in the abdominal portion of the cast or bivalving the cast may be sufficient to prevent or relieve pressure on the duodenum. Management of intestinal obstruction is the same as for any patient with this complication.

Before the cast is applied, explain the purpose of the cast and the procedure for its application. With a plaster cast, warn the patient about the heat that will be felt immediately after the wet cast is applied. Do not cover the new cast. Allow for air-drying.

! NURSING SAFETY PRIORITY
Action Alert

When moving a patient with a wet plaster cast, handle it with the palms of the hands to prevent indentations and resulting areas of pressure on the skin. Turn the patient every 1 to 2 hours to allow air to circulate and dry all parts of the cast. Be sure to remind unlicensed assistive personnel (UAP) and the family that the cast is wet and requires special handling. If the health care provider requests that the cast be elevated to reduce swelling, use a cloth-covered pillow instead of one encased in plastic, which could cause the cast to retain heat and prevent drying. Elevation of the casted extremity reduces edema but may impair arterial circulation to the affected limb. Therefore performing a neurovascular assessment of the limb distal to (below) the cast is very important.

For preventing contamination by urine or feces, the perineal area of a dry long-leg or body cast may be covered in plastic. Fracture pans are preferred over traditional bedpans because they are smaller and more comfortable. Remind UAP to take care to prevent spillage onto the cast.

Once the plaster cast is dry, inspect it at least once every 8 hours for drainage, cracking, crumbling, alignment, and fit. Plaster casts act like sponges and absorb drainage, whereas synthetic casts act like a wick pulling drainage away from the drainage site. Padding can also absorb wound drainage. Document the presence of any drainage on the cast. However, the evidence is not clear on whether drainage should be circled on the cast because it may increase anxiety and is not a reliable indicator of drainage amount. *Immediately report to the health care provider any sudden increases in the amount of drainage or change in the integrity of the cast.* After swelling decreases, it is not uncommon for the cast to become too loose and need replacement. If the patient is not admitted to the hospital, provide instructions regarding cast care.

During hospitalization, assess for other complications resulting from casting that can be serious and life threatening, such as infection, circulation impairment, and peripheral nerve damage. If the patient returns home after cast application, teach him or her how to monitor for these complications and when to notify the health care provider.

Infection most often results from the breakdown of skin under the cast (pressure necrosis). If pressure necrosis occurs, the patient typically reports a very painful "hot spot" under the cast and the cast may feel warmer in the affected area. Teach the patient or family to smell the area for mustiness or an unpleasant odor that would indicate infected material. If the infection progresses, a fever may develop.

Circulation impairment and *peripheral nerve damage* can result from tightness of the cast. Teach the patient to assess for circulation at least daily, including the ability to move the area distal to the extremity, numbness, and increased pain.

The patient with a cast may be immobilized for a prolonged period, depending on the extent of the fracture and the type of cast. Assess for complications of immobility, such as skin breakdown, pneumonia, atelectasis, thromboembolism, and constipation. Before the cast is removed, inform the patient that the cast cutter will not injure the skin but that heat may be felt during the procedure.

Because of prolonged immobilization, a joint may become contracted, usually in a fixed state of flexion. Osteoarthritis and osteoporosis may develop from lack of weight bearing. Muscle can also atrophy from lack of exercise during prolonged immobilization of the affected body part, usually an extremity.

Traction. Traction is the application of a pulling force to a part of the body to provide reduction, alignment, and rest. It is also used as a last resort to decrease muscle spasm (thus relieving pain) and prevent or correct deformity and tissue damage. A patient in traction is often hospitalized, but in some cases, home care is possible even for skeletal traction.

Mechanical traction can be either:
- Continuous, as in fracture treatment
- Intermittent, for relief of muscle spasm in other types of musculoskeletal/neurologic trauma, such as cervical nerve root compression

TABLE 54-2 TYPES OF TRACTION USED FOR MUSCULOSKELETAL TRAUMA

TYPE AND CHARACTERISTICS OF TRACTION	USE
Upper Extremity Traction	
Sidearm skin or skeletal traction (the forearm is flexed and extended 90 degrees from the upper part of the body)	Fractures of the humerus with or without involvement of the shoulder and clavicle
Overhead or 90-90 traction, skin or skeletal (the elbow is flexed and the arm is at a right angle to the body over the upper chest)	Same as above (depends on the physician's preference)
Plaster traction (pins inserted through the bone are fixed in the cast)	Fractures of the wrist
Lower Extremity Traction	
Buck's extension traction (skin) (the affected leg is in extension)	Fractures of the hip or femur preoperatively Prevention of hip flexion contractures Hip dislocation
Russell's traction (similar to Buck's traction, but a sling under the knee suspends the leg)	Fractures of the hip or distal end of the femur
Balanced skin or skeletal traction (the limb is usually elevated in a Thomas splint with Pearson's attachment, or a Böhler-Braun splint is used)	Fractures of the femur or pelvis (acetabulum)
Spinal Column and Pelvic Traction	
Cervical halter (a strap under the chin)	Cervical muscle spasms, strain/sprain, or arthritis
Cervical skeletal (e.g., halo brace, Crutchfield tongs)	Cervical fractures of the spine; muscle spasms
Pelvic belt (a strap around the hips at the iliac crests is attached to weights at the foot of the bed)	Pain, strain, sprain, or muscle spasms in the lower back
Pelvic sling (a wide strap around the hips is attached to an overhead bar to keep the pelvis off the bed)	Pelvic fractures; other pelvic injuries

Traction may also be classified as running traction or balanced suspension. In *running* traction, the pulling force is in one direction and the patient's body acts as countertraction. Moving the body or bed position can alter the countertraction force. *Balanced suspension* provides the countertraction so that the pulling force of the traction is not altered when the bed or patient is moved. This allows for increased movement and facilitates care (Table 54-2).

The two most common types of traction are skin and skeletal traction. *Skin traction* involves the use of a Velcro boot (Buck's traction) (Fig. 54-5), belt, or halter, which is usually secured around the affected leg. The primary purpose of skin traction is to decrease painful muscle spasms that accompany hip fractures. The weight is used as a pulling force and is limited to 5 to 10 pounds (2.3 to 4.5 kg) to prevent injury to the skin.

In *skeletal traction*, pins, wires, tongs (e.g., Crutchfield), or screws are surgically inserted directly into bone. These allow the use of longer traction time and heavier weights—usually 15 to 30 pounds (6.8 to 13.6 kg). Skeletal traction aids in bone

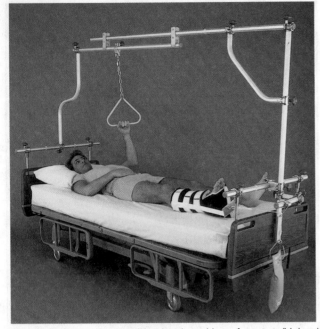

FIG. 54-5 Skin traction with a hook-and-loop fastener (Velcro) boot, commonly used for hip fractures.

realignment. Pin site care is an important part of nursing management to prevent infection.

The nurse may set up or assist in the setup of traction if specially educated. In larger or specialty hospitals or units, orthopedic technicians or physician assistants often set up traction. Once traction is applied, maintain the correct balance between traction pull and countertraction force.

⚠ NURSING SAFETY PRIORITY

Action Alert

When patients are in traction, weights usually are not removed without a prescription. They should not be lifted manually or allowed to rest on the floor. Weights should be freely hanging at all times. Teach this important point to UAP on the unit, to other personnel such as those in the radiology department, and to visitors. Inspect the skin at least every 8 hours for signs of irritation or inflammation. When possible, remove the belt or boot that is used for skin traction every 8 hours to inspect under the device.

Check traction equipment frequently to ensure its proper functioning. Inspect all ropes, knots, and pulleys at least every 8 to 12 hours for loosening, fraying, and positioning. Check the weight for consistency with the health care provider's prescription. Sometimes one of the weights is accidentally removed by a staff member or visitor who bumps into it. Replace the weights if they are not correct, and notify the health care provider or orthopedic technician.

If the patient reports severe pain from muscle spasm, the weights may be too heavy or the patient may need realignment. Report the pain to the health care provider if body realignment fails to reduce the discomfort. Assess neurovascular status of the affected body part to detect circulatory compromise and tissue damage. The circulation is usually monitored every hour for the first 24 hours after traction is applied and every 4 hours thereafter.

❓ NCLEX EXAMINATION CHALLENGE

Physiological Integrity

A client has a new synthetic arm cast for a radial fracture. What health care teaching does the nurse include for the client's home care? **Select all that apply.**
A. "Apply heat on the cast for the first 24 hours to increase blood flow for healing."
B. "Keep your arm elevated, preferably above your heart, as much as possible."
C. "Report severe numbness or inability to move your fingers to your physician."
D. "Take your pain medication as needed according to the prescription directions."
E. "Don't cover the cast with anything because it will stay wet for 24 hours."

Drug Therapy. After fracture treatment, the patient often has pain for a prolonged time during the healing process. The health care provider commonly prescribes opioid and non-opioid analgesics, anti-inflammatory drugs, and muscle relaxants.

For patients with chronic, severe pain, opioid and non-opioid drugs are alternated or given together to manage pain both centrally in the brain and peripherally at the site of injury. For severe or multiple fractures, patient-controlled analgesia (PCA) with morphine, fentanyl, or other drug is used. *Meperidine (Demerol) should never be used for older adults because it has toxic metabolites that can cause seizures and other complications. Many hospitals no longer use this drug for patients of any age. Oxycodone and oxycodone with acetaminophen (Percocet) are common oral opioid drugs that are very effective for most patients with fracture pain. NSAIDs are given to decrease associated tissue inflammation.*

For patients who have less severe injury, the analgesic may be given on an as-needed basis. Collaborate with the patient regarding the best times for the strong pain relievers to be given (e.g., before a complex dressing change, after physical therapy sessions, and at bedtime). Assess the effectiveness of the analgesic and its side effects. Constipation is a common side effect of opioid therapy, especially for older adults. Assess for frequency of bowel movements, and administer stool softeners as needed. Encourage fluids and activity as tolerated. Chapter 5 discusses the various methods of pain management, including epidural analgesia and patient-controlled analgesia.

Some patients experience a long-term, intense burning pain and edema that are associated with *complex regional pain syndrome (CRPS)*, formerly called *reflex sympathetic dystrophy (RSD)*. This syndrome often results from fractures and other musculoskeletal trauma and is discussed on p. 1168 later in this chapter.

Complementary and Alternative Therapies. With long-term, severe pain, the patient cannot depend solely on drugs for relief. Recommend temporary pain relief measures, such as ice or heat, depending on the cause of the pain. If swelling causes pressure on the affected area, ice and elevation of the affected body part may be appropriate. Teach the patient to plan activities that allow for rest and quiet periods. Some patients like soft music playing while resting. Muscle spasms are best relieved by application of heat and massage. Other physical measures include a warm, soothing bath, a back rub, and the use of therapeutic touch.

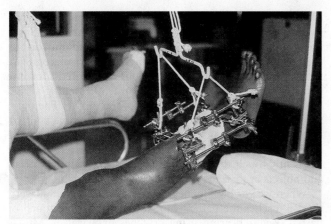

FIG. 54-6 The Hex-Fix external fixation system for tibia-fibula fractures.

If these measures are not effective in reducing pain, distraction, imagery, or music therapy may be used as an alternative. Teach the patient relaxation techniques, such as deep breathing, for use during periods of severe pain. Chapters 2 and 5 discuss these techniques in detail.

Surgical Management. For some types of fractures, closed reduction is not appropriate or sufficient. Surgical intervention may be needed to realign the bone for the healing process.

Preoperative Care. Teach the patient and family what to expect during and after the surgery. The preoperative care for a patient undergoing orthopedic surgery is similar to that for anyone having surgery with general or epidural anesthesia. (See Chapter 16 for a thorough discussion of preoperative nursing care.)

Operative Procedures. Open reduction with internal fixation (ORIF) is one of the most common methods of reducing and immobilizing a fracture. External fixation with closed reduction is used when patients have soft-tissue injury (open fracture). Although nurses do not decide which surgical technique is used, understanding the procedures enhances patient teaching and care.

Because ORIF permits early mobilization, it is often the preferred surgical method. Open reduction allows the surgeon to directly view the fracture site. Internal fixation uses metal pins, screws, rods, plates, or prostheses to immobilize the fracture during healing. The surgeon makes one or more incisions to gain access to the broken bone(s) and implants one or more devices into bone tissue after each fracture is reduced. A cast, boot, or splint is placed to maintain immobilization during the healing process.

After the bone achieves union, the metal hardware may be removed, depending on the location and type of fracture. Hardware is removed most frequently in ankle fractures, depending on the severity of the injury. If the metal implants are not bothersome, they may remain in place. Specific types of internal fixation devices are discussed later in the Fractures of Specific Sites section.

An alternative modality for the management of fractures is the external fixation apparatus, as shown in Fig. 54-6. External fixation is a system in which pins or wires are inserted through the skin and affected bone and then connected to a rigid external frame. The system may be used for upper or lower extremity fractures or for fractures of the pelvis, especially for open fractures when wound management is needed. After a fixator is removed, the patient may be placed in a cast or splint until healing is complete.

External fixation has several advantages over other surgical techniques:

- There is minimal blood loss compared with internal fixation.
- The device allows early ambulation and exercise of the affected body part while relieving pain.
- The device maintains alignment in closed fractures that will not maintain position in a cast and stabilizes comminuted fractures that require bone grafting.

In open fractures, in which skin and tissue trauma accompany the fracture, the device permits easy access to the wound while the bone heals. This method is usually preferred over the use of a window in a cast for wound care.

A disadvantage of external fixation is an increased risk for pin site infection. Pin site infections can lead to osteomyelitis, which is serious and difficult to treat (see Chapter 53).

Postoperative Care. The postoperative care for a patient undergoing ORIF or external fixation is similar to that provided for any patient undergoing surgery (see Chapter 18). Because bone is a vascular, dynamic body tissue, the patient is at risk for complications specific to fractures and musculoskeletal surgery. IV ketorolac (Toradol) is often given in the postanesthesia care unit (PACU) or soon after discharge to the post-surgical area to reduce inflammation and pain. Aggressive pain management starts as soon as possible after surgery to prevent the development of chronic pain and promote early mobility.

Additional information about postoperative care is found beginning on p. 1159 in the Fractures of Specific Sites section. Depending on the fractures that are repaired, some ORIF procedures are performed as same-day surgeries. Patients stay in the hospital up to 23 hours after surgery.

For patients with an external fixator, pay particular attention to the pin sites for signs of inflammation or infection. In the first 48 to 72 hours, *clear* fluid drainage or weeping is expected. Although no standardized method or evidence-based protocol for pin care has been established, recommendations have been made based on the evidence available regarding pin site care. Because the pins go through the skin and into bone, the risk for infection is high. Monitor the pin sites at least every 8 to 12 hours for drainage, color, odor, and severe redness, which indicate inflammation and possible infection. Follow agency policy for how to clean the pin site areas, and ensure that it follows the evidence-based guidelines from the National Association of Orthopaedic Nurses (www.naon.org) (Holmes & Brown, 2005).

The patient with an external fixator may have a disturbed body image. The frame may be large and bulky, and the affected area may have massive tissue damage with dressings. Be sensitive to this possibility in planning care. Teach about alterations to clothing that may be required while the fixator is in place.

The Ilizarov technique of circular external fixation is sometimes used to treat new fractures (closed, comminuted fractures and open fractures with bone loss), as well as malunion or nonunion of fractures. It may also be used to treat congenital bone deformities, especially in children and "little people" (e.g., dwarfs).

The circular external fixation device is used to gently pull apart the cortex of the bone and stimulate new bone growth. Unlike the traditional fixator, the Ilizarov external fixator promotes rotation, angulation, lengthening, or widening of bone to correct bony defects and allows for healing of any soft-tissue defect. The nursing care associated with this device is similar to the care of the patient with other external fixation systems with one major exception. If the device is being used for filling bone gaps using bone transport or distraction, teach the patient how to manually turn the four-sided nuts (also called *clickers*) up to four times a day. Daily distraction rates vary, but 1 mm daily is common. Screening and teaching are particularly important because the patient adjusts and cares for the apparatus over a long period of up to 6 months to 1 year. Pain control is a priority outcome for patients using this device.

Procedures for Nonunion. Some management techniques are not successful because the bone does not heal. Several additional options are available to the physician to promote bone union, such as electrical bone stimulation, bone grafting, and ultrasound fracture treatment.

For selected patients, *electrical bone stimulation* may be successful. This procedure is based on research showing that bone has electrical properties that are used in healing. The exact mechanism of action is unknown. A noninvasive, external electrical bone stimulation system delivers a small continuous electrical charge directed toward the non-healed bone. There are no known risks with this system, although patients with pacemakers cannot use this device on an arm. Implanted direct-current stimulators are placed directly in the fracture site and have no external apparatus. Both systems require several months of treatment.

Another method of treating nonunion is *bone grafting*. A bone graft may also replace diseased bone or increase bone tissue for joint replacement. In most cases, chips of bone are taken from the iliac crest or other site and are packed or wired between the bone ends to facilitate union. Allografts from cadavers may also be used. These grafts are frozen or freeze-dried and stored under sterile conditions in a bone bank.

Bone banking from living donors is becoming increasingly popular. If qualified, patients undergoing total hip replacement may donate their femoral heads to the bank for later use as bone grafts for others. Careful screening ensures that the bone is healthy and that the donor has no communicable disease. The bone cannot be donated without written consent.

One of the newest modalities for fracture healing is low-intensity pulsed ultrasound (Exogen therapy). Used for slow-healing fractures or for new fractures as an alternative to surgery, ultrasound treatment has had excellent results. The patient applies the treatment for about 20 minutes each day. It has no contraindications or adverse effects.

Physical Therapy. Many patients with musculoskeletal trauma, including fractures, are referred by their health care provider for rehabilitation therapy with a physical therapist (PT). The timing for this referral depends on the nature, severity, and treatment modality of the fracture(s).

For example, some patients who have an ORIF for one or more ankle fractures may begin therapy when the incisional staples or Steri-Strips are removed and an orthopedic knee boot is fitted. Based on the initial evaluation, the PT performs gentle manipulative exercises to increase range of motion.

The therapist may also begin to help the patient with laterality, a concept to help the brain identify the injured foot from the uninjured foot. Computer programs and mirror-box therapy can help reprogram the brain as part of cognitive retraining. In mirror-box therapy for an injured foot, the patient covers his or her affected foot while looking at and moving the uninjured foot in front of the mirror. The brain perceives the foot in the mirror as the injured foot.

Stimulation by touch also helps the brain acknowledge the injured foot. The PT teaches the patient to have someone frequently touch the injured area and use various materials and objects against the skin to desensitize it.

When weight bearing begins about 6 weeks after surgery, the PT teaches the patient how to begin with toe-touch or partial weight bearing using crutches or a walker. Muscle strengthening exercises of the affected leg help with ambulation because atrophy begins shortly after injury.

The PT also assists with pain control and edema reduction by using ice/heat packs, electrical muscle stimulation ("e-stim"), and special treatments such as dexamethasone iontophoresis. Iontophoresis is a method for absorbing dexamethasone, a synthetic steroid, through the skin near the painful area to decrease inflammation and edema. A small device delivers a minute amount of electricity via electrodes that are placed on the skin. The patient may describe the sensation as a pinch or slight sting. The current increases the ability of the skin to absorb the drug from a topical patch into the affected soft tissue.

The success of rehabilitation is affected by the patient's motivation and willingness to perform prescribed exercises and activities between PT visits. Rehabilitation for ankle surgery, for example, may take several months, depending on the severity of the injury and the age and general health condition of the patient.

Preventing and Monitoring for Neurovascular Compromise

Planning: Expected Outcomes. The patient with a fracture is expected to have no compromise in neurovascular status as evidenced by adequate circulation, movement, and sensation (CMS). If severe compromise occurs, the patient is expected to have early and prompt emergency treatment to prevent severe tissue damage.

Interventions. Perform neurovascular (NV) assessments (also known as "circ checks" or CMS assessments) frequently before and after fracture treatment. Patients who have extremity casts, splints with elastic bandage wraps, and open reduction with internal fixation (ORIF) or external fixation are especially at risk for NV compromise. If blood flow to the distal extremity is impaired, the patient reports increased pain and decreased sensation and movement. If these symptoms are allowed to progress, patients are at risk for acute compartment syndrome (ACS).

Early recognition of the signs and symptoms of ACS can prevent loss of function or loss of a limb. Identify patients who may be at risk, and monitor them closely. ACS can begin in 6 to 8 hours after an injury or take up to 2 days to appear. If it is suspected, notify the health care provider immediately, and if possible, implement interventions to relieve the pressure. For example, for the patient with tight, bulky dressings, loosen the bandage or tape. If the patient has a cast, follow agency protocol about who may cut the cast.

In a few cases, compartment pressure may be monitored on a one-time basis with a handheld device with a digital display or pressure can be monitored continuously. Monitoring is recommended for comatose or unresponsive high-risk patients with multiple trauma and fractures.

If ACS is verified, the surgeon may perform a fasciotomy, or opening in the fascia, by making an incision through the skin and subcutaneous tissues into the fascia of the affected compartment. This procedure relieves the pressure and restores circulation to the affected area. No consensus exists on what pressure requires fasciotomy (normal is 0 to 8 mm Hg). Compartment pressures must be considered in relation to the patient's hemodynamic status. After fasciotomy, the open wound is packed and dressed daily or more often until secondary closure occurs, usually in 4 to 5 days, depending on the patient's healing ability. At that time, the surgeon usually débrides the wound and may apply a skin graft to promote healing.

Preventing Infection

Planning: Expected Outcomes. The patient with a fracture is expected to be free of wound or bone infection as evidenced by no fever, no increase in white blood cell count, and negative wound culture (if wound is present).

Interventions. When caring for a patient with an open fracture, use clean or aseptic technique for dressing changes and wound irrigations. Check agency policy for specific protocols. *Immediately notify the health care provider if you observe inflammation and purulent drainage.* Other infections, such as pneumonia and urinary tract infection, may occur several days after the fracture. Monitor the patient's vital signs every 4 to 8 hours because increases in temperature and pulse often indicate systemic infection.

CONSIDERATIONS FOR OLDER ADULTS

Older adults may not have a temperature elevation even in the presence of severe infection. An acute onset of confusion (delirium) often suggests an infection in the older adult patient.

For most patients with an open fracture, the health care provider prescribes one or more broad-spectrum antibiotics prophylactically and performs surgical débridement of any wounds as soon as possible after the injury. First-generation cephalosporins, clindamycin (Cleocin), and ciprofloxacin (Cipro) are commonly used. In addition to systemic antibiotics, local antibiotic therapy through wound irrigation is commonly prescribed, especially during débridement.

A very effective wound therapy is the vacuum-assisted closure (VAC) system as a method of increasing the rate of wound healing for open fractures. This device allows quicker wound closure, which decreases the risk for infection.

When the bone is surgically repaired, hardware and/or bone grafts have typically been implanted. However, they are limited in their use. The U.S. Food and Drug Administration (FDA) approved the use of recombinant human bone morphogenetic protein-2 (rhBMP-2) for tibial and spinal fractures. This implanted genetically engineered substance increases wound healing, decreases hardware failure, and decreases the risk for infection.

Improving Physical Mobility

Planning: Expected Outcomes. The patient with a fracture is expected to increase physical mobility and be free of complications associated with impaired mobility. The patient is also expected to move purposefully in his or her own environment independently with or without an ambulatory device unless restricted by traction or other modality.

Interventions. The interventions necessary for this diagnosis can be grouped into two types: those that help increase mobility and those that prevent complications of impaired mobility.

Promoting Mobility. The use of crutches or a walker increases mobility and assists in ambulation. The patient may progress to using a walker or cane after crutches.

Crutches are the most commonly used ambulatory aid for many types of lower extremity musculoskeletal trauma (e.g., fractures, sprains, amputations). In most agencies, the physical therapist or emergency department/ambulatory care nurse fits the patient for crutches and teaches him or her how to ambulate with them. Reinforce those instructions, and evaluate whether the patient is using the crutches correctly.

Walking with crutches requires strong arm muscles, balance, and coordination. For this reason, crutches are not often used for older adults. Walkers and canes are preferred for the older adult. Crutches can cause upper extremity bursitis or axillary nerve damage if they are not fitted or used correctly. For that reason, the top of each crutch is padded. To prevent pressure on the axillary nerve, there should be two to three finger breadths between the axilla and the top of the crutch when the crutch tip is at least 6 inches (15 cm) diagonally in front of the foot. The crutch is adjusted so that the elbow is flexed no more than 30 degrees when the palm is on the handle (Fig. 54-7). The distal tips of each crutch are rubber to prevent slipping.

There are several types of gaits for walking with crutches. The most common one for musculoskeletal injury is the three-point gait, which allows little weight bearing on the affected leg. The procedure for these gaits is discussed in fundamentals of nursing books.

A *walker* is most often used by the older patient who needs additional support for balance. The physical therapist assesses the strength of the upper extremities and the unaffected leg. Strength is improved with prescribed exercises as needed.

A *cane* is sometimes used if the patient needs only minimal support for an affected leg. The straight cane offers the least support. A hemi-cane or quad-cane provides a broader base for the cane and therefore more support. The cane is placed on the *unaffected* side and should create no more than 30 degrees of flexion of the elbow. The top of the cane should

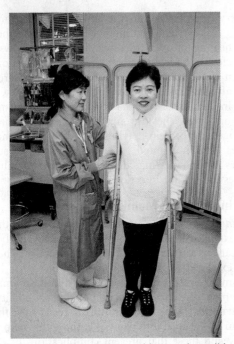

FIG. 54-7 Assisting the patient with crutch walking. Note how the therapist guards the patient and how the patient's elbows are at no more than 30 degrees of flexion.

be parallel to the greater trochanter of the femur or stylus of the wrist. Chapter 8 describes these ambulatory devices in more detail.

Preventing Complications of Immobility. The nurse plays a vital role in preventing and assessing for complications in immobilized patients with fractures. Additional information about nursing care for preventing problems associated with immobility is found in Chapter 8.

Community-Based Care

The patient with an *uncomplicated* fracture is usually discharged to home from the emergency department or urgent care center. Older adults with hip or other fractures or patients with multiple traumas are hospitalized and then transferred to home, a rehabilitation setting, or a long-term care facility for rehabilitation. Collaborate with the case manager or the discharge planner in the hospital to ensure continuity of care. Be sure to communicate the plan of care clearly to the health care agency receiving the patient.

Home Care Management

If the patient is discharged to home, the nurse, therapist, or case manager (CM) may assess the home environment for structural barriers to mobility, such as stairs. Be sure that the patient has easy access to the bathroom. Ask about scatter rugs, waxed floors, and walkway areas that could increase the risk for falls. If the patient needs to use a wheelchair or ambulatory aid, make sure that he or she can use it safely and that there is room in the house to ambulate with these devices. The physical therapist may teach the patient how to use stairs, but older adults or those using crutches may experience difficulty performing this task. Depending on the age and condition of the patient, a home health care nurse may make one or two visits to check that the home is safe and that the

---

CHART 54-5   PATIENT AND FAMILY EDUCATION: PREPARING FOR SELF-MANAGEMENT

Care of the Extremity After Cast Removal

- Remove scaly, dead skin carefully by soaking; do not scrub.
- Move the extremity carefully. Expect discomfort, weakness, and decreased range of motion.
- Support the extremity with pillows or your orthotic device until strength and movement return.
- Exercise slowly as instructed by your physical therapist.
- Wear support stockings or elastic bandages to prevent swelling (for lower extremity).

---

patient and family are able to follow the interdisciplinary plan of care.

Teaching for Self-Management

The patient with a fracture may be discharged from the hospital, emergency department, office, or clinic with a bandage, splint, cast, or external fixator. Provide verbal and written instructions on the care of these devices. Chart 54-5 describes care of the affected extremity after removal of the cast.

The patient may also need to continue wound care at home. Instruct the patient and family about how to assess and dress the wound to promote healing and prevent infection. Teach them how to recognize complications and when and where to seek professional health care if complications occur. Additional educational needs depend on the type of fracture and fracture repair.

Encourage patients and their families to ensure adequate foods high in protein and calcium that are needed for bone and tissue healing. For patients with lower extremity fractures, less weight bearing on long bones can cause anemia. The red bone marrow needs weight bearing to simulate red blood cell production. Encourage foods high in iron content. Teach the patient to take a daily iron-added multivitamin (take with food to prevent possible nausea).

Health Care Resources

Arrange for follow-up care at home. A social worker may need to help the patient apply for funds to pay medical bills. If there is severe bone and tissue damage, be realistic and help the patient and family understand the long-term nature of the recovery period. Multiple treatment techniques and surgical procedures required for complications can be mentally and emotionally draining for the patient and family. A vocational counselor may be needed to help the patient find a different type of job, depending on the extent of the fracture.

An older or incapacitated patient may need assistance with ADLs, which can be provided by home care aides if family or other caregiver is not available. In collaboration with the case manager, anticipate the patient's needs and arrange for these services.

▌EVALUATION: OUTCOMES

Evaluate the care of the patient with one or more fractures based on the identified priority patient problems. The expected outcomes include that the patient:

- States that he or she has adequate pain control
- Has adequate blood flow to maintain tissue perfusion and function
- Is free of infection
- Is free of physiologic consequences of impaired mobility
- Ambulates or moves independently with or without an assistive device (if not restricted by traction or other device)

? DECISION-MAKING CHALLENGE

Safety; Evidence-Based Practice; Informatics

The 68-year-old patient with multiple fractures of her ankle presented in the Decision-Making Challenge on p. 1149 needs a joint reduction for her dislocated tibia and fibula. As her nurse, you explain the procedure and assure her that she will not have pain during the procedure. You apply a pulse oximeter, nasal oxygen, and capnography monitoring system in preparation for the procedure.

1. What is the purpose of the capnography system?
2. While the patient receives moderate sedation, you note that her respiratory rate drops to 8 breaths/min and her capnography reading is 18. What do these values mean? What evidence-based action will you take first as a result of these values? What will you document in the electronic patient record about the patient's response during the procedure?
3. After the joint is reduced, a splint and large bulky dressing with elastic wraps are applied. The patient will be going home with her daughter, using crutches. What crutch-walking technique will you teach her?
4. What other health teaching will she need and why?

FRACTURES OF SPECIFIC SITES ✂

Upper Extremity Fractures

In addition to the general care discussed in the previous section, management of upper extremity fractures includes specific interventions related to the location and nature of the injury. Unless multiple fractures or massive soft-tissue damage occurs, upper extremity fractures do not usually require hospitalization. However, they often take many months to heal. In some cases, patients may not regain complete function for up to a year, even after extensive rehabilitation in occupational therapy. Assess neurovascular status in the affected arm and hand before and after fracture treatment. Monitor for numbness and tingling distal to (below) the injury, which may indicate peripheral nerve damage.

Fractures of the *clavicle* typically result from a fall on an outstretched hand, a fall on the shoulder, or a direct blow to the upper chest and shoulder area. Most clavicular fractures are self-healing. A splint or bandage is used for immobilization. Complicated open fractures, although uncommon, may require open reduction with internal fixation (ORIF) by pins, wires, or screws.

Scapular fractures are not common and are usually caused by direct impact to the area. Serious internal trauma, including pneumothorax, pulmonary contusion, and fractured ribs, can accompany these fractures. The shoulder is kept in position with a commercial immobilizer until the fracture heals, usually in 2 to 4 weeks. Intra-articular neck and glenoid fractures may require surgical intervention with plate and screw fixation.

Fractures of the *proximal humerus,* particularly impacted or displaced fractures, are common in the older adult. As persons age, fractures of the humerus occur more frequently in the area closer to the shoulder joint. This makes treatment more difficult in the older adult. An impacted injury is usually treated with a sling or other device for immobilization. A displaced fracture often requires ORIF with pins or a prosthesis.

Humeral shaft fractures are generally corrected by closed reduction and a hanging-arm cast or splint. If necessary, the fracture is repaired surgically (with an intramedullary rod or metal plate and screws) or with external fixation. Nonunion of the bone and radial nerve palsy are frequent complications of this fracture. Bone grafting helps promote union. Prolonged splinting is necessary while the radial nerve regenerates.

A direct blow to the condyles of the distal humerus can cause either or both condyles to fracture, usually in a T- or Y-shaped configuration. The most serious complication is damage to the brachial or median nerve. Condylar fracture is usually treated by ORIF with a series of screws, although skeletal traction and casting can be used.

Fractures of the *elbow (olecranon)* are common in adults and typically result from a fall on the elbow. Many are successfully treated by closed reduction and application of a cast. ORIF is performed for displaced fractures, and a splint is worn during the healing phase.

Forearm fractures of the ulna without accompanying injury to the radius are rare. As with other fractures of long bones, closed reduction with casting may be the appropriate treatment. If the fracture is displaced, ORIF with intramedullary rods or plates and screws is required.

One or more of the bones in the *wrist and hand* can break, but the most common fracture is of the carpal scaphoid bone in young adult men. This is also one of the most misdiagnosed fractures because it is poorly visualized on an x-ray film. Closed reduction and casting for 6 to 12 weeks is the treatment of choice. If the bone does not heal, ORIF with bone grafting is performed.

A *Colles'* (wrist) fracture is common in older adults, particularly women with osteoporosis. A Colles' fracture occurs in the last inch of the distal radius and often is the result of a fall on an outstretched hand. These fractures can usually be treated by splinting or casting for 6 to 8 weeks.

Fractures of the *metacarpals* and *phalanges (fingers)* are usually not displaced, which makes their treatment less difficult than that of other fractures. Metacarpal fractures are immobilized for 3 to 4 weeks. Phalangeal fractures are immobilized in finger splints for 10 to 14 days.

Lower Extremity Fractures
Fractures of the Hip

Hip fracture is the most common injury in older adults and one of the most frequently seen injuries in any health care setting or community. It has a high mortality rate as a result of multiple complications related to surgery, depression, and prolonged immobility. Between 25% and 40% of patients who had a hip fracture die within 1 year after surgery.

Hip fractures include those involving the upper third of the femur and are classified as intracapsular (within the joint capsule) or extracapsular (outside the joint capsule). These types are further divided according to fracture location (Fig. 54-8). In the area of the femoral neck there is concern with

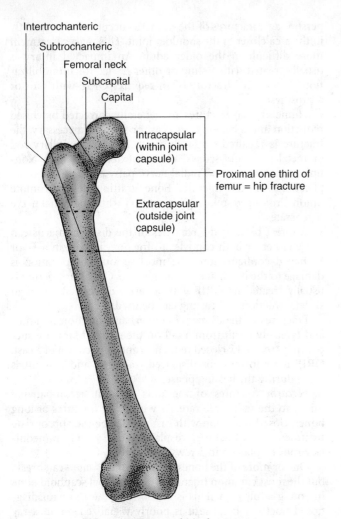

FIG. 54-8 Types of hip fractures.

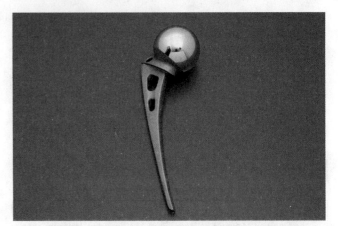

FIG. 54-9 A hip prosthesis used for fractures.

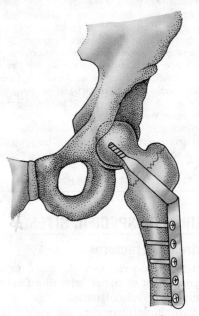

FIG. 54-10 A compression hip screw used for open reduction with internal fixation (ORIF) of the hip.

disruption of the blood supply to the head of the femur, which can result in ischemic or avascular necrosis (AVN) of the femoral head. AVN causes death and necrosis of bone tissue and results in pain and decreased mobility. This problem is most likely in patients with displaced fractures.

Osteoporosis is the biggest risk factor for hip fractures (see Chapter 53). This disease weakens the upper femur (hip), breaks, and then causes the person to fall. The number of

people with hip fracture is expected to continue to increase as the population ages, and the associated health care costs will be tremendous.

The treatment of choice is surgical repair (open reduction, internal fixation, or ORIF), when possible, to reduce pain and allow the older patient to be out of bed and ambulatory. Skin (Buck's) traction may be applied before surgery to help decrease pain associated with muscle spasm. Depending on the exact location of the fracture, an ORIF may include an intramedullary rod, pins, prostheses (for femoral head or neck fractures), or a compression screw. Epidural or general anesthesia is used. Figs. 54-9 and 54-10 illustrate examples of these devices. Occasionally a patient will be so debilitated that surgery cannot be done. In these cases, nonsurgical options include pain management and bedrest to allow natural fracture healing.

Patients usually receive IV morphine after admission to the emergency department and PCA morphine or epidural analgesia after surgery (Herr & Titler, 2009). Meperidine (Demerol) should not be used due to its toxic metabolites that can cause seizures and other adverse drug events, especially in the older adult population (see the Evidence-Based

Do ED Nurses Follow Best Practices for Acute Pain Management for Older Adults with a Fractured Hip?

Herr, K., & Titler, M. (2009). Acute pain assessment and pharmacological management practices for the older adult with a hip fracture: Review of ED trends. *Journal of Emergency Nursing, 35*(4), 312-320.

The researchers conducted a retrospective review of 1454 older adult patients with hip fractures admitted through the emergency department in 12 acute care hospitals over a 3-year period after The Joint Commission issued new pain assessment and management standards for this population. Pain assessment and management practices were examined for trends over time. Almost all patients had some documentation of pain assessment using either a numeric scale or non-numeric scale (e.g., verbal descriptor or faces scale).

The mean intensity of pain was between 6.8 and 7.2 on a 1-to-10 pain scale. Yet, only 60% of patients had an order for an analgesic. Of those orders, about 90% received an opioid. Practice improvements showed a decline in IM opioid administration and meperidine administration and an increase in IV morphine as the drug of choice. These trends are in line with current best practices but need improvement, especially the need for pain control for patients who have fractures.

Level of Evidence: 4
The study was a large descriptive study that examined medical records for trends in practice.

Commentary: Implications for Practice and Research
This study demonstrates the need for nurses to advocate for their patients for pain control. Pain is the priority problem that patients have when they sustain a fracture. Many health care providers are hesitant to prescribe pain medication for older adults for fear of respiratory depression or other negative outcome. Titrated opioid drugs are safe for older adults when given in the health care setting. Uncontrolled pain can cause delirium and increased anxiety among older adults. If a patient cannot state his or her pain intensity, nonverbal descriptors like grimacing or yelling out validate the presence of pain.

Practice box above). Chapter 5 discusses the nursing care associated with pain management in detail.

After a hip repair, older adults frequently experience acute confusion, or delirium. They may pull at tubes or the surgical dressing or attempt to climb out of bed, possibly falling and causing self-injury. Other patients stay awake all night and sleep during the day. Keep in mind that some patients have a quiet delirium. Monitor the patient frequently to prevent falls. Ask the family or other visitors to let staff know if the patient is attempting to get out of bed. Chapter 3 describes fall prevention strategies and delirium management in detail.

! NURSING SAFETY PRIORITY

Action Alert

Patients who have an ORIF are at risk for hip dislocation or subluxation. Be sure to prevent hip adduction and rotation to keep the operative leg in proper alignment. Regular pillows or abduction devices can be used for patients who are confused or restless. If straps are used to hold the device in place, check the skin for signs of pressure. Perform neurovascular assessments to ensure that the device is not interfering with arterial circulation or peripheral nerve conduction.

The patient begins ambulating with assistance the day after surgery to prevent complications associated with immobility (e.g., pressure ulcers, atelectasis, venous thromboembolism). Early movement and ambulation also decrease the chance of infection and increase surgical site healing.

Special considerations for the patient having a hip repair also include careful inspection of skin including areas of pressure, especially the heels. Use of skin traction to reduce muscle spasms may increase the period of bedrest before surgery. Decreased mobility after surgery can increase the risk for pressure injury in this area within 24 hours.

! NURSING SAFETY PRIORITY

Action Alert

Be sure that the patient's heels are up off the bed at all times. Inspect the heels and other high-risk bony prominence areas every 8 to 12 hours. Delegate turning and repositioning every 1 to 2 hours to unlicensed assistive personnel (UAP), and supervise this nursing activity.

Other postoperative interventions to prevent complications, such as venous thromboembolism, are similar to those for total hip replacement (see Chapter 20).

Many patients recover fully from hip fracture repair and regain their functional ability. They are typically discharged to their home, rehabilitation unit or center, or a skilled nursing facility for physical and occupational therapy. However, some patients are not able to return to their pre-fracture ADLs and mobility level. These patients usually do not return to their homes and are placed in long-term care facilities. A classic pilot study by Folden and Tappen (2007) identified predictors for patients who are likely to fully recover. They found that balance and cognitive ability were the best predictors.

Other Fractures of the Lower Extremity

Other fractures of the lower extremity may or may not require hospitalization. However, if the patient has severe or multiple fractures, especially with soft-tissue damage, hospital admission is usually required. Patients who have surgery to repair their injury may also be hospitalized. Coordinate care with the physical therapist regarding mobility, transfers, positioning, and ambulation. Collaborate with the case manager regarding placement after discharge. Most patients go home unless there is no support system or additional rehabilitation is needed. Health teaching and ensuring continuity of care are essential.

Fractures of the *lower two thirds of the femur* usually result from trauma often from a motor vehicle crash. A femur fracture is seldom immobilized by casting because the powerful muscles of the thigh become spastic, which causes displacement of bone ends. Extensive hemorrhage can occur with femur fracture.

Surgical treatment is ORIF with nails, rods, or a compression screw. In a few cases in which extensive bone fragmentation or severe tissue trauma is found, external fixation may be employed. Healing time for a femur fracture may be 6 months or longer. Skeletal traction, followed by a full-leg brace or cast, may be used in nonsurgical treatment.

Like most other fractures, *patellar* (knee cap) fractures result from direct impact. The surgeon typically repairs the fracture by closed reduction and casting or internal fixation with screws. A knee immobilizer is used so that the fracture can heal properly.

Trauma to the lower leg most often causes fractures of both the *tibia* and the *fibula*, particularly the lower third, and is often referred to as a "tib-fib" fracture. The major treatment techniques are closed reduction with casting, internal fixation, and external fixation. If closed reduction is used, the patient wears a cast for at least 8 to 10 weeks. Because of poor blood supply to parts of the tibia and fibula, delayed union is not unusual with this type of fracture. Internal fixation with nails or a plate and screws, followed by a long-leg cast for 4 to 6 weeks, is another option. When the fractures cause extensive skin and soft-tissue damage, the initial treatment may be external fixation, often for 6 to 10 weeks, usually followed by application of a cast until the fracture is completely healed. The patient uses ambulatory aids, usually crutches.

Ankle fractures are described by their anatomic place of injury. For example, a bimalleolar (Pott's) fracture involves the medial malleolus of the tibia and the lateral malleolus of the fibula. The small talus that makes up the rest of the ankle joint may also be broken. An ORIF is usually performed using two incisions—one on the medial (inside) aspect of the ankle and one on the lateral (outer) side. Several screws or nails are placed into the tibia, and a compression plate with multiple screws keeps the fibula in alignment. Weight bearing is restricted until the bone heals.

Treatment of fractures of the foot or phalanges (toes) is similar to that of other fractures, with either closed or open reduction. Phalangeal fractures are more painful than but not as serious as most other types of fractures. Crutches are used for ambulation.

Fractures of the Chest and Pelvis

Chest trauma may cause fractures of the ribs or sternum. The most commonly fractured ribs are numbers 4 through 8. The major concern with rib and sternal fractures is the potential for puncture of the lungs, heart, or arteries by bone fragments or ends. Assess airway, breathing, and circulation status **first** for any patient having chest trauma. Fractures of the lower ribs may damage underlying organs, such as the liver, spleen, or kidneys. These fractures tend to heal on their own without surgical intervention. Patients are often uncomfortable during the healing process and require analgesia. They also have a high risk for pneumonia because of shallow breathing caused by pain on inspiration. Encourage them to breathe normally if possible.

Because the pelvis is very vascular and is close to major organs and blood vessels, associated internal damage is the major focus in fracture management. After head injuries, pelvic fractures are the second most common cause of death from trauma. In young adults, pelvic fractures typically result from motor vehicle crashes or falls from buildings. Falls are the most common cause in older adults. The major concern related to pelvic injury is venous oozing or arterial bleeding. Loss of blood volume leads to hypovolemic shock.

Assess for internal abdominal trauma by checking for blood in the urine and stool and by monitoring the abdomen for the development of rigidity or swelling. The trauma team may use peritoneal lavage, computed tomography (CT) scanning, or ultrasound for assessment of hemorrhage. Ultrasound is noninvasive, rapid, reliable, and cost-effective and can be done at the bedside.

There are many classification systems for pelvic fractures. A system that is particularly useful divides fractures of the pelvis into two broad categories: non–weight-bearing fractures and weight-bearing fractures.

When a *non–weight-bearing* part of the pelvis is fractured, such as one of the pubic rami or the iliac crest, treatment can be as minimal as bedrest on a firm mattress or bed board. This type of fracture can be quite painful, and the patient may need stool softeners to facilitate bowel movements because of hesitancy to move. Well-stabilized fractures usually heal in 2 months.

A *weight-bearing* fracture, such as multiple fractures of the pelvic ring creating instability or a fractured acetabulum, necessitates external fixation or open reduction with internal fixation (ORIF) or both. Progression to weight bearing depends on the stability of the fracture after fixation. Some patients can fully bear weight within days of surgery, whereas others managed with traction may not be able to bear weight for as long as 12 weeks.

Compression Fractures of the Spine

Most vertebral fractures are associated with osteoporosis, metastatic bone cancer, and multiple myeloma. Compression fractures result when trabecular or cancellous bone within the vertebra becomes weakened and causes the vertebral body to collapse. The patient has severe pain, deformity (kyphosis), and occasional neurologic compromise. As discussed in the Osteoporosis section of Chapter 53, the patient's quality of life is reduced by the impact of this problem.

Nonsurgical management includes bedrest, analgesics, nerve blocks, and physical therapy to maintain muscle strength. Vertebral compression fractures (VCFs) that remain painful and impair mobility may be surgically treated with vertebroplasty or kyphoplasty. These procedures are minimally invasive techniques in which bone cement is injected through the skin (percutaneously) directly into the fracture site to provide stability and immediate pain relief. Kyphoplasty includes the additional step of inserting a small balloon into the fracture site and inflating it to contain the cement and to restore height to the vertebra. This procedure is preferred because it reduces the complication of leaking of bone cement outside the vertebral body and it may restore height to decrease kyphosis.

Minimally invasive surgeries can be done in an operating or interventional radiology suite by a surgeon or interventional radiologist. They can be done with moderate sedation or general anesthesia. IV ketorolac (Toradol) may be given before the procedure to reduce inflammation. Large-bore needles are placed into the fracture site using fluoroscopy or computed tomography guidance. Then the deflated balloon is inserted through the needles and inflated in the fracture site, and the cement is injected.

Patients may have the procedures in an ambulatory care setting and return home after 2 to 4 hours or be admitted to the hospital for an overnight stay. Chart 54-6 describes the preoperative and postoperative care for percutaneous interventions for vertebral compression devices.

Before discharge, teach the patient to report any signs or symptoms of infection from puncture sites. Remind him or her to not soak in a bath for 1 week, use analgesics as needed, resume activity, and contact the health care provider for questions or concerns.

Nursing Care for Patients Having Vertebroplasty or Kyphoplasty

Provide *preoperative care* including:
- Check the patient's coagulation laboratory test results; platelet count should be more than 100,000/mm³.
- Make sure that all anticoagulant drugs were discontinued as requested by the physician.
- Assess and document the patient's neurologic status, especially extremity movement and sensation.
- Assess the patient's pain level.
- Assess the patient's ability to lie prone for at least 1 hour.
- Establish an IV line, and take vital signs.

Provide *postoperative care* including:
- Place the patient in a flat supine position for 1 to 2 hours or as requested by the physician.
- Monitor and record vital signs and frequent neurologic assessments; report any change immediately to the physician.
- Apply an ice pack to the puncture site if needed to relieve pain.
- Assess the patient's pain level, and compare it with the preoperative level; give mild analgesic as needed.
- Monitor for complications such as bleeding at the puncture site or shortness of breath; report these findings immediately if they occur.
- Assist the patient with ambulation.

Before discharge, teach the patient and family the following:
- The patient should avoid driving or operating machinery for the first 24 hours because of drugs used during the procedure.
- Monitor the puncture site for signs of infection, such as redness, pain, swelling, or drainage.
- Keep the dressing dry, and remove it the next day.
- The patient should begin usual activities, including walking the next day, and should slowly increase activity level over the next few days.

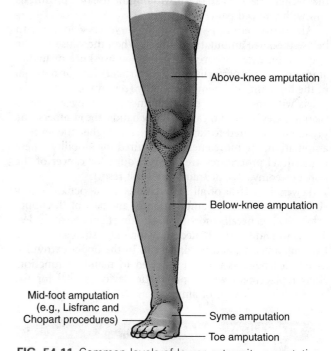

FIG. 54-11 Common levels of lower extremity amputation.

Fractures at Other Sites

Because the skull and vertebral column protect the brain and spinal cord, these fractures are described in Chapters 45 and 47. Fractures of the mandible or nose and other facial trauma are also discussed elsewhere in the text.

AMPUTATIONS

An amputation is the removal of a part of the body. Advances in microvascular surgical procedures, better use of antibiotic therapy, and improved surgical techniques for traumatic injury and bone cancer all help reduce the number of amputations. The psychosocial aspects of the procedure are as devastating as the physical impairments that result. The loss is complete and permanent and causes a change in body image and often in self-esteem. Collaborate with members of the health care team, including prosthetists, rehabilitation therapists, psychologists, case managers, and physiatrists (rehabilitation physicians), when providing care to the patient who has an amputation.

Pathophysiology
Types of Amputation

Amputations may be elective or traumatic. Most are *elective* and are related to complications of peripheral vascular disease and arteriosclerosis. These complications result in ischemia in distal areas of the *lower extremity*. Diabetes mellitus is often

an underlying cause. Amputation is considered only after other interventions have not restored circulation to the lower extremity, sometimes referred to as *limb salvage procedures* (e.g., percutaneous transluminal angioplasty [PTA]). These procedures are discussed elsewhere in this text.

Traumatic amputations most often result from accidents and are the primary cause of *upper extremity* amputation. A person may clean lawn mower blades or a snow blower without disconnecting the machine. A motor vehicle crash or industrial machine accident may also cause an amputation. The number of traumatic amputations also increases during war as a result of hidden land mines and bombs (e.g., in Iraq), and typically, one or both legs are affected. Thousands of veterans of war in the United States are amputees and have had to adjust to major changes in their lifestyles.

Injury that causes severe crushing of tissues or significant blood vessel damage usually results in amputation to preserve function of the residual limb. The ability to salvage limbs injured related to trauma, however, is increasing. Some body parts that are severed can be reattached or replanted.

Levels of Amputation

Lower extremity (LE) amputations are performed much more frequently than upper extremity amputations. Five types of lower extremity amputations may be performed (Fig. 54-11).

The loss of any or all of the small toes presents a minor disability. Loss of the great toe is significant because it affects balance, gait, and "push off" ability during walking. Midfoot amputations (e.g., the Lisfranc and the Chopart amputations) and the Syme amputation are common procedures for peripheral vascular disease. In the Syme amputation, most of the foot is removed but the ankle remains. The advantage of this surgery over traditional amputations below the knee is that weight bearing can occur without the use of a prosthesis and with reduced pain.

An intense effort is made to preserve knee joints with below-the-knee amputation (BKA). When the cause for the amputation extends beyond the knee, above-knee or higher amputations are performed. Hip disarticulation, or removal of the hip joint, and hemipelvectomy (removal of half of the pelvis with the leg) are more common in younger patients than in older ones who cannot easily handle the cumbersome prostheses required for ambulation. The higher the level of amputation, the more energy is required for mobility. These higher-level procedures are typically done for cancer of the bone, osteomyelitis, or trauma as a last resort.

Fewer than 10% of all amputations are upper extremity (UE) amputations. An amputation of any part of the upper extremity is generally more incapacitating than one of the leg. The arms and hands are necessary for ADLs such as feeding, bathing, dressing, and driving a car. In the upper extremity, as much length as possible is saved to maintain function. Early replacement with a prosthetic device is vital for the patient with this type of amputation.

🌐 CULTURAL AWARENESS

The incidence of lower extremity amputations is greater in black and Hispanic populations because the incidence of major diseases leading to amputation, such as diabetes and arteriosclerosis, is greater in these populations (Lowe & Tariman, 2008). Limited access to health care for these minority groups may also play a major role in limb loss. Language barriers may also be an obstacle to seeking health care providers.

Complications of Amputation

The most common complications of elective or traumatic amputations are:
- Hemorrhage
- Infection
- Phantom limb pain
- Neuroma
- Flexion contractures

When a person loses part or all of an extremity either by surgery or by trauma, major blood vessels are severed, which causes *bleeding*. If the bleeding is uncontrolled, the patient is at risk for hypovolemic shock and possibly death.

As with any surgical procedure or trauma, *infection* can occur in the wound or the bone (osteomyelitis). The older adult who is malnourished and confused is at the greatest risk because excreta may soil the wound or he or she may remove the dressing and pick at the incision. Preventing infection is a major emphasis in hospitals and other health care settings. In some cases, Medicare will not reimburse for acquired infections.

Phantom limb pain is a frequent complication of amputation. Sensation is felt in the amputated part immediately after surgery and usually diminishes over time. When this sensation persists and is unpleasant or painful, it is referred to as phantom limb pain (PLP). PLP is more common in patients who had chronic limb pain before surgery and less common in those who have traumatic amputations. The patient reports pain in the removed body part shortly after surgery, usually after an above-the-knee amputation (AKA). The pain is often described as intense burning, crushing, or cramping. Some

patients report that the removed part is in a distorted, uncomfortable position. They experience numbness and tingling, referred to as *phantom limb sensation,* as well as pain. Others state that the most distal area of the removed part feels as if it is retracted into the residual limb end. For most patients, the pain is triggered by touching the residual limb or by temperature or barometric pressure changes, concurrent illness, fatigue, anxiety, or stress. Routine activities such as urination can trigger the pain. If pain is long-standing, especially if it existed before the amputation, any stimulus can cause it, including touching any part of the body.

❗ NURSING SAFETY PRIORITY
Action Alert

Recognize the patient's phantom limb pain as real, and treat it aggressively. A combination of drug therapy and complementary and alternative therapies is the best approach for pain management.

Neuroma—a sensitive tumor consisting of damaged nerve cells—forms most often in amputations of the upper extremity but can occur anywhere. The patient may or may not have pain. It is diagnosed by sonography and can be treated either surgically or nonsurgically. Surgery to remove the neuroma may be performed, but it often regrows and is more painful than before the surgery. Nonsurgical modalities include nerve blocks (e.g., with phenol), steroid injections, and cognitive therapies such as hypnosis.

Flexion contractures of the hip or knee are seen in patients with amputations of the lower extremity. This complication must be avoided so that the patient can ambulate with a prosthetic device. Proper positioning and active range-of-motion exercises help prevent this complication.

❓ NCLEX EXAMINATION CHALLENGE
Psychosocial Integrity

A client who had an elective below-the-knee amputation reports pain in the part of his leg that was amputated. What is the nurse's best response to his pain?
A. "The pain will go away in a few days or so."
B. "That's phantom limb pain and every amputee has that."
C. "On a scale of 0 to 10, how would you rate your pain?"
D. "The pain is not real, so we don't treat it."

Health Promotion and Maintenance

The typical patient undergoing elective amputation is a middle-aged or older man with diabetes and a lengthy history of smoking. He most likely has not cared for his feet properly, which has resulted in a nonhealing, infected foot ulcer and possibly gangrene. Therefore adherence to the disease management plan may help prevent the need for later amputation. Lifestyle habits like maintaining a healthy weight, regular exercise, and avoiding smoking can help prevent chronic diseases like diabetes and poor blood circulation.

The second largest group who have amputations comprise young men who have motorcycle or other vehicular crashes or who are injured by industrial equipment or by combat or accidents in war. These men may either experience a traumatic amputation or undergo a surgical amputation because of a severe crushing injury and massive soft-tissue damage. Teach young male adults the importance of taking safety precautions to prevent injury at work and to avoid speeding or driving while drinking alcohol. An increasing number of young women also tend to speed and drive while drinking, which endangers themselves and others around them.

PATIENT-CENTERED COLLABORATIVE CARE

ASSESSMENT

Physical Assessment/Clinical Manifestations

Monitor neurovascular status in the affected extremity that will be amputated. When the patient has peripheral vascular disease, also check circulation in both legs. Assess skin color, temperature, sensation, and pulses in both affected and unaffected extremities. Capillary refill can be difficult to determine in the older adult related to thickened and opaque nails. In this situation, the skin near the nail bed can be used (see Chart 54-3). Capillary refill may not be as reliable as other indicators. Observe and document any discoloration of the skin, edema, ulcerations, presence of necrosis, and hair distribution on the lower extremities.

Psychosocial Assessment

People react differently to the loss of a body part. Be aware that an amputation of a portion of one finger, especially the thumb, can be traumatic to the patient. The thumb is needed for hand activities. Therefore the loss must not be underestimated. Patients undergoing amputation face a complete, permanent loss. Evaluate their psychological preparation for a planned amputation, and expect them to go through the grieving process. Adjustment to a traumatic, unexpected amputation is often more difficult than accepting a planned one. The young patient may be bitter, hostile, and depressed. In addition to loss of a body part, the patient may lose a job, the ability to participate in favorite recreational activities, or a social relationship if other people cannot accept the body change.

The patient has an altered self-concept. The physical alteration that results from an amputation affects body image and self-esteem. For example, a patient may think that an intimate relationship with a partner is no longer possible. An older adult may feel a loss of independence. Assess the patient's feelings about himself or herself to identify areas in which he or she needs emotional support. Refer the patient to the certified hospital chaplain, other spiritual leader, or social worker if he or she is hospitalized. Counseling resources are also available in the community.

Attempt to determine the patient's willingness and motivation to withstand prolonged rehabilitation after the amputation. Asking questions about how he or she has dealt with previous life crises can provide clues. Adjustment to the amputation and rehabilitation is less difficult if the patient is willing to make needed changes.

In addition to assessing the patient's psychosocial status, assess the family's reaction to the surgery or trauma. Their response usually correlates directly with the patient's progress during recovery and rehabilitation. Expect the family to grieve for the loss, and they must be allowed to adjust to the change.

Assess the patient's and family's coping abilities, and help them identify personal strengths and weaknesses. Assess the patient's religious, spiritual, and cultural beliefs. Certain groups require that the amputated body part be stored for later burial with the rest of the body or be buried immediately. Other cultural customs and rituals may apply depending on the group with which the patient associates.

Diagnostic Assessment

The surgeon determines which tests are performed to assess for viability of the limb based on blood flow. A large number of noninvasive techniques are available for this evaluation. For complete accuracy, the health care provider does not rely on any single test.

One procedure is measurement of segmental limb blood pressures, which can also be used by the nurse at the bedside. In this test, an ankle-brachial index (ABI) is calculated by dividing ankle systolic pressure by brachial systolic pressure. A normal ABI is 1 or higher.

Blood flow in an extremity can also be assessed by other noninvasive tests, including Doppler ultrasonography or laser Doppler flowmetry and transcutaneous oxygen pressure ($TcPO_2$). The ultrasonography and laser Doppler measure the speed of blood flow in the limb. The $TcPO_2$ measures oxygen pressure to indicate blood flow in the limb and has proved reliable for predicting healing.

INTERVENTIONS

A traumatic amputation requires rapid emergency care to possibly save the severed body part for reattachment and prevent hemorrhage.

Emergency Care: Traumatic Amputation

For a person who has a traumatic amputation in the community, first call 911. Assess the patient for airway or breathing problems. Examine the amputation site, and apply direct pressure with layers of dry gauze or other cloth, using clean gloves if available. Many nurses carry gloves and first aid kits for this type of emergency. Elevate the extremity above the patient's heart to decrease the bleeding. Do not remove the dressing to prevent dislodging the clot.

The fingers are the most likely part to be amputated and replanted. The current recommendation for prehospital care is to wrap the completely severed finger in dry sterile gauze (if available) or a clean cloth. Put the finger in a watertight, sealed plastic bag. *Place the bag in ice water, never directly on ice, at 1 part ice and 3 parts water* (Laskowski-Jones, 2006). Avoid contact between the finger and the water to prevent tissue damage. Do not remove any semidetached parts of the digit. Be sure that the part goes with the patient to the hospital.

Collaborative Care for the Patient with an Amputation

Patient care depends on the type and location of the amputation. For example, an above-the-knee amputation (AKA) has the potential for more postoperative complications than does a partial foot amputation. Regardless of where the amputation occurs, collaborate with the rehabilitation therapists to improve ambulation and/or enable the patient to be independent in ADLs. For many amputations, prostheses can be used to substitute for the missing body part.

Patients undergoing lower extremity amputation today are not confined to a wheelchair. Advancements in the design of prosthetics have enabled them to become independent. Therefore complications from extended bedrest are not common, even for older adults.

Assessing Tissue Perfusion and Managing Pain. The nurse's primary focus is to monitor for signs indicating that there is sufficient tissue perfusion but no hemorrhage. The skin flap at the end of the residual (remaining) limb should be pink in a light-skinned person and not discolored (lighter or darker than other skin pigmentation) in a dark-skinned patient. The area should be warm but not hot. Assess the closest proximal pulse for presence and strength, and compare it with that in the other extremity. If the patient has bilateral vascular disease, however, comparison of limbs may not be an accurate way of measuring blood flow. Use a Doppler device to determine if the affected side is being perfused.

All patients experience pain as a result of either a traumatic or surgical (elective) amputation. Some patients also report pain in the missing body part, often called phantom limb pain (PLP). Be sure to determine which type the patient has, because they are managed very differently.

! NURSING SAFETY PRIORITY

Action Alert

> If the patient reports PLP, recognize that the pain is real and should be managed promptly and completely! It is not therapeutic to remind the patient that the limb cannot be hurting because it is missing. To prevent increased pain, handle the residual limb carefully when assessing the site or changing the dressing.

Opioid analgesics are not as effective for PLP as they are for residual limb pain. IV infusions of calcitonin (Miacalcin, Calcimar) during the week after amputation can reduce phantom limb pain. The health care provider prescribes other drugs on the basis of the type of PLP the patient experiences. For instance, beta-blocking agents such as propranolol (Inderal, Apo-Propranolol ✤, Detensol ✦) are used for constant, dull, burning pain. Antiepileptic drugs such as carbamazepine (Tegretol) and gabapentin (Neurontin) may be used for knifelike or sharp burning pain. Antispasmodics such as baclofen (Lioresal) may be prescribed for muscle spasms or cramping. Some patients improve with antidepressant drugs.

Teach patients about other modalities for managing PLP, including:

- Ultrasound therapy
- Massage
- Heat
- Biofeedback
- Relaxation therapy
- Hypnosis
- Psychotherapy

Most of these modalities are described in Chapters 2 or 5. Incorporate them into the plan of care if agreeable with the patient by collaborating with specialists who are trained to perform them. For example, physical therapists often use massage, heat, transcutaneous electrical nerve stimulation (TENS), and ultrasound therapy for pain control. Collaborate with the certified hospital chaplain to provide emotional support or a social worker or psychologist to provide psychotherapy, as needed.

Preventing Infection

The surgeon typically prescribes a broad-spectrum prophylactic antibiotic immediately before elective surgery. These may be continued in patients with traumatic amputations or those who have open wounds on the residual limb. The initial pressure dressing and drains are usually removed by the surgeon 48 to 72 hours after surgery. Inspect the incision or wound for signs of infection. Record the appearance, amount, and odor of drainage, if present. The surgeon may want the incision open to air until staples or sutures are removed or may want the residual limb to have a continuous soft or rigid dressing made of fiberglass. A soft dressing is secured by an elastic bandage wrapped firmly around the residual limb.

Promoting Mobility and Preparing for Prosthesis

Collaborate with the physical therapist to begin exercises as soon as possible after surgery. If the amputation is planned, the therapist may work with the patient before surgery to start muscle-strengthening exercises and evaluate the need for ambulatory aids, such as crutches. If the patient can practice with these devices before surgery, learning how to ambulate after surgery is much easier.

For patients with AKAs or BKAs, teach range-of-motion (ROM) exercises for prevention of flexion contractures, particularly of the hip and knee. A trapeze and an overhead frame aid in strengthening the arms and allow the patient to move independently in bed. Teach the patient how to perform range-of-motion exercises. Be sure to turn the patient every 2 hours, or teach the patient to turn independently. Move the patient slowly to prevent muscle spasms (Pullen, 2010).

A firm mattress is essential for preventing contractures with a leg amputation. Assist the patient into a prone position every 3 to 4 hours for 20- to 30-minute periods if tolerated and not contraindicated. This position may be uncomfortable initially but is necessary to prevent hip flexion contractures. Instruct the patient to pull the residual limb close to the other leg and contract the gluteal muscles of the buttocks for muscle strengthening. After staples are removed, the physical therapist may begin resistive exercises, which should also be done at home.

For above- and below-the-knee amputations, teach the patient how to push the residual limb down toward the bed while supporting it on a soft pillow at first. Then instruct him or her to continue this activity using a firmer pillow and then progress to a harder surface. This activity helps prepare the residual limb for prosthesis and reduces the incidence of phantom limb pain and sensation (Pullen, 2010).

Elevation of a lower-leg residual limb on a pillow while the patient is in a supine position is controversial. Some practitioners advocate avoiding this practice at all times because it promotes hip or knee flexion contracture. Others allow elevation for the first 24 to 48 hours to reduce swelling and subsequent discomfort. Inspect the residual limb daily to ensure that it lies completely flat on the bed.

Before an elective amputation, the patient often sees a certified prosthetist-orthotist (CPO) so that planning can begin for the postoperative period. Arrangements for replacing an arm part are especially important so that the patient can achieve self-management. Some patients are fitted with a temporary prosthesis at the time of surgery. Others, particularly older patients with vascular disease, are fitted after the residual limb has healed.

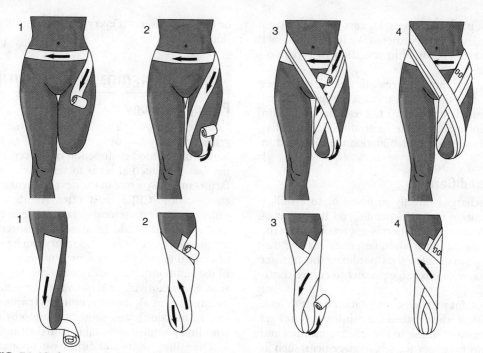

FIG. 54-12 A common method of wrapping an amputation stump. *Top,* Wrapping for above-knee amputation. *Bottom,* Wrapping for below-knee amputation.

The patient being fitted for a leg prosthesis should bring a sturdy pair of shoes to the fitting. The prosthesis will be adjusted to that heel height.

Several devices help shape and shrink the residual limb in preparation for the prosthesis. Rigid, removable dressings are preferred because they decrease edema, protect and shape the limb, and allow easy access to the wound for inspection. The Jobst air splint, a plastic inflatable device, is sometimes used for this purpose. One of its disadvantages is air leakage and loss of compression. Wrapping with elastic bandages can also be effective in reducing edema, shrinking the limb, and holding the wound dressing in place.

For wrapping to be effective, reapply the bandages every 4 to 6 hours or more often if they become loose. *Figure-eight wrapping prevents restriction of blood flow. Decrease the tightness of the bandages while wrapping in a distal-to-proximal direction.* After wrapping, anchor the bandages to the highest joint, such as above the knee for BKAs (Fig. 54-12).

The design of and materials for prostheses have improved dramatically over the years. Computer-assisted design and manufacturing (CAD-CAM) is used for a custom fit. One of the most important developments in lower extremity prosthetics is the ankle-foot prosthesis, such as the Flex-Foot for more active amputees.

Promoting Body Image and Lifestyle Adaptation

The patient often experiences feelings of inadequacy as a result of losing a body part, especially the older adult who was in poor health before surgery and men who are often the main providers for their families. If possible, arrange for him or her to meet with a rehabilitated amputee who is about the same age as the patient.

Use of the word *stump* for referring to the remaining portion of the limb (residual limb) continues to be controversial. Patients have reported feeling as if they were part of

a tree when the term was used. However, some rehabilitation specialists who routinely work with amputees believe the term is appropriate because it forces the patient to realize what has happened and promotes adjustment to the amputation. *Assess the patient to determine what term he or she prefers.*

Assess the patient's verbal and nonverbal references to the affected area. Some patients behave euphorically (extremely happy) and seem to have accepted the loss. *Do not jump to the conclusion that acceptance has occurred.* Ask the patient to describe his or her feelings about changes in body image and self-esteem. He or she may verbalize acceptance but refuse to look at the area during a dressing change. This inconsistent behavior is not unusual and should be documented and shared with other health care team members.

A patient who seems to adjust to the amputation during hospitalization may realize that it is difficult to cope with the loss after discharge from the hospital. Teach the patient and family about available resources and support from organizations such as the Amputee Coalition of America (ACA) (www.amputee-coalition.org) and the National Amputation Foundation (NAF) (www.nationalamputation.org). The NAF was originally started for veterans but has since expanded to offer services to civilians.

With advancements in prostheses and surgical techniques, most patients can return to their jobs and other activities. Professional athletes who use prostheses are often quite successful in sports. Patients with amputations ski, hike, golf, bowl, and participate in other physically demanding activities. Many amputees participate actively in organized and recreational sports.

If a job or career change is necessary, collaborate with a social worker or vocational rehabilitation specialist to evaluate the patient's skills. A supportive family or significant other is important for the adjustment to this change. The patient may also think that an intimate relationship is no longer possible because of physical changes. Discuss sexuality issues with the patient and his or her partner as needed. Professional assistance from a sex therapist, intimacy coach, or psychologist may be needed.

Help the patient and family set realistic desired outcomes and take one day at a time. Help them recognize personal strengths. If the desired outcomes are not realistic, frustration and disappointment may decrease motivation during rehabilitation. Basic principles of rehabilitation are discussed in Chapter 8.

Community-Based Care

The patient is discharged directly to home or to a skilled facility or rehabilitation facility, depending on the extent of the amputation. When rehabilitation is not feasible as in the debilitated or demented older adult, he or she may be discharged to a long-term care facility. Coordinate this transfer with the case manager or discharge planner to ensure continuity of care.

At home, the patient with a leg amputation needs to have enough room to use a wheelchair if the prosthesis is not yet available. He or she must be able to use toileting facilities and have access to areas necessary for self-management, such as the kitchen. Structural home modifications may be required before the patient goes home.

After the sutures or staples are removed, the patient begins residual limb care. A home care nurse may be needed to teach the patient and/or family how to care for the limb and the prosthesis if it is available (Chart 54-7). The limb should be rewrapped three times a day with an elastic bandage applied in a figure-eight manner (see Fig. 54-12). For many patients, a shrinker stocking or sock is easier to apply. After the limb is healed, it is cleaned each day with the rest of the body during bathing with soap and water. Teach the patient and/

⚠ NURSING SAFETY PRIORITY

Action Alert

Collaborate with the prosthetist to teach the patient about prosthesis care after amputation to ensure its reliability and proper function. These devices are custom made, taking into account the patient's level of amputation, lifestyle, and occupation. Proper teaching regarding correct cleansing of the socket and inserts, wearing the correct liners, assessing shoe wear, and a schedule of follow-up care is essential before discharge. This information may need to be reviewed by the home care nurse.

CHART 54-7   HOME CARE ASSESSMENT

The Patient with a Lower Extremity Amputation in the Home

- Assess the residual limb for:
  - Adequate circulation
  - Infection
  - Healing
  - Flexion contracture
  - Dressing/elastic wrap
- Assess the patient's ability to perform ADLs in the home.
- Evaluate the patient's ability to use ambulatory aids and to care for the prosthetic device (if available).
- Assess the patient's nutritional status.
- Assess the patient's ability to cope with body image change.

---

or family to inspect it every day for signs of inflammation or skin breakdown.

COMPLEX REGIONAL PAIN SYNDROME

Pathophysiology

Complex regional pain syndrome (CRPS), formerly called reflex sympathetic dystrophy (RSD) and causalgia, is a poorly understood dysfunction of the central and peripheral nervous systems that leads to severe, chronic pain. Genetic factors may play a role in the development of this devastating complication. CRPS most often results from fractures or other traumatic musculoskeletal injury and commonly occurs in the feet and hands. In some cases, specific nerve injuries are present, but in others, no injury can be identified. A triad of clinical manifestations is present, including abnormalities of the autonomic nervous system (changes in color, temperature, and sensitivity of skin over the affected area, excessive sweating, edema), motor symptoms (paresis, muscle spasms, loss of function), and sensory symptoms (intense burning pain that becomes intractable [unrelenting]).

Over time, spotty and diffuse osteoporosis can be seen on x-ray examination. Timing of diagnosis is important because the syndrome is more difficult to treat when diagnosed in the later stages.

PATIENT-CENTERED COLLABORATIVE CARE

The first priority of management is pain relief. Little research has been done to demonstrate the best practices for caring for a patient with CRPS (Hsu, 2009). Therefore a combination of interventions is used. Nurses play an important role in patient management, which includes drug therapy and a variety of nonpharmacologic modalities. Many classes of drugs may be used to manage the intense pain. These include topical analgesics, antiepileptic drugs, antidepressants, corticosteroids, bisphosphonates, and analgesics. Chapter 5 discusses pain management in detail.

In collaboration with the physical and occupational therapists, assist in maintaining adequate range of motion (ROM) and function. The skin of a patient with CRPS tends to alternate between warm, swollen, and red to cool, clammy, and bluish. Skin care needs to be gentle with minimal stimulation.

Peripheral or spinal cord neurostimulation using an external or internal implanted device delivers electrical pulses to block pain from getting to the brain where pain is perceived. The external or acupuncture method requires weekly sessions or a short-term continuous trial before the device is surgically implanted. Complications of implantable neurostimulators include spinal cord damage from hematoma or edema formation or other neurologic dysfunction.

A chemical sympathetic nerve block may be used. This procedure can be done by an IV infusion of phentolamine, a drug that blocks sympathetic receptors, or by injecting an anesthetic agent next to the spine to block sympathetic nerves.

Minimally invasive surgical sympathectomy, or cutting of the sympathetic nerve branches via endoscopy through a small axillary incision, may be required. Topical skin adhesive is used to close the very small incision. The patient is discharged to home a few hours later with a follow-up examination the next day with the health care provider. Usual activities can resume a few days later.

Assist the patient in coping with CRPS because it often has a profound psychological effect. A referral for psychological counseling or psychotherapy may be indicated. The Reflex Sympathetic Dystrophy Syndrome Association (RSDSA) (www.rsds.org) and National Pain Association (www.national painassociation.org) are available to help patients and their families organize or locate support groups and other resources.

? NCLEX EXAMINATION CHALLENGE

Physiological Integrity

> The nurse is concerned that a client who had an open reduction, internal fixation of his tibia and fibula is at risk for complex regional pain syndrome. What assessment findings at the affected area are common when a client has this complication? **Select all that apply.**
> A. Dull, aching pain
> B. Decrease in sweating
> C. Muscle spasms
> D. Skin discoloration
> E. Paresis
> F. Edema

SPORTS-RELATED INJURIES

In addition to the bone and muscle problems already discussed, trauma can cause cartilage, ligament, and tendon injury. Many musculoskeletal injuries are the result of playing sports (professional and recreational) or doing other strenuous physical activities. The popularity of all-terrain vehicles (ATVs) and skateboarding has increased injuries in younger patients. Sports injuries have become so common that large metropolitan hospitals have sports medicine clinics and physicians who specialize in this field.

Although the specific types of injury are numerous, this chapter includes only the most common ones seen in a hospital or ambulatory care setting. The principles of injury to one part of the body are similar to those of other sports injuries. For example, a tendon rupture in a knee is cared for in the same manner as a tendon rupture in the wrist. Chart 54-8 lists general emergency measures for sports-related injuries. All patients require frequent neurovascular monitoring.

Because the knee is most often injured, it is discussed as a typical example of other areas of the body. Trauma to the

CHART 54-8   BEST PRACTICE FOR PATIENT SAFETY & QUALITY CARE

Emergency Care of Patients with Sports-Related Injuries

- Do not move the victim until spinal cord injury is ascertained (see Chapter 45 for assessment of spinal cord injury).
- Rest the injured part; immobilize the joint above and below the injury by applying a splint if needed.
- Apply ice intermittently for the first 24 to 48 hours (heat may be used thereafter).
- Elevate the affected limb to decrease swelling.
- Use compression for the first 24 to 48 hours (e.g., elastic wrap).
- Always assume the area is fractured until x-ray studies are done.
- Assess neurovascular status in the area distal to the injury.

knee results in internal derangement, a broad term for disturbances of an injured knee joint. When surgery is required to resolve the problem, most surgeons prefer to perform the procedure through an arthroscope when possible. A description of arthroscopy is presented in Chapter 53.

KNEE INJURIES: PATELLOFEMORAL PAIN SYNDROME

Patellofemoral pain syndrome (PFPS) is the most common diagnosis in patients who have knee pain. It occurs most often in people who are runners or who overuse their knee joints. For that reason, it is sometimes referred to as "runner's knee." Patients with this problem describe pain as being behind or around their patella (knee cap) in one or both knees. Swelling is not common although stiffness may be present, especially when the knee is flexed.

Management usually involves rest, physical therapy, bracing or splinting, and mild analgesics. For patients who have pain lasting for more than 12 months, arthroscopic surgery is performed.

KNEE INJURIES: MENISCUS

Pathophysiology

There are two semilunar cartilaginous structures, or menisci, in the knee joint: the medial meniscus and the lateral meniscus. These pads act as shock absorbers, but they can tear. Tearing is usually a result of twisting the leg when the knee is flexed and the foot is placed firmly on the ground. The medial meniscus is much more likely to tear than the lateral meniscus because it is less mobile. Internal rotation causes a tear in the medial meniscus. External rotation causes a tear in the lateral meniscus.

Tears can be anterior or posterior, longitudinal or transverse. In the medial meniscus, a longitudinal tear, or "bucket handle" injury, often causes the knee to lock (i.e., the torn cartilage jams between the femur and the tibia and prevents extension of the knee). Surgery is often required for this type of injury. In transverse tears, the knee does not lock and surgery may not be required.

PATIENT-CENTERED COLLABORATIVE CARE

The patient with a torn meniscus typically has pain, swelling, and tenderness in the knee. A clicking or snapping sound can often be heard when the knee is moved.

A common diagnostic technique is the McMurray test. The examiner flexes and rotates the knee and then presses on the medial aspect while slowly extending the leg. The test result is positive if clicking is palpated or heard. A negative finding, however, does not rule out a tear.

For a locked knee, the treatment may be manipulation followed by splinting or casting for 3 to 6 weeks. If the problem recurs, a partial or total meniscectomy is performed. An *open* meniscectomy requires a surgical incision for removal of all or part of the meniscus and is rarely performed. Most surgeons prefer to remove only the affected portion during a *closed* meniscectomy, which can be done through an arthroscope as a same-day surgical procedure. As described in Chapter 53, an arthroscope is a metal tubular

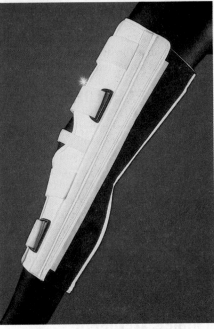

FIG. 54-13 A knee immobilizer.

instrument used for examination or surgery of joints. One or more small incisions (less than ¼-inch [0.6-cm] long) are made in the knee for insertion of the arthroscope. The surgeon threads a cutting device through the arthroscope for removal of the torn cartilage while the knee is irrigated. The surgeon may use a laser during the procedure, depending on the type and severity of the injury. A bulky pressure dressing is applied after the procedure, and the affected leg is wrapped in elastic bandages.

As for any postoperative patient, check the surgical dressing for bleeding and monitor vital signs after the patient is admitted to the same-day surgical unit. Perform neurovascular checks as outlined in Chart 54-3, usually every hour for the first few hours and then every 4 hours. Teach the patient and family what signs and symptoms to watch for after surgery and when to notify the health care provider.

The patient begins exercises immediately after surgery to strengthen the leg, prevent venous thromboembolism, and reduce swelling. Quadriceps setting, in which the patient straightens the leg while pushing the knee against the bed, is done in sets of 10 or more. Straight-leg raises are also performed. Range-of-motion (ROM) exercises are usually not started for several days.

To prevent bending the affected knee, the physician may request a knee immobilizer, such as the one shown in Fig. 54-13. Elevate the leg on one or two pillows according to the physician's preference, and apply ice to reduce postoperative swelling. Full weight bearing is restricted for several weeks, depending on the amount of cartilage removed. The patient is usually discharged from the hospital with crutches in less than 23 hours.

KNEE INJURIES: LIGAMENTS

The cruciate and collateral ligaments in the knee are predisposed to injury, often from sports or vehicular crashes. The anterior cruciate ligament (ACL) is the most commonly torn ligament in the knee. Athletes often get these injuries during skiing, skating, or gymnastics. Women have ACL tears more often than men, possibly related to hormonal influences, biomechanical factors, and anatomic differences. Proper athletic shoes and learning how to land when jumping can help prevent this injury.

When the ACL is torn, the patient feels a snap and the knee gives way because of ACL laxity. Within hours, the knee is swollen, stiff, and painful. Examination by the health care provider shows positive ligament laxity. The diagnosis of an ACL tear is best confirmed by magnetic resonance imaging (MRI).

Treatment may be nonsurgical or surgical, depending on the severity of the injury and the activity of the patient. Exercises, bracing, and limits on activities while the ligament heals may be sufficient. If medical management is not effective or the tear is severe, surgery may be needed.

The surgeon repairs the tear by reattaching the torn portions of the ligament through arthroscopy. The leg is placed in a brace or immobilizer. If the ligament cannot be repaired, reconstructive surgery may be performed with autologous grafts. A ligament from another part of the body is used to replace the torn knee ligament. Another option is artificial knee implants such as the GORE-TEX ligament.

Complete healing of knee ligaments after surgery can take 6 to 9 months or longer. These patients may use a continuous passive motion (CPM) machine at home. Teach the patient how to use and care for the machine. CPM use is discussed with the postoperative care of the total knee patient in Chapter 20.

OTHER INJURIES

CARPAL TUNNEL SYNDROME

Pathophysiology

Carpal tunnel syndrome (CTS) is a common condition in which the median nerve in the wrist becomes compressed, causing pain and numbness. The carpal tunnel is a rigid canal that lies between the carpal bones and a fibrous tissue sheet. A group of tendons surrounds the synovium and shares space with the median nerve in the carpal tunnel. When the synovium becomes swollen or thickened, this nerve is compressed.

The median nerve supplies motor, sensory, and autonomic function for the first three fingers of the hand and the palmar aspect of the fourth (ring) finger. Because the median nerve is close to other structures, wrist flexion causes nerve impingement, and extension causes increased pressure in the lower portion of the carpal tunnel.

CTS usually presents as a chronic problem. Acute cases are rare. Excessive hand exercise, edema or hemorrhage into the carpal tunnel, or thrombosis of the median artery can lead to acute CTS. *Patients with hand burns or a Colles' fracture of the wrist are particularly at risk for this problem.* In most cases, the cause may not result in nerve deficit for years.

CTS is also a common complication of certain metabolic and connective tissue diseases. For example, synovitis (inflammation of the synovium) occurs in patients with rheumatoid arthritis (RA). The hypertrophied synovium compresses the median nerve. In other chronic disorders such as diabetes mellitus, inadequate blood supply can cause median nerve neuropathy or dysfunction, resulting in CTS.

CTS is the most *common* type of repetitive stress injury (RSI). RSIs are the fastest growing type of occupational injury. People whose jobs require repetitive hand activities such as pinching or grasping during wrist flexion (e.g., factory workers, computer operators, jackhammer operators) are predisposed to CTS. It can also result from overuse in sports activities such as golf, tennis, or racquetball.

In a few cases, CTS may be a familial or congenital problem that manifests in adulthood. Space-occupying growths such as ganglia, tophi, and lipomas can also result in nerve compression.

Women, especially those older than 50 years, are much more likely than men to experience CTS, most likely due to the higher prevalence of diseases such as RA in women. The problem most often affects the dominant hand but can occur in both hands simultaneously. CTS is beginning to be found in children and adolescents as a result of the increased use of computers in everyday life.

Health Promotion and Maintenance

Most businesses recognize the hazards of repetitive motion as a primary cause of occupational injury and disability. Both men and women in the labor force are experiencing increasing numbers of RSIs. Occupational health nurses have played an important role in ergonomic assessments and in the development of ergonomically designed furniture and various aids to decrease CTS and other musculoskeletal injuries.

U.S federal and state legislation has been passed to ensure that all businesses, including health care organizations (HCOs), provide *ergonomically appropriate workstations* for their employees (Occupational Safety and Health Administration). The Joint Commission also requires that hospitals and other HCOs provide a safe work environment for all staff. In Canada, each province requires the work setting to have joint health and safety committees in which employees are actively involved in setting safety standards (Canadian Centre for Occupational Health and Safety). Chart 54-9 lists best practices for preventing CTS in the health care setting.

PATIENT-CENTERED COLLABORATIVE CARE

ASSESSMENT

A medical diagnosis is often made based on the patient's history and report of hand pain and numbness and without further assessment. Ask about the nature, intensity, and location of the pain. Patients often state that the pain is worse at night as a result of flexion or direct pressure during sleep. The pain may radiate to the arm, shoulder and neck, or chest.

In addition to reports of numbness, patients with carpal tunnel syndrome (CTS) may also have paresthesia (painful tingling). *Sensory* changes usually occur weeks or months before *motor* manifestations.

The health care provider performs several tests for abnormal sensory findings. Phalen's wrist test, sometimes called Phalen's maneuver, produces paresthesia in the median nerve distribution (palmar side of the thumb, index and middle fingers, and half of the ring finger) within 60 seconds due to increased internal carpal pressure. The patient is asked to relax the wrist into flexion or to place the back of the hands together and flex both wrists at the same time. The Phalen's test is positive in most patients with CTS.

The same sensation can be created by tapping lightly over the area of the median nerve in the wrist (Tinel's sign). If the test is unsuccessful, a blood pressure cuff can be placed on the upper arm and inflated to the patient's systolic pressure (tourniquet). This often causes pain and tingling.

The newest pain-provoking diagnostic test being used is the Okutsu position test. The patient is asked to place the hands in a palm-to-palm position with thumbs extended. Then he or she is asked to move the wrist toward the radial side as far as it can be done and hold that position for 1 minute. Pain and tingling occur more often than from the Tinel's and Phalen's tests.

Motor changes in carpal tunnel syndrome (CTS) begin with a weak pinch, clumsiness, and difficulty with fine movements. These changes progress to muscle weakness and wasting, which can impair self-management. If desired, test for pinching ability and ask the patient to perform a fine-movement task, such as threading a needle. Strenuous hand activity worsens the pain and numbness.

In addition to inspecting for muscle atrophy and task performance, observe the wrist for swelling. Gently palpate the area and note any unusual findings. Autonomic changes may be evidenced by skin discoloration, nail changes (e.g., brittleness), and increased or decreased hand sweating.

When a definitive diagnosis is uncertain, the health care provider may request routine x-rays, electromyography (EMG) and nerve conduction studies (NCS), and/or ultrasonography. MRI is generally not very helpful in diagnosis. NCS testing reveals nerve dysfunction before muscle atrophy is observed. An ultrasound scan may be done to view the cause of the problem. The most common finding is an enlarged median nerve within the carpal tunnel.

INTERVENTIONS

The health care provider uses conservative measures before surgical intervention. However, CTS can recur with either type of treatment. Management depends on the patient, but established best practices have not been determined (Uchiyama et al., 2010).

Nonsurgical Management

Aggressive drug therapy and immobilization of the wrist are the major components of nonsurgical management. Teach the patient the importance of these modalities in the hope of preventing surgical intervention.

NSAIDs are the most commonly prescribed drugs for the relief of pain and inflammation, if present. In addition to or instead of systemic medications, the physician may inject corticosteroids directly into the carpal tunnel. If the patient responds to the injection, several additional weekly or monthly injections are given. Teach him or her to take NSAIDs with or after meals to reduce gastric irritation.

A splint or hand brace may be used to immobilize the wrist during the day, during the night, or both. Many patients experience temporary relief with these devices. The occupational therapist places the wrist in the neutral position or in slight extension.

Laser or ultrasound therapy may also be helpful. Some patients report fewer symptoms after beginning yoga or other exercise routine.

Surgical Management

Surgery is necessary in about half of patients with CTS. Surgery can relieve the pressure on the median nerve by providing nerve decompression. Major surgical complications are rare after CTS surgery. In some cases, however, CTS recurs months to years after surgery.

The nurse in the physician's office or same-day surgical center reinforces the teaching provided by the surgeon regarding the nature of the surgery. Postoperative care is reviewed so the patient knows what to expect. Chapter 16 describes general preoperative care in detail.

Whatever the cause of nerve compression, the surgeon removes it either by cutting or by the newer laser technique. The two most common surgeries are the open carpal tunnel release (OCTR) and the newer endoscopic carpal tunnel release (ECTR). When CTS is a complication of rheumatoid arthritis, a synovectomy (removal of excess synovium) through a small inner-wrist incision may resolve the problem. Removal of a space-occupying growth, if present, also decompresses the nerve. A recent systematic review showed that surgical treatment seems to be more effective than conservative measures over the long term. However, there was no evidence that one type of procedure, open or endoscopic, was more effective than the other (Huisstede et al., 2010).

ECTR, the endoscopic technique, is a common alternative to OCTR, the open technique. The surgeon makes a very small incision (less than ½ inch [1.2 cm]) through which the endoscope is inserted. The surgeon then uses special instruments, which may include a laser, to free the trapped median nerve. Although ECTR is less invasive and costs less than the open procedure, the patient may have a longer period of postoperative pain and numbness compared with recovery from OCTR.

After surgery, monitor vital signs and check the dressing carefully for drainage and tightness. If ECTR has been performed, the dressing is very small. The surgeon may require that the patient's affected hand and arm be elevated above heart level for several days to reduce postoperative swelling. Check the neurovascular status of the fingers every hour during the immediate postoperative period, and encourage the patient to move them frequently. Offer pain medication

and assure him or her that a prescription for analgesics will be provided before discharge.

Hand movements, including lifting heavy objects, may be restricted for 4 to 6 weeks after surgery. The patient can expect weakness and discomfort for weeks or perhaps months. Teach him or her to report any changes in neurovascular status, including increased pain and numbness, to the surgeon's office immediately.

Remind the patient and family that the surgical procedure might not be a cure. For instance, synovitis may recur with rheumatoid arthritis and may recompress the median nerve. Multiple surgeries and other treatments are common with CTS.

The patient may need assistance with self-management activities during recovery. Ensure that assistance in the home is available before discharge; this is usually provided by the family or significant others.

TENDINOPATHY AND JOINT DISLOCATION

Other injuries can affect any synovial joint. The nursing management of each of these is similar to the collaborative care previously discussed for knee injuries. One of the most common injuries seen in general and sports medicine is Achilles tendon–related injuries (tendinopathy). *Rupture of the Achilles tendon* is common in adults who participate in strenuous sports or in women who wear high heels regularly. It can also occur after taking fluoroquinolone antibiotics, such as levofloxacin (Levoquin) and ciprofloxacin (Cipro) (Barry, 2010).

In the older adult, quadriceps tendon rupture may occur from a fall down several steps. Most cases of Achilles tendinopathy can be treated with RICE (see Chart 54-8):

- **R**est
- **I**ce
- **C**ompression
- **E**levation

Some evidence supports the use of NSAIDs, and changes in activity and shoes may be helpful (Chang et al., 2010). Ultrasound treatments may also be effective.

For severe damage and as a last resort, the tendon is surgically repaired and the leg is immobilized in a cast or brace for at least 6 to 8 weeks. If the tendon is beyond repair, a tendon transplant (also known as *tendon reconstruction*) may be performed. A tendon is removed from one part of the body and transplanted to the affected area, or a cadaver donor is used.

Dislocation of a joint occurs when the ends of two or more bones are moved away from each other. If the dislocation is not complete, the joint is partially dislocated, or subluxed. It can occur in any diarthrodial (synovial) joint but is most common in the shoulder, hip, knee, and fingers. This injury is usually the result of trauma but can be congenital or pathologic and can result from joint disease, such as arthritis.

The typical manifestations of dislocation are:

- Pain
- Immobility
- Alteration in contour of the joint
- Deviation in length of the extremity
- Rotation of the extremity

The health care provider performs a closed reduction of the joint and moves the joint surfaces back into their normal anatomic position. The patient requires light anesthetic or moderate sedation. The joint is immobilized by a cast, splint, brace, or immobilizer until healing occurs.

Recurrent dislocations are common in the knee and shoulder. For this problem, the joint may be fixed with wires or other device to prevent further displacement. A cast, splint, or traction is applied for 3 to 6 weeks.

STRAINS AND SPRAINS

A strain is excessive stretching of a muscle or tendon when it is weak or unstable. Strains are sometimes referred to as *muscle pulls*. Falls, lifting a heavy item, and exercise often cause this injury.

Strains are classified according to their severity:

- A first-degree (mild) strain causes mild inflammation but little bleeding. Swelling, ecchymosis (bruising), and tenderness are usually present.
- A second-degree (moderate) strain involves tearing of the muscle or tendon fibers without complete disruption. Muscle function may be impaired.
- A third-degree (severe) strain involves a ruptured muscle or tendon with separation of muscle from muscle, tendon from muscle, or tendon from bone. Severe pain and disability result from severe strains.

Management usually involves cold and heat applications, exercise, and activity limitations. The health care provider may prescribe anti-inflammatory drugs to decrease inflammation and pain. Muscle relaxants may also be used. In third-degree strains, surgical repair of the ruptured muscle or tendon may be needed.

A sprain is excessive stretching of a ligament. Twisting motions from a fall or sports activity typically cause the injury. Sprains are also classified according to severity. Pain and swelling result from ligament injuries. The treatment for *mild (first-degree)* sprains includes RICE (see Chart 54-8).

Second-degree sprains require immobilization, such as elastic bandage and an air stirrup ankle brace or splint, and partial weight bearing while the tear heals. For severe ligament damage (*third-degree* sprain), immobilization for 4 to

6 weeks is necessary. Arthroscopic surgery may be done, particularly for chronic joint instability.

ROTATOR CUFF INJURIES

The musculotendinous, or rotator, cuff of the shoulder functions to stabilize the head of the humerus in the glenoid cavity during shoulder abduction. Young adults usually sustain a tear of the cuff by substantial trauma, such as may occur during a fall, while throwing a ball, or with heavy lifting. Older adults tend to have small tears related to aging, repetitive motions, or falls, and the tears are usually painless.

The patient with a torn rotator cuff has shoulder pain and cannot easily abduct the arm at the shoulder. When the arm is abducted, he or she usually drops the arm because abduction cannot be maintained (drop arm test). Pain is more intense at night and with overhead activities. Partial-thickness tears are more painful that full-thickness tears, but full-thickness tears result in more weakness and loss of function. Muscle atrophy is commonly seen. Diagnosis is confirmed with x-rays, MRI, ultrasonography, and/or CT scans.

The health care provider usually treats the patient with partial-thickness tears conservatively with NSAIDs, intermittent steroid injections, physical therapy, and activity limitations while the tear heals. Physical therapy treatments may include ultrasound, electrical stimulation, ice, and heat (Smith & Smith, 2010).

For patients who do not respond to conservative treatment in 3 to 6 months or for those who have a complete (full-thickness) tear, the surgeon repairs the cuff using open, mini-open, or arthroscopic procedures. After surgery, the affected arm is usually immobilized for several weeks. Pendulum exercises are started on the third or fourth postoperative day and progress to active exercises in about 2 weeks. If the surgery is extensive, the patient's arm may be immobilized for a longer time before exercises begin. Patients then begin outpatient rehabilitation in the occupational therapy department. Teach them that they may not have full function for several months.

NURSING CONCEPT REVIEW

What might you NOTICE if the patient has impaired mobility and sensation as a result of acute musculoskeletal trauma?

- Extremity swelling, bleeding, bruising, shortening, malalignment, and/or rotation
- Report of severe pain
- Break in skin integrity
- Report of decreased or unusual sensation in extremity
- Inability or decreased ability to move extremity
- Difficulty breathing (rib trauma)
- Severe kyphosis (compression fractures)

What should you INTERPRET and how should you RESPOND to a patient with impaired mobility and sensation as a result of acute musculoskeletal trauma?

Perform and interpret focused physical assessment findings, including:

- ABC (**a**irway, **b**reathing, **c**irculation) ability
- Pain intensity and quality
- Vital signs
- Neurovascular assessment ("circ check")

Respond:

- First, establish ABCs if problem exists.
- If skin is not intact, cover wound with dry, sterile dressing, if available; use clean cloth as an option. Apply pressure to proximal pulse if patient is bleeding; for traumatic amputation, apply direct pressure to the residual body part.
- Implement measures to prevent hypovolemic shock if patient is bleeding, including lying patient flat, keeping him or her warm, and elevating the bleeding part.

NURSING CONCEPT REVIEW—cont'd

- Splint the extremity (in community setting) to prevent movement and further damage.
- If in hospital setting, assist health care provider in splinting.
- Provide pain control interventions by drug therapy as soon as possible.
- Provide emotional assurance for the patient by being present and comforting.

On what should you REFLECT?
- Monitor the patient's response to pain control interventions.
- Think about what else you could do to prevent complications.
- Determine what health teaching will be needed, depending on the treatment that is provided (e.g., surgery, cast).

GET READY FOR THE NCLEX® EXAMINATION!

KEY POINTS

Review these Key Points for each NCLEX Examination Client Needs Category.

Safe and Effective Care Environment
- Collaborate with physical and occupational therapists for care of patients with extremity fractures.
- Collaborate with the prosthetist, physical and occupational therapists, psychologist, and sex therapist or intimacy coach for care of patients with amputations.
- Several community organizations, such as the Amputee Coalition of America, are available to help patients and their families cope with the loss of a body part.
- Use strict aseptic technique when caring for wounds in patients with compound fractures to help prevent infection; give antibiotic therapy as prescribed.
- Assess the risk for and implement interventions to prevent complications of immobility in patients having musculoskeletal injury or surgery (e.g., pressure ulcers, venous thromboembolism [VTE]).

Health Promotion and Maintenance
- Teach patients and their family members and significant others how to care for casts or traction at home.
- Reinforce teaching for ambulating with crutches, walkers, or canes.
- Provide special care for older adults with hip fractures, including preventing heel pressure ulcers and promoting early ambulation to prevent complications of immobility.
- Teach exercises to patients with leg amputation to prevent hip flexion contractures.

Psychosocial Integrity
- Be aware that patients with severe musculoskeletal trauma may have a prolonged hospitalization and recovery period.
- For patients with severe trauma or amputation, assess coping skills and encourage verbalization.
- Recognize that the patient having an amputation may need to adjust to an altered lifestyle; however, new custom prosthetics improve mobility.

- Help the patient with an amputation or other musculoskeletal trauma and family to set realistic expected outcomes and take one day at a time.

Physiological Integrity
- Be aware that open fractures cause a higher risk for infection than do closed fractures.
- Assess patients with fractures for complications, such as VTE, infection, and acute compartment syndrome.
- Recognize that fat embolism syndrome is different from pulmonary (blood clot) embolism as outlined in Chart 54-2.
- Provide emergency care of the patient with a fracture as described in Chart 54-4.
- Identify the patient at risk for acute compartment syndrome; loosen bandages, or request that the patient's cast be cut if neurovascular compromise is noted.
- As a priority, assess neurovascular status frequently in patients with musculoskeletal injury, traction, or cast as described in Chart 54-3.
- Provide appropriate cast care, depending on the type of cast (plaster or synthetic); check for pressure necrosis under the cast by feeling for heat, assessing the patient's pain level, and smelling the cast for an unpleasant odor.
- Provide pin care for patients with skeletal traction or external fixation; assess for manifestations of infection at the pin sites.
- Provide postoperative care for the patient having a fracture repair, including promoting mobility and monitoring for complications of immobility.
- Provide care for patients having a vertebroplasty or kyphoplasty as described in Chart 54-6.
- Observe for hemorrhage and infection in the patient having an amputation.
- Postoperatively, assess for and promptly manage phantom limb pain in the patient who has an amputation; collaborate with specialists to incorporate complementary and alternative therapies into the patient's plan of care.
- Provide emergency care for patients with a sports-related injury as outlined in Chart 54-8.

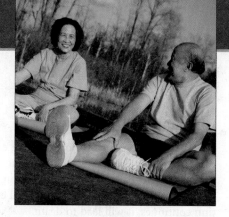

Nutrition, Metabolism, and Bowel Elimination

Why do we eat, and how are nutrition, metabolism, and bowel elimination related? Within the human body, as in all living systems, energy is required to perform any function. The word *metabolism* means to change or transform. Humans transform the energy stored within food into the types of energy needed to make the body work.

As shown in Fig. 1, *nutrition* involves ingesting many types of foods that contain proteins, carbohydrates, fats, vitamins, and minerals. Once inside the GI tract, the processes of digestion break down food into its basic elements, which then are absorbed into the blood and delivered to cells. Through metabolism, cells convert these basic elements into chemical energy, mostly adenosine triphosphate (ATP). Different cells then use metabolism to further transform ATP into heat energy, mechanical energy, chemical energy, and electrical energy. The transformation of chemical energy into other types of energy within the human body is *irreversible*. It is lost from the body in the form of heat and work. Thus bringing food into the body on a daily basis is important in meeting the human needs of nutrition and metabolism.

Heat energy helps maintain the core body temperature at or near 98.6° F—the ideal temperature for important physiologic reactions. When environmental temperatures are low, more food is needed to maintain body temperature. When environmental temperatures are high, less food is needed to maintain body temperature. Therefore, in general,

more calories need to be consumed per day in the winter than in the summer.

Mechanical energy is used for cell and tissue movement, cell shape changes, and whole body movement. *Electrical energy* generates the action potentials that allow nerves to transmit impulses and muscles to contract. *Chemical energy* is used to drive every chemical reaction in the body. As long as it remains alive, the body continuously needs to change food into these different energies.

Bowel elimination is the way the body rids itself of those food components that cannot be absorbed into the blood and converted into energy, such as fiber and cellulose. If these components remained in the GI tract, they would soon fill it to the point that no nutrients could be ingested.

Consider Fig. 1 as representing the entire nutrition, metabolism, and bowel elimination of a person throughout his or her lifetime. The energy ingested in the form of food exactly matches the energy transformed by metabolism and is used for all the different types of internal and external "work" of the body. When this ideal situation exists, the person always has the right amount of nutrients and neither stores excess nutrients nor breaks down body tissues to use for energy.

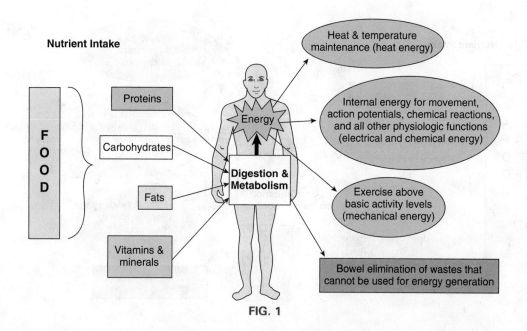

Nutrient Intake

FOOD
- Proteins
- Carbohydrates
- Fats
- Vitamins & minerals

Energy

Digestion & Metabolism

- Heat & temperature maintenance (heat energy)
- Internal energy for movement, action potentials, chemical reactions, and all other physiologic functions (electrical and chemical energy)
- Exercise above basic activity levels (mechanical energy)
- Bowel elimination of wastes that cannot be used for energy generation

FIG. 1

In Fig. 2, the person is not ingesting enough nutrients to meet metabolic energy needs. As a result, the different types of work are less efficient and the person metabolizes his or her own body tissues to provide needed energy. If this situation continues, it will lead to death.

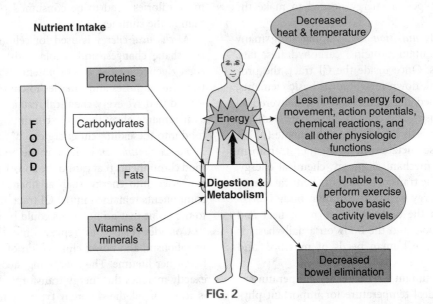

Nutrient Intake

FOOD

- Proteins
- Carbohydrates
- Fats
- Vitamins & minerals

Digestion & Metabolism → Energy

- Decreased heat & temperature
- Less internal energy for movement, action potentials, chemical reactions, and all other physiologic functions
- Unable to perform exercise above basic activity levels
- Decreased bowel elimination

FIG. 2

In Fig. 3, the person is ingesting more nutrients than are needed to meet energy needs. As a result, these extra energy compounds are converted first into glycogen and eventually into fat. Although fat represents stored energy, excessive fat can harm the body. In addition, when food is ingested to excess, metabolism and work energies are not increased. Only heat and bowel elimination increase.

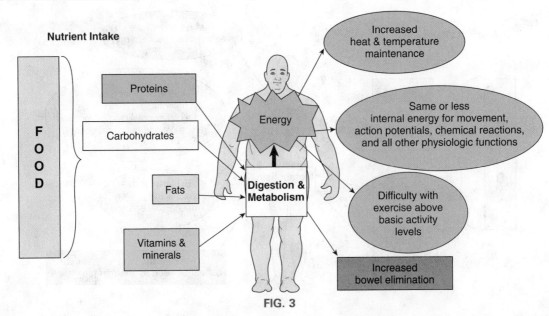

Nutrient Intake

FOOD

- Proteins
- Carbohydrates
- Fats
- Vitamins & minerals

Digestion & Metabolism → Energy

- Increased heat & temperature maintenance
- Same or less internal energy for movement, action potentials, chemical reactions, and all other physiologic functions
- Difficulty with exercise above basic activity levels
- Increased bowel elimination

FIG. 3

Problems of Digestion, Nutrition, and Elimination
Management of Patients with Problems of the Gastrointestinal System

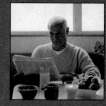

CHAPTER
55

Assessment of the Gastrointestinal System

Donna D. Ignatavicius

evolve WEBSITE

http://evolve.elsevier.com/Iggy/

Animation: Digestion
Animation: Rectal Examination
Answer Key for NCLEX Examination Challenges and
    Decision-Making Challenges
Audio Glossary
Key Points

Review Questions for the NCLEX® Examination
Video Clip: Abdomen, Bowel Sounds
Video Clip: Palpation of Abdomen
Video Clip: Percussion, Abdomen
Video Clip: Percussion, Liver, Spleen

LEARNING OUTCOMES

Safe and Effective Care Environment

1. Assess patients for complications of diagnostic tests.
2. Prioritize post-test care for patients having endoscopic procedures.

Health Promotion and Maintenance

3. Identify factors that place patients at risk for GI problems.
4. Teach pre-test and post-test care for diagnostic GI testing to patients and families.

Psychosocial Integrity

5. Identify general psychological responses to GI health problems.

Physiological Integrity

6. Briefly review the anatomy and physiology of the GI system.
7. Describe GI system changes associated with aging.
8. Perform a GI history using selected Gordon's Functional Health Patterns.
9. Perform focused physical assessment for patients with suspected or actual GI health problems.
10. Explain and interpret common laboratory tests for a patient with a GI health problem.

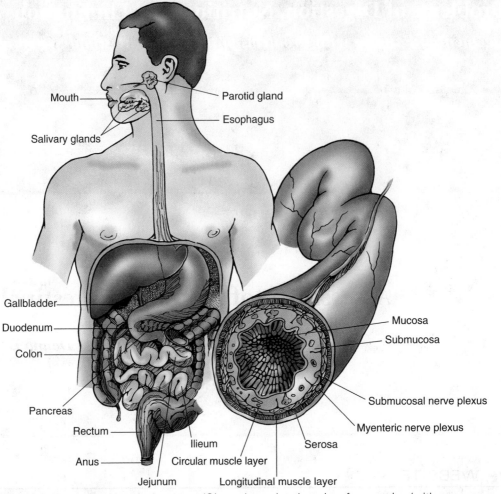

FIG. 55-1 The gastrointestinal system (GI tract) can be thought of as a tube (with necessary structures) extending from the mouth to the anus for a 25-foot length. The structure of this tube *(shown enlarged)* is basically the same throughout its length.

The GI system includes the GI tract (alimentary canal), consisting of the mouth, esophagus, stomach, small and large intestines, and rectum. The salivary glands, liver, gallbladder, and pancreas secrete substances into this tract to form the GI system (Fig. 55-1). The main function of the GI tract, with the aid of organs such as the pancreas and the liver, is the *digestion* of food to meet the body's *nutritional* needs and the *elimination* of waste resulting from digestion. Adequate nutrition is required for proper functioning of the body's organs and other cells (see the Concept Overview). The GI tract is susceptible to many health problems, including structural or mechanical alterations, impaired motility, infection, and cancer.

ANATOMY AND PHYSIOLOGY REVIEW

Overview of the Gastrointestinal System
Structure
The GI tract is a hollow muscular tube surrounded by four tissue layers. The lumen, or inner wall, of the GI tract consists of four layers: mucosa, submucosa, muscularis, and serosa. The *mucosa,* the innermost layer, includes a thin layer of smooth muscle and specialized exocrine gland cells. It is surrounded by the submucosa, which is made up of connective tissue. The *submucosa* layer is surrounded by the muscularis. The *muscularis* is composed of both circular and longitudinal smooth muscles, which work to keep contents moving through the tract. The outermost layer, the *serosa,* is composed of connective tissue. Although the GI tract is continuous from the mouth to the anus, it is divided into specialized regions. The mouth, pharynx, esophagus, stomach, and small and large intestines each perform a specific function. In addition, the secretions of the salivary, gastric, and intestinal glands; liver; and pancreas empty into the GI tract to aid digestion.

Function
The functions of the GI tract include secretion, digestion, absorption, motility, and elimination. Food and fluids are ingested, swallowed, and propelled along the lumen of the GI tract to the anus for elimination. The smooth muscles contract to move food from the mouth to the anus. Before food can be absorbed, it must be broken down to a liquid, called chyme. Digestion is the mechanical and chemical process in which complex foodstuffs are broken down into simpler forms that can be used by the body. During digestion, the stomach

secretes hydrochloric acid, the liver secretes bile, and digestive enzymes are released from accessory organs, aiding in food breakdown. After the digestive process is complete, absorption takes place. Absorption is carried out as the nutrients produced by digestion move from the lumen of the GI tract into the body's circulatory system for uptake by individual cells.

Oral Cavity

The oral cavity (mouth) includes the buccal mucosa, lips, tongue, hard palate, soft palate, teeth, and salivary glands. The buccal mucosa is the mucous membrane lining the inside of the mouth. The tongue is involved in speech, taste, and mastication (chewing). Small projections called *papillae* cover the tongue and provide a roughened surface, permitting the movement of food in the mouth during chewing. The hard palate and the soft palate together form the roof of the mouth.

Adults have 32 permanent teeth: 16 each in upper and lower arches. The different types of teeth function to prepare food for digestion by cutting, tearing, crushing, or grinding the food. Swallowing begins after food is taken into the mouth and chewed. Saliva is secreted in response to the presence of food in the mouth and begins to soften the food. Saliva contains mucin and an enzyme called *salivary amylase* (also known as *ptyalin*), which begins the breakdown of carbohydrates.

Esophagus

The esophagus is a muscular canal that extends from the pharynx (throat) to the stomach and passes through the center of the diaphragm. Its primary function is to move food and fluids from the pharynx to the stomach. At the upper end of the esophagus is a sphincter referred to as the upper esophageal sphincter (UES). When at rest, the UES is closed to prevent air into the esophagus during respiration. The portion of the esophagus just above the gastroesophageal (GE) junction is referred to as the lower esophageal sphincter (LES). When at rest, the LES is normally closed to prevent reflux of gastric contents into the esophagus. If the LES does not work properly, gastroesophageal reflux disease (GERD) can develop (see Chapter 57).

Stomach

The stomach is located in the midline and left upper quadrant (LUQ) of the abdomen and has four anatomic regions. The *cardia* is the narrow portion of the stomach that is below the gastroesophageal (GE) junction. The *fundus* is the area nearest to the cardia. The main area of the stomach is referred to as the *body* or *corpus*. The *antrum* (pylorus) is the distal (lower) portion of the stomach and is separated from the duodenum by the pyloric sphincter. Both ends of the stomach are guarded by sphincters (cardiac and pyloric), which aid in the transport of food through the GI tract and prevent backflow.

Smooth muscle cells that line the stomach are responsible for gastric motility. The stomach is also richly innervated with intrinsic and extrinsic nerves. Parietal cells lining the wall of the stomach secrete hydrochloric acid, whereas chief cells secrete pepsinogen (a precursor to pepsin, a digestive enzyme). Parietal cells also produce intrinsic factor, a substance that aids in the absorption of vitamin B_{12}. Absence of the intrinsic factor causes pernicious anemia.

After ingestion of food, the stomach functions as a food reservoir where the digestive process begins, using mechanical movements and chemical secretions. The stomach mixes or churns the food, breaking apart the large food molecules and mixing them with gastric secretions to form chyme, which then empties into the duodenum. The *intestinal phase* begins as the chyme passes from the stomach into the duodenum, causing distention. It is assisted by secretin, a hormone that inhibits further acid production and decreases gastric motility.

Pancreas

The pancreas is a fish-shaped gland that lies behind the stomach and extends horizontally from the duodenal C-loop to the spleen. The pancreas is divided into portions known as the *head*, the *body*, and the *tail* (Fig. 55-2).

Two major cellular bodies (exocrine and endocrine) within the pancreas have separate functions. The *exocrine* part is about 80% of the organ and consists of cells that secrete enzymes needed for digestion of carbohydrates, fats, and proteins (trypsin, chymotrypsin, amylase, and lipase). The *endocrine* part of the pancreas is made up of the islets of Langerhans, with alpha cells producing glucagon and beta cells producing insulin. These hormones produced are essential in the regulation of *metabolism*. Chapter 67 describes the endocrine function of the pancreas in detail.

Liver and Gallbladder

The *liver* is the largest organ in the body (other than skin) and is located mainly in the right upper quadrant (RUQ) of the abdomen. The right and left hepatic ducts transport bile from the liver. It receives its blood supply from the hepatic artery and portal vein, resulting in about 1500 mL of blood flow through the liver every minute.

The *liver* performs more than 400 functions in three major categories: storage, protection, and metabolism. It *stores* many minerals and vitamins, such as iron, magnesium, and the fat-soluble vitamins A, D, E, and K.

The *protective* function of the liver involves phagocytic Kupffer cells, which are part of the body's reticuloendothelial system. They engulf harmful bacteria and anemic red blood cells. The liver also detoxifies potentially harmful compounds (e.g., drugs, chemicals, alcohol). Therefore the risk for drug toxicity increases with aging because of decreased liver function.

The liver functions in the *metabolism* of proteins considered vital for human survival. It breaks down amino acids to remove ammonia, which is then converted to urea and is excreted via the kidneys. In addition, it synthesizes several plasma proteins, including albumin, prothrombin, and fibrinogen. The liver's role in carbohydrate metabolism involves storing and releasing glycogen as the body's energy requirements change. The organ also synthesizes, breaks down, and temporarily stores fatty acids and triglycerides.

The liver forms and continually secretes bile, which is essential for the breakdown of fat. The secretion of bile increases in response to gastrin, secretin, and cholecystokinin. Bile is secreted into small ducts that empty into the common bile duct and into the duodenum at the sphincter of Oddi. However, if the sphincter is closed, the bile goes to the gallbladder for storage.

The *gallbladder* is a pear-shaped, bulbous sac that is located underneath the liver. It is drained by the cystic duct, which joins with the hepatic duct from the liver to form the

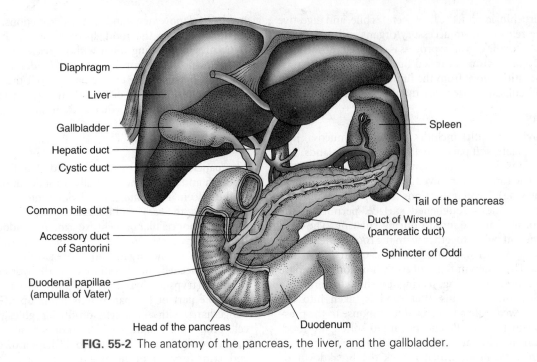

FIG. 55-2 The anatomy of the pancreas, the liver, and the gallbladder.

common bile duct (CBD). The gallbladder collects, concentrates, and stores the bile that has come from the liver. It releases the bile into the duodenum via the CBD when fat is present.

Small Intestine

The small intestine is the longest and most convoluted portion of the digestive tract, measuring 16 to 19 feet (5 to 6 m) in length in an adult. It is composed of three different regions: duodenum, jejunum, and ileum. The *duodenum* is the first 12 inches (30 cm) of the small intestine and is attached to the distal end of the pylorus. The common bile duct and pancreatic duct join to form the ampulla of Vater, emptying into the duodenum at the duodenal papilla. This papillary opening is surrounded by muscle known as the sphincter of Oddi. The 8-foot (2.5-m) portion of the small intestine that follows the sphincter of Oddi is the *jejunum*. The last 8 to 12 feet (2.5 to 4 m) of the small intestine is called the *ileum*. The ileocecal valve separates the entrance of the ileum from the cecum of the large intestine.

The inner surface of the small intestine has a velvety appearance because of numerous mucous membrane finger-like projections. These projections are called *intestinal villi*. In addition to the intestinal villi, the small intestine has circular folds of mucosa and submucosa, which increase the surface area for digestion and absorption.

The small intestine has three main *functions*: movement (mixing and peristalsis), digestion, and absorption. Because the intestinal villi increase the surface area of the small intestine, it is the major organ of absorption of the digestive system. The small intestine mixes and transports the chyme to mix with many digestive enzymes. It takes an average of 3 to 10 hours for the contents to be passed by peristalsis through the small intestine. Intestinal enzymes aid in the digestion of proteins, carbohydrates, and lipids.

Large Intestine

The large intestine extends about 5 to 6 feet in length from the ileocecal valve to the anus and is lined with columnar epithelium that has absorptive and mucous cells. It begins with the *cecum,* a dilated, pouchlike structure that is inferior to the ileocecal opening. At the base of the cecum is the vermiform appendix, which has no known digestive function. The large intestine then extends upward from the cecum as the colon. The colon consists of four divisions: ascending colon, transverse colon, descending colon, and sigmoid colon. The sigmoid colon empties into the rectum.

Following the sigmoid colon, the large intestine bends downward to form the rectum. The last 1 to 1½ inches (3 to 4 cm) of the large intestine is called the *anal canal,* which opens to the exterior of the body through the anus. Sphincter muscles surround the anal canal.

The large intestine's *functions* are movement, absorption, and elimination. Movement in the large intestine consists mainly of segmental contractions, like those in the small intestine, to allow enough time for the absorption of water and electrolytes. In addition, peristaltic contractions are triggered by colonic distention to move the contents toward the rectum, where the material is stored until the urge to defecate occurs. Absorption of water and some electrolytes occurs in the large intestine to reduce the fluid volume of the chyme. This process creates a more solid material, the feces, for elimination.

GASTROINTESTINAL CHANGES ASSOCIATED WITH AGING

Physiologic changes occur as people age, especially ages 65 years and older. Changes in digestion and elimination that can affect nutrition are common. For example, decreased gastric hydrochloric acid (HCl) can lead to decreased absorption of essential minerals like iron. Chart 55-1 lists common

CHART 55-1	NURSING FOCUS ON THE OLDER ADULT

Changes in the Gastrointestinal System Related to Aging

PHYSIOLOGIC CHANGE	DISORDERS RELATED TO CHANGE	NURSING INTERVENTIONS	RATIONALES
Stomach Atrophy of the gastric mucosa is characterized by a decrease in the ratio of gastrin-secreting cells to somatostatin-secreting cells. This change leads to decreased hydrochloric acid levels (hypochlorhydria).	Decreased hydrochloric acid levels lead to decreased absorption of iron and vitamin B_{12} and to proliferation of bacteria. Atrophic gastritis occurs as a consequence of bacterial overgrowth.	Encourage bland foods high in vitamins and iron. Assess for epigastric pain.	Bland foods help prevent gastritis. Assessment helps detect gastritis.
Large Intestine Peristalsis decreases, and nerve impulses are dulled.	Decreased sensation to defecate can result in postponement of bowel movements, which leads to constipation and impaction.	Encourage a high-fiber diet and 1500 mL of fluid intake daily (if not contraindicated). Encourage as much activity as tolerated.	These interventions increase the sensation of needing to defecate.
Pancreas Distention and dilation of pancreatic ducts change. Calcification of pancreatic vessels occurs with a decrease in lipase production.	Decreased lipase level results in decreased fat absorption and digestion. Steatorrhea, or excess fat in the feces, occurs because of decreased fat digestion.	Encourage small, frequent feedings. Assess for diarrhea.	Small, frequent feedings help prevent steatorrhea. Diarrhea may be steatorrhea. Excessive diarrhea can lead to dehydration.
Liver A decrease in the number and size of hepatic cells leads to decreased liver weight and mass. This change and an increase in fibrous tissue lead to decreased protein synthesis and changes in liver enzymes. Enzyme activity and cholesterol synthesis are diminished.	Decreased enzyme activity depresses drug metabolism, which leads to accumulation of drugs—possibly to toxic levels.	Assess for adverse effects of all drugs.	Assessment can help detect drug toxicity.

GI changes and nursing implications when caring for older adults.

ASSESSMENT METHODS

Patient History

The purpose of the health history is to determine the events related to the current health problem. One tool for assessing GI function is the nutritional-metabolic pattern and the elimination pattern assessment found in Chart 55-2. Focus questions about changes in appetite, weight, and stool. Determine the patient's pain experience.

Collect data about the patient's age, gender, and culture. This information can be helpful in assessing who is likely to have particular GI system disorders. For instance, older adults are more at risk for stomach cancer than are younger adults. Younger adults are more at risk for inflammatory bowel disease (IBD). The exact reasons for these differences continue to be studied.

Question the patient about previous GI disorders or abdominal surgeries. Ask about prescription medications being taken, including how much, when the drugs are taken, and why they have been prescribed. Inquire if the patient takes over-the-counter (OTC) drugs, herbs, and/or supplements. In particular, ask whether aspirin, NSAIDs (e.g., ibuprofen), laxatives, herbal preparations, or enemas are routinely taken. Large amounts of aspirin or NSAIDs can predispose the patient to peptic ulcer disease and GI bleeding.

Long-term use of laxatives or enemas can cause dependence and result in constipation and electrolyte imbalance. Some herbal preparations, especially ayurvedic herbs, can affect appetite, absorption, and elimination. Determine if the patient smokes or has ever smoked cigarettes, cigars, or pipes. Smoking is a major risk factor for most GI cancers. Chewing tobacco is a major cause of oral cancer.

Finally, investigate the patient's travel history. Ask whether he or she has traveled outside of the country recently. This information may provide clues about the cause of symptoms like diarrhea.

Nutrition History

A nutrition history is important when assessing GI system function. Many conditions manifest themselves as a result of alterations in intake and absorption of nutrients. The purpose of a nutritional assessment is to gather information about

> ### 🌐 CULTURAL AWARENESS
>
> Cultural and religious patterns are important in obtaining a complete nutritional history. Ask if certain foods pose a problem for the patient. For example, the spices or hot pepper used in cooking in many cultures can aggravate or precipitate GI tract symptoms such as indigestion. Note religious patterns such as fasting or abstinence.
>
> About 80% to 90% of black people are lactose intolerant. A much smaller percentage of white people also have this problem. Lactose intolerance causes bloating, cramping, and diarrhea as a result of lack of the enzyme *lactase*. Lactase is needed to convert lactose in milk and other dairy products to glucose and galactose.

Using Gordon's Functional Health Patterns

Nutritional-Metabolic Pattern
- What is your typical daily food intake? Describe a day's meals, snacks, and vitamins.
- How much salt do you typically add to your food? Do you use salt substitutes?
- How is your appetite? Any recent change?
- Do you have any difficulty chewing or swallowing?
- Do you wear dentures? How well do they fit?
- Do you ever experience indigestion or "heartburn"? How often? What seems to cause it? What helps it?
- Do you have pain, diarrhea, gas, or any other problems? Do any specific foods cause this for you?
- What is your typical daily fluid intake? What types of fluids (water, juices, soft drinks, coffee, tea)? How much?
- Have you had any recent change in your weight? Weight gain? Weight loss? How much?
- Have you noticed a change in the tightness of your rings or shoes? Tighter? Looser?
- Have you noticed any difference in the size of your abdomen?

Elimination Pattern
- What is your usual bowel elimination pattern? Frequency? Character? Discomfort? Laxatives?
- Do you have any pain or bleeding associated with bowel movements?
- Have you experienced any changes in your usual bowel pattern?
- When was your last rectal examination?
- Have you ever had an endoscopy or a colonoscopy?
- What is your usual urinary elimination pattern? Frequency? Amount? Color? Odor? Control?
- Have you noticed a change in the amount of urine?

Based on Gordon, M. (2011). *Manual of nursing diagnosis* (12th ed.). New York: Jones & Bartlett.

how well the patient's nutritional needs are being met. Inquire about any special diet and whether there are any known food allergies. Ask the patient to describe the usual foods that are eaten daily and the times that meals are taken.

Health problems can also affect nutritional intake, so explore any changes that have occurred in eating habits as a result of illness. Anorexia (loss of appetite for food) can occur with GI disease. Assess changes in taste and any difficulty or pain with swallowing (dysphagia) that could be associated with esophageal disorders. Also ask if abdominal pain or discomfort occurs with eating and whether the patient has experienced any nausea, vomiting, or dyspepsia (indigestion or heartburn). Unknown food allergies often cause these symptoms. Inquire about any unintentional weight loss, because some cancers of the GI tract may present in this manner. Assess for alcohol and caffeine consumption, because both substances are associated with many GI disorders, such as gastritis and peptic ulcer disease.

The patient's socioeconomic status may have a profound impact on his or her nutritional status. For example, people who have limited budgets, such as some older adults or the unemployed, may not be able to purchase foods required for a balanced diet. In addition, they may substitute less expensive and perhaps less effective OTC medications or herbs for prescription drugs. Necessary medical care may be delayed, and patients may not seek health care until conditions are well advanced.

Family History and Genetic Risk

Ask about a family history of GI disorders. Some GI health problems have a genetic predisposition. For example, familial adenomatous polyposis (FAP) is an inherited autosomal dominant disorder that predisposes the patient to colon cancer (McCance et al., 2010). Specific genetic risks are discussed with the GI problems in later chapters.

Current Health Problems

Because GI clinical manifestations are often vague and difficult for the patient to describe, it is important to obtain a chronologic account of the current problem, symptoms, and any treatments taken. Furthermore, ask about the location, quality, quantity, timing (onset, duration), and factors that may aggravate or alleviate each symptom (see Chart 55-2).

For example, a change in bowel habits is a common assessment finding. Obtain this information from the patient:
- Pattern of bowel movements
- Color and consistency of the feces
- Occurrence of diarrhea or constipation
- Effective action taken to relieve diarrhea or constipation
- Presence of frank blood or tarry stools
- Presence of abdominal distention or gas

An unintentional weight gain or loss is another symptom that needs further investigation. Assess the patient's:
- Normal weight
- Weight gain or loss
- Period of time for weight change
- Changes in appetite or oral intake

Pain is a common concern of patients with GI tract disorders. The mnemonic PQRST may be helpful in organizing the current problem assessment (Jarvis, 2012):

P: Precipitating or palliative. What brings it on? What makes it better? Worse? When did you first notice it?

Q: Quality or quantity. How does it look, feel, or sound? How intense/severe is it?

R: Region or radiation. Where is it? Does it spread anywhere?

S: Severity scale. How bad is it (on a scale of 1 to 10)? Is it getting better, worse, or staying the same?

T: Timing. Onset—Exactly when did it first occur? Duration—How long did it last? Frequency—How often does it occur?

Abdominal pain is often vague and difficult to evaluate. Ask the patient to describe the type of pain, such as burning, gnawing, or stabbing. The location of the pain can be determined by asking him or her to point to the involved site. Ask about the relationship of food intake to the onset or worsening of pain. For example, a high-fat meal may cause gallbladder pain.

Changes in the skin may result from several GI tract disorders, such as liver and biliary system obstruction. Ask about whether these clinical manifestations have occurred, or assess whether they are present:
- Skin discolorations or rashes
- Itching
- Jaundice (yellowing of skin caused by bilirubin pigments)
- Increased bruising
- Increased tendency to bleed

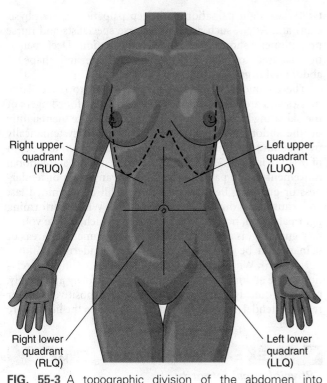

FIG. 55-3 A topographic division of the abdomen into quadrants.

Physical Assessment

Physical assessment involves a comprehensive examination of the patient's nutritional status, mouth, and abdomen. Nutritional assessment is discussed in detail in Chapter 63. Oral assessment is described in Chapter 56.

In preparation for examination of the *abdomen,* ask the patient to empty his or her bladder and then to lie in a supine position with knees bent, keeping the arms at the sides to prevent tensing of the abdominal muscles.

The abdominal examination usually begins at the patient's right side and proceeds in a systematic fashion (Fig. 55-3):
- Right upper quadrant (RUQ)
- Left upper quadrant (LUQ)
- Left lower quadrant (LLQ)
- Right lower quadrant (RLQ)

Table 55-1 lists the organs that lie in each of these areas.

If areas of pain or discomfort are noted from the history, this area is examined last in the examination sequence. This sequence should prevent the patient from tensing abdominal muscles because of the pain, which would make the examination difficult. Examine any area of tenderness cautiously, and instruct the patient to state whether it is too painful. Observe his or her face for signs of distress or pain.

The abdomen is assessed by using the four techniques of examination, but in a sequence different from that used for other body systems: inspection, auscultation, percussion, and then palpation. This sequence is preferred so that palpation and percussion do not increase intestinal activity and bowel sounds. As a nurse generalist, perform inspection, auscultation, and light palpation. Percussion and deep palpation may be done by health care providers, including advanced practice nurses (APNs), or specialty nurses. If appendicitis or an abdominal aneurysm is suspected, palpation is not done.

TABLE 55-1	LOCATION OF BODY STRUCTURES IN EACH ABDOMINAL QUADRANT

Right Upper Quadrant (RUQ)
- Most of the liver
- Gallbladder
- Duodenum
- Head of the pancreas
- Hepatic flexure of the colon
- Part of the ascending and transverse colon

Right Lower Quadrant (RLQ)
- Cecum
- Appendix
- Right ureter
- Right ovary and fallopian tube
- Right spermatic cord

Midline
- Abdominal aorta
- Uterus (if enlarged)
- Bladder (if distended)

Left Upper Quadrant (LUQ)
- Left lobe of the liver
- Stomach
- Spleen
- Body and tail of the pancreas
- Splenic flexure of the colon
- Part of the transverse and descending colon

Left Lower Quadrant (LLQ)
- Part of the descending colon
- Sigmoid colon
- Left ureter
- Left ovary and fallopian tube
- Left spermatic cord

Inspection

Inspect the skin, and note any of these findings:
- Overall symmetry of the abdomen
- Presence of discolorations or scarring
- Abdominal distention
- Bulging flanks
- Taut, glistening skin

Observe the shape of the abdomen by observing its contour and symmetry. The contour of the abdomen can be rounded, flat, concave, or distended. It is best determined when standing at the side of the bed or treatment table and looking down on the abdomen. View the abdomen at eye level from the side. Note whether the contour is symmetric or asymmetric.

! NURSING SAFETY PRIORITY

Action Alert

If a bulging, pulsating mass is present during assessment of the abdomen, do not touch the area because the patient may have an abdominal aortic aneurysm, a life-threatening problem. Notify the health care provider of this finding immediately! Peristaltic movements are rarely seen unless the patient is thin and has increased peristalsis. If these movements are observed, note the quadrant of origin and the direction of peristaltic flow. Report this finding to the health care provider because it may indicate an intestinal obstruction.

Asymmetry of the abdomen can indicate problems affecting the underlying body structures (see Table 55-1). Note the shape and position of the umbilicus for any deviations. The presence of ecchymosis around the umbilicus (Cullen's sign) is an indication of intra-abdominal bleeding.

Finally, observe the patient's abdominal movements, including the normal rising and falling with inspiration and expiration, and note any distress during movement. Occasionally, pulsations may be visible, particularly in the area of the abdominal aorta.

Auscultation

Auscultation of the abdomen is performed with the diaphragm of the stethoscope, because bowel sounds are usually high pitched. Place the stethoscope lightly on the abdominal wall while listening for bowel sounds in all four quadrants, beginning in the RLQ at the ileocecal valve area.

Bowel sounds are created as air and fluid move through the GI tract. They are normally heard as relatively high-pitched, irregular gurgles every 5 to 15 seconds, with a normal frequency range of 5 to 30 per minute. Bowel sounds are characterized as normal, hypoactive, or hyperactive. They are diminished or absent after abdominal surgery or in the patient with peritonitis or paralytic ileus.

For many years, nurses have been taught to count the number of bowel sounds in each quadrant as part of routine and postoperative abdominal assessment to assess for peristalsis. However, a classic study showed that the best, most reliable method for assessing the return of peristalsis after abdominal surgery is to ask the patient if he or she has passed flatus within the past 8 hours or a stool within the past 12 to 24 hours (Madsen et al., 2005).

Increased bowel sounds, especially loud, gurgling sounds, result from increased motility of the bowel (borborygmus). These sounds are usually heard in the patient with diarrhea or gastroenteritis or above a complete intestinal obstruction.

When auscultating the abdomen, also listen for vascular sounds or bruits ("swooshing" sounds) over the abdominal aorta, the renal arteries, and the iliac arteries. A bruit heard over the aorta usually indicates the presence of an aneurysm. *If this sound is heard, do not percuss or palpate the abdomen. Notify the health care provider of your findings!*

Percussion

Percussion may be used by APNs and other health care providers to determine the size of solid organs; to detect the presence of masses, fluid, and air; and to estimate the size of the liver and spleen. The percussion notes normally heard in the abdomen are termed tympanic (the high-pitched, loud, musical sound of an air-filled intestine) or dull (the medium-pitched, softer, thudlike sound over a solid organ, such as the liver).

The liver and spleen can be percussed. An enlarged liver is called hepatomegaly. Dullness heard in the left anterior axillary line indicates enlargement of the spleen (splenomegaly). Mild to moderate splenomegaly can be detected before the spleen becomes palpable.

Palpation

The purpose of palpation is to determine the size and location of abdominal organs and to assess for the presence of masses or tenderness. Palpation of the abdomen consists of

two types: light palpation and deep palpation. Only physicians and APNs, such as clinical nurse specialists and nurse practitioners, should perform deep palpation. Deep palpation is used to further determine the size and shape of abdominal organs and masses.

The technique of *light palpation* is used to detect large masses and areas of tenderness. Place the first four fingers of the palpating hand close together and then place them lightly on the abdomen and proceed smoothly and systematically from quadrant to quadrant. Depress the abdomen to a depth of $\frac{1}{2}$ to 1 inch (1.25 to 2.5 cm). Proceed with a rotational movement of the palpating hand. Note any areas of tenderness or guarding because these areas will be examined last and cautiously during deep palpation. While performing light palpation, notice signs of rigidity, which, unlike voluntary guarding, is a sign of peritoneal inflammation. Areas of pain should be evaluated for rebound tenderness (Blumberg's sign). With fingers placed at a 90-degree angle in relation to the abdomen, the examiner pushes slowly and deeply, releasing quickly. Pain felt on release is a positive sign for rebound tenderness and should be reported to the health care provider.

❓ NCLEX EXAMINATION CHALLENGE

Physiological Integrity

A client is seen in the emergency department with reports of nausea, anorexia, and diarrhea. In what sequence will the nurse assess the client's abdomen? (Select in order of priority.)
A. Auscultation
B. Percussion
C. Inspection
D. Light palpation

Psychosocial Assessment

Psychosocial assessment focuses on how the GI health problem affects the patient's life and lifestyle. Remember that patients are often reluctant to discuss elimination problems, which may be very personal and embarrassing. The interview focus is on whether usual activities have been interrupted or disturbed, including employment. Question the patient about recent stressful events. Emotional stress has been associated with the development or exacerbation (flare-up) of irritable bowel syndrome (IBS) and other GI disorders. If the patient is diagnosed with cancer, he or she is expected to experience the phases of the grieving process. Patients may be depressed, angry, or in denial. More specific psychosocial assessments are included in later GI chapters as part of each disease discussion.

Diagnostic Assessment
Laboratory Assessment

To make an accurate assessment of the many possible causes of GI system abnormalities, laboratory testing of blood, urine, and stool specimens may be performed.

Serum Tests. A complete blood count (CBC) *aids in the diagnosis of anemia and infection. It also detects changes in the blood's formed elements. In adults, GI bleeding is the most frequent cause of anemia. It is associated with GI cancer, peptic ulcer disease, and inflammatory bowel disease.*

Because the liver is the main site of all proteins involved in coagulation, prothrombin time (PT) is useful in evaluating the levels of these clotting factors. *PT* measures the rate at which prothrombin is converted to thrombin, a process that depends on vitamin K–associated clotting factors. Severe acute or chronic liver damage leads to a prolonged PT secondary to impaired synthesis of clotting proteins.

Many *electrolytes* are altered in GI tract dysfunction. For example, calcium is absorbed in the GI tract and may be measured to detect malabsorption. Excessive vomiting or diarrhea causes sodium or potassium depletion, thus requiring replacement.

Assays of serum enzymes are important in the evaluation of liver damage. Aspartate aminotransferase (AST) and alanine aminotransferase (ALT) are two enzymes found in the liver and other organs. These enzymes are elevated in most liver disorders, but they are highest in conditions that cause necrosis, such as severe viral hepatitis and cirrhosis.

Elevations in serum *amylase* and *lipase* may indicate acute pancreatitis. In this disease, serum amylase levels begin to elevate within 24 hours of onset and remain elevated for up to 5 days. Serum amylase and lipase are not elevated when *extensive* pancreatic necrosis is present because there are few pancreatic cells manufacturing the enzymes.

Bilirubin is the primary pigment in bile, which is normally conjugated and excreted by the liver and biliary system. It is measured as total serum bilirubin, conjugated (direct) bilirubin, and unconjugated (indirect) bilirubin. These measurements are important in the evaluation of jaundice and in the evaluation of liver and biliary tract functioning. Elevations in direct and indirect bilirubin levels can indicate impaired secretion.

The serum level of *ammonia* may also be measured to evaluate hepatic function. Ammonia is normally used to rebuild amino acids or is converted to urea for excretion. Elevated levels are seen in conditions that cause severe hepatocellular injury, such as cirrhosis of the liver or fulminant hepatitis (Pagana & Pagana, 2010).

Two primary *oncofetal antigens*—CA19-9 and *CEA*—are evaluated to diagnose cancer, monitor the success of cancer therapy, and assess for the recurrence of cancer in the GI tract. These antigens may also be increased in benign GI conditions. New tests, such as ECCO 15 and ESMO 34, have been developed in Europe and are undergoing clinical trials. Chart 55-3 lists blood tests commonly used by the health care provider in the diagnosis of GI disorders.

Urine Tests. The presence of amylase can be detected in the urine. In acute pancreatitis, renal clearance of amylase is increased. Amylase levels in the urine remain high even after serum levels return to normal. This becomes an important finding in patients who are symptomatic for 3 days or longer (Pagana & Pagana, 2010).

Urine *urobilinogen* is a form of bilirubin that is converted by the intestinal flora and excreted in the urine. Its measurement is useful in the evaluation of hepatic and biliary obstruction, because the presence of bilirubin in the urine often occurs before jaundice is seen.

Stool Tests. The 2010 American Cancer Society Screening Guidelines recommend yearly fecal occult blood test (FOBT), yearly fecal immunochemical test (FIT), or stool DNA (sDNA) at unspecified intervals to detect colorectal cancer early when it can be treated. These tests use a take-home, multi-sample method rather than having the test done during a digital rectal examination.

The traditionally used FOBT (e.g., Hemoccult II) requires an active component of guaiac and is therefore more likely than the FIT (e.g., HemeSelect or InSure) to yield false-positive results. In addition, patients having the guaiac-based test must avoid certain foods before the test, such as raw fruits and vegetables and red meat. Vitamin C–rich foods, juices, and tablets must also be avoided. Anticoagulants, such as warfarin (Coumadin), and NSAIDs should be discontinued for 7 days before testing begins. Patient compliance is likely to be higher with the FIT method because drugs and food do not interfere with the test results (Heseltine, 2007).

The newest test for detection of colorectal cancer is stool DNA (ColoSure). This test examines stool DNA to detect changes in the vimentin gene. Most patients with colorectal cancer have genetic changes that can be detected by this simple test.

Stool samples may also be collected to test for *ova and parasites* to aid in the diagnosis of parasitic infection. They may also be tested for *fecal fats* when steatorrhea (fatty stools) or malabsorption is suspected. Fat is normally absorbed in the small intestine in the presence of biliary and pancreatic secretions. In malabsorption, fat is abnormally excreted in the stool.

Other common stool tests, stool cytotoxic assay and stool culture, detect the presence of infectious agents, especially *Clostridium difficile.* Patients who are suspected of having *C. difficile* are usually symptomatic. Prolonged antibiotic therapy, especially in older adults, depresses the natural intestinal flora, causing an overgrowth of the pathogen. The bacterium releases a toxin that causes colonic epithelium necrosis resulting in severe diarrhea that is easily transmitted from person to person via the fecal-oral route.

A stool culture takes a longer time to get results and is not the test of choice. Instead, the cytotoxic assay is considered the most reliable because it has a high sensitivity (Keske & Letizia, 2010). However, the results may not be available for up to 3 days. The most common test to detect *C. difficile* is the enzyme-linked immunosorbent assay (ELISA) toxin A+B. It is easy to use, and the results are usually available in 2 to 6 hours (Keske & Letizia, 2010).

Imaging Assessment

Radiographic examinations and similar diagnostic procedures are useful in detecting structural and functional disorders of the GI system. Teach the patient how to prepare for the examination, provide an explanation of the procedure, and teach the required postprocedure care.

A *plain film of the abdomen* may be the first x-ray study that the health care provider requests when diagnosing a GI problem. This film can reveal abnormalities such as masses, tumors, and strictures or obstructions to normal movement. Patterns of bowel gas appear light on the abdominal film and can be useful in detecting an obstruction (ileus). No preparation is required except to wear a hospital gown and remove any jewelry or belts, which may interfere with the film.

When abdominal pain is severe or when bowel perforation is suspected, an *acute abdomen series* may be requested. This procedure consists of a chest x-ray, supine abdomen film, and an upright abdomen film. The chest x-ray may reveal a hiatal hernia, and an upright abdomen film may show air in the peritoneum from a bowel perforation. Today computed tomography (CT) and magnetic resonance imaging (MRI)

CHART 55-3 **LABORATORY PROFILE**

Gastrointestinal Assessment

TEST (SERUM)	NORMAL RANGE FOR ADULTS	SIGNIFICANCE OF ABNORMAL FINDINGS
Calcium (total)	9.0-10.5 mg/dL (values decrease in older adults)	*Decreased* values indicate possible: Malabsorption Renal failure Acute pancreatitis
Potassium	3.5-5.0 mEq/L or 3.5-5.0 mmol/L	*Decreased* values indicate possible: Vomiting Gastric suctioning Diarrhea Drainage from intestinal fistulas
Albumin	3.5-5.0 g/dL	*Decreased* values indicate possible: Hepatic disease
Alanine aminotransferase (ALT)	3-35 international units/L or 8-20 units/L	*Increased* values indicate possible: Liver disease Hepatitis Cirrhosis
Aspartate aminotransferase (AST)	5-40 units/L	*Increased* values indicate possible: Liver disease Hepatitis Cirrhosis
Alkaline phosphatase	30-85 international units/L or 42-128 units/L	*Increased* values indicate possible: Hepatic disease Biliary obstruction
Bilirubin (total)	0.1-1.0 mg/dL	*Increased* values indicate possible: Hemolysis Biliary obstruction Hepatic damage
Conjugated (direct) bilirubin	0.1-0.3 mg/dL	*Increased* values indicate possible: Biliary obstruction
Unconjugated (indirect) bilirubin	0.2-0.8 mg/dL	*Increased* values indicate possible: Hemolysis Hepatic damage
Ammonia	15-110 mg/dL	*Increased* values indicate possible: Hepatic disease such as cirrhosis
Xylose absorption	*5-g dose in 2 hr:* >20 mg/dL or >1.3 mmol/L *25-g dose in 2 hr:* >25 mg/dL or >1.7 mmol/L	*Decreased* values in blood and urine indicate possible: Malabsorption in the small intestine
Serum amylase	56-90 international units/L or 25-125 units/L	*Increased* values indicate possible: Acute pancreatitis
Serum lipase	0-110 units/L	*Increased* values indicate possible: Acute pancreatitis
Cholesterol	<200 mg/dL	*Increased* values indicate possible: Pancreatitis Biliary obstruction *Decreased* values indicate possible: Liver cell damage
Carbohydrate antigen 19-9 (CA19-9)	<37 units/mL	*Increased* values indicate possible: Cancer of the pancreas, stomach, colon Acute pancreatitis Inflammatory bowel disease
Carcinoembryonic antigen (CEA)	*Nonsmoker:* <2.5 ng/mL *Smoker:* up to 5 ng/mL	*Increased* values indicate possible: Colorectal, stomach, pancreatic cancer Ulcerative colitis Crohn's disease Hepatitis Cirrhosis

scans or ultrasound scans are used more often than abdominal x-rays.

An upper GI radiographic series is an x-ray visualization from the mouth to the duodenojejunal junction. It is used to detect disorders of structure or function of the esophagus (barium swallow), stomach, or duodenum. An extension of the upper GI series, the *small bowel follow-through* (SBFT), continues tracing the barium through the small intestine—up to and including the ileocecal junction—to detect disorders of the jejunum or ileum. These tests are not performed as commonly today because endoscopy procedures allow for direct visualization of the internal GI tract.

Remind the patient to withhold foods and liquids for 8 hours before the test. If possible, opioid analgesics and anticholinergic medications are withheld for 24 hours before the test because they decrease intestinal tract motility. Instruct the patient about the barium preparation and the need to drink about 16 ounces of the barium. The radiology nurse or technician explains that a rotating examination table will be used to assist the patient in assuming the vertical, supine, prone, and lateral positions required for this test.

The initial procedure takes about 30 minutes. Fluoroscopy is used to trace the barium through the esophagus and stomach. The patient stands against the x-ray table for this part of the test. The table then moves to a lying position for more views of the stomach and duodenum. The patient then drinks more barium as quickly as possible while x-rays are taken. To attempt to make him or her as comfortable as possible, a pillow for the head and a sheet to prevent chilling are supplied whenever possible. The position changes help coat the mucosa and identify gastroesophageal reflux and hiatal hernia.

If a small bowel radiographic series is included, the patient drinks additional barium and more x-rays are taken at specific intervals. This series can take several hours, depending on how long it takes the barium to reach the cecum.

After either of these series, teach the patient to drink plenty of fluids to help eliminate the barium. A mild laxative or stool softener may be given to assist in its elimination. The radiology nurse or technician instructs the patient that stools may be chalky white for 24 to 72 hours as barium is excreted. When all barium is passed, brown stools return. If the patient is at home, he or she is instructed to report abdominal fullness, pain, or a delay in return to brown stools.

A barium enema examination, also known as a lower GI series, is an x-ray of the large intestine. The 2010 American Cancer Society Screening Guidelines include this test as an option to determine the presence of colorectal cancer or polyps for people older than 50 years. The options include:
- Double-contrast barium enema every 5 years
- Flexible sigmoidoscopy every 5 years
- CT colonography (virtual colonoscopy) every 5 years
- Colonoscopy every 10 years

Patient preparation is similar to that for colonoscopy. After the study is completed, the patient expels the barium. The radiology nurse or technician teaches the patient to drink plenty of fluids to assist in eliminating the barium and prevent an intestinal obstruction. A laxative is given to help remove the barium from the intestinal tract. Stools are chalky white for about 24 to 72 hours, until all barium is passed. If the patient has positive results, he or she is scheduled for a colonoscopy.

Percutaneous transhepatic cholangiography (PTC) is an x-ray of the biliary duct system using an iodinated dye instilled via a percutaneous needle inserted through the liver into the intrahepatic ducts. This procedure may be performed when a patient has jaundice or persistent upper abdominal pain, even after cholecystectomy, but is rarely done as a diagnostic procedure today. Better information about dilated biliary ducts can be obtained using ultrasound scans and endoscopic retrograde cholangiopancreatography (ERCP) (discussed on p. 1188).

Computed tomography (CT), also referred to as a *CT scan*, provides a noninvasive cross-sectional x-ray view that can detect tissue densities and abnormalities in the abdomen, including the liver, pancreas, spleen, and biliary tract. It may be performed with or without contrast medium.

For the CT scan, the patient is told that he or she will need to lie still in a rather enclosed space of the machine. He or she must remove all jewelry and metal. If contrast medium is to be used, ask about allergies to seafood and iodine. The patient is NPO for at least 4 hours before the test if a contrast medium is to be used. IV access will be required for injection of the contrast medium. Advise the patient that he or she may feel warm and flushed upon injection. The patient who is mildly claustrophobic may require a mild sedative to tolerate the study. The radiologic technician instructs the patient to lie still and to hold his or her breath when asked, as the technician takes a series of images. The test takes about 30 minutes.

Like other parts of the body, the abdomen and its organs may also be evaluated by *magnetic resonance imaging (MRI)*, *such as magnetic resonance cholangiopancreatography (MRCP)*. For many patients with abdominal symptoms, this may be the first diagnostic test requested by the health care provider.

❓ NCLEX EXAMINATION CHALLENGE
Health Promotion and Maintenance

An older adult is scheduled for a double-contrast barium enema. What is the priority health teaching the nurse will provide?
A. "Be sure to take the laxative as prescribed after the test."
B. "Drink a gallon of GoLYTELY the day before the test."
C. "Do not take food or fluids for 24 hours before the test."
D. "Tell the nurse if you have flatus after the test is completed."

Other Diagnostic Assessment

Endoscopy. Endoscopy is direct visualization of the GI tract using a flexible fiberoptic endoscope. It is commonly requested to evaluate bleeding, ulceration, inflammation, tumors, and cancer of the esophagus, stomach, biliary system, or bowel. Obtaining specimens for biopsy and cell studies (e.g., *Helicobacter pylori*) is also possible through the endoscope. There are several types of endoscopic examinations. The patient must sign an informed consent form before having these invasive studies.

Esophagogastroduodenoscopy. Esophagogastroduodenoscopy (EGD) is a visual examination of the esophagus, stomach, and duodenum. This procedure has significantly reduced the number of upper GI series that are done. If GI bleeding is found during an EGD, the physician can inject a sclerotherapy agent into the affected area to stop the bleeding. If the patient has an esophageal stricture, it can be dilated during an EGD.

Teach the patient preparing for an upper GI endoscopic examination to remain NPO for 6 to 8 hours before the procedure. Usual drug therapy for hypertension or other diseases may be taken the morning of the test. However, diabetic patients should consult their health care provider for special instructions. Patients are also usually asked to avoid anticoagulants, aspirin, or NSAIDs for several days before the test unless it is absolutely necessary. Tell the patient that a flexible tube will be passed down the esophagus while he or she is under moderate sedation. Midazolam hydrochloride (Versed),

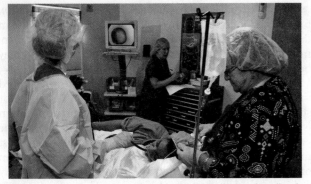

FIG. 55-4 Esophagogastroduodenoscopy allows visualization of the esophagus, the stomach, and the duodenum. If the esophagus is the focus of the examination, the procedure is called *esophagoscopy*. If the stomach is the focus, the procedure is called *gastroscopy*.

fentanyl (Fentanyl, Sublimaze), and/or propofol (Diprivan) are commonly used drugs for sedation. Atropine may be administered to dry secretions. In addition, a local anesthetic is sprayed to inactivate the gag reflex and facilitate passage of the tube. Explain that this anesthetic will depress the gag reflex and that swallowing will be difficult. If the patient has dentures, they are removed.

After the drugs are given, the patient is placed in the left lateral decubitus (Sims', or left side-lying) position with a towel or basin at the mouth for secretions. A bite block is inserted to prevent biting down on the endoscope and to protect the teeth. The physician passes the tube through the mouth and into the esophagus (Fig. 55-4). The procedure takes about 20 to 30 minutes.

After the test, the endoscopy nurse or technician checks vital signs frequently (usually every 30 minutes) until the sedation wears off. The siderails of the bed are raised during this time. The patient remains NPO until the gag reflex returns (usually in 1 to 2 hours).

> ### ! NURSING SAFETY PRIORITY
>
> **Action Alert**
>
> *The priority for care after esophagogastroduodenoscopy is to prevent aspiration. Do not offer fluids or food by mouth until you are sure that the gag reflex is intact! Monitor for signs of perforation, such as pain, bleeding, or fever.*

Remind the patient to not drive for at least 12 hours after the procedure because of sedation. Teach him or her that a hoarse voice or sore throat may persist for several days after the test. Throat lozenges can be used to relieve throat discomfort.

Endoscopic Retrograde Cholangiopancreatography. Endoscopic retrograde cholangiopancreatography (ERCP) includes visual and radiographic examination of the liver, gallbladder, bile ducts, and pancreas to identify the cause and location of obstruction. It is commonly used today for therapeutic purposes rather than for diagnosis. After a cannula is inserted into the common bile duct, a radiopaque dye is instilled and then several x-ray images are obtained. The

physician may perform a papillotomy (a small incision in the sphincter around the ampulla of Vater) to remove gallstones. If a biliary duct stricture is found, plastic or metal stents may be inserted to keep the ducts open. Biopsies of tissue are also frequently taken during this test.

The patient prepares for this test in the same manner as for an EGD, including being NPO for 6 to 8 hours before the test. The patient requires IV access for moderate sedation drugs. Ask about prior exposure to x-ray contrast media and any sensitivities or allergies. If the patient has dentures, they are removed.

Ask the patient if he or she has an implantable medical device, such as a cardiac pacemaker. Electrocautery cannot be used with this type of device (Bruesehoff, 2010). Perform medication reconciliation to determine if the patient is taking anticoagulants, NSAIDs, antiplatelet drugs, or antihyperglycemic agents. The physician decides which of these drugs are safe to take and whether any will need to be stopped before the test.

The endoscopic portion of an ERCP is similar to that of an EGD, except that the endoscope is advanced farther to the duodenum and into the biliary tract. Once the cannula is in the common duct, contrast medium is injected and x-rays are taken to view the biliary tract. A tilt table assists in distributing the contrast medium to all areas to be assessed. The patient is placed in a left lateral position for viewing the common bile duct. Once the cannula is placed, he or she is put in a prone position. After examination of the biliary tree, the cannula is directed into the pancreatic duct for examination. The ERCP lasts from 30 minutes to 2 hours, depending on the treatment that may be done.

After the test, assess vital signs frequently, usually every 15 minutes, until the patient is stable. To prevent aspiration, check to ensure that the gag reflex has returned before offering fluids or food. *Teach the patient and family to monitor for severe postprocedure complications at home, including cholangitis (gallbladder inflammation), bleeding, perforation, sepsis, and pancreatitis. The patient has severe pain if any of these complications occur. Fever is present in sepsis. These problems do not occur immediately after the procedure; they may take several hours to 2 days to develop.*

Colicky abdominal pain can result from air instilled during the procedure. Instruct the patient to report abdominal pain, fever, nausea, or vomiting that fails to resolve after returning home. Be sure that the patient has someone to drive him or her home if the test was done on an ambulatory basis.

Small Bowel Capsule Endoscopy. Small bowel endoscopy, or enteroscopy, provides a view of the small intestine. Capsule video endoscopy (M2A) is a small bowel enteroscopy that visualizes the entire small bowel, including the distal ileum. It is used to evaluate and locate the source of GI bleeding. Before the development of the M2A Capsule Endoscope, viewing the small intestine was inadequate. The capsule battery lasts around 8 hours so it is not used to view the colon.

Prepare the patient by explaining the procedure, the purpose, and what to expect during the testing. The patient must fast (water only) for 8 to 10 hours before the test and be NPO for the first 2 hours of the testing.

At the time of the procedure, the patient's abdomen is marked for the location of the sensors, and the eight-lead sensors (Sensor Array) are applied. The patient wears an abdominal belt that houses a data recorder to capture the transmitted images. After the capsule is taken with a glass of water, the patient may return to normal activity for the remainder of the study. He or she can resume a normal diet 4 hours after swallowing the capsule. At the end of the procedure, the patient returns to the facility with the capsule equipment for downloading to a central computer. The procedure lasts about 8 hours.

Because the M2A Capsule Endoscope is a single-use device that moves through the GI tract by peristalsis and is excreted naturally, explain to the patient that the capsule will be seen in the stool. No other follow-up is necessary.

Colonoscopy. Colonoscopy is an endoscopic examination of the entire large bowel. The American Cancer Society recommends that, beginning at age 50 years, all men and women should have a colonoscopy every 10 years or choose another equally effective recommended screening option (ACS, 2010). Those at high risk for cancer (e.g., family history) or those who had polyps removed should have the test more often. The physician may also obtain tissue biopsy specimens or remove polyps through the colonoscope. A colonoscopy can also evaluate the cause of chronic diarrhea or locate the source of GI bleeding. A sclerotherapy drug may be injected at the site of any bleeding. An alternative to this invasive procedure is the *CT colonography (virtual colonoscopy)*, which is not invasive and uses a CT scanner to view the colon. Patient preparation for this alternative is the same as that for the traditional colonoscopy.

Patient Preparation. Teach the patient to stay on a clear liquid diet the day before the scheduled colonoscopy. Instruct him or her to avoid red, orange, or purple (grape) beverages, and drink an abundant amount of Gatorade or other sports drink to replace electrolytes that are lost during bowel preparation. The patient should be NPO (except water) 4 to 6 hours before the procedure.

Remind patients to avoid aspirin, anticoagulants, and antiplatelet drugs for several days before the procedure. Diabetic patients should check with their health care provider about drug therapy requirements on the day of the test because they are NPO.

The patient drinks an oral liquid preparation for cleaning the bowel (e.g., sodium phosphate [Phospho-Soda]) the evening before the examination and may repeat that procedure the morning of the study. Some physicians prescribe a gallon of GoLYTELY to cleanse the bowel the day before. This regimen should not be used for older adults to prevent excessive fluid and electrolyte loss. All solutions should be chilled to improve their taste. Remind the patient to drink them quickly to prevent nausea. Watery diarrhea usually begins in about an hour after starting the bowel preparation process. In some cases, the patient may require laxatives, suppositories (e.g., bisacodyl [Dulcolax]), or one or more small-volume cleansing enemas (e.g., Fleet's).

Procedure. IV access is necessary for the administration of moderate sedation. The physician prescribes drugs to aid in relaxation, usually IV midazolam hydrochloride (Versed), propofol (Diprivan), and/or an opiate, such as Fentanyl. Complementary and alternative therapies, such as reiki, are being studied to determine if they reduce the amount of sedation needed (see the Evidence-Based Practice box above).

EVIDENCE-BASED PRACTICE

Does Modified Reiki Decrease Pain and Anxiety in Patients Undergoing a Colonoscopy?

Hulse, R.S., Stuart-Shor, E.M., & Russo, J. (2010). Endoscopic procedure with a modified Reiki intervention: A pilot study. *Gastroenterology Nursing, 33*(1), 20-26.

This pilot study examined the use of Reiki before colonoscopy to reduce anxiety and intra-procedure medications compared with usual care. A prospective, nonblinded, partially randomized patient preference design was used for 21 first-time colonoscopy patients. There were no differences in the makeup of the control (n = 10) and experimental groups (n = 11): about half were woman, and the mean age was 58 years.

The Reiki intervention reduced the patients' blood pressure, pulse, and respirations, but the drug regimen used during the procedure was the same in both groups. The experimental group did not require additional medication during the procedure. The researchers concluded that adjunctive therapy may help reduce anxiety and pain in patients having a colonoscopy.

Level of Evidence: 5
This pilot study is very small and needs to be replicated using a more rigorous, randomized, controlled trial.

Commentary: Implications for Practice and Research
The use and study of complementary and alternative medicine (CAM) have increased in the past decade. A number of therapies have been shown to decrease pain and anxiety. Nurses need to consider using these modalities as part of holistic patient care. Many patients employ CAM and would prefer it be a part of their care. Assess the patient's use of adjunctive therapies, and ask the patient what he or she prefers.

Initially, the patient is placed on the left side with the knees drawn up while the endoscope is placed into the rectum and moved to the cecum. Air may be instilled for better visualization. The entire procedure lasts about 30 to 60 minutes. Atropine sulfate is kept available in case of bradycardia resulting from vasovagal response.

Follow-up Care. Check vital signs every 15 minutes until the patient is stable. Keep the siderails up until the patient is fully alert, and maintain NPO status. Observe for signs of perforation (causes severe pain) and hemorrhage, such as a rapid drop in blood pressure. Reassure the patient that a feeling of fullness, cramping, and passage of flatus are expected for several hours after the test. Fluids are permitted after the patient passes flatus to indicate that peristalsis has returned.

If a polypectomy or tissue biopsy was performed, there may be a *small* amount of blood in the first stool after the colonoscopy. *However, report excessive bleeding or severe pain to the health care provider immediately* (Chart 55-4).

As with other endoscopic procedures, the patient will need someone to provide transportation home. Remind the patient to avoid driving for 12 hours after the procedure because of the effects of sedation.

Virtual Colonoscopy. A noninvasive imaging procedure to obtain multi-dimensional views of the entire colon is the *CT colonography,* most popularly known as the virtual colonoscopy. The bowel preparation and dietary restrictions are

DECISION-MAKING CHALLENGE

Safety; Evidence-Based Practice

A 55-year-old woman has her first screening colonoscopy today, and you are assigned as her preprocedure and postprocedure nurse. When you take her vital signs before the procedure, her blood pressure is 156/88 mm Hg. She does not have a history of hypertension or diabetes mellitus. Upon further observation, you notice that the patient seems very anxious. She states that her sister had a colonoscopy last year and was diagnosed with stage 3 colorectal cancer for which she is being treated.

1. How will you respond to the patient at this time?
2. What other preprocedure care will you provide before she has her colonoscopy?
3. After the procedure, the patient seems very drowsy and asks for something to drink. How will you respond to her and why? What evidence supports this decision?
4. The patient tells you that she had two polyps removed but there is no sign of cancer. In view of her polyps and her family history of colorectal cancer, what health teaching about colorectal cancer screening will you provide?

similar to those for traditional colonoscopy. However, if a polyp is detected during a virtual colonoscopy or bleeding is found, the patient must have a follow-up invasive colonoscopy for treatment. Therefore the advantage of the traditional colonoscopy is that both diagnostic testing and minor surgical procedures can be done at the same time.

Sigmoidoscopy. Proctosigmoidoscopy, often referred to as a *sigmoidoscopy*, is an endoscopic examination of the rectum and sigmoid colon using a flexible scope. The purpose of this test is to screen for colon cancer, investigate the source of GI bleeding, or diagnose or monitor inflammatory bowel disease. If sigmoidoscopy is used as an alternative to colonoscopy for colorectal cancer screening, it is recommended that screening begin at 50 years of age and should be done every 5 years thereafter (American Cancer Society, 2010). Patients at high risk for cancer may require more frequent screening.

The patient should have a clear liquid diet for at least 24 hours before the test. A cleansing enema or sodium biphosphate (Fleet's) enema is usually required the morning of the procedure. A laxative may also be prescribed the evening before the test.

The patient is placed on the left side in the knee-chest position. No moderate sedation is required. The endoscope is lubricated and inserted into the anus to the required depth for viewing. Tissue biopsy may be performed during this procedure, but the patient cannot feel it. The examination usually lasts about 30 minutes.

Inform the patient that mild gas pain and flatulence may be experienced from air instilled into the rectum during the examination. If a biopsy was obtained, a small amount of bleeding may be observed. Instruct the patient that excessive bleeding should be reported immediately to the health care provider.

Gastric Analysis. Gastric analysis measures the hydrochloric acid and pepsin content for evaluation of aggressive gastric and duodenal disorders (e.g., Zollinger-Ellison syndrome). There are two tests in gastric analysis: basal gastric secretion and gastric acid stimulation. Basal gastric secretion measures the secretion of hydrochloric acid between meals. If only small amounts of secretion are collected, a follow-up gastric stimulation test is given.

The patient is NPO for at least 12 hours before the test. Teach patients to avoid alcohol, tobacco, and drugs that may affect gastric secretion for 24 hours before the study. A nasogastric (NG) tube is inserted, and gastric residual contents are aspirated and discarded.

The NG tube is attached to suctioning equipment for collecting the contents at 15-minute intervals for 1 hour. Samples are collected and labeled with basal acid output (BAO), time, and volume of each specimen.

For the gastric acid stimulation test, the NG tube is left in place and a drug that stimulates gastric acid secretion (e.g., pentagastrin or betazole dihydrochloride [Histalog]) is given. Fifteen minutes after injection of the drug, specimens are again collected at 15-minute intervals for 1 hour. Samples are collected and labeled with maximal acid output (MAO), time, and volume of each specimen. Depressed levels of gastric secretion suggest the presence of gastric cancer. Increased levels of gastric secretion indicate Zollinger-Ellison syndrome and duodenal ulcers (see Chapter 58).

After the test is completed, the NG tube is removed and the patient can resume normal eating patterns. No other follow-up is necessary.

Ultrasonography. Ultrasonography (US) is a technique in which high-frequency, inaudible vibratory sound waves are passed through the body via a transducer. The echoes of the sound waves created are then recorded and converted into images for analysis. US is commonly used to view soft tissues, such as the liver, the spleen, the pancreas, and the biliary system. The advantages of this test are that it is painless and noninvasive and requires no radiation.

The patient may be fasting, depending on the abdominal organs to be examined. Inform the patient that it will be necessary to lie still during the study. He or she is instructed to drink 1 to 2 L of fluid just before the test, because a full bladder is necessary for accurate visualization.

The patient is usually placed in a supine position. The technician applies insulating gel to the end of the transducer and on the area of the abdomen under study. This gel allows airtight contact of the transducer with the skin. The technician moves the transducer back and forth over the skin until the desired images are obtained. The study takes about 15 to 30 minutes. No follow-up care is necessary.

Endoscopic Ultrasonography. Endoscopic ultrasonography (EUS) provides images of the GI wall and high-resolution images of the digestive organs. The ultrasonography is performed through the endoscope. This procedure is useful in diagnosing the presence of lymph node tumors, mucosal tumors, and tumors of the pancreas, stomach, and rectum. The patient preparation and follow-up care are similar to the preparation and follow-up care for both endoscopy and ultrasonography.

Liver-Spleen Scan. A liver-spleen scan uses IV injection of a radioactive material that is taken up primarily by the liver and secondarily by the spleen. The scan evaluates the liver and the spleen for tumors or abscesses, organ size and location, and blood flow.

Teach the patient about the need to lie still during the scanning. Assure the patient that the injection has only small amounts of radioactivity and is not dangerous. Ask female patients of childbearing age if they may be pregnant or are currently breast-feeding. The radionuclide can be found in breast milk, and radiation from x-rays or scans should be avoided in pregnancy.

The technician or the physician gives the radioactive injection through an IV line, and a wait of about 15 minutes is necessary for uptake. The patient is placed in many different positions while the scanning takes place. Tell the patient that the radionuclide is eliminated from the body through the urine in 24 hours. Careful handwashing after toileting decreases the exposure to any radiation present in the urine.

NURSING CONCEPT REVIEW

What should you NOTICE in a patient with adequate digestion and elimination related to the GI system?

Physical Assessment
- No nausea or vomiting
- Sufficient appetite
- No intentional weight loss
- No dyspepsia (indigestion)
- No jaundice
- Abdomen soft and not tender
- Normoactive bowel sounds present is all quadrants
- No change in bowel habits

- No abdominal pain
- Normal brown, formed stool
- No frequent diarrhea or constipation

Diagnostic Assessment
- No occult blood in stool
- Normal liver enzymes, such as ALT
- Normal bilirubin levels
- Serum and urine amylase within normal limits
- Serum ammonia level within normal limit
- Serum albumin within normal limit
- Electrolytes within normal limits

GET READY FOR THE NCLEX® EXAMINATION!

KEY POINTS

Review these Key Points for each NCLEX Examination Client Needs Category.

Safe and Effective Care Environment
- Remember that the priority for care is to check for the return of the gag reflex after an upper endoscopic procedure before offering fluids or food; aspiration may occur if the gag reflex is not intact.

Health Promotion and Maintenance
- If an endoscopic procedure on an ambulatory basis is scheduled, remind the patient to have someone available to drive him or her home because of the effects of moderate sedation.
- Teach patients having invasive colon diagnostic procedures to follow instructions carefully for the bowel preparation before testing; the bowel must be clear to allow visualization of the colon.
- Instruct the patient to drink plenty of fluids and take a laxative as prescribed to eliminate barium if used during diagnostic testing.

Psychosocial Integrity
- Remember that problems of digestion, nutrition, and elimination can markedly affect lifestyle.

Physiological Integrity
- Perform a focused abdominal assessment using inspection, auscultation, and light palpation.
- Do not palpate or auscultate any abdominal pulsating mass because it could be a life-threatening aortic aneurysm.
- Assess and report any major complications of GI testing to the health care provider.
- Review and interpret laboratory results, and report abnormal findings to the health care provider (see Chart 55-3).
- Monitor vital signs carefully for the patient having any endoscopic procedure and moderate sedation.
- Assess patients who have endoscopies for bleeding, fever, and severe pain.
- For patients having a colonoscopy, check for passage of flatus before allowing fluids or food.

56

Care of Patients with Oral Cavity Problems

Cherie R. Rebar

LEARNING OUTCOMES

Safe and Effective Care Environment

1. Plan continuity of care between the hospital and community-based agencies for patients having oral surgery.
2. Identify appropriate community resources for patients with oral cavity health problems.

Health Promotion and Maintenance

3. Teach patients ways to prevent oral cancer and maintain good oral health.
4. Develop a teaching plan for patients who have stomatitis to promote digestion and nutrition.
5. Develop a teaching plan for community-based care of patients with oral cancer.

Psychosocial Integrity

6. Identify the patient's response to an oral cancer diagnosis.

7. Refer patients with oral cancer to appropriate support groups.

Physiological Integrity

8. Prioritize postoperative care for patients undergoing surgery for oral cancer to maintain a patent airway and prevent aspiration.
9. Describe collaborative interventions to promote nutrition for postoperative patients having extensive oral surgery.
10. Identify methods to help patients communicate effectively after oral surgery.
11. Plan care for patients who have disorders of the salivary glands.
12. State best practices for teaching or providing oral care for patients.

The oral cavity, or mouth, is where *digestion* of food begins. The teeth tear, grind, and crush food into small particles to promote swallowing. The enzymes in saliva begin the breakdown of carbohydrates. If a person cannot take food or fluid into the mouth, cannot chew food, or cannot swallow, the basic *human need for nutrition* may not be met by use of the GI tract. Adequate intake of fluids and nutrients into the body is vital to promote function of every body organ and system.

The pharynx (throat) is located just behind the mouth and has a role in both *digestion* and oxygenation. The pharynx is the portal between the mouth and the GI tract, where nutrients are broken down for utilization within the body. The pharynx also is a portal for oxygenation, as inhaled air passes through the nose, into the pharynx, and down into the trachea. A blockage of the posterior oral cavity, for example, by a tumor, can interfere with oxygenation and digestion.

Oral cavity disorders, then, can severely affect *nutrition* and oxygenation, as well as speech, body image, and self-esteem. Although there are many oral health problems, this chapter discusses the most common disorders. Nurses play an important role in maintaining and restoring oral health through nursing interventions, including patient and family

CHART 56-1 PATIENT AND FAMILY EDUCATION: PREPARING FOR SELF-MANAGEMENT

Maintaining a Healthy Oral Cavity

- Perform self-examination of your mouth every week; report any unusual finding or any noted change.
- Be sure to eat a well-balanced diet.
- Brush and floss your teeth every day. Set a routine, and keep to it. Keeping floss where you can see it (such as on the countertop by the sink) will encourage you to stick to your routine.
- Manage your stress as much as possible; learn how to maintain your emotional health by using healthy coping mechanisms.
- Avoid contact with agents that may cause inflammation of the mouth, such as mouthwashes that contain alcohol.
- If possible, avoid drugs that may cause inflammation of the mouth or reduce the flow of saliva.
- Be aware of any changes in the occlusion of your teeth, mouth pain, or swelling; seek medical attention promptly.
- See your dentist regularly; have problems attended to promptly.
- If you wear dentures, make sure they are in good repair and fit properly.

education. Chart 56-1 lists ways to help maintain a healthy oral cavity.

STOMATITIS

Pathophysiology

Stomatitis is a broad term that refers to inflammation within the oral cavity and may present in many different ways. Painful single or multiple ulcerations (called *aphthous ulcers* or "canker sores") that appear as inflammation and erosion of the protective lining of the mouth are one of the most common forms of stomatitis. The sores cause pain, and open areas place the person at risk for bleeding and infection. Mild erythema (redness) may respond to topical treatments. Extensive stomatitis may require treatment with opioid analgesics. Stomatitis is classified according to the cause of the inflammation. *Primary stomatitis,* the most common type, includes aphthous (noninfectious) stomatitis, herpes simplex stomatitis, and traumatic ulcers. *Secondary stomatitis* generally results from infection by opportunistic viruses, fungi, or bacteria in patients who are immunocompromised. It can also result from drugs, such as chemotherapy. (See Chapter 24 for discussion of chemotherapy-induced stomatitis.)

A common type of secondary stomatitis is caused by *Candida albicans. Candida* is sometimes present in small amounts in the mouth, especially in older adults. Long-term antibiotic therapy destroys other normal flora and allows the *Candida* to overgrow. The result can be candidiasis, also called *moniliasis,* a fungal infection that is very painful. Candidiasis is also common in those undergoing immunosuppressive therapy, such as chemotherapy, radiation, and steroids.

In addition, the mouth is susceptible to the effects of human immune deficiency virus (HIV) infection. Other systemic diseases that can cause stomatitis include chronic kidney disease and inflammatory bowel disease. Poor oral

EVIDENCE-BASED PRACTICE

What Are Best Practices When Providing Oral Hygiene to Critically Ill Older Adults Who Are Orally Intubated?

Feider, L., Mitchell, P., & Bridges, E. (2010). Oral care practices for orally intubated critically ill adults. *American Journal of Critical Care,* 19(2), 175-183.

Evidence shows that when proper oral care is provided as a nursing intervention for older adults, infections such as aspiration pneumonia and ventilator-associated pneumonia (VAP) decrease. In this study, a survey of 347 respondents was conducted to determine the type of oral care provided by critical care nurses for older adults who were orally intubated. These data were compared with the recommendations for oral care found in the *AACN Procedure Manual for Critical Care Nurses* and the Centers for Disease Prevention and Control (CDC) oral care guidelines.

Survey results demonstrated that there was a variety of facility policies for oral care and therefore various interpretations of how oral care should be given. Methods included a mix of brushing, swabbing, suctioning, and rinsing with chlorhexidine gluconate. Nurses were not aware that facility policies were often not consistent with national oral care standards based on current evidence.

Level of Evidence: 2

The study was a large descriptive, cross-sectional survey, with results compared against national recommendations for best practice.

Commentary: Implications for Practice and Research

The findings of this research clearly indicate that nurses recognize and practice facility-based policies but are not aware of published best practices, such as those from the CDC. Because proper oral care has been associated with a decrease in complications associated with VAP, nurses must become aware of these evidence-based standards of care and bridge the gap that exists between those standards and facility policy.

CONSIDERATIONS FOR OLDER ADULTS

Older adults are especially at high risk for candidiasis because aging causes a decrease in immune function. The risk increases for patients who are diabetic, malnourished, or under emotional stress. Those who wear dentures may use soft denture liners that provide comfort but can also be colonized by *C. albicans,* contributing to denture stomatitis. In addition, it is now known that older adults who have poor oral hygiene are at high risk for mouth infections and aspiration pneumonia. All health care professionals in any health care setting should be trained in and aware of best practices for oral care for geriatric populations; this could greatly improve patient outcomes, especially for older intubated adults in critical care settings. (See the Evidence-Based Practice box above.)

health is a risk factor for certain infections, such as ventilator-associated pneumonia.

Stomatitis can result from infection, allergy, vitamin deficiency, systemic disease, and irritants such as tobacco and alcohol. Infectious agents, such as bacteria and viruses, may have a role in the development of recurrent stomatitis.

Certain foods may trigger allergic responses that cause aphthous ulcers. Foods such as coffee, potatoes, cheese, nuts, citrus fruits, and gluten may be causative factors. In some cases, strict diets have resulted in the improvement of ulcers. Deficiencies in complex B vitamins, folate, zinc, and iron associated with malnutrition can contribute to the formation of recurrent stomatitis.

PATIENT-CENTERED COLLABORATIVE CARE

ASSESSMENT

When performing an oral assessment, ask about a history of recent infections, nutritional changes, oral hygiene habits, oral trauma, or stress. A drug history should also be collected, including over-the-counter (OTC) drugs and nutritional and herbal supplements. Document the course of the current outbreak, and determine if stomatitis has occurred frequently. Ask the patient if the lesions interfere with swallowing, eating, or communicating.

The symptoms of stomatitis range in severity from a dry, painful mouth to open ulcerations, predisposing the patient to infection. These ulcerations can alter *nutritional* status because of difficulty with eating or swallowing. When they are severe, stomatitis and edema have the potential to obstruct the airway.

In oral candidiasis, a type of yeast infection, white plaque-like lesions appear on the tongue, palate, pharynx (throat), and buccal mucosa (inside the cheeks) (Fig. 56-1). When these patches are wiped away, the underlying surface is red and sore. Patients may report pain, but others describe the lesions as dry or hot. The older adult patient who has systemic illness or is taking antibiotics or chemotherapy is particularly susceptible to oral candidiasis.

While examining the mouth, wear nonsterile gloves. Use adequate lighting, using a penlight and tongue blade. Assess the mouth for lesions, coating, and cracking. Document characteristics of the lesions including their location, size, shape, odor, color, and drainage.

If lesions are seen along the pharynx and the patient reports dysphagia (pain on swallowing), suspect that the lesions might extend down the esophagus. Additional swallowing studies may be prescribed by the health care provider to establish a firm diagnosis.

The physical assessment should also include palpating the cervical and submandibular lymph nodes for swelling.

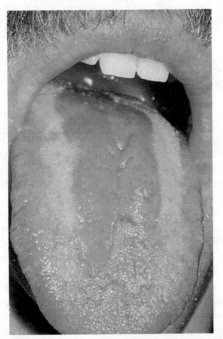

FIG. 56-1 Oral candidiasis.

Advanced practice nurses and other health care providers usually perform this part of the examination.

> ## ! NURSING SAFETY PRIORITY
> ### Action Alert
>
> When assessing the patient with stomatitis, be alert for signs and symptoms of dysphagia, such as coughing or choking when swallowing, a sensation of food "sticking" in the pharynx, or difficulty initiating the swallowing process. If dysphagia is suspected based on the patient's subjective description or the objective assessment, document all findings and report these to the health care provider. Dysphagia can cause numerous problems, including airway obstruction, aspiration pneumonia, and malnutrition.

INTERVENTIONS

Interventions for stomatitis are targeted toward health promotion through careful *oral hygiene* and food selection. When providing mouth care for the patient, the nurse may delegate oral care to unlicensed assistive personnel (UAP). Because the accountability for the delegated task is the nurse's, remind UAP to use a soft-bristled toothbrush or disposable foam swabs to stimulate gums and clean the oral cavity. Toothpaste should be free of sodium lauryl sulfate (SLS), if possible, because this ingredient has been associated with various types of stomatitis. Teach the patient to rinse the mouth every 2 to 3 hours with a sodium bicarbonate solution or warm saline solution (may be mixed with hydrogen peroxide). He or she should avoid most commercial mouthwashes because they have high alcohol content, causing a burning sensation in irritated or ulcerated areas. Health food stores sell more natural mouthwashes that are not alcohol-based. Teach the patient to check the labels for alcohol content. Frequent, gentle mouth care promotes débridement of ulcerated lesions and can prevent superinfections. Chart 56-2 lists measures for special oral care.

Drug therapy used for stomatitis includes antimicrobials, immune modulators, and symptomatic topical agents. Complementary and alternative therapies may also be tried.

Antimicrobials, including antibiotics, antivirals, and antifungals, may be necessary for control of infection. Tetracycline syrup (swish/swallow) 250 mg/10 mL four times daily for 10 days may be prescribed, especially for recurrent

> ## CHART 56-2   BEST PRACTICE FOR PATIENT SAFETY & QUALITY CARE
>
> ### Care of the Patient with Problems of the Oral Cavity
>
> - Remove dentures if the patient has severe stomatitis or oral pain.
> - Encourage the patient to perform oral hygiene or provide it after each meal and as often as needed.
> - Increase mouth care to every 2 hours or more frequently if stomatitis is not controlled.
> - Use a soft toothbrush or gauze for oral care.
> - Encourage frequent rinsing of the mouth with warm saline or sodium bicarbonate (baking soda) solution, or a combination of these solutions.
> - Teach the patient to avoid commercial mouthwashes, particularly those with high alcohol content, and lemon-glycerin swabs.
> - Assist the patient in selecting soft, bland, and nonacidic foods.
> - Apply topical analgesics or anesthetics as prescribed by the health care provider, and monitor their effectiveness.

aphthous ulcers (RAUs). The patient rinses for 2 minutes and swallows the syrup, thus obtaining both topical and systemic therapy. Minocycline swish/swallow and chlorhexidine mouthwashes may also be used.

A regimen of IV acyclovir (Zovirax) is prescribed for immunocompromised patients who contract herpes simplex stomatitis. Acyclovir is typically administered to those with normal kidney function at a dose of 5 mg/kg, infused at a constant rate over a 1-hour period every 8 hours for 7 days. Patients with healthy immune systems may be given acyclovir in oral or topical form.

For fungal infections like yeast, nystatin (Mycostatin) oral suspension 600,000 units four times daily for 7 to 10 days is the drug most often used. The patient swishes and swallows the topical preparation. Ice pop troches (lozenges) of the antifungal preparation allow the drug to slowly dissolve, and the cold provides an analgesic effect. Topical triamcinolone in benzocaine (Kenalog in Orabase) and oral dexamethasone elixir used as a swish/expectorate preparation are commonly used for stomatitis, especially RAU.

Immune modulating agents that may be prescribed include:

- Oral levamisole
- Topical amlexanox (Aphthasol)
- Topical granulocyte-macrophage colony-stimulating factor (GM-CSF)
- Thalidomide

The exact mechanism for how these drugs work is not clear. However, they may inhibit release of mediators that contribute to the inflammation seen in patients with RAU.

Other drugs can be used to control pain, such as OTC benzocaine anesthetics (e.g., Orabase, Anbesol) and camphor phenol (Campho-Phenique). Fifteen mL of 2% viscous lidocaine every 3 hours (maximum of 8 doses per day) can be used as a gargle or mouthwash. Teach patients to use this drug with extreme caution because its anesthetizing effect may cause burns from hot liquids in the mouth. Patients may also become more susceptible to choking when using viscous lidocaine.

Dietary changes may also help decrease pain. Cool or cold liquids can be very soothing. Teach patients to avoid hard, spicy, salty, and acidic foods or fluids that can further irritate the ulcers. Include foods high in protein and vitamin C to promote healing, including scrambled eggs, bananas, custards, puddings, and ice cream, unless the patient has lactose intolerance.

❓ NCLEX EXAMINATION CHALLENGE

Physiological Integrity

Nystatin (Mycostatin) suspension is prescribed for a client who is diagnosed with oral candidiasis. What instructions does the nurse provide to the client when using this drug?
A. "Take the drug when your mouth hurts or seems dry."
B. "Swish the drug around in your mouth before swallowing it."
C. "Spit the drug out after you rinse your mouth with it."
D. "Use the drug once a day for 7 to 10 days."

ORAL TUMORS

Oral cavity tumors can be benign, precancerous, or cancerous. Whether benign or malignant, tumors of the mouth affect many daily functions, including swallowing, chewing, and speaking. Pain accompanying the tumor can also limit daily activities and self-care. Oral tumors affect body image, especially if treatment involves removal of the tongue or part of the mandible (jaw) or requires a tracheostomy.

PREMALIGNANT LESIONS

Leukoplakia

Leukoplakia presents as slowly developing changes in the oral mucous membranes causing thickened, white, firmly attached patches that cannot easily be scraped off. These patches appear slightly raised and sharply rounded. Most of these lesions are benign. However, a small percentage of them become cancerous. Although leukoplakia can be found anywhere on the oral mucosa, lesions on the lips or tongue are more likely to progress to cancer.

Leukoplakia results from mechanical factors that cause long-term oral mucous membrane irritation, such as poorly fitting dentures, chronic cheek nibbling, or broken or poorly repaired teeth. In addition, oral hairy leukoplakia (OHL) can be found in patients with HIV infection. Tobacco products (smoked, dipped, or chewed) have also been implicated in the development of leukoplakia, sometimes referred to as "smoker's patch." Oral leukoplakia can be confused with oral candidal infection. However, unlike candidal infection, leukoplakia cannot be removed by scraping.

Leukoplakia is the most common oral lesion among adults. OHL is associated with Epstein-Barr virus (EBV) and can be an early manifestation of HIV infection. When associated with HIV infection, the appearance of OHL is highly correlated with progression from HIV infection to acquired immune deficiency syndrome (AIDS). Leukoplakia not associated with HIV infection is more often seen in people older than 40 years. Men have twice the incidence of leukoplakia that women have, but this ratio is changing because increasing numbers of women are smoking.

Erythroplakia

Erythroplakia presents as a red, velvety mucosal lesion on the surface of the oral mucosa. There are more malignant changes in erythroplakia than in leukoplakia; therefore erythroplakia is often considered "precancerous" in presentation. As such, these lesions should be regarded with suspicion and analyzed by biopsy. Erythroplakia is most commonly found on the floor of the mouth, tongue, palate, and mandibular mucosa. It can be difficult to distinguish from inflammatory or immune reactions.

ORAL CANCER

In the past decade, dentists and physicians have begun systematically screening their patients for oral cancer. Oral assessment has become a part of the routine dental examination. People should visit a dentist at least twice a year for professional dental hygiene and oral cancer screening, which includes inspecting and palpating the mouth for lesions.

Prevention strategies for oral cancer include minimizing sun and tanning bed exposure, tobacco cessation, and decreasing alcohol intake. Most dentists now use digital technology instead of x-rays when performing the annual or biannual dental examination. Excessive, prolonged radiation from x-rays has been associated with head and neck cancer (Oral Cancer Foundation, 2010). Teach patients to follow the guidelines in Chart 56-1 to maintain oral health.

Pathophysiology

Squamous Cell Carcinoma

More than 90% of oral cancers are squamous cell carcinomas that begin on the surface of the epithelium. Over a period of many years, premalignant (or dysplastic) changes begin. Cells begin to vary in size and shape. Alterations in the thickness of the lining of the epithelium develop, resulting in atrophy. These tumors usually grow slowly, and the lesions may be large before the onset of symptoms unless ulceration is present. *Mucosal erythroplasia is the earliest sign of oral carcinoma. Oral lesions that appear as red, raised, eroded areas are suspicious for cancer. A lesion that does not heal within 2 weeks or a lump or thickening in the cheek is a symptom that warrants further assessment* (Oral Cancer Foundation, 2010).

Squamous cell cancer can be found on the lips, tongue, buccal mucosa, and oropharynx. The major risk factors in its development are increasing age, tobacco use, and alcohol use. Most oral cancers occur in people older than 40 years. Tobacco use in any form (e.g., smoking or chewing tobacco) can increase the risk for cancer. A person who frequently consumes alcohol and uses tobacco in any form is at the highest risk. Genetic changes in patients with oral cancer have been found, especially the mutation of the *TP53* gene (McCance et al., 2010).

An increased rate of oral cancer is found in people with occupations such as textile workers, plumbers, and coal and metal workers. Additional factors, such as sun exposure, poor nutritional habits, poor oral hygiene, and infection with the human papilloma virus (HPV16) may also contribute to oral cancer (Oral Cancer Foundation, 2010). People with periodontal (gum) disease in which mandibular (jaw) bone loss has occurred are especially at risk for cancer of the mouth.

Mouth cancers account for about 3% of all cancers in men and 2% of all cancers in women in the United States. Over 37,000 new cases are diagnosed each year, with almost 8000 deaths (Oral Cancer Foundation, 2010). Most cancers occur in middle-aged and older people, although in recent years, younger adults have been affected, probably as a result of sun exposure.

Basal Cell Carcinoma

Basal cell carcinoma of the mouth occurs primarily on the lips. The lesion is asymptomatic and resembles a raised scab. With time, it evolves into a characteristic ulcer with a raised, pearly border. Basal cell carcinomas do not metastasize (spread) but can aggressively involve the skin of the face. The major risk factor for this type of cancer is excessive sunlight exposure.

Basal cell carcinoma occurs as a result of the failure of basal cells to mature into keratinocytes. It is the second most common type of oral cancer, but it is much less common than squamous cell carcinoma.

Kaposi's Sarcoma

Kaposi's sarcoma is a malignant lesion in blood vessels. It is usually painless and appears as a raised, purple nodule or plaque. In the mouth, the hard palate is the most common site of Kaposi's sarcoma, but it can be found also on the gums, tongue, or tonsils. It is most often associated with AIDS. (See Chapter 21 for a complete discussion of Kaposi's sarcoma.)

PATIENT-CENTERED COLLABORATIVE CARE

ASSESSMENT

Begin by assessing the patient's routine oral hygiene regimen and use of dentures or oral appliances, which might add to discomfort or mechanically irritate the mucosa. Ask about oral bleeding, which might indicate an ulcerative lesion or periodontal (gum) disease. Determine the patient's past and current appetite and nutritional state, including difficulty with chewing or swallowing. A continuing trend of weight loss may be related to metastasis, heavy alcohol intake, difficulty in eating or chewing, or an underlying health problem (Chart 56-3).

An examination of the oral cavity requires adequate lighting. Thoroughly inspect the oral cavity for any lesions, evidence of pain, or restriction of movement. Gently using a tongue blade and penlight, examine all areas of the mouth. Carefully note any change in speech caused by tongue movement. Notice any change in voice or swallowing, and assess for thick or absent saliva. After inspection, the advanced practice nurse, specialty nurse, or other health care provider uses bimanual palpation of any visible nodules to determine size and fixation. The cervical lymph nodes should also be palpated (Fig. 56-2).

The functioning and appearance of the mouth are strongly linked with body image and quality of life. Therefore it is

CHART 56-3	KEY FEATURES

Oral Cancer

- Bleeding from the mouth
- Poor appetite
- Difficulty chewing
- Difficulty swallowing
- Poor nutritional status and weight loss
- Thick or absent saliva
- Painless oral lesion that is red, raised, or eroded
- Thickening or lump in cheek

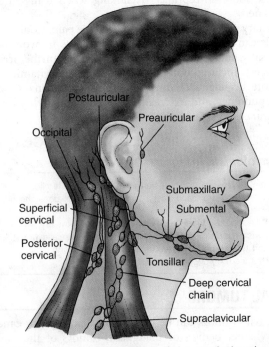

FIG. 56-2 The lymph nodes of the cervical region.

important to assess the impact of oral lesions on the patient's self-concept. In addition, assess for any educational or cultural needs that might affect health teaching or treatment. Evaluate the patient's support system and past coping mechanisms.

Oral CDx brushing of a lesion is helpful in determining whether it is precancerous. This procedure is usually performed by a dentist during a routine dental examination (Oral CDx, 2008). However, biopsy is the definitive method for diagnosis of oral cancer. The physician obtains a needle biopsy specimen of the abnormal tissue to assess for malignant or premalignant changes. Incisional biopsies may also be performed. An intraoral biopsy can be done under local anesthesia. In very small lesions, an excisional biopsy can permit complete tumor removal. Magnetic resonance imaging (MRI) is useful in detecting perineural involvement and in evaluating thickness in cancers of the tongue. Both computed tomography (CT) and MRI can be used to determine spread to the liver or lungs if further staging of the disease is warranted.

An aqueous solution of toluidine blue 1% can be applied to oral lesions to determine if they are malignant. This preparation stains malignant lesions, leaving normal tissue unaffected. However, a lesion that is the result of an inflammatory process may also absorb the stain, leading to a false-positive result. Although a biopsy is still needed to confirm a cancer diagnosis, toluidine blue may be useful for screening high-risk patients (National Institute of Dental and Craniofacial Research, 2008).

INTERVENTIONS

Both the presence of tumors of the oral cavity and the effects of their treatment threaten the integrity of the oral mucosa and the patient's airway. Oral cavity lesions can be treated by surgical excision, by nonsurgical treatments such as radiation or chemotherapy, or by a combination of treatments (referred to as *multimodal therapy*). Chemotherapy is currently not used independently in the treatment of oral cancers but is used in addition to other modes of treatment to sensitize malignant cells to radiation, to shrink a malignancy before surgery, or to decrease the potential for malignancy (Oral Cancer Foundation, 2010). Multimodal therapy is the most costly treatment option, yet more frequently used (Oral Cancer Foundation, 2010). *If the patient has extensive tumor involvement and copious, tenacious (thick and "stringy") secretions, maintaining an open airway is the nurse's priority for care.* Other nursing interventions focus on restoring and maintaining oral health

Nonsurgical Management

Implement interventions to *manage the patient's airway* by increasing air exchange, removing secretions, and preventing aspiration as needed. Assess for dyspnea resulting from the tumor obstruction or from excessive secretions. Assess the quality, rate, and depth of respirations. Auscultate the lungs for adventitious sounds, such as wheezes caused by aspiration. Listen for stridor caused by partial airway obstruction. Promote deep breathing to help produce an effective cough to mobilize the patient's secretions.

To increase air exchange, place the patient in a semi-Fowler's or high-Fowler's position. Encourage fluids to help liquefy secretions. Chest physiotherapy also increases air exchange as well as promotes effective coughing. If available,

collaborate with the respiratory therapist about performing this procedure. If needed, use oral suction equipment with a dental tip or a tonsil tip (Yankauer catheter) to remove secretions that obstruct the airway. Teach the patient and family to use the catheters as needed.

If edema occurs with oral cavity lesions, the patient may receive steroids to reduce inflammation. Antibiotics may be prescribed if infection is present because it can increase inflammation and edema. A cool mist supplied by a face tent may assist with oxygen transport and control of edema.

> ### ! NURSING SAFETY PRIORITY
> #### Action Alert
>
> Aspiration precautions prevent or reduce the risk factors for aspiration. Assess the patient's level of consciousness (LOC), gag reflex, and ability to swallow. To prevent aspiration, place the patient sitting upright at 90 degrees (high-Fowler's position). As a precaution, keep suction equipment nearby. For patients at high risk, assess the gag reflex before giving any fluids. Remind UAP to feed patients at risk for aspiration in small amounts. Teach visitors to speak with the nurse before offering any type of food or drink to the patient. Provide thickened liquids as an aid to prevent aspiration.

It is important to work with the patient to *establish an oral hygiene routine.* Perform oral hygiene every 2 hours for ulcerated lesions, infection, or in the immediate postoperative period. Modifications might be needed because of oral discomfort, bleeding, or edema. Oral care with a soft-bristled toothbrush is preferred. If the platelet count falls below 40,000/mm^3, switch the patient to an ultrasoft "chemobrush." The use of "toothettes" or a disposable foam brush is discouraged because these products may not adequately control bacteremia-promoting plaque and may further dry the oral mucosa. Lubricant can be applied to moisten the lips and oral mucosa as needed.

Teach patients and their families that the patient should avoid using commercial mouthwashes and lemon-glycerin swabs. Commercial mouthwashes contain alcohol, and lemon-glycerin swabs are acidic. These substances can cause a burning sensation and contribute to dry oral mucous membranes. Encourage frequent rinsing of the mouth with sodium bicarbonate solution or warm saline (see also Chart 56-2). Follow hospital or health care provider protocol if available.

Radiation therapy for oral cancers can be given by external beam or interstitial implantation to reduce the size of the tumor before surgery. *External-beam* radiation passes through the skin or mucous membrane to the tumor site. Typically, treatments are given as five daily treatments per week, with a 2-day break each week, over a 6- to 9-week period. Each treatment lasts only about 10 to 15 minutes, with more time being dedicated to undertaking special precautions to minimize the dose of radiation to the brain or spinal cord (Oral Cancer Foundation, 2010).

Another option is the implantation of radioactive substances (*interstitial radiation* therapy or brachytherapy) either to boost the dosage or to deliver a radiation dose close to the tumor bed. This form of implant therapy can be curative in early-stage lesions in the floor of the mouth or anterior tongue. It may also add a boost of radiation to a tumor that received external-beam radiation.

With the exception of radioactive seeds, which have a low level of emission, patients receiving interstitial radiation are usually hospitalized for the duration of treatment. *Place patients on radiation transmission precautions while the materials are active or in place.* A tracheostomy may be required with interstitial implants because of edema and increased oral secretions. (See Chapter 24 for general nursing care of patients undergoing radiation therapy.)

Teach the patient undergoing *chemotherapy* and family members about the side effects of these agents, which vary with each drug. Give antiemetics as prescribed, and provide other comfort measures as needed. (See Chapter 24 for general care of patients receiving chemotherapy.)

! NURSING SAFETY PRIORITY

Drug Alert

Patients who are undergoing radiation and/or chemotherapy treatment may experience a decreased ability to tolerate prescribed and over-the-counter medications. Teach patients about expected side effects, and remind them to not take any medication (including over-the-counter medications, herbs, or vitamin supplements) without first discussing them with their health care provider.

One of the most recent advances in the use of drugs for oral cancer is targeted therapy. Hormone-like substances known as *growth factors (GFs)* occur in the body's cells. Oral tumor cells, along with other types of cancers, grow quickly because they have more GF receptors than normal healthy tissue. One of these GFs is called *epidermal growth factor (EGF)*, which has been associated with oral cancers. Newer drugs that can target and block EGF receptors (EGF-R) are being tested, and more than a dozen have been approved, including cetuximab (Erbitux), erlotinib (Tarceva), and panitumumab (Vectibix). Chapter 24 describes targeted molecular therapy.

Surgical Management

The physician can often remove small, noninvasive lesions of the oral cavity in an ambulatory setting with local anesthesia. The surgical defect is usually small enough to be closed by sutures. These smaller lesions may also be responsive to carbon dioxide laser therapy or cryotherapy (extreme cold application), as well as photodynamic therapy. These procedures can be performed as an ambulatory care procedure in a surgical center but may require general anesthesia.

Small oral cancers are equally responsive to radiation or photodynamic therapy and to surgery. More invasive lesions (stages III and IV) require more extensive surgical excision and result in a greater loss of function and disfigurement. Not all lesions can be excised by the peroral approach (through the mouth). The goal of surgical resection is removal of the tumor with a surgical margin that is free of cancer cells.

Preoperative Care. Before excision of a lesion in the oral cavity, assess and document the patient's level of understanding of the disease process, the rationale for the surgery, and the planned intervention. Problems associated with cancer therapy can be reduced or optimally managed by collaborating with the patient and family regarding preparation and instruction. Reinforce information as needed. Include family members or other caregivers in the health teaching unless culturally inappropriate.

For small, local excisions, postoperative restrictions include a liquid diet for a day and then advancing as tolerated.

There are no activity limitations, and postoperative analgesics are prescribed.

Instructions for the patient undergoing large surgical resections may include but are not limited to these expectations after surgery:

- Placement of a temporary tracheostomy, oxygen therapy, and suctioning
- Temporary loss of speech because of the tracheostomy
- Frequent monitoring of postoperative vital signs
- NPO status until intraoral suture lines are healed
- Need to have IV lines in place for drug delivery and hydration
- Postoperative drug therapy and activity (out of bed on the first postoperative day)
- Possibility of surgical drains

Because communication is interrupted, assess the patient's ability to read, write, and draw pictures to communicate. In coordination with the patient, select the method of communication to use after surgery with staff and family members (e.g., Magic Slate, computer, picture board, or pad and pencil). Preprinted flashcards may be used to communicate the patient's needs, such as "I am tired," "I am in pain," or "I am hungry." Urge the patient to practice the chosen method before surgery to reduce frustration after surgery.

Operative Procedures. Three factors influence the extent of surgery performed for oral cancers: the size and location of the tumor, tumor invasion into the bone, and whether there has been metastasis (cancer spread) to neck lymph nodes. Small, noninvasive tumors can be removed perorally (through the mouth). Otherwise, an external approach may be used. The most extensive oral operations are composite resections, which combine partial or total glossectomy (tongue removal) and partial mandibulectomy (jaw removal). In the commando (co-mandible) procedure (**COM**bined neck dissection, **MAND**ibulectomy, and **O**ropharyngeal resection), the surgeon removes a segment of the mandible with the oral lesion and performs a radical neck dissection (see Chapter 31).

Metastasis to cervical lymph nodes usually indicates a poor prognosis for patients with cancer of the oral cavity. In those with cervical node metastasis, a neck dissection may also be performed. A radical neck dissection usually involves the removal of all cervical lymph nodes on the affected side, along with cranial nerve XI (the accessory nerve), the internal jugular vein, and the sternocleidomastoid (front neck) muscle. Modified and selective neck dissections may be performed in patients with minimal lymph node involvement.

Postoperative Care. The patient may have a temporary or permanent tracheostomy, requiring intensive nursing care to promote airway clearance. In addition, care must be taken to protect the surgical incision site from mechanical damage and infection (see Chapter 31). Nursing interventions to relieve pain or discomfort and promote nutrition are also important. Older adults are a special risk for surgery and need to be monitored very carefully (Chart 56-4).

Ensure that the predetermined method of communication is available for the patient, family members, and staff. When the patient has an adequate airway and can effectively clear secretions by coughing, the tracheostomy tube may be removed. When the tube is removed, an airtight dressing is placed over the site and the tracheostomy incision heals without the need for sutures.

The Postoperative Older Adult with Oral Cancer

- Assess the mouth and surrounding tissues for candidiasis, mucositis, and pain; assess for loss of appetite and taste.
- Monitor the patient's weight.
- Monitor nutritional and fluid intake.
- Assess for difficulty in eating or speech.
- Assess pain status and measures used to control pain.
- Monitor the patient's response to medications.
- Identify psychosocial problems, such as depression, anxiety, and fear.
- Assess the patient's overall physiological condition and how this may affect pharmacologic therapy.

! NURSING SAFETY PRIORITY

Action Alert

After extensive excision or resection for oral cancer, the most important nursing intervention is maintaining the patient's airway! Upon awakening from anesthesia, the patient may not recall, or realize, that a tracheostomy tube is in place and may initially panic because of the inability to speak. Remind the patient why he or she cannot speak, and provide reassurance that the vocal cords are intact (unless a total laryngectomy has been performed, in which case the loss of voice is permanent).

Patients who have undergone extensive resection may have slurred speech or difficulty in speaking as a result of nerve damage or tongue removal. Collaborate with the speech-language pathologist if speech is altered.

Protect the incision site to avoid infection. Provide gentle mouth care for cleaning away thick secretions and stimulating the flow of saliva. The delivery of oral care depends on the nature and extent of the surgical procedure. Give oral care at least every 4 hours in the early postoperative phase. The presence of unusual odors from the mouth can indicate infection; therefore continual assessment of the oral cavity is very important. In the early postoperative phase, take care to avoid disruption of the suture line during oral hygiene.

Elevate the head of the bed to assist in decreasing edema by gravity. If skin grafting was done, inspect the donor site (generally on the anterior thigh) every 8 hours for bleeding or signs of infection. (See Chapter 31 for specific nursing care of the patient with a radical neck dissection.)

To provide optimal *pain relief* in the postoperative period, rely on subjective and objective data to assess the need for analgesics and their effectiveness. The desired outcome of drug therapy during this period is relief of pain while allowing the patient to function at an optimal level. Those who have undergone surgery for oral cancer describe their pain as throbbing or pounding. IV morphine is usually the initial pain medication given. Tylox or Percocet (oxycodone plus acetaminophen) may be used for systemic relief of moderate pain after the IV morphine is discontinued.

Patients who have undergone extensive resections of the oral cavity remain on NPO status for several days. This time allows healing in the oral cavity before food comes in contact with the incision. Nasogastric feeding or total parenteral nutrition may be needed until oral nutrition can begin (see Chapter 63).

When oral fluid intake is started, assess for and document signs of difficulty swallowing, aspiration, or leakage of saliva or fluids from the suture line. Monitor daily weights and hydration. Nutritional supplementation may be used to improve the patient's quality of life. Patients who have weight loss or who are having difficulty maintaining hydration may be candidates for the placement of a gastrostomy tube. Coordinate nutritional care with the dietitian.

Encourage the patient to perform swallowing exercises. Collaborate with the speech-language pathologist to assist with swallowing techniques. Thickened fluids may be needed to prevent aspiration. A swallowing impairment may be temporary or permanent.

? DECISION-MAKING CHALLENGE

Teamwork and Collaboration; Patient-Centered Care

A 40-year-old homeless woman is admitted to the emergency department with difficulty breathing and swallowing. On assessment, the triage nurse finds that she has very poor dental hygiene and a large oral tumor. After a thorough evaluation, the patient is scheduled for oral surgery to remove as much of the tumor as possible.

1. As the patient's nurse, what is your priority for her care immediately after surgery?
2. As you develop her plan of care, for what complications is this patient most at risk?
3. With what members of the health care team will you collaborate?
4. In view of her homelessness, what support systems might you seek?
5. What follow-up care is realistic for this patient?

Community-Based Care

Continuing care for the patient with an oral tumor depends on the severity of the tumor, its collaborative care, and available support systems. Most patients are maintained at home during follow-up care. Ongoing nutritional management remains a vital part of the treatment plan. In addition, the patient and family may benefit from a community-based support group for cancer victims.

Home Care Management

If radiation therapy is part of the patient's treatment plan, home care considerations include health teaching and management strategies. Complications due to radiation to the head or neck can be acute or delayed. Acute effects include treatment-related mucositis, stomatitis, and alterations in taste. Long-term effects such as xerostomia (excessive mouth dryness) and dental decay require ongoing oral care, the use of saliva substitutes, and follow-up dental visits. Although ongoing dental care is important, the possible adverse effects that radiation has on bone make elective oral surgical procedures, such as tooth extraction, impossible in the area of the radiation. Fatigue is a common side effect of radiation and chemotherapy.

The patient whose tracheostomy tube has been removed is often placed on a soft diet by mouth before discharge. Occasionally, however, patients are discharged from the hospital while still requiring tracheostomy suction, oral suction, and nasogastric feedings. Suction equipment, nutritional supplies, and nursing care can be provided by home care companies. (See Chapter 63 for home care preparation for the patient receiving home parenteral nutrition and Chapter 31 for home care preparation for the patient with a tracheostomy.)

CHART 56-5 PATIENT AND FAMILY EDUCATION: PREPARING FOR SELF-MANAGEMENT

Care of the Patient with Oral Cancer at Home

- Follow the treatment plan for cancer therapies.
- Remember that taste sensation may be decreased; add seasonings to food to better enjoy it.
- Use a thickening agent for liquids if dysphagia is present.
- Eat soft foods if stomatitis occurs.
- Inspect the mouth every day for changes, such as redness.
- Continue meticulous oral hygiene at home using a chemobrush and frequent rinsing; clean after every use.
- Use saliva substitute as prescribed.
- Avoid sun or tanning bed exposure if radiation is part of therapy.
- Clean with a gentle, nondeodorant soap, such as Ivory.

Teaching for Self-Management

Teach the patient and family about drug therapy, nutritional therapies, any treatments (e.g., tracheostomy care, suture line care, dressing changes), and early symptoms of infection before hospital discharge (Chart 56-5). Alterations in taste and dysphagia make maintaining adequate nutrition a challenge for the oral cancer patient. Alterations in taste occur when the taste buds are included in the radiation treatment field. Taste sensation may begin to return several weeks after the completion of treatment. Some types of chemotherapy can also affect the patient's taste. Sometimes the loss of taste is permanent.

Changes in taste include dislike of meat, such as beef or pork, and metallic tastes in the mouth. Teach patients to add seasonings to foods, to use gravies or sauces to make foods more palatable, and to use high-protein foods such as cheeses, milk, eggs, puddings, and legumes in place of meat. Instruct patients with dysphagia in swallowing exercises. Recommend thickened liquids because thin liquids, such as water, are difficult to control during swallowing. Collaborate with the dietitian to teach the family how to assess the nutritional intake of the patient who is just beginning to eat. Liquid dietary supplements are usually recommended at this time. If bleeding or stomatitis is present, recommend soft foods to prevent further injury to the mucous membranes.

Teach the patient or family members to inspect the oral cavity daily for areas of redness, which can indicate the onset of stomatitis. Meticulous oral hygiene should be continued at home, especially with adjuvant chemotherapy or radiation. Reinforce the oral hygiene routine, emphasizing the need for frequent mouth rinsing to reduce the number of microorganisms and to maintain adequate hydration. The patient should use a chemobrush (an extra-soft type of toothbrush), rinse the chemobrush with hydrogen peroxide and water or with a diluted bleach solution after each use, and change chemobrushes weekly. The brush may also be cleaned in a dishwasher.

Saliva production is greatly reduced as a consequence of radiation. The resulting xerostomia (dry mouth) causes the inability to eat dry foods and may be permanent. Teach the patient regarding the use of saliva substitutes.

Skin reactions are also a common side effect of radiation. Instruct the patient to avoid sun exposure, to avoid perfumed lotions and powders, and to cleanse the face and neck area with a gentle nondeodorant soap. Teach male patients to use an electric razor for shaving and to avoid alcohol-based aftershave lotions to prevent further skin irritation.

NCLEX EXAMINATION CHALLENGE

Safe and Effective Care Environment

A client who has completed radiation therapy for an oral tumor is being discharged to home. What health teaching should the nurse provide? **Select all that apply.**

A. "Eat any foods that appeal to you."
B. "Rinse your mouth several times daily with Listerine."
C. "Use saliva substitutes as prescribed."
D. "Avoid exposure to the sun and tanning beds."
E. "Use a nondeodorant soap like Ivory."
F. "Use a firm-bristled toothbrush to remove plaque."

Health Care Resources

Patients who have undergone composite resection often require community services because they have both physical and psychosocial needs. Depression related to a change in body image is common. Excision of a portion of the jaw can leave a facial defect that may be difficult to hide. Assess for depression and other behavioral responses. A social worker or other health care professional may be needed for patient and family counseling. Those who have undergone a total glossectomy may be able to speak with special training and the use of an intraoral prosthesis created by a maxillofacial prosthodontist. The prosthesis is similar to dentures.

Collaborate with the case manager to provide assistance in obtaining special equipment or nutritional resources needed by the patient at home. The case manager assesses the patient's financial needs and makes referrals to government, community, and religious organizations as needed. Refer the patient to the American Cancer Society (ACS) (www.cancer.org) or the Oral Cancer Foundation (www.oralcancerfoundation.org) for local support groups and resources, including additional information. The ACS often provides dressing supplies and transportation to and from follow-up visits or medical treatments.

DISORDERS OF THE SALIVARY GLANDS

ACUTE SIALADENITIS

Pathophysiology

Acute sialadenitis, the inflammation of a salivary gland, can be caused by infectious agents, irradiation, or immunologic disorders. Salivary gland inflammation can have a bacterial or viral cause, such as infection with cytomegalovirus (CMV). The most common bacterial organisms are *Staphylococcus aureus, Staphylococcus pyogenes, Streptococcus pneumoniae,* and *Escherichia coli.* This disorder most commonly affects the parotid or submandibular gland in adults.

A decrease in the production of saliva (as in dehydrated or debilitated patients or in those who are on NPO status postoperatively for an extended time) can lead to acute sialadenitis. The bacteria or viruses enter the gland through the ductal opening in the mouth. Systemic drugs, such as phenothiazines and the tetracyclines, can also trigger an episode of acute sialadenitis. Untreated infections of the salivary glands can evolve into abscesses, which can rupture and spread infection into the tissues of the neck and the mediastinum.

Patients who receive radiation for the treatment of cancers of the head and neck or thyroid may develop decreased salivary flow, predisposing them to acute or persistent sialadenitis. The effect of radiation on the salivary glands is rapid and dose related. Immunologic disorders such as HIV infection can cause enlargement of the parotid gland that result from secondary infection. Sjögren's syndrome, an autoimmune disorder, is characterized by chronic salivary gland enlargement and inflammation (see Chapter 20).

PATIENT-CENTERED COLLABORATIVE CARE

During the initial interview, assess for any predisposing factors for sialadenitis, such as ionizing radiation to the head or neck area. Collect a thorough drug history, and ask about systemic illnesses, such as HIV infection.

Dehydration can be assessed by examining the oral membrane for dryness and the skin for turgor. Other assessment findings include pain and swelling of the face over the affected gland. Assess facial function because the branches of cranial nerve VII (the facial nerve) lie close to the salivary glands. Fever and general malaise also occur, and purulent drainage can often be massaged from the affected duct in the oral cavity.

Collaborative care includes the administration of IV fluids and measures such as these to treat the underlying cause and increase the flow of saliva:
- Hydration
- Application of warm compresses
- Massage of the gland
- Use of a saliva substitute
- Use of sialagogues (substances that stimulate the flow of saliva)

Sialagogues include lemon slices and citrus-flavored and other fruit-flavored candy. Massage is accomplished by milking the edematous gland with the fingertips toward the ductal opening. Elevation of the head of the bed promotes gravity drainage of the edematous gland.

Acute sialadenitis is best prevented by adherence to routine oral hygiene. This practice prevents infections from ascending to the salivary glands from the mouth.

POST-IRRADIATION SIALADENITIS

The salivary glands are sensitive to ionizing radiation, such as from radiation therapy or radioactive iodine treatment of thyroid cancers. Exposure of the glands to radiation produces a type of sialadenitis known as xerostomia (very dry mouth caused by a severe reduction in the flow of saliva) within 24 hours. Radiation to the salivary glands can also produce pain and edema, which generally abate after several days.

Xerostomia may be temporary or permanent, depending on the dose of radiation and the percentage of total salivary gland tissue irradiated. Little can be done to relieve the patient's dry mouth during the course of radiation therapy. Frequent sips of water and frequent mouth care, especially before meals, are the most effective interventions. After the course of radiation therapy has been completed, saliva substitutes may provide moisture for 2 to 4 hours at a time. Over-the-counter solutions are available, or methylcellulose (Cologel), glycerin, and saline may be mixed to form a solution.

SALIVARY GLAND TUMORS

Of all oral tumors, those of the salivary glands are relatively rare. Initially, malignant tumors present as slow-growing, painless masses. Involvement of the facial nerve results in facial weakness or paralysis (partial or total) on the affected side.

Collect information about any prior radiation exposure, because radiation to the head and neck areas is associated with the occurrence of salivary gland tumors. Salivary gland tumors present as localized, firm masses. Large tumors may cause facial nerve paralysis. Submandibular and minor salivary gland tumors may be tender or painful. Tumor invasion of the hypoglossal nerve causes impaired movement of the tongue, and a loss of sensation can follow. *Pay particular attention to assessment of the facial nerve because of its proximity to the salivary glands.* Assess the patient's ability to:
- Wrinkle the brow
- Raise the eyebrows
- Squeeze and hold the eyes shut, while the nurse gently pulls upwards on the eyebrows and cheeks beneath the orbit to check for symmetry
- Wrinkle the nose
- Pucker the lips
- Puff out the cheeks
- Grimace or smile

Be aware of any asymmetry when the patient performs these motions. The treatment of choice for both benign and malignant tumors of the salivary glands is surgical excision. However, radiation therapy is often used for salivary gland cancers that are large, have recurred, show evidence of residual disease after excision, or are highly malignant.

Patients who have undergone parotidectomy (surgical removal of the parotid glands) or submandibular gland surgery are at risk for weakness or loss of function of the facial nerve because the nerve courses directly through the gland. Facial nerve repair with grafting can be done at the time of surgery. A combination of surgery followed by radiation is common for advanced disease. Care for patients after parotidectomy is similar to that required for those having oral cancer surgery, described on p. 1197.

NURSING CONCEPT REVIEW

What might you NOTICE if the patient has inadequate digestion and oxygenation as a result of oral cavity problems?
- Dysphagia (difficulty swallowing)
- Dyspnea
- Stridor or wheezes
- Changes in speech or voice
- Copious, thickened oral secretions
- Excessive coughing during meals

What should you INTERPRET and how should you RESPOND to a patient experiencing inadequate digestion and oxygenation as a result of oral cavity problems?
Perform and interpret focused physical assessment findings, including:
- Breath sounds
- Oxygen saturation by pulse oximetry
- Ability to cough and clear the airway

NURSING CONCEPT REVIEW—cont'd

- Ability to manage excessive oral secretions
- Ability to chew food and swallow

Respond:
- Place the patient with the head elevated to at least 30 degrees.
- Apply oxygen as needed.
- Suction the oral cavity as needed.
- Encourage deep breathing and coughing every 2 hours.
- Increase fluids to liquefy secretions, depending on swallowing ability.
- Notify the respiratory therapist or Rapid Response Team if interventions are not successful in restoring oxygenation.

On what should you REFLECT?
- Observe patient for evidence of increased oxygenation, including increased ease of breathing.
- Observe patient for evidence of increased ability to swallow.
- Observe patient for evidence of increased ability to manage oral secretions.
- Consider follow-up interventions to manage patient, including coordinating care with dietitian and speech-language pathologist.
- Think about what else you might do to promote digestion and nutrition.

GET READY FOR THE NCLEX® EXAMINATION!

KEY POINTS

Review these Key Points for each NCLEX Examination Client Needs Category.

Safe and Effective Care Environment
- Be aware that airway management is the priority for care for patients having surgery for oral cancer.
- Place patients having oral cancer surgery in a high-Fowler's position to facilitate breathing and prevent aspiration.
- Be sure to assess for swallowing ability to prevent aspiration by checking the gag reflex before offering liquids or food to the patient who has had oral cancer surgery.
- Plan continuity of care to meet patients' needs when they are transferred from the hospital to community-based agencies.

Health Promotion and Maintenance
- Teach patients to seek medical or dental attention for oral lesions that do not heal; these lesions could be oral carcinomas.
- Remind patients to visit their dentist regularly for dental hygiene and oral examination.
- Follow the best practice recommendations for maintaining oral health as listed in Chart 56-1.
- Instruct patients to avoid harsh commercial mouthwashes if they have oral lesions.
- Teach patients to avoid tobacco, alcohol, and sun exposure to decrease their chance of having oral cancer.
- Instruct patients with acute sialadenitis to use sialagogues to stimulate saliva, such as citrus foods or candies.

Psychosocial Integrity
- Assist the patient and family in identifying and using coping mechanisms to deal with possible changes in body image and altered self-esteem.

- Recognize that patients with stomatitis are often unable to eat or swallow without discomfort.
- Refer patients with oral cancer to support groups, such as those available through the American Cancer Society.

Physiological Integrity
- Remember that stomatitis usually manifests as painful single or multiple ulcerations within the mouth.
- Recognize that stomatitis can be caused by a variety of organisms; *Candida* infections are very common in patients who receive antibiotic therapy and in those who are immunocompromised.
- Provide gentle oral care for patients with oral lesions, including chemobrushes and warm saline or sodium bicarbonate solution.
- Be aware that patients with stomatitis receive antimicrobials, anti-inflammatory agents, immune modulators, and topical agents for relief of symptoms, including pain.
- Differentiate leukoplakia and erythroplakia: leukoplakia presents as thin, white patches, and erythroplakia presents as red, velvety lesions.
- Be aware that patients with oral cancer may have chemotherapy, radiation, surgery, or a combination of these treatment methods.
- Be aware that sialadenitis can occur as result of radiation therapy.
- For patients with salivary gland tumors, assess for facial nerve involvement.
- Remember that a parotidectomy involves the removal of the salivary glands; postoperative care is similar to that for patients who have oral cancer surgery.

Care of Patients with Esophageal Problems

Donna D. Ignatavicius

℮volve WEBSITE

http://evolve.elsevier.com/Iggy/

Answer Key for NCLEX Examination Challenges and
   Decision-Making Challenges
Audio Glossary

Concept Map Creator
Key Points
Review Questions for the NCLEX® Examination

LEARNING OUTCOMES

Safe and Effective Care Environment

1. Explain the importance of collaborating with the health care team when providing care to patients with esophageal health problems that impair swallowing or limit nutrition.

Health Promotion and Maintenance

2. Teach the patient and family about lifestyle changes to decrease gastroesophageal reflux disease (GERD) and the discomfort of hiatal hernias.
3. Describe special considerations for the older adult with GERD.

Psychosocial Integrity

4. Identify the need for psychosocial support to patients and their families through diagnosis and treatment of esophageal cancer.

Physiological Integrity

5. Evaluate the impact of esophageal cancer on the patient's nutritional status, including the risk for aspiration.
6. Perform focused assessments for patients with esophageal health problems.
7. Apply knowledge of pathophysiology to anticipate complications of GERD.
8. Plan how to teach patients with GERD about drug therapy.
9. Develop a teaching plan for the patient and family about postoperative care after esophageal surgery.
10. Apply knowledge of pathophysiology to recognize complications of esophageal surgical procedures.
11. Plan community-based care for patients diagnosed with esophageal cancer.

The esophagus moves partially digested food from the mouth to the stomach. If food cannot reach the stomach, the patient cannot meet the *human need for nutrition*. Nutrients in food are necessary for normal body cell function. Common problems of the esophagus that can interfere with *digestion* and *nutrition* are caused by inflammation, structural defects or obstruction, and cancer. Patient-centered collaborative care requires dietary and lifestyle changes, as well as medical and surgical therapies.

GASTROESOPHAGEAL REFLUX DISEASE

Pathophysiology

Gastroesophageal reflux disease (GERD) is the most common upper GI disorder in the United States. It occurs most often in middle-aged and older adults but can affect people of any age. GERD occurs as a result of reflux (backward flow) of GI contents into the esophagus. The incidence of GERD is increasing throughout the world (Chait, 2010).

Reflux produces symptoms by exposing the esophageal mucosa to the irritating effects of gastric or duodenal contents, resulting in inflammation. A person with acute symptoms of inflammation is often described as having reflux esophagitis, which may be mild or severe (McCance et al., 2010).

The reflux of gastric contents into the esophagus is normally prevented by the presence of two high-pressure areas that remain contracted at rest. A 1.2-inch (3-cm) segment at the proximal end of the esophagus is called the *upper esophageal sphincter (UES)*. Another small portion at the gastroesophageal junction (near the cardiac sphincter) is called the lower esophageal sphincter (LES). The function of the LES is supported by its anatomic placement in the abdomen, where the surrounding pressure is significantly higher than in the low-pressure thorax. Sphincter function is also supported by the acute angle (angle of His) that is formed as the esophagus enters the stomach.

The most common cause of GERD is excessive relaxation of the LES, which allows the reflux of gastric contents into the esophagus and exposure of the esophageal mucosa to acidic gastric contents. Nighttime reflux tends to cause prolonged exposure of the esophagus to acid because the supine position decreases peristalsis and the benefit of gravity. Although controversial, *Helicobacter pylori* may contribute to reflux as well (McCance et al., 2010).

A person having reflux may be asymptomatic and not aware that reflux is occurring. However, the esophagus has only limited resistance to the damaging effects of the acidic GI contents. The pH of acid secreted by the stomach ranges from 1.5 to 2.0, whereas the pH of the distal esophagus is normally neutral (6.0 to 7.0).

Refluxed material is returned to the stomach by a combination of gravity, saliva, and peristalsis. The inflamed esophagus cannot eliminate the refluxed material as quickly as a healthy one, and therefore the length of exposure increases with each reflux episode. Hyperemia (increased blood flow) and erosion (ulceration) occur in the esophagus in response to the chronic inflammation. Gastric acid and pepsin injure tissue. Minor capillary bleeding often occurs with the erosion, but hemorrhage is rare.

During the process of healing, the body may substitute Barrett's epithelium (columnar epithelium) for the normal squamous cell epithelium of the lower esophagus. Although this new tissue is more resistant to acid and therefore supports esophageal healing, it is considered premalignant. It is associated with an increased risk for cancer in patients with prolonged GERD. The fibrosis and scarring that accompany the healing process can produce esophageal stricture (narrowing of the esophageal opening). The stricture leads to progressive difficulty in swallowing. Uncontrolled esophageal reflux also creates a risk for other serious complications, such as hemorrhage and aspiration pneumonia. GERD may be one of the causes of adult-onset asthma, laryngitis, and dental decay. It has also been associated with cardiac disease.

Gastric distention caused by eating very large meals or delayed gastric emptying predisposes the patient to reflux. A number of individual factors, including certain foods and drugs, influence the function of the LES (Table 57-1). Smoking and alcohol also weaken the tone of the LES.

Patients who have a nasogastric tube also have decreased esophageal sphincter function. The tube keeps the cardiac

TABLE 57-1	FACTORS CONTRIBUTING TO DECREASED LOWER ESOPHAGEAL SPHINCTER PRESSURE
• Fatty foods • Caffeinated beverages, such as coffee, tea, and cola • Chocolate • Citrus fruits • Tomatoes and tomato products • Smoking and use of other tobacco products	• Calcium channel blockers • Nitrates • Peppermint, spearmint • Alcohol • Anticholinergic drugs • High levels of estrogen and progesterone • Nasogastric tube placement

CHART 57-1	KEY FEATURES
Gastroesophageal Reflux Disease	
• Dyspepsia (heartburn) • Regurgitation (may lead to aspiration or bronchitis) • Coughing, hoarseness, or wheezing at night • Water brash (hypersalivation) • Dysphagia • Odynophagia (painful swallowing)	• Epigastric pain • Belching • Flatulence • Nausea • Pyrosis (retrosternal burning) • Globus (feeling of something in back of throat) • Pharyngitis • Dental caries (severe cases)

sphincter open and allows acidic contents from the stomach to enter the esophagus. Other factors that increase intra-abdominal and intragastric pressure (e.g., pregnancy, wearing tight belts or girdles, bending over, ascites) overcome the gastroesophageal pressure gradient maintained by the LES and allow reflux to occur. Many patients with obstructive sleep apnea report frequent episodes of GERD. People with hiatal hernias often have reflux because the upper portion of the stomach protrudes through the diaphragm into the thorax to allow acid to reach the esophagus (see later discussion of hiatal hernia).

Overweight and obese patients are at an increased risk for the disease. Increased weight increases intra-abdominal pressure, which contributes to reflux of stomach contents into the esophagus.

PATIENT-CENTERED COLLABORATIVE CARE

ASSESSMENT

Ask the patient about a history of heartburn or atypical chest pain associated with the reflux of GI contents. Ask whether he or she has been newly diagnosed with asthma or has experienced morning hoarseness or pneumonia. These symptoms are suggestive of severe reflux reaching the pharynx or mouth or pulmonary aspiration.

Physical Assessment/Clinical Manifestations

The clinical manifestations of reflux vary in severity, depending on the patient (Chart 57-1). Dyspepsia, *also known as "heartburn," and regurgitation are the main symptoms of GERD.* The pain is described as a substernal burning sensation that tends to move up and down the chest in a wavelike fashion. Because heartburn might not be viewed as a serious concern, patients may delay seeking treatment. If the heartburn is severe, the pain may radiate to the neck or jaw or may be referred to the back. The pain typically worsens when the patient bends over, strains, or lies down. Patients may come to the emergency department (ED) fearing that they are having a myocardial infarction ("heart attack").

With severe GERD, the pain occurs after each meal and lasts for 20 minutes to 2 hours. Patients usually obtain prompt relief by drinking fluids, taking antacids, or maintaining an upright posture.

Regurgitation (backward flow into the throat) of food particles or fluids is common. The patient feels warm fluid traveling up the throat without nausea. If the fluid reaches the level of the pharynx, he or she notes a sour or bitter taste in the mouth. This problem can even occur in an upright position. The danger of aspiration is increased if regurgitation occurs when the patient is lying down.

Eructation (belching), flatulence (gas), and bloating after eating are other common manifestations. Nausea and vomiting rarely occur, and unplanned weight loss is not common.

Assess for crackles in the lung, which can be an indication of associated aspiration. Assess the patient for coughing, hoarseness, or wheezing at night. Bronchitis may occur in those who have long-term regurgitation.

A reflex salivary hypersecretion known as water brash occurs in response to reflux. Water brash is different from regurgitation. The patient reports a sensation of fluid in the throat, but unlike with regurgitation, there is no bitter or sour taste.

Chronic GERD can cause dysphagia (difficulty swallowing). Dysphagia usually indicates a narrowing of the esophagus because of stricture or inflammation. Assess the patient for:
- The degree of dysphagia
- Whether dysphagia occurs when ingesting solids, liquids, or both
- Whether dysphagia is intermittent or occurs with each swallowing effort

Odynophagia (painful swallowing) can also occur with chronic GERD, but it is rare in people with uncomplicated reflux disease. Severe and long-lasting chest pain may be present if spasms occurring in the esophagus cause the muscle to contract with excess force. The resulting pain can be agonizing and may last for hours.

Other manifestations include chronic cough that occurs mostly at night or when the patient is lying down, asthma, and atypical chest pain. Cough and symptoms of asthma occur when refluxed acid is spilled over into the tracheobronchial tree. *Atypical chest pain* is thought to be caused by stimulation of pain receptors in the esophageal wall and by esophageal spasm. This type of chest pain can mimic angina and needs to be carefully distinguished from cardiac pain.

CONSIDERATIONS FOR OLDER ADULTS

In the older adult, the incidence of heartburn decreases in those with gastroesophageal reflux (GERD). Instead, the more severe complications of the disease are more frequent in this population, including atypical chest pain; ear, nose, and throat infections; and pulmonary problems, such as aspiration pneumonia, sleep apnea, and asthma. Barrett's esophagus and esophageal erosions are also more common in older adults. The cause for these differences is not known (Chait, 2010).

Diagnostic Assessment

The most accurate method of diagnosing GERD is *24-hour ambulatory esophageal pH monitoring*. This test involves placing a small catheter through the nose into the distal esophagus. The patient is asked to keep a diary of activities and symptoms, and the pH is continuously monitored and recorded. Ambulatory pH monitoring is especially useful in diagnosing patients with atypical symptoms. A wireless monitoring device may be used to promote patient comfort.

Esophagogastroduodenoscopy (EGD) is useful in diagnosing or evaluating reflux esophagitis or in monitoring complications such as Barrett's esophagus. This test requires the use of moderate sedation during the procedure, and patients must have someone accompany them home after recovery. During the procedure, tissue samples can be obtained for biopsy and strictures can be dilated (see Chapter 55).

Although not as common, *esophageal manometry*, or motility testing, may be performed when the diagnosis is uncertain. Water-filled catheters are inserted in the patient's nose or mouth and slowly withdrawn while measurements of LES pressure and peristalsis are recorded. When used alone, manometry is not sensitive or specific enough to establish a diagnosis of GERD.

❚ INTERVENTIONS

Nonsurgical Management

The purpose of treatment for GERD is to relieve symptoms, treat esophagitis, and prevent complications such as strictures or Barrett's esophagus. For most patients, GERD can be controlled by nutrition therapy, lifestyle changes, and drug therapy. *The most important role of the nurse is patient and family education. Teach the patient that GERD is a chronic disorder that requires ongoing management. The disease should be treated more aggressively in older adults (Chait, 2010).*

Nonpharmacologic Interventions. Nutrition therapy is used to relieve symptoms in patients with relatively mild GERD. Ask about the patient's basic meal patterns and food preferences. Coordinate with the dietitian, patient, and family about how to adapt to changes in eating that may decrease reflux symptoms.

Teach the patient to limit or eliminate foods that decrease LES pressure, such as chocolate, alcohol, fatty foods (especially fried), caffeine, and carbonated beverages. The patient should also restrict spicy and acidic foods (e.g., orange juice, tomatoes) until esophageal healing can occur, because these foods irritate the inflamed tissue and cause heartburn. Peppermint may also aggravate symptoms.

Large meals increase the volume of and pressure in the stomach and delay gastric emptying. Therefore remind the patient to eat four to six small meals each day rather than three large ones. Encourage patients to eat no food for at least 3 hours before going to bed. Reflux episodes are most damaging at night. Patients may have the most difficulty restricting evening snacks. Advise the patient to eat slowly and chew thoroughly to facilitate digestion and prevent eructation (belching).

The control of GERD involves *lifestyle changes* to promote health and control reflux (Chart 57-2). Teach the patient to elevate the head by 6 to 12 inches for sleep to prevent nighttime reflux. This can be done by placing blocks under the head of the bed or by using a large, wedge-style pillow instead of a standard pillow.

Teach the patient to sleep in the right side-lying position to decrease the effects of nighttime episodes of reflux. Nighttime reflux is extremely common, and infrequent swallowing in combination with a supine position impairs esophageal clearance. Smoking and alcohol cause decreased LES pressure. Explore the possibility and methods for smoking cessation, and make appropriate referrals. Ask the patient about his or her use of alcoholic beverages. If appropriate, assist the patient in finding alcohol-cessation programs.

Assist the patient in examining approaches to weight reduction. Decreasing intra-abdominal pressure often reduces reflux symptoms. Teach the patient to avoid wearing constrictive clothing, lifting heavy objects or straining, and working in a bent-over or stooped position. Emphasize that these general adaptations are an essential and effective part of disease management and can produce prompt results in uncomplicated cases.

Obese patients often have obstructive sleep apnea, as well as GERD. Those who receive continuous positive airway pressure (CPAP) treatment report improved sleeping and decreased episodes of reflux at night. See Chapter 31 for a discussion of CPAP.

Some drugs lower LES pressure and *cause* reflux, such as oral contraceptives, anticholinergic agents, sedatives, NSAIDs (e.g., ibuprofen), nitrates, and calcium channel blockers. The possibility of eliminating those drugs causing reflux should be explored with the health care provider.

Drug Therapy. Drug therapy for GERD management includes three major types—antacids, histamine blockers, and proton pump inhibitors. These drugs have one or more of these functions (Chart 57-3):

- Inhibit gastric acid secretion
- Accelerate gastric emptying
- Protect the gastric mucosa

In uncomplicated cases of GERD, *antacids* may be effective for *occasional* episodes of heartburn. Antacids act by elevating the pH level of the gastric contents, thereby deactivating pepsin. They are not helpful in controlling frequent symptoms because their length of action is too short and their nighttime effectiveness is minimal. These drugs also *increase* LES pressure and therefore are not given for long-term use.

Antacids containing aluminum hydroxide or magnesium hydroxide may be used. Maalox and Mylanta consist of a combination of these two agents. Patients often tolerate them better because they produce fewer side effects, such as constipation and diarrhea. Teach the patient to take the antacid 1 hour before and 2 to 3 hours after each meal. Some antacids are prepared as double-strength (DS) suspensions or tablets. The advantage of DS preparations is that a smaller amount of the drug is required. For example, 30 mL of regular Mylanta equals 15 mL of Mylanta-II (DS preparation).

Gaviscon, a combination of alginic acid and sodium bicarbonate, is often a very effective drug for GERD. It forms a thick foam that floats on top of the gastric contents and theoretically decreases the incidence of reflux. If reflux occurs, the foam enters the esophagus first and buffers the acid in the refluxed material. Remind the patient to take this drug when food is in the stomach.

Histamine receptor antagonists, commonly called *histamine blockers,* such as famotidine (Pepcid), ranitidine (Zantac), and nizatidine (Axid), decrease acid. With low-dose forms of these drugs available over the counter (OTC) and widely advertised for heartburn, many patients self-medicate before seeking professional assistance from their health care provider. When patients who have self-medicated with OTC preparations have uncontrolled symptoms, the health care provider usually prescribes a *higher* dose.

Ranitidine and the other preparations are long acting, allowing less-frequent dosing. They also appear to produce fewer side effects and may be safe for long-term use. Although these drugs do not affect the occurrence of reflux directly, they do reduce gastric acid secretion, improve symptoms, and promote healing of inflamed esophageal tissue.

Proton pump inhibitors (PPIs), such as omeprazole (Prilosec), rabeprazole (Aciphex), pantoprazole (Protonix), and esomeprazole (Nexium), are the *main* treatment for more severe GERD. Some PPIs are available as OTC drugs. These agents provide effective, long-acting inhibition of gastric acid secretion by affecting the proton pump of the gastric parietal cell. PPIs reduce gastric acid secretion and can be given in a single daily dose. If once-a-day dosing fails to control symptoms, twice-daily dosing may be used. A newer PPI, omeprazole/sodium bicarbonate (Zegerid), is the first immediate-release PPI and is designed for short-term use. Another newer PPI, dexlansoprazole (Kapidex), is a dual-release (delayed-release) drug that is available in several dosages but tends to be associated with more side and adverse effects than some of the other PPIs.

Some PPIs, such as Nexium and Protonix, may be administered in IV form for short-term use to treat or to prevent stress ulcers that can result from surgery. PPIs promote rapid tissue healing, but recurrence is common when the drug is stopped. Long-term use may mask reflux symptoms, and stopping the drug determines if reflux has been resolved. Long-term use may also cause community-acquired pneumonia and GI infections.

Research has also found that long-term use of proton pump inhibitors may increase the risk for hip fracture, especially in older adults. PPIs can interfere with calcium

CHART 57-3 COMMON EXAMPLES OF DRUG THERAPY

Gastroesophageal Reflux Disease (GERD)

DRUG/USUAL DOSAGE	PURPOSE FOR DRUG	NURSING INTERVENTIONS	RATIONALES
Antacids			
Aluminum or magnesium salts (Mylanta, Maalox) 30 mL orally between meals and as needed (PRN) throughout the day and at bedtime (Also see Chart 58-3 in Chapter 58)	Increases pH of gastric contents by deactivating pepsin	Give 1 hr before meals, 2-3 hr after meals, and at bedtime. Observe the patient for constipation or diarrhea. Suggest the use of combination mixtures or alternating use of aluminum and magnesium products.	These drugs work best if the stomach is empty. If given after meals, hydrogen ion load is high in food. Aluminum products produce constipation, and magnesium products induce diarrhea. Balancing their effects is important for patient adherence.
Alginic acid and sodium bicarbonate (Gaviscon), 1 tablet or 10-20 mL orally throughout the day and at bedtime	Buffers acid in stomach	Give after meals and at bedtime.	Alginic acid forms a viscous foam that floats on top of the gastric contents, impeding reflux or buffering its effects when it occurs.
Histamine Receptor Antagonists			
Ranitidine (Zantac) 150 mg orally twice daily Famotidine (Pepcid) 40 mg orally daily or 20 mg orally twice daily	Decreases gastric acid secretions by blocking histamine receptors in parietal cells	Administer with meals and at bedtime.	Ranitidine and famotidine are more potent, longer-acting drugs but produce fewer side effects.
Nizatidine (Axid) 150 mg orally twice daily		Use cautiously and in reduced dosages in patients with renal disease. Observe for dysrhythmias. Do not mix with tomato-based, mixed-vegetable juices; apple juice is the preferred choice.	Patients need an adequate creatinine clearance to prevent drug toxicity. Dysrhythmias are common adverse effects of the drug. Nizatidine may be less potent when mixed with tomato-based, mixed-vegetable juices.
Prokinetic Drugs			
Metoclopramide (Reglan) 10 mg orally three or four times daily	Increases gastric emptying	Instruct the patient to take the drug before meals. Teach the patient to report any neurologic or psychotropic side effects, such as restlessness, anxiety, ataxia, or hallucinations.	This drug increases the rate of gastric emptying. Long-term drug use produces adverse effects in up to one third of patients. *Therefore this drug is not commonly used.*
Proton Pump Inhibitors			
Omeprazole (Prilosec, Losec ✦) 20-30 mg orally daily	Decreases gastric acid production (long-acting)	Instruct the patient to take the drug before meals. Observe the patient for typical side effects: abdominal cramping, diarrhea, headache.	Gastric acid suppression is greater than 90%. Action is prolonged, but GI effects are severe in some patients.
Lansoprazole (Prevacid) 15 mg orally daily for gastroesophageal reflux disease (GERD); up to 60 mg orally for GI ulcers or Zollinger-Ellison syndrome		Instruct the patient to take the drug before meals. For the patient who has difficulty swallowing or has a nasogastric tube, open the capsule and mix granules in apple juice (or applesauce if not tube-fed).	Same as for omeprazole. The drug is safe to administer by opening (not crushing) the capsule.
Rabeprazole (Aciphex) 60 mg orally daily (may increase to 120 mg in two divided doses)		Do not crush, break, or chew delayed-release tablets. Teach patient to wear sunscreen.	This form of the drug is released slowly into the body throughout the day. The drug predisposes the patient to burns.
Pantoprazole (Protonix, Protonix IV) 40 mg orally daily or 40 mg IV daily for 7-10 days given in 15-min or 2-min infusions		Do not crush, break, or chew delayed-release tablets. Do not give Protonix IV with other IV drugs.	This form of the drug is released slowly into the body throughout the day. Protonix IV is not compatible with most other IV drugs.
Esomeprazole (Nexium) 20-40 mg orally daily; 20-40 mg IV daily for 7-10 days given between 10 and 30 min (do not run less than 3 minutes)		Do not administer with digoxin, rabeprazole, or iron salts. Do not crush, break, or chew this delayed-release oral drug. Do not give IV Nexium with other IV drugs.	This drug may alter the effect and absorption of these agents. The oral form of the drug is released slowly throughout the day. IV Nexium is not compatible with most other IV drugs.

Postoperative Instructions for Patients Having Endoscopic Therapies for Gastroesophageal Reflux Disease (e.g., Stretta Procedure)

- Remain on clear liquids for 24 hours after the procedure.
- After the first day, consume a soft diet, such as custard, pureed vegetables, mashed potatoes, and applesauce.
- Avoid nonsteroidal anti-inflammatory drugs and aspirin for 10 days.
- Continue drug therapy as prescribed, usually proton pump inhibitors.
- Use liquid medications whenever possible.
- Do not allow nasogastric tubes for at least 1 month because the esophagus could be perforated.
- Contact the health care provider immediately if these problems occur:
  - Chest or abdominal pain
  - Bleeding
  - Dysphagia
  - Shortness of breath
  - Nausea or vomiting

absorption and protein digestion and therefore reduce available calcium to bone tissue. Decreased calcium makes bones more brittle and likely to fracture, especially as people age (Chait, 2010).

? NCLEX EXAMINATION CHALLENGE

Physiological Integrity

A client with gastroesophageal reflux disease (GERD) is newly diagnosed by the nurse practitioner, who prescribes pantoprazole (Protonix) 40 mg. What teaching will the nurse provide for this client about this drug?
A. "Be sure to take this drug every day until you feel better."
B. "Do not take the drug with tomato-based foods or drinks."
C. "Be aware that this drug can cause anxiety and restlessness."
D. "Do not crush the drug because it has a delayed release."

Endoscopic Therapies. In the past 15 years, several noninvasive endoscopic procedures have been approved for severe GERD. Two techniques used are the Stretta procedure and endoluminal gastroplication. These nonsurgical methods are becoming more popular and may often replace surgery for GERD when other measures are not effective. Patients who are very obese or have severe symptoms may not be candidates for these procedures.

In the Stretta procedure, the physician applies radiofrequency (RF) energy through the endoscope using needles placed near the gastroesophageal junction. The RF energy decreases vagus nerve activity, thus reducing discomfort for the patient. This nonsurgical procedure has also been approved for patients with Barrett's esophagus (Bulsiewicz & Shaheen, 2011).

In the gastroplication procedure, the physician tightens the LES through the endoscope using sutures near the sphincter. Chart 57-4 outlines discharge instructions for endoscopic therapies.

The advantages of endoscopic therapies compared with surgery include:

- Use of light or moderate sedation (rather than general anesthesia)
- Ambulatory care procedure (rather than an inpatient stay)
- Short procedure (45 minutes versus several hours)
- 1 to 2 days absence from work (rather than 2 to 3 weeks)
- No antibiotics and lower complication rate, including fewer deaths

Surgical Management

A very small percentage of patients with GERD require anti-reflux surgery. It is usually indicated for otherwise healthy patients who have failed to respond to medical treatment or have developed complications related to GERD. Various surgical procedures may be used through conventional open techniques or laparoscope.

Laparoscopic Nissen fundoplication (LNF) is a minimally invasive surgery (MIS) and is the gold standard for surgical management. A discussion of this procedure can be found in the next section (Hiatal Hernia) in the Surgical Management discussion. Patients who have surgery are encouraged to continue following the basic anti-reflux regimen of antacids and nutritional therapy because the rate of recurrence is high.

HIATAL HERNIA

Hiatal hernias, also called *diaphragmatic hernias,* involve the protrusion of the stomach through the esophageal hiatus of the diaphragm into the chest. The esophageal hiatus is the opening in the diaphragm through which the esophagus passes from the thorax to the abdomen. Most patients with hiatal hernias are asymptomatic, but some may have daily symptoms similar to those with GERD (McCance et al., 2010).

Pathophysiology

The two major types of hiatal hernias are sliding hernias and paraesophageal (rolling) hernias. *Sliding hernias* are the most common type. The esophagogastric junction and a portion of the fundus of the stomach slide upward through the esophageal hiatus into the chest, usually as a result of weakening of the diaphragm (Fig. 57-1). The hernia generally moves freely and slides into and out of the chest during changes in position or intra-abdominal pressure. Although volvulus (twisting) and obstruction do occur rarely, the major concern for a sliding hernia is the development of esophageal reflux and its complications (see Gastroesophageal Reflux Disease section earlier in this chapter). The development of reflux is related to chronic exposure of the lower esophageal sphincter (LES) to the low pressure of the thorax, which significantly reduces the effectiveness of the LES. Symptoms associated with decreased LES pressure are worsened by positions that favor reflux, such as bending or lying supine. Coughing, obesity, and ascites also increase reflux symptoms.

With *rolling hernias,* also known as *paraesophageal hernias,* the gastroesophageal junction remains in its normal intra-abdominal location but the fundus (and possibly portions of the stomach's greater curvature) rolls through the esophageal hiatus and into the chest beside the esophagus (see Fig. 57-1). The herniated portion of the stomach may be small or quite large. In rare cases, the stomach completely inverts into the chest. Reflux is not usually present because the LES remains

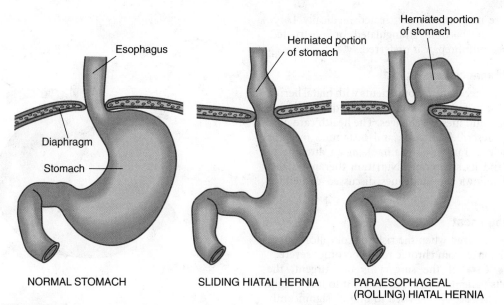

Esophagus

Diaphragm

Stomach

Herniated portion of stomach

Herniated portion of stomach

NORMAL STOMACH

SLIDING HIATAL HERNIA

PARAESOPHAGEAL (ROLLING) HIATAL HERNIA

FIG. 57-1 A comparison of the normal stomach and sliding and paraesophageal (rolling) hiatal hernias.

anchored below the diaphragm. However, the risks for volvulus (twisting), obstruction (blockage), and strangulation (stricture) are high. The development of iron deficiency anemia is common because slow bleeding from venous obstruction causes the gastric mucosa to become engorged and ooze. Significant bleeding or hemorrhage is rare.

Rolling hernias are thought to develop from an anatomic defect occurring when the stomach is not properly anchored below the diaphragm rather than from muscle weakness. They can also be caused by previous esophageal surgeries, including sliding hernia repair.

PATIENT-CENTERED COLLABORATIVE CARE

ASSESSMENT

Ask the patient if he or she has heartburn, regurgitation (backward flow of food into the throat), pain, dysphagia (difficulty swallowing), and eructation (belching). Assess general physical appearance and nutritional status. Note the location, onset, duration, and quality of pain, as well as factors that relieve it or make it worse. The primary symptoms of sliding hiatal hernias are associated with reflux. Auscultate the lungs because pulmonary symptoms similar to asthma may be triggered by episodes of aspiration, particularly at night. A detailed history is crucial in attempting to differentiate angina from noncardiac chest pain caused by reflux. Symptoms resulting from hiatal hernia typically worsen after a meal or when the patient is in a supine position (Chart 57-5).

In those with rolling hernias, assess for symptoms related to the stretching or displacement of thoracic contents by the hernia. Patients may report a feeling of fullness after eating or have breathlessness or a feeling of suffocation if the hernia interferes with breathing. Some may experience chest pain associated with reflux that mimics angina.

The *barium swallow study with fluoroscopy* is the most specific diagnostic test for identifying hiatal hernia. Rolling

---

CHART 57-5	**KEY FEATURES**

Hiatal Hernias

Sliding Hiatal Hernias	**Paraesophageal Hernias**
• Heartburn	• Feeling of fullness after eating
• Regurgitation	• Breathlessness after eating
• Chest pain	• Feeling of suffocation
• Dysphagia	• Chest pain that mimics angina
• Belching	• Worsening of manifestations in a recumbent position

hernias are usually clearly visible, and sliding hernias can often be observed when the patient moves through a series of positions that increase intra-abdominal pressure. To visualize sliding hernias, an esophagogastroduodenoscopy (EGD) may be performed to view both the esophagus and gastric lining (see Chapter 55).

INTERVENTIONS

Patients with hiatal hernias may be managed either medically or surgically. Collaborative care is based on the severity of symptoms and the risk for serious complications. Sliding

❗ NURSING SAFETY PRIORITY

Action Alert

The most important role of the nurse in caring for a patient with a hiatal hernia is health teaching. Encourage the patient to avoid eating in the late evening and to avoid foods associated with reflux. Teach the patient and family that the patient should follow a restricted diet and exercise to reduce body weight if overweight. Obesity increases intra-abdominal pressure and worsens both the hernia and the symptoms of reflux. Teach about positioning, including:

• Sleep at night with the head of the bed elevated 6 inches
• Remain upright for several hours after eating
• Avoid straining or excessive vigorous exercise
• Refrain from wearing clothing that is tight or constrictive around the abdomen

hiatal hernias are most commonly treated medically. Large rolling hernias can become strangulated or obstructed. Therefore early surgical repair is preferred.

Nonsurgical Management

The collaborative interventions for patients with hiatal hernia are similar to those for GERD and include drug therapy, nutrition therapy, and lifestyle changes. The health care provider typically prescribes antacids and histamine receptor antagonists, such as ranitidine (Zantac), in an attempt to control reflux and its symptoms. Nutrition therapy is also important and follows the guidelines discussed earlier for GERD.

Surgical Management

Surgery may be required when the risk for complications is high or when damage from chronic reflux becomes severe.

Preoperative Care. If the surgery is not urgent, the surgeon instructs patients who are overweight to lose weight before surgery. They are also advised to quit or significantly reduce smoking. As part of preoperative teaching, reinforce the surgeon's instructions and prepare the patient for what to expect after surgery.

Laparoscopic Nissen fundoplication (LNF) is the minimally invasive surgery commonly used for hiatal hernia repair. Complications after LNF occur less frequently compared with those seen in patients having the more traditional open surgical approach.

A small percentage of patients are not candidates for LNF and therefore require a conventional open fundoplication. Teach patients having this procedure what to expect after surgery. For example, for the trans-thoracic surgical approach, teach the patient about chest tubes. Inform the patient that a nasogastric tube will be inserted during surgery and will remain in place for several days. Oral intake is started gradually with clear liquids after peristalsis is re-established or to stimulate peristalsis. Instruct the patient how to deep breathe and use the incentive spirometer. These measures are essential to prevent postoperative respiratory complications. The high incision makes deep breathing extremely painful. Teach the patient about postoperative pain, and assure him or her that adequate postoperative analgesic will be given promptly. Pain levels must be continuously monitored.

Operative Procedures. Although several hiatal hernia repair procedures are used, each involves reinforcement of the lower esophageal sphincter (LES) by fundoplication. The surgeon wraps a portion of the stomach fundus around the distal esophagus to anchor it and reinforce the LES (Fig. 57-2). In laparoscopic surgery, the repair is performed through several $\frac{1}{2}$-inch incisions in the abdomen. For the conventional open procedure, the surgeon typically uses a high trans-thoracic approach that requires a large chest incision for access to the surgical area.

Postoperative Care. Patients having the *LNF procedure* are at risk for bleeding and infection, although these problems are not common. *The nursing care priority is to observe for these complications and provide health teaching as described in Chart 57-6.*

Postoperative care after *conventional open repair* closely follows that required after any esophageal surgery. Complications after open surgery are more common and potentially serious. Carefully assess for complications of open

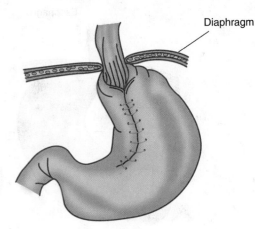

FIG. 57-2 Open surgical approach for Nissen fundoplication for gastroesophageal reflux disease or hiatal hernia repair.

CHART 57-6 **PATIENT AND FAMILY EDUCATION: PREPARING FOR SELF-MANAGEMENT**

Postoperative Instructions for Patients Having Laparoscopic Nissen Fundoplication (LNF)

- Stay on a soft diet for about a week, including mashed potatoes, puddings, custard, and milkshakes; avoid carbonated beverages, tough foods, and raw vegetables that are difficult to swallow.
- Remain on antireflux medications as prescribed for at least a month.
- Do not drive for a week after surgery; do not drive if taking opioid pain medication.
- Walk every day, but do not do any heavy lifting.
- Remove small dressings 2 days after surgery, and shower; do not remove Steri-Strips until 10 days after surgery.
- Wash incisions with soap and water, rinse well, and pat dry; report any redness or drainage from the incisions to your surgeon.
- Report fever above 101° F (38.3° C), nausea, vomiting, or uncontrollable bloating or pain. For patients older than 65 years, report elevations above 100° F (37.8° C).
- Schedule an appointment for follow-up with your surgeon in 3 to 4 weeks.

---

fundoplication surgery, described next, and report any complications to the health care provider (Chart 57-7).

! NURSING SAFETY PRIORITY

Action Alert

The primary focus of care after conventional surgery for a hiatal hernia repair is the prevention of respiratory complications. Elevate the head of the patient's bed at least 30 degrees to lower the diaphragm and promote lung expansion. Assist the patient out of bed and begin ambulation as soon as possible. Be sure to support the incision during coughing to reduce pain and to prevent excessive strain on the suture line, especially with obese patients.

CHART 57-7 BEST PRACTICE FOR PATIENT SAFETY & QUALITY CARE

Assessment of Postoperative Complications Related to Fundoplication Procedures

COMPLICATION	ASSESSMENT FINDINGS
Temporary dysphagia	The patient has difficulty swallowing when oral feeding begins.
Gas bloat syndrome	The patient has difficulty belching to relieve distention.
Atelectasis, pneumonia	The patient experiences dyspnea, chest pain, or fever.
Obstructed nasogastric tube	The patient experiences nausea, vomiting, or abdominal distention. The nasogastric tube does not drain.

Incentive spirometry and deep breathing are routinely used after surgery to maintain patency of the airways and lung expansion. Adequate pain control with analgesics is essential for postoperative deep breathing and coughing. Patients with a smoking history or chronic airway limitation (e.g., chronic obstructive pulmonary disease, asthma) require more aggressive management by the respiratory therapist to prevent atelectasis and pneumonia. Patients with large hiatal hernias are at the highest risk for developing respiratory complications.

The patient having the conventional surgery usually has a large-bore (diameter) nasogastric (NG) tube to prevent the fundoplication wrap from becoming too tight around the esophagus. Initially the NG drainage should be dark brown with old blood but should become normal yellowish green within the first 8 hours after surgery. Check the NG tube every 4 to 8 hours for proper placement in the stomach. The tube should be properly anchored so it is not displaced, because re-insertion could perforate the fundoplication. Follow the surgeon's requests for care of the patient with an NG tube.

Monitor patency of the NG tube to keep the stomach decompressed. This prevents retching or vomiting, which can strain or rupture the stomach sutures. The NG tube is irritating. Therefore provide frequent oral hygiene to increase comfort. Assess the patient's hydration status regularly, including accurate measures of intake and output. Adequate fluid replacement helps thin respiratory secretions.

After open fundoplication, the patient may begin clear fluids when peristalsis is re-established or in an effort to stimulate peristalsis. Some surgeons create a temporary gastrostomy for feeding to allow for undisturbed healing of the repair. The patient gradually progresses to a near-normal diet during the first 4 to 6 weeks. Some foods, especially caffeinated or carbonated beverages and alcohol, are either restricted or eliminated. The food storage area of the stomach is reduced by the surgery, and meals need to be both smaller and more frequent.

Carefully supervise the first oral feedings because temporary dysphagia is common. Continuous dysphagia usually indicates that the fundoplication is too tight, and dilation may be required.

Another common complication of this surgery is the gas bloat syndrome, in which patients are unable to voluntarily eructate (belch). The syndrome is usually temporary but may persist, even in those who have the laparoscopic approach. Teach the patient to avoid drinking carbonated beverages and to avoid eating gas-producing foods (especially high-fat foods), chewing gum, and drinking with a straw.

Other patients have aerophagia (air swallowing) from attempting to reverse or clear acid reflux. Teach them to relax consciously before and after meals, to eat and drink slowly, and to chew all food thoroughly. Air in the stomach that cannot be removed by belching can be extremely uncomfortable. Frequent position changes and ambulation are often effective interventions for eliminating air from the GI tract. If gas pain is still present, patients are taught to take simethicone, 80 mg four times daily as needed. Be sure to remind the patient to crush and dissolve the medication in water before taking.

Community-Based Care

Patients undergoing one of the open surgical repairs require activity restrictions during the 3- to 6-week postoperative recovery period. For laparoscopic surgery, activity is typically restricted for a shorter time and the patient can return to his or her usual lifestyle more quickly, usually in a few days to a week.

For long-term management, teach the patient and family about appropriate nutritional modifications. The use of stool softeners or bulk laxatives is recommended for the first postoperative weeks until healing is complete. Instruct the patient to avoid straining and to prevent constipation. Teach him or her to inspect the healing incision daily and to notify the health care provider if swelling, redness, tenderness, discharge, or fever occurs. Advise the patient to avoid contact with people with respiratory infections and to contact the health care provider if symptoms of a cold or influenza develop. Continuous coughing can cause the incision or the fundoplication to dehisce ("break open"). Advise the patient to avoid smoking. Provide information about smoking-cessation methods, if appropriate.

If needed, collaborate with the dietitian to educate the patient and family about dietary changes. Encourage the patient to eat smaller and more frequent meals. Few ongoing diet restrictions are needed, but overeating or eating the wrong types of foods can produce discomfort if the patient cannot belch. Instruct the patient to report reflux symptoms to the health care provider.

Although severe surgical complications are rare, conditions such as gas bloat syndrome and dysphagia may continue. Prepare the patient for these problems and for the potential that reflux may not be completely controlled or may occur again. Although surgery controls the condition, a cure is rare and lifestyle modifications need to be ongoing.

ESOPHAGEAL TUMORS

Pathophysiology

Although esophageal tumors can be benign, most are usually malignant (cancerous) and the majority arise from the epithelium. Squamous cell carcinomas of the esophagus are located in the upper two thirds of the esophagus. Adenocarcinomas are more commonly found in the distal third and at the gastroesophageal junction and are now the most common type of esophageal cancer (McCance et al., 2010). Esophageal tumors grow rapidly because there is no serosal layer to limit their extension. Because the esophageal mucosa is richly supplied with lymph tissue, there is early spread of tumors to lymph nodes. Esophageal tumors can protrude into the esophageal lumen and can cause thickening or invade deeply into surrounding tissue. In rare cases, the lesion may be confined to the epithelial layer (in situ). In most cases, the tumor is large and well established on diagnosis. More than half of esophageal cancers metastasize (spread throughout the body).

The two primary risk factors associated with the development of squamous cell carcinoma of the esophagus are tobacco use and heavy alcohol intake. The compounds in tobacco smoke may be responsible for the genetic mutations seen in many esophageal tumors. A smoker has two to six times the risk for eventually developing esophageal cancer than does a nonsmoker (American Cancer Society [ACS], 2010). Many alcoholic beverages contain potent carcinogens that may be responsible for the development of esophageal tumors. Smoking and excessive alcohol can act together in causing esophageal cancer. Obesity and malnutrition are also risk factors.

Long-term, untreated *gastroesophageal reflux disease (GERD)* can lead to esophageal adenocarcinoma. For people with Barrett's esophagus, the risk for developing esophageal cancer also greatly increases. Barrett's esophagus results from exposure to acid and pepsin, which leads to the replacement of normal distal squamous mucosa with columnar epithelium as a response to tissue injury. This tissue undergoes dysplasia (cell appearance changes) and, ultimately, becomes cancerous. In parts of the world where esophageal cancer is more common, the incidence of squamous cell carcinoma appears to be linked to high levels of nitrosamines (which are found in pickled and fermented foods) and foods high in nitrate. Diets that are chronically deficient in fresh fruits and vegetables have also been implicated in the development of squamous cell carcinoma.

GENETIC/GENOMIC CONSIDERATIONS

Certain genetic factors may have a role in the development of esophageal cancers. It is thought that these cancers result from mutations in tumor suppressor genes. Tumor suppressor genes are normal genes that control cell growth and division. When this type of gene is mutated and does not work properly, cells are unable to stop growing and dividing and tumors can result. (See Chapter 23 for a more complete discussion.)

Overexpression and mutations of the *Tp53, Tp16, and Tp17* tumor suppressor genes have been found in people with esophageal cancer (Nussbaum et al., 2007). In addition, the presence of the mutated Tp53 gene may be an indication of advanced disease, especially in patients with adenocarcinomas.

Overexpression of *cyclin D1*, a protein that promotes cell growth and division, has also been found in patients with esophageal squamous cell cancers. Cyclins are products of oncogenes, which are normal genes involved in cell division and are controlled by suppressor genes. Prolonged exposure to carcinogens, such as tobacco, can cause oncogenes to escape the control of suppressor genes, leading to overexpression of cyclins and uncontrolled cell growth (cancer).

⚡ NCLEX EXAMINATION CHALLENGE

Health Promotion and Maintenance

A client has a history of gastroesophageal reflux disease and is worried about getting cancer of the esophagus. What health teaching about ways to decrease the risk for cancer will the nurse provide? **Select all that apply.**
A. "Consider dieting and exercise because you are overweight."
B. "Drink a glass of red wine every night because it provides antioxidants."
C. "Join a good smoking-cessation program as soon as possible."
D. "Eat plenty of fruits and vegetables instead of so much junk food."
E. "Sleep with two pillows every night to prevent reflux when sleeping."

PATIENT-CENTERED COLLABORATIVE CARE

▮ ASSESSMENT

History

Assess for risk factors related to the development or symptoms of esophageal cancer, such as racial and ethnic background, age, gender, history of alcohol consumption, tobacco use, dietary habits, and other esophageal problems (e.g., dysphagia, reflux). Esophageal cancer (squamous cell) occurs most often in middle-aged and older adults and tends to occur more in black males, although the exact cause for racial differences is not known. White males are more predisposed to esophageal adenocarcinoma. Ask the patient about consumption of smoked pickled foods, changes in appetite, changes in taste, or weight loss. *Cancer of the esophagus is a silent tumor in its early stages, with few observable signs. By the time the tumor causes symptoms, it usually has spread extensively.*

Physical Assessment/Clinical Manifestations

Dysphagia *(difficulty swallowing) is the most common symptom of esophageal cancer, but it may not be present until the esophageal opening has gotten much smaller.* Dysphagia is both persistent and progressive when stricture (narrowing) occurs. It is initially associated with swallowing solids, particularly meat, and then progresses rapidly over a period of weeks or months to difficulty in swallowing soft foods and liquids. Late in the disease, even saliva can induce choking. Patients usually report a sensation that food is sticking in the throat or in the substernal area. Careful assessment of the dysphagia is an important part of the diagnosis because dysphagia associated with other esophageal disorders is not usually continuous. Weight loss often accompanies dysphagia and can be more than 20 pounds over several months.

Odynophagia (painful swallowing) is reported by many patients as a steady, dull, substernal pain that may radiate. It occurs most often when the patient drinks cold liquids. The presence of severe or persistent pain often indicates tumor invasion of the mediastinal structures. Assess for regurgitation, vomiting, halitosis (foul breath), and chronic hiccups, which often accompany advanced disease. In most patients, pulmonary problems develop. Assess for chronic cough, increased secretions, and a history of recent infections. Tumors in the upper esophagus may involve the larynx and thus cause hoarseness. Chart 57-8 summarizes the common clinical manifestations of esophageal tumors.

Psychosocial Assessment

The diagnosis of esophageal cancer causes high patient anxiety. The disease is accompanied by distressing symptoms and is often terminal. The fear of choking can place unusual stress, especially at mealtimes. The loss of pleasure and social aspects of eating may affect relationships with family and friends. Assess the patient's response to the diagnosis and prognosis. Ask about his or her usual coping strengths and resources. Assess the impact of the disease on the patient's usual daily activity routine. Determine the availability of support systems and the potential financial impact of the disease and its treatment. Refer the patient and family members to psychological counseling, pastoral care, and/or the social worker or case manager as needed. Chapter 9 describes end-of-life care for patients in the terminal stage of the disease.

Diagnostic Assessment

A barium swallow study with fluoroscopy is usually the first diagnostic test requested to evaluate dysphagia. In a barium swallow, the margins of a tumor may be seen. The definitive diagnosis of esophageal cancer is made by *esophageal ultrasound (EUS)* with fine needle aspiration to examine the tumor tissue. An esophagogastroduodenoscopy (EGD) may also be performed to inspect the esophagus and obtain tissue specimens for cell studies and disease staging. A complete cancer staging workup is performed to determine the extent of the disease and plan appropriate therapy.

Positron emission tomography (PET) may identify metastatic disease with more accuracy than a computed tomography (CT) scan. PET can also help evaluate response to chemotherapy to treat the cancer.

ANALYSIS

The most specific common problem for patients with esophageal cancer is *decreased nutritional intake related to impaired swallowing and possible metastasis.* Many patients with cancer also have pain and are fearful due to the diagnosis of cancer. Chapter 24 describes problems that are typically seen with any patient with cancer.

PLANNING AND IMPLEMENTATION

Promoting Nutrition

Planning: Expected Outcomes. The major concern for a patient with esophageal cancer is weight loss secondary to dysphagia. Therefore he or she is expected to maintain adequate nutrient intake and weight either orally or via an alternative method.

Interventions. Interventions to maintain or improve nutritional status focus on treatments that remove or shrink the obstructive tumor. Methods to reduce the effects of

---

treatment that can impact nutrition are also a priority. Surgery is the most definitive intervention for esophageal cancer.

Nonsurgical treatment options for cancer of the esophagus that can assist in both disease and nutrition management include:

- Nutrition therapy
- Swallowing therapy
- Chemotherapy
- Radiation therapy
- Chemoradiation
- Targeted therapies
- Photodynamic therapy
- Esophageal dilation
- Endoscopic therapies

Nonsurgical Management. The treatment of esophageal cancer often involves a combination of the therapies just mentioned. Patients with cancer of the esophagus experience many physical problems, and symptom management becomes essential.

The purpose of nutrition therapy is to administer food and fluids to support the patient who is malnourished or at high risk for becoming malnourished. Conduct a screening assessment to provide information about the patient's nutritional status. The dietitian determines the caloric needs of the patient to meet daily requirements. Be sure the patient is weighed daily. Careful positioning is essential for a patient who is experiencing frequent reflux or who has tubes to keep the esophagus patent. Teach the patient to remain upright for several hours after meals and to avoid lying completely flat. Remind unlicensed assistive personnel (UAP) and other health care team members to keep the head of the bed elevated to a 30-degree angle or more to prevent reflux.

Semisoft foods and thickened liquids are preferred because they are easier to swallow. Record the amount of food and fluid intake every day to monitor progress in meeting desired nutritional outcomes. Liquid nutritional supplements (e.g., Boost, Ensure) are used between feedings to increase caloric intake. Ongoing efforts are made to preserve the ability to swallow, but enteral feedings (tube feedings) may be needed temporarily when dysphagia is severe. In patients with complete esophageal obstruction or life-threatening fistulas, the surgeon may create a gastrostomy or jejunostomy for feeding. Encourage the patient and family to meet with the dietitian for diet teaching and planning. Chapter 63 describes care for patients receiving enteral feeding.

Collaborate with the speech-language pathologist (SLP) to assist the patient with oral exercises to improve swallowing *(swallowing therapy)*. Ask the patient to suck on a lollipop to enhance tongue strength. Teach the patient to reach for food particles on the lips or chin using the tongue. In preparation

---

CHART 57-8   KEY FEATURES

Esophageal Tumors

- Persistent and progressive dysphagia (most common feature)
- Feeling of food sticking in the throat
- Odynophagia (painful swallowing)
- Severe, persistent chest or abdominal pain or discomfort
- Regurgitation
- Chronic cough with increasing secretions
- Hoarseness
- Anorexia
- Nausea and vomiting
- Weight loss (often more than 20 pounds)
- Changes in bowel habits (diarrhea, constipation, bleeding)

! NURSING SAFETY PRIORITY

Critical Rescue

When the patient with an esophageal tumor is eating or drinking, monitor for signs and symptoms of aspiration, such as choking or coughing! Food aspiration can cause airway obstruction, pneumonia, or both, especially in older adults. In coordination with the SLP, teach family members and caregivers how to feed the patient, if needed. Teach them how to monitor for aspiration and implement appropriate measures if choking occurs.

for swallowing, remind the patient to position the head in forward flexion (chin tuck). Then tell him or her to place food at the back of the mouth. Monitor him or her for sealing of the lips and for tongue movements while eating. Check for pocketing of food in the cheeks after swallowing.

The use of *chemotherapy* in the treatment of esophageal cancer has been only moderately effective. It can be given as a primary treatment if the patient is not a candidate for surgery or for palliation (control of symptoms). In most cases, though, chemotherapy is given in combination with radiation therapy to provide the patient the best chance of cure. The rationale for this approach is to shrink the tumor and eliminate any other tumor that may be in the local lymph nodes, improving the odds for a complete surgical resection. The two most commonly used chemotherapeutic agents have traditionally been 5-fluorouracil (5-FU) and a platinum-based agent, such as cisplatin (Platinol), carboplatin (Paraplatin), and oxaliplatin (Eloxatin). These drugs make the tumor cells more sensitive to the effects of radiation. Other drugs have been tried successfully for treatment of esophageal cancer, including paclitaxel (Taxol), docetaxel (Taxotere), and irinotecan (Camptosar). Because chemotherapeutic drugs affect healthy cells as well as cancer cells, they have many side effects that cause discomfort to the patient. Chapter 24 describes chemotherapy in detail and discusses the role of the nurse in caring for patients receiving these drugs.

Radiation therapy to manage esophageal cancer is only moderately effective and can be used alone or in combination with other treatments. Radiation alone can provide palliation of symptoms by shrinking the tumor. It is contraindicated for patients with tracheoesophageal fistula, mediastinitis, mediastinal hemorrhage, or infiltration of the cancer to the trachea or bronchus. Normal esophageal tissue is very sensitive to the effects of radiation. Although high doses of radiation demonstrate the best results for tumor shrinkage, esophageal stricture or stenosis can result in many patients, which then requires esophageal dilation. Chapter 24 describes radiation methods and the general nursing care for the patient having radiation therapy.

Chemoradiation is a treatment for esophageal cancer that involves the use of chemotherapy at the same time as radiation therapy. One cycle of chemotherapy is given during the first week of radiation and another is delivered during the fifth week of radiation. Additional drug cycles are given after radiation therapy is complete.

The newest addition to the treatment of esophageal cancer is targeted therapies, used in combination with radiation and chemotherapy. Unlike chemotherapy, these therapies interfere with cancer cell growth in a variety of ways with less impact on healthy cells. Many of these drugs focus on proteins that are involved in signaling cells when to grow and divide. A key to success with targeted therapy is that the cancer cells must overexpress the targeted protein. Thus each patient's cancer cells are first examined for the overexpression to determine if targeted therapy is appropriate and which drug to use. A number of agents have been approved for other GI cancers but are still used experimentally for esophageal cancer. For example, cetuximab (Erbitux) is a monoclonal antibody that targets the epithelial growth factor receptor (EGFR) on the surface of cancer cells. EGRF is often overexpressed in esophageal tumors. Other targeted therapies, such as trastuzumab (Herceptin), gefitinib (Iressa), and erlotinib (Tarceva), have also been used. Chapter 24 describes targeted therapies in detail, including nursing implications for patient safety and quality care.

Photodynamic therapy (PDT) was originally used for the treatment of skin cancer but is now used also as a palliative treatment for patients with advanced esophageal cancer who are not candidates for surgery. It may be used also as a cure for patients who have very small, localized tumors. The patient is injected with porfimer sodium (Photofrin), a light-sensitive drug that collects in cancer cells. Two days after the injection, a fiberoptic probe with a light at the tip is threaded into the esophagus through an endoscope. The light activates the Photofrin, destroying only cancer cells. PDT is far less invasive than surgery and is performed on an ambulatory care basis under moderate sedation.

The side effects of Photofrin are rare but include nausea, fever, and constipation. Before the procedure, the patient is given written guidelines concerning photosensitivity measures. Remind the patient to avoid exposure to sunlight for 1 to 3 months. Sunglasses and protective clothing that covers all exposed body areas are essential. The patient may experience chest pain secondary to tissue damage and will require pain relief with opioid analgesics for a short time. Teach the patient to follow a clear liquid diet for 3 to 5 days after the procedure and advance to full liquids as tolerated. Warn the patient that tissue particles may release from the tumor site and be present in the sputum. Chapter 24 describes in detail the health teaching needed to promote patient safety associated with PDT.

Esophageal dilation may be performed as necessary throughout the course of the disease to achieve temporary but immediate relief of dysphagia. It is usually performed on an ambulatory care basis. Dilators are used to tear soft tissue, thereby widening the esophageal lumen (opening). In most cases, malignant tumors can be dilated safely, but perforation remains a significant risk. Large metal stents may be used to keep the esophagus open for longer periods. A stent covered with graft material can be used to seal a perforation. Bacteremia can also occur. To reduce the risk for endocarditis, antibiotics are given. The treatment is repeated as often as needed to preserve the patient's ability to swallow.

When patients are not candidates for surgery or the tumor is too large to remove surgically, laser therapy or electrocoagulation using endoscopy may be performed as a palliative measure. Both of these methods destroy some cancer cells and reduce tumor size to improve swallowing. The procedures are done in ambulatory care settings or same-day surgery centers using moderate sedation.

Surgical Management. The purposes of surgical resection vary from palliation to cure. **Esophagectomy** is the removal of all or part of the esophagus. An **esophagogastrostomy** involves the removal of part of the esophagus and proximal stomach. The remaining stomach may be "pulled up" to take the place of the esophagus, or a section of the jejunum or colon may be placed as a conduit. Conventional open surgical techniques are lengthy and are associated with many complications or death. Fistula formation between the trachea and esophagus, abscess, and respiratory complications are common.

For patients with early-stage cancer, a laparoscopic-assisted minimally invasive esophagectomy (MIE) may be

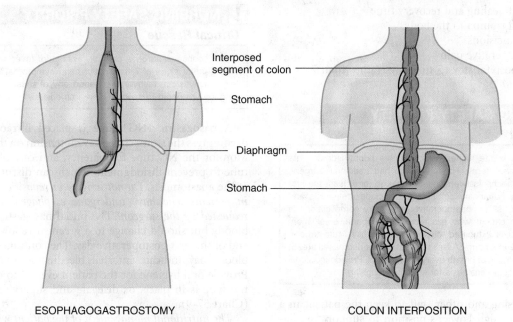

Interposed
segment of colon

Stomach

Diaphragm

Stomach

ESOPHAGOGASTROSTOMY   COLON INTERPOSITION

FIG. 57-3 Open surgical approaches to the treatment of esophageal cancer.

performed. However, most patients require the conventional open surgery because of tumor size and metastasis by the time they are diagnosed with the disease.

Preoperative Care. Preoperative preparation for patients undergoing esophagectomy or esophagogastrostomy can be quite extensive, especially before conventional techniques. Advise the patient to stop smoking 2 to 4 weeks before surgery to enhance pulmonary function. Patient preparation may include 5 days to 2 to 3 weeks of nutritional support to decrease the risk for postoperative complications. Ideally this supplementation is given orally, but many patients require tube feeding or parenteral nutrition. Teach the patient and family to monitor the patient's weight and intake and output. A preoperative evaluation may be required to treat dental disease. Teach the patient to use meticulous oral care four times daily to decrease the risk for postoperative infection.

Preoperative nursing care focuses on teaching and on psychological support regarding the surgical procedure and preoperative and postoperative instructions. Teach the patient about:

- The number and sites of all incisions and drains
- The placement of a jejunostomy tube for initial enteral feedings
- The need for chest tubes if the pleural space is entered
- The purpose of the nasogastric tube
- The need for IV infusion

Teach the patient about routines for turning, coughing, deep breathing, and chest physiotherapy. Emphasize the crucial nature of postoperative respiratory care. If colon interposition (resecting a piece of colon and creating an esophagus) is planned, the patient also has a complete bowel preparation before surgery.

The patient facing a serious illness and extensive surgery can be expected to have feelings of grief and anxiety. Encourage the patient to talk about personal feelings and fears, and involve the family or significant others in all preoperative teaching and discussions. A social worker or case manager can be extremely helpful in providing continuity of care and support to the entire family.

Operative Procedures. In the MIE procedure, the surgeon makes four or five small incisions in the chest and abdomen using a video-assisted thoracoscope and laparoscope. The lower esophagus and gastric fundus are removed. The remaining portion of the esophagus is then anastomosed (reconnected) to the stomach.

For most patients, the surgeon performs an open subtotal or total esophagectomy because tumors are often large and involve distant lymph nodes. For a subtotal (partial) removal, the diseased portion of the esophagus is removed and the cervical portion is anastomosed (connected) to the stomach (Fig. 57-3). A pyloromyotomy is done by cutting and suturing the pylorus. Finally, a jejunostomy tube may be placed for postoperative enteral feeding.

For patients with early-stage tumors of the lower third of the esophagus, a transhiatal esophagectomy is the preferred surgical approach. The surgery is performed through an upper midline cervical incision. With this approach, the pleural space is not entered, reducing respiratory complications. For patients with tumors in the upper esophagus, a radical neck dissection and laryngectomy may also be needed if the disease has spread to the larynx. Chapter 31 discusses the care of patients having these procedures.

The surgeon may perform a colon interposition when the tumor involves the stomach or the stomach is otherwise unsuitable for anastomosis. A section of right or left colon is removed and brought up into the thorax to substitute for the esophagus (see Fig. 57-3).

Postoperative Care. The patient requires intensive postoperative care and is at risk for multiple serious complications. The patient having an MIE has the same risk for postoperative complications as one having the open procedure. The advantages of MIE, though, include:

- Less blood loss during surgery; fewer blood transfusions

- Decreased healing and recovery time
- Decreased trauma to the body
- No large incisions
- Less postoperative pain
- Shorter hospital stay (5 to 7 days rather than 7 to 10 days)

! NURSING SAFETY PRIORITY

Action Alert

Respiratory care is the highest postoperative priority for patients having an esophagectomy. For those who had traditional surgery, intubation with mechanical ventilation is needed for at least the first 16 to 24 hours. Pulmonary complications include atelectasis and pneumonia. The risk for postoperative pulmonary complications is increased in the patient who has received preoperative radiation. Once the patient is extubated, begin deep breathing, turning, and coughing every 1 to 2 hours. Assess the patient for decreased breath sounds and shortness of breath every 1 to 2 hours. Provide incisional support and adequate analgesia for effective coughing.

Remind nursing and other staff to keep the patient in a semi-Fowler's or high Fowler's position to support ventilation and prevent reflux. The health care provider prescribes prophylactic antibiotics and supplemental oxygen. *Ensure the patency of the chest tube drainage system, and monitor for changes in the volume or color of the drainage.*

Cardiovascular complications, particularly hypotension during surgery, can occur as a result of pressure placed on the posterior heart and usually respond well to IV fluid administration.

! NURSING SAFETY PRIORITY

Action Alert

Monitor for manifestations of fluid volume overload, particularly in older patients and in those who have undergone lymph node dissection. Assess for edema, crackles in the lungs, and increased jugular venous pressure. In the immediate postoperative phase, the patient is often admitted to the intensive care unit. Critical care nurses assess hemodynamic parameters such as cardiac output, cardiac index, and systemic vascular resistance every 2 hours to monitor for myocardial ischemia. Observe for atrial fibrillation that results from irritation of the vagus nerve during surgery, and manage according to agency protocol.

The patient with poor nutrition or prior radiation or chemotherapy is at risk for infection. For those who undergo more radical surgical procedures, there is a serious risk for leakage at the anastomosis (surgical connection) sites. This situation is especially true with colon interpositions because several sites are stressed by the effects of tension, poor blood supply, and delayed healing. *Mediastinitis* (inflammation of the mediastinum) resulting from an anastomotic leak can lead to fatal sepsis.

Wound management is another major postoperative concern for conventional surgery because the patient typically has multiple incisions and drains. *Provide direct support to the incision during turning and coughing to prevent dehiscence.* Wound infection can occur 4 to 5 days after surgery. Leakage from the site of anastomosis is a dreaded complication that can appear 2 to 10 days after surgery. If an anastomotic leak occurs, all oral intake is discontinued and is not resumed until the site of the leak has healed.

! NURSING SAFETY PRIORITY

Critical Rescue

After esophageal surgery, carefully assess for fever, fluid accumulation, general signs of inflammation, and symptoms of early shock (e.g., tachycardia, tachypnea). Report any of these findings to the surgeon OR Rapid Response Team immediately!

A nasogastric (NG) tube is placed intraoperatively to decompress the stomach to prevent tension on the suture line. Monitor the NG tube for patency, and carefully secure the tube to prevent dislodgment, which can disrupt the sutures at the anastomosis. *Do not irrigate or reposition the NG tube in patients who have undergone esophageal surgery unless requested by the surgeon!* The initial nasogastric drainage is bloody but should change to a greenish yellow color by the end of the first postoperative day. The continued presence of blood may indicate internal bleeding at the suture line. Provide oral hygiene for the patient every 2 to 4 hours while the tube is in place, or delegate and supervise this activity (Chart 57-9).

The nutritional management of the patient who has undergone esophageal surgery is an early postoperative concern. After conventional surgery, on the second postoperative day, initial feedings usually begin through the jejunostomy tube (J tube). The feedings are slowly increased over the next several days. Feeding by this method can be discontinued once the patient is taking adequate oral nutrition. However, some patients may require J-tube feedings for about 1 month if large amounts of residual feeding are aspirated.

Before beginning oral feedings, a cine-esophagram study is performed to detect any anastomotic leaks, strictures, or signs of aspiration. If no leaks are seen, a liquid diet is started. If liquids are well tolerated, the patient's diet is advanced to include semisolid foods and then solid foods.

Place the patient in an upright position, and supervise all initial swallowing efforts. The food storage area of the stomach has been radically decreased, and gravity is the only defense against reflux. *Teach the patient and/or family the importance of the patient eating six to eight small meals per day. Fluids should be taken between, rather than with, meals to*

CHART 57-9 BEST PRACTICE FOR PATIENT SAFETY & QUALITY CARE

Managing the Patient with a Nasogastric Tube After Esophageal Surgery

- Check for tube placement every 4 to 8 hours.
- Ensure that the tube is patent (open) and draining; drainage should turn from bloody to yellowish green by the end of the first postoperative day.
- Secure the tube well to prevent dislodgment.
- Do not irrigate or reposition the tube without a physician's request.
- Provide meticulous oral and nasal hygiene every 2 to 4 hours.
- Keep the head of the bed elevated to at least 30 degrees.
- When the patient is permitted to have a small amount of water, place him or her in an upright position and observe for dysphagia (difficulty swallowing).
- Observe for leakage from the anastomosis site, as indicated by fever, fluid accumulation, and manifestations of early shock (tachycardia, tachypnea, altered mental status).

prevent diarrhea. Diarrhea can occur 20 minutes to 2 hours after eating and can be managed with loperamide (Imodium) before meals. The diarrhea is thought to be the result of vagotomy syndrome, which develops as a result of interrupted vagal fibers to the abdominal organs during surgery.

Community-Based Care

Patients with esophageal cancer have many challenges to face once they are discharged home. The combination treatment regimens cause long-lasting side effects, such as fatigue and weakness. These complex treatments also require the patient and family to be knowledgeable about symptom management and to know when to report concerns to the health care provider.

Home Care Management

Once the patient is discharged to home, ongoing respiratory care remains a priority. Give the patient and family instructions for ambulation and incentive spirometer use. Encourage the patient to be as active as possible and to avoid excessive bedrest because this can lead to complications of immobility. Teach the family to protect the patient from infection and to contact the health care provider immediately if signs of respiratory infection develop. Patients should stay away from people with infections and avoid large crowds.

Teaching for Self-Management

Remind the patient and family to wash their hands frequently, and teach them to inspect the incisions daily for redness, tenderness, swelling, odor, and discharge because proper wound healing is still a concern at the time of discharge. Instruct them to report a temperature greater than 101° F (38.3° C), or 100° F (37.8° C) for older adults. Prepare written instructions about the signs of anastomosis leakage. *Teach the patient or family to immediately report to the health care provider the presence of fever and a swollen, painful neck incision.*

Nutritional support also remains a concern. Encourage the patient to continue increasing oral feedings as tolerated. Remind him or her to eat small, frequent meals containing high-calorie, high-protein foods that are soft and easily swallowed. Teach the value of using supplemental eggnogs and milkshakes between meals, and instruct the patient to eat slowly. Lactose-free products should be used if the patient cannot tolerate dairy foods. Patients who have undergone esophageal resection can lose up to 10% of their body weight. Teach the patient to monitor his or her weight at home and to report a weight loss of 5 pounds or more in 1 month. If sufficient oral intake is not possible, the family may need instruction about tube feedings or parenteral nutrition at home.

Emphasize the importance of remaining upright after meals. Dysphagia or odynophagia may recur because of stricture, reflux, or cancer recurrence. These symptoms should be promptly reported to the health care provider. Despite radical surgery, the patient with cancer of the esophagus often still has a terminal illness and a relatively short life expectancy. Emphasis is placed on maximizing quality of life. Realistic planning is important as the patient's condition eventually worsens, and the patient and family are assisted to plan for the future together. Assist family members in exploring formal and informal sources of support. Help the family or significant others arrange for hospice care when it is needed. Chapter 9 describes end-of-life care, including hospice.

Health Care Resources

Referrals to community or home care organizations assist the family in providing care in the home. The patient may need transportation to the radiation treatment center five times per week for up to 6 weeks. Oncology nursing care may be needed to monitor and evaluate the patient who is receiving chemotherapy at home through venous access devices or portable infusion pumps. Inform the patient and family about the services available through the American Cancer Society (www.cancer.org), including support groups and transportation. Familiarize the family with area hospice services for future planning. Coordinate resource referrals with the case manager or home care agency.

▌EVALUATION: EXPECTED OUTCOMES

Evaluate the care of the patient with esophageal cancer based on the identified priority patient problems. The major expected outcome is that the patient will be able to consume adequate nutrition and maintain a stable weight.

▌DECISION-MAKING CHALLENGE

Teamwork and Collaboration; Safety; Evidence-Based Practice

A 58-year-old patient is admitted for a partial esophagectomy. He has a history of alcoholism and says he quit drinking when he found out about his diagnosis. He has not smoked in 35 years. You are assigned to care for the patient after he returns from the postanesthesia care unit (PACU).

1. What is the priority for care for this patient after surgery? What position will you place the patient in and why? Locate one or two sources of current evidence supporting your answer.
2. For what postoperative complications will you monitor, and why could they occur after this surgery?
3. The patient has a nasogastric (NG) tube in place after surgery. What nursing care will you provide for the patient related to the NG tube?
4. The patient's life partner tells you that he is worried that the patient may not be able to return to his job as a family practice physician. How might you respond to his concern?
5. With what members of the health care team might you collaborate and why?

ESOPHAGEAL DIVERTICULA

Diverticula are sacs resulting from the herniation of esophageal mucosa and submucosa into surrounding tissue. They may develop anywhere along the length of the esophagus. No environmental risk factors are known to be involved in their development. The incomplete or late opening of swallowing muscles can cause high pressure in the hypopharynx and lead to *Zenker's diverticula,* the most common form. This type occurs most often in older adults. Patients report dysphagia (difficulty swallowing), regurgitation (reflux), nocturnal cough, and halitosis (bad breath). They can also be at risk for perforation because the mucosa is without the protection of the normal esophageal muscle layer.

Esophageal diverticula are diagnosed most often by esophagogastroduodenoscopy (EGD). This procedure must be performed with strict care because of the risk for perforation. Nutrition therapy and positioning are the major interventions for controlling symptoms related to diverticula. Collaborate with the dietitian to assist the patient in exploring variations in the size and frequency of meals and in food texture and consistency. Semisoft foods and smaller meals are often best tolerated and may reduce or relieve the symptoms of pressure and reflux. Nocturnal reflux associated with diverticula is managed by teaching the patient to sleep with the head of the bed elevated and to avoid the supine position for at least 2 hours after eating. Advise the patient to avoid vigorous exercise after meals. Teach him or her to avoid restrictive clothing and frequent stooping or bending.

Surgical management is aimed at removing the diverticula. Postoperatively, the patient is NPO for several days to promote healing. During that period, the patient receives IV fluids for hydration, tube feedings, and then oral fluid and food. Provide pain relief measures, and monitor for complications such as bleeding or perforation. *A nasogastric (NG) tube is placed during surgery for decompression and is not irrigated or repositioned unless specifically requested by the surgeon.*

Community-based care includes teaching the patient and family about:

- Nutritional therapy
- Positioning guidelines to prevent reflux
- Warning signs of complications, such as bleeding or infection

ESOPHAGEAL TRAUMA

Trauma to the esophagus can result from blunt injuries, chemical burns, surgery or endoscopy, or the stress of continuous severe vomiting (Table 57-2). Trauma may affect the esophagus directly, impairing swallowing and nutrition, or it may create problems in related structures such as the lungs or mediastinum. The incidence of most forms of esophageal trauma is low in adults. When excessive force is exerted on the esophageal mucosa, it may perforate or rupture, allowing the caustic acid secretions to enter the mediastinal cavity. These tears are associated with a high mortality rate related to shock, respiratory impairment, or sepsis.

Chemical injury is usually a result of the accidental or intentional ingestion of caustic substances. The damage to the mouth and esophagus is rapid and severe. Acid burns tend to affect the superficial mucosal lining, whereas alkaline substances cause deeper penetrating injuries. Strong alkalis can cause full perforation of the esophagus within 1 minute. Additional problems may include aspiration pneumonia and hemorrhage. Esophageal strictures may develop as scar tissue forms.

Patients with esophageal trauma are initially evaluated and treated in the emergency department. Assessment focuses on the nature of the injury and the circumstances surrounding it. *Assess for airway patency, breathing, chest pain, dysphagia, vomiting, and bleeding as the priorities for patient care.* If the risk for extending the damage is not excessive, an x-ray or endoscopic study may be requested to evaluate tears or perforation. A CT scan of the chest can be done to assess for the presence of mediastinal air.

After the injury, keep the patient NPO to prevent further leakage of esophageal secretions. Esophageal and gastric suction can be used for drainage and to rest the esophagus. Esophageal rest is maintained for more than a week after injury to allow for initial healing of the mucosa. Total parenteral nutrition (TPN) is prescribed to provide calories and protein for wound healing while the patient is not eating.

To prevent sepsis, the health care provider prescribes broad-spectrum antibiotics. High-dose corticosteroids may be administered to suppress inflammation and prevent strictures (esophageal narrowing). In addition, opioid and nonopioid analgesics are prescribed for pain management. When caustic burns involve the mouth, topical agents such as lidocaine (Xylocaine Viscous) may be used for analgesia and local anti-inflammatory action.

If nonsurgical management is not effective in healing traumatized esophageal tissue, the patient may need surgery to remove the damaged tissue. Those with severe injuries may require resection of part of the esophagus with a gastric pull-through and repositioning or replacement by a bowel segment.

TABLE 57-2	COMMON CAUSES OF ESOPHAGEAL PERFORATION
• Straining	• Instrument or tubes
• Seizures	• Chemical injury
• Trauma	• Complications of esophageal surgery
• Foreign objects	• Ulcers

NURSING CONCEPT REVIEW

What might you NOTICE if the patient has inadequate digestion and nutrition as a result of chronic esophageal problems?

- Dysphagia (difficulty swallowing)
- Odynophagia (painful swallowing)
- Dyspepsia (indigestion or "heartburn")
- Regurgitation (reflux)
- Eructation (belching)
- Chronic cough
- Choking
- Halitosis (foul breath)
- Weight loss

What should you INTERPRET and how should you RESPOND to a patient experiencing inadequate digestion and nutrition as a result of chronic esophageal problems?

Perform and interpret focused physical findings, including:

- Assess ability to chew and swallow food.
- Assess chest pain (dyspepsia) for quality, location, and intensity.
- Assess body weight change.
- Auscultate lungs.
- Assess readiness to learn.

Respond by:

- Providing semi-solid or thickened liquids if solid foods cannot be swallowed comfortably
- Collaborating with the dietitian and occupational therapist (OT) for swallowing evaluation and training
- Monitoring for aspiration of secretions or food

NURSING CONCEPT REVIEW—cont'd

- Teaching lifestyle changes, such as foods to avoid, smoking and alcohol cessation, weight reduction (if obese), and importance of drug therapy to control symptoms
- Monitoring weight
- Monitoring for increased dysphagia

On what should you REFLECT?
- Evaluate for rapid weight changes (decrease if obese, and increase if severe weight loss has occurred).

- Monitor for manifestations of aspiration.
- Observe patient for improvement in GI symptoms.
- Evaluate effectiveness of health teaching.
- Think about what else you might do to promote digestion and nutrition.

GET READY FOR THE NCLEX® EXAMINATION!

KEY POINTS

Review these Key Points for each NCLEX Examination Client Needs Category.

Safe and Effective Care Environment
- Consult with the dietitian, patient, and family regarding nutritional restrictions for patients with GERD.
- Collaborate with the health care team for the patient with impaired swallowing and/or limited nutrition.
- Teach the patient and family to recognize the symptoms of dysphagia.
- Remain with the dysphasic patient during meals to prevent or assist with choking episodes.

Health Promotion and Maintenance
- Teach the patient oral exercises aimed at improving swallowing.
- Stress the importance of recognizing and controlling reflux through nutrition therapy and medications to avoid further esophageal damage that could lead to Barrett's esophagus.
- Teach the patient to elevate the head of the bed by 6 inches for sleep to prevent nighttime reflux.
- Instruct the patient to sleep in the right side-lying position to minimize the effects of nighttime episodes of reflux.
- Teach the patient with esophageal cancer to monitor his or her body weight and to notify the health care provider for a loss of 5 pounds or greater within 1 month.
- Teach the patient to avoid alcoholic beverages, smoking, and other substances as listed in Chart 57-2 because they lead to increased gastroesophageal reflux.
- Teach the patient to prevent gas bloat syndrome by avoiding drinking carbonated beverages, eating gas-producing foods, chewing gum, and drinking with a straw.
- Review postprocedure instructions for patients having endoscopic therapies for GERD as outlined in Chart 57-4.

Psychosocial Integrity
- Allow the patient the opportunity to express fear or anxiety regarding the diagnosis of esophageal cancer and related treatment regimen of surgery, chemotherapy, and radiation.
- Explain all procedures, restrictions, drug therapy, and follow-up care to the patient and family.
- Refer the patient or family members to psychological counseling, hospice, pastoral care, and the case manager as needed.

Physiological Integrity
- For patients with GERD, teach the importance of strict adherence to antireflux agents in preventing esophageal damage (see Chart 57-3).
- Be aware that laparoscopic Nissen fundoplication (LNF) is the most common surgical procedure for patients with GERD and hiatal hernia.
- Assess for complications and provide postoperative care for patients having the LNF procedure, as described in Charts 57-6 and 57-7.
- Be sure to frequently monitor the nutritional status of the patient with esophageal cancer.
- Teach the patient having open conventional esophageal surgery about incisions, drains, and jejunostomy tube placement before he or she undergoes surgery for esophageal cancer.
- For the patient with a nasogastric (NG) tube, check the NG tube every 4 to 8 hours for proper placement and anchorage; follow guidelines as outlined in Chart 57-9.
- Assess the patient after esophageal surgery for pulmonary and cardiac complications of surgery, and report changes to the health care provider.
- Assess patients for key features of esophageal tumors as listed in Chart 57-8.

Care of Patients with Stomach Disorders

Donna D. Ignatavicius

evolve WEBSITE

http://evolve.elsevier.com/Iggy/

Animation: Bleeding Ulcer, Pathophysiology
Answer Key for NCLEX Examination Challenges and
    Decision-Making Challenges
Audio Glossary

Concept Map Creator
Key Points
Review Questions for the NCLEX® Examination

LEARNING OUTCOMES

Safe and Effective Care Environment

1. Describe the importance of collaborating with members of the health care team when caring for patients with stomach disorders.
2. Identify community resources for patients with gastric disorders.

Health Promotion and Maintenance

3. Develop a teaching plan for patients about complementary and alternative therapies that have been used to help manage gastritis and peptic ulcer disease (PUD).
4. Plan interventions to promote GI health and prevent gastritis.

Psychosocial Integrity

5. Identify the need for end-of-life care for patients with advanced gastric cancer.

Physiological Integrity

6. Compare etiologies and assessment findings of acute and chronic gastritis.

7. Identify risk factors for gastritis.
8. Compare and contrast assessment findings associated with gastric and duodenal ulcers.
9. Identify the most common medical complications that can result from PUD.
10. Describe the purpose and adverse effects of drug therapy for gastritis and PUD.
11. Monitor patients with PUD and gastric cancer for signs of upper GI bleeding.
12. Prioritize interventions for patients with upper GI bleeding.
13. Plan individualized care for the patient having gastric surgery.
14. Explain the purpose and procedure for gastric lavage.
15. Evaluate the impact of gastric disorders on the nutrition status of the patient.
16. Develop a preoperative and postoperative plan of care for the patient undergoing gastric surgery.
17. Identify risk factors for gastric cancer.

Although only a few diseases affect the stomach, they can be very serious and in some cases life threatening. The most common disorders include gastritis, peptic ulcer disease, and gastric cancer. Each of these health problems can result in impaired or altered *digestion* and *nutrition*. The stomach is part of the upper GI system that is responsible for a large part of the digestive process. Patient-centered collaborative care for stomach disorders often includes therapies to meet the patient's *need for adequate nutrition.*

GASTRITIS

Gastritis is the inflammation of gastric mucosa (stomach lining). It can be scattered or localized and can be classified according to cause, cellular changes, or distribution of the lesions. Gastritis can be erosive (causing ulcers) or non-erosive. Although the mucosal changes that result from *acute* gastritis typically heal after several months, this is not true for *chronic* gastritis.

Pathophysiology

Prostaglandins provide a protective mucosal barrier that prevents the stomach from digesting itself by a process called acid autodigestion. If there is a break in the protective barrier, mucosal injury occurs. The resulting injury is worsened by histamine release and vagus nerve stimulation. Hydrochloric acid can then diffuse back into the mucosa and injure small vessels. This back-diffusion causes edema, hemorrhage, and erosion of the stomach's lining. The pathologic changes of gastritis include vascular congestion, edema, acute inflammatory cell infiltration, and degenerative changes in the superficial epithelium of the stomach lining.

Types of Gastritis

Inflammation of the gastric mucosa or submucosa after exposure to local irritants or other cause can result in acute gastritis. The early pathologic manifestation of gastritis is a thickened, reddened mucous membrane with prominent rugae, or folds. Various degrees of mucosal necrosis and inflammatory reaction occur in acute disease. The diagnosis cannot be based solely on clinical symptoms. Complete regeneration and healing usually occur within a few days. If the stomach muscle is not involved, complete recovery usually occurs with no residual evidence of gastric inflammatory reaction. If the muscle is affected, hemorrhage may occur during an episode of acute gastritis.

Chronic gastritis appears as a patchy, diffuse (spread out) inflammation of the mucosal lining of the stomach. As the disease progresses, the walls and lining of the stomach thin and atrophy. With progressive gastric atrophy from chronic mucosal injury, the function of the parietal (acid-secreting) cells decreases and the source of intrinsic factor is lost. The intrinsic factor is critical for absorption of vitamin B_{12}. When body stores of vitamin B_{12} are eventually depleted, pernicious anemia results. The amount and concentration of acid in stomach secretions gradually decrease until the secretions consist of only mucus and water.

Chronic gastritis is associated with an increased risk for gastric cancer. The persistent inflammation extends deep into the mucosa, causing destruction of the gastric glands and cellular changes. Chronic gastritis may be categorized as type A, type B, or atrophic.

Type A (nonerosive) chronic gastritis refers to an inflammation of the glands, as well as the fundus and body of the stomach. Type B chronic gastritis usually affects the glands of the antrum but may involve the entire stomach. In atrophic chronic gastritis, diffuse inflammation and destruction of deeply located glands accompany the condition. Chronic atrophic gastritis affects all layers of the stomach, thus decreasing the number of cells. The muscle thickens, and inflammation is present. Chronic atrophic gastritis is characterized by total loss of fundal glands, minimal inflammation, thinning of the gastric mucosa, and intestinal metaplasia (abnormal tissue development). These cellular changes can lead to peptic ulcer disease (PUD) and gastric cancer (McCance et al., 2010).

Etiology and Genetic Risk

Acute Gastritis. The onset of infection with Helicobacter pylori can result in acute gastritis. *H. pylori* is a gram-negative bacterium that penetrates the mucosal gel layer of the gastric epithelium. Although less common, other forms of bacterial gastritis from organisms such as staphylococci, streptococci, *Escherichia coli,* or salmonella can cause life-threatening problems such as sepsis and extensive tissue necrosis (death).

Long-term NSAID use creates a high risk for acute gastritis. NSAIDs inhibit prostaglandin production in the mucosal barrier. Other risk factors include alcohol, caffeine, and corticosteroids. Acute gastritis is also caused by local irritation from radiation therapy and accidental or intentional ingestion of corrosive substances, including acids or alkalis (e.g., lye and drain cleaners). Emotional stress and acute anxiety may also contribute to gastritis.

Chronic Gastritis. Type A gastritis has been associated with the presence of antibodies to parietal cells and intrinsic factor. Therefore an autoimmune cause for this type of gastritis is likely. Parietal cell antibodies have been found in most patients with pernicious anemia and in more than one half of those with type A gastritis. A genetic link to this disease, with an autosomal dominant pattern of inheritance, has been found in the relatives of patients with pernicious anemia (McCance et al., 2010).

The most common form of the disease is type B gastritis, caused by *H. pylori* infection. A direct correlation exists between the number of organisms and the degree of cellular abnormality present. The host response to the *H. pylori* infection is activation of lymphocytes and neutrophils. Release of inflammatory cytokines, such as interleukin (IL)-1, IL-8, and tumor necrosis factor (TNF)–alpha, damages the gastric mucosa (McCance et al., 2010).

Chronic local irritation and toxic effects caused by alcohol ingestion, radiation therapy, and smoking have been linked to chronic gastritis. Surgical procedures that involve the pyloric sphincter, such as a pyloroplasty, can lead to gastritis by causing reflux of alkaline secretions into the stomach. Other systemic disorders such as Crohn's disease, graft-versus-host disease, and uremia can also precipitate the development of chronic gastritis.

Atrophic gastritis is a type of chronic gastritis that is seen most often in older adults. It can occur after exposure to toxic substances in the workplace (e.g., benzene, lead, nickel) or *H. pylori* infection, or it can be related to autoimmune factors.

Health Promotion and Maintenance

Gastritis is a very common health problem in the United States. Yet, a balanced diet, regular exercise, and stress-reduction techniques can help prevent it (Chart 58-1). A balanced diet includes following the recommendations of the U.S. Department of Agriculture (USDA) and limiting intake of foods and spices that can cause gastric distress, such as caffeine, chocolate, mustard, pepper, and other strong or hot spices. Alcohol and tobacco consumption should also be avoided. Regular exercise maintains peristalsis, which helps prevent gastric contents from irritating the gastric mucosa. Stress-reduction techniques can include aerobic exercise, meditation, reading, and/or yoga, depending on individual preferences. Psychotherapy may also be considered.

Excessive use of aspirin and other NSAIDs should also be avoided. If a family member has *H. pylori* infection or has had

---

CHART 58-1   PATIENT AND FAMILY EDUCATION: PREPARING FOR SELF-MANAGEMENT

Gastritis Prevention

- Eat a well-balanced diet.
- Avoid drinking excessive amounts of alcoholic beverages.
- Use caution in taking large doses of aspirin, other NSAIDs (e.g., ibuprofen), and corticosteroids.
- Avoid excessive intake of caffeine-containing beverages, especially coffee and tea.
- Be sure that foods and water are safe, to avoid contamination.
- Manage stress levels using complementary and alternative therapies, such as relaxation and meditation techniques.
- Stop smoking.
- Protect yourself against exposure to toxic substances in the workplace, such as lead and nickel.
- Seek medical treatment if you are experiencing symptoms of esophageal reflux (see Chapter 57).

CHART 58-2   KEY FEATURES

Gastritis

Acute Gastritis	Chronic Gastritis
• Rapid onset of epigastric pain or discomfort	• Vague report of epigastric pain that is relieved by food
• Nausea and vomiting	• Anorexia
• Hematemesis (vomiting blood)	• Nausea or vomiting
• Gastric hemorrhage	• Intolerance of fatty and spicy foods
• Dyspepsia (heartburn)	• Pernicious anemia
• Anorexia	

---

it in the past, patient testing should be considered. This test can identify the bacteria before they cause gastritis.

PATIENT-CENTERED COLLABORATIVE CARE

ASSESSMENT

Symptoms of *acute* gastritis range from mild to severe. The patient may report epigastric discomfort, anorexia, cramping, nausea, and vomiting (Chart 58-2). Assess for abdominal tenderness and bloating, hematemesis (vomiting blood), or melena (traces of blood in the stool). Symptoms last only a few hours or days and vary with the cause. Aspirin/NSAID–related gastritis may result in dyspepsia (heartburn). Gastritis or food poisoning caused by endotoxins, such as staphylococcal endotoxin, has an abrupt onset. Severe nausea and vomiting often occur within 5 hours of ingestion of the contaminated food. *In some cases, gastric hemorrhage is the presenting symptom, which is a life-threatening emergency.*

Chronic gastritis causes few symptoms unless ulceration occurs. Patients may report nausea, vomiting, or upper abdominal discomfort. Periodic epigastric pain may occur after a meal. Some patients have anorexia (see Chart 58-2).

Several blood tests are available to detect *H. pylori* if gastritis or an ulcer is suspected. Examples of these tests are described on p. 1228 in the Peptic Ulcer Disease section of this chapter. One of the most common methods is a blood test to detect *IgG or IgM anti–H. pylori* antibodies.

Esophagogastroduodenoscopy (EGD) via an endoscope with biopsy is the gold standard for diagnosing gastritis. The physician takes a biopsy to establish a definitive diagnosis of the type of gastritis. If lesions are patchy and diffuse, biopsy of several suspicious areas may be necessary to avoid misdiagnosis. A *cytologic examination* of the biopsy specimen is performed to confirm or rule out gastric cancer. Tissue samples can also be taken to detect *H. pylori* using *rapid urease testing*. As the name implies, this test provides quick results unlike the more traditional tissue culture that takes several weeks to determine if the bacteria are present. The results of these tests are more reliable if the patient has discontinued taking antacids for at least a week (Pagana & Pagana, 2010).

INTERVENTIONS

Patients with gastritis are not often seen in the acute care setting unless they have an exacerbation ("flare up") of acute or chronic gastritis that results in fluid and electrolyte imbalance or bleeding. Collaborative care is directed toward supportive care for relieving the symptoms and removing or reducing the cause of discomfort.

Acute gastritis is treated symptomatically and supportively because the healing process is spontaneous, usually occurring within a few days. When the cause is removed, pain and discomfort usually subside. If bleeding is severe, a blood transfusion may be necessary. Fluid replacement is prescribed for patients with severe fluid loss. Surgery, such as partial gastrectomy, pyloroplasty, and/or vagotomy, may be needed for patients with major bleeding or ulceration. Treatment of *chronic* gastritis varies with the cause. The approach to management includes the elimination of causative agents, treatment of any underlying disease (e.g., uremia, Crohn's disease), avoidance of toxic substances (e.g., alcohol, tobacco), and health teaching.

Eliminating the causative factors, such as *H. pylori* infection if present, is the primary treatment approach. Drugs and nutritional therapy are also used. In the *acute* phase, the health care provider prescribes drugs that block and buffer gastric acid secretions to relieve pain.

H_2-receptor antagonists, such as famotidine (Pepcid) and nizatidine (Axid), are typically used to block gastric secretions. Sucralfate (Carafate, Sulcrate ✦), a *mucosal barrier fortifier*, may also be prescribed. *Antacids* used as buffering agents include aluminum hydroxide combined with magnesium hydroxide (Maalox) and aluminum hydroxide combined with simethicone and magnesium hydroxide (Mylanta). Antisecretory agents (proton pump inhibitors [PPIs]) such as omeprazole (Prilosec) or pantoprazole (Protonix) may be prescribed to suppress gastric acid secretion (Chart 58-3).

⚠ NURSING SAFETY PRIORITY

Drug Alert

Teach the patient to monitor for symptom relief and side effects of drugs to treat gastritis and to notify the health care provider of any adverse effects or worsening of gastric distress. The dose, frequency, or type of drug may need to be changed if symptoms of gastric irritation appear or persist. *Remind patients not to take additional over-the-counter (OTC) drugs such as Pepcid AC if they are taking similar prescribed drugs.*

CHART 58-3 COMMON EXAMPLES OF DRUG THERAPY

Peptic Ulcer Disease

DRUG AND USUAL DOSAGE	PURPOSE OF DRUG	NURSING INTERVENTIONS	RATIONALES
Antacids			
Magnesium hydroxide with aluminum hydroxide (Maalox, Mylanta) 50-80 mEq orally 1 hr and 3 hr after meals and at bedtime	Increases pH of gastric contents by deactivating pepsin	Give 2 hr after meals and at bedtime. Use liquid rather than tablets. Do not give other drugs within 1-2 hr of antacids. Assess patients for a history of renal disease. Assess the patient for a history of heart failure. Observe the patient for the side effect of diarrhea.	Hydrogen ion load is high after ingestion of foods. Suspensions are more effective than chewable tablets. Antacids interfere with absorption of other drugs. Hypermagnesemia may result. These antacids have a high sodium content. These antacids contain magnesium, which cannot be excreted by poorly functioning kidneys, thus causing toxicity. Inadequate renal perfusion from heart failure decreases the ability of the kidneys to excrete magnesium, thus causing toxicity. Magnesium often causes diarrhea.
Aluminum hydroxide (Amphojel) 50-80 mEq orally 1 hr and 3 hr after meals and at bedtime		Give 1 hr after meals and at bedtime. Use liquid rather than tablets if palatable. Do not give other drugs within 1-2 hr of antacids. Observe patients for the side effect of constipation. If constipation occurs, consider alternating with magnesium antacid. Use for patients with renal failure.	Hydrogen ion load is high after ingestion of food. Suspensions are more effective than chewable tablets. Antacids interfere with absorption of other drugs. Aluminum causes constipation, and magnesium has a laxative effect. Aluminum binds with phosphates in the GI tract. This antacid does not contain magnesium.
H₂ Antagonists			
Ranitidine (Zantac) 150 mg orally twice daily or 300 mg orally at bedtime; 50 mg IV every 6 hr or 8 mg/hr IV (continuous) Famotidine (Pepcid) 40 mg orally once daily or in two divided doses; 20 mg IV every 12 hr Nizatidine (Axid) 150 mg orally twice daily or 300 mg at bedtime	Decreases gastric acid secretions by blocking histamine receptors in parietal cells	Give single dose at bedtime for treatment of GI ulcers. **NOTE:** IV ranitidine may also be given to prevent surgical stress ulcers. **NOTE:** IV famotidine may also be given to prevent surgical stress ulcers.	Bedtime administration suppresses nocturnal acid production.

Continued

CHART 58-3   COMMON EXAMPLES OF DRUG THERAPY

Peptic Ulcer Disease—cont'd

DRUG AND USUAL DOSAGE	PURPOSE OF DRUG	NURSING INTERVENTIONS	RATIONALES
Mucosal Barrier Fortifiers			
Sucralfate (Carafate, Sulcrate ✦) 1 g orally four times daily or 2 g twice daily	Binds with bile acids and pepsin to protect stomach mucosa	Give 1 hr before and 2 hr after meals, and at bedtime. Do not give within 30 min of giving antacids or other drugs.	Food may interfere with drug's adherence to mucosa. Antacids may interfere with effect.
Proton Pump Inhibitors			
Omeprazole (Prilosec, Losec ✦) 20 mg orally twice daily or 40 mg at bedtime	Suppresses H,K–ATPase enzyme system of gastric acid secretion	Have patients take capsule whole; do not crush (unless giving Zegerid, a fast-acting form of the drug). Give single dose at bedtime for ulcer disease.	Delayed-release capsules allow absorption after granules leave the stomach. Bedtime administration suppresses nocturnal acid production.
Lansoprazole (Prevacid) 15 or 30 mg orally at bedtime		Give single dose at bedtime for ulcer disease; do not crush.	Bedtime administration suppresses nocturnal acid production.
Rabeprazole (Aciphex) 20 mg orally once daily		Take after the morning meal. Do not crush capsule.	Drug promotes healing and symptom relief of duodenal ulcers. Drug is a sustained-release capsule.
Pantoprazole (Protonix) 40 mg orally or IV daily for 7-10 days		Do not crush. IV form must be given with filter and in a separate line. Do not give Protonix IV with other IV drugs.	Drug is enteric-coated. Given IV, drug precipitates easily. The IV form is not compatible with most other drugs.
Esomeprazole (Nexium) 20 or 40 mg orally daily (or IV daily for 7-10 days)		Give 1 hr before meals. Assess for hepatic impairment. Do not give Nexium IV with other IV drugs.	Food decreases absorption. Patients with severe hepatic problems need a low dose. The IV form is not compatible with most other drugs.
Prostaglandin Analogs			
Misoprostol (Cytotec) 200 mcg orally four times daily	Decreases gastric secretions and enhances resistance to mucosal injury when patient is taking NSAIDs	Take with food. Avoid magnesium-containing antacids.	Drug protects against NSAID-induced ulcers. Both misoprostol and magnesium-containing antacids can cause diarrhea.
Antimicrobials			
Clarithromycin (Biaxin) 500 mg orally three times daily	Treats *Helicobacter pylori*	Antimicrobials should be given as part of therapy to eradicate *H. pylori* infection. The selection of the specific drug depends on its effectiveness, side effects, and drug interactions.	*H. pylori* is a gram-negative bacterium implicated in the development of peptic ulcer disease (PUD).
Amoxicillin (Amoxil) 1 g orally twice daily			
Tetracycline 500 mg orally four times daily			
Metronidazole (Flagyl) 250 mg orally three times daily and at bedtime			

Patients with *chronic* gastritis may require vitamin B$_{12}$ for prevention or treatment of pernicious anemia. If *H. pylori* is found, the health care provider treats the infection. Current practice for infection treatment is described on p. 1229 in the discussion of Drug Therapy in the Peptic Ulcer Disease section.

The nurse, health care provider, or pharmacist teaches patients to avoid drugs and other irritants that are associated with gastritis episodes, if possible. These drugs include corticosteroids, erythromycin (E-Mycin, Erythromid ✚), and NSAIDs, such as naproxen (Naprosyn) and ibuprofen (Motrin, Advil, Amersol ✚, Novo-Profen ✚). NSAIDs are also available as OTC drugs and should not be used. Teach patients to read all OTC drug labels because many preparations contain aspirin or other NSAID.

Instruct the patient to limit intake of any foods and spices that cause distress, such as those that contain caffeine or high acid content (e.g., tomato products, citrus juices) or those that are heavily seasoned with strong or hot spices. Bell peppers and onions are also commonly irritating foods. Most patients seem to progress better with a bland, non-spicy diet and smaller, more frequent meals. Alcohol and tobacco should also be avoided.

Assist the patient with various techniques that reduce stress and discomfort, such as progressive relaxation, cutaneous stimulation, guided imagery, and distraction. Other complementary and alternative therapies that have been used are listed in Table 58-1. Chapter 2 describes these therapies in detail.

❓ NCLEX EXAMINATION CHALLENGE

Health Promotion and Maintenance

A client with a recent diagnosis of acute gastritis needs health teaching about nutrition therapy. Which foods and beverages should the nurse teach the client to avoid? **Select all that apply.**
A. Potatoes
B. Onions
C. Apples
D. Milk
E. Orange juice
F. Tomato juice

TABLE 58-1 COMMONLY USED COMPLEMENTARY AND ALTERNATIVE THERAPIES FOR GASTRITIS AND PEPTIC ULCER DISEASE (PUD)

Herbs and Vitamins
- Gamma-linolenic acid (GLA)
- Probiotics
- Vitamin B$_{12}$
- Bromelain
- Vitamin A
- Vitamin C
- Astragalus
- Barberry
- Chamomile
- Cranberry
- Dandelion
- Ginger
- Green tea
- Licorice
- Slippery elm
- Tumeric
- Yarrow

Homeopathy
- Pulsatilla
- Ipecacuanha
- Carbo vegetabilis
- Nux vomica

PEPTIC ULCER DISEASE

A **peptic ulcer** is a mucosal lesion of the stomach or duodenum. **Peptic ulcer disease** (PUD) results when mucosal defenses become impaired and no longer protect the epithelium from the effects of acid and pepsin.

Pathophysiology

Types of Ulcers

Three types of ulcers may occur: gastric ulcers, duodenal ulcers, and stress ulcers (less common). Most gastric and duodenal ulcers are caused by *H. pylori* infection, which is transmitted via the fecal-oral route and thought to be acquired in childhood. It can also be transmitted from contaminated endoscopic equipment (Pagana & Pagana, 2010). About half of the world's population is infected with the bacterium (Fromm, 2009).

As a response to the bacteria, cytokines, neutrophils, and other substances are activated and cause epithelial cell necrosis. Urease, a substance secreted by the *H. pylori* bacterium, produces ammonia and creates a more alkaline environment (McCance et al., 2010). Hydrogen ions are then released in response to the presence of ammonia and contribute further to mucosal damage. Urease can be detected through laboratory testing to confirm the *H. pylori* infection.

Gastric ulcers usually develop in the antrum of the stomach near acid-secreting mucosa. When a break in the mucosal barrier occurs (such as that caused by *H. pylori* infection), hydrochloric acid injures the epithelium. Gastric ulcers may then result from back-diffusion of acid or dysfunction of the pyloric sphincter (Fig. 58-1). Without normal functioning of the pyloric sphincter, bile refluxes (backs up) into the stomach. This reflux of bile acids may break the integrity of the mucosal barrier and produce hydrogen ion back-diffusion, which leads to mucosal inflammation. Toxic agents and bile then destroy the membrane of the gastric mucosa.

Gastric emptying is often delayed in patients with gastric ulceration. This causes regurgitation of duodenal contents, which worsens the gastric mucosal injury. Decreased blood flow to the gastric mucosa may also alter the defense barrier and thereby allow ulceration to occur. Gastric ulcers are deep and penetrating, and they usually occur on the lesser curvature of the stomach, near the pylorus (Fig. 58-2).

Most *duodenal ulcers* occur in the upper portion of the duodenum. They are deep, sharply demarcated lesions that penetrate through the mucosa and submucosa into the muscularis propria (muscle layer). The floor of the ulcer consists of a necrotic area residing on granulation tissue and surrounded by areas of fibrosis.

The main feature of a duodenal ulcer is high gastric acid secretion, although a wide range of secretory levels is found. In patients with duodenal ulcers, pH levels are low (excess acid) in the duodenum for long periods. Protein-rich meals, calcium, and vagus nerve excitation stimulate acid secretion. Combined with hypersecretion, a rapid emptying of food from the stomach reduces the buffering effect of food and delivers a large acid bolus to the duodenum (see Fig. 58-1). Inhibitory secretory mechanisms and pancreatic secretion may be insufficient to control the acid load.

Many patients with duodenal ulcer disease have confirmed *H. pylori* infection. These bacteria produce substances that

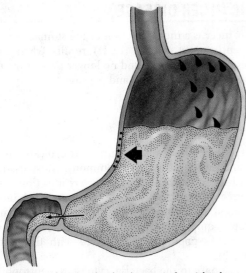

Conditions favoring the development of **gastric ulcers** are normal gastric acid secretion and delayed stomach emptying with *increased diffusion of gastric acid back into the stomach tissues.*

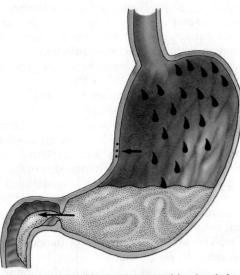

Conditions favoring the development of **duodenal ulcers** are normal diffusion of acid back into stomach tissues with *increased secretion of gastric acid* and *increased stomach emptying.*

FIG. 58-1 The pathophysiology of peptic ulcer.

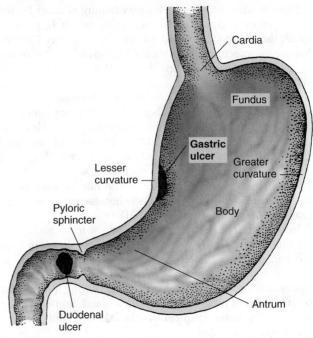

FIG. 58-2 The most common sites for peptic ulcers.

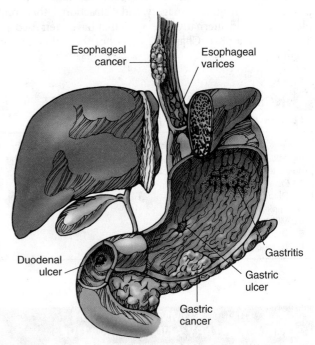

FIG. 58-3 Common causes of upper GI bleeding.

damage the mucosa. Urease produced by *H. pylori* breaks down urea into ammonia.

Stress ulcers are acute gastric mucosal lesions occurring after an acute medical crisis or trauma, such as head injury and sepsis. In the patient who is NPO for major surgery, gastritis may lead to stress ulcers, which are multiple shallow erosions of the stomach and occasionally the proximal duodenum. Patients who are critically ill, especially those with extensive burns (Curling's ulcer), sepsis (ischemic ulcer), or increased intracranial pressure (Cushing's ulcer), are also susceptible to these ulcers.

Bleeding caused by gastric erosion is the main manifestation of acute stress ulcers. Multifocal lesions associated with stress ulcers occur in the stomach and proximal duodenum. These lesions begin as areas of ischemia and evolve into erosions and ulcerations that may progress to massive hemorrhage. Little is known of the exact etiology of stress ulcers. However, in the presence of elevated levels of hydrochloric acid, ischemic areas can progress to erosive gastritis and subsequent ulcerations. Stress ulcers are associated with lengthened hospital stay and increased mortality rates.

Complications of Ulcers

The most common complications of PUD are hemorrhage, perforation, pyloric obstruction, and intractable disease. *Hemorrhage is the most serious complication* (Fig. 58-3). It

---

tends to occur more often in patients with *gastric* ulcers and in older adults. Many patients have a second episode of bleeding if underlying infection with *H. pylori* remains untreated or if therapy does not include an H_2 antagonist. With massive bleeding, the patient vomits bright red or coffee-ground blood (hematemesis). Hematemesis usually indicates bleeding at or above the duodenojejunal junction (upper GI bleeding) (Chart 58-4).

Minimal bleeding from ulcers is manifested by occult blood in a tarry stool (melena). Melena may occur in patients with gastric ulcers but is more common in those with duodenal ulcers. Gastric acid digestion of blood typically results in a granular dark vomitus *(coffee-ground appearance)*. The digestion of blood within the duodenum and small intestine may result in a black stool.

Gastric and duodenal ulcers can perforate and bleed. *Perforation* occurs when the ulcer becomes so deep that the entire thickness of the stomach or duodenum is worn away. The stomach or duodenal contents can then leak into the peritoneal cavity. Sudden, sharp pain begins in the mid-epigastric region and spreads over the entire abdomen. The amount of pain correlates with the amount and type of GI contents spilled. The classic pain causes the patient to be apprehensive. The abdomen is tender, rigid, and boardlike (peritonitis). The patient assumes the knee-chest ("fetal") position to decrease the tension on the abdominal muscles. He or she can become severely ill within hours. Bacterial septicemia and hypovolemic shock follow. Peristalsis diminishes, and paralytic ileus develops. *Peptic ulcer perforation is a surgical emergency and can be life threatening!*

Pyloric (gastric outlet) obstruction (blockage) occurs in a small percentage of patients and is manifested by vomiting caused by stasis and gastric dilation. Obstruction occurs at the pylorus (the gastric outlet) and is caused by scarring, edema, inflammation, or a combination of these factors.

Symptoms of obstruction include abdominal bloating, nausea, and vomiting. When vomiting persists, the patient may have hypochloremic (metabolic) alkalosis from loss of large quantities of acid gastric juice (hydrogen and chloride ions) in the vomitus. Hypokalemia may also result from the vomiting or metabolic alkalosis.

Many patients with ulcers have a single episode with no recurrence. However, *intractability* may develop from complications of ulcers, excessive stressors in the patient's life, or an inability to adhere to long-term therapy. He or she no longer responds to conservative management, or recurrences of symptoms interfere with ADLs. In general, the patient continues to have recurrent pain and discomfort despite treatment. Those who fail to respond to traditional treatments or who have a relapse after discontinuation of therapy are referred to a gastroenterologist.

Etiology and Genetic Risk

Peptic ulcer development is associated primarily with bacterial infection with *H. pylori and NSAIDs*. NSAIDs (e.g., ibuprofen) break down the mucosal barrier and disrupt the mucosal protection mediated systemically by cyclooxygenase (COX) inhibition. COX-2 inhibitors (celecoxib [Celebrex]) are less likely to cause mucosal damage but place patients at high risk for cardiovascular events, such as myocardial infarction. In addition, NSAIDs cause decreased endogenous prostaglandins, resulting in local gastric mucosal injury. GI complications from NSAID use can occur at any time, even after long-term uncomplicated use. NSAID-related ulcers are difficult to treat, even with long-term therapy, because these ulcers have a high rate of recurrence.

Certain substances may contribute to gastroduodenal ulceration by altering gastric secretion, producing localized damage to mucosa and interfering with the healing process. For example, corticosteroids (e.g., prednisone), theophylline (Theo-Dur), and caffeine stimulate hydrochloric acid production. Patients receiving radiation therapy may also develop GI ulcers. Other risk factors for PUD are the same as for gastritis (see Chart 58-1).

Genetic factors may be important. *H. pylori* infection tends to occur in people who are genetically susceptible. Those with a family history of PUD are at higher risk for having PUD than those without a family history (McCance et al., 2010).

Incidence/Prevalence

PUD affects millions of people across the world. However, health care provider visits, hospitalizations, and the mortality rate for PUD have decreased in the past few decades. The use of proton pump inhibitors and *H. pylori* treatment may explain these declines. Duodenal ulcers are increasing in "baby boomers," however, which may be the result of increased NSAID use for arthritic pain as they age.

Health Promotion and Maintenance

Health promotion and illness prevention practices are the same as for gastritis (see Chart 58-1). For critically ill patients, health care providers prescribe drug therapy to prevent stress ulcers as described on p. 1229 in the Drug Therapy section.

PATIENT-CENTERED COLLABORATIVE CARE

ASSESSMENT

History

Collect data related to the causes and risk factors for peptic ulcer disease (PUD). Question the patient about factors that can influence the development of PUD, including alcohol intake and tobacco use. Note if certain foods such as tomatoes or caffeinated beverages precipitate or worsen symptoms. Information regarding actual or perceived daily stressors should also be obtained.

A history of current or past medical conditions focuses on GI problems, particularly any history of diagnosis or treatment for *H. pylori* infection. Review all prescription and OTC drugs that the patient is taking. Specifically inquire whether the patient is taking corticosteroids, chemotherapy, or NSAIDs. Also ask whether he or she has ever undergone radiation treatments. Assess whether the patient has had any GI surgeries, especially a partial gastrectomy, which can cause chronic gastritis.

A history of GI upset, pain and its relationship to eating and sleep patterns, and actions taken to relieve pain are also important. Inquire about any changes in the character of the pain, because this may signal the development of complications. For example, if pain that was once intermittent and relieved by food and antacids becomes constant and radiates to the back or upper quadrant, the patient may have ulcer perforation. However, many people with active duodenal or gastric ulcers report having no ulcer symptoms.

Physical Assessment/Clinical Manifestations

Physical assessment findings may reveal epigastric tenderness, usually located at the midline between the umbilicus and the xiphoid process. *If perforation into the peritoneal cavity is present, the patient has a rigid, boardlike abdomen accompanied by rebound tenderness and pain.* Initially, auscultation of the abdomen may reveal hyperactive bowel sounds, but these may diminish with progression of the disorder.

Dyspepsia (indigestion) is the most commonly reported symptom associated with PUD. It is typically described as sharp, burning, or gnawing. Some patients may perceive discomfort as a sensation of abdominal pressure or of fullness or hunger. Specific differences between gastric and duodenal ulcers are listed in Table 58-2.

Gastric ulcer pain often occurs in the upper epigastrium with localization to the left of the midline and is aggravated by food. *Duodenal* ulcer pain is usually located to the right of the epigastrium. The pain associated with a duodenal ulcer occurs 90 minutes to 3 hours *after* eating and often awakens the patient at night. Pain may also be exacerbated (made worse) by certain foods (e.g., tomatoes, hot spices, fried foods, onions, alcohol, caffeine drinks) and certain drugs (e.g., NSAIDs, corticosteroids). Perform a comprehensive pain assessment that includes:

- Location
- Characteristics
- Onset/duration
- Frequency
- Quality
- Severity
- All precipitating and alleviating factors

Nausea and vomiting may be symptoms accompanying ulcer disease, most commonly with pyloric sphincter dysfunction. It results from gastric stasis associated with pyloric obstruction. Appetite is generally maintained in patients with a peptic ulcer unless pyloric obstruction is present. Some health care agencies use a 0-to-5 nausea scale to rate the degree of the patient's report of nausea (Halpin et al., 2010).

To assess for fluid volume deficit that occurs from bleeding, take orthostatic blood pressures and monitor for signs and symptoms of dehydration. Orthostatic changes are present if there is a decrease of more than 20 mm Hg in systolic blood pressure, a decrease of 10 mm Hg in diastolic blood pressure, and/or an increase in pulse when the patient rises from a lying to an erect (sitting or, if possible, standing) position. Also assess for dizziness, especially when the patient

TABLE 58-2	DIFFERENTIAL FEATURES OF GASTRIC AND DUODENAL ULCERS	
FEATURE	**GASTRIC ULCER**	**DUODENAL ULCER**
Age	Usually 50 yr or older	Usually 50 yr or older
Gender	Male/female ratio of 1.1:1	Male/female ratio of 1:1
Blood group	No differentiation	Most often type O
General nourishment	May be malnourished	Usually well nourished
Stomach acid production	Normal secretion or hyposecretion	Hypersecretion
Occurrence	Mucosa exposed to acid-pepsin secretion	Mucosa exposed to acid-pepsin secretion
Clinical course	Healing and recurrence	Healing and recurrence
Pain	Occurs 30-60 min after a meal; at night: rarely. Worsened by ingestion of food	Occurs 1½-3 hr after a meal; at night: often awakens patient between 1 and 2 AM. Relieved by ingestion of food
Response to treatment	Healing with appropriate therapy	Healing with appropriate therapy
Hemorrhage	Hematemesis more common than melena	Melena more common than hematemesis
Malignant change	Perhaps in less than 10%	Rare
Recurrence	Tends to heal, and recurs often in the same location	60% recur within 1 yr; 90% recur within 2 yr
Surrounding mucosa	Atrophic gastritis	No gastritis

is upright, because this is a symptom of fluid volume deficit. Older adults often experience dizziness when they get out of bed and are at risk for falls.

NCLEX EXAMINATION CHALLENGE

Physiological Integrity

When taking a history of a client diagnosed with a duodenal ulcer, which assessment finding does the nurse expect?
A. Severe weight loss
B. Pain while eating
C. Hematemesis after eating
D. Waking at night with pain

Psychosocial Assessment

Assess the impact of ulcer disease on the patient's lifestyle, occupation, family, and social and leisure activities. Evaluate the impact that lifestyle changes will have on the patient and family. This assessment may reveal information about the patient's ability to adhere to the prescribed treatment regimen and to obtain the needed social support to alter his or her lifestyle.

Laboratory Assessment

Serologic testing for IgG anti–*H. pylori* antibody is the most common noninvasive method to confirm *H. pylori* infection. IgA and IgM anti–*H. pylori* antibody testing may also be performed. Serologic immune testing methods, such as the enzyme-linked immunosorbent assay (ELISA), may be done several months after the diagnosis of infection to determine the effectiveness of treatment. A negative result indicates that treatment was successful.

Although *H. pylori* does not survive in the stool, an ELISA may detect its presence. A breath test to detect urease may also be performed as a screening tool, but it is not reliable as the serologic testing method.

Patients who have venous bleeding from a peptic ulcer may have *decreased hemoglobin and hematocrit* values. The *stool* may also be positive for occult (not seen) blood if bleeding is present.

Imaging Assessment

In the past, upper GI series with barium follow-through was the typical test for diagnosing peptic ulcers. However, this procedure is not the most reliable way to visualize any lesions. If perforation is suspected, the health care provider may request a chest and abdomen x-ray series.

Other Diagnostic Assessment

The major diagnostic test for PUD is esophagogastroduodenoscopy (EGD), which is the most accurate means of establishing a diagnosis. Direct visualization of the ulcer crater by EGD allows the health care provider to take specimens for *H. pylori* testing and for biopsy and cytologic studies for ruling out gastric cancer. The rapid urease test can confirm a quick diagnosis because urease is produced by the bacteria in the gastric mucosa. EGD may be repeated at 4- to 6-week intervals while the health care provider evaluates the progress of healing in response to therapy. Chapter 55 describes this test in more detail.

GI bleeding may be tested using a nuclear medicine GI bleeding study. No special preparation is required for this scan. The patient is injected with a contrast medium (usually Tc99m), and the GI system is scanned for the presence of bleeding after a waiting period. A second scan may be done 1 to 2 days after the bleeding is treated to determine if the interventions were effective.

ANALYSIS

The priority patient problems for patients with peptic ulcer disease (PUD) are:
1. Acute or Chronic Pain related to gastric and/or duodenal ulceration
2. Potential for upper GI bleeding

PLANNING AND IMPLEMENTATION

Managing Acute Pain or Chronic Pain

Planning: Expected Outcomes. The patient with PUD is expected to report pain control as evidenced by no more than a 3 on a 0-10 pain intensity scale.

Interventions. PUD causes significant discomfort that impacts many aspects of daily living. Interventions to manage pain focus on drug therapy and dietary changes. One of the primary purposes for drug therapy is to decrease pain by eliminating *H. pylori* infection and promoting healing of gastric mucosa.

Drug Therapy. The primary purposes of drug therapy in the treatment of PUD are to (1) provide pain relief, (2) eliminate *H. pylori* infection, (3) heal ulcerations, and (4) prevent recurrence. Several different regimens can be used. In selecting a therapeutic drug regimen, the health care provider must consider the efficacy of the treatment, the anticipated side effects, the ability of the patient to adhere to the regimen, and the cost of the treatment.

Although numerous drugs have been evaluated for the treatment of *H. pylori* infection, no single agent has been used successfully against the organism. A common drug regimen for *H. pylori* infection is PPI-triple therapy, which includes a proton pump inhibitor (PPI) such as lansoprazole (Prevacid) plus two antibiotics such as metronidazole (Flagyl, Novonidazol ✦) and tetracycline (Ala-Tet, Panmycin, Nu-Tetra ✦) or clarithromycin (Biaxin, Biaxin XL) and amoxicillin (Amoxil, Amoxi ✦) for 7 to 14 days. Seven-day therapy is also effective when a PPI, levofloxacin (Levaquin), and either amoxicillin or clarithromycin are used (Schrauwen et al., 2009).

> ### CONSIDERATIONS FOR OLDER ADULTS
>
> Many older adults have *H. pylori* infection that is undiagnosed because of vague symptoms associated with physiologic changes of aging and comorbidities that mask dyspepsia. Teach older adults about the importance of *H. pylori* screening because early detection and aggressive treatment can prevent PUD and gastric cancer (Fromm, 2009).

Hyposecretory drugs reduce gastric acid secretions and are therefore used for both peptic ulcer disease (PUD) and gastritis management. The primary prescribed drugs include proton pump inhibitors and H₂-receptor antagonists (see Chart 58-3).

Proton pump inhibitors (PPIs) are the drug class of choice for treating patients with acid-related disorders. Examples include omeprazole (Prilosec), lansoprazole (Prevacid), rabeprazole (Aciphex), pantoprazole (Protonix), and esomeprazole (Nexium). These drugs suppress the H,K–ATPase enzyme system of gastric acid production, and several of them are available as over-the-counter (OTC) drugs.

Omeprazole, lansoprazole, and esomeprazole are each available as delayed-release capsules designed to release their contents after they pass through the stomach. Omeprazole and lansoprazole may be dissolved in a sodium bicarbonate solution and given through any feeding tube. Bicarbonate protects the dissolved omeprazole and lansoprazole granules in gastric acid. Therefore the drugs are still absorbed correctly. These capsules can also be opened. The enteric-coated capsules can be put in apple juice or orange juice and given through a large-bore feeding tube. Rabeprazole (Aciphex) and pantoprazole (Protonix) are enteric-coated tablets that quickly dissolve after the tablet has moved through the stomach and should not be crushed before giving them. Several of the PPIs are also available in an IV form, which may be helpful for patients who are NPO. A new faster-acting form of omeprazole combined with sodium bicarbonate (Zegerid) can be purchased OTC and is prescribed most often for active duodenal ulcers for a 4- to 8-week period.

Some patients use these PPIs for years and perhaps a lifetime. However, these drugs should not be used for a prolonged period because, over time, they may contribute to osteoporotic-related fractures, especially spinal fractures in older women (Kwok et al., 2010). Omeprazole (Prilosec and Prilosec OTC) reduce the effect of clopidogrel (Plavix), an antiplatelet drug. Teach patients to tell their health care provider if they are taking clopidogrel.

H2-receptor antagonists are drugs that block histamine-stimulated gastric secretions. These drugs may also be used for indigestion and gastritis. Lower-dose forms are available in over-the-counter (OTC) products. H2-receptor antagonists block the action of the H2 receptors of the parietal cells, thus inhibiting gastric acid secretion. Two of the most common drugs are famotidine (Pepcid) and nizatidine (Axid) and are available as Pepcid OTC and Axid AR in OTC form. These drugs are typically administered in a single dose at bedtime and are used for 4 to 6 weeks in combination with other therapy.

Antacids buffer gastric acid and prevent the formation of pepsin. They may help small duodenal ulcers heal but are usually not used alone as drug therapy. Liquid suspensions are the most therapeutic form, but tablets may be more convenient and enhance adherence. The most widely used preparations are mixtures of aluminum hydroxide and magnesium hydroxide. This combination overcomes the unpleasant GI side effects of either of these preparations when used alone. Mylanta and Maalox are examples of this type of combination antacid formulation. The aluminum and magnesium hydroxide combination products neutralize well at small doses. These products must be administered cautiously to patients with renal impairment because elimination is reduced and excessive amounts are retained in the body.

> ## ! NURSING SAFETY PRIORITY
> ### *Drug Alert*
>
> Teach the patient that to achieve a therapeutic effect, sufficient antacid must be ingested to neutralize the hourly production of acid. For optimal effect, take antacids about 2 hours after meals to reduce the hydrogen ion load in the duodenum. Antacids may be effective from 30 minutes to 3 hours after ingestion. If taken on an empty stomach, they are quickly evacuated. Thus the neutralizing effect is reduced.

Calcium carbonate (Tums) is a potent antacid, but it triggers gastrin release, causing a rebound acid secretion. Therefore its use in acid inhibition is not recommended.

Antacids can interact with certain drugs such as phenytoin (Dilantin), tetracycline (Ala-Tet, Nu-Tetra ✤), and ketoconazole (Nizoral) and interfere with their effectiveness. Ask what other drugs the patient is using before a specific antacid is prescribed. Other drugs are given 1 to 2 hours before or after the antacid. Inform the patient that flavored antacids, especially wintergreen, should be avoided. The flavoring increases the emptying time of the stomach. Thus the desired effect of the antacid is negated.

Teach the patient with past or present heart failure to avoid antacids with high sodium content, such as aluminum hydroxide, magnesium hydroxide, sodium bicarbonate, and simethicone combination products (Gelusil and Mylanta). Magaldrate (Riopan) has the lowest sodium concentration.

Sucralfate (Carafate) is a *mucosal barrier fortifier* (protector) that forms complexes with proteins at the base of a peptic ulcer. This protective coat prevents further digestive action of both acid and pepsin. Sucralfate does not inhibit acid secretion. Rather, it binds bile acids and pepsins, reducing injury from these substances. The drug may be used in conjunction with H2-receptor antagonists and antacids but should not be administered within 1 hour of the antacid. Sucralfate is given on an empty stomach 1 hour before each meal and at bedtime. The main side effect of this drug is constipation.

Nutrition Therapy. The role of diet in the management of ulcer disease is controversial. There is no evidence that dietary restriction reduces gastric acid secretion or promotes tissue healing, although a bland diet may assist in relieving symptoms. Food itself acts as an antacid by neutralizing gastric acid for 30 to 60 minutes. An increased rate of gastric acid secretion, called *rebound*, may follow.

> ## ! NURSING SAFETY PRIORITY
> ### *Action Alert*
>
> Teach the patient with peptic ulcer disease to avoid substances that increase gastric acid secretion. This includes caffeine-containing beverages (coffee, tea, cola). Both caffeinated and decaffeinated coffees should be avoided, because coffee contains peptides that stimulate gastrin release.

Teach the patient to exclude any foods that cause discomfort. A bland, nonirritating diet is recommended during the acute symptomatic phase. Bedtime snacks are avoided because they may stimulate gastric acid secretion. Eating six smaller daily meals may help, but this regimen is no longer a regular part of therapy. No evidence supports the theory that eating six daily meals promotes healing of the ulcer. This practice may actually stimulate gastric acid secretion. Patients should avoid alcohol and tobacco because of their stimulatory effects on gastric acid secretion.

Complementary and Alternative Therapies. Teach patients about complementary and alternative therapies that can reduce stress, including hypnosis and imagery. For example, the use of yoga and meditation techniques has demonstrated a beneficial effect on anxiety disorders. Many have suggested that GI disorders result from the dysfunction of both the GI tract itself and the brain. This means that emotional stress is thought to worsen GI disorders such as peptic ulcer disease. Yoga is thought to alter the activities of the central and autonomic nervous systems.

Many herbs, such as powders of slippery elm and marshmallow root, quercetin, and licorice, are used commonly by patients with gastritis and PUD. These herbs are thought to heal inflamed tissue and increase blood flow to the gastric mucosa. Other substances include zinc, vitamin C, essential fatty acids, acidophilus, vitamins E and A, and glutamine. All of these substances enhance healing. Table 58-1 provides a more complete list of therapies that have been used. Many of them have been scientifically supported in animal studies. Additional research using humans is being conducted.

Managing Upper GI Bleeding

Planning: Expected Outcomes. The patient with upper GI bleeding (often called *upper GI hemorrhage* or *UGH*) is expected to have vital signs within normal limits.

Interventions. Blood loss from PUD results in high morbidity and mortality. Fluid volume loss secondary to vomiting can lead to dehydration and electrolyte imbalances. Monitoring and early recognition of complications are critical to the successful management of PUD. Interventions aimed at managing complications associated with PUD include prevention and/or management of bleeding, perforation, and gastric outlet obstruction. In some cases, surgical treatment of complications becomes necessary.

Nonsurgical Management. Because prevention or early detection of complications is needed to obtain a positive clinical outcome, monitor the patient carefully and immediately report changes to the health care provider. The type of intervention selected will depend on the type and severity of the complication.

Emergency: Upper GI Bleeding. The patient who is actively bleeding has a life-threatening emergency. He or she needs supportive therapy to prevent hypovolemic shock and possible death.

! NURSING SAFETY PRIORITY

Critical Rescue

*The first priority for care of the patient with upper GI bleeding is to maintain **a**irway, **b**reathing, and **c**irculation (ABCs). Provide oxygen and other ventilatory support as needed. Start two large-bore IV lines for replacing fluids and blood. Monitor vital signs, hematocrit, and oxygen saturation.*

The purpose of managing hypovolemia is to expand intravascular fluid in a patient who is volume depleted. Carefully monitor the patient's fluid status, including intake and output. *Fluid replacement in older adults should be closely monitored to prevent fluid overload.* Serum electrolytes are also assessed because depletions from vomiting or nasogastric suctioning must be replaced. Volume replacement with isotonic solutions (e.g., 0.9% normal saline solution, lactated Ringer's solution) should be started immediately. The health care provider may prescribe blood products such as packed red blood cells to expand volume and correct a low hemoglobin and hematocrit. For patients with active bleeding, fresh frozen plasma may be given if the prothrombin time is 1.5 times higher than the midrange control value.

Continue to monitor the patient's hematocrit, hemoglobin, and coagulation studies for changes from the baseline measurements. With mild bleeding (less than 500 mL), slight feelings of weakness and mild perspiration may be present. When blood loss exceeds 1 L/24 hr, manifestations of shock may occur, such as hypotension, chills, palpitations, diaphoresis, and a weak, thready pulse.

A combination of several different treatments, including nasogastric tube (NGT) placement and lavage, endoscopic therapy, interventional radiologic procedures, and acid suppression, can be used to control acute bleeding and prevent rebleeding. If the patient is actively bleeding at home, he or she is usually admitted to the emergency department for GI lavage. If the patient is already a patient in the hospital, lavage can be done at the bedside. After the bleeding has stopped, H$_2$-receptor antagonists, proton pump inhibitors, and antacids are the primary drugs used.

Nasogastric Tube Placement and Lavage. Upper GI bleeding often requires the health care provider or nurse to insert a large-bore nasogastric tube (NGT) to:

- Determine the presence or absence of blood in the stomach
- Assess the rate of bleeding
- Prevent gastric dilation
- Administer lavage

Patients who have upper GI bleeding often have discomfort, nausea, and/or vomiting, which can be worsened by inserting an NGT. Therefore several methods are available to prevent these problems, such as applying lidocaine gel or spray before the tube is placed. Some health care providers do not use any

of these methods to promote patient comfort, even though they have been shown to be effective.

Once the NGT is placed, proper positioning of the tube is confirmed by x-ray examination. Irrigate the NGT to maintain its patency and prevent obstruction with clotted blood (Chart 58-5).

Gastric lavage requires the insertion of a large-bore NGT with instillation of a room-temperature solution in volumes of 200 to 300 mL. There is no evidence that sterile saline or sterile water is better than tap water for this procedure. Follow agency protocol for the solution that is required. The solution and blood are repeatedly withdrawn manually until returns are clear or light pink and without clots. Instruct the patient to lie on the left side during this procedure to limit the flow of the lavage solution out of the stomach. The NGT may remain in place for a few days or be removed after lavage.

Endoscopic Therapy. Endoscopic therapy via an esophagogastroduodenoscopy (EGD) can assist in achieving homeostasis during an acute hemorrhage by isolating the bleeding artery to embolize (clot) it. Octreotide (Sandostatin) or terlipressin (Novapressin) may be given IV as adjuvant therapy. These drugs are synthetic GI hormones (somatostatin analogs) that suppress gastric acid secretion.

Pre-EGD nursing care involves inserting one or two large-bore IV catheters if they are not in place. A large catheter allows the patient to receive IV moderate sedation (e.g., midazolam [Versed] and an opioid) and possibly a blood transfusion. Keep the patient NPO 4 to 6 hours before the procedure. This prevents the risk for aspiration and allows the endoscopist to view and treat the ulcer. A patient must sign a consent form before the EGD *after* the physician informs him or her about the procedure. During the EGD, a specialized endoscopy nurse and technician assist the physician with the procedure.

! NURSING SAFETY PRIORITY

Action Alert

After esophagogastroduodenoscopy (EGD), monitor vital signs, heart rhythm, and oxygen saturation frequently until they return to baseline. In addition, frequently assess the patient's ability to swallow saliva. The patient's gag reflex may initially be absent after an EGD because of anesthetizing (numbing) the throat with a spray before the procedure. *After the procedure, do not allow the patient to have food or liquids until the gag reflex is intact!*

Endoscopic therapy is beneficial for most patients with active bleeding. However, ulcers that continue to bleed or continue to rebleed despite endoscopic therapy may require an interventional radiologic procedure or surgical repair.

Interventional Radiologic Procedures. For patients with persistent, massive upper GI bleeding or those who are not surgical candidates, catheter-directed embolization may be performed. This endovascular procedure is usually done if endoscopic procedures are not successful or available. A femoral approach is most often used, but brachial access may be used. An arteriogram is performed to identify the arterial anatomy and find the exact location of the bleeding. A liquid substance is used to clot the bleeding artery. Nursing care of patients having this procedure is similar to the care required for patients undergoing arteriography (Loffroy & Guiu, 2009).

Acid Suppression. Aggressive acid suppression is used to prevent rebleeding. When acute bleeding is stopped and clot

CHART 58-5   BEST PRACTICE FOR PATIENT SAFETY & QUALITY CARE

Nasogastric Tubes

1. Inform the patient about the procedure and its potential discomfort.
2. Position the patient with pillows behind the shoulders.
3. Lubricate the tube with a water-soluble lubricant.
4. Measure the length of the tube to be passed:
   a. Measure from the bridge of the nose to the earlobe to the xiphoid process.
   b. Indicate this length with a piece of tape on the tube.

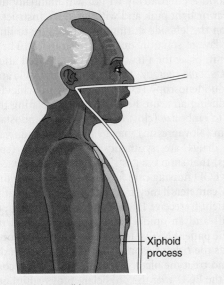

Xiphoid process

5. Determine which nostril is more patent.
6. Encourage the patient to swallow or drink water if the level of consciousness and treatment plan permit.
7. Insert the tube:
   a. Pass the tube gently into the nasopharynx. Ask the patient to swallow repeatedly while the tube is advanced.
   b. If resistance is met, rotate the tube slowly, aiming downward and toward the closer ear.
   c. In the intubated or semiconscious patient, flex the head toward the chest while passing the tube.
8. Withdraw the tube immediately if any change is noted in respiratory status.
9. Test for tube placement by using these techniques:
   a. Obtain a sample of the gastric contents by aspirating with a 50-mL catheter-tipped syringe.
   b. Test the pH of the gastric contents (should be between 1 and 3.5).
   c. Obtain a request for an x-ray study to confirm placement.
10. Connect the tube to suction at low pressure:
    a. The Levin tube is connected to intermittent low suction.
    b. The Salem sump or Anderson tube is connected to continuous low suction.
11. Secure the tube to the patient's nose and to his or her gown:
    a. Tie a slipknot around the tube with a rubber band.
    b. Pin the rubber band to the gown.
12. Check intake and output every 4 hr or more often, as indicated.
13. Observe the patient for nausea, vomiting, abdominal fullness, or distention.
14. If irrigation is indicated, use only a normal saline solution.
15. Observe the patient for alterations in fluid and electrolyte balance.
16. If indicated, instruct the patient about movement that will not dislodge the tube and cause nasal irritation.
17. Remove the tape securing the tube to the nose daily and PRN to clean skin; reapply tape.

formation has taken place within the ulcer crater, the clot remains in contact with gastric contents. Acid-suppressive agents are used to stabilize the clot by raising the pH level of gastric contents. Several types of drugs are used. H_2-receptor antagonists prevent acid from being produced by parietal cells. Proton pump inhibitors prevent the transport of acid across the parietal cell membrane, whereas antacids buffer acid produced in the stomach.

Perforation is managed by immediately replacing fluid, blood, and electrolytes, administering antibiotics, and keeping the patient NPO. Maintain nasogastric suction to drain gastric secretions and thus prevent further peritoneal spillage. Carefully monitor intake and output and check vital signs at least hourly. Monitor the patient for clinical manifestations of septic shock, such as fever, pain, tachycardia, lethargy, or anxiety.

Pyloric obstruction is caused by edema, spasm, or scar tissue. Symptoms of obstruction related to difficulty in emptying the stomach include feelings of fullness, distention, or nausea after eating, as well as vomiting copious amounts of undigested food.

Treatment of obstruction is directed toward restoring fluid and electrolyte balance and decompressing the dilated stomach. Obstruction related to edema and spasm generally responds to medical therapy. First, the stomach must be decompressed with nasogastric suction. Next, interventions are directed at correcting metabolic alkalosis and dehydration. The NGT is clamped after about 72 hours. Check the patient for retention of gastric contents. If the amount retained is not more than 50 mL in 30 minutes, the health care provider may allow oral fluids. In some cases, surgical intervention may be required to treat PUD.

Surgical Management.   Evidence-based guidelines for the treatment of PUD that include *H. pylori* treatment and the development of nonsurgical means of controlling bleeding have led to a decline in the need for surgical intervention. In PUD, surgical intervention may be used to:

- Treat patients who do not respond to medical therapy or other nonsurgical procedures
- Treat a surgical emergency that develops as a complication of PUD, such as perforation

Two general surgical approaches are available for PUD—minimally invasive surgery and conventional open surgery.

Minimally invasive surgery (MIS) via laparoscopy (a type of endoscope) is occasionally used to remove a chronic gastric ulcer or treat hemorrhage from perforation. Several small incisions allow access to the stomach and duodenum. The patient may have partial stomach removal (subtotal gastrectomy), pyloroplasty (to open the pylorus) and/or a vagotomy (vagus nerve cutting) to control acid secretion (Fig. 58-4). The advantages of MIS over traditional procedures include a shorter hospital stay, fewer complications, less pain, and better, quicker recovery. MIS is discussed in more detail in Chapter 17. Conventional surgery is performed using an open approach. This procedure is discussed on p. 1235 under Surgical Management in the Gastric Cancer section.

Community-Based Care

Patients may be discharged from the hospital as long as there is no evidence of ongoing bleeding, orthostatic changes, or cardiopulmonary distress or compromise. Those discharged after treatment for peptic ulcer disease (PUD) and/

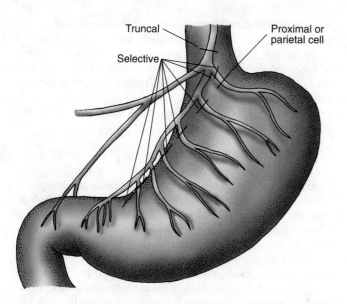

FIG. 58-4 Various types of vagotomies.

CHART 58-6 HOME CARE ASSESSMENT

The Patient with Ulcer Disease

Assess gastrointestinal and cardiovascular status, including:
- Vital signs, including orthostatic vital signs
- Skin color
- Presence of abdominal pain (location, severity, character, duration, precipitating factors, and relief measures)
- Character, color, and consistency of stools
- Changes in bowel elimination pattern
- Hemoglobin and hematocrit
- Bowel sounds; palpate for areas of tenderness

Assess nutritional status, including:
- Dietary patterns and habits
- Intake of caffeine and alcohol
- Relationship of food to symptoms

Assess medication history:
- Use of steroids
- Use of NSAIDs
- Use of over-the-counter medications

Assess patient's coping style:
- Recent stressors
- Past coping style

Assess patient's understanding of illness and ability to adhere to the therapeutic regimen:
- Symptoms to report to health care provider
- Expected and side effects of medications
- Food and drug interactions
- Need for smoking cessation

or complications secondary to the disease must face several challenges to manage the disease successfully. Long-term adherence to drug therapy may require the patient to take several drugs each day. Permanent lifestyle alterations in nutrition habits must also be made.

Home Care Management

Most patients are discharged to the home to continue their recovery. Those who have had major surgery or have had complications, such as hemorrhage, may require one or two visits from a home care nurse to assess clinical progress, especially if the patient is an older adult (Chart 58-6).

Teaching for Self-Management

The primary focus of home care preparation is patient and family teaching regarding risk factors for the recurrence of PUD. Teach them how to recognize new complications and what to do if they occur, especially abdominal pain; nausea and vomiting; black, tarry stools; and weakness or dizziness.

Teach the patient and family about risk factors for recurring peptic ulcers. Help them plan ways to make needed lifestyle changes. For postsurgical patients, especially those who have undergone partial stomach removal, a smaller meal may be required. Other postoperative nutrition changes are described on p. 1238 in the discussion of Teaching for Self-Management in the Gastric Cancer section.

⚠ NURSING SAFETY PRIORITY

Action Alert

Teach the patient who has had surgery for PUD to avoid any OTC product containing aspirin or other NSAID. Emphasize the importance of following the treatment regimen for treating *H. pylori* infection and healing the ulcer. Emphasize the importance of keeping all follow-up appointments. Help the patient identify situations that cause stress, describe feelings during stressful situations, and develop a plan for coping with stressors. Encourage the patient to learn and use relaxation techniques, such as exercise, biofeedback, humor, and imagery. Psychotherapy may be indicated to cope with excessive anxiety or stress.

Health Care Resources

If needed, refer the patient and family to the National Digestive Diseases Information Clearinghouse (www.acg.gi.org/patients/gitract/nddic.asp). This group provides information and support to patients who have digestive disorders.

EVALUATION: OUTCOMES

Evaluate the care of the patient with peptic ulcer disease (PUD) based on the identified priority patient problems. The expected outcomes are that the patient:
- Does not have active PUD or associated complications
- Verbalizes pain relief or control
- Adheres to the drug regimen and lifestyle changes to prevent recurrence and heal the ulcer

ZOLLINGER-ELLISON SYNDROME

Zollinger-Ellison syndrome (ZES) is a rare disease that is manifested by upper GI tract ulceration, increased gastric acid secretion, and one or more duodenal or pancreatic tumors, called gastrinomas. About two thirds of these tumors are malignant. Although most of these tumors grow slowly, a small portion of patients have tumors that develop rapidly and metastasize widely. Metastasis occurs mainly in the liver and regional lymph nodes.

Pathophysiology

ZES is caused by gastrin-secreting tumors that stimulate the acid-secreting cells of the stomach to maximal activity. This large quantity of acid causes GI ulceration. In the early course of the disease, symptoms are similar to those of peptic ulcer disease (PUD). However, these symptoms tend to progress and respond poorly to traditional ulcer therapy. Diarrhea occurs in almost half of patients. It may be associated with large amounts of hydrochloric acid secreted into the proximal duodenum. Steatorrhea (an excessive amount of fat in the feces) results from the inactivation of pancreatic lipase secondary to the large concentrations of acid and decreased amounts of bile acids.

In some patients, gastrinoma results from an autosomal dominant disorder called *multiple endocrine neoplasia type 1 (MEN-1) syndrome,* in which there is a mutation in the *MEN-1* suppressive gene. Gastrinomas contain multiple hormones, but adrenocorticotropic hormone (ACTH) is most commonly found (McCance et al., 2010).

PATIENT-CENTERED COLLABORATIVE CARE

Patients may report PUD symptoms and may have diarrhea and/or steatorrhea. Ask whether any relatives have had ZES. Radiographic and endoscopic findings for ZES are similar to those for PUD. *However, infection with H. pylori is usually absent.* The diagnosis is usually made by radioimmunoassay studies that reveal *increased serum gastrin levels* in conjunction with the clinical features of the disease.

The aim of therapy is to suppress acid secretion to control symptoms. Proton pump inhibitors (PPIs), such as lansoprazole (Prevacid) and omeprazole (Prilosec, Losec ✦), are the drugs of choice to reduce gastric acid secretion and heal the ulcers. High doses of H2-receptor antagonists are also effective in reducing gastric acid and providing symptom relief.

The tumor requires complete surgical resection as a curative treatment. In some patients, a radical pancreaticoduodenectomy (Whipple procedure) is performed. Chapter 62 in the discussion of Surgical Management in the Pancreatic Cancer section describes this procedure and nursing care in detail. Patients with aggressive disease can also be treated with chemotherapeutic agents such as 5-fluorouracil, doxorubicin, and streptozocin to reduce tumor size and control symptoms before surgery. Octreotide (Sandostatin) may also be used.

GASTRIC CANCER

Most cancers of the stomach are adenocarcinomas. This type of cancer develops in the mucosal cells that form the innermost lining of any portion or all of the stomach. Often there are no symptoms in the early stages and the disease is advanced when detected.

Pathophysiology

Gastric cancer usually begins in the glands of the stomach mucosa. Atrophic gastritis and intestinal metaplasia (abnormal tissue development) are precancerous conditions. Inadequate acid secretion in patients with atrophic gastritis creates an alkaline environment that allows bacteria (especially *H. pylori*) to multiply. This infection causes mucosa-associated lymphoid tissue (MALT) lymphoma, which starts in the stomach (McCance et al., 2010).

Gastric cancers spread by direct extension through the gastric wall and into regional lymphatics, which carry tumor deposits to lymph nodes. Direct invasion of and adherence to adjacent organs (e.g., the liver, pancreas, and transverse colon) may also result. Hematogenous spread via the portal vein to the liver and via the systemic circulation to the lungs and bones is the most common mode of metastasis. Peritoneal seeding of cancer cells from the tumor areas to the omentum, peritoneum, ovary, and pelvic cul-de-sac can also occur.

In people with *advanced* gastric cancer, there is invasion of the muscularis (stomach muscle) or beyond. These lesions are not cured by surgical resection. The overall 5-year survival rate of people with stomach cancer in the United States is poor because most patients have no symptoms until the disease advances.

Etiology and Genetic Risk

Infection with H. pylori is the largest risk factor for gastric cancer because it carries the cytotoxin-associated antigen A (CagA) gene. Patients with pernicious anemia, gastric polyps, chronic atrophic gastritis, and achlorhydria (absence of secretion of hydrochloric acid) are two to three times more likely to develop gastric cancer.

The disease also seems to be positively correlated with eating pickled foods, nitrates from processed foods, and salt added to food. The ingestion of these foods over a long period can lead to atrophic gastritis, a precancerous condition. A low intake of fruits and vegetables is also a risk factor for cancer (McCance et al., 2010).

Gastric surgery seems to increase the risk for gastric cancer because of the eventual development of atrophic gastritis, which results in changes to the mucosa. Patients with Barrett's esophagus from prolonged or severe gastroesophageal reflux disease (GERD) have an increased risk for cancer in the cardia (at the point where the stomach connects to the esophagus).

Incidence/Prevalence

Men appear to have a slightly greater risk than women. Asians and Asian Americans are at an especially high risk because of preferences for salted and smoked fish. The average age for developing gastric cancer is 70 years (National Cancer Institute, 2010).

⊕ CULTURAL AWARENESS

Minority groups in the United States have a greater incidence of gastric cancer than Euro-Americans (whites), probably because of diets higher in salt and pickled foods. Asian/Pacific Islanders, American Indians/Alaska Natives, and blacks are the most at-risk groups (National Cancer Institute, 2010).

Health Promotion and Maintenance

Teach patients with gastritis and/or *H. pylori* infection to follow the treatment regimen to ensure that gastritis heals and *H. pylori* infection is eliminated. *Stress the need for eating a well-balanced diet and limiting pickled foods, salted foods, and processed foods to help prevent gastric cancer.*

? NCLEX EXAMINATION CHALLENGE
Health Promotion and Maintenance

The nurse assesses a client for the risk for gastric cancer. Which of these factors would likely increase the client's risk? **Select all that apply.**
A. Having a history of untreated gastroesophageal reflux disease
B. Being an adult between 20 and 40 years of age
C. Eating a diet high in smoked and pickled foods
D. Eating a diet with high-fiber foods
E. Eating a diet high in salt and adding salt to food

PATIENT-CENTERED COLLABORATIVE CARE

ASSESSMENT

Question the patient about known risk factors for the development of gastric cancer. Ask about preferred foods, especially pickled, salted, or smoked foods. Inquire whether the patient has ever been diagnosed with or treated for *H. pylori* infection, gastritis, or pernicious anemia. Note whether he or she has a history of gastric surgery or polyps. Also ask whether any of the patient's immediate relatives have gastric cancer.

Although patients with *early* gastric cancer may be asymptomatic, indigestion (heartburn) and abdominal discomfort are the *most* common symptoms (Chart 58-7). These symptoms are often ignored, however, or a change in diet or use of antacids relieves them. As the tumor grows, these symptoms become more severe and do not respond to nutrition changes or antacids. Epigastric or back pain is also an early symptom that may go unrecognized.

In *advanced* gastric cancer, progressive weight loss, nausea, and vomiting can occur. Vomiting represents pronounced dilation, thickening of the stomach wall, or pyloric obstruction. Obstructive symptoms appear earlier with tumors located near the pylorus than with fundic lesions. Patients with advanced disease may have weakness, fatigue, and anemia. Physical assessment findings in advanced disease may be absent, or a palpable epigastric mass may suggest hepatomegaly (liver enlargement) from metastatic disease. Hard, enlarged lymph nodes in the left supraclavicular chain, left axilla, or umbilicus result from metastasis from gastric cancer. Masses on the right suggest metastasis in the perigastric lymph nodes or liver.

In patients with advanced disease, anemia is evidenced by *low hematocrit* and hemoglobin values. Patients may have macrocytic or microcytic anemia associated with decreased iron or vitamin B_{12} absorption. *The stool may be positive for occult blood. Hypoalbuminemia* and *abnormal results of liver tests* (e.g., bilirubin and alkaline phosphatase) occur with advanced disease and with hepatic metastasis. *The level of carcinoembryonic antigen (CEA) is elevated in advanced cancer of the stomach.*

The health care provider uses esophagogastroduodenoscopy (EGD) with biopsy for definitive diagnosis of gastric cancer. The lesion can be viewed directly, and biopsies of all visible lesions can be obtained to determine the presence of cancer cells. During the endoscopy, an endoscopic (endoluminal) ultrasound (EUS) of the gastric mucosa can also be performed. This technology allows the health care provider to evaluate the depth of the tumor and the presence of lymph node involvement, which permits more accurate staging of the disease. Computed tomography (CT), positron emission tomography (PET), and magnetic resonance imaging (MRI) scans of the chest, abdomen, and pelvis are used in determining the extent of the disease and planning therapy.

INTERVENTIONS

Management of gastric cancer includes drug therapy, radiation, and/or surgery. Drug therapy and radiation may be used instead of surgery or as an adjunct before and/or after surgery.

Nonsurgical Management

The treatment of gastric cancer depends highly on the stage of the disease. Radiation and chemotherapy commonly prolong survival of patients with advanced gastric disease.

Combination *chemotherapy* with multiple cycles of drugs such as cisplatin and epirubicin before and after surgery may be given. Bone marrow suppression, nausea, and vomiting are common adverse drug effects. Chapter 24 discusses the general nursing care of patients receiving chemotherapy.

Although gastric cancers are somewhat sensitive to the effects of radiation, the use of this treatment is limited because the disease is often widely spread to other abdominal organs on diagnosis. Organs such as the liver, kidneys, and spinal cord can endure only a limited amount of radiation. Intraoperative radiotherapy (IORT) is available in large tertiary care health care systems. Radiation may be used for palliative management when surgery is not an option.

The most common side effects of radiation include impaired skin integrity, fatigue, and anorexia. Nausea, vomiting, and diarrhea may occur about 1 week after treatment is initiated and diminish a month or more after treatment ends. (See Chapter 24 for more information on radiation therapy.)

Surgical Management

Surgical resection by removing the tumor is the preferred method for treating gastric cancer. The primary surgical procedures for the treatment of gastric cancer are total gastrectomy and subtotal (partial) gastrectomy. In early stages, laparoscopic surgery (minimally invasive surgery [MIS]) plus adjuvant chemotherapy or radiation may be curative. Patients having MIS have less pain, shorter hospital stays, rare postoperative complications, and quicker recovery. However, MIS is seldom performed because very few patients are diagnosed in the early stage of the disease.

Most patients with advanced disease are candidates for palliative surgical treatment. Metastasis in the supraclavicular lymph nodes, inguinal lymph nodes, liver, umbilicus, or perirectal wall indicates that the opportunity for cure by resection has been lost. Palliative resection may significantly improve

---

CHART 58-7	KEY FEATURES

Early Versus Advanced Gastric Cancer

Early Gastric Cancer*
- Indigestion
- Abdominal discomfort initially relieved with antacids
- Feeling of fullness
- Epigastric, back, or retrosternal pain

Advanced Gastric Cancer
- Nausea and vomiting
- Obstructive symptoms
- Iron deficiency anemia
- Palpable epigastric mass
- Enlarged lymph nodes
- Weakness and fatigue
- Progressive weight loss
- Signs of distant metastasis:
  - Virchow's nodes
  - Blumer's shelf
  - "Sister Mary Joseph nodes"
  - Krukenberg's tumor

***Note:** Many patients with early gastric cancer have no clinical manifestations.

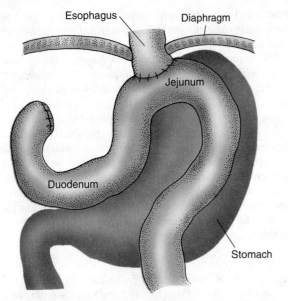

FIG. 58-5 Total gastrectomy with anastomosis of the esophagus to the jejunum (esophagojejunostomy) is the principal surgical intervention for extensive gastric cancer.

the quality of life for a patient suffering from obstruction, hemorrhage, or pain.

Preoperative Care. Before conventional open-approach surgery, a nasogastric tube (NGT) is inserted and connected to suction to remove secretions and empty the stomach. This allows surgery to take place without contamination of the peritoneal cavity by gastric secretions. Chart 58-5 describes the procedure for inserting the NGT and nursing care associated with maintenance. The NGT remains in place for a few days *postoperatively* to prevent the accumulation of secretions, which may lead to vomiting or GI distention and pressure on the incision.

Because weight loss is problematic for patients with gastric cancer, nutrition therapy is a vital aspect of preoperative and postoperative management. Preoperatively, compression by the tumor can prevent adequate nutritional intake. To correct malnutrition before surgery, the health care provider may prescribe enteral supplements to the diet and/or total parenteral nutrition (TPN). Vitamin, mineral, iron, and protein supplements are essential to correct nutritional deficits.

Other preoperative nursing measures for the patient undergoing open gastric surgery are the same as those for any patient undergoing abdominal surgery and general anesthesia (see Chapter 16).

Operative Procedures. The surgeon usually removes part or all of the stomach to take out the tumor. When the tumor is located in the mid-portion or distal (lower) portion of the stomach, a subtotal (partial) gastrectomy is typically performed. The omentum, spleen, and relevant nodes are also removed.

For the patient with a removable growth in the proximal (upper) third of the stomach, a total gastrectomy is performed (Fig. 58-5). In this procedure the surgeon removes the entire stomach along with the lymph nodes and omentum. The surgeon sutures the esophagus to the duodenum or jejunum to reestablish continuity of the GI tract. More radical surgery involving removal of the spleen and distal pancreas

is controversial, although the Whipple procedure may be used to prolong life. However, the complications of this drastic surgery are very serious and common. For patients with advanced disease, total gastrectomy is performed only when gastric bleeding or obstruction is present.

Patients with tumors at the gastric outlet who are not candidates for subtotal or total gastrectomy may undergo gastroenterostomy for palliation. The surgeon creates a passage between the body of the stomach and the small bowel, often the duodenum.

Postoperative Care. Provide the usual postoperative care for patients who have had general anesthesia to prevent atelectasis, paralytic ileus, and wound infection (see Chapter 18). In addition, monitor the patient for the development of complications that are specific to gastric surgery.

Auscultate the lungs for adventitious sounds (crackles or reduced breath sounds), and monitor for the return of bowel sounds. Take vital signs as appropriate to detect signs of infection or bleeding. Aggressive pulmonary exercises and early ambulation can help prevent respiratory complications and deep vein thrombosis. Also inspect the operative site every shift for the presence of redness, swelling, or drainage, which indicates wound infection. Keep the head of the bed elevated to prevent aspiration from reflux.

Decreased patency caused by a clogged NGT can result in *acute gastric dilation* after surgery. This problem is manifested by epigastric pain and a feeling of fullness, hiccups, tachycardia, and hypotension. Irrigation or replacement of the NGT by request of the surgeon can relieve these symptoms.

Dumping syndrome is a term that refers to a group of vasomotor symptoms that occur after eating. This syndrome is believed to occur as a result of the rapid emptying of food contents into the small intestine, which shifts fluid into the gut causing abdominal distention. Observe for *early* manifestations of this syndrome, which typically occurs within 30 minutes of eating. Symptoms include vertigo, tachycardia, syncope, sweating, pallor, palpitations, and the desire to lie down. Report these manifestations to the surgeon, and encourage the patient to lie down. Monitor the patient for late symptoms.

Late dumping syndrome, which occurs 90 minutes to 3 hours after eating, is caused by a release of an excessive amount of insulin. The insulin release follows a rapid rise in the blood glucose level that results from the rapid entry of high-carbohydrate food into the jejunum. Observe for manifestations, including dizziness, light-headedness, palpitations, diaphoresis, and confusion.

Dumping syndrome is managed by nutrition changes that include decreasing the amount of food taken at one time and eliminating liquids ingested with meals. In collaboration with the dietitian, teach the patient to eat a high-protein, high-fat, low- to moderate-carbohydrate diet (Table 58-3). Acarbose may be used to decrease carbohydrate absorption. A somatostatin analog, octreotide (Sandostatin), 50 mcg subcutaneously 2 to 3 times daily 30 minutes before meals may be prescribed in severe cases. This drug decreases gastric and intestinal hormone secretion and slows stomach and intestinal transit time.

Alkaline reflux gastropathy, also known as *bile reflux gastropathy,* is a complication of gastric surgery in which the pylorus is bypassed or removed. Endoscopic examination reveals regurgitated bile in the stomach and mucosal

TABLE 58-3	DIET FOR DUMPING SYNDROME		
FOOD GROUP	**FOODS ALLOWED OR ENCOURAGED**	**FOODS TO USE WITH CAUTION**	**FOODS THAT MUST BE EXCLUDED**
Soups		Fluids 1 hr before and after meals	Spicy soups
Meat and meat substitutes	8 oz or more per day: fish, poultry, beef, pork, veal, lamb, eggs, cheese, and peanut butter		Spicy meats or meat substitutes
Potato and substitutes	Potato, rice, pasta, starchy vegetables (small amount)		Highly spiced potatoes or substitutes
Bread and cereal	White bread, rolls, muffins, crackers, and cereals (small amount)	Whole-grain bread, rolls, crackers, and cereals	Breads with frosting or jelly, sweet rolls, and coffee cake
Vegetables	Two or more cooked vegetables	Gas-producing vegetables, such as cabbage, onions, broccoli, or raw vegetables	
Fruits	Limit three per day: unsweetened cooked or canned fruits	Unsweetened juice or fruit drinks 30-45 min after meals; fresh fruit	Sweetened fruit or juice
Beverages	Dietetic drinks	Limit to 1 hr after meals; caffeine-containing beverages, such as coffee, tea, and cola; if tolerated, diet carbonated beverages	Milk shakes, malts, and other sweet drinks; regular carbonated beverages and alcohol
Fats	Margarine, oils, shortening, butter, bacon, and salad dressings	Mayonnaise	Any fats with milk products
Desserts	Fruit (see Fruits)	Sugar-free gelatin, pudding, and custard	All sweets, cakes, pies, cookies, candy, ice cream, and sherbet
Seasonings and miscellaneous	Diet jelly, diet syrups, sugar substitutes	Excessive amounts of salt	Excessive amounts of spices, sugar, jelly, honey, syrup, or molasses

General Principles
- Several small meals daily
- Relatively high fat and protein content
- Low roughage
- Relatively low carbohydrate content
- No milk, sweets, or sugars
- Liquid between meals *only*

hyperemia. Symptoms include early satiety (satisfied quickly with little food), abdominal discomfort, and vomiting.

Delayed gastric emptying is often present after gastric surgery and usually resolves within 1 week. Edema at the anastomosis (surgical connection areas) or adhesions (scar tissue) obstructing the distal loop may cause mechanical blockage. Metabolic causes (e.g., hypokalemia, hypoproteinemia, or hyponatremia) should be considered. The edema is resolved with nasogastric suction, maintenance of fluid and electrolyte balance, and proper nutrition.

Afferent loop syndrome may occur when the duodenal loop is partially obstructed after radical surgery. Pancreatic and biliary secretions fill the intestinal loop, which becomes distended. Painful contractions attempt to propel these secretions from the loop. Teach patients to report abdominal bloating and pain 20 to 60 minutes after eating, often followed by nausea and vomiting. Treatment consists of surgical correction of the incomplete loop obstruction.

Several problems related to *nutrition* develop as a result of partial removal of the stomach, including deficiencies of vitamin B_{12}, folic acid, and iron; impaired calcium metabolism; and reduced absorption of calcium and vitamin D. These problems are caused by a reduction of intrinsic factor. The decrease results from the resection and from inadequate absorption because of rapid entry of food into the bowel. In the absence of intrinsic factor, clinical manifestations of pernicious anemia may occur. Assess for the development of atrophic glossitis secondary to vitamin B_{12}

deficiency. In atrophic glossitis, the tongue takes on a shiny, smooth, and "beefy" appearance. The patient may also have signs of anemia secondary to folic acid and iron deficiency. Monitor the complete blood count (CBC) for signs of megaloblastic anemia and leukopenia (low red blood cell [RBC] and white blood cell [WBC] levels). These manifestations are corrected by the administration of vitamin B_{12}. The health care provider may also prescribe folic acid or iron preparations.

❓ DECISION-MAKING CHALLENGE

Patient-Centered Care

A 58-year-old patient had a partial gastrectomy for gastric cancer yesterday and has a nasogastric tube connected to suction. When you meet him to perform your initial assessment, he tells you that he is a family physician who is one of few health care providers in a rural town and is worried about who will care for his patients during his postoperative recovery and treatment. He is also concerned about who will "look after" his older life partner who has been living with him for 21 years.

1. How will you respond to the patient's concerns?
2. What priority care will you plan to provide for him today and why?
3. For what complications is he at risk and why? How would you know if he has abdominal bleeding?
4. Conduct an electronic data-based search for current evidence related to health teaching for this patient. How will you determine the strength of the evidence? How will you conduct an analysis and draw conclusions about the data you find?

Community-Based Care

Patients who have undergone total gastrectomy and those who are debilitated with advanced gastric cancer are discharged to home with maximal assistance and support or to a transitional care unit or skilled nursing facility. Patients who have undergone subtotal gastrectomy and are not debilitated may be discharged to home with partial assistance for ADLs. Recurrence of cancer is common, and patients need regular follow-up examinations and imaging assessments. Collaborate with the case manager (CM) to ensure continuity of care and thorough follow-up with diagnostic testing.

Home Care Management

Gastric cancer is a life-threatening illness. Therefore the patient and family members require physical and emotional care. Assess their ability to cope with the disease and the possible need for end-of-life care. The adverse effects of gastric cancer treatment can be debilitating, and patients need to learn symptom management strategies. Hospice programs can help both the patient and the family cope with these physical and emotional needs.

Patients may fear returning home because of their inability for self-management. Enlisting family and health care resources for the patient may ease some of this anxiety. Provide the family with adequate information about community support systems to make the transition to home care easier. If the prognosis is poor, they need continued professional support from case managers, social workers, and/or nurses to cope with death and dying. (See Chapter 9 for a discussion of end-of-life care.)

Teaching for Self-Management

Educate the patient and family about any continuing needs, drug therapy, and nutrition therapy. If patients are discharged to home with surgical dressings, teach the patient and family how to change them. Review the manifestations of incisional infection (e.g., fever, redness, and drainage) that they should report to their surgeon.

Patients who will be receiving radiation therapy or chemotherapy require instructions related to the side effects of these treatments. Nausea and vomiting are common side effects of chemotherapy, and instruction in the use of prescribed antiemetics may be needed. (See Chapter 24 for health teaching for patients receiving chemotherapy or radiation therapy.)

In collaboration with the dietitian, teach the patient and family about the type and quantity of foods that will provide optimal nutritional value. Interventions to minimize dumping syndrome and decrease gastric stimulants are also emphasized (see Table 58-3). Remind the patient to:

- Eat small, frequent meals
- Avoid drinking liquids with meals
- Avoid foods that cause discomfort
- Eliminate caffeine and alcohol consumption
- Begin a smoking-cessation program, if needed
- Receive B_{12} injections, as prescribed
- Lie flat after eating for a short time

Health Care Resources

A home care referral provides continued assessment, assistance, and encouragement to the patient and family. A home care nurse can help with care procedures and provide valuable psychological support. Additional referrals to a dietitian, professional counselor, or clergy/spiritual leader may be necessary. Referral to a hospice agency can be of great assistance for the patient with advanced disease. Hospice care may be delivered in the home or in an institutional setting. Appropriate support groups (e.g., I Can Cope, provided by the American Cancer Society) can be a major resource.

NURSING CONCEPT REVIEW

What might you NOTICE if the patient is experiencing impaired digestion and nutrition as a result of a stomach disorder?

- Report of epigastric pain or indigestion before or after a meal
- Report of inability to tolerate certain foods
- Nausea and/or vomiting (with or without blood)
- Melena or frank blood in stools

What should you INTERPRET and how should you RESPOND to a patient experiencing impaired digestion and nutrition as a result of a stomach disorder?

Perform and interpret physical assessment, including:
- Taking vital signs
- Observing and documenting assessment findings
- Preparing for gastric lavage if hematemesis is present

- Interpreting laboratory values and other diagnostic findings:
  - Presence of *H. pylori*
  - Decreased hemoglobin and hematocrit

Respond by:
- Maintaining **a**irway, **b**reathing, and **c**irculation (ABCs)
- Placing patient in sitting position or on left side to prevent aspiration if vomiting
- Preparing to assist with gastric lavage if hematemesis is present

On what should you REFLECT?
- Think about what else you could do to care for this patient.
- Consider with whom you should collaborate to improve or maintain digestion and nutrition for this patient.
- After patient interventions, monitor for changes in vital signs, hematocrit, and hemoglobin.

GET READY FOR THE NCLEX® EXAMINATION!

KEY POINTS

Review these Key Points for each NCLEX Examination Client Needs Category.

Safe and Effective Care Environment

- Provide information about organizations for digestive disorders to receive information and support; refer the patient to the American Cancer Society if gastric cancer is the diagnosis.

Health Promotion and Maintenance

- Identify patients at risk for gastritis and PUD, especially older adults who take large amounts of NSAIDs and those with *H. pylori.*
- Teach patients behaviors to prevent PUD, such as avoiding large consumption of caffeine, alcohol, coffee, aspirin, and other NSAIDs. Also teach them to avoid contaminated foods and water and smoking (see Chart 58-1).
- Teach patients about various complementary and alternative therapies that are currently used for gastritis and PUD.

Psychosocial Integrity

- Allow patients with gastric cancer to express feelings of grief, fear, and anxiety.
- For patients with advanced gastric cancer, identify the need for end-of-life care, including referral to hospice care.

Physiological Integrity

- Teach patients the importance of adhering to *H. pylori* treatment to prevent the risk for gastric cancer.
- For patients who have undergone a gastrectomy, collaborate with the dietitian and instruct the patient regarding diet changes to avoid abdominal distention and dumping syndrome.
- Teach patients with abnormal symptoms (e.g., abdominal tenderness, abdominal pain that is relieved by food or pain

that becomes worse 3 hours after eating, dyspepsia, melena, and/or distention) to consult with their physician immediately for a prompt diagnosis and treatment.
- Teach patients that hematemesis is a medical emergency and that they should go to the emergency department for prompt treatment.
- Teach the proper administration of antacids (one to two after meals). Tell patients that antacids can interfere with the effectiveness of certain drugs, such as phenytoin (Dilantin).
- Teach the proper administration of H_2 antagonists. Explain that they should be given on an empty stomach (see Chart 58-3).
- Teach the proper administration of antisecretory agents, noting that most cannot be crushed because they are sustained-release or enteric-coated tablets.
- Assess patients for clinical manifestations of gastritis.
- Monitor patients with ulcers for any of the signs and symptoms of GI bleeding that are listed in Chart 58-4. Report any of these symptoms if noted to a physician immediately.
- Insert a nasogastric tube (NGT) as outlined in Chart 58-5.
- After an EGD, monitor the patient's vitals signs, heart rhythm, and oxygen saturation frequently until they return to baseline. To prevent aspiration, assess the gag reflex and ensure that it is intact before giving the patient food.
- Observe the patient for signs and symptoms of dumping syndrome after gastric surgery; teach the manifestations and management of this syndrome. Advise the patient to eat six small meals per day and to consume a diet high in protein and fat but low in carbohydrate-rich foods. Liquids should not be taken with meals.

Care of Patients with Noninflammatory Intestinal Disorders

Donna D. Ignatavicius

evolve WEBSITE

http://evolve.elsevier.com/Iggy/

Animation: Nasogastric Tube Placement
Answer Key for NCLEX Examination Challenges and
  Decision-Making Challenges
Audio Glossary

Key Points
Concept Map Creator
Review Questions for the NCLEX® Examination

LEARNING OUTCOMES

Safe and Effective Care Environment

1. Prioritize nursing care for the patient with abdominal trauma.
2. Identify community-based resources for patients with colorectal cancer (CRC).
3. Describe the importance of collaborating with health care team members to provide care for patients with CRC.

Health Promotion and Maintenance

4. Teach patients health promotion practices to prevent CRC.
5. Plan health teaching for patients to promote self-management when caring for a colostomy.

Psychosocial Integrity

6. Assess patient and family response to a diagnosis of CRC.

Physiological Integrity

7. Develop a teaching-learning plan for patients with irritable bowel syndrome (IBS).
8. Differentiate the most common types of hernias.
9. Develop a plan of care for a patient undergoing a minimally invasive inguinal hernia repair.
10. Identify risk factors for CRC.
11. Interpret assessment findings for patients with CRC.
12. Explain the role of the nurse in managing the patient with CRC.
13. Develop a perioperative plan of care for a patient undergoing a colon resection and colostomy.
14. Explain the differences between small-bowel and large-bowel obstructions.
15. Develop a plan of care for a patient with an intestinal obstruction to promote elimination.
16. Describe the postoperative care for a patient having a hemorrhoid surgical procedure.
17. Explain the pathophysiology of malabsorption syndrome.

Intestinal health problems may be inflammatory or non-inflammatory. This chapter describes those disorders that are noninflammatory in origin. Noninflammatory intestinal problems often cause rectal bleeding, changing bowel patterns, and abdominal pain. If not diagnosed and managed early, some intestinal problems can lead to inadequate absorption of vital nutrients and therefore affect the need for *nutrition* and *elimination*.

IRRITABLE BOWEL SYNDROME

Pathophysiology

Irritable bowel syndrome (IBS) is a functional GI disorder that causes chronic or recurrent diarrhea, constipation, and/or abdominal pain and bloating. It is sometimes referred to as *spastic colon, mucous colon,* or *nervous colon* (Fig. 59-1). *IBS is the most common digestive disorder seen in clinical*

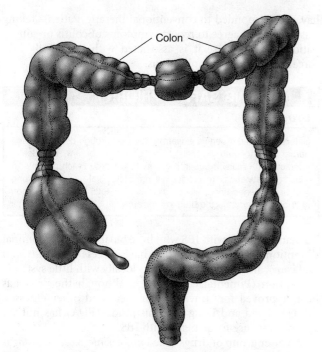

Colon

FIG. 59-1 Spastic contractions of the colon as they occur with irritable bowel syndrome.

practice and may affect as many as one in five people in the United States.

In most patients, no actual pathophysiologic bowel changes occur. However, microscopic inflammatory changes have recently been found in some patients with the disease due to bacterial overgrowth and subsequent infection.

In patients with IBS, bowel motility changes and increased or decreased bowel transit times result in changes in the normal *bowel elimination* pattern to one of these classifications: diarrhea (IBS-D), constipation (IBS-C), alternating diarrhea and constipation (IBS-A), or a mix of diarrhea and constipation (IBS-M). Symptoms of the disease typically begin to appear in young adulthood and continue throughout the patient's life.

The etiology of IBS remains unclear. Recent research suggests that a combination of environmental, immunologic, genetic, hormonal, and stress factors play a role in the development and course of the disease. Examples of environmental factors include foods and fluids like caffeinated or carbonated beverages and dairy products. Infectious agents have also been identified. Several recent studies have found that patients with IBS often have small-bowel bacterial overgrowth, which causes bloating and abdominal distention. Multiple normal flora and pathogenic agents have been identified, including *Pseudomonas aeruginosa* (Kerckhoffs et al., 2011). Other researchers believe that these agents are less causative and serve as measurable biomarkers for the disease (Malinen et al., 2010).

Immunologic and genetic factors have also been associated with IBS, especially cytokine genes, including pro-inflammatory interleukins (IL) such as IL-6 and tumor necrosis factor (TNF)–alpha (Barkhordari et al., 2010). These findings may provide the basis of targeted drug therapy for the disease.

In the United States, women are two times more likely to have IBS than men. This difference may be the result of hormonal differences. However, in other areas of the world, this distribution pattern may not occur. For example, researchers found that there is not a female predominance for the disease in Asian countries (Gwee et al., 2010).

Considerable evidence relates the role of stress and mental or behavioral illness, especially anxiety and depression, to IBS. Many patients diagnosed with IBS meet the criteria for at least one primary mental health disorder. Some researchers suggest that psychosocial problems may be a cause for IBS (Nicholl et al., 2008). However, the pain and other chronic symptoms of the disease may lead to secondary mental health disorders. For example, when diarrhea is predominant, patients fear that there will be no bathroom facilities available and can become very anxious. The long-term nature of dealing with a chronic disease for which there is no cure can lead to secondary depression in some patients.

PATIENT-CENTERED COLLABORATIVE CARE

ASSESSMENT

Ask the patient about a history of weight change, fatigue, malaise, abdominal pain, changes in the bowel pattern (constipation, diarrhea, or an alternating pattern of both) or consistency of stools, and the passage of mucus. Patients with IBS do not usually lose weight. Ask whether the patient has had any GI infections. Collect information on all drugs the patient is taking, because some of them can cause symptoms similar to those of IBS. Ask about the nutrition history, including the use of caffeinated drinks or beverages sweetened with sorbitol or fructose, which can cause bloating or diarrhea.

The course of the illness is specific to each patient. Most patients can identify factors that cause exacerbations, such as diet, stress, or anxiety. Food intolerance may be associated with IBS. Dairy products (e.g., lactose intolerance), raw fruits, and grains can contribute to bloating, flatulence (gas), and abdominal distention.

A flare-up of worsening cramps, abdominal pain, and diarrhea and/or constipation may bring the patient to the health care provider. One of the *most common concerns of patients with IBS is pain in the left lower quadrant of the abdomen.* Assess the location, intensity, and quality of the pain. Some patients have internal visceral (organ) hypersensitivity that can cause or contribute to the pain. Nausea may be associated with mealtime and defecation. The constipated stools are small and hard and are generally followed by several softer stools. The diarrheal stools are soft and watery, and mucus is often present in the stools. Patients with IBS often report belching, gas, anorexia, and bloating.

The patient generally appears well, with a stable weight, and nutritional and fluid status are within normal ranges. Inspect and auscultate the abdomen. Bowel sounds vary but are generally within normal range. With constipation, bowel sounds may be hypoactive; with severe diarrhea, they may be hyperactive.

Routine laboratory values (including a complete blood count [CBC], serum albumin, erythrocyte sedimentation rate [ESR], and stools for occult blood) are normal in IBS. Some health care providers request a *hydrogen breath test*

(Lindberg, 2009). When small-intestinal bacterial overgrowth or malabsorption of nutrients is present, excess hydrogen is produced. Some of this hydrogen is absorbed into the bloodstream and travels to the lungs where it is exhaled. Patients with IBS often have an increased amount of hydrogen during exhalation.

Teach the patient that he or she will need to be NPO (may have water) for at least 12 hours before the hydrogen breath test. At the beginning of the test, the patient blows into a hydrogen analyzer. Then, small amounts of test sugar are ingested, depending on the purpose of the test, and additional breath samples are taken every 15 minutes for 1 hour or longer. If lactose tolerance is evaluated, lactose is ingested. If bacterial overgrowth is tested, lactulose is given (Pagana & Pagana, 2010).

INTERVENTIONS

The patient with IBS is usually cared for in an ambulatory care setting and learns self-management strategies. Interventions include health teaching, drug therapy, and stress reduction. Some patients also use complementary and alternative therapies. A holistic approach to patient care is essential for positive outcomes (Bengtsson et al., 2010).

Keeping a symptom diary in which the patient records potential triggers and bowel habits for a period of time can assist in identifying triggers for disease symptoms. Assist patients to identify and avoid specific foods that they cannot tolerate. These foods may include caffeine, alcohol, egg, wheat products, beverages that contain sorbitol or fructose, and other gastric irritants. Milk and milk products should be avoided if lactose intolerance is suspected. In this case, teach patients to use lactose-free or soy products as substitutes. Patients who are lactose intolerant need to increase intake of calcium-rich, lactose-free foods or take a calcium supplement because they are at high risk for osteoporosis.

Dietary fiber and bulk help produce bulky, soft stools and establish regular bowel habits. The patient should ingest about 30 to 40 g of fiber each day. Eating regular meals, drinking 8 to 10 cups of liquid each day, and chewing food slowly help promote normal bowel function. If needed, collaborate with the dietitian to help the patient and family with meal planning.

Drug therapy depends on the predominant symptom of IBS. The health care provider may prescribe bulk-forming or antidiarrheal agents and/or newer drugs to control symptoms.

For the treatment of *constipation-predominant IBS (IBS-C)*, bulk-forming laxatives, such as *psyllium* hydrophilic mucilloid (Metamucil), are generally taken at mealtimes with a glass of water. The hydrophilic properties of these drugs help prevent dry, hard, or liquid stools. *Lubiprostone* (Amitiza) is a new oral drug available for women with IBS-C. The drug is not effective for men. Lubiprostone is classified as a locally acting chloride channel activator that increases intestinal chloride without affecting intestinal sodium and potassium concentrations. Teach the patient to take the drug with food and water.

Diarrhea-predominant IBS (IBS-D) may be treated with antidiarrheal agents, such as loperamide (Imodium), and psyllium (a bulk-forming agent). *Alosetron* (Lotronex), a selective serotonin (5-HT3) receptor antagonist, may be used with caution in women with IBS-D as a last resort when they

have not responded to conventional therapy. Patients taking this drug must agree to report symptoms of colitis or constipation early because it is associated with potentially life-threatening bowel complications.

> ### ! NURSING SAFETY PRIORITY
> #### Drug Alert
>
> Before the patient begins alosetron, take a thorough drug (including herbs) history, both prescribed and over the counter, because it interacts with many drugs in a variety of classes. Teach patients to report constipation, fever, increasing abdominal pain, increasing fatigue, darkened urine, bloody diarrhea, or rectal bleeding as soon as it occurs and stop the drug immediately.

Many patients with IBS who have bloating and abdominal distention without constipation have success with *rifaximin* (Xifaxan), an antibiotic that works locally with little systemic absorption (Pimental et al., 2011). Although the drug has been approved for "traveler's diarrhea" and other illnesses, the U.S. Food and Drug Administration (FDA) has not yet approved its use for patients with IBS.

A newer group of drugs called *muscarinic-receptor antagonists* also inhibit intestinal motility. Some of these agents have been approved for people with overactive bladders but have not yet received FDA approval for IBS. Examples in this group currently undergoing clinical trials are darifenacin (Enablex) and fesoterodine (Toviaz).

For IBS in which pain is the predominant symptom, tricyclic antidepressants such as amitriptyline (Elavil) have also been successfully used. It is unclear whether their effectiveness is due to the antidepressant or anticholinergic effects of the drugs. If patients have postprandial (after eating) discomfort, they should take these drugs 30 to 45 minutes before mealtime.

Complementary and Alternative Therapies

For patients with increased intestinal bacterial overgrowth, recommend daily probiotic supplements. *Probiotics* have been shown to be effective for reducing bacteria and successfully alleviating GI symptoms of IBS (Lyra et al., 2010). There is also evidence that peppermint oil capsules may be effective in reducing symptoms for patients with IBS (Pirotta, 2009).

Acupuncture and moxibustion (Acu-Moxa) treatment has helped some patients by reducing flatulence and bloating and improving stool consistency (Anastasi et al., 2009). Moxibustion is the use of herbs to facilitate healing. Encourage patients to try these therapies, especially if they can be reimbursed by insurance companies. Third-party payers are becoming more sensitive to the use of these proven therapies as adjuncts in holistic disease management.

Stress management is also an important part of holistic care. Suggest relaxation techniques, meditation, and/or yoga to help the patient decrease GI symptoms. If the patient is in a stressful work or family situation, personal counseling may be helpful. Based on patient preference, make appropriate referrals or assist in making appointments, if needed. The opportunity to discuss problems and attempt creative problem solving is often helpful. Teach the patient that regular exercise is important for managing stress and promoting regular bowel elimination.

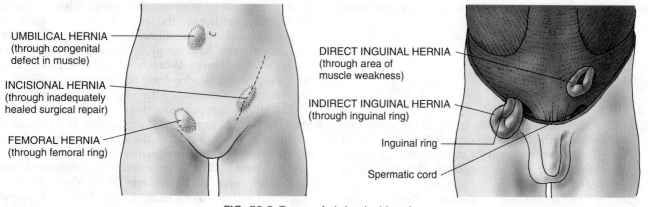

FIG. 59-2 Types of abdominal hernias.

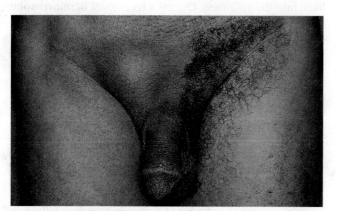

FIG. 59-3 A right direct inguinal hernia.

HERNIATION

Pathophysiology

A **hernia** is a weakness in the abdominal muscle wall through which a segment of the bowel or other abdominal structure protrudes. Hernias can also penetrate through any other defect in the abdominal wall, through the diaphragm, or through other structures in the abdominal cavity.

The most common types of abdominal hernias (Fig. 59-2) are indirect, direct, femoral, umbilical, and incisional.

- An **indirect inguinal hernia** is a sac formed from the peritoneum that contains a portion of the intestine or omentum. The hernia pushes downward at an angle into the inguinal canal. In males, indirect inguinal hernias can become large and often descend into the scrotum.
- **Direct inguinal hernias,** in contrast, pass through a weak point in the abdominal wall (Fig. 59-3).
- **Femoral hernias** protrude through the femoral ring. A plug of fat in the femoral canal enlarges and eventually pulls the peritoneum and often the urinary bladder into the sac.
- **Umbilical hernias** are congenital or acquired. Congenital umbilical hernias appear in infancy. Acquired umbilical hernias directly result from increased intra-abdominal pressure. They are most commonly seen in obese people.

- **Incisional, or ventral, hernias** occur at the site of a previous surgical incision. These hernias result from inadequate healing of the incision, which is usually caused by postoperative wound infections, inadequate nutrition, and obesity.

Hernias may also be classified as reducible, irreducible (incarcerated), or strangulated. A hernia is **reducible** when the contents of the hernial sac can be placed back into the abdominal cavity by gentle pressure. An **irreducible** (incarcerated) hernia cannot be reduced or placed back into the abdominal cavity. *Any hernia that is not reducible requires immediate surgical evaluation.*

A hernia is **strangulated** when the blood supply to the herniated segment of the bowel is cut off by pressure from the hernial ring (the band of muscle around the hernia). If a hernia is strangulated, there is ischemia and obstruction of the bowel loop. This can lead to necrosis of the bowel and possibly bowel perforation. *Signs of strangulation are abdominal distention, nausea, vomiting, pain, fever, and tachycardia.*

The most important elements in the development of a hernia are congenital or acquired muscle weakness and increased intra-abdominal pressure. The most significant factors contributing to increased intra-abdominal pressure are obesity, pregnancy, and lifting heavy objects.

Indirect inguinal hernias, the most common type, are most common in men because they follow the tract that develops when the testes descend into the scrotum before birth. Direct hernias occur more often in older adults. Femoral and adult umbilical hernias are most common in obese or pregnant women. Incisional hernias can occur in people who have undergone abdominal surgery.

Defects in the muscle wall result from weakened collagen or widened spaces at the inguinal ligament. These muscle weaknesses can be inherited or acquired as part of the aging process. Increases in intra-abdominal pressure as a result of pregnancy, obesity, abdominal distention, ascites, heavy lifting, or coughing can contribute to their occurrence.

Health Promotion and Maintenance

Even though the muscle weakness cannot be prevented, exercises can strengthen muscles. Obesity is considered a contributing factor because it causes increased intra-abdominal pressure. Weight control helps decrease the likelihood of hernias by decreasing pressure on the abdominal muscles.

Heavy lifting and straining also increase intra-abdominal pressure and should be avoided.

PATIENT-CENTERED COLLABORATIVE CARE

ASSESSMENT

The patient with a hernia typically comes to the health care provider's office or the emergency department with a report of a "lump" or protrusion felt at the involved site. The development of the hernia may be associated with straining or lifting.

Perform an abdominal assessment inspecting the abdomen when the patient is lying and again when he or she is standing. If the hernia is reducible, it may disappear when the patient is lying flat. The advanced practice nurse or other health care provider asks the patient to strain or perform the Valsalva maneuver and observes for bulging. Auscultate for active bowel sounds. *Absent bowel sounds may indicate obstruction and strangulation, which is a medical emergency!*

To palpate an inguinal hernia, the health care provider gently examines the ring and its contents by inserting a finger in the ring and noting any changes when the patient coughs. *The hernia is never forcibly reduced; that maneuver could cause strangulated intestine to rupture.*

If a male patient suspects a hernia in his groin, the health care provider has him stand for the examination. Using the right hand for the patient's right side and the left hand for the patient's left side, the examiner pushes in the loose scrotal skin with the index finger, following the spermatic cord upward to the external inguinal cord. At this point, the patient is asked to cough, and any palpable herniation is noted.

INTERVENTIONS

The type of treatment selected depends on patient factors such as age, as well as the type and severity of the hernia.

Nonsurgical Management

If the patient is not a surgical candidate, often an older adult with multiple health problems, the health care provider may prescribe a truss for an inguinal hernia, most often for men. A truss is a pad made with firm material. It is held in place over the hernia with a belt to help keep the abdominal contents from protruding into the hernial sac. If a truss is used, it is applied only after the physician has reduced the hernia if it is not incarcerated. The patient usually applies the truss upon awakening. Teach him to assess the skin under the truss daily and to protect it with a light layer of powder.

Surgical Management

Most hernias are inguinal. Surgical repair of a hernia is the treatment of choice. Surgery is usually performed on an ambulatory care basis for patients who have no pre-existing health conditions that would complicate the operative course. In same-day surgery centers, anesthesia may be regional or general and the surgery is typically laparoscopic. More extensive surgery, such as a bowel resection or temporary colostomy, may be necessary if strangulation results in a gangrenous section of bowel. Patients undergoing extensive surgery are hospitalized for a longer period.

A minimally invasive inguinal hernia repair (MIIHR) through a laparoscope, also called herniorrhaphy, is the surgery of choice. A conventional open herniorrhaphy may be performed when laparoscopy is not appropriate. Patients having minimally invasive surgery (MIS) recover more quickly, have less pain, and develop fewer postoperative complications compared with those having the conventional surgery.

In addition to patient education about the procedure, the most important preoperative preparation is to teach the patient to remain NPO for the number of hours before surgery that the surgeon specifies. If same-day surgery is planned, remind the patient to arrange for someone to take him or her home and be available for the rest of the day at home. For patients having an open surgical approach, provide general preoperative care as described in Chapter 16.

During an MIIHR, the surgeon makes several small incisions, identifies the defect, and places the intestinal contents back into the abdomen. During a traditional herniorrhaphy, the surgeon makes an abdominal incision to perform this procedure. When a hernioplasty is also performed, the surgeon reinforces the weakened outside abdominal muscle wall with a mesh patch.

The patient who has had MIIHR is discharged from the surgical center in 3 to 5 hours, depending on recovery from anesthesia. Teach him or her to rest for several days before returning to work and a normal routine. Caution patients who are taking oral opioids for pain management to not drive or operate heavy machinery. Teach them to observe incisions for redness, swelling, heat, drainage, and increased pain and promptly report their occurrence to the surgeon. Remind patients that soreness and discomfort rather than severe, acute pain are common after MIS. Be sure to make a follow-up telephone call on the day after surgery to check on the patient's status.

General postoperative care of patients having a hernia repair is the same as that described in Chapter 18 *except that they should avoid coughing.* To promote lung expansion, encourage deep breathing and ambulation. With repair of an indirect inguinal hernia, the physician may suggest a scrotal support and ice bags applied to the scrotum to prevent swelling, which often contributes to pain. Elevation of the scrotum with a soft pillow helps prevent and control swelling.

In the immediate postoperative period, male patients who have had an inguinal hernia repair may experience difficulty voiding. Encourage them to stand to allow a more natural position for gravity to facilitate voiding and bladder emptying. Urine output of less than 30 mL per hour should be reported to the surgeon. Techniques to stimulate voiding such as allowing water to run may also be used. A fluid intake of at least 1500 to 2500 mL daily prevents dehydration and maintains urinary function. A "straight" or intermittent catheterization is required if the patient cannot void.

Most patients have uneventful recoveries after a hernia repair. Surgeons generally allow them to return to their usual activities after surgery, with avoidance of straining and lifting for several weeks while subcutaneous tissues heal and strengthen.

Provide oral instructions and a written list of symptoms to be reported, including fever, chills, wound drainage, redness or separation of the incision, and increasing incisional pain. Teach the patient to keep the wound dry and clean with antibacterial soap and water. Showering is usually permitted in a few days.

COLORECTAL CANCER

Pathophysiology

Colorectal refers to the colon and rectum, which together make up the large intestine, also known as the *large bowel.* Colorectal cancer (CRC) is cancer of the colon or rectum and is a major health problem worldwide. In the United States, it is one of the most common malignancies.

Most CRCs are **adenocarcinomas,** which are tumors that arise from the glandular epithelial tissue of the colon. They develop as a multi-step process, resulting in a number of molecular changes, such as loss of key tumor suppressor genes and activation of certain oncogenes that alter colonic mucosa cell division. The increased proliferation of the colonic mucosa forms polyps that can transform into malignant tumors. Most CRCs are believed to arise from adenomatous polyps that present as a visible protrusion from the mucosal surface of the bowel (McCance et al., 2010).

Tumors occur in different areas of the colon, with about two thirds occurring within the rectosigmoid region. The percentages in Fig. 59-4 indicate an increased incidence of cancer in the proximal sections of the large intestine over the past 35 years.

Colorectal cancer (CRC) can metastasize by direct extension or by spreading through the blood or lymph. The tumor may spread locally into the four layers of the bowel wall and into neighboring organs. It may enlarge into the lumen of the bowel or spread through the lymphatics or the circulatory system. The circulatory system is entered directly from the primary tumor through blood vessels in the bowel or via the lymphatics. The liver is the most frequent site of metastasis from circulatory spread. Metastasis to the lungs, brain, bones, and adrenal glands may also occur. Colon tumors can also spread by peritoneal seeding during surgical resection of the tumor. Seeding may occur when a tumor is excised and cancer cells break off from the tumor into the peritoneal cavity. For this reason, special techniques are used during surgery to decrease this possibility.

Complications related to the increasing growth of the tumor locally or through metastatic spread include bowel obstruction or perforation with resultant peritonitis, abscess formation, and fistula formation to the urinary bladder or the vagina. The tumor may invade neighboring blood vessels and cause frank bleeding. Tumors growing into the bowel lumen can gradually obstruct the intestine and eventually block it completely. Those extending beyond the bowel wall may place pressure on neighboring organs (uterus, urinary bladder, and ureters) and cause symptoms that mask those of the cancer. Chapter 23 discusses cancer pathophysiology in more detail.

Etiology and Genetic Risk

The major risk factors for the development of colorectal cancer (CRC) include being older than 50 years, genetic predisposition, personal or family history of cancer, and/or diseases that predispose the patient to cancer such as familial adenomatous polyposis (FAP), Crohn's disease, and ulcerative colitis (McCance et al., 2010). Only a small percentage of colorectal cancers are familial and transmitted genetically.

GENETIC/GENOMIC CONSIDERATIONS

People with a first-degree relative (sister, sibling, or child) diagnosed with colorectal cancer (CRC) have three to four times the risk for developing the disease. An autosomal dominant inherited genetic disorder known as *familial adenomatous polyposis (FAP)* accounts for 1% of CRCs. FAP is the result of one or more mutations in the adenomatous polyposis coli (APC) gene (McCance et al., 2010). In these very young patients, thousands of adenomatous polyps develop over the course of 10 to 15 years and have nearly a 100% chance of becoming malignant. By 20 years of age, most patients require surgical intervention, usually a colectomy with ileostomy or ileoanal pullthrough, to prevent cancer. Chemotherapy may also be used for cancer prevention.

Hereditary nonpolyposis colorectal cancer (HNPCC) is another autosomal dominant disorder and accounts for a small percentage of all colorectal cancers. HNPCC is also caused by gene mutations, including *MLH1* and *MLH2.* People with these mutations have an 80% chance of developing CRC at an average of 45 years of age. They also tend to have a higher incidence of endometrial, ovarian, stomach, and ureteral cancers (Nussbaum et al., 2007). Genetic testing is available for both of these familial CRC syndromes. Refer patients for genetic counseling and possible testing if the patient prefers.

The role of infectious agents in the development of colorectal and anal cancer continues to be investigated. Some lower GI cancers are related to *Helicobacter pylori, Streptococcus bovis,* JC virus, and human papilloma virus (HPV) infections.

There is also strong evidence that long-term smoking, increased body fat, physical inactivity, and heavy alcohol

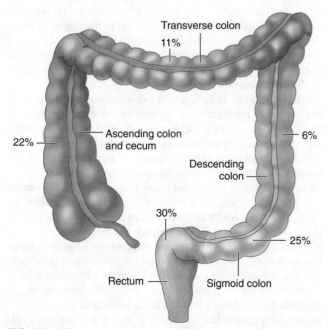

FIG. 59-4 The incidence of cancer in relation to colorectal anatomy.

Transverse colon
11%
Ascending colon and cecum
22%
6%
Descending colon
30%
25%
Rectum
Sigmoid colon

consumption are risk factors for colorectal cancer (American Cancer Society [ACS], 2010). A high-fat diet, particularly animal fat from red meats, increases bile acid secretion and anaerobic bacteria, which are thought to be carcinogenic within the bowel. Diets with large amounts of refined carbohydrates that lack fiber decrease bowel transit time.

Incidence/Prevalence

Colorectal cancer (CRC) is the third most common cause of cancer death in the United States (ACS, 2010). It is not common before 40 years of age, but the incidence in younger adults is slowly increasing, most likely due to increases in HPV infections (Stubenrauch, 2010). The overall incidence of CRC has decreased over the past 10 years, most likely as a result of increased cancer screenings. The disease is most common in African Americans, and their survival rate is lower than that of Euro-Americans (Caucasians). The possible reasons for this difference include less use of diagnostic testing (especially colonoscopy), decreased access to health care, cultural beliefs, and lack of education about the need for early cancer detection (Good et al., 2010; Hamlyn, 2008).

Health Promotion and Maintenance

People at risk can take action to decrease their chance of getting CRC and/or increase their chance of surviving it. For example, those whose family members have had hereditary CRC should be genetically tested for FAP and HNPCC. If gene mutations are present, the person at risk can collaborate with the health care team to decide what prevention or treatment plan to implement.

Teach people about the need for diagnostic screening. When an adult turns 40 years of age, he or she should discuss with the health care provider about the need for colon cancer screening. The interval depends on level of risk. People of average risk who are 50 years of age and older, without a family history, should undergo regular CRC screening. The screening includes fecal occult blood testing (FOBT) and colonoscopy every 10 years or double-contrast barium enema every 5 years. People who have a personal or family history of the disease should begin screening earlier and more frequently (National Comprehensive Cancer Network, 2008). Teach all patients to follow the American Cancer Society recommendations for CRC screening listed in Chart 59-1.

Teach patients, regardless of risk, to modify their diets as needed to decrease fat, refined carbohydrates, and low-fiber foods. Encourage baked or broiled foods, especially those high in fiber and low in animal fat. Teach people the hazards of smoking, excessive alcohol, and physical inactivity. Refer patients as needed for smoking- or alcohol-cessation programs, and recommend ways to increase regular physical exercise.

PATIENT-CENTERED COLLABORATIVE CARE

ASSESSMENT

History

When taking a history, ask the patient about major risk factors, such as a personal history of breast, ovarian, or endometrial cancer (which can spread to the colon); ulcerative colitis; Crohn's disease; familial polyposis or adenomas;

CHART 59-1   BEST PRACTICE FOR PATIENT SAFETY & QUALITY CARE

Screening Recommendations for Men and Women Ages 50 Years and Older at Average Risk for Colorectal Cancer

PROCEDURE: CHOICE OF ONE OF THE FOLLOWING	INTERVAL AFTER SCREENING INITIATED AT AGE 50 YEARS	COMMENTS
FOBT and sigmoidoscopy	Every 5 years	FOBT procedure: two or three samples from three consecutive bowel movements obtained at home; tested by physician or nurse
OR Double-contrast barium enema	Every 5 years	
OR Colonoscopy	Every 10 years	

FOBT, Fecal occult blood testing.

---

polyps, or a family history of CRC. Also assess the patient's participation in age-specific cancer screening guidelines. Ask about whether the patient uses tobacco and/or alcohol. Assess the patient's usual physical activity level.

Ask whether vomiting and changes in bowel habits, such as constipation or change in shape of stool with or without blood, have been noted. The patient may also report fatigue (related to anemias), abdominal fullness, vague abdominal pain, or unintentional weight loss. These symptoms suggest advanced disease.

Physical Assessment/Clinical Manifestations

The clinical manifestations of CRC depend on the location of the tumor. *However, the most common signs are rectal bleeding, anemia, and a change in stool consistency or shape.* Stools may contain microscopic amounts of blood that are not noticeably visible, or the patient may have mahogany (dark)-colored or bright red stools (Fig. 59-5). Gross blood is not usually detected with tumors of the right side of the colon but is common (but not massive) with tumors of the left side of the colon and the rectum.

Tumors in the transverse and descending colon result in symptoms of obstruction as growth of the tumor blocks the passage of stool. The patient may report "gas pains," cramping, or incomplete evacuation. Tumors in the rectosigmoid colon are associated with hematochezia (the passage of red blood via the rectum), straining to pass stools, and narrowing of stools. Patients may report dull pain. Right-sided tumors can grow quite large without disrupting bowel patterns or appearance because the stool consistency is more liquid in this part of the colon. These tumors ulcerate and bleed intermittently, so stools can contain dark or mahogany-colored blood. A mass may be palpated in the lower right quadrant, and the patient often has anemia secondary to blood loss.

Examination of the abdomen begins with assessment for obvious distention or masses. Visible peristaltic waves accompanied by high-pitched or "tinkling" bowel sounds may indicate a partial bowel obstruction from the tumor. Total absence

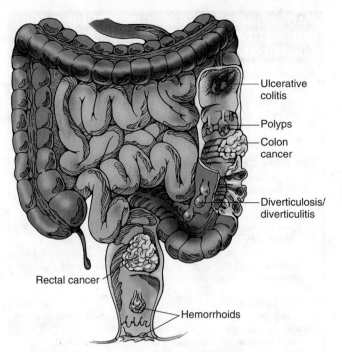

FIG. 59-5 Common causes of lower gastrointestinal bleeding.

of bowel sounds indicates a complete bowel obstruction. Palpation and percussion are performed by the advanced practice nurse or other health care provider to determine whether the spleen or liver is enlarged or whether masses are present along the colon. The examiner may also perform a digital rectal examination to palpate the rectum and lower sigmoid colon for masses. Fecal occult blood screening should not be done with a specimen from a rectal examination because it is not reliable.

Psychosocial Assessment

The psychological consequences associated with a diagnosis of colorectal cancer (CRC) are many. Patients must cope with a diagnosis that instills fear and anxiety about treatment, feelings that life has been disrupted, a need to search for ways to deal with the diagnosis, and concern about family. They also have questions about why colon cancer affected them, as well as concerns about pain, possible disfigurement, and possible death. In addition, if the cancer is believed to have a genetic origin, there is anxiety concerning implications for immediate family members.

Laboratory Assessment

Hemoglobin and hematocrit values are often decreased as a result of the intermittent bleeding associated with the tumor. For some patients, that may be the first indication that a tumor is present. CRC that has metastasized to the liver causes liver function tests to be elevated.

A positive test result for occult blood in the stool (fecal occult blood test [FOBT]) indicates bleeding in the GI tract. These tests can yield false-positive results if certain vitamins or drugs are taken before the test. Remind the patient to avoid aspirin, vitamin C, and red meat for 48 hours before giving a stool specimen. Also assess whether the patient is taking anti-inflammatory drugs (e.g., ibuprofen, corticosteroids, or

salicylates). These drugs should be discontinued for a designated period before the test. Two or three separate stool samples should be tested on 3 consecutive days. Negative results do not completely rule out the possibility of CRC.

Carcinoembryonic antigen (CEA), an oncofetal antigen, is elevated in many people with CRC. The normal value is less that 5 ng/mL or 5 mcg/L (SI units) (Pagana & Pagana, 2010). This protein is not specifically associated with the colorectal cancer, and it may be elevated in the presence of other benign or malignant diseases and in smokers. CEA is often used to monitor the effectiveness of treatment and to identify disease recurrence.

Imaging Assessment

A double-contrast barium enema (air and barium are instilled into the colon) or colonoscopy provides better visualization of polyps and small lesions than a barium enema alone. These tests may show an occlusion in the bowel where the tumor is decreasing the size of the lumen.

Computed tomography (CT) or magnetic resonance imaging (MRI) of the chest, abdomen, pelvis, lungs, or liver helps confirm the existence of a mass, the extent of disease, and the location of distant metastases. CT-guided virtual colonoscopy is growing in popularity and may be more thorough than traditional colonoscopy. However, treatments or surgeries cannot be performed when a virtual colonoscopy is used.

Other Diagnostic Assessment

A sigmoidoscopy provides visualization of the lower colon using a fiberoptic scope. Polyps can be visualized, and tissue samples can be taken for biopsy. Polyps are usually removed during the procedure. A colonoscopy provides views of the entire large bowel from the rectum to the ileocecal valve. As with sigmoidoscopy, polyps can be seen and removed, and tissue samples can be taken for biopsy. *Colonoscopy is the definitive test for the diagnosis of colorectal cancer. These procedures and associated nursing care are discussed in Chapter 55.*

▌ANALYSIS

The priority problems for patients with colorectal cancer (CRC) include:
1. Potential for colorectal cancer metastasis
2. Grieving related to cancer diagnosis

▌PLANNING AND IMPLEMENTATION

The primary approach to treating CRC is to remove the entire tumor or as much of the tumor as possible to prevent or slow metastatic spread of the disease. A patient-centered collaborative care approach is essential to meet the desired outcomes.

Preventing or Controlling Metastasis

Planning: Expected Outcomes. The patient with colorectal cancer (CRC) is expected to not have the cancer spread to vital organs. Thus the patient's life expectancy will be increased and the quality of life will be improved. However, if metastasis is present, the desired outcome is to ensure that the patient is as comfortable as possible and pain is well-managed.

Interventions. Although surgical resection is the primary means used to control the disease, several adjuvant (additional) therapies are used. Adjuvant therapies are administered before or after surgery to achieve a cure, if possible, and to prevent recurrence.

Nonsurgical Management. The type of therapy used is based on the pathologic staging of the disease. Several staging systems may be used. The American Joint Committee on Cancer (AJCC) system uses this broad staging classification and description:

- Stage I—Tumor invades up to muscle layer
- Stage II—Tumor invades up to other organs or perforates peritoneum
- Stage III—Any level of tumor invasion and up to 4 regional lymph nodes
- Stage IV—Any level of tumor invasion; many lymph nodes affected with distant metastases

Radiation Therapy. The administration of preoperative radiation therapy has not improved overall survival rates for colon cancer, but it has been effective in providing local or regional control of the disease. Postoperative radiation has not demonstrated any consistent improvement in survival or recurrence. However, as a palliative measure, radiation therapy may be used to control pain, hemorrhage, bowel obstruction, or metastasis to the lung in advanced disease. For rectal cancer, unlike colon cancer, radiation therapy is almost always a part of the treatment plan. Reinforce information about the radiation therapy procedure to the patient and family, and monitor for possible side effects (e.g., diarrhea, fatigue). Chapter 24 describes the general care of patients undergoing radiation therapy.

Drug Therapy. Adjuvant *chemotherapy* after primary surgery is recommended for patients with stage II or stage III disease to interrupt the DNA production of cells and improve survival. The drugs of choice are IV 5-fluorouracil (5-FU) with leucovorin (LV) (folinic acid), capecitabine (Xeloda), or a combination of drugs referred to as *FOLFOX.* The most frequently used FOLFOX combination for metastatic CRC is 5-FU (fluorouracil), leucovorin, and oxaliplatin (Eloxatin), a platinum analog. These drugs cannot discriminate between cancer and healthy cells. Therefore common side effects are diarrhea, mucositis, leukopenia, mouth ulcers, and peripheral neuropathy.

Bevacizumab (Avastin) is the first antiangiogenesis drug to be approved for advanced CRC. This type of drug reduces blood flow to the growing tumor cells, thereby depriving them of necessary nutrients needed to grow. It is usually given in combination with other chemotherapeutic agents.

Cetuximab (Erbitux), a monoclonal antibody, may also be given for advanced disease. This drug works by blocking factors that promote cancer cell growth. Cetuximab is usually given in combination with another drug.

Intrahepatic arterial chemotherapy, often with 5-FU, may be administered to patients with liver metastasis. Patients with CRC also receive drugs for relief of symptoms, such as opioid analgesics and antiemetics.

Surgical Management. Surgical removal of the tumor with margins free of disease is the best method of ensuring removal of CRC. The size of the tumor, its location, the extent of metastasis, the integrity of the bowel, and the condition of the patient determine which surgical procedure is performed for colorectal cancer (Table 59-1). Many regional lymph nodes are removed and examined for presence of cancer. The number of lymph nodes that contain cancer is a strong predictor of prognosis. The most common surgeries performed

---

TABLE 59-1   SURGICAL PROCEDURES FOR COLORECTAL CANCERS IN VARIOUS LOCATIONS

Right-Sided Colon Tumors
- Right hemicolectomy for smaller lesions
- Right ascending colostomy or ileostomy for large, widespread lesions
- Cecostomy (opening into the cecum with intubation to decompress the bowel)

Left-Sided Colon Tumors
- Left hemicolectomy for smaller lesions
- Left descending colostomy for larger lesions

Sigmoid Colon Tumors
- Sigmoid colectomy for smaller lesions
- Sigmoid colostomy for larger lesions
- Abdominoperineal resection for large, low sigmoid tumors (near the anus) with colostomy (the rectum and the anus are completely removed, leaving a perineal wound)

Rectal Tumors
- Resection with anastomosis or pull-through procedure (preserves anal sphincter and normal elimination pattern)
- Colon resection with permanent colostomy
- Abdominoperineal resection with colostomy

---

are colon resection (removal of the tumor and regional lymph nodes) with reanastomosis, colectomy (colon removal) with *colostomy (temporary or permanent) or ileostomy/ileoanal pull-through,* and abdominoperineal (AP) resection. A colostomy is the surgical creation of an opening of the colon onto the surface of the abdomen. An AP resection is performed when rectal tumors are present. The surgeon removes the sigmoid colon, rectum, and anus through combined abdominal and perineal incisions.

For patients having a colon resection, minimally invasive surgery (MIS) via laparoscopy is commonly performed today. This procedure results in shorter hospital stays, less pain, fewer complications, and quicker recovery compared with the conventional open surgical approach.

Preoperative Care. Reinforce the physician's explanation of the planned surgical procedure. The patient is told as accurately as possible what anatomic and physiologic changes will occur with surgery. The location and number of incision sites and drains are also discussed.

Before evaluating the tumor and colon during surgery, the surgeon may not be able to determine whether a colostomy (or less commonly, an ileostomy) will be necessary. The patient is told that a colostomy is a possibility. If a colostomy is planned, the surgeon consults a certified wound, ostomy, continence nurse (CWOCN) or an enterostomal therapist (ET) (ostomy nurse) to recommend optimal placement of the ostomy. He or she teaches the patient about the rationale and general principles of ostomy care. In many settings, the CWOCN marks the patient's abdomen to indicate a potential ostomy site that will decrease the risk for complications such as interference of the undergarments or a prosthesis with the ostomy appliance. Table 59-2 describes the role of the CWOCN or ET.

The patient who requires low rectal surgery (e.g., AP resection) is faced with the risk for postoperative sexual

TABLE 59-2	**PREOPERATIVE ASSESSMENT BY THE CWOCN OR ET NURSE**

Key Points of Psychosocial Assessment
- Patient's and family's level of knowledge of disease and ostomy care
- Patient's educational level
- Patient's physical limitations (particularly sensory)
- Support available to patient
- Patient's type of employment
- Patient's involvement in activities such as hobbies
- Financial concerns regarding purchase of ostomy supplies

Key Points of Physical Assessment
- Before marking, the nurse specialist considers:
  - Contour of the abdomen in lying, sitting, and standing positions
  - Presence of skin folds, creases, bony prominences, and scars
  - Need to avoid a prosthesis
  - Location of belt line
  - Location that is easily visible to the patient
  - Possible location in the rectus muscle

Adapted from Pontieri-Lewis, V. (2006). Basics of ostomy care. *MEDSURG Nursing, 15*(4), 199-202.
ET, Enterostomal therapist; *CWOCN,* certified wound, ostomy, continence nurse.

dysfunction and urinary incontinence after surgery as a result of nerve damage during surgery. The surgeon discusses the risk for these problems with the patient before surgery and allows him or her to verbalize concerns and questions related to this risk. Reinforce teaching about abdominal surgery performed for the patient under general anesthesia, and review the routines for turning and deep breathing (see Chapter 16). Teach the patient about the method of pain management to be used after surgery such as IV patient-controlled analgesia (PCA), epidural analgesia, or other method.

If the bowel is not obstructed or perforated, elective surgery is planned. The patient may be instructed to thoroughly clean the bowel, or "bowel prep," to minimize bacterial growth and prevent complications. Mechanical cleaning is accomplished with laxatives and enemas or with "whole-gut lavage." For whole-gut lavage, the patient may drink large quantities of a sodium sulfate and polyethylene glycol solution (e.g., GoLYTELY). This solution overwhelms the absorptive capacity of the small bowel and clears feces from the colon. However, the use of bowel preps is controversial, and some surgeons do not recommend it because of patient discomfort. Older adults may become dehydrated from this process. Infection rates are not different with or without bowel preps.

To reduce the risk for infection, the surgeon may prescribe one dose of oral or IV antibiotics to be given before the surgical incision is made. Teach patients that a nasogastric tube (NGT) may be placed for decompression of the stomach after surgery. A peripheral IV or central venous catheter is also placed for fluid and electrolyte replacement while the patient is NPO after surgery. Patients having minimally invasive surgeries do not need an NGT.

The patient with colorectal cancer faces a serious illness with long-term consequences of the disease and treatment. A case manager or social worker can be very helpful in identifying patient and family needs, as well as ensuring continuity of care and support.

Operative Procedures. For the conventional open surgical approach, the surgeon makes a large incision in the abdomen and explores the abdominal cavity to determine whether the tumor can be removed. For a colon resection, the portion of the colon with the tumor is excised and the two open ends of the bowel are irrigated before anastomosis (reattachment) of the colon. If an anastomosis is not feasible because of the location of the tumor or the bowel is inflamed, a colostomy is created.

A colostomy may be created in the ascending, transverse, descending, or sigmoid colon (Fig. 59-6). One of several techniques is used to construct a colostomy. A loop stoma (surgical opening) is made by bringing a loop of colon to the skin surface, severing and everting the anterior wall, and suturing it to the abdominal wall. Loop colostomies are usually performed in the transverse colon and are usually temporary. An external rod may be used to support the loop until the intestinal tissue adheres to the abdominal wall. Care must be taken to avoid displacing the rod, especially during appliance changes.

An end stoma is often constructed, most often in the descending or sigmoid colon, when a colostomy is intended to be permanent. It may also be done when the surgeon oversews the distal stump of the colon and places it in the abdominal cavity, preserving it for future reattachment. An end stoma is constructed by severing the end of the proximal portion of the bowel and bringing it out through the abdominal wall.

The least common colostomy is the double-barrel stoma, which is created by dividing the bowel and bringing both the proximal and distal portions to the abdominal surface to create two stomas. The proximal stoma (closest to the patient's head) is the functioning stoma and eliminates stool. The distal stoma (farthest from the head) is considered nonfunctioning, although it may secrete some mucus. The distal stoma is sometimes referred to as a *mucous fistula.*

MIS colon resection or total colectomy allows complete tumor removal with an adequate surgical margin and removal of associated lymph nodes. Several small incisions are made, and a miniature video camera is placed within the abdomen to help see the area that is involved. This technique takes longer than the conventional procedure and requires specialized training. However, blood loss is less.

Postoperative Care. Patients who have an *open colon resection* without a colostomy receive care similar to that of those having any abdominal surgery (see Chapter 18). Other patients have surgeries that also require colostomy management. They typically have a nasogastric tube (NGT) after open surgery and receive IV PCA for the first 24 to 36 hours. After NGT removal, the diet is slowly progressed from liquids to solid foods as tolerated. The care of patients with an NGT is found on p. 1256 in the discussion of Interventions in the Intestinal Obstruction section.

By contrast, patients who have *laparoscopic (MIS) surgery* can progress from liquids to solids more quickly. Because they usually have less pain, they are able to ambulate earlier than those who have the conventional approach. The hospital stay is usually shorter for the patient with MIS—less than 23 hours or 1 to 2 days, depending on the patient's age and general condition.

Colostomy Management. The patient who has a colostomy may return from surgery with a clear ostomy pouch system

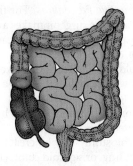

The **ascending colostomy** is done for right-sided tumors.

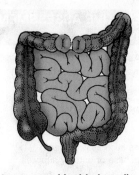

The **transverse (double-barrel) colostomy** is often used in such emergencies as intestinal obstruction or perforation because it can be created quickly. There are two stomas. The proximal one, closest to the small intestine, drains feces. The distal stoma drains mucus.

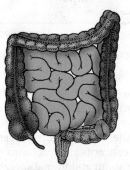

The **descending colostomy** is done for left-sided tumors.

The **sigmoid colostomy** is done for rectal tumors.

FIG. 59-6 Different locations of colostomies in the colon.

in place. A clear pouch allows the health care team to observe the stoma. If no pouch system is in place, a petrolatum gauze dressing is usually placed over the stoma to keep it moist. This is covered with a dry, sterile dressing. In collaboration with the ostomy nurse, place a pouch system as soon as possible. The colostomy pouch system, also called an *appliance,* allows more convenient and acceptable collection of stool than a dressing does.

Assess the color and integrity of the stoma frequently. A healthy stoma should be reddish pink and moist and protrude about ¾ inch (2 cm) from the abdominal wall (Fig. 59-7). During the initial postoperative period, the stoma may be slightly edematous. A small amount of bleeding at the stoma is common.

! NURSING SAFETY PRIORITY

Action Alert

Report any of these problems related to the colostomy to the surgeon:
- Signs of ischemia and necrosis (dark red, purplish, or black color; dry, firm, or flaccid)
- Unusual bleeding
- Mucocutaneous separation (breakdown of the suture line securing the stoma to the abdominal wall)

Also assess the condition of the peristomal skin (skin around the stoma), and frequently check the pouch system for proper fit and signs of leakage. The skin should be intact, smooth, and without redness or excoriation.

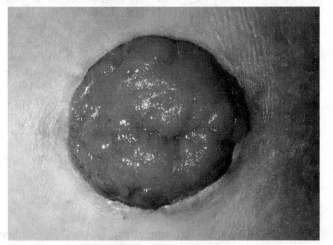

FIG. 59-7 A mature colostomy.

The colostomy should start functioning in 2 to 4 days postoperatively. When it begins to function, the pouch may need to be emptied frequently because of excess gas collection. It should be emptied when it is one-third to one-half full of stool. Stool is liquid immediately postoperatively but becomes more solid, depending on where in the colon the stoma was placed. For example, the stool from a colostomy in the ascending colon is liquid, the stool from a colostomy in the transverse colon is pasty, and the stool from a colostomy in the descending colon is more solid (similar to usual stool expelled from the rectum).

Wound Management. For an AP resection, the perineal wound is generally surgically closed and two bulb suction drains such as Jackson-Pratt drains are placed in the wound or through stab wounds near the wound. The drains help prevent drainage from collecting within the wound and are usually left in place for several days, depending on the character and amount of drainage. These drains are described in more detail in Chapter 18.

Monitoring drainage from the perineal wound and cavity is important because of the possibility of infection and abscess formation. Serosanguineous drainage from the perineal wound may be observed for 1 to 2 months after surgery. Complete healing of the perineal wound may take 6 to 8 months. This wound can be a greater source of discomfort than the abdominal incision and ostomy, and more care may be required. The patient may experience phantom rectal sensations because sympathetic innervation for rectal control has not been interrupted. Rectal pain and itching may occasionally occur after healing. However, there is no known physiologic explanation for these sensations. Interventions may include use of antipruritic drugs, such as benzocaine, and sitz baths. Continually assess for signs of infection, abscess, or other complications, and implement methods for promoting wound drainage and comfort (Chart 59-2).

❓ NCLEX EXAMINATION CHALLENGE

Physiological Integrity

A nurse is assigned to care for a client who had a partial colectomy and ascending colostomy yesterday. What assessment findings are expected for the client? **Select all that apply.**
A. The colostomy stoma is pinkish red and moist.
B. The nasogastric tube is draining bright red blood.
C. The client has pain that is controlled by analgesics.
D. The colostomy is draining solid brown stool.
E. The perineal incision is covered with a surgical dressing.

Assisting with the Grieving Process

Planning: Expected Outcomes. The expected outcomes are that the patient will verbalize feelings about the diagnosis and treatment and progress through the normal stages of grief.

Interventions. The patient and family are faced with a possible loss of or alteration in body functions. Medical and surgical interventions for the treatment of colorectal cancer may result in cure, disease control, or palliation. Interventions are designed to assist the patient in planning effective strategies for expressing feelings of grief and developing coping skills.

Observe and identify:
- The patient's and family's current methods of coping
- Effective sources of support used in past crises
- The patient's and family's present perceptions of the health problem
- Signs of anticipatory grief, such as crying, anger, and withdrawal from usual relationships

Encourage the patient to verbalize feelings about the diagnosis, treatment, and anticipated alteration in body functions if a colostomy is planned. (See discussion of Operative Procedures on p. 1248 in the Surgical Management section.)

CHART 59-2 BEST PRACTICE FOR PATIENT SAFETY & QUALITY CARE

Perineal Wound Care

Wound Care
- Place an absorbent dressing (e.g., abdominal pad) over the wound.
- Instruct the patient that he or she may:
  - Use a feminine napkin as a dressing
  - Wear jockey-type shorts rather than boxers

Comfort Measures
- If prescribed, soak the wound area in a sitz bath for 10 to 20 minutes three or four times per day.
- Administer pain medication as prescribed, and assess its effectiveness.
- Instruct the patient about permissible activities. The patient should:
  - Assume a side-lying position in bed; avoid sitting for long periods
  - Use foam pads or a soft pillow to sit on whenever in a sitting position
  - Avoid the use of air rings or rubber donut devices

Prevention of Complications
- Maintain fluid and electrolyte balance by monitoring intake and output and by monitoring output from the perineal wound.
- Observe incision integrity, and monitor wound drains; watch for erythema, edema, bleeding, drainage, unusual odor, and excessive or constant pain.

Sadness, anger, feelings of loss, and depression are normal responses to this change in body function.

If a colostomy is planned, instruct the patient on what to expect about the appearance and care of the colostomy. Postoperatively, encourage him or her to look at and touch the stoma. When the patient is physically able, ask him or her to participate in colostomy care. Participation helps restore the patient's sense of control over his or her lifestyle and thus facilitates improved self-esteem.

Assist the patient in identifying the nature of and reaction to the loss. Encourage the patient to verbalize feelings and identify fears to help move him or her through the appropriate phases of the grief process. Establish a trusting, ongoing relationship with the patient, and provide support through the personal grieving stages.

In collaboration with the social worker or chaplain, and when appropriate, assist the patient in identifying personal coping strategies. Encourage him or her to implement cultural, religious, and social customs associated with the loss, and identify sources of community support. Modifications in lifestyle are needed for patients with CRC. Help the patient and family identify these changes and how best to make them.

❗ NURSING SAFETY PRIORITY

Action Alert

Refer patients who are at risk for or have familial CRC for genetic counseling. Specially trained nurses can discuss the purposes and goals of genetic testing. Ensure privacy and confidentiality. A review of the family history may provide important information concerning the pattern of colorectal cancer inheritance. To make an informed decision, the patient and family need information about the advantages, risks, and costs of appropriate genetic tests. Monitor the patient's response regarding genetic risk factors.

The chaplain, social worker, or case manager assists in discussions and decisions with them concerning treatment, the prognosis, and end-of-life decisions, as appropriate.

Community-Based Care

Patients undergoing an uncomplicated colon resection by open approach are typically hospitalized for 3 days or longer, depending on the age of the patient and any complications or concurrent health problems. Collaborate with the case manager to assist patients and their families in coping with the immediate postoperative phase of recovery. After hospitalization for surgery, the patient is usually managed at home. Radiation therapy or chemotherapy is typically done on an ambulatory care basis. For the patient with advanced cancer, hospice care may be an option (see Chapter 9).

Home Care Management

Assess all patients for their ability for self-management within limitations. For those requiring assistance with care, home care visits by nurses or assistive nursing personnel can be provided.

For the patient who has undergone a colostomy, review the home situation to aid the patient in arranging for care. Ostomy products should be kept in an area (preferably the bathroom) where the temperature is neither hot nor cold (skin barriers may become stiff or melt in extreme temperatures) to ensure proper functioning. The home care nurse or CWOCN or ET may serve as a consultant after the patient is discharged home to ensure continuity of care (per The Joint Commission's National Patient Safety Goals).

No changes are needed in sleeping accommodations. A moisture-proof covering may initially be placed over the bed mattress if patients feel insecure about the pouch system. They may consume their usual diet on discharge.

Teaching for Self-Management

Before discharge, teach the patient to avoid lifting heavy objects or straining on defecation to prevent tension on the anastomosis site. If he or she had the open surgical approach, the patient should avoid driving for 4 to 6 weeks while the incision heals. Patients who have had laparoscopy can usually return to all usual activities in 1 to 2 weeks.

> **! NURSING SAFETY PRIORITY**
>
> *Action Alert*
>
> A stool softener may be prescribed to keep stools at a soft consistency for ease of passage. Teach patients to note the frequency, amount, and character of the stools. In addition to this information, teach those with colon resections to watch for and report clinical manifestations of intestinal obstruction and perforation (e.g., cramping, abdominal pain, nausea, vomiting). Advise the patient to avoid gas-producing foods and carbonated beverages. Four to six weeks may be required to establish the effects of certain foods on bowel patterns.

Colostomy Care. Rehabilitation after surgery requires that patients and family members learn how to perform colostomy care. Provide adequate opportunity before discharge for patients to learn the psychomotor skills involved in this care. Plan sufficient practice time for learning how to handle, assemble, and apply all ostomy equipment. Teach patients and families or other caregivers about:

- The normal appearance of the stoma
- Signs and symptoms of complications
- Measurement of the stoma
- The choice, use, care, and application of the appropriate appliance to cover the stoma
- Measures to protect the skin adjacent to the stoma
- Nutrition changes to control gas and odor
- Resumption of normal activities, including work, travel, and sexual intercourse

The appropriate pouch system must be selected and fitted to the stoma. Patients with flat, firm abdomens may use either flexible (bordered with paper tape) or nonflexible (full skin barrier wafer) pouch systems. A firm abdomen with lateral creases or folds requires a flexible system. Patients with deep creases, flabby abdomens, a retracted stoma, or a stoma that is flush or concave to the abdominal surface benefit from a convex appliance with a stoma belt. This type of system presses into the skin around the stoma, causing the stoma to protrude. This protrusion helps tighten the skin and prevents leaks around the stoma opening onto the peristomal skin.

Measurement of the stoma is necessary to determine the correct size of the stomal opening on the appliance. The opening should be large enough not only to cover the peristomal skin but also to avoid stomal trauma. The stoma will shrink within 6 to 8 weeks after surgery. Therefore it needs to be measured at least once weekly during this time and as needed if the patient gains or loses weight. Teach the patient and family caregiver to trace the pattern of the stomal area on the wafer portion of the appliance and to cut an opening about 1/8- to 1/16-inch larger than the stomal pattern to ensure that stomal tissue will not be constricted.

Skin preparation may include clipping peristomal hair or shaving the area (moving from the stoma outward) to achieve a smooth surface, prevent unnecessary discomfort when the wafer is removed, and minimize the risk for infected hair follicles. Advise the patient to clean around the stoma with mild soap and water before putting on an appliance. He or she should avoid using moisturizing soaps to clean the area because the lubricants can interfere with adhesion of the appliance.

> **! NURSING SAFETY PRIORITY**
>
> *Action Alert*
>
> Teach the patient and family to apply a skin sealant (preferably without alcohol) and allow it to dry before application of the appliance (colostomy bag) to facilitate less painful removal of the tape or adhesive. If peristomal skin becomes raw, stoma powder or paste or a combination may also be applied. The paste or other filler cream is also used to fill in crevices and creases to create a flat surface for the faceplate of the colostomy bag. If the patient develops a fungal rash, an antifungal cream or powder should be used.

Control of gas and odor from the colostomy is often an important outcome for patients with new ostomies. Although a leaking or inadequately closed pouch is the usual cause of odor, flatus can also contribute to the odor. Remind the patient that although generally no foods for ostomates are forbidden, certain foods and habits can cause flatus or contribute to odor when the pouch is open. Broccoli, beans, spicy foods, onions, brussels sprouts, cabbage, cauliflower, cucumbers, mushrooms, and peas often cause flatus, as does chewing gum, smoking, drinking beer, and skipping meals. Crackers,

CHART 59-3 HOME CARE ASSESSMENT

The Patient with a Colostomy

Assess gastrointestinal status, including:
- Dietary and fluid intake and habits
- Presence or absence of nausea and vomiting
- Weight gain or loss
- Bowel elimination pattern and characteristics and amount of effluent (stool)
- Bowel sounds

Assess condition of stoma, including:
- Location, size, protrusion, color, and integrity
- Signs of ischemia, such as dull coloring or dark or purplish bruising

Assess peristomal skin for:
- Presence or absence of excoriated skin, leakage underneath drainage system
- Fit of appliance and effectiveness of skin barrier and appliance

Assess patient's and family's coping skills, including:
- Self-care abilities in the home
- Acknowledgment of changes in body image and function
- Sense of loss

EVIDENCE-BASED PRACTICE

What Are the Sexuality Challenges That Men with Intestinal Ostomies Have?

Symms, M.R., Rawl, S.M., Grant, M., Wendel, C.S., Coons, S.J., Hickey, S., et al. (2008). Sexual health and quality of life among male veterans with intestinal ostomies. *Clinical Nurse Specialist, 22*(1), 30-40.

The researchers conducted this study of 481 male veterans in three Veterans Administration sites to determine the effect of intestinal ostomies on their sexual health. The design was case-controlled, and both quantitative and qualitative data were collected. The study group was compared with another group who had other surgeries. Quality of life was determined by responses on the modified City of Hope Quality of Life-Ostomy questionnaire.

Compared with sexual activity before surgery, the study group reported more problems with intimacy and sexuality than the control group. They had less sexual activity and more erectile dysfunction than men in the control group. For study group subjects, those who had successful sexual relationships felt less isolation and less trouble adjusting to their ostomies.

Level of Evidence: 2
The study used a large sample and a control group for comparison.

Commentary—Implications for Practice and Research
Although the researchers used a convenience sample of one group of men, they had a large sample and obtained both quantitative and qualitative data. Nurses need to include a sexual health assessment in their care of patients with ostomies. They need to be open to discussion about sexual issues and refer patients to other resources, such as intimacy or sexual counselors, as needed. Additional studies should be conducted with non-veterans and include women of various ethnicities.

---

toast, and yogurt can help prevent gas. Asparagus, broccoli, cabbage, turnips, eggs, fish, and garlic contribute to odor when the pouch is open. Buttermilk, cranberry juice, parsley, and yogurt will help prevent odor. Charcoal filters, pouch deodorizers, or placement of a breath mint in the pouch will help eliminate odors. The patient should be cautioned to not put aspirin tablets in the pouch because they may cause ulceration of the stoma. Vents that allow release of gas from the ostomy bag through a deodorizing filter are available and may decrease the patient's level of self-consciousness about odor.

The patient with a sigmoid colostomy may benefit from colostomy irrigation to regulate elimination. However, most patients with a sigmoid colostomy can become regulated through diet. An irrigation is similar to an enema but is administered through the stoma rather than the rectum.

In addition to teaching the patient about the clinical manifestations of obstruction and perforation, ask the patient to report any fever or sudden onset of pain or swelling around the stoma. Other home care assessment is listed in Chart 59-3.

Psychosocial Concerns. The diagnosis of cancer can be emotionally immobilizing for the patient and family or significant others, but treatment may be welcomed because it may provide hope for control of the disease. Explore reactions to the illness and perceptions of planned interventions.

The patient's reaction to ostomy surgery may include:
- Fear of not being accepted by others
- Feelings of grief related to disturbance in body image
- Concerns about sexuality

Symms et al. (2008) found in their study of male veterans with intestinal ostomies that problems related to sexual activity and intimacy were their greatest challenge. (See the Evidence-Based Practice box above.)

Allow the patient to verbalize his or her feelings. By teaching how to physically manage the ostomy, help him or her begin to restore self-esteem and improve body image. Inclusion of family and significant others in the rehabilitation process may help maintain relationships and raise self-esteem. Anticipatory instruction includes information on leakage accidents, odor control measures, and adjustments to resuming sexual relationships.

Health Care Resources

Several resources are available to maintain continuity of care in the home environment and provide for patient needs that the nurse is not able to meet. Make referrals to community-based case managers or social workers, who can provide further emotional counseling, aid in managing financial concerns, or arrange for services in the home or long-term care as needed.

Provide information about the United Ostomy Associations of America, Inc. (www.uoaa.org), a self-help group of people who have ostomies. This group has literature such as the organization's publication *(Ostomy Quarterly)* and information about local chapters. The organization conducts a visitor program that sends specially trained visitors (who have an ostomy [ostomate]) to talk with patients. After obtaining consent, make a referral to the visitor program so that the volunteer ostomate can see the patient both preoperatively and postoperatively. A physician's consent for visitation may be necessary.

The local division or unit of the American Cancer Society (ACS) (www.cancer.org) can help provide necessary medical equipment and supplies, home care services, travel accommodations, and other resources for the patient who is having cancer treatment or surgery. Inform the patient and family of the programs available through the local division or unit.

Because of short hospital stays, patients with new ostomies receive much health teaching from nurses working for home care agencies. This resource also helps provide physical care needs, medication management, and emotional support. If the patient has advanced colorectal cancer, a referral for hospice services in the home, nursing home, or other long-term care setting may be appropriate. The home care nurse informs the patient and family about what ostomy supplies are needed and where they can be purchased. Price and location are considered before recommendations are made.

EVALUATION: OUTCOMES

Evaluate the care of the patient with colorectal cancer based on the identified priority patient problems. The expected outcomes are that the patient:

- Adjusts to actual or impending loss
- Is free of complications or metastasis associated with CRC
- States he or she has well-controlled pain and is as comfortable as possible (if metastasis is present)

INTESTINAL OBSTRUCTION

Pathophysiology

Intestinal obstructions can be partial or complete and are classified as mechanical or nonmechanical. In mechanical obstruction, the bowel is physically blocked by problems outside the intestine (e.g., adhesions), in the bowel wall (e.g., Crohn's disease), or in the intestinal lumen (e.g., tumors). Nonmechanical obstruction (also known as paralytic ileus or *adynamic ileus*) does not involve a physical obstruction in or outside the intestine. Instead, peristalsis is decreased or absent as a result of neuromuscular disturbance, resulting in a slowing of the movement or a backup of intestinal contents.

Intestinal contents are composed of ingested fluid, food, and saliva; gastric, pancreatic, and biliary secretions; and swallowed air. In both mechanical and nonmechanical obstructions, the intestinal contents accumulate at and above the area of obstruction. Distention results from the intestine's inability to absorb the contents and move them down the intestinal tract. To compensate for the lag, peristalsis increases in an effort to move the intestinal contents forward. This increase stimulates more secretions, which then leads to additional distention. The bowel then becomes edematous, and increased capillary permeability results. Plasma leaking into the peritoneal cavity and fluid trapped in the intestinal lumen decrease the absorption of fluid and electrolytes into the vascular space. Reduced circulatory blood volume (hypovolemia) and electrolyte imbalances typically occur. Hypovolemia ranges from mild to extreme (hypovolemic shock).

Specific fluid and electrolyte problems result, depending on the part of the intestine that is blocked. An obstruction high in the small intestine causes a loss of gastric hydrochloride, which can lead to *metabolic alkalosis*. Obstruction below the duodenum but above the large bowel results in loss of both acids and bases, so that acid-base imbalance is usually not compromised. Obstruction at the end of the small intestine and lower in the intestinal tract causes loss of alkaline fluids, which can lead to *metabolic acidosis*.

If hypovolemia is severe, renal insufficiency or even death can occur. Bacterial peritonitis with or without actual perforation can also result. Bacteria in the intestinal contents lie stagnant in the obstructed intestine. This is not a problem unless the blood flow to the intestine is compromised.

However, with so-called *closed-loop obstruction* (blockage in two different areas) or a strangulated obstruction (obstruction with compromised blood flow), the risk for peritonitis is greatly increased. Bacteria without blood supply can form and release an endotoxin into the peritoneal or systemic circulation and cause septic shock. With a strangulated obstruction, major blood loss into the intestine and the peritoneum can result.

Etiology

Intestinal obstruction is a common and serious disorder caused by a variety of conditions and is associated with significant morbidity. It can occur anywhere in the intestinal tract, although the ileum in the small intestine (the narrowest part of the intestinal tract) is the most common site.

Mechanical obstruction can result from:

- Adhesions (scar tissue from surgeries or pathology)
- Benign or malignant tumor
- Complications of appendicitis
- Hernias
- Fecal impactions (especially in older adults)
- Strictures due to Crohn's disease or previous radiation therapy
- Intussusception (telescoping of a segment of the intestine within itself) (Fig. 59-8)
- Volvulus (twisting of the intestine) (see Fig. 59-8)
- Fibrosis due to disorders such as endometriosis
- Vascular disorders (e.g., emboli and arteriosclerotic narrowing of mesenteric vessels)

In people ages 65 years or older, diverticulitis, tumors, and fecal impaction are the most common causes of obstruction.

Paralytic ileus, or nonmechanical obstruction, is most commonly caused by handling of the intestines during abdominal surgery; intestinal function is lost for a few hours

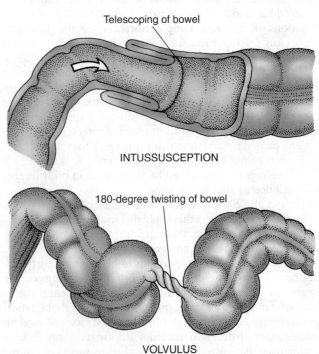

FIG. 59-8 Two types of mechanical obstruction.

Telescoping of bowel

INTUSSUSCEPTION

180-degree twisting of bowel

VOLVULUS

to several days. Electrolyte disturbances, especially hypokalemia, predispose the patient to this problem. The ileus can also be a consequence of peritonitis, because leakage of colonic contents causes severe irritation and triggers an inflammatory response. Vascular insufficiency to the bowel, also referred to as *intestinal ischemia*, is another potential cause of an ileus. It results when arterial or venous thrombosis or an embolus decreases blood flow to the mesenteric blood vessels surrounding the intestines, as in heart failure or severe shock. Severe insufficiency of blood supply can result in infarction of surrounding organs (e.g., bowel infarction).

Incidence/Prevalence

Obstruction of the intestines is the most common reason for surgery of the small intestine. Because bowel obstruction is a result of other disorders, statistics on the incidence of bowel obstruction are not readily available.

Obstruction of the intestines occurs in all age-groups, but the incidence differs with age. In adults, most obstructions occur in the small intestine.

PATIENT-CENTERED COLLABORATIVE CARE

ASSESSMENT

History

Collect information about a history of:
- Abdominal surgery
- Radiation therapy
- Inflammatory bowel disease
- Gallstones
- Hernias
- Trauma
- Peritonitis
- Tumors

Question the patient about recent nausea and vomiting and the color of emesis. Perform a thorough pain assessment with particular attention to the onset, aggravating factors, alleviating factors, and patterns or rhythms of the pain. Severe pain that then stops and changes to tenderness on palpation may indicate perforation and should be reported promptly to the physician. Ask about the passage of flatus and the time, character, and consistency of the last bowel movement. Singultus (hiccups) is common with all types of intestinal obstruction. When an obstruction is suspected, keep the patient NPO and contact the physician promptly for further guidance.

Assess for a family history of colorectal cancer (CRC), and ask about blood in the stool or a change in bowel pattern. Body temperature with uncomplicated obstruction is rarely higher than 100° F (37.8° C). A temperature higher than this, with or without guarding and tenderness, and a sustained elevation in pulse could indicate a strangulated obstruction or peritonitis. A fever, tachycardia, hypotension, increasing abdominal pain, abdominal rigidity, or change in color of skin overlying the abdomen should be reported to the attending physician immediately.

Physical Assessment/Clinical Manifestations

The patient with *mechanical* obstruction in the *small intestine* often has mid-abdominal pain or cramping. The pain can be sporadic, and the patient may feel comfortable between episodes. If strangulation is present, the pain becomes more localized and steady. Vomiting often accompanies obstruction and is more profuse with obstructions in the proximal small intestine. The vomitus may contain bile and mucus or be orange-brown and foul smelling as a result of bacterial overgrowth with low ileal obstruction. Obstipation (no passage of stool) and failure to pass flatus accompany complete obstruction. Diarrhea may be present in partial obstruction.

Mechanical colonic obstruction causes a milder, more intermittent colicky abdominal pain than is seen with small-bowel obstruction. Lower abdominal distention and obstipation may be present, or the patient may have ribbon-like stools if obstruction is partial. Alterations in bowel patterns and blood in the stools accompany the obstruction if colorectal cancer or diverticulitis is the cause.

On examination of the abdomen, observe for abdominal distention, which is common in all forms of intestinal obstruction. Peristaltic waves may also be visible. Auscultate for proximal high-pitched bowel sounds (borborygmi), which are associated with cramping early in the obstructive process as the intestine tries to push the mechanical obstruction forward. In later stages of mechanical obstruction, bowel sounds are absent, especially distal to the obstruction. Abdominal tenderness and rigidity are usually minimal. The presence of a tense, fluid-filled bowel loop mimicking a palpable abdominal mass may signal a closed-loop, strangulating small-bowel obstruction.

In most types of *nonmechanical* obstruction, the pain is described as a constant, diffuse discomfort. Colicky cramping is not characteristic of this type of obstruction. Pain associated with obstruction caused by vascular insufficiency or infarction is usually severe and constant. On inspection, abdominal distention is typically present. On auscultation of the abdomen, note and document decreased bowel sounds in early obstruction and absent bowel sounds in later stages. Vomiting of gastric contents and bile is frequent, but the vomitus rarely has a foul odor and is rarely profuse. Obstipation may or may not be present. Chart 59-4 compares small-bowel and large-bowel obstructions.

CHART 59-4	KEY FEATURES

Small-Bowel and Large-Bowel Obstructions

SMALL-BOWEL OBSTRUCTIONS	LARGE-BOWEL OBSTRUCTIONS
Abdominal discomfort or pain possibly accompanied by visible peristaltic waves in upper and middle abdomen	Intermittent lower abdominal cramping
Upper or epigastric abdominal distention	Lower abdominal distention
Nausea and early, profuse vomiting (may contain fecal material)	Minimal or no vomiting
Obstipation	Obstipation or ribbon-like stools
Severe fluid and electrolyte imbalances	No major fluid and electrolyte imbalances
Metabolic alkalosis	Metabolic acidosis (not always present)

Laboratory Assessment

There is no definitive laboratory test to confirm a diagnosis of mechanical or nonmechanical obstruction. White blood cell (WBC) counts are normal unless there is a strangulated obstruction, in which case there may be leukocytosis (increased WBCs). Hemoglobin, hematocrit, creatinine, and blood urea nitrogen (BUN) values are often elevated, indicating dehydration. Serum sodium, chloride, and potassium concentrations are reduced because of loss of fluid and electrolytes. Elevations in serum amylase levels may be found with strangulating obstructions, which can damage the pancreas.

Patients with high obstruction in the small intestine have arterial blood gas (ABG) values indicative of metabolic alkalosis. Obstruction in the large intestine may show values suggestive of metabolic acidosis. Chapter 14 describes ABGs and these acid-base imbalances in detail.

Imaging Assessment

The health care provider obtains supine and upright abdominal x-rays and a CT scan as soon as an obstruction is suspected. Distention with fluid and gas in the small intestine with the absence of gas in the colon indicates an obstruction in the small intestine. X-ray findings are often normal when a strangulated obstruction actually exists in the small intestine.

Other Diagnostic Assessment

The diagnostic examination chosen depends on the suspected location of the obstruction. As an initial assessment, the physician may choose to do an abdominal ultrasound to evaluate the potential cause of the obstruction. The physician may perform endoscopy (sigmoidoscopy or colonoscopy) to determine the cause of the obstruction, except when perforation or complete obstruction is suspected.

INTERVENTIONS

Interventions are aimed at uncovering the cause and relieving the obstruction. Intestinal obstructions can be relieved by nonsurgical or surgical means. If the obstruction is partial and there is no evidence of strangulation, nonsurgical management is the treatment of choice.

Nonsurgical Management

Paralytic ileus responds well to nonsurgical methods of relieving obstruction. Nonsurgical approaches are also preferred in the treatment of patients with terminal disease associated with bowel obstruction. In addition to being NPO, patients typically have a nasogastric tube (NGT) inserted to decompress the bowel by draining fluid and air. The tube is attached to suction.

Nasogastric Tubes. Most patients with an obstruction have an NGT unless the obstruction is mild.

A Salem sump tube is inserted through the nose and placed into the stomach. It is attached to low continuous suction. This tube has a vent ("pigtail") that prevents the stomach mucosa from being pulled away during suctioning. Levin tubes do not have a vent and therefore should be connected to low intermittent suction. They are used less often than the Salem sump tubes. Chart 58-5 in Chapter 58 describes how to insert an NGT.

Question the patient about the passage of flatus, and record flatus and the character of bowel movements daily. Flatus or stool means that peristalsis has returned. Assess for nausea, and ask the patient to report this manifestation.

> ## ! NURSING SAFETY PRIORITY
> ### *Action Alert*
>
> *At least every 4 hours, assess the patient with an NGT for proper placement of the tube, tube patency, and output (quality and quantity).* Monitor the nasal skin around the tube for irritation. Use a device that secures the tube to the nose to prevent accidental removal. Clean the nose with the same type of skin protectant used for ostomy skin care before applying the NGT securing device. Assess for peristalsis by auscultating for bowel sounds with the suction disconnected (suction masks peristaltic sounds).

Monitor any NGT for proper functioning. Occasionally, NGTs move out of optimal drainage position or become plugged. In this case, note a decrease in gastric output or stasis of the tube's contents. Assess the patient for nausea, vomiting, increased abdominal distention, and placement of the tube. If the NGT is repositioned or replaced, confirmation of proper placement is obtained by x-ray examination before use. After appropriate placement is established, aspirate the contents and irrigate the tube with 30 mL of normal saline every 4 hours or as requested by the health care provider.

Other Nonsurgical Interventions. Most types of nonmechanical obstruction respond to nasogastric decompression in conjunction with medical treatment of the primary disorder. Incomplete mechanical obstruction can sometimes be successfully treated without surgery. Obstruction caused by lower fecal impaction usually resolves after disimpaction and enema administration. Intussusception may respond to hydrostatic pressure changes during a barium enema.

IV fluid replacement and maintenance are indicated for all patients with intestinal obstruction because the patient is NPO and fluids and electrolytes are lost (particularly potassium) through vomiting and nasogastric suction. On the basis of serum electrolytes and blood urea nitrogen (BUN) levels, the health care provider prescribes aggressive fluid replacement with 2 to 4 L of normal saline or lactated Ringer's solution with potassium added. Use care with patients who are susceptible to fluid overload (e.g., older adults with a history of heart or kidney failure). Monitor lung sounds, weight, and intake and output daily. Blood replacement may be indicated in strangulated obstruction because of blood loss into the bowel or peritoneal cavity.

Monitor vital signs and other measures of fluid status (e.g., urine output, skin turgor, mucous membranes) every 2 to 4 hours depending on the severity of the patient's symptoms. In collaboration with the dietitian, the physician may prescribe total parenteral nutrition (TPN), especially if the patient has had chronic nutritional problems and has been NPO for an extended period. Chapter 63 discusses the nursing care of patients receiving TPN.

The patient with intestinal obstruction is usually thirsty, although older adults have a decreased thirst response as they age. Delegate frequent mouth care to unlicensed assistive personnel (UAP) to help maintain moist mucous membranes. Be sure to supervise this activity. A few ice chips may be allowed if the patient is not having surgery. Follow agency protocol or the physician's request regarding ice chips.

Abdominal distention can cause a great deal of discomfort, especially when it is severe. The colicky, crampy pain that comes and goes with mechanical obstruction and the nausea, vomiting, dry mucous membranes, and thirst contribute to the patient's discomfort. Continually assess the character and location of the pain, and immediately report any pain that significantly increases or changes from a colicky, intermittent type to a constant discomfort. These changes can indicate perforation of the intestine or peritonitis.

Opioid analgesics may be temporarily withheld in the diagnostic workup period so that clinical manifestations of perforation or peritonitis are not masked. Explain to the patient and family the rationale for not giving analgesics. In addition, if analgesics such as morphine are given, they may slow intestinal motility and can cause vomiting. Be alert to this side effect because nausea and vomiting are also signs of NG tube obstruction or worsening bowel obstruction.

Help the patient obtain a position of comfort with frequent position changes to promote increased peristalsis. A semi-Fowler's position helps alleviate the pressure of abdominal distention on the chest. This position is for comfort and promotion of thoracic excursion to facilitate breathing.

Discomfort is generally less with nonmechanical obstruction than with mechanical obstruction. With both types of obstruction, discomfort is aggravated by taking in food or fluids.

If strangulation is thought to be likely, the health care provider prescribes IV broad-spectrum antibiotics. In addition, in cases of partial obstruction or paralytic ileus, drugs that enhance gastric motility such as octreotide acetate (Sandostatin) may be used.

Surgical Management

In patients with complete mechanical obstruction and in some cases of incomplete mechanical obstruction, surgical intervention is necessary to relieve the obstruction. A strangulated obstruction is complete, and surgical intervention is always required. An exploratory laparotomy (a surgical opening of the abdominal cavity to investigate the cause of the obstruction) is initially performed for many patients with obstruction. More specific surgical procedures depend on the cause of the obstruction.

Preoperative Care. Provide general preoperative teaching for both the patient and family as discussed in Chapter 16. In cases of complete obstruction, the patient may feel too ill to want the information. Reinforce the information with the family or other caregiver. Depending on the cause and severity of the obstruction, as well as the expertise of the surgeon, patients have either minimally invasive surgery (MIS) via laparoscopy or a conventional open approach.

Operative Procedures. In the *conventional open surgical approach,* the surgeon makes a large incision, enters the abdominal cavity, and explores for obstruction and its cause, if possible (exploratory laparotomy). If adhesions are found, they are lysed (cut and released). Obstruction caused by a tumor or diverticulitis requires a colon resection with primary anastomosis or a temporary or permanent colostomy. If obstruction is caused by intestinal infarction, an embolectomy, thrombectomy, or resection of the gangrenous small or large bowel may be necessary. In severe cases, a colectomy (removal of the entire colon) may be needed.

For the *MIS* approach, the specially trained surgeon makes several small incisions in the abdomen and places a video camera to view the abdominal contents to determine the extent of the obstruction. A laparoscope (type of endoscope) with a lighted end is inserted along with various surgical instruments to remove the problem. This procedure takes longer than the open approach, but blood loss is less.

Postoperative Care. General postoperative care for the patient undergoing an *exploratory laparotomy* with lysis of adhesions, colon resection, thrombectomy, or embolectomy is similar to that described in Chapter 18. In addition, patients have an NGT in place until peristalsis resumes. A clear liquid diet may be prescribed to encourage peristalsis return. As liquids are started, the NGT can be disconnected from suction and capped for 1 to 2 hours after the patient has taken clear liquids to determine if he or she is able to tolerate them. If the patient vomits after liquids, the suction is resumed. When the patient has return of peristalsis, the NGT is removed slowly by first discontinuing suction and then clamping the tube for a scheduled amount of time. Residual drainage is checked at each stage to assess peristalsis without decompression before removing the tube entirely.

Most patients today have laparoscopic surgery (MIS) for mechanical intestinal obstructions. They usually do *not* have an NGT and can recover more quickly than those with the open surgical approach. The hospital stay for those having MIS to remove tumors, adhesions, and other obstructions may be as short as 1 to 2 days compared with 3 days or longer for the conventional surgical patients. Recovery is much quicker because there is less pain and fewer postoperative complications among those who had laparoscopic surgery.

🅠 DECISION-MAKING CHALLENGE

Patient-Centered Care; Teamwork and Collaboration

> A 91-year-old woman is admitted from an independent living facility with a diagnosis of complete intestinal obstruction due to a severe fecal impaction. She has been vomiting for 2 days and is extremely dehydrated. Her serum electrolytes are abnormal, and she is very weak. Her daughter and granddaughter are in the emergency department and tell you that they are very concerned about her health. They ask you what is wrong with her and what her prognosis is.
>
> 1. What is your best response to the family members at this time?
> 2. What evidence-based collaborative interventions are appropriate for this patient immediately?
> 3. What information do you need to better care for the patient?
> 4. What electrolyte imbalances would you expect? What clinical manifestations of dehydration do you expect this patient to have? How might her presentation be somewhat different from that of a younger adult and why?
> 5. What safety concerns do you have for this patient? What interventions are needed to ensure her safety?

Community-Based Care

All patients with intestinal obstruction are hospitalized for monitoring and treatment. The length of stay varies according to the type of obstruction, the treatment, and the presence of complications. Patients who have complicated obstruction, such as strangulation or incarceration, are at greater risk for peritonitis, sepsis, and shock.

Patients with nonmechanical (adynamic) intestinal obstruction are less likely to require a lengthy hospitalization because of the obstruction alone. Adynamic obstruction generally responds to NG intubation and suction within a few days. However, if the ileus occurs as a complication of an abdominal surgery, the hospital stay could be lengthy.

CHART 59-5   NURSING FOCUS ON THE OLDER ADULT

Preventing Fecal Impaction

- Teach the patient to eat high-fiber foods, including plenty of raw fruits and vegetables and whole-grain products.
- Encourage the patient to drink adequate amounts of fluids, especially water.
- Do not routinely administer a laxative; teach the patient that laxative abuse decreases abdominal muscle tone and contributes to an atonic colon.
- Encourage the patient to exercise regularly, if possible. Walking every day is an excellent exercise for promoting intestinal motility.
- Use natural foods to stimulate peristalsis, such as warm beverages and prune juice.
- Take bulk-forming products, such as Metamucil, to provide fiber.
- Check the patient's stool for amount and frequency; oozing of soft or diarrheal stool often indicates a fecal impaction.
- Have the patient sit on a toilet or bedside commode, rather than on a bedpan, for elimination.

Home Care Management

For the patient who has had an intestinal obstruction, preparation for home care depends on the cause of the obstruction and the treatment required. Those who have resolution of obstruction without surgical intervention are assessed for their knowledge of strategies to avoid recurrent obstruction. For example, if fecal impaction was the cause of the obstruction, assess the patient's ability to carry out a bowel regimen independently (Chart 59-5). For those who have had surgery, evaluate their ability to function at home with the added tasks of incision care and possibly colostomy care.

Teaching for Self-Management

Instruct the patient to report any abdominal pain or distention, nausea, or vomiting, with or without constipation, because these symptoms might indicate recurrent obstruction. The patient should be reassured, however, that recurrent paralytic ileus is not common.

Teach the patient who has had surgery about incision care, drug therapy, and activity limitations. Drug therapy consists of an oral opioid analgesic, such as oxycodone hydrochloride with acetaminophen (Tylox, Percocet, Endocet ✦), to be taken as needed for incisional discomfort. As with any opioid therapy, scheduled doses of a laxative with a softener (e.g., Docusate with Senna) may be added to prevent constipation and possible recurrent obstruction.

The patient who had curative treatment of the underlying cause most likely requires less support than one who had treatment of obstruction related to a serious disease that will require further management. Encourage the patient to express fears and concerns about the future. Assess the patient's understanding and needs with regard to treatment plans.

Health Care Resources

The need for follow-up appointments depends on the cause of the obstruction and the treatment required. In collaboration with the case manager, make arrangements for a home care nurse if the patient needs help with incision or colostomy care.

ABDOMINAL TRAUMA

Pathophysiology

Abdominal trauma is defined as injury to the structures located between the diaphragm and the pelvis, which occurs when the abdomen is subjected to blunt or penetrating forces. Organs injured may include the large or small bowel, liver, spleen, duodenum, pancreas, kidneys, and urinary bladder.

At least one half of all *blunt abdominal traumas* occur from motor vehicle crashes. Other causes of blunt trauma include falls, aggravated assaults, and contact sports. The spleen is the most commonly injured organ from *blunt* abdominal trauma. *Penetrating abdominal trauma* is caused by gunshot wounds, stabbing, or impalement with an object. The liver is the most commonly injured organ from penetrating abdominal trauma. Most penetrating injuries are caused by gunshot wounds (GSWs). *Trauma is the leading cause of death in young adults (younger than 40 years) in the United States.*

PATIENT-CENTERED COLLABORATIVE CARE

ASSESSMENT

First, assess any patient experiencing trauma for airway, breathing, and circulation (ABCs).

! NURSING SAFETY PRIORITY

Critical Rescue

Once the patient with abdominal trauma has been assessed for airway, breathing, and circulation, focus on the risks for hemorrhage, shock, and peritonitis. Mental status, vital signs, and skin perfusion are *priority* nursing assessments, with skin perfusion being the most reliable clinical guide in assessing hypovolemic shock:

- In a person with mild shock, the skin is pale, cool, and moist.
- With moderate shock, diaphoresis is more marked and urine output ceases.
- With severe shock, changes in mental status are manifested by agitation, disorientation, and recent memory loss.

Assess for abdominal trauma by asking the patient about the presence, location, and quality of pain. Inspect the abdomen, flanks, back, genitalia, and rectum for contusions, abrasions, lacerations, ecchymosis, penetrating injuries, and symmetry. All of the patient's clothes must be removed for this examination.

Inspection of the abdomen may reveal distention. To perform an adequate inspection, turn the patient while maintaining spinal immobilization. *Ecchymosis (bruising) may indicate internal bleeding. Ecchymosis present in the distribution of a lap seat belt should be reported to the health care provider immediately because the bowel or other major organ may be injured.*

Auscultate the abdomen for bowel sounds. Absent or diminished bowel sounds may be caused by the presence of blood, bacteria, or a chemical irritant in the abdominal cavity. Also auscultate for bruits in the abdomen, which could indicate renal artery injury.

Injury to the spleen is present in many people with left lower rib fractures. Liver injury may be present in those with right lower rib fractures. Dullness over hollow organs that normally contain gas, such as the stomach and the large and small intestines, may indicate the presence of blood or fluid. Light abdominal palpation identifies areas of tenderness, rebound tenderness, guarding, rigidity, and spasm. A palpated mass may be blood or a fluid collection.

The patient without obvious significant bleeding or definite signs of peritoneal irritation undergoes abdominal ultrasound, diagnostic peritoneal lavage (DPL), and CT. For DPL, the physician inserts a large-bore catheter into the abdomen and allows fluid to enter the abdominal cavity. If the return drainage from the abdomen is pink or grossly bloody, the health care team prepares for surgery. Abdominal ultrasound or focused abdominal sonography for trauma (FAST) is used to diagnose blunt abdominal trauma and may replace CT and DPL for diagnosis. Patients with hemodynamic instability or peritonitis are candidates for immediate laparotomy.

INTERVENTIONS

Nonsurgical and surgical interventions are aimed at preserving or restoring hemodynamic stability, preventing or decreasing blood loss, and preventing complications. Patients with abdominal trauma from a vehicle crash often have other injuries such as multiple fractures. *The priority for care is to establish and maintain the ABCs.*

Emergency Care: Abdominal Trauma

Nursing interventions include placement of at least two large-bore IV catheters in the upper extremities. IV catheters are not used in the lower extremities; if the vasculature has been injured, fluid can pool in the abdomen. The health care provider may insert a central venous catheter to assist with rapid fluid volume infusion. IV fluids include saline, crystalloids, and possibly blood. Be sure to type and cross-match the patient for as many as 4 to 8 units of packed red blood cells.

These laboratory values are monitored:

- Arterial blood gases
- Complete blood count (CBC)
- Serum electrolyte, glucose and amylase, and blood urea nitrogen (BUN) determinations
- Liver function tests
- Coagulation studies

Measuring arterial blood gases may help determine the severity of shock. Hemoglobin and hematocrit values do not initially reflect true blood loss; values can be skewed because of hemoconcentration from volume loss or the dilutional effects of IV fluids. Serial hemoglobin and hematocrit measurements may be more accurate in determining true blood loss. An elevated white blood cell (WBC) count may indicate a ruptured spleen or intestinal injury. Elevated levels of serum transaminases may indicate liver injury. Elevation of serum amylase activity may signal injury to the pancreas or the bowel. All laboratory work is compiled so that values can be compared and subtle changes noted.

Continuous hemodynamic monitoring is begun in the emergency department. Insert an indwelling urinary (Foley) catheter unless there is blood at the urinary meatus. Initially and hourly thereafter, evaluate urine output for bleeding and specific gravity. Laboratory tests indicate the amount of blood and protein in the urine. If there is an open abdominal wound or evisceration, cover it with a sterile dry dressing unless the physician requests otherwise. Unless it is contraindicated, as in the case of a skull fracture, the physician or nurse inserts a nasogastric tube (NGT) to identify bleeding

and minimize the risk for vomiting and aspiration. Antibiotics are administered as prescribed to reduce the risk for peritonitis.

If the patient with known abdominal trauma has no definite clinical manifestations of active bleeding or organ injury, he or she is admitted to the hospital for observation. Many patients are admitted to the critical care unit. Blunt trauma can cause active, but often not obvious, damage.

> **⚠ NURSING SAFETY PRIORITY**
>
> *Critical Rescue*
>
> For the patient who has sustained abdominal trauma, assess for abdominal or referred pain and nausea. Every 15 to 30 minutes in the early postinjury period and then hourly, evaluate:
> - Mental status
> - Vital signs
> - Clinical findings, such as vomiting, guarding, rigidity, or rebound tenderness
> - Bowel sounds
> - Urine output
>
> Report any change immediately to the health care provider! It is more important to recognize the high risk for an active abdominal injury and assess for general signs of organ injury (e.g., hemorrhage and peritonitis) than to identify the exact nature of the abdominal injury. Opioid analgesics are given for pain after the physician's initial assessment is complete. Explain to the patient and family the rationale for delaying analgesics.

Intra-abdominal Pressure Monitoring

Some patients are monitored for intra-abdominal pressure (IAP) using a continuous monitoring system. As the name implies, intra-abdominal pressure is pressure within the abdominal cavity. The normal IAP in healthy adults is 0 to 5 mm Hg, but obese patients often have a higher normal value. In patients with abdominal injury (especially blunt trauma), IAP may increase to the point that major body organs are damaged.

When IAP becomes higher than the central venous pressure, the inferior vena cava and other abdominal vessels are compressed. This leads to impaired venous return, increased afterload, and decreased preload. The patient is then at risk for deep vein thrombosis and pulmonary embolism (PE). The patient has tachycardia and hypotension. As the IAP increases further (over 20 mm Hg), acidosis and ischemia occur. *If elevated IAP is left untreated, damage to the intestine increases the risk for sepsis, multiple organ dysfunction syndrome (MODS), and death.* Renal, cardiac, and respiratory damage are the most likely to occur, although the central nervous system can be affected.

The health care provider may request continuous or intermittent IAP monitoring in the critical care unit. It is usually done by inserting a urinary catheter and using a stopcock, pressure transducer system, clamp, IV tubing, and bag of saline. *Report any increase in IAP immediately to the physician. A sustained or repeated IAP of 12 mm Hg or higher is considered* intra-abdominal hypertension (IAH) *or* acute compartment syndrome (ACS). Acute IAH has a rapid onset after abdominal trauma (especially blunt trauma) and must be treated immediately using either a nonsurgical (vasopressor drugs and fluids) or surgical approach (fasciotomy). Surgery is risky because it increases the chance of embolic stroke and PE.

Surgical Management

For the patient with severe abdominal trauma, the surgeon performs an *exploratory laparotomy* and repairs abdominal injuries immediately if there are definite signs of peritoneal irritation. These signs include rebound tenderness, significant blood loss, evisceration, or a gunshot wound (GSW) with possible peritoneal involvement. After surgery, many of these patients are admitted to a critical care unit and mechanically ventilated.

Most stab wounds and GSWs require exploratory laparotomy. Using local anesthesia, the surgeon explores and cleans superficial penetrating wounds. The patient does not require an exploratory laparotomy for superficial wounds.

Patients with multiple trauma stay in the hospital for a prolonged period. Before discharge from the hospital, teach the patient and family the signs and symptoms of abdominal bleeding whether or not surgery has been performed. Instruct them to report abdominal pain, nausea, vomiting, bloody or black stools, fever, weakness, and dizziness.

Hemorrhage can occasionally occur weeks after blunt abdominal trauma, despite medical evaluation or treatment. For the patient who has surgery or exploration of wounds, provide instructions on wound care before discharge from the hospital. Provide additional health teaching as the patient's overall condition requires.

POLYPS

Pathophysiology

Polyps in the intestinal tract are small growths covered with mucosa and attached to the surface of the intestine. Although most are benign, they are significant because some have the potential to become malignant.

Polyps are identified by their tissue type. Although only a very small number of adenomas progress to cancer, almost all colorectal cancers develop from an adenoma. Adenomas are further classified as villous or tubular. Of these, villous adenomas pose a greater cancer risk.

Familial adenomatous polyposis (FAP) and hereditary nonpolyposis colorectal cancer (HNPCC) are inherited syndromes characterized by progressive development of colorectal adenomas. Unless these syndromes are treated, colorectal cancer (CRC) inevitably occurs by the fourth to fifth decade of life. These conditions were discussed on p. 1245 in the Genetic/Genomic Considerations feature in the Colorectal Cancer section.

In addition to being classified by their tissue type, polyps are described according to their appearance (Fig. 59-9).

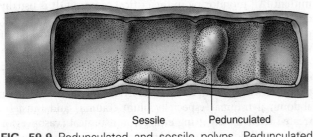

Sessile   Pedunculated

FIG. 59-9 Pedunculated and sessile polyps. Pedunculated polyps, such as tubular adenomas, are stalk-like. Sessile polyps, such as villous adenomas, are broad based.

Pedunculated polyps are stalk-like; a thin stem attaches them to the intestinal wall. They become elongated as peristalsis pulls them into the lumen of the intestine. Polyps attached to the intestinal walls by a broad base are described as sessile. A malignant polyp may be pedunculated or sessile.

PATIENT-CENTERED COLLABORATIVE CARE

Polyps are usually asymptomatic and are discovered during routine colonoscopy screening. However, they can cause gross rectal bleeding, intestinal obstruction, or intussusception (telescoping of the bowel). Biopsy specimens of polyps can be obtained and the entire polyp can be removed (polypectomy) with the use of a snare that fits through the sigmoidoscope or colonoscope. This often eliminates the need for abdominal surgery to remove a suspicious or definitely malignant polyp. The patient with FAP often requires a total colectomy (colon removal) to prevent the development of cancer.

Nursing care focuses on patient education. Instruct the patient about:

- The nature of the polyp
- Clinical manifestations to report to the health care provider
- The need for regular, routine monitoring or screening

If the patient has had a polypectomy, follow-up sigmoidoscopic or colonoscopic examinations are needed because there is an increased risk for developing multiple polyps.

Nursing care of the patient after a polypectomy of the colorectal area includes monitoring for abdominal distention and pain, rectal bleeding, mucopurulent drainage from the rectum, and fever. A small amount of blood might appear in the stool after a polypectomy, but this should be temporary.

HEMORRHOIDS

Pathophysiology

Hemorrhoids are unnaturally swollen or distended veins in the anorectal region. The veins involved in the development of hemorrhoids are part of the normal structure in the anal region. With limited distention, the veins function as a valve overlying the anal sphincter that assists in continence. Increased intra-abdominal pressure causes elevated systemic and portal venous pressure, which is transmitted to the anorectal veins. Arterioles in the anorectal region shunt blood directly to the distended anorectal veins, which increases the pressure. With repeated elevations in pressure from increased intra-abdominal pressure and engorgement from arteriolar shunting of blood, the distended veins eventually separate from the smooth muscle surrounding them. The result is prolapse of the hemorrhoidal vessels.

Hemorrhoids can be internal or external (Fig. 59-10). Internal hemorrhoids, which cannot be seen on inspection of the perineal area, lie above the anal sphincter. External hemorrhoids lie below the anal sphincter and can be seen on inspection of the anal region. Prolapsed hemorrhoids can become thrombosed or inflamed, or they can bleed.

Hemorrhoids are common and not significant unless they cause pain or bleeding. Caused by increased abdominal pressure, the condition worsens during pregnancy, constipation

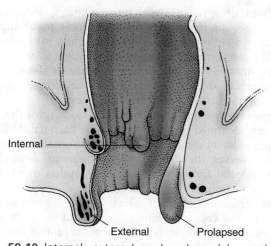

FIG. 59-10 Internal, external, and prolapsed hemorrhoids. *Internal hemorrhoids* lie above the anal sphincter and cannot be seen on inspection of the anal area. *External hemorrhoids* lie below the anal sphincter and can be seen on inspection of the anal region. Hemorrhoids that enlarge, fall down, and protrude through the anus are called *prolapsed hemorrhoids.*

with straining, obesity, heart failure, prolonged sitting or standing, and strenuous exercise and weight lifting. Decreased fluid intake can also cause hemorrhoids because of the development of hard stool and subsequent constipation. Straining while evacuating stool causes them to enlarge.

Health Promotion and Maintenance

Prevention of constipation is the most important preventive measure. It can be prevented by increasing fiber in the diet, such as eating more whole grains and raw vegetables and fruits. Encourage patients to drink plenty of water unless otherwise contraindicated (e.g., kidney disease, heart disease). Remind the patient to avoid straining at stool. Remind him or her to exercise regularly with a gradual buildup in intensity. Maintaining a healthy weight also helps prevent hemorrhoids.

PATIENT-CENTERED COLLABORATIVE CARE

ASSESSMENT

The most common symptoms of hemorrhoids are bleeding, swelling, and prolapse (bulging). Blood is characteristically bright red and is present on toilet tissue or streaked in the stool. Pain is a common symptom and is often associated with thrombosis, especially if thrombosis occurs suddenly. Other symptoms include itching and a mucous discharge. Diagnosis is usually made by inspection and digital examination, although anoscopy, proctoscopy, or proctoscopic ultrasonography can be performed.

INTERVENTIONS

Interventions are typically conservative and are aimed at reducing symptoms with a minimum of discomfort, cost, and time lost from usual activities. Local treatment and nutrition therapy are used when symptoms begin. Cold packs applied

to the anorectal region for a few minutes at a time beginning with the onset of pain and tepid sitz baths three or four times per day are often enough to relieve discomfort, even if the hemorrhoids are thrombosed.

Topical anesthetics, such as lidocaine (Xylocaine), are useful for severe pain. Dibucaine (Nupercainal) ointment and similar products are available over the counter and may be applied for mild to moderate pain and itching. This ointment should be used only temporarily, however, because it can mask worsening symptoms and delay diagnosis of a severe disorder. If itching or inflammation is present, the health care provider prescribes a steroid preparation, such as hydrocortisone. Cleansing the anal area with moistened cleansing tissues rather than standard toilet tissue helps avoid irritation. The anal area should be cleansed gently by dabbing, rather than by wiping.

Diets high in fiber and fluids are recommended to promote regular bowel movements without straining. Stool softeners, such as docusate sodium (Colace), can be used temporarily. Irritating laxatives are avoided, as are foods and beverages that can make hemorrhoids worse. Spicy foods, nuts, coffee, and alcohol can be irritating. Remind patients to avoid sitting for long periods. The health care provider may prescribe mild oral analgesics for pain if the hemorrhoids are thrombosed.

Conservative treatment should alleviate symptoms in 3 to 5 days. If symptoms continue or recur frequently, the patient may require surgical intervention.

The surgeon can perform several procedures for symptomatic internal hemorrhoids on an ambulatory care basis. Current recommended therapies include ultrasound coagulation, rubber band ligation, circular stapling, and laser-assisted or simple resection of the hemorrhoids. The type of surgery depends on the degree of prolapse, whether there is thrombosis, and the overall condition of the patient.

The harmonic scalpel is an ultrasonically activated instrument that vibrates to coagulate small and medium-size vessels. In rubber band ligation, a rubber ring is placed around the internal hemorrhoid that constricts blood flow to the hemorrhoid, resulting in shrinking of the hemorrhoid. The rubber band usually causes a feeling of tightness in the area until the rubber band falls off in 2 to 4 days. Complications of these procedures include pain, thrombosis of other hemorrhoids, infection, and abscess formation. Bleeding may occur after the band falls off. If the hemorrhoid is prolapsed, a circular stapling device is used to excise a band of mucosa above the prolapse and restore the hemorrhoidal tissue back into the anal canal.

Hemorrhoidectomy, or resection of the hemorrhoid, tends to cause more pain than the other procedures. Urinary retention can also occur because of rectal spasms and anorectal tenderness. Hemorrhage, which may be internal and not visible or external, is a rare but potential complication.

Teach patients with hemorrhoids about the need to eat high-fiber, high-fluid diets to promote regular bowel patterns before and after surgery. Advise them to avoid stimulant laxatives, which can be habit forming.

For patients who undergo any type of surgical intervention, monitor for bleeding and pain postoperatively and teach them to report these problems to their health care provider. Using moist heat (e.g., sitz baths) three or four times per day can help promote comfort.

The physician usually prescribes stool softeners such as docusate sodium (Colace) to begin preoperatively and continue after surgery. Analgesics and anti-inflammatory drugs are prescribed. A mild laxative should be administered if the patient has not had a bowel movement by the third postoperative day.

MALABSORPTION SYNDROME

Pathophysiology

Malabsorption is a syndrome associated with a variety of disorders and intestinal surgical procedures. It interferes with the ability to absorb nutrients and is a result of a generalized flattening of the mucosa of the small intestine. With various disorders, physiologic mechanisms limit absorption of nutrients because of one or more of these abnormalities:

- Bile salt deficiencies
- Enzyme deficiencies
- Presence of bacteria
- Disruption of the mucosal lining of the small intestine
- Altered lymphatic and vascular circulation
- Decrease in the gastric or intestinal surface area

The nutrient involved in malabsorption depends on the type and location of the abnormality in the intestinal tract.

Deficiencies of bile salts can lead to malabsorption of fats and fat-soluble vitamins. Bile salt deficiencies can result from decreased synthesis of bile in the liver, bile obstruction, or alteration of bile salt absorption in the small intestine.

Enzymes normally found in the intestine split disaccharides (complex sugars) to monosaccharides (simple sugars). Examples of these enzymes are lactase, sucrase, maltase, and isomaltase. Lactase deficiency is the most common disaccharide enzyme deficiency. Without sufficient amounts of this enzyme, the body is not able to break down lactose. Lactase deficiency can be due to genetic inheritance, injury to intestinal mucosa from viral hepatitis, bacterial proliferation in the intestine, or sprue. Deficiencies of the other disaccharide enzymes are rare.

Pancreatic enzymes are also necessary for absorption of vitamin B_{12}. With destruction or obstruction of the pancreas or insufficient pancreatic stimulation, this nutrient is not well absorbed. Chronic pancreatitis, pancreatic carcinoma, resection of the pancreas, and cystic fibrosis can cause these malabsorption problems.

Loops of bowel can accumulate intestinal contents, resulting in bacterial overgrowth, when peristalsis is decreased. Bacteria at these sites break down bile salts, and fewer salts are available for fat absorption. They can also ingest vitamin B_{12}, which contributes to vitamin B_{12} deficiency. This process can occur after a gastrectomy.

Disruption of the mucosal lining of the intestine is responsible for the malabsorption that occurs with celiac

(nontropical) sprue, tropical sprue, Crohn's disease, and ulcerative colitis. In celiac (nontropical) sprue, the absorptive surface area in the small intestine is lost; there is malabsorption of most nutrients. Celiac sprue is thought to be due to a genetic immune hypersensitivity response to gluten or its breakdown products or to result from the accumulation of gluten in the diet with peptidase deficiency.

Tropical sprue is caused by an infectious agent that has not been identified but is thought to be bacterial. Mucosal changes occur in a more widespread manner than in celiac sprue. However, the changes are not as severe as in celiac sprue. Tropical sprue results in malabsorption of fat, folic acid, and vitamin B_{12} in later stages of the disease.

The inflammation in Crohn's disease interferes with the surface of cells absorbing bile salts and therefore leads to fat malabsorption. In ulcerative colitis, protein loss may occur.

Obstruction to lymphatic flow in the intestine can lead to loss of plasma proteins along with loss of minerals (e.g., iron, copper, calcium), vitamin B_{12}, folic acid, and lipids. Lymphatic obstruction can be caused by many conditions. Certain cancers such as lymphoma, inflammatory states, radiation enteritis, Crohn's disease, heart failure, and constrictive pericarditis are causes of lymphatic obstruction.

Interference with blood flow to the intestinal mucosa results in malabsorption. With intestinal surgery, there is loss of the surface area needed to facilitate absorption. Resection of the ileum results in vitamin B_{12}, bile salt, and other nutrient deficiencies. Gastric surgery is one of the most common causes of malabsorption and maldigestion. Other conditions associated with poor digestion and malabsorption include small-bowel ischemia and radiation enteritis.

PATIENT-CENTERED COLLABORATIVE CARE

ASSESSMENT

Chronic diarrhea is a classic symptom of malabsorption. It occurs as a result of unabsorbed nutrients, which add to the bulk of the stool, and unabsorbed fat. Steatorrhea (greater than normal amounts of fat in the feces) is a common sign. It is a result of bile salt deconjugation, nonabsorbed fats, or bacteria in the intestine. Not all patients with malabsorption have diarrhea. Instead, some have an increased stool mass. Other clinical manifestations include:

- Unintentional weight loss
- Bloating and flatus (carbohydrate malabsorption)
- Decreased libido
- Easy bruising (purpura)
- Anemia (with iron and folic acid or vitamin B_{12} deficiencies)
- Bone pain (with calcium and vitamin D deficiencies)
- Edema (caused by hypoproteinemia)

Laboratory studies reveal a decrease in mean corpuscular volume (MCV), mean corpuscular hemoglobin (MCH), and mean corpuscular hemoglobin concentration (MCHC). These decreases indicate hypochromic microcytic anemia resulting from iron deficiency. Increased MCV and variable MCH and MCHC values indicate macrocytic anemia resulting from vitamin B_{12} and folic acid deficiencies. Serum iron levels are low in protein malabsorption because of insufficient gastric acid for use of iron. Serum cholesterol levels may be low from decreased absorption and digestion of fat. Low serum calcium levels may indicate malabsorption of vitamin D and amino acids. Low levels of serum vitamin A (retinol) and carotene, its precursor, indicate a bile salt deficiency and malabsorption of fat. Serum albumin and total protein levels are low if protein is lost. A quantitative fecal fat analysis is elevated in either malabsorption or maldigestion.

A *lactose tolerance test* result that shows less than a 20% rise in the blood glucose level over the fasting blood glucose level indicates lactose intolerance. A hydrogen breath test can also be performed to detect this problem. The xylose absorption test can reveal low urine and serum D-xylose levels if malabsorption in the small intestine is present, a common finding in celiac sprue. An abnormal D-xylose test can indicate bacterial overgrowth in the small intestine.

The *Schilling test* measures urinary excretion of vitamin B$_{12}$ for diagnosis of pernicious anemia and a variety of other malabsorption syndromes. The *bile acid breath test* assesses the absorption of bile salt. If the patient has bacterial overgrowth, the bile salts will become deconjugated and the carbon dioxide level in the breath will peak earlier than expected.

Biopsy of the small intestine is performed for diagnosis of tropical sprue or celiac sprue. Ultrasonography is used to diagnose pancreatic tumors and tumors in the small intestine that are causing malabsorption. X-rays of the GI tract reveal pancreatic calcifications, tumors, or other abnormalities that cause malabsorption. A CT scan may also be done.

INTERVENTIONS

Interventions for most malabsorption syndromes focus on (1) avoidance of substances that aggravate malabsorption and (2) supplementation of nutrients. Surgical management of the primary disease may be indicated. Drug therapy may also improve or resolve malabsorption.

Nutrition management includes a low-fat diet for patients who have gallbladder disease, severe steatorrhea, or cystic fibrosis. A low-fat diet may or may not be indicated for pancreatic insufficiency because this disorder improves with enzyme replacement. Some clinicians believe that limitation of fat intake is not necessary with enzyme replacement. Dietary intake of fat is actually beneficial to the patient because it has a high number of calories. After a total gastrectomy, a high-protein, high-calorie diet and small, frequent meals are recommended. Lactose-free or lactose-restricted diets are available for patients with lactase deficiency, and gluten-free diets are available for those with celiac sprue.

The health care provider prescribes nutritional supplements according to the specific deficiency. Common supplements include:

Special Skin Care for Patients with Chronic Diarrhea

- Use medicated wipes or premoistened disposable wipes rather than toilet tissue to clean the perineal area.
- Clean the perineal area well with mild soap and warm water after each stool; rinse soap from the area well.
- If the physician allows, provide a sitz bath several times per day.
- Apply a thin coat of A+D Ointment or other medicated protective barrier, such as aloe products, after each stool.
- Keep the patient off the affected buttock area.
- For open areas, cover with thin DuoDerm or Tegaderm occlusive dressing to promote rapid healing.
- Observe for fungal or yeast infections, which appear as dark red rashes with "satellite" lesions. Obtain prescription for medication if this problem occurs.

- Water-soluble vitamins, such as folic acid and vitamin B complex
- Fat-soluble vitamins, such as vitamin A, vitamin D, and vitamin K
- Minerals, such as calcium, iron, and magnesium
- Pancreatic enzymes, such as pancrelipase (Pancrease, Viokase)

Antibiotics are used to treat tropical sprue, Whipple's disease, and other disorders involving bacterial overgrowth. Tropical sprue is treated with trimethoprim/sulfamethoxazole (Bactrim, Septra). Bacterial overgrowth can be caused by a variety of disorders but is often treated with tetracycline and metronidazole (Flagyl, Novonidazol ✦). Steroids are sometimes given in celiac disease to decrease inflammation.

Drug therapy is used to control the clinical manifestations of malabsorption. Antidiarrheal agents, such as diphenoxylate hydrochloride and atropine sulfate (Lomotil), are often used to control diarrhea and steatorrhea. Anticholinergics, such as dicyclomine hydrochloride (Bentyl, Bentylol ✦), may be given before meals to inhibit gastric motility. IV fluids may be necessary to replenish fluid losses associated with diarrhea.

Provide special measures to protect the skin when chronic diarrhea occurs (Chart 59-6). Conduct an ongoing assessment for clinical manifestations of malabsorption, and relate these to activities and dietary intake. For example, patients with steatorrhea are monitored for fluid and electrolyte imbalances and are encouraged to drink electrolyte-rich liquids liberally. Teach them the rationale for dietary, drug, and surgical management of nutritional deficiencies, and evaluate interventions on the basis of changes in or resolution of clinical manifestations.

NURSING CONCEPT REVIEW

What might you NOTICE if the patient has impaired absorption and inadequate nutrition as a result of non-inflammatory intestinal disorders?

- Rectal bleeding
- Report of change in bowel habits
- Diarrhea or report of constipation
- Fatigue
- Vomiting
- Abdominal pain
- Change in bowel sounds (decreased or increased)
- Weight loss

NURSING CONCEPT REVIEW—cont'd

What should you INTERPRET and how should you RESPOND to a patient with impaired absorption and inadequate nutrition as a result of noninflammatory intestinal disorders?

Perform and interpret focused physical assessment findings, including:

- Vital signs
- Complete pain assessment
- Abdominal assessment
- Current weight compared with previous weight

Respond:

- Decrease abdominal pain by placing patient in sitting position.
- Start IV (large-bore) to replace fluids and electrolytes, and give blood transfusion as prescribed.
- Provide rest.
- Provide privacy and dignity.

- Assist with hygiene as needed.
- Insert nasogastric tube and connect to low suction as needed.
- Check laboratory values of hemoglobin and hematocrit.
- Check stool for occult or frank blood.
- Give antidiarrheal drugs if prescribed.
- Record intake and output.
- Assist with ADLs and ambulation as needed.

On what should you REFLECT?

- Continue to monitor for vomiting and diarrhea and for changes in pain.
- Think about what you need to document. Decide when you might need to call the health care provider or Rapid Response Team.
- Determine what health teaching and community resources may be needed for the patient and family.
- Think about what you can do to help prevent complications of the health problem.

GET READY FOR THE NCLEX® EXAMINATION!

KEY POINTS

Review these Key Points for each NCLEX Examination Client Needs Category.

Safe and Effective Care Environment

- Refer patients with familial CRC syndromes for genetic counseling and testing.
- Refer ostomy patients to the United Ostomy Associations of America, Inc. and the American Cancer Society for additional information and support groups.
- Consult with the certified wound, ostomy, continence nurse (CWOCN) or enterostomal therapist (ET) when a patient is scheduled for or has a new colostomy.
- Prioritize care for patients experiencing abdominal trauma: first assess <u>a</u>irway, <u>b</u>reathing, and <u>c</u>irculation (ABCs), and then monitor mental status, vital signs, and skin perfusion to assess for hypovolemic shock.

Health Promotion and Maintenance

- Teach patients with irritable bowel syndrome (IBS) to avoid GI stimulants, such as caffeine, alcohol, and milk and milk products, and to manage stress.
- Instruct patients on dietary modifications to decrease the occurrence of colorectal cancer (CRC).
- Teach adults 50 years and older to have routine screening for CRC as listed in Chart 59-1; people with genetic predispositions should have earlier and more frequent screening.
- Teach patients and caregivers how to provide colostomy care, including dietary measures, skin care, and ostomy products.

- Teach people measures for preventing constipation to minimize hemorrhoid occurrence.

Psychosocial Integrity

- Assess effects of IBS on patient lifestyle; recommend stress management techniques.
- Assist the patient with CRC with the anticipatory grieving process.
- Be aware that having a colostomy is a life-altering event that can severely impact one's body image; issues related to sexuality and fear of acceptance should be discussed.

Physiological Integrity

- Assess patients with IBS for elimination pattern, abdominal pain, and nausea.
- Be aware that minimally invasive inguinal hernia repair is an ambulatory procedure done via laparoscopy; postoperative management requires health teaching regarding rest for a few days and inspection of incisions for signs of infection.
- Be aware that a strangulated hernia can cause ischemia and bowel obstruction, requiring immediate intervention.
- Monitor patients who have conventional open herniorrhaphy for ability to void.
- Recognize that surgical procedures for CRC vary depending on tumor location as specified in Table 59-1.
- Keep the peristomal skin clean and dry; observe for leakage around the pouch seal.

GET READY FOR THE NCLEX® EXAMINATION!—cont'd

- Provide meticulous perineal wound care for patients having an abdominoperineal (AP) resection, as described in Chart 59-2.
- Assess the characteristics of the colostomy stoma, which should be reddish pink and moist; report abnormalities such as ischemia and necrosis (purplish or black) or unusual bleeding to the surgeon.
- Recall that bowel sounds are altered in patients with obstruction; absent bowel sounds imply total obstruction.

- Assess the patient's nasogastric tube for proper placement, patency, and output at least every 4 hours.
- Monitor patients with bowel obstruction for signs and symptoms of fluid, electrolyte, and acid-base imbalances.
- Teach patients having hemorrhoid surgery to take stool softeners before and after surgery to decrease discomfort during defecation.
- Be aware that intestinal polyps are usually benign but can become malignant if not removed.

60

Care of Patients with Inflammatory Intestinal Disorders

Donna D. Ignatavicius

LEARNING OUTCOMES

Safe and Effective Care Environment

1. Describe the importance of collaborating with health care team members to provide care for patients with chronic inflammatory bowel disease (IBD).

Health Promotion and Maintenance

2. Differentiate care for older adults with acute and chronic inflammatory bowel disorders.
3. Develop a health teaching plan for patients to promote self-management when caring for ileostomy or other surgical diversion.
4. Identify community resources for patients and families regarding chronic IBD.
5. Discuss ways that food poisoning can be prevented.

Psychosocial Integrity

6. Identify expected body image changes associated with having an ileostomy or other surgical diversion.
7. Describe patient and family response to chronic IBD.

Physiological Integrity

8. Differentiate common types of acute inflammatory bowel disease.
9. Develop a collaborative plan of care for the patient who has appendicitis and peritonitis.
10. Discuss the common causes of gastroenteritis.
11. Compare and contrast the pathophysiology and clinical manifestations of ulcerative colitis and Crohn's disease.
12. Identify priority problems for patients with ulcerative colitis.
13. Explain the purpose of and nursing implications related to drug therapy for patients with IBD.
14. Plan priority postoperative care for a patient undergoing surgery for IBD.
15. Develop a hospital discharge teaching plan for patients having surgery for IBD.
16. Explain the role of nutrition therapy in managing the patient with diverticular disease.
17. Describe the comfort measures that the nurse can use for the patient with anal disorders.

Inflammatory bowel health problems affect the small intestine, large intestine (colon), or both. Together, these organs are called the *intestinal tract*. Continued digestion of food and absorption of nutrients occur primarily in the small intestine (bowel) to meet the body's needs for energy. Water is reabsorbed in the large intestine to help maintain a fluid balance and promote the passage of waste products. When the intestinal tract and its nearby structures become inflamed, *digestion and nutrition* may be inadequate to meet a patient's needs.

ACUTE INFLAMMATORY BOWEL DISORDERS

Appendicitis, gastroenteritis, and peritonitis are the most common acute inflammatory bowel problems. These disorders are potentially life threatening and can have major systemic complications if not treated promptly.

APPENDICITIS

Pathophysiology

Appendicitis is an acute inflammation of the vermiform appendix that occurs most often among young adults. It is the most common cause of right lower quadrant (RLQ) pain. The appendix usually extends off the proximal cecum of the colon just below the ileocecal valve. Inflammation occurs when the lumen (opening) of the appendix is obstructed (blocked), leading to infection as bacteria invade the wall of the appendix. The initial obstruction is usually a result of fecaliths (very hard pieces of feces) composed of calcium phosphate–rich mucus and inorganic salts. Less common causes are malignant tumors, helminthes (worms), or other infections.

When the lumen is blocked, the mucosa secretes fluid, increasing the internal pressure and restricting blood flow, resulting in pain. If the process occurs slowly, an abscess may develop, but a rapid process may result in peritonitis (inflammation of the peritoneum). *All complications of peritonitis are serious. Gangrene can occur within 24 to 36 hours, is life threatening, and is one of the most common indications for emergency surgery. Perforation may develop within 24 hours, but the risk rises rapidly after 48 hours.* Perforation of the appendix also results in peritonitis with a temperature of greater than 101° F (38.3° C) and a rise in pulse rate.

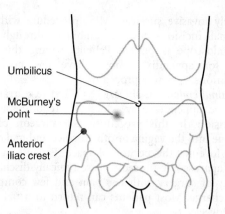

FIG. 60-1 McBurney's point is located midway between the anterior iliac crest and the umbilicus in the right lower quadrant. This is the classic area for localized tenderness during the later stages of appendicitis.

Umbilicus	
McBurney's point	
Anterior iliac crest	

CONSIDERATIONS FOR OLDER ADULTS

Appendicitis is relatively rare at extremes in age. However, perforation is more common in older people, causing a higher mortality rate. The diagnosis of appendicitis is difficult to establish in older adults because symptoms of pain and tenderness may not be as pronounced in this age-group. This difference results in treatment delay and an increased risk for perforation, peritonitis, and death.

PATIENT-CENTERED COLLABORATIVE CARE

ASSESSMENT

History taking and tracking the sequence of symptoms are important because nausea or vomiting before abdominal pain can indicate gastroenteritis. Abdominal pain followed by nausea and vomiting can indicate appendicitis. Ask about risk factors such as age, familial tendency, and intra-abdominal tumors. Classically, patients with appendicitis have cramplike pain in the epigastric or periumbilical area. Anorexia is a frequent symptom with nausea and vomiting occurring in many cases.

Perform a complete pain assessment. Initially, pain can present anywhere in the abdomen or flank area. As the inflammation and infection progress, the pain becomes more severe and steady and shifts to the RLQ between the anterior iliac crest and the umbilicus. This area is referred to as *McBurney's point* (Fig. 60-1). *Abdominal pain that increases with cough or movement and is relieved by bending the right hip or the knees suggests perforation and peritonitis.* An advanced practice nurse or other health care provider assesses for muscle rigidity and guarding on palpation of the abdomen. The patient

may report pain after release of pressure. This is referred to as "rebound" tenderness.

Laboratory findings do not establish the diagnosis, but often there is a moderate elevation of the white blood cell (WBC) count (leukocytosis) to 10,000 to 18,000/mm^3 with a "shift to the left" (an increased number of immature WBCs). A WBC elevation to greater than 20,000/mm^3 may indicate a perforated appendix. An ultrasound study may show the presence of an enlarged appendix. If symptoms are recurrent or prolonged, a computed tomography (CT) scan can be used for diagnosis and may reveal the presence of a fecalith.

INTERVENTIONS

All patients with suspected or confirmed appendicitis are hospitalized and examined by a surgeon. When the diagnosis is not clear, the health care team observes the patient before surgical exploration.

Nonsurgical Management

Keep the patient with suspected or known appendicitis on NPO to prepare for the possibility of emergency surgery and to avoid making the inflammation worse.

! NURSING SAFETY PRIORITY

Action Alert

For the patient with suspected appendicitis, administer IV fluids as prescribed to prevent fluid and electrolyte imbalance and to replace fluid volume. If tolerated, advise the patient to maintain a semi-Fowler's position so that abdominal drainage, if any, can be contained in the lower abdomen. Once the diagnosis of appendicitis is confirmed and surgery is scheduled, administer opioid analgesics and antibiotics as prescribed. *The patient with suspected or confirmed appendicitis should not receive laxatives or enemas, which can cause perforation of the appendix. Heat should never be applied to the abdomen because this may increase circulation to the appendix and result in increased inflammation and perforation!*

Surgical Management

Surgery is required as soon as possible. An appendectomy is the removal of the inflamed appendix by one of several surgical approaches. Uncomplicated appendectomy procedures are usually done via laparoscopy. A laparoscopy is a minimally invasive surgical (MIS) procedure with one or more small incisions near the umbilicus through which a small endoscope is placed. Patients having this type of surgery for appendix removal have few postoperative complications. A newer procedure known as *natural orifice transluminal endoscopic surgery* (NOTES) (e.g., transvaginal endoscopic appendectomy) does not require an external skin incision. In this procedure, the surgeon places the endoscope into the vagina or other orifice and makes a small incision to enter the peritoneal space. Patients having any type of laparoscopic procedures are typically discharged the same day of surgery with less pain and few complications after discharge. Most patients can return to usual activities in 1 to 2 weeks.

If the diagnosis is not definitive but the patient is at high risk for complications from suspected appendicitis, the surgeon may perform an exploratory laparotomy to rule out appendicitis. A laparotomy is an open surgical approach with a larger abdominal incision for complicated or atypical appendicitis or peritonitis.

Preoperative teaching is often limited because the patient is in pain or may be transferred quickly to the operating suite for emergency surgery. The patient is prepared for general anesthesia and surgery, as described in Chapter 16. After surgery, care of the patient who has undergone an appendectomy is the same as that required for anyone who has received general anesthesia (see Chapter 18).

If peritonitis or abscesses are found, wound drains are inserted and a nasogastric tube may be placed to decompress the stomach and prevent abdominal distention. Administer IV antibiotics and opioid analgesics as prescribed. Help the patient out of bed on the evening of surgery to help prevent respiratory complications, such as atelectasis. He or she may be hospitalized for as long as 3 to 5 days and return to normal activity in 4 to 6 weeks.

PERITONITIS

Peritonitis is a life-threatening, acute inflammation of the visceral/parietal peritoneum and endothelial lining of the abdominal cavity. Primary peritonitis is rare and indicates the peritoneum is infected via the bloodstream. This problem is not discussed here.

Pathophysiology

Normally the peritoneal cavity contains about 50 mL of sterile fluid (transudate), which prevents friction in the abdominal cavity during peristalsis. When the peritoneal cavity is contaminated by bacteria, the body first begins an inflammatory reaction walling off a localized area to fight the infection. This local reaction involves vascular dilation and increased capillary permeability, allowing transport of leukocytes and subsequent phagocytosis of the offending organisms. If this walling off process fails, the inflammation spreads and contamination becomes massive, resulting in diffuse (widespread) peritonitis.

Peritonitis is most often caused by contamination of the peritoneal cavity by bacteria or chemicals. Bacteria gain entry into the peritoneum by perforation (from appendicitis, diverticulitis, peptic ulcer disease) or from an external penetrating wound, a gangrenous gallbladder, bowel obstruction, or ascending infection through the genital tract. Less common causes include perforating tumors, leakage or contamination

during surgery, and infection by skin pathogens in patients undergoing continuous ambulatory peritoneal dialysis (CAPD). Common bacteria responsible for peritonitis include *Escherichia coli, Streptococcus, Staphylococcus, Pneumococcus,* and *Gonococcus.* Chemical peritonitis results from leakage of bile, pancreatic enzymes, and gastric acid.

When diagnosis and treatment of peritonitis are delayed, blood vessel dilation continues. The body responds to the continuing infectious process by shunting extra blood to the area of inflammation (hyperemia). Fluid is shifted from the extracellular fluid compartment into the peritoneal cavity, connective tissues, and GI tract (*"third spacing"*). This shift of fluid can result in a significant decrease in circulatory volume and *hypovolemic shock.* Severely decreased circulatory volume can result in insufficient perfusion of the kidneys, leading to kidney failure with electrolyte imbalance. Assess for clinical manifestations of these life-threatening problems.

Peristalsis slows or *stops* in response to severe peritoneal inflammation, and the lumen of the bowel becomes distended with gas and fluid. Fluid that normally flows to the small bowel and the colon for reabsorption accumulates in the intestine in volumes of 7 to 8 L daily. The toxins or bacteria responsible for the peritonitis can also enter the bloodstream from the peritoneal area and lead to bacteremia or septicemia (bacterial invasion of the blood).

Respiratory problems can occur as a result of increased abdominal pressure against the diaphragm from intestinal distention and fluid shifts to the peritoneal cavity. Pain can interfere with respirations at a time when the patient has an increased oxygen demand because of the infectious process.

PATIENT-CENTERED COLLABORATIVE CARE

ASSESSMENT

Ask the patient about abdominal pain, and determine the character of the pain (e.g., cramping, sharp, aching), location of the pain, and whether the pain is localized or generalized. Ask about a history of a low-grade fever or recent spikes in temperature.

Physical findings of peritonitis (Chart 60-1) depend on several factors: the stage of the disease, the ability of the body to localize the process by walling off the infection, and whether the inflammation has progressed to generalized

---

CHART 60-1   KEY FEATURES

Peritonitis

- Rigid, boardlike abdomen (classic)
- Abdominal pain (localized, poorly localized, or referred to the shoulder or chest)
- Distended abdomen
- Nausea, anorexia, vomiting
- Diminishing bowel sounds
- Inability to pass flatus or feces

- Rebound tenderness in the abdomen
- High fever
- Tachycardia
- Dehydration from high fever (poor skin turgor)
- Decreased urine output
- Hiccups
- Possible compromise in respiratory status

peritonitis. The patient most often appears acutely ill, lying still, possibly with the knees flexed. Movement is guarded, and he or she may report and show signs of pain (e.g., facial grimacing) with coughing or movement of any type. During inspection, observe for progressive abdominal distention, often seen when the inflammation markedly reduces intestinal motility. Auscultate for bowel sounds, which usually disappear with progression of the inflammation.

The cardinal signs of peritonitis are abdominal pain and tenderness. In the patient with *localized* peritonitis, the abdomen is tender on palpation in a well-defined area with rebound tenderness in this area. With *generalized* peritonitis, tenderness is widespread.

! NURSING SAFETY PRIORITY

Action Alert

> *For patients with peritonitis, assess for abdominal wall rigidity, which is a classic finding that is sometimes referred to as a "boardlike" abdomen.* Monitor the patient for a high fever because of the infectious process. Assess for tachycardia occurring in response to the fever and decreased circulating blood volume. Observe whether he or she has dry mucous membranes and a low urine output seen with third spacing. Nausea and vomiting may also be present. Hiccups may occur as a result of diaphragmatic irritation. Be sure to document all assessment findings.

White blood cell (WBC) counts are often elevated to 20,000/mm³ with a high neutrophil count. Blood culture studies may be done to determine whether septicemia has occurred and to identify the causative organism to enable appropriate therapy. The health care provider requests laboratory tests to assess fluid and electrolyte balance and renal status, including electrolytes, blood urea nitrogen (BUN), creatinine, hemoglobin, and hematocrit. Oxygen saturation and end–carbon dioxide monitoring may be obtained to assess respiratory function and acid-base balance.

Abdominal x-rays can assess for free air or fluid in the abdominal cavity, indicating perforation. The x-rays may also show dilation, edema, and inflammation of the small and large intestines. An abdominal sonogram may be useful in locating the problem.

▌INTERVENTIONS

Patients with peritonitis are hospitalized because of the severe nature of the illness. If complications are extensive, the patients are often admitted to a critical care unit. Nursing interventions focus on the early identification of complications.

Nonsurgical Management

The physician prescribes IV fluids and broad-spectrum antibiotics immediately after establishing the diagnosis of peritonitis. IV fluids are used to replace fluids collected in the peritoneum and bowel. Monitor daily weight and intake and output carefully. A nasogastric tube (NGT) decompresses the stomach and the intestine, and the patient is NPO. Apply oxygen as prescribed and according to the patient's respiratory status and oxygen saturation via pulse oximetry. Administer analgesics, and monitor for pain control. Document pain assessments thoroughly. A surgical consultation is requested in case surgery should become necessary.

Surgical Management

Abdominal surgery is the usual treatment for identifying and repairing the cause of the peritonitis. If the patient is so critically ill that surgery would be life threatening, it may be delayed. Surgery focuses on controlling the contamination, removing foreign material from the peritoneal cavity, and draining collected fluid.

Exploratory laparotomy (surgical opening into the abdomen) or laparoscopy is used to remove or repair the inflamed or perforated organ (e.g., appendectomy for an inflamed appendix; a colon resection, with or without a colostomy, for a perforated diverticulum). Before the incision(s) is closed, the surgeon irrigates the peritoneum with antibiotic solutions. Several catheters may be inserted to drain the cavity and provide a route for irrigation after surgery.

The preoperative care is similar to that described in Chapter 16 for patients having general anesthesia. Chapter 18 describes general postoperative care for exploratory laparotomy. Multi-system complications can occur with peritonitis. Loss of fluids from the extracellular space to the peritoneal cavity, NGT suctioning, and NPO status require that the patient receives IV fluid replacement. Be sure that unlicensed assistive personnel (UAP) carefully measure intake and output. Fluid rates may be changed frequently based on laboratory values and patient condition.

! NURSING SAFETY PRIORITY

Action Alert

> Monitor the patient's level of consciousness, vital signs, respiratory status (respiratory rate and breath sounds), and intake and output at least hourly immediately after abdominal surgery. Maintain the patient in a semi-Fowler's position to promote drainage of peritoneal contents into the lower region of the abdominal cavity. This position helps increase lung expansion.

The patient has one or more incisions and drains. If an open surgical procedure is needed, the infection may slow healing of an incision or the incision may be partially open to heal by second or third intention. These wounds require special care involving manual irrigation or packing as prescribed by the surgeon. If the surgeon requests peritoneal irrigation through a drain, *maintain sterile technique during manual irrigation.* Assess whether the patient retains the fluid used for irrigation by comparing the amount of fluid returned with the amount of fluid instilled. Fluid retention could cause abdominal distention or pain.

Community-Based Care

The length of hospitalization depends on the extent and severity of the infectious process. Patients who have a localized abscess drained and who respond to antibiotics and IV fluids without multi-system complications are discharged in several days. Others may require mechanical ventilation or hemodialysis with longer hospital stays. Some patients may be transferred to a transitional care unit to complete their antibiotic therapy and recovery. Convalescence is often longer than for other surgeries because of multi-system involvement.

When discharged home, assess the patient's ability for self-management at home with the added task of incision care and a reduced activity tolerance. Provide the patient and family with written and oral instructions to report these problems to the health care provider immediately:

- Unusual or foul-smelling drainage
- Swelling, redness, or warmth or bleeding from the incision site
- A temperature higher than 101° F (38° C)
- Abdominal pain
- Signs of wound dehiscence or ileus

Patients with an incision healing by second or third intention may require dressings, solution, and catheter-tipped syringes to irrigate the wound. A home care nurse may be needed to assess, irrigate, or pack the wound and change the dressing as needed until the patient and family feel comfortable with the procedure. If the patient needs assistance with ADLs, a home care aide or temporary placement in a skilled care facility may be indicated. Collaborate with the case manager (CM) to determine the most appropriate setting for seamless continuing care in the community.

Review information about antibiotics and analgesics. For patients taking oral opioid analgesics such as oxycodone with acetaminophen (Tylox, Percocet, Endocet ✦) for any length of time, a stool softener such as docusate sodium (Colace, Regulex ✦) may be prescribed. Older adults are especially at risk for constipation from codeine-based drugs.

Teach patients to refrain from any lifting for *at least* 6 weeks. Other activity limitations are made on an individual basis with the physician's recommendation.

❓ NCLEX EXAMINATION CHALLENGE

Physiological Integrity

An older adult has a perforated appendix and is scheduled for emergent surgery. What assessment findings will the nurse expect the client to have before surgery? **Select all that apply.**
A. Bradycardia
B. Dizziness
C. Distended abdomen
D. Fever
E. Diarrhea
F. Fistulas
G. Incontinence

GASTROENTERITIS

Pathophysiology

Gastroenteritis is an increase in the frequency and water content of stools and/or vomiting as a result of inflammation of the mucous membranes of the stomach and intestinal tract. It affects mainly the small bowel and can be caused by either viral or bacterial infections, which have similar manifestations. They are considered self-limiting in their course unless complications occur. All organisms implicated in gastroenteritis can cause diarrhea. However, the organisms discussed in this section have distinguishing characteristics.

Some clinicians include shigellosis when discussing gastroenteritis. Others consider shigellosis separately as a dysentery type of illness. Dysenteries affect the *large* bowel. Gastroenteritis affects the *small* bowel. Other clinicians classify infectious disease of the intestine as bacterial, viral, or parasitic, without using the term *gastroenteritis*.

Food poisoning is sometimes described in conjunction with gastroenteritis with specific reference to the organism causing the food poisoning. Gastroenteritis, however, differs from food poisoning with regard to transmission in the body, incubation time, and effect on immunity.

The following discussion of gastroenteritis includes the epidemic viral form and the bacterial forms (*Campylobacter, Escherichia coli,* and shigellosis) (Table 60-1). Organisms associated with food poisoning are discussed later in this chapter.

Infection with viral and bacterial organisms can produce GI illnesses that cause watery diarrhea. These disorders may be caused by noninflammatory, inflammatory, or penetrating mechanisms. Organisms such as enterotoxigenic *E. coli* can release enterotoxin (a noninflammatory toxic substance specific to the intestinal mucosa), which results in diarrhea. *Shigella* or *Campylobacter* can attach itself to mucosal epithelium without penetrating it, resulting in destruction of the intestinal villi and malabsorption. Infections that are caused by bacterial toxins reduce the absorptive capacity of the distal small bowel and proximal colon, resulting in diarrhea. Finally, the organism can penetrate the intestine, causing cellular destruction, necrosis, and a potential for ulceration. Diarrhea occurs often with white blood cells (WBCs) or red blood cells (RBCs) present in the stool.

All of these organisms are transmitted via the oral-fecal route and result in *increased* GI motility, with fluids and electrolytes being secreted into the intestine at rapid rates. Invading organisms more easily attach to the intestinal mucosa if the normal intestinal flora is altered. This can occur in patients who are receiving antibiotics, are malnourished, or are debilitated. Two groups of viruses, the rotaviruses (which usually affect young children) and Norwalk virus, as well as bacterial pathogens, are the most common causes of

TABLE 60-1	COMMON TYPES OF GASTROENTERITIS AND THEIR CHARACTERISTICS
TYPE	**CHARACTERISTICS**
Viral Gastroenteritis	
Epidemic viral	Caused by many parvovirus-type organisms
	Transmitted by the fecal-oral route in food and water
	Incubation period 10-51 hrs
	Communicable during acute illness
Rotavirus and Norwalk virus	Transmitted by the fecal-oral route and possibly the respiratory route
	Incubation in 48 hrs
	Rotavirus is most common in infants and young children
	Norwalk virus affects young children and adults
Bacterial Gastroenteritis	
Campylobacter enteritis	Transmitted by the fecal-oral route or by contact with infected animals or infants
	Incubation period 1-10 days
	Communicable for 2-7 weeks
Escherichia coli diarrhea	Transmitted by fecal contamination of food, water, or fomites
Shigellosis	Transmitted by direct and indirect fecal-oral routes
	Incubation period 1-7 days
	Communicable during the acute illness to 4 wk after the illness
	Humans possibly carriers for months

gastroenteritis. Rotaviruses can also affect older adults in group settings, such as long-term care facilities.

The three most common types of *bacterial* gastroenteritis are *E. coli* diarrhea ("traveler's diarrhea"), *Campylobacter* enteritis (another "traveler's diarrhea"), and *Shigellosis* (bacillary dysentery). The reservoirs of *E. coli* are humans, who are often asymptomatic.

Diarrhea caused by *E. coli* and *Campylobacter* occurs worldwide, commonly in epidemic outbreaks. *E. coli* epidemics are highest in areas of poor sanitation during warm months. *Campylobacter* incidence is highest during warm months. Shigellosis occurs in every age-group but most frequently in children (younger than 10 years) and older adults because of their depressed immune systems. Outbreaks of shigellosis are common in areas with crowded living conditions, such as in correctional facilities.

PATIENT-CENTERED COLLABORATIVE CARE

ASSESSMENT

The patient history can provide information related to the potential cause of the illness. Ask about recent travel, especially to tropical regions of Asia, Africa, or Central or South America. Some areas of Mexico may also be the source of gastroenteritis. Newcomers (immigrants) from these countries often have gastroenteritis. Traveler's diarrhea can begin 3 days to 2 weeks after the patient's arrival.

The patient who has gastroenteritis usually looks ill. Nausea and vomiting can occur with all types of gastroenteritis but are usually limited to the first 1 or 2 days. Patients have diarrhea, which varies in consistency and amount with the causative organism.

In patients with epidemic viral gastroenteritis, myalgia (muscle aches), headache, and malaise are often reported. Weakness and cardiac dysrhythmias may be the result of loss of potassium (hypokalemia) from diarrhea. Monitor for and document manifestations of hypokalemia.

! NURSING SAFETY PRIORITY

Action Alert

For patients with gastroenteritis, note any abdominal distention and listen for hyperactive bowel sounds. Depending on the amount of fluids lost through diarrhea and vomiting, patients may have varying degrees of dehydration manifested by:

- Poor skin turgor
- Fever
- Dry mucous membranes
- Orthostatic blood pressure changes (which can cause falls, especially for older adults)
- Hypotension
- Oliguria

In some cases, dehydration may be severe, and shock may occur if diarrhea is prolonged. *Dehydration occurs rapidly in older adults and may require hospitalization. Monitor mental status changes, such as acute confusion, that result from hypoxia in the older adult. These changes may be the only clinical manifestation of dehydration in older adults.*

Diarrhea associated with epidemic viral gastroenteritis is commonly limited to 24 to 48 hours. Infection with the Norwalk virus has a rapid onset of nausea, abdominal cramps, vomiting, and diarrhea. This enteritis is usually mild. *Campylobacter* enteritis is a more severe disease with foul-smelling stools containing blood, which can number 20 to 30 per day for up to 7 days. *E. coli* gastroenteritis may or may not have blood or mucus in the stool. Diarrhea can last for up to 10 days. *Shigella* causes stools to have blood and mucus, which can continue for up to 5 days. Monitor for and document the number of stools daily for the patient who is hospitalized.

As part of the laboratory assessment, Gram stain of stool is usually done before culture. Cultures positive for the organism are diagnostic (Pagana & Pagana, 2010). Many WBCs on Gram stain suggest shigellosis. The presence of WBCs and RBCs in the stool may indicate *Campylobacter* gastroenteritis.

■ INTERVENTIONS

For any type of gastroenteritis, encourage fluid replacement. The amount and route of fluid administration are determined by the patient's hydration status and overall health condition.

Fluid Replacement

Teach patients to drink extra fluids to replace fluid lost through vomiting and diarrhea. Depending on the patient's age and severity of dehydration, he or she may be admitted to the hospital for gastroenteritis or may stay in the emergency department or urgent care center until adequate hydration is restored.

Obtain a weight, orthostatic blood pressure, and other vital sign measurements at admission. IV fluids such as half-strength normal saline (0.45% sodium chloride) to replace sodium lost in vomitus, with or without potassium supplements, are infused as prescribed. *Potassium is usually needed for patients with excessive diarrhea.* Continue to monitor the patient's vital signs, intake and output, and weight. A rapid gain or loss of 1 kg (2.2 lbs) of body weight is equivalent to the gain or loss of 1 L of fluid. Advise the patient to alternate periods of rest and activity.

Depending on the type of gastroenteritis, especially if the geographic area is experiencing epidemic infections, the local health department may need to be notified. For example, it is mandatory that every case of shigellosis be reported. In some endemic areas, *Campylobacter* enteritis must be reported.

Drug Therapy

Drugs that suppress intestinal motility may not be given for bacterial or viral gastroenteritis. *Use of these drugs can prevent the infecting organisms from being eliminated from the body.* If the health care provider determines that antiperistaltic agents are necessary, an initial dose of loperamide (Imodium) 4 mg can be administered orally, followed by 2 mg after each loose stool, up to 16 mg daily.

! NURSING SAFETY PRIORITY

Drug Alert

Diphenoxylate hydrochloride with atropine sulfate (Lomotil, Lomanate) reduces GI motility but is used sparingly because of its habit-forming ability. *The drug should not be used for older adults because it also causes drowsiness and could contribute to falls.*

Treatment with antibiotics may be needed if the gastroenteritis is due to bacterial infection with fever and severe diarrhea. Depending on the type and severity of the illness, examples of drugs that may be prescribed include ciprofloxacin (Cipro), levofloxacin (Levaquin), or azithromycin (Zithromax). If the gastroenteritis is due to shigellosis, anti-infective agents such as trimethoprim/sulfamethoxazole (Septra DS, Bactrim DS, Roubac ✦) or ciprofloxacin are prescribed.

For relatively short-term diarrhea of 24 to 48 hours' duration, the diagnosis is based primarily on the patient's history and clinical manifestations, not by a stool examination. When diarrhea is severe or persists for long periods, the stool is examined to determine the causative organism and to begin specific treatment. It should be determined whether the diarrhea is caused by *Salmonella* or by parasites because these organisms respond to specific medications (see p. 1289 in the Parasitic Infection section). Diarrhea that continues longer than 10 days, especially if associated with nocturnal diarrhea, is probably *not* due to gastroenteritis.

Skin Care

Frequent stools that are rich in electrolytes and enzymes, as well as frequent wiping and washing of the anal region, can irritate the skin. Teach the patient to avoid toilet paper and harsh soaps. Ideally, he or she can gently clean the area with warm water or an absorbent material, followed by thorough but gentle drying. Cream, oil, or gel can be applied to a damp, warm washcloth to remove stool that sticks to open skin. Special prepared skin wipes can also be used. Protective barrier cream can be applied to the skin between stools. Sitz baths for 10 minutes two or three times daily can also relieve discomfort.

If leakage of stool is a problem, the patient can use absorbent cotton or panty liner and keep it in place with snug underwear. For patients who are incontinent, remind unlicensed assistive personnel (UAP) to keep the perineal and buttock areas clean and dry. The use of incontinent pads at night instead of briefs allows air to circulate to the skin and prevents irritation.

Teaching for Self-Management

During the acute phase of the illness, teach the patient and family about the importance of fluid replacement. Teaching the patient and family about reducing the risk for transmission of gastroenteritis is also important (Chart 60-2). Adhere to these precautions for up to 7 weeks after the illness or up to several months if *Shigella* was the offending organism.

CHRONIC INFLAMMATORY BOWEL DISEASE

Ulcerative colitis and Crohn's disease are the two most common inflammatory bowel diseases (IBDs) that affect adults. Comparisons and differences are listed in Table 60-2. Viral and bacterial dysenteries can cause symptoms similar to those of IBD, and other problems must be ruled out before a definitive diagnosis is made.

The approach to each patient is individualized. Encourage patients to self-manage their disease by learning about the illness, treatment, drugs, and complications.

CHART 60-2 PATIENT AND FAMILY EDUCATION: PREPARING FOR SELF-MANAGEMENT

Preventing Transmission of Gastroenteritis

Advise the patient to:
- Wash hands well for at least 30 seconds with an antibacterial soap, especially after a bowel movement, and maintain good personal hygiene.
- Restrict the use of glasses, dishes, eating utensils, and tubes of toothpaste for their own use. In severe cases, disposable utensils may be wise.
- Maintain clean bathroom facilities to avoid exposure to stool.
- Inform the health care provider if symptoms persist beyond 3 days.
- Do not prepare or handle food that will be consumed by others. If the patient is employed as a food handler, the public health department should be consulted for recommendations about the return to work.

TABLE 60-2 DIFFERENTIAL FEATURES OF ULCERATIVE COLITIS AND CROHN'S DISEASE

FEATURE	ULCERATIVE COLITIS	CROHN'S DISEASE
Location	Begins in the rectum and proceeds in a continuous manner toward the cecum	Most often in the terminal ileum, with patchy involvement through all layers of the bowel
Etiology	Unknown	Unknown
Peak incidence at age	15-25 yr and 55-65 yr	15-40 yr
Number of stools	10-20 liquid, bloody stools per day	5-6 soft, loose stools per day, non-bloody
Complications	Hemorrhage Nutritional deficiencies	Fistulas (common) Nutritional deficiencies
Need for surgery	Infrequent	Frequent

ULCERATIVE COLITIS

Pathophysiology

Ulcerative colitis (UC) creates widespread inflammation of mainly the rectum and rectosigmoid colon but can extend to the entire colon when the disease is extensive. Distribution of the disease can remain constant for years. UC is a disease that is associated with periodic remissions and exacerbations (flare-ups) (McCance et al., 2010). Many factors can cause exacerbations, including intestinal infections.

The intestinal mucosa becomes hyperemic (has increased blood flow), edematous, and reddened. In more severe inflammation, the lining can bleed and small erosions, or ulcers, occur. Abscesses can form in these ulcerative areas and result in tissue necrosis (cell death). Continued edema and mucosal thickening can lead to a narrowed colon and possibly a partial bowel obstruction. Table 60-3 lists the categories of the severity of UC.

The patient's stool typically contains blood and mucus. Patients report tenesmus (an unpleasant and urgent sensation to defecate) and lower abdominal colicky pain relieved with defecation. Malaise, anorexia, anemia, dehydration,

TABLE 60-3 AMERICAN COLLEGE OF GASTROENTEROLOGISTS CLASSIFICATION OF UC SEVERITY

SEVERITY	STOOL FREQUENCY	SIGNS/SYMPTOMS
Mild	<4 stools/day with/ without blood	Asymptomatic Laboratory values usually normal
Moderate	>4 stools/day with/ without blood	Minimal symptoms Mild abdominal pain Mild intermittent nausea Possible increased C-reactive protein* or ESR†
Severe	>6 bloody stools/ day	Fever Tachycardia Anemia Abdominal pain Elevated C-reactive protein* and/or ESR†
Fulminant	>10 bloody stools/ day	Increasing symptoms Anemia may require transfusion Colonic distention on x-ray

Adapted from Present, D.H. (2006). *Current and investigational approaches in the management of ulcerative colitis.* Secaucus, NJ: Thomson Professional Postgraduate Services/Shire Pharmaceuticals, Inc.
UC, Ulcerative colitis.
*C-reactive protein is a sensitive acute-phase serum marker that is evident in the first 6 hours of an inflammatory process.
†ESR (erythrocyte sedimentation rate) may be helpful but is less sensitive than C-reactive protein.

TABLE 60-4 COMPLICATIONS OF ULCERATIVE COLITIS AND CROHN'S DISEASE

COMPLICATION	DESCRIPTION
Hemorrhage/ perforation	Lower gastrointestinal bleeding results from erosion of the bowel wall.
Abscess formation	Localized pockets of infection develop in the ulcerated bowel lining.
Toxic megacolon	Paralysis of the colon causes dilation and subsequent colonic ileus, possibly perforation.
Malabsorption	Essential nutrients cannot be absorbed through the diseased intestinal wall, causing anemia and malnutrition (most common in Crohn's disease).
Nonmechanical bowel obstruction	Obstruction results from toxic megacolon or cancer.
Fistulas	In Crohn's disease in which the inflammation is transmural, fistulas can occur anywhere but usually track between the bowel and bladder resulting in pyuria and fecaluria.
Colorectal cancer	Patients with ulcerative colitis with a history longer than 10 years have a high risk for colorectal cancer. This complication accounts for about one third of all deaths related to ulcerative colitis.
Extraintestinal complications	Complications include arthritis, hepatic and biliary disease (especially cholelithiasis), oral and skin lesions, and ocular disorders, such as iritis. The cause is unknown.
Osteoporosis	Osteoporosis occurs especially in patients with Crohn's disease.

fever, and weight loss are common. Extraintestinal manifestations such as migratory polyarthritis, ankylosing spondylitis, and erythema nodosum are present in a large number of patients. The common complications of UC, including extraintestinal manifestations, are listed in Table 60-4.

Etiology and Genetic Risk

The exact cause of UC is unknown, but genetic and immunologic factors have been suspected. A genetic basis of the disease has been supported because it is often found in families and twins. Immunologic causes, including autoimmune dysfunction, are likely the etiology of extraintestinal manifestations of the disease. Epithelial antibodies in the IgG class have been identified in the blood of some patients with UC (McCance et al., 2010).

With long-term disease, cellular changes can occur that increase the risk for colon cancer. Damage from proinflammatory cytokines, such as specific interleukins (e.g., IL-1, IL-6, IL-8) and tumor necrosis factor (TNF)–alpha, have cytotoxic effects on the colonic mucosa (McCance et al., 2010).

Incidence/Prevalence

Chronic inflammatory bowel disease (IBD) affects about 1.4 million people in the United States and is split about equally between ulcerative colitis (UC) and Crohn's disease

CULTURAL AWARENESS

Ulcerative colitis is more common among Jewish persons than among those who are not Jewish, and among whites more than non-whites (Crohn's and Colitis Foundation of America, 2008). The reasons for these cultural differences are not known.

(discussed later). Peak age for being diagnosed with UC is between 30 and 40 years and again at 55 to 65 years. Women are more often affected than men in their younger years, but men have the disease more often as middle-aged and older adults (Crohn's and Colitis Foundation of America, 2008).

PATIENT-CENTERED COLLABORATIVE CARE

ASSESSMENT

History

Collect data on family history of IBD, previous and current therapy for the illness, and dates and types of surgery. Obtain a nutrition history, including intolerance of milk and milk products and fried, spicy, or hot foods. Ask about usual bowel elimination pattern (color, number, consistency, and character of stools), abdominal pain, tenesmus, anorexia, and fatigue. Note any relationship between diarrhea, timing of meals, emotional distress, and activity. Inquire about recent (past 2 to 3 month) exposure to antibiotics suggesting *Clostridium difficile* infection. Has the patient traveled to or emigrated from tropical areas? Ask about recent use of NSAIDs that can either present with the initial diagnosis or cause a flare-up of the disease. Ask about any extraintestinal symptoms such as arthritis, mouth sores, vision problems, and skin disorders.

Physical Assessment/Clinical Manifestations

Symptoms vary with an acuteness of onset. Vital signs are usually within normal limits in mild disease. In more severe cases, the patient may have a low-grade fever (99° to 100° F [37.2° to 37.8° C]). The physical assessment findings are usually nonspecific, and in milder cases the physical examination may be normal. Viral and bacterial infections cause symptoms similar to those of UC.

Note any abdominal distention along the colon. Patients with fever associated with tachycardia may indicate peritonitis, dehydration, and bowel perforation. Assess for clinical manifestations associated with extraintestinal complications, such as inflamed joints and lesions inside the mouth.

Psychosocial Assessment

Many patients are very concerned about the frequency of stools and the presence of blood. *The inability to control the disease symptoms, particularly diarrhea, can be disruptive and stress producing.* Severe illness may limit the patient's activities outside the home with fear of fecal incontinence resulting in feeling "tied to the toilet." Severe anxiety and depression may result. Eating may be associated with pain and cramping and an increased frequency of stools. Mealtimes may become unpleasant experiences. Frequent visits to health care providers and close monitoring of the colon mucosa for abnormal cell changes can be anxiety provoking.

Assess the patient's understanding of the illness and its impact on his or her lifestyle. Encourage and support the patient while exploring:

- The relationship of life events to disease exacerbations
- Stress factors that produce symptoms
- Family and social support systems
- Concerns regarding the possible genetic basis and associated cancer risks of the disease
- Internet access for reliable education information

Laboratory Assessment

As a result of chronic blood loss, hematocrit and hemoglobin levels may be low, which indicates anemia and a chronic disease state. *An increased WBC count, C-reactive protein, or erythrocyte sedimentation rate (ESR) is consistent with inflammatory disease.* Blood levels of sodium, potassium, and chloride may be *low* as a result of frequent diarrheal stools and malabsorption through the diseased bowel (Pagana & Pagana, 2010). Hypoalbuminemia (decreased serum albumin) is found in patients with extensive disease from losing protein in the stool.

Other Diagnostic Assessment

A colonoscopy is the most definitive test for diagnosing UC. Annual colonoscopies are recommended when the patient has longer than a 10-year history of UC involving the entire colon. In some cases, a *computed tomography (CT) scan* may be done to confirm the disease or its complications. *Barium enemas* with air contrast can show differences between UC and Crohn's disease and identify complications, mucosal patterns, and the distribution and depth of disease involvement. In early disease, the barium enema may show incomplete filling as a result of inflammation and fine ulcerations along the bowel contour, which appear deeper in more advanced disease.

ANALYSIS

The priority problems for patients with ulcerative colitis are:

1. Diarrhea and incontinence related to inflammation of the bowel mucosa
2. Pain related to inflammation and ulceration of the bowel mucosa and skin irritation
3. Potential for lower GI bleeding and resulting anemia

PLANNING AND IMPLEMENTATION

Decreasing Diarrhea and Bowel Incontinence

Planning: Expected Outcomes. The major concern for a patient with ulcerative colitis is the occurrence of frequent, bloody diarrhea and fecal incontinence from tenesmus. Therefore, with treatment, the patient is expected to have decreased diarrhea, formed stools, and control of bowel movements.

Interventions. Many measures are used to relieve symptoms and to reduce intestinal motility, decrease inflammation, and promote intestinal healing. Nonsurgical and/or surgical management may be needed.

Nonsurgical Management. Nonsurgical management includes drug and nutrition therapy. The use of physical and emotional rest is also an important consideration. Teach the patient to record color, volume, frequency, and consistency of stools to determine severity of the problem.

Monitor the skin in the perianal area for irritation and ulceration resulting from loose, frequent stools. Stool cultures may be sent for analysis if diarrhea continues. Have the patient weigh himself or herself one or two times per week. If the patient is hospitalized, remind unlicensed assistive personnel to weigh him or her on admission and daily and document all weights.

? NCLEX EXAMINATION CHALLENGE

Physiological Integrity

The nurse is caring for a client with an exacerbation of ulcerative colitis. Which laboratory finding for the client will the nurse expect?

A. Decreased erythrocyte sedimentation rate
B. Decreased serum potassium
C. Decreased C-reactive protein
D. Decreased platelet count

Drug Therapy. Common drug therapy for UC includes aminosalicylates, glucocorticoids, antidiarrheal drugs, and immunomodulators. Teach patients about side effects and adverse drug events (ADEs) and when to call their health care provider.

The *aminosalicylates* are drugs commonly used to treat mild to moderate UC and/or maintain remission. Several aminosalicylic acid compounds are available. These drugs, also called *5-ASAs,* are thought to have an anti-inflammatory effect by inhibiting prostaglandins and are usually effective in 2 to 4 weeks.

Sulfasalazine (Azulfidine, Azulfidine EN-tabs), the first aminosalicylate approved for UC, is metabolized by the intestinal bacteria into 5-ASA, which delivers the beneficial effects of the drug, and sulfapyridine, which is responsible for unwanted side effects.

Mesalamine (Asacol, Pentasa, Rowasa, Apriso, Canasa) is better tolerated than sulfasalazine because none of its

	TABLE 60-5	RECOMMENDED DOSES FOR 5-ASA MEDICATIONS		
GENERIC NAME	**TRADE NAME**		**DOSAGE AVAILABLE**	**RECOMMENDED DOSE**
Sulfasalazine	Azulfidine		500 mg tablets	3-4 g daily in divided doses
	Azulfidine En-tabs			Children >2 yr: 30 mg/kg/day
	Azulfidine oral suspension (50 mg/mL)		250 mg/5 mL liquid	not to exceed 2 g/day
Mesalamine	Asacol		400 mg tablets	800 mg three times daily
	Pentasa		500 mg tablets	1 g four times daily
	Rowasa enemas		4 g/60 mL	At bedtime
	Rowasa suppository		1000 mg/supp	Twice daily or at bedtime
Olsalazine (rarely used)	Dipentum		250 mg tablets	1 g daily in two divided doses
Balsalazide	Colazal		750 mg tablets	3 tablets three times daily

5-ASA, 5-aminosalicylic acid.

! NURSING SAFETY PRIORITY

Drug Alert

Teach patients taking sulfasalazine to report nausea, vomiting, anorexia, rash, and headache to the health care provider. With higher doses, hemolytic anemia, hepatitis, male infertility, or agranulocytosis can occur. This drug is in the same family as sulfonamide antibiotics. Therefore assess the patient for an allergy to sulfonamide or other drugs that contain sulfur *before* the patient takes the drug. The use of a thiazide diuretic is also a contraindication for sulfasalazine.

preparations contain sulfapyridine. Asacol is an enteric-coated drug and is released in the terminal ileum and right side of the colon. Pentasa and Apriso are delayed- and extended-release drugs that work throughout the colon and rectum. Rowasa can be given as an enema, and Canasa can be given as a suppository. These preparations have minimal systemic absorption and therefore have fewer side effects. Table 60-5 lists commonly used 5-ASA drugs.

Glucocorticoids, such as prednisone and prednisolone, are corticosteroid therapies prescribed during exacerbations of the disease. Prednisone (Deltasone, Winpred) 40 to 65 mg daily is typically prescribed, but the dose may be increased as acute flare-ups occur. Once clinical improvement occurs, the corticosteroids are tapered because of the adverse effects that commonly occur with long-term steroid therapy (e.g., hyperglycemia, osteoporosis, peptic ulcer disease, increased risk for infection). For patients with rectal symptoms, topical steroids in the form of small retention enemas may be prescribed.

To provide symptomatic management of diarrhea, *antidiarrheal drugs* may be prescribed. These drugs are given very cautiously, however, because they can cause colon dilation and toxic megacolon. Common antidiarrheal drugs include diphenoxylate hydrochloride and atropine sulfate (Lomotil) and loperamide (Imodium).

Immunomodulators are drugs that alter a person's immune response. Alone, they are often not effective in the treatment of ulcerative colitis. However, in combination with steroids, they may offer a synergistic effect to a quicker response, thereby decreasing the amount of steroids needed. Immunosuppressants used with UC (and Crohn's disease, discussed later in this chapter) include infliximab (Remicade) and adalimumab (Humira).

Although not approved as a first-line therapy for ulcerative colitis, *infliximab* (Remicade) may be used for refractory disease or for severe complications, such as toxic megacolon (massive dilation of the colon that can lead to gangrene and

peritonitis) and extraintestinal manifestations. Remicade is an immunoglobulin G (IgG) monoclonal antibody that reduces the activity of tumor necrosis factor (TNF) to decrease inflammation. Adalimumab (Humira) is another monoclonal antibody approved for refractory (not responsive to other therapies) cases. They are used more commonly in management of Crohn's disease. These drugs cause immunosuppression and should be used with caution. Teach the patient to report any signs of a beginning infection, including a cold, and to avoid large crowds or others who are sick.

Nutrition Therapy and Rest. Patients with severe symptoms are kept NPO to ensure bowel rest. The physician may prescribe total parenteral nutrition (TPN) for severely ill and malnourished patients during severe exacerbations. Chapter 63 describes this therapy in detail. Patients with less severe symptoms may drink elemental formulas such as Vivonex PLUS or Vivonex T.E.N, which are absorbed in the small bowel and reduce bowel stimulation.

Diet is not a major factor in the inflammatory process, but some patients with ulcerative colitis (UC) find that caffeine and alcohol increase diarrhea and cramping. For some patients, raw vegetables and other high-fiber foods can cause GI symptoms. Lactose-containing foods may be poorly tolerated and should be reduced or eliminated. Teach patients that carbonated beverages, pepper, nuts and corn, dried fruits, and smoking are common GI stimulants that could cause discomfort. Each patient differs in their food and fluid tolerances.

During an exacerbation of the disease, activity is generally restricted because rest can reduce intestinal activity, provide comfort, and promote healing. Ensure that the patient has easy access to a bedpan, bedside commode, or bathroom in case of urgency or tenesmus.

Complementary and Alternative Therapies. In addition to dietary changes, complementary and alternative therapies may be used to supplement traditional management of ulcerative colitis. Examples include herbs (e.g., flaxseed), selenium, and vitamin C. Biofeedback, hypnosis, yoga, acupuncture, and ayurveda (a combination of diet, yoga, herbs, and breathing exercises) may also be helpful. These therapies need further study to validate their effectiveness, but some patients find them helpful.

Surgical Management. Some patients with ulcerative colitis require surgery to help manage their disease when medical therapies alone are not effective. In some cases, surgery is performed for complications of UC such as toxic megacolon, hemorrhage, dysplastic biopsy results, and colon cancer.

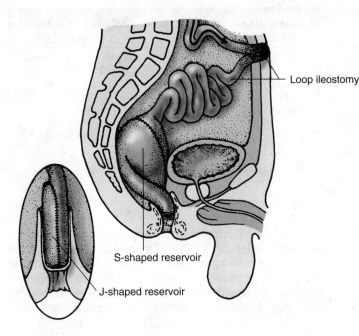

Stage 1.
After removal of the colon, a temporary loop ileostomy is created and an ileo-anal reservoir is formed. The reservoir is created in an S-shaped reservoir (using three loops of ileum) or a J-shaped reservoir (suturing a portion of ileum to the rectal cuff, with an upward loop).

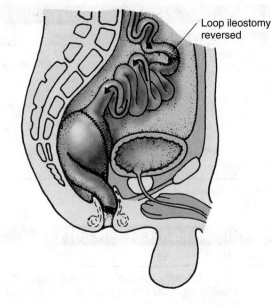

Stage 2.
After the reservoir has had time to heal—usually several months—the temporary loop ileostomy is reversed and stool is allowed to drain into the reservoir.

FIG. 60-2 The creation of an ileo-anal reservoir.

Preoperative Care. General preoperative teaching related to abdominal surgery is described in Chapter 16. If a temporary or permanent ileostomy is planned, provide an in-depth explanation to the patient and family. An **ileostomy** is a procedure in which a loop of the ileum is placed through the abdominal wall (**stoma**) for drainage of fecal material into a pouching system worn on the abdomen. The external pouching system consists of a solid skin barrier (wafer) to protect the skin and a fecal collection device (pouch), similar to the system used for patients with colostomies (discussed in Chapter 61).

If an ileostomy is planned, the surgeon consults with a certified wound, ostomy, continence nurse (CWOCN) or enterostomal therapist (ET) (sometimes called an *ostomy nurse*) before surgery for recommendations on the best location of the stoma. A visit from an **ostomate** (a patient with an ostomy) may be helpful before surgery. Parenteral antibiotics are given within 1 hour of surgical opening based on current best evidence and per The Joint Commission's National Patient Safety Goals.

In the past, patients have been required to follow a bowel preparation process before surgery using laxatives, enemas, and/or oral antibiotics to cleanse the bowel of normal flora to help reduce the risk for infection. Current research indicates that mechanical (enemas) and antibiotic bowel preparation does not affect the incidence of surgical site infections and is therefore not typically required (Howard et al., 2009).

Operative Procedures. Any one of several surgical approaches may be used for the patient with UC. Minimally invasive procedures, such as laparoscopic, laparoscopic-assisted, hand-assisted, and robotic-assisted surgery, are becoming common for patients with ulcerative colitis in large tertiary care centers (Kessler et al., 2011). Laparoscopic surgery usually involves one or several small incisions but often takes longer to perform than the open surgical approach. A newer procedure, natural orifice transluminal endoscopic surgery (NOTES), can be performed via the anus or vagina for select patients. Patients may have moderate sedation or general anesthesia for minimally invasive surgical procedures and are often *not* admitted to critical care units for continuing postoperative care.

Patients who are obese, have had previous abdominal surgeries, or have dense scar tissue (adhesions) may not be candidates for laparoscopic procedures. The conventional open surgical approach involves an abdominal incision and is done under general anesthesia. Patients with open procedures are typically admitted to critical care units for stabilization.

Restorative Proctocolectomy with Ileo Pouch–Anal Anastomosis (RPC-IPAA). This procedure has become the gold standard for patients with UC. In some centers, the surgery is performed via laparoscopy (laparoscopic RPC-IPAA). It is usually a two-stage procedure that *first* includes the removal of the colon and most of the rectum (Fig. 60-2). The anus and anal sphincter remain intact. The surgeon surgically creates an internal pouch (reservoir) using the last 1½ feet of the small intestine. The pouch, sometimes called a *J-pouch, S-pouch,* or *pelvic pouch,* is then connected to the anus. A temporary ileostomy through the abdominal skin is created to allow healing of the internal pouch and all anastomosis sites. It also allows for an increase in the capacity of the internal pouch. In the *second* surgical stage, the loop ileostomy is closed. The time interval between the first and second stage varies, but

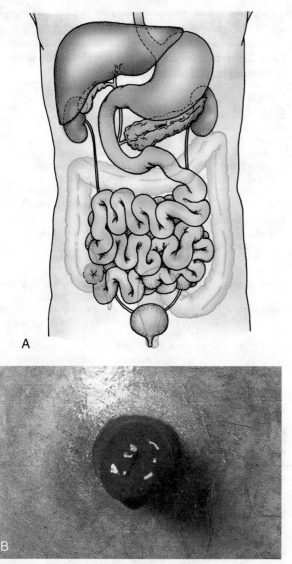

FIG. 60-3 A, Total proctocolectomy with a permanent ileostomy. This involved removal of the colon, the rectum, and the anus with closure of the anus. Note the missing colon, rectum, and anus with the resultant stoma **(B)** in the right lower quadrant.

many patients have the second surgical stage to close the ileostomy within 1 to 2 months of the first surgery.

Usually bowel continence is excellent after this procedure, but some patients have leakage of stool during sleep. They may take antidiarrheal drugs to help control this problem.

Total Proctocolectomy with a Permanent Ileostomy. Total proctocolectomy with a permanent ileostomy is done for patients who are not candidates or do not want the ileo-anal pouch. The procedure involves the removal of the colon, rectum, and anus with surgical closure of the anus (Fig. 60-3, *A*). The surgeon brings the end of the ileum out through the abdominal wall and forms a stoma, or ostomy.

With an ileostomy, initially after surgery the output is a loose, dark green liquid that may contain some blood. Over time, a process called "ileostomy adaptation" occurs. The small intestine begins to perform some of the functions that had previously been done by the colon, including the

absorption of increased amounts of sodium and water. Stool volume decreases, becomes thicker (pastelike), and turns yellow-green or yellow-brown. The effluent (fluid material) usually has little odor or a sweet odor. Any foul or unpleasant odor may be a symptom of a problem such as blockage or infection.

The ostomy drains frequently, and the stool is irritating. *The patient must wear a pouch system at all times.* The stool from the small intestine contains many enzymes and bile salts, which can quickly irritate and excoriate the skin. *Skin care around the stoma is a priority!* A pouch system with a skin barrier (gelatin or pectin) provides sufficient protection for most patients. Other products are also available.

Postoperative Care. Provide general postoperative care after surgery, as described in Chapter 18. All patients requiring open approach surgery for ulcerative colitis have a large abdominal incision. At first, most patients are NPO and a nasogastric tube (NGT) is used for suction. The tube is removed in 1 to 2 days as the drainage decreases, and fluids and food are slowly introduced. The patient having minimally invasive surgery (MIS) usually does not have an NGT.

In collaboration with the ostomy nurse, help the patient adjust and learn the required care. The ileostomy begins to drain within 24 hours after surgery at more than 1 L per day. Be sure that fluids are replaced by adding an additional 500 mL or more each day to prevent dehydration. After about a week of high-volume output, the drainage slows and becomes thicker. During this period, some patients need antidiarrheal drugs.

The hospital stay is usually from 2 to 5 days, depending on whether the patient has laparoscopic or conventional open surgery. Patients having MIS have less pain from surgery and faster restoration of bowel function when compared with other surgical patients, but the incidence of complications is about the same (Fajardo et al., 2010).

For those who have the RPC-IPAA procedure, remind them that the internal pouch can become inflamed. This problem is usually effectively treated with metronidazole (Flagyl) for 7 to 10 days. Teach patients that after the second stage of surgery, they might have burning during bowel elimination because gastric acid cannot be well absorbed by the ileum. Also instruct them to omit foods that can cause odors or gas, such as cabbage, asparagus, and beans. Teach patients to eliminate foods that cannot be well digested, such as nuts and corn. Each patient differs in which foods he or she can tolerate.

Surgery for UC may result in altered body image. However, it may be viewed as positive because the patient will have fewer symptoms and feel more comfortable than before the procedure. Patients have to adjust to having an ostomy before they can resume their presurgery activities.

NCLEX EXAMINATION CHALLENGE

Safe and Effective Care Environment

The health care provider prescribes sulfasalazine (Azulfidine) for a client with ulcerative colitis. What nursing action is most important before the client begins the medication?
A. Determine if the client's insurance pays for the drug.
B. Ask the client if he smokes or drinks alcohol.
C. Ask the client if he has any allergies to sulfa-type drugs.
D. Teach the client the importance of avoiding crowds.

Minimizing Pain

Planning: Expected Outcomes. The desired outcome for the patient is that he or she will verbalize decreased pain as a result of evidence-based pain management collaborative interventions.

Interventions. Pain control requires pharmacologic and nonpharmacologic measures. Physical discomfort can contribute to emotional distress. A variety of symptom-reducing interventions and supportive measures are used. Surgery also reduces pain for many patients.

The purpose of pain management is alleviation of pain or a reduction in pain to a level of comfort that is acceptable to the patient. Increases in pain may indicate the development of complications such as peritonitis (see earlier discussion in this chapter). Assist the patient in reducing or eliminating factors that can cause or increase the pain experience. For example, he or she may benefit from nutrition changes to decrease abdominal discomfort such as cramping and bloating.

Antidiarrheal drugs may be needed to control diarrhea, thus reducing the discomfort. However, they must be used with caution and for a short time because toxic megacolon can develop.

Perineal skin can be irritated by contact with loose stools and frequent cleaning. Explain special measures for skin care. Use of medicated wipes is soothing if the rectal area is tender or sensitive from the use of toilet tissue (Chart 60-3). Various manufacturers of ostomies (Hollister, ConvaTec) produce a system for skin care that may help prevent and heal perineal skin irritation. These systems usually include a skin-cleaning solution, a moisturizing and healing cream, and a petroleum jelly–like barrier that prevents contact of moisture and stool with the skin.

Monitoring for Lower GI Bleeding

Planning: Expected Outcomes. For patients who experience GI bleeding, the patient with UC is expected to have a reduction in or cessation of bleeding with prompt collaborative care. If possible, patients are expected to remain free of complications of the disease that can cause bleeding, such as perforation.

Interventions. The primary nursing priority is to monitor the patient closely for signs and symptoms of GI bleeding resulting from the disease or its complications.

If the patient has lower GI bleeding of more than 0.5 mL per minute, a GI bleeding scan may be useful to localize the site of the bleeding (Pagana & Pagana, 2010). This test cannot indicate the cause of the bleeding, however, and may take several hours to administer. Patients in the critical care unit are not candidates for the test because they must leave the unit for the test.

CHART 60-3   BEST PRACTICE FOR PATIENT SAFETY & QUALITY CARE

Pain Control and Skin Care for Patients with Inflammatory Bowel Disease

PATIENT PROBLEM	INTERVENTIONS
Abdominal pain (particularly with exacerbations of the disease)	Administer analgesics. Assist with frequent positioning. Identify foods that increase pain. Perform a comprehensive pain assessment. Observe for signs and symptoms of peritonitis. Evaluate effectiveness of pain management. Teach music therapy, guided imagery.
Skin excoriation and/or irritation from frequent bowel movements	Encourage good skin care with a mild soap and water after each bowel movement. Gently pat the area dry. Identify foods that increase diarrhea. Sitz baths may be of benefit. Apply a thin coat of A+D Ointment or aloe cream. Use medicated wipes instead of tissue. Ensure appropriate ostomy supplies that fit well. Antidiarrheal medications may help, but use with caution. Observe for symptoms related to megacolon (fever, leukocytosis, tachycardia, distended abdomen with 3-view abdominal x-ray noting an enlarged colon).

NURSING SAFETY PRIORITY

Critical Rescue

For the patient with ulcerative colitis, monitor stools for blood loss. The blood may be bright red (frank bleeding) or black and tarry (melena). Monitor hematocrit, hemoglobin, and electrolyte values, and assess vital signs. Prolonged slow bleeding can lead to anemia. Observe for fever, tachycardia, and signs of fluid volume depletion. Changes in mental status may occur, especially among older adults, and may be the first indication of dehydration or anemia.

If symptoms of GI bleeding begin, notify the health care provider immediately. Blood products are often prescribed for patients with severe anemia. Prepare for the blood transfusion by inserting a large-bore IV catheter if it is not already in place. Chapter 42 outlines nursing actions during blood transfusion.

Community-Based Care

Home Care Management

The patient with ulcerative colitis provides self-management at home but usually requires hospitalization during severe exacerbations and surgery. In addition, those who have extraintestinal problems often need ongoing collaborative care for joint and/or skin problems.

Home care management focuses on controlling clinical manifestations and monitoring for complications. For patients returning home or transferring to nursing home or transitional care after surgery, ongoing respiratory care, incision care (if applicable), ostomy care, and pain management should be continued.

Teaching for Self-Management

Teach the patient about the nature of ulcerative colitis, including its acute episodes, remissions, and symptom management. Also stress that even though the cause is unknown, relapses can be resolved with proper health care. Teach patients taking immunosuppressive drugs, such as corticosteroids and monoclonal antibodies, to report signs of possible infection, such as sore throat, to the health care provider. Remind them to avoid crowds and anyone who has an infection. Review the purpose of drug therapy, when drugs should be taken, side effects, and adverse drug events. Any signs and symptoms of an infection need to be reported to the health care provider.

Instruct the patient about measures to reduce or control abdominal pain, cramping, and diarrhea. Also teach the patient and family about symptoms associated with disease exacerbation that should be reported to the health care provider, such as fever higher than 101° F (38° C), tachycardia, palpitations, and an increase in diarrhea, abdominal pain, or nausea/vomiting. Provide written information and contact numbers for the health care provider.

There is no special diet for a patient with an ileostomy. However, teach the patient to avoid any foods that cause gas or make the stool thicker. Examples include high-fiber foods like nuts, raw cabbage, corn, celery, apples with peels, and popcorn. The patient needs to learn what foods he or she tolerates best and adjust the diet accordingly.

If he or she has undergone a temporary or permanent surgical diversion, collaborate with the ostomy nurse to explain and demonstrate required care so that the patient can self-manage. Also teach the importance of including adequate amounts of salt and water in the diet because the ileostomy increases the loss of these substances. Urge the patient to be cautious in situations that lead to heavy sweating or fluid loss, such as strenuous physical activity, high environmental heat, and episodes of diarrhea and vomiting.

Finding the best ostomy pouching system is a major issue for many patients. An effective system is one that:

- Protects the skin
- Contains the effluent (drainage) and reduces odor, if any
- Remains securely attached to the skin for a dependable period of time

Most patients desire an adhesive barrier that will last for 3 to 7 days. The barrier must create a solid seal to prevent the enzymes in the drainage from irritating the skin. Solid barriers are classified as "regular wear" or "extended wear." A person with a high output may want an extended-wear barrier. A special cream can be used to help fill any uneven skin surfaces and provide a consistent seal. Pouches are also individualized by the patient. Large pouches can hold more but are heavy when full. Patients also have to consider the costs of the various systems and how much their insurance (if they have it) will pay for them. Chart 60-4 describes the main aspects of ileostomy care, including skin care.

A patient with an ileostomy may have many concerns about management at home and about sexual and social adjustments. Considering possible sexual issues helps the patient identify and discuss these concerns with the sex partner. For example, a change in positioning during intercourse may alleviate apprehension. Social situations may cause anxiety related to decreased self-esteem and a disturbance in body image. Encourage the patient to discuss possible concerns in addressing and resolving these potentially stressful events. Clinical depression is common among patients with ulcerative colitis. Refer patients to appropriate mental health resources if depression is suspected.

CHART 60-4 **PATIENT AND FAMILY EDUCATION: PREPARING FOR SELF-MANAGEMENT**

Ileostomy Care

Skin Protection
- Use a skin barrier to protect your skin from contact with contents from the ostomy.
- Use skin care products, such as skin sealants and ostomy skin creams. If your skin continues to come into contact with ostomy contents, select a product to fill in problem areas and provide an even skin surface.
- Watch your skin for any irritation or redness.

Pouch Care
- Empty your pouch when it is one-third to one-half full.
- Change the pouch during inactive times, such as before meals, before retiring at night, on waking in the morning, and 2 to 4 hours after eating.
- Change the entire pouch system every 3 to 7 days.

Nutrition
- Chew food thoroughly.
- Be cautious of high-fiber and high-cellulose foods. You may need to eliminate these from the diet if they cause severe problems (diarrhea, constipation, or blockage). Examples include corn, peanuts, coconut, Chinese vegetables, string beans, tough-fiber meats, shrimp and lobster, rice, bran, and vegetables with skins (tomatoes, corn, and peas).

Drug Therapy
- Avoid taking enteric-coated and capsule medications.
- Inform any health care provider who is prescribing medications for you that you have an ostomy. Before having prescriptions filled, inform your pharmacist that you have an ostomy.
- Do not take any laxative or enemas. You should usually have loose stool and should contact a physician if no stool has passed in 6 to 12 hours.

Symptoms to Watch for
- Report any drastic increase or decrease in drainage to your health care provider.
- If stomal swelling, abdominal cramping, or distention occurs or if ileostomy contents stop draining:
  - Remove the pouch with faceplate.
  - Lie down, assuming a knee-chest position.
  - Begin abdominal massage.
  - Apply moist towels to the abdomen.
  - Drink hot tea.
  - If none of these maneuvers is effective in resuming ileostomy flow or if abdominal pain is severe, call your health care provider right away.

Health Care Resources

If the patient needs assistance with self-management at home, collaborate with the case manager or social worker to arrange the services of a home care aide or nurse. A home care nurse can provide assessment and guidance in integrating ostomy care into the patient's lifestyle. The nurse may also teach about wound care, including the monitoring of wound healing, if needed (Chart 60-5). The patient and family need to know where to purchase ostomy supplies, along with the name, size, and manufacturer's order number.

For patients with a permanent ileostomy, locate a community ostomy support group by contacting the United Ostomy Associations of America (www.uoaa.org). The United

Ostomy Association of Canada serves the needs of Canadian patients (www.ostomycanada.ca). A local support group or the Crohn's and Colitis Foundation of America (www.ccfa.org) may be helpful in obtaining supplies and providing education for ostomates. Inform the patient and family of available ostomy ambulatory care clinics and ostomy specialists. If the patient agrees, a visit from an ostomate can be continued after discharge to home.

EVALUATION: OUTCOMES

Evaluate the care of the patient with ulcerative colitis based on the identified priority patient problems. Expected outcomes may include that the patient will:

- Verbalize decreased pain
- Gain control over bowel elimination

CHART 60-5   HOME CARE ASSESSMENT

The Patient with Inflammatory Bowel Disease

Assess gastrointestinal function and nutritional status, including:
- Abdominal cramping or pain
- Bowel elimination pattern, specifically frequency, characteristics, and amount of stools and presence or absence of blood in stools
- Food and fluid intake (include relationship of specific foods to cramping and stools)
- Weight gain or loss
- Signs and symptoms of dehydration
- Presence or absence of fever, rectal tenesmus, or urgency
- Bowel sounds
- Condition of perianal skin, including presence or absence of perianal fistula or abscess

Assess patient's and family's coping skills, including:
- Current and ongoing stress level and coping style
- Availability of support system

Assess home environment, including:
- Adequacy and availability of bathroom facilities
- Opportunity for rest and relaxation

Assess ability to self-manage therapeutic regimen, including:
- Drug therapy
- Signs and symptoms to report
- Nutrition therapy
- Availability of community resources
- Importance of follow-up care

- Not experience lower GI bleeding
- Self-manage the ileostomy (temporary or permanent)
- Maintain peristomal skin integrity
- Demonstrate behaviors that integrate ostomy care into his or her lifestyle if a permanent ileostomy is performed

CROHN'S DISEASE

Pathophysiology

Crohn's disease (CD) is an inflammatory disease of the small intestine (most often), the colon, or both. It can affect the GI tract from the mouth to the anus but most commonly affects the terminal ileum. CD is a slowly progressive and unpredictable disease with involvement of multiple regions of the intestine with normal sections in between (called "skip lesions" on x-rays). Like ulcerative colitis (UC), this disease is recurrent with remissions and exacerbations.

Unlike UC, Crohn's disease presents as transmural inflammation that causes a thickened bowel wall. Strictures and deep ulcerations (cobblestone appearance) also occur, which put the patient at risk for developing bowel fistulas. The result is severe diarrhea and malabsorption of vital nutrients. Anemia is common, usually from iron deficiency or malabsorption issues.

The complications associated with Crohn's disease are similar to those of ulcerative colitis (see Table 60-4). Hemorrhage is more common in ulcerative colitis, but it can occur in CD as well. Severe malabsorption by the small intestine is more common in patients with CD because UC does not involve the small bowel to any significant extent. *Therefore patients with CD can become very malnourished and debilitated.*

Rarely, cancer of the small bowel and colon develop but can occur after the disease has been present for 15 to 20 years. Fistula formation is a common complication of CD but is rare in UC. Fistulas can occur between segments of the intestine or manifest as cutaneous fistulas (opening to the skin) or perirectal abscesses. They can also extend from the bowel to other organs and body cavities, such as the bladder or vagina (Fig. 60-4). Some patients develop intestinal obstruction, which, at first, is secondary to inflammation and edema.

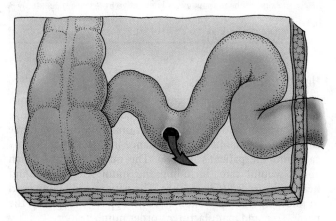

External enterocutaneous
(between skin and intestine)

Enteroenteric
(between intestine and intestine)

FIG. 60-4 The types of fistulas that are complications of Crohn's disease.

Over time, fibrosis and scar tissue develop and obstruction results from a narrowing of the bowel. Most patients with CD require surgery at some time.

The exact cause of CD is not known, but it seems to include a combination of genetic, immune, and environmental factors. About 10% to 20% of patients have a positive family history for the disease, but no predominant inheritance pattern is present (Nussbaum et al., 2007). The discovery of a mutation in the *NOD2/CARD15* gene on chromosome 16 seems to be associated with some patients who have CD. This gene is found in monocytes that normally recognize and destroy bacteria. Other gene mutations that may contribute to the pathogenesis of CD are *IBD3*, *IBD5*, and *IBD10.*

Proinflammatory cytokines, such as tumor necrosis factor–alpha (TNF-alpha) and interleukins (e.g., IL-6 and IL-8), are immunologic factors that contribute to the etiology of CD. Many of the drugs used for the disease inhibit or block one or more of these factors.

Other risk factors include tobacco use, Jewish ethnicity, and living in urban areas (McCance et al., 2010). The reasons for these factors have not been established. It was once thought that stress and nutrition play a role in the *development* of CD, but these factors have not been proven. However, inadequate nutrition can worsen the patient's symptoms.

Almost a million people in the United States have Crohn's disease. Most have symptoms and are diagnosed as adolescents or young adults. It is more common in people of Ashkenazi Jewish background than in any other group (Nussbaum et al., 2007).

PATIENT-CENTERED COLLABORATIVE CARE

ASSESSMENT

Crohn's disease is made worse by bacterial infection and inflammation. A detailed history is needed to identify manifestations specific to the disease. Ask about recent unintentional weight loss, the frequency and consistency of stools, the presence of blood in the stool, fever, and abdominal pain.

Perform a thorough abdominal examination, assess for manifestations of the disease, and evaluate the patient's nutritional and hydration status.

When inspecting the abdomen, assess for distention, masses, or visible peristalsis. Inspection of the perianal area may reveal ulcerations, fissures, or fistulas. During auscultation, bowel sounds may be decreased or absent with severe inflammation or obstruction. An increase in high-pitched or rushing sounds may be present over areas of narrowed bowel loops. Muscle guarding, masses, rigidity, or tenderness may be noted on palpation by the advanced practice nurse or other health care provider.

The clinical presentation of Crohn's disease varies greatly from person to person. Most patients report diarrhea, abdominal pain, and low-grade fever. Fever is common with fistulas, abscesses, and severe inflammation. If the disease occurs in only the ileum, diarrhea occurs five or six times per day, often with a soft, loose stool. Steatorrhea (fatty diarrheal stools) is common. Rarely, stools may contain bright red blood.

Abdominal pain from the inflammatory process is usually constant and often located in the right lower quadrant. The patient also may have pain around the umbilicus before and after bowel movements. If the lower colon is diseased, pain is common in both lower abdominal quadrants.

Most patients with Crohn's disease have *weight loss.* Nutritional problems are the result of increased catabolism from chronic inflammation, anorexia, malabsorption, or self-imposed dietary restrictions. These problems result in fluid and electrolyte imbalances and vital nutrient deficiencies.

The inflammatory bowel changes decrease the small bowel's ability to absorb nutrients, which may be made worse by surgery and fistulas.

! NURSING SAFETY PRIORITY
Action Alert

> For the patient with Crohn's disease, be especially alert for manifestations of peritonitis (discussed earlier in this chapter), small-bowel obstruction, and nutritional and fluid imbalances. Early detection of a change in the patient's status helps reduce these life-threatening complications.

The patient who has Crohn's disease (CD) needs a complete psychosocial assessment. The chronic nature of the problem and the associated complications can greatly affect patients and their families. Lifestyle changes are necessary to cope with such a disruptive and painful chronic illness. Assess the patient's coping skill, and help identify support systems. Clinical depression and severe anxiety disorders are common among patients with CD.

The health care provider requests many laboratory studies for patients with Crohn's disease. The results of laboratory tests often indicate the extent and severity of inflammation or complications that occur with the disease.

Anemia is common as a result of slow bleeding and poor nutrition. Serum levels of folic acid and vitamin B_{12} are generally low because of malabsorption, further contributing to anemia. Amino acid malabsorption and protein-losing enteropathy may result in *decreased albumin* levels. C-reactive protein and ESR may be elevated to indicate inflammation. White blood cells (WBCs) in the urine may show infection (pyuria), which is caused by ureteral obstruction or an enterovesical (bowel to bladder) fistula. If severe diarrhea or fistula is present, the patient may have electrolyte losses, particularly potassium and magnesium. Assess the patient for clinical manifestations that can occur as a result of electrolyte losses (see Chapter 13).

X-rays show the narrowing, ulcerations, strictures, and fistulas common with Crohn's disease. An abdominal ultrasound or CT scan may also be performed. In acute illness, these tests may be deferred until the risk for perforation lessens. If the patient has lower GI bleeding of more than 0.5 mL per minute, a gastrointestinal bleeding scan may be useful to localize the site of the bleeding (Pagana & Pagana, 2010).

INTERVENTIONS

Collaborative care for patients with Crohn's disease is similar to that described on p. 1274 in the Nonsurgical Management discussion in the Ulcerative Colitis section. Specific interventions vary with the severity of disease and the complications that are present.

Drug Therapy

Drugs used to manage Crohn's disease (CD) are similar to those used in the treatment of ulcerative colitis (UC). For mild to moderate disease, 5-ASA drugs may be very effective (see p. 1274 in the Drug Therapy discussion in the Ulcerative Colitis section).

Most patients have moderate to severe disease and need stronger drug therapy to control their symptoms. Two agents that may be prescribed for CD are azathioprine (Imuran) and mercaptopurine (Purinethol). These drugs suppress the immune system but can lead to serious infections. Methotrexate (MTX) may also be given to suppress immune activity of the disease.

More recently, a group of monoclonal antibody drugs has been approved for use in Crohn's disease when other drugs have been ineffective. These drugs inhibit tumor necrosis factor (TNF)–alpha, which decreases the inflammatory response. Examples of commonly used drugs for patients with CD include infliximab (Remicade), adalimumab (Humira), natalizumab (Tysabri), and certolizumab pegol (Cimzia). These agents are not given to patients with a history of cancer, heart disease, or multiple sclerosis.

> ### ! NURSING SAFETY PRIORITY
> #### *Drug Alert*
>
> Both infliximab and certolizumab pegol must be given in a health care setting, such as a physician's office via parenteral routes. Adalimumab (Humira) is self-administered by subcutaneous injection every other week. If needed, instruct patients on how to give themselves a subcutaneous injection. Teach patients to report injection site reactions, including redness and swelling. Remind them that headache, abdominal pain, and nausea and vomiting are common side effects. Teach them to avoid crowds, such as malls and large shopping centers, and people with infection. Reinforce the need to report any infection, including a cold or sore throat, to the health care provider immediately.
>
> Natalizumab is given IV under medical supervision every 4 weeks for moderate to severe CD and is given when other drugs are not effective. Although the use of this drug has decreased the length of hospital stays (Dudley-Brown et al., 2009), natalizumab can cause progressive multifocal leukoencephalopathy (PML), a deadly infection that affects the brain. Before giving the drug, be sure that patient is free of all infections. Teach patients the importance of reporting any cognitive, motor, or sensory changes immediately to the health care provider.

Although glucocorticoids can be effective for patients with Crohn's disease, sepsis can result from abscesses or fistulas that may be present. These drugs mask the symptoms of infection. Therefore they must be used with caution. Monitor the patient closely for signs of infection. Metronidazole (Flagyl, Novonidazole ✦) has also been helpful in patients with fistulas.

Nutrition Therapy

Long-standing nutritional deficits can have severe consequences for the patient with Crohn's disease. Malnutrition can lead to poor fistula and wound healing, loss of lean muscle mass, decreased immune responses, and increased morbidity and mortality. During severe exacerbations of the disease, the patient may be hospitalized to provide bowel rest and nutritional support with total parenteral nutrition (TPN). For less severe exacerbations, an elemental or semi-elemental product such as Vivonex PLUS may be prescribed to induce remission. These products are absorbed in the jejunum and therefore permit the distal small intestine and colon to rest. Nutritional supplements, such as Ensure or Sustacal, can be added then to provide nutrients and more calories. Teach the patient to avoid GI stimulants, such as caffeinated beverages and alcohol.

Fistula Management

Fistulas (abnormal tracts between two or more body areas) are common with acute exacerbations of Crohn's disease. They can be between the bowel and bladder (enterovesical), between two segments of bowel (enteroenteric), between the skin and bowel (enterocutaneous), or between the bowel and vagina (enterovaginal) (see Fig. 60-4). The patient with one or more fistulas often has complications such as systemic infections, skin problems, malnutrition, and fluid and electrolyte imbalances. Treatment of the patient with a fistula is complicated and includes nutrition and electrolyte therapy, skin care, and prevention of infection.

> ### ! NURSING SAFETY PRIORITY
> #### *Action Alert*
>
> Adequate nutrition and fluid and electrolyte balance are priorities in the care of the patient with a fistula. GI secretions are high in volume and rich in electrolytes and enzymes. The patient is at high risk for malnutrition, dehydration, and hypokalemia (decreased serum potassium). Assess for these complications, and collaborate with the health care team to manage them. Monitor urinary output. A decrease indicates possible dehydration, which should be treated immediately by providing additional fluids.

The patient requires at least 3000 calories daily to promote healing of the fistula. If he or she cannot take adequate oral fluids and nutrients, total enteral nutrition (TEN) or TPN may be prescribed. For patients who do not require TEN or TPN, collaborate with the dietitian to:

- Carefully monitor the patient's tolerance to the prescribed diet.
- Assist the patient in selecting high-calorie, high-protein, high-vitamin, low-fiber meals.
- Offer enteral supplements, such as Ensure and Vivonex PLUS.
- Record food intake for accurate calorie counts.

Providing enteral supplements, recording intake and output, and taking daily weights may be delegated to unlicensed assistive personnel (UAP) under the supervision of the RN.

Collaborate with the wound or ostomy nurse to select the most appropriate wound management for each patient.

> ### ! NURSING SAFETY PRIORITY
> #### *Action Alert*
>
> For patients with fistulas, preserving and protecting the skin is the nursing priority. *Be sure that wound drainage is not in direct contact with skin because intestinal fluid enzymes are caustic!* Clean the skin promptly to prevent skin breakdown or fungal infection, which can cause major discomfort for the patient.

Enzymes and bile in the stool contribute to the problem of skin irritation and excoriation. Skin irritation needs to be prevented. This may be accomplished through the use of skin

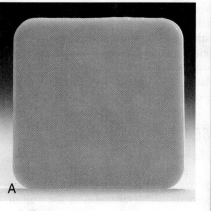

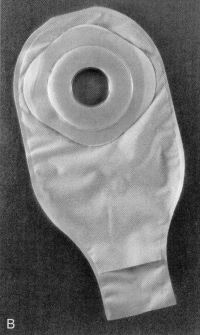

FIG. 60-5 Skin barriers, such as wafers **(A)** are cut to fit ⅛ inch around the fistula. A drainable pouch **(B)** is applied over the wafer and clamped **(C)** until the pouch is to be emptied. Effluent should drain into the bag and not contact the skin.

barriers, pouching systems, and insertion of drains (Fig. 60-5). Skin barriers or dressings are used when the fistula drainage is less than 100 mL in 24 hours. A pouch is used for heavily draining fistulas to reduce the risk for skin breakdown and measure the effluent (drainage). However, they are very challenging because of location and drainage amount. Treatment with an antifungal powder applied to the skin around the fistula is often very helpful to prevent or treat *Candida* infection.

For some fistulas, pouching may not be possible because of their location. Drainage may need to be managed using regulated wall suction or a vacuum-assisted closure (VAC) device. Continuous low wall suction is attached to a suction catheter in the wound bed of the fistula, not into the fistula tract. These systems are not meant for long-term management.

VAC therapy promotes wound healing by secondary intention as it prepares the wound bed for closure, reduces edema, promotes granulation and perfusion, and removes exudate and infectious material. It should not be used for patients who are at risk for bleeding or only for the purpose of drainage containment. Chapter 27 describes this therapy in detail.

Patients with fistulas are also at high risk for intra-abdominal abscesses and sepsis. Antibiotic therapy is commonly prescribed. Observe for signs of systemic infection or sepsis, such as fever, abdominal pain, or a change in mental status. Monitor for increased WBC levels that could indicate a systemic infection.

Other helpful interventions for the patient with CD are those that relax the patient and soothe the GI tract. Such therapies may include naturopathy, herbs (e.g., ginger), acupuncture, hypnotherapy, and ayurveda (a combination of diet, herbs, yoga, breathing exercises). The evidence supporting the use of these substances for CD is lacking, but many patients find them helpful for overall physical and emotional health. Teach patients about the availability of these therapies, and recommend that they include them in their collaborative plan of care.

? DECISION-MAKING CHALLENGE

Patient-Centered Care; Teamwork and Collaboration; Informatics

A 29-year-old woman who practices as a licensed practical nurse in a long-term care setting is admitted to the hospital with a draining enterocutaneous fistula as a result of long-term Crohn's disease. She has been taking infliximab (Remicade) for about 10 months but has noticed a return in her symptoms over the past week. The patient tells you that she is very upset about her condition and that she needs to go back to work as soon as she can. She is single but works extra shifts to help support her mother, who has advanced colon cancer.

1. What is your best response to the patient at this time?
2. What patient assessments will you perform on admission and why?
3. Based on the patient data provided, what priority problems do you identify?
4. Using best, current evidence, how will you plan care with other members of the health care team? What members of the health care team will be involved in this patient's care and why?

Surgical Management

Surgery for Crohn's disease may be performed for those patients who have not improved with medical management or for those who have complications from the disease. Surgery to manage CD is not as successful as that for ulcerative colitis due to the extent of the disease. The patient with a fistula may undergo resection of the diseased area. Other indications for surgical treatment include perforation, massive hemorrhage, intestinal obstruction or strictures, abscesses, or cancer.

In some cases, a resection (removal of part of the small bowel) can be performed as minimally invasive surgery (MIS) via laparoscopy. This surgery involves one or more small incisions, less pain, and a quicker surgical recovery. Both small-bowel resection (usually the ileum) and ileocecal resection can be done using this procedure. For other patients, an open surgical approach is used to allow for better visual access to the bowel.

Stricturoplasty may be performed for bowel strictures related to Crohn's disease. This procedure increases the bowel diameter. Care before and after each of these surgical procedures is similar to care for patients undergoing other types of abdominal surgery (see Chapters 16 and 18).

Community-Based Care

The discharge care plan for the patient with Crohn's disease is similar to that for the patient with ulcerative colitis (see p. 1278 in the discussion of Community-Based Care in the Ulcerative Colitis section). Collaborate with the case manager and wound nurse to help the patient plan self-management.

The interventions that were started in the hospital to manage the disease should be continued in the home. Reinforce measures to control the disease and related symptoms and manage nutrition. Teach the patient and family to make arrangements for the patient to have easy access to the bathroom, as well as privacy to perform fistula care, if needed.

The teaching plan for Crohn's disease is similar to that for the patient with ulcerative colitis. Teach the patient about the usual course of the disease, symptoms of complications, and when to notify the health care provider. Provide health teaching for drug therapy, including purpose, dose, and side effects. In addition to other drugs, vitamin supplements, including monthly vitamin B_{12} injections, may be needed because of the inability of the ileum to absorb these nutrients. In collaboration with the dietitian, instruct the patient to follow a low-residue, high-calorie diet and to avoid foods that cause discomfort, such as milk, gluten, and other GI stimulants like caffeine.

Remind the patient to take rest periods, especially during exacerbations of the disease. If stress appears to increase symptoms of the disease, recommend stress management techniques, counseling, and/or physical activity to improve quality of life (Crumbock et al., 2009). For long-term follow-up, teach the patient about the increased risk for bowel cancer and the importance of having frequent colonoscopies.

If a patient has a fistula, explain and demonstrate fistula care. Provide the opportunity for the patient to practice this care in the hospital. Ideally, he or she should be independent in fistula care before leaving the hospital. However, because of location of the fistula (perirectal or vaginal) or a large abdomen, assistance may be needed. If this is the case, teach a family member or other caregiver how to manage the fistula. Patients may be transferred to a transitional or skilled nursing unit for collaborative care.

Patients who are discharged to home after undergoing resection and anastomosis may require visits from a home care nurse to assess the surgical wound and monitor for complications (see Chart 60-5). Assess the patient's and family's ability to monitor the progress of fistula healing and to watch for indications of infection and sepsis. A home care aide or other service might be helpful for the patient who cannot meet nutritional needs or who needs help with grocery shopping and meal preparation.

In collaboration with the CM, assist with obtaining the equipment and supplies for fistula care, such as skin barriers and wound drainage bags. A support group sponsored by the United Ostomy Associations of America (www.uoaa.org) or a local hospital in the community may also be available to help with meeting physical and psychosocial needs.

DIVERTICULAR DISEASE

Diverticula are pouchlike herniations of the mucosa through the muscular wall of any portion of the gut but most commonly the colon. Diverticulosis is the presence of many abnormal pouchlike herniations (diverticula) in the wall of the intestine. Diverticulitis is the inflammation of one or more diverticula.

Pathophysiology

Diverticula can occur in any part of the small or large intestine but usually occur in the sigmoid colon (Fig. 60-6). The muscle of the colon hypertrophies, thickens, and becomes rigid, and herniation of the mucosa and submucosa through the colon wall is seen. Diverticula seem to occur at points of weakness in the intestinal wall, often at areas where blood vessels interrupt the muscle layer. Muscle weakness develops as part of the aging process or as a result of a lack of fiber in the diet.

Without inflammation, diverticula cause few problems. If undigested food or bacteria become trapped in a diverticulum, however, blood supply to that area is reduced. Bacteria invade the diverticulum, resulting in diverticulitis, which then can perforate and develop a local abscess. A perforated diverticulum can progress to an intra-abdominal perforation with peritonitis (inflammation of the peritoneum).

Bleeding from diverticula can range from minor local bleeding to massive hemorrhage. Minor bleeding is often due to inflammation in areas of new blood vessel tissue at the base of the diverticulum. Hemorrhage can result when a blood

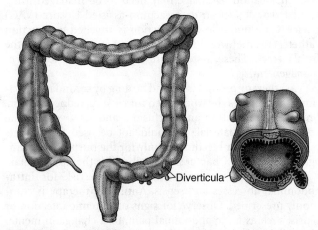

FIG. 60-6 Several abnormal outpouchings, or herniations, in the wall of the intestine, which are diverticula. These can occur anywhere in the small or large intestine but are found most often in the sigmoid colon, as shown in this figure. Diverticulitis is the inflammation of a diverticulum that occurs when undigested food or bacteria become trapped in the diverticulum.

vessel breaks down within a diverticulum. Inflammation from recurrent diverticulitis can lead to scarring and narrowing of the bowel lumen, which may then result in obstruction. Inflammation can also result in fistulas to other organs, such as the bladder and the vagina.

High intraluminal pressure forces the formation of a pouch in the weakened area of the mucosa, frequently near blood vessels. Diets low in fiber that cause less bulky stool and constipation have been implicated in the formation of diverticula. Retained undigested food in diverticula is suggested to be one cause of diverticulitis. The retained food reduces blood flow to that area and makes bacterial invasion of the sac easier.

The exact incidence of diverticulosis is unknown, but millions of people are affected by the problem. Diverticulitis is found in one half of adults older than 60 years, with more men than women affected. The cause for this difference is not known. Although diverticulosis is common, only one of five people with this disease has noticeable symptoms.

PATIENT-CENTERED COLLABORATIVE CARE

ASSESSMENT

The patient with *diverticulosis* usually has no symptoms. Unless pain or bleeding develops, the condition may go undiagnosed. Occasionally, diverticulosis will cause symptoms. For the patient with uncomplicated diverticulosis, ask about intermittent pain in the left lower quadrant and a history of constipation. If diverticulitis is suspected, ask about a history of low-grade fever, nausea, and abdominal pain. Inquire about recent bowel elimination patterns because constipation may develop as a result of intestinal inflammation. Also ask about any bleeding from the rectum.

On physical examination, uncomplicated *diverticulosis* may produce no clinical manifestations. Occasionally, tenderness occurs on abdominal palpation.

The patient with *diverticulitis* may have abdominal pain, most often localized to the left lower quadrant. It is intermittent at first but becomes progressively steady. Occasionally, pain may be just above the pubic bone or may occur on one side. Abdominal pain is generalized if peritonitis has occurred. Nausea and vomiting are common. The patient's temperature is elevated, ranging from a low-grade fever to 101° F (38.3° C). Chills may be present. Often an increased heart rate (tachycardia) occurs with fever.

CONSIDERATIONS FOR OLDER ADULTS

The first sign of peritonitis in older adults may be a sudden change in mental status (e.g., acute confusion). For those who have dementia, the confusion worsens. Fever and chills may not be present due to normal physiologic changes associated with aging.

On examination of the abdomen, observe for distention. The patient may report tenderness over the involved area. Localized muscle spasm, guarded movement, and rebound tenderness may be present with peritoneal irritation. If generalized peritonitis is present, profound guarding occurs; rebound tenderness is more widespread; and sepsis, hypotension, or hypovolemic shock can occur. If the perforated

diverticulum is close to the rectum, the health care provider may palpate a tender mass during the rectal examination. Blood pressure checks may show orthostatic changes. *If bleeding is massive, the patient may have hypotension and dehydration that result in shock.*

For the patient with uncomplicated diverticulosis, laboratory studies are not indicated. The patient with diverticulitis, however, has an *elevated white blood cell (WBC) count. Decreased hematocrit and hemoglobin* values are common if chronic or severe bleeding occurs. Stool tests for occult blood, if requested, are sometimes positive. Urinalysis may show a few red blood cells (RBCs) if the left ureter is near a perforated diverticulum.

X-rays of the intestinal tract with barium contrast may show diverticula. An upper GI series with small-bowel follow-through shows diverticula of the small intestine, and barium enema shows diverticula of the large intestine. Diverticula are most often diagnosed during routine colonoscopy.

The patient with diverticulitis usually does *not* undergo a barium enema procedure in the acute phase of the illness because of the risk for rupture of the inflamed diverticulum. A barium enema may be completed after the patient has been treated with antibiotics and the inflammation has resolved. Abdominal x-rays may be done to evaluate for free air and fluid indicating perforation. A computed tomography (CT) scan may be performed to diagnose an abscess or thickening of the bowel related to diverticulitis.

Abdominal ultrasonography, a noninvasive test, may also reveal bowel thickening or an abscess. The physician may recommend a colonoscopy 4 to 8 weeks *after the acute phase* of the illness to rule out a tumor in the large intestine, particularly if the patient has rectal bleeding.

INTERVENTIONS

Patients are managed on an ambulatory care basis if the symptoms are mild. Monitor the patient for any prolonged or increased fever, abdominal pain, or blood in the stool.

The patient with moderate to severe diverticulitis may be hospitalized, especially if the patient is older. Manifestations suggesting the need for admission are a temperature higher than 101° F (38.3° C), persistent and severe abdominal pain for more than 3 days, and/or lower GI bleeding.

Nonsurgical Management

A combination of drug and nutrition therapy with rest is used to decrease the inflammation associated with diverticular disease. Broad-spectrum antimicrobial drugs, such as metronidazole (Flagyl) plus trimethoprim/sulfamethoxazole (TMZ) (Bactrim or Bactrim DS, Septra) or ciprofloxacin (Cipro) are often prescribed. A mild analgesic may be given for pain. Chart 60-6 lists nursing interventions needed for care of older adults with diverticulitis.

The patient with more severe pain may be admitted to the hospital for IV fluids to correct dehydration and IV drug therapy. For patients with moderate to severe diverticulitis, an opioid analgesic, such as morphine sulfate, may alleviate pain.

Laxatives and enemas are avoided because they increase intestinal motility. Assess the patient on an ongoing basis for manifestations of fluid and electrolyte imbalance.

Teach the patient to rest during the acute phase of illness. Remind him or her to refrain from lifting, straining,

CHART 60-6   NURSING FOCUS ON THE OLDER ADULT

Diverticulitis

- Provide antibiotics, analgesics, and anticholinergics as prescribed. Observe older patients carefully for side effects of these drugs, especially confusion (or increased confusion), urinary retention or failure, and orthostatic hypotension.
- Do not give laxatives or enemas. Teach the patient and the family about the importance of avoiding these measures.
- Encourage the patient to rest and to avoid activities that may increase intra-abdominal pressure, such as straining and bending.
- While diverticulitis is active, provide a *low*-fiber diet. When the inflammation resolves, provide a *high*-fiber diet. Teach the patient and family about these diets and when they are appropriate.
- Because older patients do not always experience the typical pain or fever expected, observe carefully for other signs of active disease, such as a sudden change in mental status.
- Perform frequent abdominal assessments to determine distention and tenderness on palpation.
- Check stools for occult or frank bleeding.

coughing, or bending to avoid an increase in intra-abdominal pressure, which can result in perforation of the diverticulum. Nutrition therapy should be restricted to low fiber or clear liquids based on symptoms. The patient with more severe symptoms is NPO. A nasogastric tube (NGT) is inserted if nausea, vomiting, or abdominal distention is severe. Infuse IV fluids as prescribed for hydration. In collaboration with the dietitian, the patient increases dietary intake slowly as symptoms subside. When inflammation has resolved and bowel function returns to normal, a fiber-containing diet is introduced gradually.

Surgical Management

Diverticulitis can result in rupture of the diverticulum with peritonitis, pelvic abscess, bowel obstruction, fistula, persistent fever or pain, or uncontrolled bleeding. The surgeon performs emergency surgery if peritonitis, bowel obstruction, or pelvic abscess is present. Colon resection, with or without a colostomy, is the most common surgical procedure for patients with diverticular disease. The surgeon removes the portion that is inflamed or diseased and, if possible, creates an anastomosis of the colon to restore patency. Inflammation and infection, however, may prevent an anastomosis. If this is the case, the surgeon may perform a colostomy (see Fig. 60-3, *B* for appearance of a stoma). Some patients may have colostomy closure and anastomosis after the bowel has been allowed to rest for 3 to 6 months.

Preparation of the patient for surgery depends on the severity of the condition and whether it is an emergency or is performed a few weeks after the acute stage. The surgeon informs the patient whether a temporary or permanent colostomy might be required. If a colostomy is a possible outcome, collaborate with the certified wound, ostomy, and continence nurse (CWOCN) or an enterostomal therapist (ET) (ostomy nurse) to describe its function and care.

The patient may have one of two surgical approaches: conventional open approach or minimally invasive surgery (MIS) via a laparoscopy. The advantage of MIS is that patients are discharged from the hospital quicker, have less pain after surgery, and have fewer postoperative complications. They are able to resume normal activities much faster than patients having the conventional open surgery.

The nursing care for patients after an open colon resection for diverticulitis is the same as that for any patient who has undergone open abdominal surgery. The patient may have a drain in place at the abdominal incision site for several days. If a colostomy has been performed, the stoma may be covered with a petroleum gauze dressing because the colostomy does not drain for about 2 days, or a colostomy bag may be placed over the stoma. If the stoma is visible, monitor for color and integrity. The stoma should be pinkish to cherry red without retraction into the abdomen or prolapse.

The patient may be NPO with an NGT until peristalsis returns if open surgery is performed. Clear liquids are then introduced; the diet is advanced to solids, depending on the return of peristalsis and bowel function. Patients who had laparoscopic surgery usually do not have an NGT.

Most patients with a colostomy for diverticulitis have a sigmoid colostomy because the sigmoid colon is the most common site of diverticulitis. Drainage from a sigmoid colostomy at first consists of loose stool, but eventually the stool becomes formed. A tight seal around the stoma is essential to avoid contact of feces with the skin. Colostomy care is detailed in Chapter 59.

Give the patient an opportunity to express feelings about the ostomy if it was created. Discuss these feelings with the patient, reinforcing that anger and depression are normal responses. When he or she is physically able, encourage the patient to look at the stoma and touch the pouching system. Collaborate with the ostomy nurse to teach the patient how to self-manage ostomy care.

Community-Based Care

The length of stay for patients hospitalized for diverticulitis ranges from 1 to 4 days, depending on the response to treatment and the surgical procedure performed. Discharge plans vary according to the treatment. The patient who has surgical intervention has the added responsibilities of incision care and possibly colostomy care with temporary limitations placed on activities.

Patients with diverticular disease need education regarding a high-fiber diet. Encourage the patient with *diverticulosis* to eat a diet high in cellulose and hemicellulose types of fiber. These substances can be found in wheat bran, whole-grain breads, and cereals. Teach the patient to eat at least 25 to 35 g of fiber per day. Fresh fruits and vegetables with high fiber content are added to add bulk to stools.

If not accustomed to eating high-fiber foods, teach the patient to add them to the diet gradually to avoid flatulence and abdominal cramping. If he or she cannot tolerate the recommended fiber requirement, a bulk-forming laxative, such as psyllium hydrophilic mucilloid (Metamucil), can be taken to increase fecal size and consistency. Teach the patient to drink plenty of fluids to help prevent bloating that may occur with a high-fiber diet. Alcohol should be avoided because it irritates the bowel. Foods containing seeds or indigestible material that may block a diverticulum, such as nuts, corn, popcorn, cucumbers, tomatoes, figs, and strawberries, may be eliminated. Teach the patient that dietary fat intake should not exceed 30% of the total daily caloric intake.

Teach the patient to avoid all fiber when symptoms of *diverticulitis* are present, because high-fiber foods are then irritating. As inflammation resolves, fiber can gradually be added until progression to a high-fiber diet is established. The patient who has undergone surgery is usually taking solid food by the time of discharge from the hospital.

Provide oral and written instructions on incision care and the signs and symptoms to report to the health care provider for the patient who had abdominal surgery. If a colostomy was created, reinforce ostomy care as needed. Encourage the patient to express concerns about body image. Allow time and address sexual concerns regarding the changed body image.

Instruct the patient with any type of diverticular disease, orally and in writing, about the manifestations of acute diverticulitis, including fever, abdominal pain, and bloody, mahogany, or tarry stools. Advise patients to avoid the use of laxatives (other than bulk-forming types) and enemas. Reassure them that this disorder should not cause problems if a proper diet is followed.

In collaboration with the case manager, arrange for a home care nurse, if needed, to assess wound healing and proper functioning of the ostomy and the appliance. If the patient is interested, arrange for a visit from an ostomy volunteer (ostomate) or an ostomy nurse. For information about other community resources, remind the patient to contact the United Ostomy Associations of America (www.uoaa.org).

? NCLEX EXAMINATION CHALLENGE

Physiological Integrity

An older adult with a history of diverticulitis is admitted to the emergency department stating that she has severe abdominal pain and has not had a bowel movement in 6 days. What priority assessment will the nurse perform?
A. Listen to the client's breath sounds.
B. Take the client's height and weight.
C. Auscultate the client's bowel sounds.
D. Perform a rectal examination.

ANAL DISORDERS

Anorectal Abscess

Anorectal abscess is a localized area of induration and pus caused by inflammation of the soft tissue near the rectum or anus. It is most often the result of obstruction of the ducts of glands in the anorectal region. Feces, foreign bodies, or trauma can be the cause of the obstruction and stasis, leading to infection that spreads into nearby tissue.

Rectal pain is often the first symptom. There may be no other manifestations at first, but local swelling, redness, and tenderness are present within a few days after the onset of pain. If the abscess becomes chronic, discharge, bleeding, and pruritus (itching) may exist. Fever occurs if larger abscesses are present.

Anorectal abscesses are managed by surgical incision and drainage (I&D). The physician can often incise (surgically remove) simple perianal and ischiorectal abscesses using a local anesthetic. For patients with more extensive abscesses, a regional or general anesthetic may be needed. Systemic antibiotics are given only for patients who are immunocompromised, are diabetic, have valvular disease or a prosthetic valve, or are obese.

CHART 60-7 BEST PRACTICE FOR PATIENT SAFETY & QUALITY CARE

Promoting Perineal Comfort

- Keep the perineal area clean with mild soap.
- Pat the perineal area dry instead of rubbing it.
- Provide warm sitz baths, or apply warm compresses to the area.
- If the area is acutely inflamed, apply cold packs.
- Provide a chair cushion for the seated patient. For the older or debilitated patient, monitor the skin carefully to prevent pressure sores.
- Use absorbent pads for drainage, if any, and change them often.
- Use premoistened wipes for cleaning the perineal area after a bowel movement.
- Use witch hazel wipes (e.g., Tucks) to relieve pain.
- Give bulk-forming agents, such as psyllium mucilloid (Metamucil), as prescribed, to reduce pain associated with defecation.
- Apply a topical anesthetic cream to the perineal area, as prescribed.
- Give oral analgesics, as prescribed, for pain relief.
- Do not administer enemas or give potent laxatives.

! NURSING SAFETY PRIORITY

Action Alert

For patients with an anorectal abscess, nursing interventions are focused on comfort and helping the patient maintain optimal perineal hygiene (Chart 60-7). Encourage the use of warm sitz baths, analgesics, bulk-producing agents, and stool softeners after the surgery until healing occurs. *Stress the importance of good perineal hygiene after all bowel movements and the maintenance of a regular bowel pattern with a high-fiber diet.*

Patients are often embarrassed about having anal problems. Provide privacy and maintain the patient's dignity during the examination and treatment.

Anal Fissure

An anal fissure is a tear in the anal lining, which can be very painful. Smaller fissures occur with straining to have a stool, such as with diarrhea or constipation. Larger, deeper fissures may occur as a result of another disorder (e.g., Crohn's disease, tuberculosis, leukemia, neoplasm) or from trauma (e.g., from a foreign body, rough anal intercourse, perirectal surgery).

An *acute* anal fissure is superficial and usually resolves on its own or heals quickly with conservative treatment. *Chronic* fissures recur, and surgical treatment may be needed. Pain during and after defecation and bright red blood in the stool are the most common symptoms. Other manifestations include pruritus, urinary frequency or retention, dysuria, and dyspareunia (painful intercourse).

The diagnosis is made by stretching and inspecting the perianal skin. If the patient is having pain at the time of the examination, diagnostic testing is usually limited to inspection. If he or she is not in severe pain, a digital examination and possibly a sigmoidoscopy are performed. When painless or multiple fissures are present, a colonoscopy may be performed to rule out any inflammatory bowel disorder.

Management of an acute fissure is usually aimed at local pain relief and softening of stools to reduce trauma to the area. Teach the patient to use warm sitz baths, analgesics, and bulk-producing agents (e.g., psyllium hydrophilic mucilloid [Metamucil]) to help minimize the pain from defecation. Topical anti-inflammatory agents (hydrocortisone creams and suppositories) may be helpful for some patients.

Explain pain control measures to the patient. Remind him or her to notify the health care provider if pain is not relieved within a few days. If fissures do not respond to management within several days to weeks, surgical repair under a local anesthetic may be needed. Teach the patient to report any drainage or bleeding from the rectum to the health care provider.

Anal Fistula

An anal fistula, or *fistula in ano,* is an abnormal tract leading from the anal canal to the perianal skin. Most anal fistulas result from anorectal abscesses, which are caused by obstruction of anal glands (see Anorectal Abscess, p. 1287). Fistulas can also occur with tuberculosis, Crohn's disease, or cancer. Intermittent discharge is usually noted over the perianal area.

The patient with an anal fistula has pruritus (itching), purulent discharge, and tenderness or pain that is worsened by bowel movements. A proctoscope may be used to identify the source of symptoms and to locate the fistula. Because fistulas do not heal spontaneously, surgery is necessary. To perform a fistulotomy, the surgeon opens the tissue over the tract and scrapes the base. The incision site then heals by secondary intention. For a fistula higher in the anus, a special surgical technique is used to preserve important sphincters. After surgery, instruct the patient about sitz baths, analgesics, and the use of bulk-producing agents or stool softeners to reduce pain.

PARASITIC INFECTION

Pathophysiology

Parasites can enter and invade the GI tract and cause infections. They commonly enter through the mouth (oral-fecal transmission) from contaminated food or water, oral-anal sexual practices, or contact with feces from a contaminated person. Common parasites that cause infection in humans are *Giardia lamblia,* which causes giardiasis; *Entamoeba histolytica, which causes* amebiasis (amebic dysentery); and *Cryptosporidium. Handwashing is the best way to prevent the spread of parasitic infections.*

G. lamblia is a protozoal parasite that causes superficial invasion, destruction, and inflammation of the mucosa in the small intestine. This organism occurs in cysts and trophozoites (sporozoan parasites). Trophozoites die rapidly after they leave the body in stool. Cysts, however, can remain alive in the right type of environment for weeks or months. Humans who eliminate cysts are infectious. Flies can spread the cysts, and the problem is more common in areas that use human excrement for fertilizer. Humans are hosts to this organism, but beavers and dogs may be reservoirs for infection.

Giardiasis is a well-recognized problem in international travelers, campers, and immunosuppressed patients. In the United States, giardiasis is prevalent and is the most common parasitic infection. This disorder affects only the intestinal system, causing acute diarrhea, chronic diarrhea, or malabsorption syndrome. The acute phase usually is self-limiting, lasting days or weeks. The chronic phase can last for years.

Diarrhea is usually mild in both forms, but it can be severe. As stools increase in frequency, they become more watery, greasy, frothy, and malodorous with mucus. Weight loss and weakness are also common. Malabsorption can occur with diarrhea that continues for longer than 3 weeks. Manifestations result from malabsorption of fat, protein, and vitamin B_{12} and lactase deficiency.

Humans are the only known hosts for *E. histolytica* (also known as *amebiasis*). This organism also occurs in cysts and trophozoites. Amebiasis occurs worldwide, but it is most common in tropical areas. Prevalence rates are as high in areas with poor sanitation, crowding, and poor nutrition. Amebiasis causes tens of thousands of deaths annually worldwide. The disease causes less severe symptoms and often goes undiagnosed in temperate climates.

E. histolytica either feeds on bacteria in the intestine or invades and ulcerates the mucosa of the large intestine. The parasite can be limited to the GI tract (intestinal amebiasis), or it can extend outside the intestines (extraintestinal amebiasis). People can have intestinal amebiasis without having any symptoms, or symptoms can range from mild to severe.

Cryptosporidium is manifested by diarrhea. This infection occurs most commonly in immunosuppressed patients, particularly those with human immune deficiency virus (HIV). It can also occur in children and older adults from contaminated swimming pools. (See Chapter 21 for a discussion of HIV infection.)

PATIENT-CENTERED COLLABORATIVE CARE

ASSESSMENT

A thorough history can help determine potential sources of exposure to parasitic infection. A history of travel to parts of the world where such infections are prevalent increases suspicion for infection with parasites. GI symptoms related to travel may be delayed as long as 1 to 2 weeks after the return home. Immigrants (newcomers) may have the infection upon entering a new country. A nutrition history is especially helpful if several people in a group become ill. Common water supplies or bodies of water may be infected with *Giardia* or *Cryptosporidium*. Trichinosis should be considered if the patient has eaten pork products.

Mild to moderate *E. histolytica* infestation causes the daily passage of several strongly foul-smelling stools, possibly with mucus but without blood, accompanied by abdominal cramping, flatulence (gas), fatigue, and weight loss.

The infected patient usually experiences remissions and recurrences. Severe amebic dysentery is manifested by frequent, more liquid, and foul-smelling stools with mucus *and* blood. Fever up to 104° F (40° C), tenesmus (feeling the urge to defecate), generalized abdominal tenderness, and vomiting can also occur. The ulcerations of invading amebiasis that occur in the colon can cause pain, bleeding, and obstruction. Ulcerations can also occur in the rectum, resulting in formed stool with blood. Complications are rare but include appendicitis and bowel perforation.

Extraintestinal amebiasis can occur without symptoms of intestinal infection. The most common form is amebic liver abscess, which causes symptoms of fever, pain, and an enlarged liver. The abscess can rupture, and death can result if the infection and complications are not treated.

The diagnosis of *amebiasis* is made by examining the stool for parasites. Because *E. histolytica* is difficult to detect, serial stool examinations are needed if the disease is suspected. The use of sigmoidoscopy may detect ulcerations in the rectum or colon. Exudate obtained during sigmoidoscopic examination is studied for the parasite. The white blood cell (WBC) count can be very high when severe dysentery is present.

The diagnosis of *giardiasis* is also confirmed by the presence of parasites in the stool. Because organisms may not be detected for at least 1 week after symptoms appear, multiple stool samples should be examined.

INTERVENTIONS

Treatment for all types of *amebiasis* involves the use of amebicide drugs. Metronidazole (Flagyl, Novonidazole ✦) and diloxanide furoate (Entamide) or diloxanide furoate and tetracycline hydrochloride (Sumycin) followed by chloroquine are commonly prescribed. The patient with severe dysentery requires IV fluids replacement and possibly opiates, such as diphenoxylate hydrochloride and atropine sulfate (Lomotil), to control bowel motility. The patient with extraintestinal amebiasis or severe dehydration is hospitalized, especially the older adult. The patient with asymptomatic, mild, or moderate disease is treated with drug therapy on an ambulatory care basis. Therapy effectiveness is based on the examination of at least three stools at 2- to 3-day intervals, starting 2 to 4 weeks after drug therapy has been completed. *Teach patients the importance of keeping their follow-up appointments and taking all drugs as prescribed.*

Treatment for *giardiasis* is drug therapy. Metronidazole is the drug of choice, 250 mg orally three times daily for 5 days. Tinidazole (Fasigyn) can be used as an alternative. Stools are examined 2 weeks after treatment to assess for drug effectiveness.

Infection with *Cryptosporidium* is usually self-limiting in people who have normal immune function. Drug therapy for patients who are immunosuppressed may include paromomycin (Paromycin), an aminoglycoside antibiotic. Teach patients that this drug can cause dizziness.

FOOD POISONING

Foodborne illnesses are a common problem in the United States and all other parts of the world and can cause death. The problem results when a person ingests infectious organisms in food. Unlike gastroenteritis, food poisoning is not directly communicable from person to person and incubation periods are shorter. However, like gastroenteritis, it causes diarrhea, nausea, and vomiting. Food poisoning can be differentiated from gastroenteritis by obtaining a thorough history of common food intake in patients who have common symptoms of acute diarrhea, nausea, and vomiting.

Food poisoning is caused by over 250 pathogens. Examples include gram-negative *Salmonella, Staphylococcal aureus, Escherichia coli*, and botulism. Table 60-6 lists more information about these microbes. All cases of botulism and salmonellosis need to be reported to the local health department. Cases of staphylococcal and *E. coli* food poisoning are reported if epidemic outbreaks occur.

Salmonellosis

Salmonellosis is a bacterial infection caused by the *Salmonella* organism and affects many people each year in the United States. *Salmonella* bacteria live in the intestinal tracts of humans and animals. They can be transmitted by the "five Fs": flies, fingers, food, feces, and fomites. Incubation is 8 to 48 hours after the person has ingested the contaminated food or liquid, the most common source. Foods that are most commonly contaminated are eggs, beef, poultry, and green leafy vegetables (e.g., spinach). In 2008, contaminated jalapeno peppers from Mexico caused *Salmonella* infection in hundreds of people in the United States.

! NURSING SAFETY PRIORITY

Action Alert

Explain modes of transmission of parasitic infections and means to avoid the spread of infection and recurrent contact with parasitic organisms. *Inform the patient that the infection can be transmitted to others until amebicides effectively kill the parasites.* Teach the patient to:

- Avoid contact with stool.
- Keep toilet areas clean.
- Wash hands meticulously with an antimicrobial soap after bowel movements.
- Maintain good personal hygiene by bathing or showering daily.
- Avoid stool from dogs and beavers.

Advise the patient to avoid sexual practices that allow rectal contact until drug therapy is completed. *All household and sexual partners should have stool examinations for parasites.* If the water supply is suspected as the source, a sample is obtained and sent for analysis. Multiple infections are common in households, often as a result of contaminated water supplies. Well water and water from areas with inadequate or no filtration equipment can be sources of contamination.

TABLE 60-6	COMMON TYPES OF FOOD POISONING

Staphylococcal Infection
- Caused by contaminated meats and dairy products
- Can be transmitted by human carriers
- Causes abrupt onset of vomiting and diarrhea without fever

***Escherichia coli* Infection**
- Caused by meat contaminated with animal feces
- Causes abrupt vomiting, diarrhea, abdominal cramping, and fever

Botulism
- Commonly associated with improperly canned foods, especially fruits and vegetables
- Nausea, vomiting, diarrhea, and weakness progressing to paralysis
- Diplopia, dysphagia, and dysarthria

Salmonellosis
- Caused by contaminated food or drink but can be transmitted by the fecal-oral route
- Fever, nausea, vomiting, abdominal cramping, and diarrhea lasting for 3 to 5 days

Symptoms usually last for 4 to 7 days. Most people have fever, nausea, vomiting, cramping abdominal pain, and foul-smelling diarrhea, which may be bloody. In some patients, fever is very high.

Salmonellosis is usually self-limiting, but bacteremia that infects the joints or bone may occur later in the disease process. Diagnosis is made by stool culture. Treatment is symptomatic. If bacteremia occurs, antibiotics such as ampicillin or ciprofloxacin (Cipro) are prescribed. Unfortunately, some *Salmonella* bacteria have become resistant to antibiotics because of the use of these drugs in animals. Some patients, especially older adults, are hospitalized with severe diarrhea and dehydration.

Patients may be carriers of the bacterium for up to 1 year. Instruct those with *Salmonella* gastroenteritis and their contacts to wash their hands before meals and after defecating to avoid transmission of the organism.

Staphylococcal Infection

Staphylococcus is responsible for 25% of reported food poisoning outbreaks. It is found in meats and dairy products and can be transmitted by carriers of the organism. For staphylococcal food poisoning to occur, there must be contamination of food and a period of time (hours) during which the organisms multiply. This can take place during the slow cooling of food after it is cooked.

Symptoms of staphylococcal food poisoning include an abrupt onset of vomiting, abdominal cramping, and diarrhea. The person usually has symptoms 2 to 4 hours after ingesting the contaminated food. The patient is afebrile but weak.

A diagnosis can be made when stool culture yields 100,000 enterotoxin-producing staphylococci. However, symptoms rarely last more than 24 hours, and people do not always seek medical attention. Antimicrobial drug therapy is not usually indicated unless an agent produces progressive systemic involvement. Parenteral fluids may be needed for dehydration.

Escherichia coli Infection

Since 1992, a number of outbreaks of *E. coli* food poisoning have occurred in the United States. Many strains of *E. coli* exist, and not all of them cause harm. However, some cause disease by making a substance called *Shiga toxin*. The bacteria that make these substances are called *Shiga toxin–producing E. coli*, or *STEC* for short. The most commonly identified STEC in the United States is *E. coli* O157:H7 (sometimes called just *O157*). In 2007, prepackaged spinach processed in the United States was contaminated with these bacteria and caused hundreds of people to become ill.

Enterohemorrhagic strains of *E. coli* (EHEC) and STEC can cause serious complications, such as hemorrhagic colitis and hemolytic-uremic syndrome. These problems affect older adults most often.

The symptoms of STEC infections vary, but most people have severe abdominal cramping, vomiting, and diarrhea (often bloody). Treatment of the patient with *E. coli* food poisoning includes IV fluids and supportive therapy, possibly with antidiarrheal agents. Antibiotics are not effective. Chart 60-8 outlines best practices for preventing STEC infections.

CHART 60-8   PATIENT AND FAMILY EDUCATION: PREPARING FOR SELF-MANAGEMENT

Ways to Prevent STEC (E. coli) Infections

- Wash your hands *thoroughly* after using the bathroom and after changing diapers and before preparing or eating food.
- Wash your hands after contact with any animals or their environments (e.g., zoo).
- Cook meats thoroughly to at least 160° to 170° internal temperature; use a food thermometer to ensure doneness.
- Avoid raw milk, unpasteurized juices (like fresh apple cider), and unpasteurized dairy products.
- Avoid swallowing water when swimming.
- Prevent cross-contamination during food preparation by washing hands, counters, cutting boards, and utensils after they touch raw meat.

STEC, Shiga toxin–producing *Escherichia coli.*

Botulism

Botulism is a paralytic disease resulting from ingestion of a toxin in food contaminated with *Clostridium botulinum*. Botulism occurs most often with home-canned foods, particularly vegetables, fruits, condiments, and, less commonly, meat and fish. It can also occur in commercially prepared products and with products not adequately heated to destroy toxins before they are eaten.

Incubation is usually 18 to 36 hours. After this time, symptoms occur. Initial symptoms include diplopia (double vision), dysphagia (difficulty swallowing), and dysarthria (slurred speech). Illness may be mild or severe, with paralysis, respiratory failure, and death. Weakness can progress rapidly from the neck to the arms, chest, and legs. Paralytic ileus, severe constipation, and urinary retention can also occur. Nausea, vomiting, and abdominal pain may occur before or after the onset of paralysis. The diagnosis is made on the basis of the patient's history and a stool culture of *C. botulinum*. The blood may be positive for toxins.

Treatment with trivalent botulism antitoxin is given as soon as the diagnosis is made if the patient is not hypersensitive to it. The physician may lavage the stomach to stop absorption of toxin. All patients are hospitalized to observe for and treat respiratory paralysis. Nothing is given orally until swallowing and respiratory function are restored. The physician prescribes IV fluids as needed. If respiratory paralysis occurs, intubation and mechanical ventilation are implemented. If ventilation can be maintained, the patient can survive with no neurologic deficits after the illness.

! NURSING SAFETY PRIORITY
Action Alert

To prevent botulism, teach patients the importance of discarding cans of food that are punctured or swollen or that have defective seals. Remind them to check for expiration dates and to not use any canned food that has expired. Containers for home-canned foods must be sterilized by boiling for 20 minutes to destroy *C. botulinum* spores before canning.

NURSING CONCEPT REVIEW

What might you NOTICE if the patient has impaired digestion and inadequate nutrition as a result of inflammatory intestinal problems?

- Report of nausea
- Vomiting
- Report of epigastric or abdominal pain
- Diarrhea (sometimes bloody)
- Elevated temperature
- Weakness

What should you INTERPRET and how should you RESPOND to a patient with impaired digestion and inadequate nutrition as a result of inflammatory intestinal problems?

Perform and interpret focused physical assessment findings, including:

- Vital signs
- Complete pain assessment
- Skin turgor and mucous membrane dryness
- Abdominal assessment
- Current and previous weight
- History of recent food intake
- History of recent travel

Respond:

- Prevent pain and aspiration by placing patient in sitting position.
- Place IV catheter (large-bore) to replace fluids.
- Provide privacy, and assist with hygiene.
- Provide rest.
- Check laboratory values for hemoglobin and hematocrit (anemia).
- Check serum electrolytes (dehydration, hypokalemia).
- Give antidiarrheal drugs if prescribed.
- Record intake and output.
- Assist with ADLs and ambulation as needed.

On what should you REFLECT?

- Continue to monitor for vomiting and diarrhea and changes in pain level.
- Think about what you need to document.
- Decide when you might need to call the health care provider or Rapid Response Team (for hospitalized patients).
- Determine what health teaching and community resources may be needed for this patient and family.
- Think about what you can do to help prevent complications of the health problem.

GET READY FOR THE NCLEX® EXAMINATION!

KEY POINTS

Review these Key Points for each NCLEX Examination Client Needs Category.

Safe and Effective Care Environment

- Teach patients to use infection control measures to prevent transmission of gastroenteritis as stated in Chart 60-2.
- Collaborate with a CWOCN or ET nurse for ileostomy teaching and care; collaborate with a case manager when planning for patient discharge.

Health Promotion and Maintenance

- Teach patients with chronic IBD to avoid GI stimulants, such as alcohol and caffeine; each patient's response to foods differs.
- Instruct patients with diverticulosis about nutrition modifications, such as avoiding nuts, foods with seeds, and GI stimulants.
- Teach patients with diverticulosis to eat a high-fiber diet; diverticulitis requires a low-fiber diet.

Psychosocial Integrity

- Be aware that all inflammatory bowel diseases (acute and chronic) are very disruptive to one's daily routine; chronic IBD requires a lifetime of modifications.

- Recognize that having an ileostomy impacts the patient's body image and self-esteem; assess for coping strategies that the patient has previously used, and identify personal support systems to assist in coping.

Physiological Integrity

- Assess for the classic clinical manifestations of appendicitis, which include abdominal pain, nausea and vomiting, and abdominal tenderness upon palpation (McBurney's point); some patients also have leukocytosis.
- Assess for the key features of peritonitis as listed in Chart 60-1.
- Assess for signs and symptoms of dehydration in patients who have inflammatory bowel disease.
- Administer antidiarrheal medications as prescribed to decrease stools and therefore prevent dehydration in patients with inflammatory bowel diseases.
- Be aware that there are two major types of chronic inflammatory bowel disease (IBD): ulcerative colitis (UC) and Crohn's disease; both have similarities but also have differences (see Table 60-2).
- Recognize that perforation (rupture) of the appendix requires prompt intervention and can result in peritonitis.

GET READY FOR THE NCLEX® EXAMINATION!—cont'd

- Be alert for GI bleeding in the patient with chronic inflammatory bowel disease (IBD).
- Be aware that patients with Crohn's disease are at high risk for malnutrition as a result of an inability to absorb nutrients via the small intestine.
- Teach patients how to provide ileostomy care, paying particular attention to skin care; the effluent has a high enzyme content that can easily cause severe skin excoriation (see Chart 60-4).
- Monitor for complications of UC as listed in Table 60-4.
- Provide nursing interventions for patients with IBD as listed in Chart 60-3.
- Administer 5-aminosalicylic acid (5-ASA) drugs as prescribed (e.g., Pentasa) to decrease inflammation in patients with UC; most of these same drugs are also used for Crohn's disease management.
- Administer infliximab (Remicade) or other monoclonal antibody agent as prescribed for patients with Crohn's disease; these drugs may also be useful for those with UC in selected cases.
- Observe for manifestations of lower GI bleeding in patients with chronic inflammatory and diverticular disease.
- Instruct patients with anorectal disorders to use sitz baths, bulk-forming agents (e.g., Metamucil), and stool softeners to decrease pain.
- Be aware that GI problems, including diarrhea, may also be caused by parasites and food poisoning.

CHAPTER 61

Care of Patients with Liver Problems

Donna D. Ignatavicius

LEARNING OUTCOMES

Safe and Effective Care Environment

1. Describe the need to collaborate with health care team members to provide care for patients with liver problems.

Health Promotion and Maintenance

2. Identify community resources for patients with chronic liver disease.
3. Identify risk factors for cirrhosis and hepatitis.
4. Develop a health teaching plan for patients and families to prevent hepatitis and its spread to others.
5. Develop a health teaching plan for patients and families to prevent or slow the progress of alcohol-induced cirrhosis.

Psychosocial Integrity

6. Explain the psychosocial needs of patients with hepatitis.

Physiological Integrity

7. Explain the pathophysiology and complications associated with cirrhosis of the liver.
8. Interpret laboratory test findings commonly seen in patients with cirrhosis.

9. Analyze assessment data from patients with cirrhosis to determine priority patient problems.
10. Develop a collaborative plan of care for the patient with late-stage cirrhosis.
11. Describe the role of the nurse in monitoring for and managing potentially life-threatening complications of cirrhosis.
12. Identify emergency interventions for the patient with bleeding esophageal varices.
13. Explain the role of the nurse when assisting with a paracentesis procedure.
14. Compare and contrast the transmission of hepatitis viral infections.
15. Explain ways in which each type of hepatitis can be prevented.
16. Identify potentially life-threatening complications of liver trauma.
17. Describe treatment options for patients with cancer of the liver.
18. Describe the common complications that result from liver transplantation.

The liver is the largest and one of the most vital internal organs, performing more than 400 functions and affecting every system in the body. When the liver is diseased or damaged, it cannot provide these activities. As a result, *digestion, nutrition, and metabolism* can be severely affected. Liver diseases range in severity from mild hepatic inflammation to chronic end-stage cirrhosis.

CIRRHOSIS

Cirrhosis is extensive, irreversible scarring of the liver, usually caused by a chronic reaction to hepatic inflammation and necrosis. The disease typically develops slowly and has a progressive, prolonged, destructive course resulting in end-stage liver disease. The most common causes for cirrhosis in the

United States are hepatitis C, alcoholism, and biliary obstruction. Worldwide, hepatitis B and hepatitis D are the leading causes. Without liver transplantation, cirrhosis is usually fatal (Kelso, 2008).

Pathophysiology

Cirrhosis is characterized by widespread fibrotic (scarred) bands of connective tissue that change the liver's normal makeup. Inflammation caused by either toxins or disease results in extensive degeneration and destruction of hepatocytes (liver cells). As cirrhosis develops, the tissue becomes nodular. These nodules can block bile ducts and normal blood flow throughout the liver. Impairments in blood and lymph flow result from compression caused by excessive fibrous tissue. In early disease, the liver is usually enlarged, firm, and hard. As the pathologic process continues, the liver shrinks in size, resulting in decreased liver function, which can occur in weeks to years. Some patients with cirrhosis have no symptoms until serious complications occur. The impaired liver function results in elevated serum liver enzymes (Pagana & Pagana, 2010).

Cirrhosis of the liver can be divided into several common types, depending on the cause of the disease (McCance et al., 2010):

- Postnecrotic cirrhosis (caused by viral hepatitis [especially hepatitis C] and certain drugs or other toxins)
- Laennec's or alcoholic cirrhosis (caused by chronic alcoholism)
- Biliary cirrhosis (also called *cholestatic*; caused by chronic biliary obstruction or autoimmune disease)

Complications of Cirrhosis

Common problems and complications associated with hepatic cirrhosis depend on the amount of damage sustained by the liver. In compensated cirrhosis, the liver is scarred but can still perform essential functions without causing major symptoms. In decompensated cirrhosis, liver function is impaired with obvious manifestations of liver failure.

The loss of hepatic function contributes to the development of metabolic abnormalities. Hepatic cell damage may lead to these common complications:

- Portal hypertension
- Ascites and esophageal varices
- Coagulation defects
- Jaundice
- Portal-systemic encephalopathy (PSE) with hepatic coma
- Hepatorenal syndrome
- Spontaneous bacterial peritonitis

Portal Hypertension. Portal hypertension, a persistent increase in pressure within the portal vein greater than 5 mm Hg, is a major complication of cirrhosis (Minano & Garcia-Tsao, 2010). It results from increased resistance to or obstruction (blockage) of the flow of blood through the portal vein and its branches. The blood meets resistance to flow and seeks collateral (alternative) venous channels around the high-pressure area.

Blood flow backs into the spleen, causing splenomegaly (spleen enlargement). Veins in the esophagus, stomach, intestines, abdomen, and rectum become dilated. Portal hypertension can result in ascites (abdominal fluid), esophageal varices

(distended veins), prominent abdominal veins (caput medusae), and hemorrhoids.

Ascites and Esophageal Varices. Ascites is the collection of free fluid within the peritoneal cavity caused by increased hydrostatic pressure from portal hypertension (McCance et al., 2010). The collection of plasma protein in the peritoneal fluid reduces the amount of circulating plasma protein in the blood. When this decrease is combined with the inability of the liver to produce albumin because of impaired liver cell functioning, the serum colloid osmotic pressure is decreased in the circulatory system. The result is a fluid shift from the vascular system into the abdomen, a form of "third spacing." As a result, the patient may have hypovolemia and edema at the same time.

Massive ascites may cause renal vasoconstriction, triggering the renin-angiotensin system. This results in sodium and water retention, which increases hydrostatic pressure and the vascular volume and leads to more ascites.

As a result of portal hypertension, the blood backs up from the liver and enters the esophageal and gastric veins. Esophageal varices occur when fragile, thin-walled esophageal veins become distended and tortuous from increased pressure. The potential for varices to bleed depends on their size; size is determined by direct endoscopic observation. Varices occur most often in the distal esophagus but can also be present in the stomach and rectum.

Bleeding esophageal varices is a life-threatening medical emergency. Severe blood loss may occur, resulting in shock from hypovolemia. The bleeding may be either hematemesis (vomiting blood) or melena (black, tarry stools). Loss of consciousness may occur before any observed bleeding. Variceal bleeding can occur spontaneously with no precipitating factors. However, any activity that increases abdominal pressure may increase the likelihood of a variceal bleed, including heavy lifting or vigorous physical exercise. In addition, chest trauma or dry, hard food in the esophagus can cause bleeding.

Patients with portal hypertension may also have portal hypertensive gastropathy. This complication can occur with or without esophageal varices. Slow gastric mucosal bleeding occurs, which may result in chronic slow blood loss, occult-positive stools, and anemia.

Splenomegaly (enlarged spleen) results from the backup of blood into the spleen. The enlarged spleen destroys platelets, causing thrombocytopenia (low serum platelet count) and increased risk for bleeding. Thrombocytopenia is often the first clinical sign that a patient has liver dysfunction.

Biliary Obstruction. In patients with cirrhosis, the production of bile in the liver is decreased. This prevents the absorption of fat-soluble vitamins (e.g., vitamin K). Without vitamin K, clotting factors II, VII, IX, and X are not produced in sufficient quantities and the patient is susceptible to bleeding and easy bruising. These abnormalities are confirmed by coagulation studies.

Jaundice (yellowish coloration of the skin) in patients with cirrhosis is caused by one of two mechanisms: hepatocellular disease or intrahepatic obstruction (Table 61-1). *Hepatocellular* jaundice develops because the liver cells cannot effectively excrete bilirubin. This decreased excretion results in excessive circulating bilirubin levels. *Intrahepatic obstructive* jaundice results from edema, fibrosis, or scarring of the hepatic bile channels and bile ducts, which interferes with

TABLE 61-1	LABORATORY DIAGNOSTIC DIFFERENTIATION OF JAUNDICE		
TEST	**HEPATOCELLULAR JAUNDICE**	**OBSTRUCTIVE JAUNDICE**	**HEMOLYTIC JAUNDICE**
Serum bilirubin			
Indirect (unconjugated)	Increased	Slightly increased	Increased
Direct (conjugated)	Increased	Moderately increased	Normal
Urine bilirubin	Increased	Increased	None
Urobilinogen			
Stool	Normal to decreased	None	Increased
Urine	Normal to increased	None	Increased

TABLE 61-2   STAGES OF PORTAL-SYSTEMIC ENCEPHALOPATHY

Stage I Prodromal
- Subtle manifestations that may not be recognized immediately
- Personality changes
- Behavior changes (agitation, belligerence)
- Emotional lability (euphoria, depression)
- Impaired thinking
- Inability to concentrate
- Fatigue, drowsiness
- Slurred or slowed speech
- Sleep pattern disturbances

Stage II Impending
- Continuing mental changes
- Mental confusion
- Disorientation to time, place, or person
- Asterixis (hand flapping)

Stage III Stuporous
- Progressive deterioration
- Marked mental confusion
- Stuporous, drowsy but arousable
- Abnormal electroencephalogram tracing
- Muscle twitching
- Hyperreflexia
- Asterixis

Stage IV Comatose
- Unresponsiveness, leading to death in most patients progressing to this stage
- Unarousable, obtunded
- Usually no response to painful stimulus
- No asterixis
- Positive Babinski's sign
- Muscle rigidity
- Fetor hepaticus (characteristic liver breath—musty, sweet odor)
- Seizures

normal bile and bilirubin excretion. Patients with jaundice often report pruritus (itching).

Hepatic Encephalopathy. Hepatic encephalopathy (also called portal-systemic encephalopathy [PSE]) is a complex cognitive syndrome that results from liver failure and cirrhosis. Patients report sleep disturbance, mood disturbance, mental status changes, and speech problems early as this complication begins. Hepatic encephalopathy may be reversible with early intervention. Later neurologic symptoms include an altered level of consciousness, impaired thinking processes, and neuromuscular problems.

Hepatic encephalopathy may develop slowly in patients with chronic liver disease and go undetected until the late stages. Symptoms develop rapidly in acute liver dysfunction. Four stages of development have been identified: prodromal, impending, stuporous, and comatose (Table 61-2). The patient's symptoms may gradually progress to coma or fluctuate among the four stages.

The exact mechanisms causing hepatic encephalopathy are not clearly understood but probably are the result of the shunting of portal venous blood into the central circulation so that the liver is bypassed. As a result, substances absorbed by the intestine are not broken down or detoxified and may lead to metabolic abnormalities, such as elevated serum ammonia and gamma-aminobutyric acid (GABA) (Kelso, 2008). Elevated serum ammonia results from the inability of the liver to detoxify protein by-products and is common in patients with hepatic encephalopathy. However, it is not a clear indicator of the presence of encephalopathy. Some patients may have major impairment without high elevations of serum ammonia, and elevations of ammonia can occur without evidence of encephalopathy.

Factors that may lead to hepatic encephalopathy in patients with cirrhosis include:

- High-protein diet
- Infections
- Hypovolemia (decreased fluid volume)
- Hypokalemia (decreased serum potassium)
- Constipation
- GI bleeding (causes a large protein load in the intestines)
- Drugs (e.g., hypnotics, opioids, sedatives, analgesics, diuretics, illicit drugs)

The prognosis depends on the severity of the underlying cause, the precipitating factors, and the degree of liver dysfunction.

Other Complications. The development of hepatorenal syndrome (HRS) indicates a poor prognosis for the patient with liver failure. It is often the cause of death in these patients. This syndrome is manifested by:

- A sudden decrease in urinary flow (<500 mL/24 hr) (oliguria)
- Elevated blood urea nitrogen (BUN) and creatinine levels with abnormally decreased urine sodium excretion
- Increased urine osmolarity

HRS often occurs after clinical deterioration from GI bleeding or the onset of hepatic encephalopathy. It may also complicate other liver diseases, including acute hepatitis and fulminant liver failure.

Patients with cirrhosis and ascites may develop acute *spontaneous bacterial peritonitis* (SBP). Those who are particularly susceptible are patients with very advanced liver disease. This may be the result of low concentrations of proteins; proteins normally provide some protection against bacteria.

The bacteria responsible for SBP are typically from the bowel and reach the ascitic fluid after migrating through the bowel wall and transversing the lymphatics. Clinical manifestations vary but may include fever, chills, and abdominal pain and tenderness. However, manifestations can also be minimal with only mild symptoms in the absence of fever. Worsening encephalopathy and increased jaundice may also be present without abdominal symptoms.

The diagnosis of SBP is made when a sample of ascitic fluid is obtained by paracentesis for cell counts and culture. An ascitic fluid leukocyte count of more than 250 polymorphonuclear (PMN) leukocytes may indicate the need for treatment.

Etiology and Genetic Risk

Hepatitis C is the leading cause of cirrhosis and liver failure in the United States. It is an infectious bloodborne illness that usually causes chronic disease. Inflammation caused by infection over time leads to progressive scarring of the liver. It usually takes decades for cirrhosis to develop, although alcohol use in combination with hepatitis C may speed the process.

Hepatitis B and hepatitis D are the most common causes of cirrhosis worldwide. Hepatitis B also causes inflammation and low-grade damage over decades that can ultimately lead to cirrhosis. Hepatitis D is another virus that infects the liver but only in people who already have hepatitis B (see discussion of hepatitis on p. 1305).

Cirrhosis can occur as a result of other factors. For example, *alcohol* has a direct toxic effect on the hepatocytes and causes liver inflammation (alcoholic hepatitis). The liver becomes enlarged, with cellular degeneration and infiltration by fat, leukocytes, and lymphocytes. Over time, the inflammatory process decreases and the destructive phase increases. Early scar formation is caused by fibroblast infiltration and collagen formation. Damage to the liver tissue progresses as malnutrition and repeated exposure to the alcohol continue. If alcohol is withheld, the fatty infiltration and inflammation is reversible. If alcohol abuse continues, widespread scar tissue formation and fibrosis infiltrate the liver as a result of cellular necrosis. The long-term use of illicit drugs, such as cocaine, has similar effects on the liver.

The amount of alcohol necessary to cause cirrhosis varies widely from person to person, and there are gender differences. In women, it may take as few as two to three drinks per day over a minimum of 10 years. In men, perhaps six drinks per day over the same time period may be needed to cause disease. Binge drinking can increase risk for hepatitis and fatty liver.

Biliary cirrhosis occurs as a result of obstruction of the bile duct, usually from gallbladder disease or an autoimmune form of the disease called *primary biliary cirrhosis (PBC)*. Patients with PBC typically have a genetic predisposition to the disease and a positive antimitochondrial antibody (AMA) (Lindor et al., 2009). Table 61-3 summarizes known causes of liver cirrhosis.

Incidence/Prevalence

The incidence of cirrhosis in the United States is not well known, but about 27,000 die from it each year. The disease affects twice as many men as women (Kelso, 2008).

TABLE 61-3	COMMON CAUSES OF CIRRHOSIS
• Alcoholic liver disease	• Drugs and chemical toxins
• Viral hepatitis	• Gallbladder disease
• Autoimmune hepatitis	• Metabolic/genetic causes
• Steatohepatitis (from fatty liver)	• Cardiovascular disease

PATIENT-CENTERED COLLABORATIVE CARE

ASSESSMENT

History

Obtain data from patients with suspected cirrhosis, including age, gender, and employment history, especially history of exposure to alcohol, drugs (prescribed and illicit), and chemical toxins. Keep in mind that all exposures are important regardless of how long ago they occurred. Determine whether there has ever been a needle stick injury. Sexual history and orientation may be important in determining an infectious cause for liver disease, because men having sex with men (MSM) are at high risk for hepatitis A, hepatitis B, and hepatitis C. People with hepatitis can develop cirrhosis (American Liver Foundation, 2011).

Inquire about whether there is a family history of alcoholism and/or liver disease. Ask the patient to describe his or her alcohol intake, including the amount consumed during a given period. Is there a history of illicit drug use, including oral, IV, and intranasal forms? Is there a history of tattoos? Has the patient been in the military or in prison? Is the patient a health care worker, firefighter, or police officer? For patients previously or currently in an alcohol or drug recovery program, how long have they been sober? This information is sensitive and often difficult for the patient to answer. Be sure to establish why you are asking these questions, and accept answers in a nonjudgmental manner. Provide privacy during the interview. For many people, the behaviors causing the liver disease occurred years before the onset of their current illness and they are regretful and often embarrassed.

Ask the patient about previous medical conditions, such as an episode of jaundice or acute viral hepatitis, biliary tract disorders (such as cholecystitis), viral infections, surgery, blood transfusions, autoimmune disorders, obesity, altered lipid profile, heart failure, respiratory disorders, or liver injury.

Physical Assessment/Clinical Manifestations

Because cirrhosis has a slow onset, many of the *early* manifestations are vague and nonspecific. Assess for:
- Fatigue
- Significant change in weight
- GI symptoms, such as anorexia and vomiting
- Abdominal pain and liver tenderness (both of which may be ignored by the patient)

Liver function problems are often found during a routine physical examination or when laboratory tests are completed for an unrelated illness or problem. The patient with *compensated cirrhosis* may be completely unaware that there is a liver problem. The first sign may present before the onset of symptoms when routine laboratory tests, presurgical evaluations, or life and health insurance assessments show abnormalities. These tests could indicate abnormal liver function or thrombocytopenia, requiring a more thorough diagnostic workup.

The development of late signs of *advanced cirrhosis* (also called "end-stage liver failure") usually causes the patient to seek medical treatment. GI bleeding, jaundice, ascites, and spontaneous bruising indicate poor liver function and complications of cirrhosis.

Thoroughly assess the patient with liver dysfunction or failure because it affects every body system (Fig. 61-1). The

NEUROLOGIC FINDINGS
Asterixis
Paresthesias of feet
Peripheral nerve degeneration
Portal-systemic encephalopathy
Reversal of sleep-wake pattern
Sensory disturbances

GASTROINTESTINAL (GI)
FINDINGS
Abdominal pain
Anorexia
Ascites
Clay-colored stools
Diarrhea
Esophageal varices
Fetor hepaticus
Gallstones
Gastritis
Gastrointestinal bleeding
Hemorrhoidal varices
Hepatomegaly
Hiatal hernia
Hypersplenism
Malnutrition
Nausea
Small nodular liver
Vomiting

RENAL FINDINGS
Hepatorenal syndrome
Increased urine bilirubin

ENDOCRINE FINDINGS
Increased aldosterone
Increased antidiuretic hormone
Increased circulating estrogens
Increased glucocorticoids
Gynecomastia

IMMUNE SYSTEM DISTURBANCES
Increased susceptibility to infection
Leukopenia

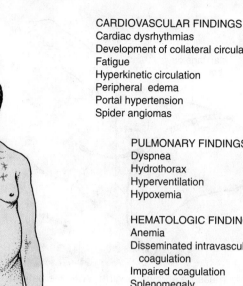

CARDIOVASCULAR FINDINGS
Cardiac dysrhythmias
Development of collateral circulation
Fatigue
Hyperkinetic circulation
Peripheral edema
Portal hypertension
Spider angiomas

PULMONARY FINDINGS
Dyspnea
Hydrothorax
Hyperventilation
Hypoxemia

HEMATOLOGIC FINDINGS
Anemia
Disseminated intravascular
   coagulation
Impaired coagulation
Splenomegaly
Thrombocytopenia

DERMATOLOGIC FINDINGS
Axillary and pubic hair changes
Caput medusae
Ecchymosis
Increased skin pigmentation
Jaundice
Palmar erythema
Pruritus
Spider angiomas

FLUID AND ELECTROLYTE
DISTURBANCES
Ascites
Decreased effective blood volume
Dilutional hyponatremia or
   hypernatremia
Hypocalcemia
Hypokalemia
Peripheral edema
Water retention

FIG. 61-1 The clinical picture of a patient with liver dysfunction. Manifestations vary according to the progression of the disease.

clinical picture and course vary from patient to patient depending on the severity of the disease. Assess for:
- Obvious yellowing of the skin (jaundice) and sclerae (icterus)
- Dry skin
- Rashes
- Purpuric lesions, such as petechiae (round, pinpoint, red-purple lesions) or ecchymosis (large purple, blue, or yellow bruises)
- Warm and bright red palms of the hands (palmar erythema)
- Vascular lesions with a red center and radiating branches, known as "spider angiomas" (telangiectases, spider nevi, or vascular spiders), on the nose, cheeks, upper thorax, and shoulders
- Ascites (abdominal fluid)
- Peripheral dependent edema of the extremities and sacrum
- Sicca syndrome (in patients with primary biliary cirrhosis [PBC]) (Lindor et al., 2009)

- Osteoporosis (especially in patients with PBC) (Lindor et al., 2009)
- Vitamin deficiency (especially fat-soluble vitamins A, D, E, and K)

Abdominal Assessment. *Massive* ascites can be detected as a distended abdomen with bulging flanks. The umbilicus may protrude, and dilated abdominal veins (caput medusae) may radiate from the umbilicus. Ascites can cause physical problems. For example, orthopnea and dyspnea from increased abdominal distention can interfere with lung expansion. The patient may have difficulty maintaining an erect body posture, and problems with balance may affect walking. Inspect and palpate for the presence of inguinal or umbilical hernias, which are likely to develop because of increased intra-abdominal pressure.

Minimal ascites is often more difficult to detect, especially in the obese patient. Advanced assessment techniques, such as the percussion test for shifting dullness and the presence of a fluid wave, may be performed by the health care provider.

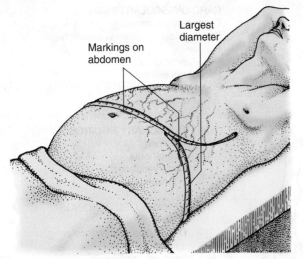

Largest diameter

Markings on abdomen

FIG. 61-2 How to measure abdominal girth. With the patient supine, bring the tape measure around the patient and take a measurement at the level of the umbilicus. Before removing the tape, mark the abdomen along the sides of the tape on the patient's flanks (sides) and midline to ensure that later measurements are taken in the same place.

When performing an assessment of the abdomen, keep in mind that hepatomegaly (liver enlargement) occurs in many cases of early cirrhosis. Splenomegaly is common in nonalcoholic causes of cirrhosis. As the liver deteriorates, it may become hard and small. The advanced practice nurse or other health care provider palpates the right upper quadrant for hepatomegaly below the costal (rib cage) border. It may also be assessed by percussing for dullness over the enlarged liver.

Measure the patient's abdominal girth to evaluate the progression of ascites (Fig. 61-2). To measure abdominal girth, the patient lies flat while the nurse or other examiner pulls a tape measure around the largest diameter (usually over the umbilicus) of the abdomen. The girth is measured at the end of exhalation. Mark the abdominal skin and flanks to ensure the same tape measure placement on subsequent readings. *Taking daily weights, however, is the most reliable indicator of fluid retention.*

Other Physical Assessment. Observe vomitus and stool for blood. This may be indicated by frank blood in the excrement or by a positive fecal occult blood test (FOBT) (Hema-Check, Hematest). Gastritis, stomach ulceration, or oozing esophageal varices may be responsible for the blood in the stool.

Note the presence of fetor hepaticus, which is the distinctive breath odor of chronic liver disease and hepatic encephalopathy and is characterized by a fruity or musty odor. Fetor hepaticus results from the inability of the damaged liver to metabolize and detoxify mercaptan, which is produced by bacterial breakdown of methionine, a sulfurous amino acid.

Amenorrhea (no menstrual period) may occur in women and men may exhibit testicular atrophy, gynecomastia (enlarged breasts), and impotence as a result of inactive hormones. Patients with problems of the hematologic system caused by hepatic failure may have bruising and petechiae (small, purplish hemorrhagic spots on the skin).

Continually assess the patient's neurologic function. Subtle changes in mental status and personality often progress to coma, a late complication of encephalopathy. Monitor for asterixis, a coarse tremor characterized by rapid, nonrhythmic extensions and flexions in the wrists and fingers.

Psychosocial Assessment

The patient with hepatic cirrhosis may undergo subtle or obvious personality, cognitive, and behavior changes, such as agitation. He or she may experience sleep pattern disturbances or may exhibit signs of emotional lability (fluctuations in emotions), euphoria (a very elevated mood), or depression. A psychosocial assessment identifies needs and helps guide care.

Repeated hospitalizations are common for patients with cirrhosis. It is a life-altering chronic disease, impacting not only the patient but also the immediate and extended family members and significant others. There are significant emotional, physical, and financial changes. Substance abuse may continue even as health worsens. It is important, whenever possible, to use resources available to these patients and their families. Collaborate with social workers, substance abuse counselors, and mental health/behavioral health care professionals as needed for patient assessment and management.

Laboratory Assessment

Laboratory study abnormalities are common in patients with liver disease (Table 61-4). Serum levels of aspartate aminotransferase (AST), alanine aminotransferase (ALT), and lactate dehydrogenase (LDH) may be elevated because these enzymes are released into the blood during hepatic inflammation. However, as the liver deteriorates, the hepatocytes may be unable to create an inflammatory response and the AST and ALT may be normal. ALT levels are more specific to the liver whereas AST can be found in muscle, kidney, brain, and heart. An AST/ALT ratio greater than 2 is usually found in alcoholic liver disease.

Increased alkaline phosphatase and gamma-glutamyl transpeptidase (GGT) levels are caused by biliary obstruction and therefore may increase in patients with cirrhosis (Kelso, 2008). However, alkaline phosphatase also increases when bone disease, such as osteoporosis, is present. Total serum bilirubin levels also rise. Indirect bilirubin levels increase in patients with cirrhosis because of the inability of the failing liver to excrete bilirubin. Therefore bilirubin is present in the urine (urobilinogen) in increased amounts. Fecal urobilinogen concentration is decreased in patients with biliary tract obstruction. These patients have light- or clay-colored stools.

Total serum protein and albumin levels are decreased in patients with severe or chronic liver disease as a result of decreased synthesis by the liver (Pagana & Pagana, 2010). Loss of osmotic "pull" proteins like albumin promotes the movement of intravascular fluid into the interstitial tissues (e.g., ascites). Prothrombin time/international normalized ratio (PT/INR) is prolonged because the liver decreases the production of prothrombin. The platelet count is low, resulting in a characteristic thrombocytopenia of cirrhosis. Anemia may be reflected by decreased red blood cell (RBC), hemoglobin, and hematocrit values. The white blood cell (WBC) count may also be decreased. Ammonia levels are usually elevated in patients with advanced liver disease. Serum creatinine may be elevated in patients with deteriorating kidney

TABLE 61-4 ASSESSMENT OF ABNORMAL LABORATORY FINDINGS IN LIVER DISEASE

ABNORMAL FINDING	SIGNIFICANCE
Serum Enzymes	
Elevated serum aspartate aminotransferase (AST)	Hepatic cell destruction, hepatitis (most specific indicator)
Elevated serum alanine aminotransferase (ALT)	Hepatic cell destruction, hepatitis
Elevated lactate dehydrogenase (LDH)	Hepatic cell destruction
Elevated serum alkaline phosphatase	Obstructive jaundice, hepatic metastasis
Bilirubin	
Elevated serum total bilirubin	Hepatic cell disease
Elevated serum direct conjugated bilirubin	Hepatitis, liver metastasis
Elevated serum indirect unconjugated bilirubin	Cirrhosis
Elevated urine bilirubin	Hepatocellular obstruction, viral or toxic liver disease
Elevated urine urobilinogen	Hepatic dysfunction
Decreased fecal urobilinogen	Obstructive liver disease
Serum Proteins	
Increased serum total protein	Acute liver disease
Decreased serum total protein	Chronic liver disease
Decreased serum albumin	Severe liver disease
Elevated serum globulin	Immune response to liver disease
Other Tests	
Elevated serum ammonia	Advanced liver disease or portal-systemic encephalopathy (PSE)
Prolonged prothrombin time (PT) or international normalized ratio (INR)	Hepatic cell damage and decreased synthesis of prothrombin

function. Dilutional hyponatremia (low serum sodium) may occur in patients with ascites.

Patients with primary biliary cirrhosis, an autoimmune disease, usually have high disease-specific AMA and antinuclear antibody (ANA) titers and elevated levels of immunoglobulin M (IgM) (Lindor et al., 2009).

Imaging Assessment

Plain x-rays of the abdomen may show hepatomegaly, splenomegaly, or massive ascites. A computed tomography (CT) scan may be requested.

Magnetic resonance imaging (MRI) is another test used to diagnose the patient with liver disease. It can reveal mass lesions, giving additional specific information. This information is helpful in determining whether the condition is malignant or benign.

Other Diagnostic Assessment

Ultrasound (US) of the liver is often the first assessment for a person with suspected liver disease to detect ascites, hepatomegaly, and splenomegaly. It can also determine the presence of biliary stones or biliary duct obstruction. Liver US is useful

in detecting portal vein thrombosis and evaluating whether the direction of portal blood flow is normal.

Some patients being assessed for liver disease require biopsies to determine the exact pathology and the extent of disease progression. This procedure can be problematic because a large number of patients are at risk for bleeding. Even a **percutaneous** (through the skin) biopsy can pose a significant risk to the patient. To minimize this risk, an interventional radiologist can perform a liver biopsy using a long sheath through a jugular vein that then is threaded into the hepatic vein and liver. A tissue sample is obtained for microscopic evaluation. If a biopsy procedure is not possible, a radioisotope liver scan may be used to identify cirrhosis or other diffuse disease.

The physician may request *arteriography* if US is not conclusive in finding portal vein thrombosis. To evaluate the portal vein and its branches, a portal venogram may be performed instead, by passing a catheter into the liver and into the portal vein. This procedure is described on p. 1302 in the Transjugular Intrahepatic Portal-Systemic Shunt section.

The physician may perform an **esophagogastroduodenoscopy (EGD)** to directly visualize the upper GI tract and to detect the presence of bleeding or oozing esophageal varices, stomach irritation and ulceration, or duodenal ulceration and bleeding. EGD is performed by introducing a flexible fiberoptic endoscope into the mouth, esophagus, and stomach while the patient is under moderate sedation. A camera attached to the scope permits direct visualization of the mucosal lining of the upper GI tract. An **endoscopic retrograde cholangiopancreatography (ERCP)** uses the endoscope to inject contrast material via the sphincter of Oddi to view the biliary tract and allow for stone removals, sphincterotomies, biopsies, and stent placements if required. These procedures are described in more detail in Chapter 55.

? NCLEX EXAMINATION CHALLENGE

Physiological Integrity

When caring for a client with advanced cirrhosis, what laboratory assessment findings will the nurse expect? **Select all that apply.**
A. Increased serum albumin
B. Decreased bilirubin in the urine
C. Increased alanine aminotransferase
D. Increased alkaline phosphatase
E. Decreased bilirubin in the stool
F. Increased platelets

ANALYSIS

The priority problems for patients with cirrhosis include:
1. Excess Fluid Volume related to third spacing of abdominal and peripheral fluid
2. Potential for hemorrhage due to portal hypertension
3. Potential for hepatic encephalopathy due to shunting of portal venous blood and/or increased serum ammonia levels

PLANNING AND IMPLEMENTATION

Managing Fluid Volume

Planning: Expected Outcomes. The patient with cirrhosis is expected to have less excess fluid volume as evidenced by decreased ascites and peripheral edema and adequate circulatory volume. If ascites continues, the patient will not have respiratory distress and will manage ascites by adhering to the collaborative plan of care (see the Concept Map for liver failure due to cirrhosis on p. 1301).

Interventions. Fluid accumulations are minimal during the early stages of ascites. Therefore interventions are aimed at preventing the accumulation of additional fluid and moving the existing fluid collection. Nonsurgical treatment measures are used to treat ascites in most cases.

Supportive measures to control abdominal ascites include nutrition therapy, drug therapy, paracentesis, and respiratory support. The patient's fluid and electrolyte status is also carefully monitored. If the patient is jaundiced, he or she will likely scratch the skin because the excess bilirubin products cause irritation and pruritus (itching).

! NURSING SAFETY PRIORITY

Action Alert

For skin irritation and pruritus associated with jaundice, teach the patient to use cool rather than warm water on the skin and to not use an excessive amount of soap. Teach unlicensed assistive personnel to use lotion to soothe the skin. Assess for open skin areas from scratching, which could become infected.

Nutrition Therapy. The health care provider usually places the patient with abdominal ascites on a low-sodium diet as an initial means of controlling fluid accumulation in the abdominal cavity. The amount of daily sodium (Na^+) intake restriction varies, but a 1- to 2-gram (2000 mg) Na^+ restriction may be tried first. In collaboration with the dietitian, explain the purpose of the restriction and advise the patient and family to read the sodium content labels on all food and beverages. Table salt should be completely excluded. Low-sodium diets may be distasteful, so suggest alternative flavoring additives such as lemon, vinegar, parsley, oregano, and pepper. Remind the patient that seasoned and salty food is an acquired taste; in time, he or she will become used to the decrease in dietary sodium.

In general, patients with late-stage cirrhosis are malnourished and have multiple dietary deficiencies. Vitamin supplements such as thiamine (due to alcohol withdrawal), folate, and multivitamin preparations are typically added to the IV fluids because the liver cannot store vitamins. For patients with biliary cirrhosis, bile may not be available for fat-soluble vitamin transport and absorption. Oral vitamins are prescribed when IV fluid administration is discontinued.

Drug Therapy. The health care provider usually prescribes a *diuretic* to reduce fluid accumulation and to prevent cardiac and respiratory problems. Monitor the effect of diuretic therapy by weighing the patient daily, measuring daily intake and output, measuring abdominal girth, documenting peripheral edema, and assessing electrolyte levels. Serious electrolyte imbalances, such as hypokalemia (decreased potassium) and hyponatremia (decreased sodium), may occur with loop diuretic therapy. Depending on the diuretic selected, the provider may prescribe an oral or IV potassium supplement. Some clinicians prescribe a combination of furosemide (Lasix) and spironolactone (Aldactone) as a combination diuretic therapy for the treatment of ascites. Because these drugs work differently, they are used for maintenance of sodium and potassium balance. For example, furosemide causes potassium loss, whereas spironolactone conserves it in the body.

CHART 61-1 BEST PRACTICE FOR PATIENT SAFETY & QUALITY CARE

The Patient with Paracentesis

- Explain the procedure, and answer patient questions.
- Obtain vital signs, including weight.
- *Ask the patient to void before the procedure to prevent injury to the bladder!*
- Position the patient in bed with the head of the bed elevated.
- Monitor vital signs per protocol or physician's request.
- Measure the drainage, and record accurately.
- Describe the collected fluid.
- Label and send the fluid for laboratory analysis; document in the patient record that specimens were sent.
- After the physician removes the catheter, apply a dressing to the site; assess for leakage.
- Maintain bedrest per protocol.
- Weigh the patient after the paracentesis; document in the patient record weight both before and after paracentesis.

All patients with ascites have the potential to develop spontaneous bacterial peritonitis (SBP) from bacteria in the collected ascitic fluid. In some patients, mild symptoms such as low-grade fever and loss of appetite occur. In others, there may be abdominal pain, fever, and change in mental status. When performing an abdominal assessment, listen for bowel sounds and assess for abdominal wall rigidity. Send a sample of ascitic fluid for a culture before drug therapy begins. Quinolones such as norfloxacin (Noroxin) are the drugs of choice for SBP. If the patient is allergic to this class of *antibiotics*, combination antibiotics like trimethoprim-sulfamethoxazole (Bactrim) are given.

Paracentesis. For some patients, abdominal paracentesis may be needed. Nursing implications associated with this procedure are described in Chart 61-1. The procedure is performed at the bedside, in an interventional radiology department, or in an ambulatory care setting. The physician inserts a trocar catheter or drain into the abdomen to remove the ascitic fluid from the peritoneal cavity. This procedure is done using ultrasound for added safety. In some situations, a short-term ascites drain catheter may be placed while the patient is awaiting surgical intervention, or new tunneled ascites drains (e.g., PleurX drains) can allow a patient or family caregiver to drain ascites at home.

If SBP is suspected, a sample of fluid is withdrawn and sent for cell count and culture. If the patient has symptoms of infection, the physician may prescribe antibiotics while awaiting the culture results.

Respiratory Support. Excessive ascitic fluid volume may cause the patient to have respiratory problems. He or she may develop *hepatopulmonary syndrome*. Dyspnea develops as a

---

! NURSING SAFETY PRIORITY

Action Alert

For the patient with hepatopulmonary syndrome, monitor his or her oxygen saturation with pulse oximetry. If needed, apply oxygen therapy to ease breathing. Elevate the head of the bed to at least 30 degrees or as high as the patient wants to improve breathing. This position, with his or her feet elevated to decrease dependent ankle edema, often relieves dyspnea. Weigh the patient daily, or delegate and supervise this activity.

Concept Map: Cirrhosis

INTERVENTIONS

1 Physical Assessment/Clinical Manifestations

Assess for jaundice and icterus; dry skin; rashes; petechiae; ecchymosis; palmar erythema; spider angiomas on the nose, cheeks, upper thorax, and shoulders; ascites; peripheral dependent edema of the extremities and sacrum.
Assesses the affect of liver dysfunction on the body systems; degree of effect varies depending on the severity of the disease.

2 Nursing Safety Priority: Action Alert

Monitor for and manage potentially life-threatening complications of cirrhosis with ascites, esophageal varices, coagulation defects, jaundice, encephalopathy, hepatic coma, hepatorenal syndrome, spontaneous bacterial peritonitis.
Prevents hemorrhage and death.

3 Lab findings

Monitor lab values closely, especially hematocrit, hemoglobin, and platelets. Administer blood products as indicated.
Checks for destroyed platelets caused by splenomegaly (which causes thrombocytopenia and increased risk for bleeding) and blood loss (causes decreased hematocrit and hemoglobin).

4 Fluid Status

Monitor fluid status (I&O and daily weight).
Tracks the hypovolemia and edema that can develop as a result of ascites from the "third spacing," which occurs as the fluid moves from the vascular system into the abdomen at the same time.

5 Abdominal Girth

Measure and record size of abdominal girth.
Determines need for parencentesis and/or drug therapy. Portal hypertension can result in ascites, esophageal varices, caput medusae, and hemorrhoids.

6 Sodium

Teach the patient about decreased sodium in the diet (1 to 2 g). Review how to read nutritional labels. Avoid table salt; use lemon, vinegar, parsley, oregano, and pepper instead. Remind the patient that he will get used to the taste of a low-sodium diet.
Low-sodium diet controls fluid accumulation in the abdominal cavity.

7 Activity

Decrease activity that increases abdominal pressure, such as heavy lifting or vigorous physical exercise, chest trauma, or dry, hard food in the esophagus.
Such increased activity can cause bleeding and increases the likelihood of a variceal bleed.

8 Nursing Safety Priority: Action Alert

Teach the patient to use cool or warm water on the skin and not to use too much soap. Teach UAP to use lotion. Assess for open areas from scratching.
Soothes and protects skin integrity; scratched areas can become infected.

9 Level of Consciousness

Monitor for decreased level of consciousness.
Decreased level of consciousness can occur before any bleeding is observed—either hematemesis or melena. Variceal bleeding can occur spontaneously with no precipitating factors.

Concept Map by Deanne A. Blach, MSN, RN

EXPECTED OUTCOMES
- Free of bleeding episodes or immediate management if bleeding occurs.
- Decreased or no LOC or ascites.
- Lab values within normal limits.
- No development of encephalopathy or immediate management if it occurs.
- Highest quality of life possible.
- Abstain successfully from alcohol or drugs.

Planning

HISTORY

Ray Crandall, a 67-year-old farm hand, has a 30-year history of heavy alcohol use. He arrives in the ED with hematemesis and melena.

CIRRHOSIS PATHOPHYSIOLOGY

A slow, progressive, irreversible destruction of hepatocytes; scarring of the liver occurs, reducing blood flow through the liver. Digestion, nutrition, and metabolism are severely affected. Eventually results in end-stage liver failure.

Perform and Interpret Physical Assessment

OBJECTIVE DATA

Mr. Crandall states he feels light-headed and dizzy when he stands up. VS on admission: BP, 100/60 mm Hg; HR, 116; T, 100.8° F; RR, 24; pulse ox, 92%; HGB, 11g/dL; HCT, 33%. Platelets, 100,000. Ascites, caput medusa, and hemorrhoids present.

result of increased intra-abdominal pressure, which limits thoracic expansion and diaphragmatic excursion. Auscultate lungs every 4 to 8 hours for crackles that could indicate pulmonary complications, depending on the patient's overall condition.

Fluid and electrolyte imbalances are common as a result of the disease or treatment. Laboratory tests, such as blood urea nitrogen (BUN), serum protein, hematocrit, and electrolytes, help determine fluid and electrolyte status. An elevated BUN, decreased serum proteins, and increased hematocrit may indicate hypovolemia.

If medical management fails to control ascites, the physician may choose to divert ascites into the venous system by creating a shunt. Patients with ascites are poor surgical risks. The transjugular intrahepatic portal-systemic shunt (TIPS) is a nonsurgical procedure that is used to control long-term ascites and to reduce variceal bleeding. This procedure is described in the discussion of Interventions in the Preventing or Managing Hemorrhage section that follows.

Preventing or Managing Hemorrhage

Planning: Expected Outcomes. The patient is expected to be free of bleeding episodes. However, if he or she has a hemorrhage, it is expected to be controlled by prompt, evidence-based interdisciplinary interventions. Esophageal variceal bleeds are the most common type of upper GI bleeding.

Interventions. All patients with cirrhosis should be screened for esophageal varices by endoscopy to detect them early *before they bleed.* If patients have varices, they are placed on preventive therapy. If acute bleeding occurs, early interventions are used to manage it. *Because massive esophageal bleeding can cause rapid blood loss, emergency interventions are needed.*

Drug Therapy. The role of early drug therapy is to *prevent* bleeding and infection in patients who have varices. A nonselective *beta-blocking agent* such as propranolol (Inderal) is usually prescribed to prevent bleeding. By decreasing heart rate and the hepatic venous pressure gradient, the chance of bleeding may be reduced.

Up to 20% of cirrhotic patients who are admitted to the hospital due to upper GI bleeding have bacterial infections, and even more patients develop health care–associated infections, usually urinary tract infections or pneumonia. Infection is one of the most common indicators that patients will have an acute variceal bleed (AVB). Therefore cirrhotic patients with GI bleeding should receive *antibiotics* on admission to the hospital. The recommended antibiotic is oral norfloxacin (Noroxin) or ciprofloxacin (Cipro). IV ceftriaxone (Cefizox) may be more effective for some patients (Augustin et al., 2010).

If bleeding occurs, the health care team intervenes quickly to control it by combining vasoactive drugs with endoscopic

! NURSING SAFETY PRIORITY

Drug Alert

Both terlipressin and somatostatin can cause ischemic complications and serious dysrhythmias. Observe patients for significant changes in cardiac rhythm, apical pulse rate, and blood pressure. Monitor for clinical manifestations of a stroke, and report any changes immediately to the physician. The patient is managed in the critical care setting.

therapies. *Vasoactive drugs* reduce portal pressure. Research shows that IV terlipressin (a synthetic vasopressin) and natural somatostatin are the most effective (Augustin et al., 2010). Octreotide, a synthetic somatostatin, and vasopressin may be used as a last resort because they have multiple side effects.

Endoscopic Therapies. Endoscopic therapies include ligation of the bleeding veins or sclerotherapy. Both procedures have been very effective in controlling bleeding and improving patient survival rates. Esophageal varices may be managed with endoscopic variceal ligation (EVL) (banding). This procedure involves the application of small "O" bands around the base of the varices to decrease the blood supply to the varices. The patient is unaware of the bands, and they cause no discomfort.

Endoscopic sclerotherapy (EST), also called injection sclerotherapy, may be done to stop bleeding. The varices are injected with a sclerosing agent via a catheter. This procedure is associated with complications such as mucosal ulceration, which could result in further bleeding.

Rescue Therapies. If rebleeding occurs, rescue therapies are used. These procedures include a second endoscopic procedure, balloon tamponade and esophageal stents, and shunting procedures. Short-term esophagogastric balloon tamponade using a Minnesota or Sengstaken-Blakemore tube with esophageal stents is a very effective way to control bleeding. However, the procedure can cause potentially life-threatening complications, such as aspiration, asphyxia, and esophageal perforation (Augustin et al., 2010). Similar to a nasogastric tube, the tube is placed through the nose and into the stomach. An attached balloon is inflated to apply pressure to the bleeding variceal area. Before this tamponade, the patient is usually intubated and placed on a mechanical ventilator to protect the airway (Kelso, 2008). This therapy is used if the patient is not able to have a second endoscopy or TIPS procedure.

Transjugular Intrahepatic Portal-Systemic Shunt. The transjugular intrahepatic portal-systemic shunt (TIPS) is a nonsurgical procedure performed in interventional radiology departments. This procedure is used for patients who have not responded to other modalities for hemorrhage or long-term ascites. If time permits, patients have a Doppler ultrasound to assess vein anatomy and patency. The patient receives heavy IV sedation or general anesthesia for this procedure. The radiologist places a large sheath through the jugular vein. A needle is guided through the sheath and pushed through the liver into the portal vein. A balloon enlarges this tract, and a stent keeps it open. Most patients also have a Doppler ultrasound study of the liver after the TIPS procedure to record the blood flow through the shunt.

Serious complications of TIPS are not common. Patients are usually discharged in 1 or 2 days and are followed up with ultrasounds for the first year after the shunt is placed. Some of them require re-opening at least once during the first year as an ambulatory care procedure.

Other Interventions. Depending on the procedure done to control esophageal bleeding, patients usually have a nasogastric tube (NGT) inserted to detect any new bleeding episodes. Patients often receive packed red blood cells, fresh frozen plasma, dextran, albumin, and platelets through large-bore IV catheters.

Monitor vital signs every hour, and check coagulation studies, including prothrombin time (PT), partial thromboplastin time (PTT), platelet count, and international normalized ratio (INR).

Additional interventions for upper GI bleeding are discussed in Chapter 58. All patients with GI bleeding from esophageal varices should be considered for liver transplantation to prevent further bleeding episodes.

Preventing or Managing Hepatic Encephalopathy

Planning: Expected Outcomes. The patient is expected to be free of encephalopathy. However, if it occurs, it is expected that the interdisciplinary team will intervene early to prevent further health problems or death.

Interventions. The mechanisms that cause hepatic encephalopathy are not completely clear, but ammonia probably plays a significant role. The poorly functioning liver cannot convert ammonia and other by-products of protein metabolism to a less toxic form. They are carried by the circulatory system to the brain, where they affect cerebral function. The aim of management is to stop or slow this process.

Because ammonia is formed in the GI tract by the action of bacteria on protein, nonsurgical treatment measures to decrease ammonia production include dietary limitations and drug therapy to reduce bacterial breakdown. Collaborate with the dietitian, pharmacist, and physician to plan and implement these interventions.

Nutrition Therapy. Patients with cirrhosis have increased nutritional requirements—high-carbohydrate, moderate-fat, and high-protein foods. However, the diet may be changed for those who have elevated serum ammonia levels with signs of encephalopathy. Patients should have a moderate amount of protein and fat foods and simple carbohydrates. Strict protein restrictions are not required because patients need protein for healing. In collaboration with the dietitian, be sure to include family members or significant others in nutrition counseling. The patient is often weak and unable to remember complicated guidelines. Brief, simple directions regarding dietary dos and don'ts are recommended. Keep in mind any financial, cultural, or personal preferences when discussing food choices, including the patient's food allergies.

When a patient with cirrhosis has GI bleeding, it can result in the formation of increased amounts of ammonia as intestinal bacteria attempt to metabolize the blood cells. GI bleeding may lead to hepatic coma.

Drug Therapy. Drugs are used sparingly because they are difficult for the failing liver to metabolize. In particular, opioid analgesics, sedatives, and barbiturates should be restricted, especially for the patient with a history of encephalopathy.

Several types of drugs, however, may eliminate or reduce ammonia levels in the body. These include lactulose (e.g., Evalose, Heptalac) or lactitol and nonabsorbable antibiotics. However, these drugs are often not effective.

The health care provider may prescribe *lactulose* (or lactitol) to promote the excretion of ammonia in the stool. This drug is a viscous, sticky, sweet-tasting liquid that is given either orally or by NG tube. The purpose is to obtain a laxative effect. Cleansing the bowels may rid the intestinal tract of the toxins that contribute to encephalopathy. It works by increasing osmotic pressure to draw fluid into the colon and prevents absorption of ammonia in the colon. The drug may be prescribed to the patient who has manifested signs of encephalopathy, regardless of the stage. The desired effect of the drug is production of two or three soft stools per day and a decrease in patient confusion caused by this complication.

Observe for response to lactulose. The patient may report intestinal bloating and cramping. Serum ammonia levels may be monitored but do not always correlate with symptoms. Hypokalemia and dehydration may result from excessive stools. Remind unlicensed nursing personnel to help the patient with skin care if needed to prevent breakdown caused by excessive stools.

Several *nonabsorbable antibiotics* may be given if lactulose does not help the patient meet the desired outcome or if he or she cannot tolerate the drug. These drugs should not be given together. Older adults can become weak and dehydrated from having multiple stools. Neomycin sulfate (Mycifradin), a broad-spectrum antibiotic, may be given to act as an intestinal antiseptic. It destroys the normal flora in the bowel, diminishing protein breakdown and decreasing the rate of ammonia production. Maintenance doses of neomycin are given orally but may also be administered as a retention enema. Long-term use has the potential for kidney toxicity and therefore is not commonly used. It cannot be used for patients with existing kidney disease.

Metronidazole (Flagyl, Novonidazole ✦) is another broad-spectrum antibiotic with similar action to neomycin, but it has less potential for renal toxicity. However, it should also be used for a short period of time and is therefore not commonly used. Rifaximin (Xifaxan) seems to be the most effective and safest for long-term use.

Frequently assess for changes in level of consciousness and orientation. Check for asterixis (liver flap) and fetor hepaticus (liver breath). These signs suggest worsening encephalopathy. Thiamine supplements and benzodiazepines may be needed if the patient is at risk for alcohol withdrawal.

Community-Based Care

If the patient with late-stage cirrhosis survives life-threatening complications, he or she is usually discharged to the home or to a long-term care facility after treatment measures have managed the acute medical problems. A home care referral may be needed if the patient is discharged to the home. These chronically ill patients are often readmitted multiple times, and community-based care is aimed at preventing rehospitalization. Patients with end-stage disease may benefit from hospice care. Collaborate with the case manager (CM) or other discharge planner to coordinate interdisciplinary continuing care.

Home Care Management

In collaboration with the patient, family, and CM, assess physical adaptations needed to prepare the patient's home for recovery. Referrals for physical therapy, nutrition therapy, and transportation for physician and laboratory follow-up may be needed. The patient's rest area needs to be close to a bathroom because diuretic and/or lactulose therapy increases the frequency of urination and stools. If the patient has difficulty reaching the toilet, additional equipment (e.g., bedside commode) is necessary. Special, adult-size incontinence pads or briefs may be helpful if the patient has an altered mental status and has incontinence. If the patient has shortness of breath from massive ascites, elevating the head of the bed and maintaining the patient in a semi-Fowler's to high Fowler's

---

CHART 61-2   PATIENT AND FAMILY EDUCATION: PREPARING FOR SELF-MANAGEMENT

Cirrhosis

Nutrition Therapy
- Consume a diet that adheres to the guidelines set by your physician, nurse, or dietitian.
- If you have excessive fluid in your abdomen, follow the low-sodium diet prescribed for you.
- Eat small, frequent meals that are nutritionally well balanced.
- Include in your diet daily supplemental liquids (e.g., Ensure or Ensure Plus) and a multivitamin.

Drug Therapy
- Take the diuretics or preventive beta blocker prescribed for you. If you experience muscle weakness, irregular heartbeat, or light-headedness, contact your health care provider right away.
- Take the medication prescribed for you that helps prevent gastro-intestinal bleeding.
- Take the lactulose syrup as prescribed to maintain two or three bowel movements every day.
- Do *not* take any other medication (prescribed or over the counter) unless specifically prescribed by your health care provider.

Alcohol Abstinence
- Do not consume any alcohol.
- Seek support services for help if needed.

position may help alleviate respiratory distress. Alternatively, a reclining chair with a foot elevator may be used.

Teaching for Self-Management

The patient is discharged to the home setting with an individualized teaching plan (Chart 61-2) that includes nutrition therapy, drug therapy, and alcohol abstinence, if needed. The patient who has a tunneled ascites drain (e.g., PleurX drain) will need teaching about how to access the drain and remove excess fluid. If needed, family teaching is also required.

In collaboration with the dietitian and in keeping with the patient's financial, cultural, and personal food preferences, provide information on eating a well-balanced diet. The patient with encephalopathy often finds that small, frequent meals are best tolerated. If the patient's nutritional intake or albumin/pre-albumin is decreased after discharge, multivitamin supplements and supplemental liquid feedings (e.g., Ensure, Boost) are usually needed. Teach patients to avoid excessive vitamins and minerals that can be toxic to the liver, such as fat-soluble vitamins, excessive iron supplements, and niacin. Remind patients to check labels for these substances before taking any vitamin supplement.

The patient is often discharged while receiving diuretics. Provide instructions regarding the health care provider's prescription for the diuretic. Teach about side effects of therapy, such as hypokalemia. The patient may need to take a potassium supplement if he or she is taking a diuretic that is not potassium-sparing.

If the patient has had problems with bleeding from gastric ulcers, the provider may prescribe an H_2-receptor antagonist agent or proton pump inhibitor to reduce acid reflux (see Chapter 57). Patients who have had episodes of spontaneous bacterial peritonitis (SBP) may be on a daily maintenance antibiotic. Because some patients may have alienated relatives

over the years because of substance abuse, it may be necessary to help them identify a friend, neighbor, or person in their recovery group for support.

Teach family members about how to recognize signs of encephalopathy and to contact the health care provider if these signs develop. Reinforce that constipation, bleeding, and infections can increase the risk for encephalopathy.

Advise the patient to avoid all over-the-counter drugs, especially NSAIDs and hepatic toxic herbs, vitamins, and minerals. Reinforce the need to keep appointments for follow-up medical care. Remind the patient and family to notify the physician immediately if any GI bleeding (overt bleeding or melena) is noted so that re-evaluation can begin quickly.

! NURSING SAFETY PRIORITY

Action Alert

One of the most important aspects of ongoing care for the patient with cirrhosis is to stress the need to avoid alcohol and illicit drugs. By avoiding alcohol and drugs, the patient may:
- *Prevent further fibrosis of the liver from scarring*
- *Allow the liver to heal and regenerate*
- *Prevent gastric and esophageal irritation*
- *Reduce the incidence of bleeding*
- *Prevent other life-threatening complications*

Health Care Resources

The patient with chronic cirrhosis may require a home care nurse for several visits after hospital discharge. The home care nurse can monitor the effectiveness of treatment in controlling ascites. The encephalopathic patient may need to be monitored for adherence to drug therapy and alcohol abstinence, if appropriate. Individual and group therapy sessions may be arranged to assist patients in dealing with alcohol abstinence if they are too ill to attend a formal treatment program. If needed, refer the patient and family to self-help groups, such as Alcoholics Anonymous and Al-Anon.

The patient with cirrhosis may also desire spiritual support. Finances are frequently a problem for the chronically ill patient and family; social support and community services need to be identified. The American Liver Foundation (www.liverfoundation.org) and American Gastroenterological Association (www.gastro.org) are excellent sources for more information about liver disease.

For patients who are not candidates for liver transplantation, address end-of-life issues. Discuss options such as hospice care with patients and their families. Be aware that they will go through a grieving process and will perhaps be in denial or very angry (see Chapter 9).

EVALUATION: OUTCOMES

Evaluate the care of the patient with cirrhosis based on the identified priority patient problems. The expected outcomes include that the patient will:
- Have a decrease in or have no ascites
- Have electrolytes within normal limits (WNL)
- Not have hemorrhage or will be managed immediately if bleeding occurs
- Not develop encephalopathy or will be managed immediately if it occurs

- Have the highest quality of life possible
- Successfully abstain from alcohol or drugs (if disease is caused by these substances)

HEPATITIS

Pathophysiology

Hepatitis is the widespread inflammation of liver cells. *Viral* hepatitis is the most common type and can be either acute or chronic. Less common types of hepatitis are caused by chemicals, drugs, and some herbs. This section discusses hepatitis caused by a virus. Viral hepatitis results from an infection caused by one of five major categories of viruses:

- Hepatitis A virus (HAV)
- Hepatitis B virus (HBV)
- Hepatitis C virus (HCV)
- Hepatitis D virus (HDV)
- Hepatitis E virus (HEV)

Some cases of viral hepatitis are not any of these viruses. These patients have non–A-E hepatitis.

Liver injury with inflammation can develop after exposure to a number of drugs and chemicals by inhalation, ingestion, or parenteral (IV) administration. Toxic and drug-induced hepatitis can result from exposure to hepatotoxins (e.g., industrial toxins, alcohol, and drugs). Hepatitis may also occur as a secondary infection during the course of infections with other viruses, such as Epstein-Barr, herpes simplex, varicella-zoster, and cytomegalovirus.

After the liver has been exposed to any causative agent (e.g., a virus), it becomes enlarged and congested with inflammatory cells, lymphocytes, and fluid, resulting in right upper quadrant pain and discomfort. As the disease progresses, the liver's normal lobular pattern becomes distorted as a result of widespread inflammation, necrosis, and hepatocellular regeneration. This distortion increases pressure within the portal circulation, interfering with the blood flow into the hepatic lobules. Edema of the liver's bile channels results in obstructive jaundice (yellowing of the skin).

Classification of Hepatitis and Etiologies

The five major types of acute viral hepatitis vary by mode of transmission, manner of onset, and incubation periods. Hepatitis cases must be reported to the local public health department, which then notifies the Centers for Disease Control and Prevention (CDC).

Hepatitis A. The causative agent of hepatitis A, hepatitis A virus (HAV), is a ribonucleic acid (RNA) virus of the enterovirus family. *It is a hardy virus and survives on human hands.* The virus is resistant to detergents and acids but is destroyed by chlorine (bleach) and extremely high temperatures.

TABLE 61-5 **EXAMPLES OF EXTRAHEPATIC MANIFESTATIONS OF HEPATITIS A**

Neurologic Findings
- Post–viral encephalitis
- Guillain-Barré syndrome
- Transverse myelitis

Hematologic Findings
- Aplastic anemia
- Autoimmune hemolysis
- Anemia

Renal Findings
- Acute tubular necrosis (ATN)
- Nephrotic syndrome

Gastrointestinal Findings
- Pancreatitis
- Acalculous cholecystitis

Other Findings
- Reactive arthritis
- Cutaneous vasculitis

HAV usually has a mild course similar to that of a typical flu-like infection and often goes unrecognized. It is spread most often by the fecal-oral route by fecal contamination either from person-to-person contact (e.g., oral-anal sexual activity) or by consuming contaminated food or water. Common sources of infection include shellfish caught in contaminated water and food contaminated by food handlers infected with HAV. The incubation period of hepatitis A is usually 15 to 50 days, with a peak of 25 to 30 days. The disease is usually not life threatening, but its course may be more severe in people older than 40 years and those with pre-existing liver disease such as hepatitis C.

In a small percentage of HAV cases, severe illness with extrahepatic manifestations can occur (Table 61-5). Advanced age and conditions such as chronic liver disease may cause widespread damage that requires a liver transplant. In some cases, death may occur from HAV.

The incidence of hepatitis A is particularly high in non-affluent countries in which sanitation is poor. However, over 35,000 cases are diagnosed each year in the United States (American Liver Foundation, 2010). Some adults have hepatitis A and do not know it. The course is similar to that of a GI illness, and the disease and recovery are usually uneventful.

Hepatitis B. The hepatitis B virus (HBV) is not transmitted like HAV. It is a double-shelled particle containing DNA composed of a core antigen (HBcAg), a surface antigen (HBsAg), and another antigen found within the core (HBeAg) that circulates in the blood. HBV may be spread through these common modes of transmission (Lok & McMahon, 2009):

- Unprotected sexual intercourse with an infected partner
- Sharing needles
- Accidental needle sticks or injuries from sharp instruments primarily in health care workers (low incidence)
- Blood transfusions (that have not been screened for the virus, before 1992)
- Hemodialysis
- Maternal-fetal route (more common in Asia)
- Close person-to-person contact by open cuts and sores

In addition, patients who are immunosuppressed either by disease or drug therapy are more likely to develop hepatitis B.

The clinical course of hepatitis B may be varied. Symptoms usually occur within 25 to 180 days of exposure and include:

- Anorexia, nausea, and vomiting
- Fever
- Fatigue
- Right upper quadrant pain
- Dark urine with light stool
- Joint pain
- Jaundice

Blood tests confirm the disease, although many people with hepatitis B have no symptoms.

Most adults who get hepatitis B recover, clear the virus from their body, and develop immunity. However, a small percentage of people do not develop immunity and become carriers. Hepatitis carriers can infect others even though they are not sick and have no obvious signs of hepatitis B. Chronic carriers are at high risk for cirrhosis and liver cancer. Because of the high number of newcomers from endemic areas, the incidence of hepatitis B has increased in the United States.

Hepatitis C. The causative virus of hepatitis C (HCV) is an enveloped, single-stranded RNA virus. Transmission is blood to blood. The rate of sexual transmission is very low in a single-couple relationship but increases with multiple sex partners.

HCV is spread most commonly by:

- Illicit IV drug needle sharing (highest incidence)
- Blood, blood products, or organ transplants received before 1992
- Needle stick injury with HCV-contaminated blood (health care workers at high risk)
- Unsanitary tattoo equipment
- Sharing of intranasal cocaine paraphernalia

The disease is **not** transmitted by casual contact or by intimate household contact. However, those infected are advised not to share razors, toothbrushes, or pierced earrings because microscopic blood may be on these items.

The average incubation period is 7 weeks. Acute infection and illness are not common. Most people are completely unaware that they have been infected. They are asymptomatic and not diagnosed until many months or years after the initial exposure when an abnormality is detected during a routine laboratory evaluation or when liver problems occur. Unlike with hepatitis B, most people infected with hepatitis C do not clear the virus and a chronic infection develops.

HCV usually does its damage over decades by causing a chronic inflammation in the liver that eventually causes the liver cells to scar. This scarring may progress to cirrhosis. Alcohol use increases the progression and severity of cirrhosis.

Hepatitis C–induced cirrhosis is the leading indication for liver transplantation in the United States. Unfortunately, the newly transplanted liver often becomes re-infected with the virus.

Hepatitis D. Hepatitis D (delta hepatitis, or HDV) is caused by a defective RNA virus that needs the helper function of HBV. It occurs only with HBV to cause viral replication. This usually develops into chronic HDV. The incubation period is about 14 to 56 days. As with HBV, the disease is transmitted primarily by parenteral routes, especially patients who are IV drug abusers. Having sexual contact with a person with HDV is also a high risk factor.

Hepatitis E. The hepatitis E virus (HEV) causes a waterborne infection associated with epidemics in the Indian subcontinent, Asia, Africa, the Middle East, Mexico, and Central and South America. Many large outbreaks have occurred after heavy rains and flooding. Like hepatitis A, HEV is caused by fecal contamination of food and water.

In the United States, hepatitis E has been found only in international travelers. It is transmitted via the fecal-oral route, and the clinical course resembles that of hepatitis A. HEV has an incubation period of 15 to 64 days. There is no evidence at this time of a chronic form of HEV. The disease tends to be self-limiting and resolves on its own.

Complications of Hepatitis

Failure of the liver cells to regenerate, with progression of the necrotic process, results in a severe acute and often fatal form of hepatitis known as fulminant hepatitis. Hepatitis is considered to be chronic when liver inflammation lasts longer than 6 months. Chronic hepatitis usually occurs as a result of hepatitis B or hepatitis C. Superimposed infection with hepatitis D (HDV) in patients with chronic HBV may also result in chronic hepatitis. Chronic hepatitis can lead to cirrhosis and liver cancer. Many patients have multiple infections, especially the combination of HBV with either HCV, HDV, or HIV infections.

Incidence/Prevalence

The incidence of hepatitis A and hepatitis B is declining as a result of CDC recommendations for vaccination. However, hepatitis B and hepatitis C are a concern because of their association with cirrhosis and liver cancer. Although exact numbers are not known, it is estimated that about 200 million people worldwide have the hepatitis C virus (HCV), making this type of hepatitis the most common type. Currently there is no vaccine for HCV. Therefore it is expected that the cases of HCV will rise over the next several decades as a result of increasing illicit drug use. This increase will require a major increase in transplantations and lead to many more deaths (Lok & McMahon, 2009).

Health Promotion and Maintenance

Hepatitis vaccines for infants, children, and adolescents have helped decrease the incidence of hepatitis A and hepatitis B. Some adults are also advised to receive these immunizations.

Measures for preventing hepatitis A (HAV) in adults include:

- Proper handwashing, especially after handling shellfish
- Avoiding contaminated food or water (including tap water in countries with high incidence)
- Receiving immunoglobulin within 14 days if exposed to the virus
- Receiving the HAV vaccine before traveling to areas where the disease is common (e.g., Mexico, Caribbean)
- Receiving the vaccine if living or working in enclosed areas with others, such as college dormitories, correctional institutions, day-care centers, and long-term care facilities

Several HAV vaccines are available (e.g., Havrix and Vaqta). Both of these vaccines are made of inactivated hepatitis A virus and are given in the deltoid muscle.

Several vaccines can also provide protection against hepatitis B (HBV) infection (e.g., Engerix-B and Recombivax-HB). Twinrix is a combination HAV and HBV vaccine that is also available for adults. Examples of groups for whom immunization against HBV should be used include (Lok & McMahon, 2009):

- People who have sexual intercourse with more than one partner
- People with sexually transmitted disease (STD) or a history of STD
- Men having sex with men (MSM)
- People with any chronic liver disease (such as hepatitis C or cirrhosis)
- Patients with human immune deficiency virus (HIV) infection
- People who are exposed to blood or body fluids in the workplace, including health care workers, firefighters, and police
- People in correctional facilities
- Patients needing immunosuppressant drugs
- Family members, household members, and sexual contacts of people with HBV infection

Additional measures to prevent viral hepatitis for health care workers and others in contact with infected patients are listed in Charts 61-3 and 61-4.

CHART 61-3   BEST PRACTICE FOR PATIENT SAFETY & QUALITY CARE

Prevention of Viral Hepatitis in Health Care Workers

- Use Standard Precautions to prevent the transmission of disease between patients or between patients and health care staff (see Chapter 25).
- Eliminate needles and other sharp instruments by substituting needleless systems. (Needle sticks are the major source of hepatitis B transmission in health care workers.)
- Take the hepatitis B vaccine (e.g., Recombivax HB), which is given in a series of three injections. This vaccine also prevents hepatitis D by preventing HBV.
- For postexposure prevention of hepatitis A, seek medical attention immediately for immunoglobulin (Ig) administration.
- Report all cases of hepatitis to the local health department.

CHART 61-4   PATIENT AND FAMILY EDUCATION: PREPARING FOR SELF-MANAGEMENT

Health Practices to Prevent Viral Hepatitis

- Maintain adequate sanitation and personal hygiene. Wash your hands before eating and after using the toilet.
- Drink water treated by a water purification system.
- If traveling in underdeveloped or nonindustrialized countries, drink only bottled water. Avoid food washed or prepared with tap water, such as raw vegetables, fruits, and soups. Avoid ice.
- Use adequate sanitation practices to prevent the spread of the disease among family members.
- Do not share bed linens, towels, eating utensils, or drinking glasses.
- Do not share needles for injection, body piercing, or tattooing.
- Do not share razors, nail clippers, toothbrushes, or Waterpiks.
- Use a condom during sexual intercourse, or abstain from this activity.
- Cover cuts or sores with bandages.
- If ever infected with hepatitis, never donate blood, body organs, or other body tissue.

PATIENT-CENTERED COLLABORATIVE CARE

ASSESSMENT

History

Begin by asking the patient whether he or she has had known exposure to a person with hepatitis. For the patient who presents with few or no symptoms of liver disease but has abnormal laboratory tests (e.g., elevated alanine aminotransferase [ALT] or aspartate aminotransferase [AST] level), the history may need to include additional questions regarding risk factors such as:

- Exposure to either inhaled or ingested chemical
- Use of herbal supplements
- Use of any new prescribed drug or over-the-counter (OTC) medication
- Recent ingestion of shellfish
- Exposure to a possibly contaminated water source
- Travel to another country
- Sexual activities with men, women, or both, and whether it was protected or unprotected
- Illicit drug use, IV or intranasal
- For health care workers, recent needle stick exposure
- Body piercing or tattooing
- Close living accommodations (e.g., military barracks, correctional institutions, overcrowded dormitories, long-term facilities, day-care centers) or employment in any such setting
- Blood or blood products or organ transplants received before 1992
- Military service
- Place of birth (United States or other country) and parents' place of birth
- History of alcohol use (how many drinks each day or week)
- Human immune deficiency virus (HIV)

Physical Assessment/Clinical Manifestations

Assess whether the patient has:

- Abdominal pain
- Changes in skin or sclera (icterus)
- Arthralgia (joint pain) or myalgia (muscle pain)
- Diarrhea/constipation
- Changes in color of urine or stool
- Fever
- Lethargy
- Malaise
- Nausea/vomiting
- Pruritus (itching)

Lightly palpate the right upper abdominal quadrant to assess for liver tenderness. The patient may report right upper quadrant pain with jarring movements. Inspect the skin, sclerae, and mucous membranes for jaundice. He or she may present for medical treatment only after jaundice appears, believing that other vague symptoms are related to an influenza-like syndrome.

Jaundice in hepatitis results from intrahepatic obstruction and is caused by edema of the liver's bile channels. Dark urine and clay-colored stools are often reported by the patient. If possible, obtain a urine and stool specimen for visual inspection and laboratory analysis. The patient may also have skin abrasions from pruritus (itching).

Psychosocial Assessment

Viral hepatitis has various presentations, but for most infected people the initial course is mild with few or no symptoms. The long-term complications of fibrosis and cirrhosis cause the more serious problem. This is especially true for patients who have chronic HBV and HCV infection.

Emotional problems for affected patients may center on their feeling sick and fatigued. General malaise, inactivity, and vague symptoms contribute to depression. Some patients often feel guilty and are remorseful about decisions made that caused the disease. These feelings are most likely to occur when the source of infection is from drug abuse. Family members may be angry that the patient caused the disease.

Infectious diseases such as hepatitis continue to have a social stigma. The patient may feel embarrassed by the precautions that are imposed in the hospital and continue to be necessary at home. This embarrassment may cause the patient to limit social interactions. Patients may be afraid that they will spread the virus to family and friends.

Family members are sometimes afraid of getting the disease and may distance themselves from the patient. Allow them to verbalize these feelings, and explore the reasons for these fears. Educate the patient and family members about modes of transmission, and clarify information as needed.

Patients may be unable to return to work for several weeks during the acute phases of illness. The loss of wages and the cost of hospitalization for a patient without insurance coverage may produce great anxiety and financial burden. This situation may last for months or years if hepatitis becomes chronic.

Laboratory Assessment

Hepatitis A, hepatitis B, and hepatitis C are usually confirmed by acute elevations in levels of liver enzymes, indicating liver cellular damage, and by specific serologic markers.

Levels of ALT and AST levels may possibly rise into the thousands in acute or fulminant cases of hepatitis. Alkaline phosphatase levels may be normal or elevated. Serum total bilirubin levels are elevated and are consistent with the clinical appearance of jaundice. Elevated levels of bilirubin are also present in the urine (Pagana & Pagana, 2010).

The presence of *hepatitis A* is established when hepatitis A virus (HAV) antibodies (anti-HAV) are found in the blood. Ongoing inflammation of the liver by HAV is indicated by the presence of immunoglobulin M (IgM) antibodies, which persist in the blood for 4 to 6 weeks. Previous infection is identified by the presence of immunoglobulin G (IgG) antibodies. These antibodies persist in the serum and provide permanent immunity to HAV.

The presence of the *hepatitis B* virus (HBV) is established when serologic testing confirms the presence of hepatitis B antigen-antibody systems in the blood and a detectable viral count (HBV polymerase chain reaction [PCR] DNA). Antigens located on the surface (shell) of the virus (HBsAg) and IgM antibodies to hepatitis B core antigen (anti-HBcAg IgM) are the most significant serologic markers. The presence of these markers establishes the diagnosis of hepatitis B. *The patient is infectious as long as HBsAg (hepatitis B surface antigen) is present in the blood.* Persistence of this serologic marker after 6 months or longer indicates a carrier state or chronic hepatitis. HBsAg levels normally decline and disappear after the acute hepatitis B episode. The presence of antibodies to hepatitis B surface antibody (HBsAb) in the blood indicates recovery and immunity to hepatitis B. *People who have been vaccinated against HBV have a positive HBsAb because they also have immunity to the disease* (Pagana & Pagana, 2010).

Enzyme-linked immunosorbent assay (ELISA) is the initial screening test for patients suspected of being infected with *hepatitis C* virus (HCV). It is also the most commonly used enzyme test for HCV antibodies (anti-HCV). The antibodies can be detected within 4 weeks of the infection (Pagana & Pagana, 2010). A more specific assay called the *recombinant immunoblot assay (RIBA)* can be used as a confirmatory test. These tests show that the patient has been exposed to HCV and has developed the antibody. To identify the actual circulating virus, the HCV PCR RNA test is used. This confirms active virus and can measure the viral load. A new diagnostic tool called the OraQuick HCV Rapid Antibody Test was approved by the Food and Drug Administration in the United States in 2010. It has the advantage of providing a quick diagnosis of the disease as a point-of-care test.

The presence of *hepatitis D* virus (HDV) can be confirmed by the identification of intrahepatic delta antigen or, more often, by a rise in the hepatitis D virus antibodies (anti-HDV) titer. This increase can be seen within a few days of infection (Pagana & Pagana, 2010).

Hepatitis E virus (HEV) testing is usually reserved for travelers in whom hepatitis is present but the virus cannot be detected. Hepatitis E antibodies (anti-HEV) are found in people infected with the virus.

Other Diagnostic Assessment

Liver biopsy may be used to confirm the diagnosis of hepatitis and to establish the stage and grade of liver damage. Characteristic changes help the pathologist distinguish among a virus, drug, toxin, fatty liver, iron, and other disease. It is usually performed in an ambulatory care setting as a percutaneous procedure (through the skin) after a local anesthetic is given. If coagulation is abnormal, however, it may be done using either a computed tomography (CT)–guided or transjugular route to reduce the risk for pneumothorax or hemothorax. Ultrasound may also be used.

▌INTERVENTIONS

The patient with viral hepatitis can be mildly or acutely ill depending on the severity of the inflammation. Most patients are not hospitalized, although older adults and those with dehydration may be admitted for a short-term stay. The plan of care for all patients with viral hepatitis is based on measures to rest the liver, promote cellular regeneration, and prevent complications, if possible.

During the acute stage of viral hepatitis, interventions are aimed at resting the inflamed liver to promote hepatic cell regeneration. *Rest* is an essential intervention to reduce the liver's metabolic demands and increase its blood supply. Collaborative care is generally supportive. The patient is usually tired and expresses feelings of general malaise. Complete bedrest is usually not required, but rest periods alternating with periods of activity are indicated and are often enough to promote hepatic healing. Individualize the patient's plan of care and change it as needed to reflect the severity of symptoms, fatigue, and the results of liver function tests and enzyme determinations. Activities such as self-care and ambulating are gradually added to the activity schedule as tolerated.

The diet should be high in carbohydrates and calories with moderate amounts of fat and protein after nausea and anorexia subside. Small, frequent meals are often preferable to three standard meals. Ask the patient about food preferences because favorite foods are tolerated better than randomly selected foods. Encourage the patient to eat foods that are appealing. High-calorie snacks may be needed. Supplemental vitamins are often prescribed.

Drugs of any kind are used sparingly for patients with hepatitis to allow the liver to rest. An antiemetic to relieve nausea may be prescribed.

For patients with chronic hepatitis B and hepatitis C, a number of drugs are given, including antiviral and immuno-modulating drugs. Examples of antiviral drugs that may be used for HBV include:

- Tenofovir or entecavir (Baraclude) (as first-line therapy for patients who develop cirrhosis, but no co-infection)
- Interferon (as a first-line drug for patients who do *not* have cirrhosis)
- Adefovir dipivoxil (Hepsera) (as second-line therapy)
- Lamivudine (Epivir-HBV)
- Telbivudine (Tyzeka)

Teach patients taking these drugs to report any muscle weakness or aching because most of them can cause myopathy (muscle weakness).

The current standard of care for hepatitis C is a combination of drugs, typically subcutaneous pegylated interferon alpha once a week and oral ribavirin (Copegus, Rebetol) daily. Ribavirin should never be given to a pregnant patient. Women of childbearing age must agree to use contraception if they are receiving treatment or if they are sexual partners of patients taking this drug. A new drug that can better achieve a sustained viral response, telaprevir (Incivek), has recently been approved by the FDA. In addition, a new protease inhibitor, boceprevir (Victrelis), has been approved by the FDA to treat chronic hepatitis C in adults who have not been treated previously or have failed the typical treatment.

The length of treatment for hepatitis C depends on genotype or strain of hepatitis. There are several different genotypes; most Americans who have hepatitis C are genotype 1. This genotype usually requires 48 weeks of treatment. Genotypes 2 and 3 have a better response rate if the viral load is low and usually need only 24 weeks of treatment.

? DECISION-MAKING CHALLENGE

Patient-Centered Care; Safety

A 27-year-old secretary is preparing to fly home to visit her mother. Her best friend, who is a nurse, notices that the woman has yellowish skin and icterus. He asks if she has noticed any changes in her urine and bowel movements. She responds that she has noticed that her urine is dark and her stool has been much lighter for the past week. He tells her that she may have hepatitis or some other liver problem and takes her to the emergency department, where she is diagnosed with hepatitis A. She is very dehydrated and weak and is admitted for overnight hydration, additional testing, and observation. You have been assigned to take care of her this AM.

1. What transmission precautions will you provide for this patient and why? Should her friend who is a nurse be treated in any way? Why or why not?
2. The patient is very upset that she is not able to fly home and see her mother, who is ill. She asks you when she will be able to take the trip. What is your best response to her concerns?
3. How will you determine when the patient is adequately rehydrated?
4. What health teaching will you provide before she goes home?

CHART 61-5 PATIENT AND FAMILY EDUCATION: PREPARING FOR SELF-MANAGEMENT

Viral Hepatitis

- Avoid all medications, including over-the-counter drugs such as acetaminophen (Tylenol, Exdol ✚), unless prescribed by your physician.
- Avoid all alcohol.
- Rest frequently throughout the day, and get adequate sleep at night.
- Eat small, frequent meals with a high-carbohydrate, moderate-fat, and moderate-protein content.
- Avoid sexual intercourse until antibody testing results are negative.
- Follow the guidelines for preventing transmission of the disease (see Chart 61-4).

Genotypes 4 and 5 are typically treated for 48 weeks. The desired outcome of treatment is to have a negative HCV PCR RNA level and to sustain a negative level after treatment has ended. The secondary expected outcome is improvement in liver function. Response rates vary, but adults who are young, have a low viral load, and have minimal scarring on liver biopsy have a better chance of clearing the virus and remaining free of hepatitis C after treatment has ended.

Community-Based Care

Home care management varies according to the type of hepatitis and whether the disease is acute or chronic. A primary focus in any case is preventing the spread of the infection. For hepatitis transmitted by the fecal-oral route, careful handwashing and sanitary disposal of feces are important. Standard Precautions are used for hepatitis transmitted percutaneously and permucosally. Education is therefore very important. Collaborate with the certified infection control practitioner and infectious disease specialist if needed in caring for these patients. These experts can also suggest resources for the patient and family.

! NURSING SAFETY PRIORITY

Action Alert

Teach the patient with viral hepatitis and the family to use measures to prevent infection transmission (see Chart 61-4). In addition, instruct the patient to avoid alcohol and to check with the health care provider before taking any medication or vitamin, supplement, or herbal preparation.

Encourage the patient to increase activity gradually to prevent fatigue. Suggest that he or she eat small, frequent meals of high-carbohydrate foods (Chart 61-5).

FATTY LIVER (STEATOSIS)

Fatty liver is caused by the accumulation of fats in and around the hepatic cells. It may be caused by alcohol abuse or other factors. Nonalcoholic fatty liver disease (NAFLD) and nonalcoholic steatohepatitis (NASH) are types of fatty liver disease. Causes include:

- Diabetes mellitus
- Obesity
- Elevated lipid profile

Fatty infiltration of the liver may result from faulty fat metabolism in the liver and the movement of fatty acids from adipose tissue (fat). Many patients are asymptomatic. The most common and typical finding is an elevated ALT and AST or normal ALT and elevated AST (part of a group of liver function tests [LFTs]).

Magnetic resonance imaging (MRI), ultrasound, and nuclear medicine examinations can be used to confirm excessive fat in the liver. A percutaneous biopsy can also confirm the diagnosis. Interventions are aimed at removing the underlying cause of the infiltration. Weight loss, glucose control, and aggressive treatment using lipid-lowering agents are recommended. Monitoring liver function tests is essential in disease management.

HEPATIC ABSCESS

Although hepatic abscesses are not common, they carry a high mortality (death) rate. Abscesses occur when the liver is invaded by bacteria or protozoa. These organisms destroy the liver tissue, producing a necrotic cavity filled with infective agents, liquefied liver cells and tissue, and leukocytes. The infectious necrotic tissue walls off the abscess from the healthy liver.

A pyogenic liver abscess occurs when bacteria invade the liver. Infecting organisms include *Escherichia coli* and *Klebsiella, Enterobacter, Salmonella, Staphylococcus,* and *Enterococcus* species. A pyogenic abscess is generally solitary and confined to the right lobe, but occasionally abscesses are multiple. The usual cause is acute cholangitis, which occurs as a complication of cholelithiasis. Pyogenic liver abscesses may also result from liver trauma, abdominal peritonitis, and sepsis, or an abscess can extend to the liver after pneumonia or bacterial endocarditis. Symptoms are usually sudden.

The protozoan *Entamoeba histolytica* causes an amebic hepatic abscess, which may occur after amebic dysentery. These abscesses usually occur in the form of a single abscess in the right hepatic lobe, and the symptoms develop slowly.

Patients with hepatic abscesses are generally quite ill. On occasion, an abscess is not diagnosed until autopsy. Common manifestations include:

- Right upper abdominal pain with a palpable, tender liver
- Anorexia
- Weight loss
- Nausea and vomiting
- Fever and chills
- Weakness and malaise
- Shoulder pain
- Dyspnea
- Pleural pain if the diaphragm is involved

A liver abscess is usually diagnosed by contrast-enhanced CT scan or ultrasound. These abscesses are usually drained under CT or ultrasound guidance. Specimens may be sent for laboratory analysis so that the optimal antibiotic can be selected.

LIVER TRAUMA

The liver is one of the most common organs to be injured in patients with abdominal trauma. Damage or injury should be suspected whenever any upper abdominal or lower chest trauma is sustained. The liver is often injured by steering

---

CHART 61-6 **KEY FEATURES**

Liver Trauma

- Right upper quadrant pain with abdominal tenderness
- Abdominal distention and rigidity
- Guarding of the abdomen
- Increased abdominal pain exaggerated by deep breathing and referred to the right shoulder (Kehr's sign)
- Indicators of hemorrhage and hypovolemic shock:
  - Hypotension
  - Tachycardia
  - Tachypnea
  - Pallor
  - Diaphoresis
  - Cool, clammy skin
  - Confusion or other change in mental state

---

wheels in vehicular accidents. Common injuries include simple lacerations, multiple lacerations, avulsions (tears), and crush injuries.

The liver is a highly vascular organ and receives almost a third of the body's cardiac output. When hepatic trauma occurs, blood loss can be massive. *Observe for early signs of hypovolemic shock* (Chart 61-6).

An ultrasound or CT scan of the abdomen is often done to determine the presence of a hematoma (blood clot). A decreased hematocrit may confirm suspected blood loss. Clinical manifestations include right upper quadrant pain with abdominal tenderness, distention, guarding, and rigidity. Abdominal pain exaggerated by deep breathing and referred to the right shoulder may indicate diaphragmatic irritation.

When organ damage is confirmed, a surgeon uses a laparoscope or performs an open exploratory laparotomy to identify and control the source and type of bleeding. Minor surgical interventions, such as suture placement, wound packing, decompression, or a combination of these procedures, are often performed to stop the bleeding. Liver lobe resection is required in some extensive liver injuries. This procedure may be done using laparoscopy. Catheter-directed embolization of an intrahepatic blood vessel as an interventional radiologic procedure may be a useful alternative to surgical resection.

Patients with hepatic trauma require multiple blood products such as packed red blood cells and fresh frozen plasma, as well as massive volume infusion to maintain adequate hydration. After surgery, the patient is admitted to a critical care unit. Monitor the patient for persistent or new bleeding. Closely monitor complete blood count and coagulation studies for trends in changes.

CANCER OF THE LIVER

Pathophysiology

Cancers may be *primary* tumors (hepatocellular carcinoma) starting in the liver, or they may be *metastatic* cancers that spread from another organ to the liver. They are most often seen in regions of Asia and the Mediterranean area. Worldwide, the disease kills about 1 million people each year and affects Vietnamese men more than any other group. Black and Hispanic populations have twice the rate of the disease as Euro-Americans, and older adults are affected more than other age-groups (Rossi et al., 2010). In the United States and worldwide, the incidence of liver cancer is increasing because there is an increase in cases of hepatitis C (HCV).

Chronic infection with HBV and HCV frequently lead to cirrhosis, which is a risk factor for developing liver cancer. It is important to remember that cirrhosis from any cause, including alcoholic liver disease, increases the risk for cancer.

PATIENT-CENTERED COLLABORATIVE CARE

ASSESSMENT

In the early stage of cancer, most patients are without symptoms. Later in the disease, they report weight loss, anorexia, and weakness. Ask the patient if he or she has or has had recent abdominal pain, the most common concern. It is most often felt in the right upper quadrant before jaundice, bleeding, ascites, and edema develop. Palpation may reveal an enlarged, nodular liver.

Elevated serum alpha-fetoprotein (AFP) (a tumor marker for cancers of the liver, testis, and ovary) and increased alkaline phosphatase are also common (Pagana & Pagana, 2010). Ultrasound (US) and contrast-enhanced CT are both useful in detecting metastasis. If the primary tumor site is not known, a CT- or ultrasound-guided liver biopsy can confirm the diagnosis, although this procedure is risky because of possible bleeding and spread of the cancer cells.

INTERVENTIONS

Surgical resection and liver transplantation offer the only treatments for long-term survival. Unfortunately, most patients are not candidates for surgical removal because their tumors are unresectable. Selective internal radiation therapy (SIRT) has been successful for some patients. Other palliative approaches include hepatic artery embolization, ablation techniques, and drug therapy.

Hepatic artery embolization causes cell death by blocking blood supply to the tumor in the liver. It is performed under moderate sedation by an interventional radiologist who threads a catheter through the femoral artery to inject small particles into the hepatic artery. The patient usually stays overnight in the hospital for observation in case of bleeding. This procedure may be followed by infusing a chemotherapy agent directly into the hepatic artery (chemoembolization).

Common *ablation* procedures include radiofrequency ablation (RFA), percutaneous ethanol injection, and cryotherapy. RFA uses energy waves to heat cancer cells and kill them. It is most often performed as an ambulatory care procedure using a percutaneous laparoscopic approach. Ethanol may also be injected directly into the tumor to destroy tumor cells, although this procedure is not as commonly done as RFA (Rossi et al., 2010). Cryotherapy uses liquid nitrogen to freeze and destroy liver tumors. The general nursing care for patients having these procedures is described in Chapter 24.

Chemotherapy may be administered orally or IV. However, it is not effective in many cases. Examples of drugs used are doxorubicin (Adriamycin), 5-fluorouracil (5-FU), and cisplatin. Sorafenib (Nexavar) is a kinase inhibitor that is approved for inoperable liver cancer. Other drugs are targeted therapies that are being investigated and used with some success.

Another drug route is a catheter-directed method directly into the hepatic artery, a procedure called *hepatic arterial infusion (HAI)*. The interventional radiologist places a catheter into the artery that supplies the tumor and injects a mixture of chemotherapy and contrast agent into the tumor. This procedure has the unique effect of depositing chemotherapeutic drugs directly into the tumor without causing major systemic effects. Examples of agents given are fluorodeoxyuridine (FUDR) with or without dexamethasone (the most commonly used), oxaliplatin, mitomycin-C, or irinotecan (Moore, 2007). Chapter 24 describes the general nursing care for patients receiving chemotherapy.

Patients with advanced liver cancer usually need end-of-life care and hospice services. Collaborate with the case manager to help patients and their families find the best community resources that meet their needs. Chapter 9 describes end-of-life care and hospice services in detail.

LIVER TRANSPLANTATION

Liver transplantation has become a common procedure worldwide. The patient with end-stage liver disease or acute liver failure who has not responded to conventional medical or surgical intervention is a potential candidate for liver transplantation. The most common reason for a liver transplant is hepatitis C. It may also be used for the patient with a *primary* liver tumor.

The patient for potential transplantation has extensive physiologic and psychological assessment and evaluation by physicians and transplant coordinators. Alternative treatment should be extensively explored before committing a patient for a liver transplant. Patients who are *not* considered candidates for transplantation are those with:

- Severe cardiovascular instability with advanced cardiac disease
- Severe respiratory disease
- Metastatic tumors
- Inability to follow instructions regarding drug therapy and self-management

Liver transplantation has become the most effective treatment for an increasing number of patients with acute and chronic liver diseases. Inclusion and exclusion criteria vary among transplantation centers and are continually revised as treatment options change and surgical techniques improve.

Donor livers are obtained primarily from trauma victims who have not had liver damage. They are distributed through a nationwide program—the United Network of Organ Sharing (UNOS). This system distributes donor livers based on regional considerations and patient acuity. Candidates with the highest level of acuity receive highest priority.

The donor liver is transported to the surgery center in a solution that preserves the organ for up to 8 hours. The diseased liver is removed through an incision made in the upper abdomen. The new liver is carefully put in its place and is attached to the patient's blood vessels and bile ducts. The procedure can take many hours to complete and requires a highly specialized team and large volumes of fluid and blood replacement.

Living donors have also been used and are usually close family members or spouse. This is done on a voluntary basis after careful psychological and physiologic preparation and testing. The donor's liver is resected (usually removal of one lobe) and implanted into the recipient after removal of the diseased liver. In both the donor and the recipient, the liver regenerates and grows in size to meet the demands of the body.

Pathophysiology

Although liver transplantations are commonly done, complications can occur. Some problems can be medically managed, whereas others require removal of the transplant. The two most common complications are acute graft rejection and infection.

The success of all transplantations has greatly improved since the introduction many years ago of cyclosporine (cyclosporin A), an immunosuppressant drug. Today, many other anti-rejection drugs are used. (See Chapter 19 for a complete discussion of rejection and preventive drug therapy.)

! NURSING SAFETY PRIORITY

Action Alert

For the patient who has undergone liver transplantation, monitor for clinical manifestations of rejection, which may include tachycardia, fever, right upper quadrant or flank pain, decreased bile pigment and volume, and increasing jaundice. Laboratory findings include elevated serum bilirubin, rising ALT and AST levels, elevated alkaline phosphatase levels, and increased prothrombin time/international normalized ratio (PT/INR).

Transplant rejection is treated aggressively with immunosuppressive drugs. As with all rejection treatments, the patient is at a greater risk for infection. If therapy is not effective, liver function rapidly deteriorates. Multi-system organ failure, including respiratory and renal involvement, develops along with diffuse coagulopathies and portal-systemic encephalopathy (PSE). The only alternative for treatment is emergency retransplantation.

Infection is another potential threat to the transplanted graft and the patient's survival. Vaccinations and prophylactic antibiotics are helpful in prevention. Immunosuppressant therapy, which must be used to prevent and treat organ rejection, significantly increases the patient's risk for infection. Other risk factors include the presence of multiple tubes and intravascular lines, immobility, and prolonged anesthesia.

In the early post-transplantation period, common infections include pneumonia, wound infections, and urinary tract infections. Opportunistic infections usually develop after the first postoperative month and include cytomegalovirus, mycobacterial infections, and parasitic infections. Latent infections such as tuberculosis and herpes simplex may be reactivated.

The physician prescribes broad-spectrum antibiotics for prophylaxis during and after surgery. Obtain culture specimens from all lines and tubes and collect specimens for culture at predetermined time intervals as dictated by the agency's policy. If an infection is detected, the physician prescribes organism-specific anti-infective agents.

The biliary anastomosis is susceptible to breakdown, obstruction, and infection. If leakage occurs or if the site becomes necrotic or obstructed, an abscess can form or peritonitis, bacteremia, and cirrhosis may develop. Observe for potential complications, which are listed in Table 61-6.

TABLE 61-6 **ASSESSMENT AND PREVENTION OF COMMON POSTOPERATIVE COMPLICATIONS ASSOCIATED WITH LIVER TRANSPLANTATION**

ASSESSMENT	PREVENTION
Acute Graft Rejection Occurs from the 4th to 10th postoperative day Manifested by tachycardia, fever, right upper quadrant (RUQ) or flank pain, diminished bile drainage or change in bile color, or increased jaundice Laboratory changes: (1) increased levels of serum bilirubin, transaminases, and alkaline phosphatase; (2) prolonged prothrombin time	Prophylaxis with immunosuppressant agents, such as cyclosporine Early diagnosis to treat with more potent anti-rejection drugs
Infection Can occur at any time during recovery Manifested by fever or excessive, foul-smelling drainage (urine, wound, or bile); other indicators depend on location and type of infection	Antibiotic prophylaxis; vaccinations Frequent cultures of tubes, lines, and drainage Early removal of invasive lines Good handwashing Early diagnosis and treatment with organism-specific anti-infective agents
Hepatic Complications (Bile Leakage, Abscess Formation, Hepatic Thrombosis) Manifested by decreased bile drainage, increased RUQ abdominal pain with distention and guarding, nausea or vomiting, increased jaundice, and clay-colored stools Laboratory changes: increased levels of serum bilirubin and transaminases	If present, keep T-tube in dependent position and secure to patient; empty frequently, recording quality and quantity of drainage Report manifestations to physician immediately May necessitate surgical intervention
Acute Renal Failure Caused by hypotension, antibiotics, cyclosporine, acute liver failure, or hypothermia Indicators of hypothermia: shivering, hyperventilation, increased cardiac output, vasoconstriction, and alkalemia Early indicators of renal failure: changes in urine output, increased blood urea nitrogen (BUN) and creatinine levels, and electrolyte imbalance	Monitor all drug levels with nephrotoxic side effects Prevent hypotension Observe for early signs of renal failure, and report them immediately to the physician

PATIENT-CENTERED COLLABORATIVE CARE

Care of the patient undergoing liver transplantation requires an interdisciplinary team approach. Receiving a transplant has a major psychosocial impact. Transplant complications cause patients to be very anxious. In collaboration with the members of the health care team, assure them and their families that these problems are common and usually successfully treated.

After the patient is identified as a candidate and a donor organ is procured, the actual liver transplantation surgical procedure usually takes many hours. The length of the procedure can vary greatly.

In the immediate postoperative period, the patient is managed in the critical care unit and requires aggressive monitoring and care. Assess for signs and symptoms of complications of surgery, and immediately report them to the surgeon (see Table 61-6).

! NURSING SAFETY PRIORITY

Action Alert

For the patient who has had a liver transplantation, monitor the temperature frequently per hospital protocol, and report elevations, increased abdominal pain, distention, and rigidity, which are indicators of peritonitis. Nursing assessment also includes monitoring for a change in neurologic status that could indicate encephalopathy from a nonfunctioning liver. Report signs of clotting problems (e.g., bloody oozing from a catheter, petechiae, ecchymosis) to the surgeon immediately because they may indicate impaired function of the transplanted liver.

NURSING CONCEPT REVIEW

What might you NOTICE if the patient is experiencing inadequate digestion, nutrition, and metabolism as a result of impaired liver function?

- Jaundice
- Icterus
- Report of nausea and anorexia
- Vomiting
- Weight loss
- Bruising or bleeding
- Ascites

What should you INTERPRET and how should you RESPOND to a patient experiencing inadequate digestion, nutrition, and metabolism as a result of impaired liver function?

Perform and interpret physical assessment findings, including:
- Assess respiratory status to check for dyspnea or shallow breathing.
- Check level of consciousness and cognition.
- Take vital signs (look for fever or decreased BP) and oxygen saturation.
- Check for blood in the vomitus.
- Perform an abdominal assessment, including measuring girth.

- Check urine for dark color and stool for clay-colored appearance.
- Take current weight, and compare with previous weight.
- Assess skin for open areas.
- Check most recent laboratory values for coagulation studies and LFTs.

Respond by:
- Applying oxygen to assist in ease of breathing
- Keeping head of bed elevated to at least 30 degrees
- Maintaining rest
- Collaborating with dietitian and pharmacist as needed
- Prioritizing and pacing activities to prevent fatigue
- Monitoring patient closely for complications, such as bleeding; call the Rapid Response Team if bleeding occurs

On what should you REFLECT?
- Monitor the patient for restored digestion and nutrition, such as increased appetite.
- Think about what may have caused the liver problem.
- Consider for what complications the patient is at risk.
- Think about what members of the health care team need to provide care for this patient.

GET READY FOR THE NCLEX® EXAMINATION!

KEY POINTS

Review these Key Points for each NCLEX Examination Client Needs Category.

Safe and Effective Care Environment
- Monitor the patient with cirrhosis for bleeding and neurologic changes.
- When caring for patients with cirrhosis, collaborate with the dietitian, physician, and pharmacist.

- Refer patients with liver disorders to the American Liver Foundation; refer dying patients to hospice and other community resources as needed.

Health Promotion and Maintenance
- Follow the guidelines listed in Chart 61-3 to prevent viral hepatitis in the workplace.

GET READY FOR THE NCLEX® EXAMINATION!—cont'd

- Teach patients to take precautions to prevent viral hepatitis in the community as described in Chart 61-4.
- For patients with viral hepatitis, instruct them to follow the guidelines listed in Chart 61-5.

Psychosocial Integrity

- Recognize that patients with cirrhosis have mental and emotional changes due to hepatic encephalopathy.
- Be aware that patients with cirrhosis and/or chronic hepatitis may feel guilty about their disease because of past habits such as drug and alcohol abuse.
- Be aware that family members and friends may fear getting hepatitis from the patient.
- Be aware that patients having liver transplantation have major concerns about the possibility of complications, such as organ rejection.

Physiological Integrity

- Be aware that cirrhosis has many causes other than alcohol abuse (see Table 61-3).
- Monitor laboratory values of patients suspected of or diagnosed with cirrhosis of the liver as listed in Tables 61-1 and 61-4.

- Observe for clinical manifestations of hepatic encephalopathy (PSE) as listed in Table 61-2.
- Assess for manifestations of cirrhosis as shown in Fig. 61-1.
- Provide care for the patient having a paracentesis as described in Chart 61-1.
- Administer drug therapy to decrease ammonia levels (which cause PSE) in patients with cirrhosis, such as lactulose and nonabsorbable antibiotics.
- Differentiate the five major types of hepatitis: A, B, C, D, and E. HDV occurs only with HBV and is transmitted most commonly by blood and body fluid exposure. Hepatitis A is transmitted via the fecal-oral route. Hepatitis C is the most common type and is also transmitted via blood and body fluids.
- Be aware that patients with chronic viral hepatitis often develop cirrhosis and cancer of the liver.
- Recognize that potent immunomodulators and antivirals are given to treat hepatitis B and hepatitis C.
- Monitor for bleeding in the patient with liver trauma; assume that any abdominal trauma has damaged the liver.
- Observe the patient having a liver transplantation for complications, such as those described in Table 61-6.

Care of Patients with Problems of the Biliary System and Pancreas

Donna D. Ignatavicius

e*volve* WEBSITE

http://evolve.elsevier.com/Iggy/

Animation: Laparoscopic Cholecystectomy; Gallbladder Removal
Answers for NCLEX Examination Challenges and Decision-Making Challenges

Audio Glossary
Concept Map Creator
Key Points
Review Questions for the NCLEX® Examination

LEARNING OUTCOMES

Safe and Effective Care Environment

1. Collaborate with health care team members to provide care for patients with pancreatic disorders.

Health Promotion and Maintenance

2. Teach people about health promotion practices to prevent gallbladder disease.
3. Teach people about health promotion practices to prevent pancreatitis.
4. Identify community-based resources for patients with pancreatic disorders.

Psychosocial Integrity

5. Describe the psychosocial needs of patients with pancreatic cancer and their families.
6. Assess patient and family response to a diagnosis of pancreatic cancer.

Physiological Integrity

7. Identify risk factors for gallbladder disease.
8. Interpret diagnostic test results associated with gallbladder disease.
9. Compare postoperative care of patients undergoing a traditional cholecystectomy with that of patients having laparoscopic cholecystectomy.
10. Compare and contrast the pathophysiology of acute and chronic pancreatitis.
11. Interpret laboratory test results associated with acute pancreatitis.
12. Interpret common assessment findings associated with acute and chronic pancreatitis.
13. Prioritize nursing care for patients with acute pancreatitis and patients with chronic pancreatitis.
14. Explain the use and precautions associated with enzyme replacement for chronic pancreatitis.
15. Develop a postoperative plan of care for patients having a Whipple procedure.

The biliary system (liver and gallbladder) and pancreas secrete enzymes and other substances that promote food digestion in the stomach and small intestine. When these organs do not work properly, the person has impaired *digestion,* which may result in inadequate *nutrition.* Collaborative care for patients with problems of the biliary system and pancreas includes the need to promote nutrition for healthy cellular function. This chapter focuses on problems of the gallbladder and pancreas. Liver disorders were described in Chapter 61.

Because of the close anatomic location of these organs, disorders of the gallbladder and pancreas may extend to other organs if the primary health problem is not treated early. Inflammation is caused by obstruction (blockage) in the biliary system from gallstones, edema, stricture, or tumors. For example, gallstones in the cystic duct cause cholecystitis.

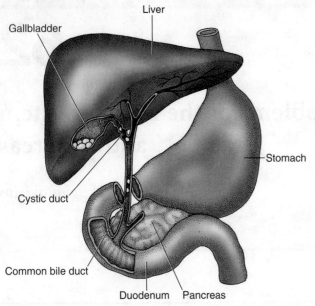

FIG. 62-1 Gallstones within the gallbladder and obstructing the common bile and cystic ducts.

Gallstones lodged in the ampulla of Vater block the flow of bile and pancreatic secretions, which can result in pancreatitis.

GALLBLADDER DISORDERS

CHOLECYSTITIS

Pathophysiology

Cholecystitis is an inflammation of the gallbladder that affects many people, most commonly in affluent countries. It may be either acute or chronic, although most patients have the acute type. Over 500,000 surgeries for this health problem are done in the United States each year (Comstock, 2008).

Acute Cholecystitis

Two types of acute cholecystitis can occur: calculous and acalculous cholecystitis. The most common type is calculous cholecystitis, in which chemical irritation and inflammation result from gallstones (cholelithiasis) that obstruct the cystic duct (most often), gallbladder neck, or common bile duct (choledocholithiasis) (Fig. 62-1). When the gallbladder is inflamed, trapped bile is reabsorbed and acts as a chemical irritant to the gallbladder wall; that is, the bile has a toxic effect. Reabsorbed bile, in combination with impaired circulation, edema, and distention of the gallbladder, causes ischemia and infection. The result is tissue sloughing with necrosis and gangrene. The gallbladder wall may eventually perforate (rupture). If the perforation is small and localized, an abscess may form. Peritonitis, infection of the peritoneum, may result if the perforation is large.

The exact pathophysiology of gallstone formation is not clearly understood, but abnormal metabolism of cholesterol and bile salts plays an important role in their formation. The gallbladder provides an excellent environment for the production of stones because it only occasionally mixes its normally abundant mucus with its highly viscous,

concentrated bile. Impaired gallbladder motility can lead to stone formation by delaying bile emptying and causing biliary stasis.

Gallstones are composed of substances normally found in bile, such as cholesterol, bilirubin, bile salts, calcium, and various proteins. They are classified as either cholesterol stones or pigment stones. Cholesterol calculi form as a result of metabolic imbalances of cholesterol and bile salts. They are the most common type found in people in the United States. Pigmented stones are associated with cirrhosis of the liver (McCance et al., 2010).

Bacteria can collect around the stones in the biliary system. Severe bacterial invasion can lead to life-threatening *suppurative* cholangitis when symptoms are not recognized quickly and pus accumulates in the ductal system.

Acalculous cholecystitis (inflammation occurring without gallstones) is typically associated with biliary stasis caused by any condition that affects the regular filling or emptying of the gallbladder. For example, a decrease in blood flow to the gallbladder or anatomic problems such as twisting or kinking of the gallbladder neck or cystic duct can result in pancreatic enzyme reflux into the gallbladder, causing inflammation. Most cases of this type of cholecystitis occur in patients with:

- Sepsis
- Severe trauma or burns
- Long-term total parenteral nutrition
- Multi-system organ failure
- Major surgery
- Hypovolemia

Chronic Cholecystitis

Chronic cholecystitis results when repeated episodes of cystic duct obstruction cause chronic inflammation. Calculi are almost always present. In chronic cholecystitis, the gallbladder becomes fibrotic and contracted, which results in decreased motility and deficient absorption.

Pancreatitis and cholangitis (bile duct inflammation) can occur as chronic complications of cholecystitis. These problems result from the backup of bile throughout the biliary tract. Bile obstruction leads to jaundice.

Jaundice (yellow discoloration of the skin and mucous membranes) and icterus (yellow discoloration of the sclerae) can occur in patients with acute cholecystitis but are most commonly seen in those with the *chronic* form of the disease. Obstructed bile flow caused by edema of the ducts or gallstones contributes to *extrahepatic obstructive jaundice.* Jaundice in cholecystitis may also be caused by direct liver involvement. Inflammation of the liver's bile channels or bile ducts may cause *intrahepatic* obstructive jaundice, resulting in an increase in circulating levels of bilirubin, the major pigment of bile.

When the concentration of bilirubin in the blood increases, jaundice can occur. In a person with obstructive jaundice, the normal flow of bile into the duodenum is blocked, allowing excessive bile salts to accumulate in the skin. This accumulation of bile salts leads to pruritus (itching) or a burning sensation. The bile flow blockage also prevents bilirubin from reaching the large intestine, where it is converted to urobilinogen. Because urobilinogen accounts for the normal brown color of feces, clay-colored stools result. Water-soluble bilirubin is normally excreted by the kidneys in the urine. When

TABLE 62-1 RISK FACTORS FOR CHOLECYSTITIS

- Women
- Aging
- American Indian, Mexican American, or Caucasian
- Obesity
- Rapid weight loss or prolonged fasting
- Increased serum cholesterol
- Women on hormone replacement therapy (HRT) or older birth control pills
- Cholesterol-lowering drugs
- Family history of gallstones
- Prolonged total parenteral nutrition
- Crohn's disease
- Gastric bypass surgery
- Sickle cell disease
- Glucose intolerance/diabetes mellitus
- Pregnancy
- Genetic factors

CHART 62-1 KEY FEATURES

Cholecystitis

- Episodic or vague upper abdominal pain or discomfort that can radiate to the right shoulder
- Pain triggered by a high-fat or high-volume meal
- Anorexia
- Nausea and/or vomiting
- Dyspepsia (indigestion)
- Eructation (belching)
- Flatulence (gas)
- Feeling of abdominal fullness
- Rebound tenderness (Blumberg's sign)
- Fever
- Jaundice, clay-colored stools, dark urine, steatorrhea (most common with chronic cholecystitis)

an excess of circulating bilirubin occurs, the urine becomes dark and foamy because of the kidneys' effort to clear the bilirubin.

Etiology and Genetic Risk

A familial or genetic tendency appears to play a role in the development of cholelithiasis, but this may be partially related to familial nutrition habits (excessive dietary cholesterol intake) and sedentary lifestyles. Genetic-environment interactions may contribute to gallstone production (Attasaranya et al., 2008).

Cholelithiasis is seen more frequently in obese patients, probably as a result of impaired fat metabolism or increased cholesterol. The risk for developing gallstones increases as people age. Patients with diabetes mellitus are also at increased risk because they usually have higher levels of fatty acids (triglycerides). American Indians have a higher incidence of the disease than other groups, which may be due to the higher incidence of diabetes mellitus and obesity in this population (McCance et al., 2010). Risk factors for cholecystitis are listed in Table 62-1.

WOMEN'S HEALTH CONSIDERATIONS

Women who are between 20 and 60 years of age are twice as likely to develop gallstones as are men. Obesity is a major risk factor for gallstone formation, especially in women. Pregnancy and drugs such as hormone replacements and birth control pills (especially the older oral contraceptives) alter hormone levels and delay muscular contraction of the gallbladder, decreasing the rate of bile emptying. The incidence of gallstones is higher in women who have had multiple pregnancies. Combinations of causative factors increase the incidence of stone formation, especially in women. Therefore some clinicians refer to the patient most at risk for cholecystitis and gallstones by the four **F**s:
- **F**emale
- **F**orty
- **F**at
- **F**ertile

PATIENT-CENTERED COLLABORATIVE CARE

ASSESSMENT

Physical Assessment/Clinical Manifestations

Patients with acute cholecystitis present with abdominal pain, although clinical manifestations vary in intensity and frequency (Chart 62-1).

Obtain the patient's height, weight, and vital signs, or delegate these activities to unlicensed assistive personnel (UAP). Ask about food preferences, and determine whether excessive fat and cholesterol are part of the diet. Inquire if any foods cause pain. Question whether any GI symptoms occur when fatty food is eaten: flatulence (gas), dyspepsia (indigestion), eructation (belching), anorexia, nausea, vomiting, and abdominal pain or discomfort.

Ask the patient to describe the pain, including its intensity and duration, precipitating factors, and any measures that relieve it. Pain may be described as indigestion of varying intensity, ranging from a mild, persistent ache to a steady, constant pain in the right upper abdominal quadrant. It may radiate to the right shoulder or scapula. In some cases, the abdominal pain of chronic cholecystitis may be vague and nonspecific. The usual pattern is episodic. Patients often refer to acute pain episodes as "gallbladder attacks."

CONSIDERATIONS FOR OLDER ADULTS

Older adults and patients with diabetes mellitus may have atypical manifestations of cholecystitis, including the absence of pain and fever. Localized tenderness may be the only presenting sign. The older patient may become acutely confused (delirium) as the first manifestation of gallbladder disease.

The severe pain of biliary colic is produced by obstruction of the cystic duct of the gallbladder or movement of one or more stones. When a stone is moving through or is lodged within the duct, tissue spasm occurs in an effort to get the stone through the small duct.

! NURSING SAFETY PRIORITY

Critical Rescue

Biliary colic may be so severe that it occurs with tachycardia, pallor, diaphoresis, and prostration (extreme exhaustion). Assess the patient for possible shock caused by biliary colic. Notify the health care provider or Rapid Response Team if these manifestations occur. Stay with the patient, and lower the head of the bed.

Ask patients to describe their daily activity or exercise routines to determine whether they are sedentary. Question whether there is a family history of gallbladder disease. If the patient is female, ask whether she takes hormone replacement therapy (HRT) or birth control pills.

Assessment for rebound tenderness (Blumberg's sign) and deep palpation are performed only by physicians and advanced practice nurses. To elicit rebound tenderness, the health care provider pushes his or her fingers deeply and steadily into the patient's abdomen and then quickly releases the pressure. Pain that results from the rebound of the palpated tissue may indicate peritoneal inflammation. Deep palpation below the liver border in the right upper quadrant may reveal a sausage-shaped mass, representing the distended, inflamed gallbladder. Percussion over the posterior rib cage worsens localized abdominal pain.

In *chronic* cholecystitis, patients may have slowly developing symptoms and may not seek medical treatment until late symptoms such as jaundice (yellowing of the skin), clay-colored stools, and dark urine occur from biliary obstruction. Yellowing of the sclerae (icterus) and oral mucous membranes may also be present. Steatorrhea (fatty stools) occurs because fat absorption is decreased because of the lack of bile. Bile is needed for the absorption of fats and fat-soluble vitamins in the intestine. As with any inflammatory process, the patient may have an elevated temperature of 99° to 102° F (37.2° to 38.9° C), tachycardia, and dehydration from fever and vomiting.

CONSIDERATIONS FOR OLDER ADULTS

Older adults become dehydrated much quicker than other age-groups, and they may not present with a fever. Monitor for a new onset of disorientation or acute confusion due to decreased blood volume available to oxygenate the cells of the brain (hypoxia).

Diagnostic Assessment

A differential diagnosis rules out other diseases that may cause similar symptoms, such as peptic ulcer disease, hepatitis, and pancreatitis. An increased white blood cell (WBC) count indicates inflammation. Serum levels of alkaline phosphatase, aspartate aminotransferase (AST), and lactate dehydrogenase (LDH) may be elevated, indicating abnormalities in liver function in patients with severe biliary obstruction. The direct (conjugated) and indirect (unconjugated) serum bilirubin levels are also elevated. If the pancreas is involved, serum amylase and lipase levels are elevated.

Calcified gallstones are easily viewed on abdominal x-ray. Stones that are not calcified cannot be seen. *Ultrasonography (US) of the right upper quadrant is the best diagnostic test for cholecystitis.* It is safe, accurate, and painless. Acute cholecystitis is seen as edema of the gallbladder wall and pericholecystic fluid. A hepatobiliary scan can be performed to visualize the gallbladder and determine patency of the biliary system.

When the cause of cholecystitis or cholelithiasis is not known or the patient has manifestations of biliary obstruction (e.g., jaundice), an *endoscopic retrograde cholangiopancreatography* (ERCP) may be performed. Some patients have the less invasive and safer *magnetic resonance cholangiopancreatography* (MRCP), which can be performed by an interventional radiologist. For this procedure, the patient is given oral or IV contrast material (gadolinium) before having a magnetic resonance imaging (MRI) scan (Daniak et al., 2008). Before the test, ask the patient about any history of urticaria (hives) or other allergy. Gadolinium does not contain iodine, which decreases the risk for an allergic response. Chapter 55 discusses these tests in more detail.

INTERVENTIONS

Most patients do not respond to nonsurgical interventions during the acute phase of cholecystitis. Surgery is the treatment of choice.

Nonsurgical Management

Many people with gallstones have no symptoms. Acute pain occurs when gallstones partially or totally obstruct the cystic or common bile duct. Most patients find that they need to avoid fatty foods to prevent further episodes of biliary colic. Withhold food and fluids if nausea and vomiting occur. IV therapy is used for hydration.

Acute biliary pain requires opioid analgesia, such as morphine or hydromorphone (Dilaudid). In the past, meperidine (Demerol) was the drug of choice because it was thought to cause fewer spasms of the sphincter of Oddi, which blocks bile flow. However, this drug breaks down into a toxic metabolite (normeperidine) and can cause seizures, especially in older adults. All opioids may cause some degree of sphincter spasm.

Ketorolac (Toradol, Acular) may be used for mild to moderate pain. The health care provider prescribes antiemetics to control nausea and vomiting. IV antibiotic therapy may also be given, depending on the cause of cholecystitis or as a one-time dose for surgery.

For some patients with small stones or for those who are not good surgical candidates, a treatment that is commonly used for kidney stones can be used to break up gallstones—*extracorporeal shock wave lithotripsy (ESWL).* This procedure can be used only for patients who have a normal weight, cholesterol-based stones, and good gallbladder function. The patient lies on a water-filled pad, and shock waves break up the large stones into smaller ones that can be passed through the digestive system. During the procedure, he or she may have pain from the movement of the stones or duct or gallbladder spasms. A therapeutic bile acid, such as ursodeoxycholic acid (UDCA), may be used after the procedure to help dissolve the remaining stone fragments.

Another treatment option in people who cannot have surgery is the insertion of a percutaneous transhepatic biliary catheter to open the blocked duct(s) so that bile can flow. Catheters can be placed several ways, depending on the condition of the biliary ducts, in an internal, external, or internal/external drain. Biliary catheters usually divert bile from the liver into the duodenum to bypass a stricture. When all of the bile enters the duodenum, it is called an *internal* drain. However, in some cases, a patient has an *internal/external* drain in which part of the bile empties into a drainage bag. Patients who need this drain for an extended period may have the external drain capped. If jaundice or leakage around the catheter site occurs, teach the patient to reconnect the catheter to a drainage bag and have a follow-up cholangiogram injection done by an interventional radiologist. An *external* only catheter is connected either temporarily or permanently to a drainage bag. A reduction in bile drainage indicates that the drain is no longer working.

Surgical Management

Cholecystectomy is a surgical removal of the gallbladder. One of two procedures is performed: the laparoscopic cholecystectomy and, far less often, the traditional open approach cholecystectomy.

Laparoscopic Cholecystectomy. Laparoscopic cholecystectomy, a minimally invasive surgery (MIS), is currently the "gold standard" and is performed far more often than the traditional open approach. The advantages of MIS include:

- Complications are not common.
- The death rate is very low.
- Bile duct injuries are rare.
- Patient recovery is quicker.
- Postoperative pain is less severe.

The laparoscopic procedure (often called a "lap chole") is commonly done on an ambulatory care basis in a same-day surgery suite. The surgeon explains the procedure. The nurse answers questions and reinforces the physician's instructions. Reinforce what to expect after surgery, and review pain management, deep-breathing exercises, and incentive spirometry use. There is no special preoperative preparation other than the routine preparation for surgery under general anesthesia described in Chapter 16. An IV antibiotic is usually given immediately before or during surgery.

During the surgery, the surgeon makes a very small midline puncture at the umbilicus. Additional small incisions may be needed, although single-incision laparoscopic cholecystectomy (SILC) using a flexible endoscope can be done (Binenbaum et al., 2009). The abdominal cavity is insufflated with 3 to 4 L of carbon dioxide. Gasless laparoscopic cholecystectomy using abdominal wall lifting devices is a more recent innovation in some centers. This technique results in improved pulmonary and cardiac function. A trocar catheter is inserted, through which a laparoscope is introduced. The laparoscope is attached to a video camera, and the abdominal organs are viewed on a monitor. The gallbladder is dissected from the liver bed, and the cystic artery and duct are closed. The surgeon aspirates the bile and crushes any large stones and then extracts the gallbladder through the umbilical port.

Removing the gallbladder with the laparoscopic technique reduces the risk for wound complications. Some patients have discomfort from carbon dioxide retention in the abdomen.

! NURSING SAFETY PRIORITY

Action Alert

After a laparoscopic cholecystectomy, assess the patient's oxygen saturation level frequently until the effects of the anesthesia have passed. Offer the patient food and water when fully awake, and monitor for nausea and vomiting. Be sure to have the head of the bed elevated in the same-day surgery unit to prevent aspiration from vomiting. Assist the patient to the bathroom to void. Early ambulation also promotes absorption of the carbon dioxide. Administer an oral opioid as needed after the laparoscopic procedure. IV pain control is usually not needed after the laparoscopic procedure because there is only one or a few small incisions that are covered with Steri-Strips and small adhesive bandages (e.g., Band-Aids).

The patient is usually discharged from the hospital or surgery center the same day, although older and obese patients may stay overnight. Provide postoperative teaching regarding pain management, incision care, and follow-up appointments. After laparoscopic surgery, the patient can return to usual activities much sooner than those having an open cholecystectomy. Most patients are able to resume usual activities within a week.

A newer procedure is *natural orifice transluminal endoscopic surgery* (NOTES) for removal of or repair of organs.

Surgery can be performed on many body organs through the mouth, vagina, and rectum. For removal of the gallbladder, the vagina is used most often in women because it can be easily decontaminated with Betadine or other antiseptic and allows easy access into the peritoneal cavity. The surgeon makes a small internal incision through the cul-de-sac of Douglas between the rectum and uterine wall to access the gallbladder. The main advantages of this procedure are the lack of visible incisions and minimal, if any, postoperative complications (Navarra et al., 2010).

Traditional Cholecystectomy. Use of the open surgical approach (abdominal laparotomy) has greatly declined during the past 20 years. Patients who have this type of surgery usually have severe biliary obstruction.

The surgical nurse provides the usual preoperative care and teaching in the operating suite on the day of surgery (see Chapter 16). The surgeon removes the gallbladder through an incision and explores the biliary ducts for the presence of stones or other cause of obstruction. If the common bile duct is explored, the surgeon may insert a T-tube drain to ensure patency of the duct, although this is not done commonly today. Trauma to the common bile duct stimulates inflammation, which can slow bile flow and contribute to bile stasis. In addition, the surgeon usually inserts a drainage tube such as a Jackson-Pratt (JP) drain. This tube is placed in the gallbladder bed to prevent fluid accumulation. The drainage is usually serosanguineous (serous fluid mixed with blood) and is stained with bile in the first 24 hours after surgery. Antibiotic therapy is given to prevent infection.

Patient care for a patient who has had a traditional open cholecystectomy is similar to the care for any patient who has had abdominal surgery under general anesthesia as described in Chapter 18. Postoperative incisional pain after a traditional cholecystectomy is controlled with opioids using a patient-controlled analgesia (PCA) pump. Encourage the patient to use coughing and deep-breathing exercises when pain is controlled and the incision is splinted.

Antiemetics may be necessary for episodes of postoperative nausea and vomiting. Administer the antiemetic early, as prescribed, to prevent retching associated with vomiting and thus to decrease pain related to muscle straining.

Provide care for the incision, the surgical drain, and possibly a T-tube to drain bile into a drainage bag via gravity flow. The surgeon typically removes the surgical dressing and drain within 24 hours after surgery.

! NURSING SAFETY PRIORITY

Action Alert

The priority for caring for the patient with a T-tube is to avoid raising the drainage system above the site of insertion to prevent backup of bile into the surgical area and causing infection. Although less commonly used today due to many complications, the T-tube may remain in place for over a week.

The patient is NPO until fully awake postoperatively. Document the patient's level of consciousness, vital signs, and pain level. Assess the surgical incision for signs of infection, such as excessive redness or purulent drainage. Report changes to the surgeon immediately. Begin ambulation as soon as possible to prevent deep vein thrombosis and promote peristalsis.

TABLE 62-2	CAUSES OF POSTCHOLECYSTECTOMY SYNDROME
• Pseudocyst • Common bile duct (CBD) leak • CBD or pancreatic duct stricture or obstruction • Sphincter of Oddi dysfunction	• Retained or new CBD gallstone • Pancreatic or liver mass • Primary sclerosing cholangitis • Diverticular compression

Advance the diet from clear liquids to solid foods as peristalsis returns. The patient usually resumes solid foods and is discharged to home 1 to 2 days after surgery, depending on any complications and the patient's general condition. In the early postoperative period, if bile flow is reduced, a low-fat diet may reduce discomfort and prevent nausea. For most patients, a special diet is not required. Advise them to eat nutritious meals and avoid excessive intake of fatty foods, especially fried food, butter, and "fast food." If the patient is obese, recommend a weight-reduction program, such as Weight Watchers.

Teach the patient to keep the incision clean and report any changes that may indicate infection. Remind him or her to report repeat abdominal or epigastric pain with vomiting that may occur several weeks to months after surgery. These symptoms indicate possible postcholecystectomy syndrome (PCS).

Although PCS occurs in a small number of patients, patients who have it are usually discouraged that they have pain after already having surgery to cure it (Comstock, 2008). Causes of PCS are listed in Table 62-2. Management depends on the exact cause but usually involves the use of endoscopic retrograde cholangiopancreatography (ERCP) to find the cause of the problem and repair it. This procedure and related nursing care are described in Chapter 55. Collaborative care includes pain management, antibiotics, nutrition and hydration therapy (possibly short-term parenteral nutrition), and control of nausea and vomiting.

❓ NCLEX EXAMINATION CHALLENGE

Physiological Integrity

A client is admitted to the same-day surgery unit after recovery from a laparoscopic cholecystectomy. Which action is the nurse's priority in caring for the client?
A. Turn the client on the right side to help the flow of bile into the drainage bag.
B. Check that the nasogastric tube is connected to low intermittent suction.
C. Document the client's use of the patient-controlled analgesia (PCA) pump.
D. Monitor the client's oxygen saturation level via pulse oximetry.

CANCER OF THE GALLBLADDER

Pathophysiology

Primary cancer of the gallbladder is rare and is more common in women than in men. Adenocarcinoma and squamous cell cancer of the gallbladder account for the majority of the cases. The tumor tends to begin in the inner layer (mucosa) of the gallbladder wall. It then grows outward to include the entire gallbladder before it begins to metastasize (spread) to close organs like the liver, small intestine, and pancreas. These rare cancers appear more frequently in patients with preexisting chronic cholecystitis and cholelithiasis. They also tend to occur more often in American Indians than in any other group, but the reason for this finding is not known (McCance et al., 2010).

PATIENT-CENTERED COLLABORATIVE CARE

▌ASSESSMENT

Early symptoms, when present, develop slowly and are similar to those of chronic cholecystitis and cholelithiasis. Assess for characteristic manifestations, which include:
- Anorexia
- Weight loss
- Nausea and vomiting
- Abdominal bloating
- Fever
- General malaise
- Jaundice (in advanced disease)
- Enlargement of the liver and spleen
- Severe abdominal pain (in advanced disease)

A moderately tender, irregularly shaped mass may be palpated. Gallbladder cancer is typically discovered during other procedures for diagnosis of suspected cholecystitis or during cholecystectomy.

The diagnosis of gallbladder cancer is usually made by ultrasonography, but other tests can be done. Some patients have a computed tomography (CT) scan or magnetic resonance cholangiopancreatography (MRCP) in which a contrast medium is injected into the bile ducts. Other more invasive tests, like endoscopic retrograde cholangiopancreatography (ERCP), may be performed. Liver function studies indicate liver involvement. Two serum tests that reveal the presence of cancer cells are carcinoembryonic antigen (CEA) assay and CA 19-9.

▌INTERVENTIONS

The prognosis for the patient with cancer of the gallbladder is poor because it is usually diagnosed in late disease due to the lack of specific manifestations. Three treatments are used: surgery, radiation therapy, and chemotherapy. Surgical intervention is either potentially curative (for an early resectable tumor) or palliative (for advanced disease with metastasis). The patient who is diagnosed with early disease has either a simple cholecystectomy (gallbladder removal) or extended cholecystectomy (removal of the gallbladder, surrounding lymph nodes, and a small margin of the liver). For palliative surgery to extend the patient's life or decrease discomfort, radical surgery is done.

Nursing care is similar to that for patients who have a cholecystectomy (see p. 1319) or Whipple procedure (see p. 1331), depending on the extent of disease. These procedures are described elsewhere in this chapter. Teach terminally ill patients and their families about end-of-life care and available hospice services (see Chapter 9).

Radiation therapy and chemotherapy alone are not effective for gallbladder cancer. However, they may be given as adjunctive procedures with surgery or instead of surgery in patients who are not surgical candidates to shrink the tumor.

Intensity-modulated radiation therapy that is much more advanced and intense than regular radiation is used. Chemotherapy with 5-fluorourical (5-FU), doxorubicin, and mitomycin may be effective in reducing tumor size. Chapter 24 describes in detail the care of the patient receiving radiation and chemotherapy.

PANCREATIC DISORDERS

ACUTE PANCREATITIS

Pathophysiology

Acute pancreatitis is a serious and, at times, life-threatening inflammatory process of the pancreas. This process is caused by a premature activation of excessive pancreatic enzymes that destroy ductal tissue and pancreatic cells, resulting in autodigestion and fibrosis of the pancreas. The pathologic changes occur in different degrees. The severity of pancreatitis depends on the extent of inflammation and tissue damage. Pancreatitis can range from mild involvement evidenced by edema and inflammation to necrotizing hemorrhagic pancreatitis (NHP). NHP is diffusely bleeding pancreatic tissue with fibrosis and tissue death.

The pancreas is unusual in that it functions as both an exocrine gland and an endocrine gland. The primary endocrine disorder is diabetes mellitus and is discussed in Chapter 67. The exocrine function of the pancreas is responsible for secreting enzymes that assist in the breakdown of starches, proteins, and fats. These enzymes are normally secreted in the inactive form and become activated once they enter the small intestine. Early activation (i.e., activation within the pancreas rather than the intestinal lumen) results in the inflammatory process of pancreatitis. Direct toxic injury to the pancreatic cells and the production and release of pancreatic enzymes (e.g., trypsin, lipase, elastase) result from the obstructive damage. After pancreatic duct obstruction, increased pressure may contribute to ductal rupture allowing spillage of trypsin and other enzymes into the pancreatic parenchymal tissue. Autodigestion of the pancreas occurs as a result (Fig. 62-2). In acute pancreatitis, four major pathophysiologic processes occur: lipolysis, proteolysis, necrosis of blood vessels, and inflammation.

The hallmark of pancreatic necrosis is enzymatic fat necrosis of the endocrine and exocrine cells of the pancreas caused by the enzyme lipase. Fatty acids are released during this lipolytic process and combine with ionized calcium to form a soaplike product. The initial rapid lowering of serum calcium levels is not readily compensated for by the parathyroid gland. Because the body needs ionized calcium and cannot use bound calcium, hypocalcemia occurs.

Proteolysis involves the splitting of proteins by hydrolysis of the peptide bonds, resulting in the formation of smaller polypeptides. Proteolytic activity may lead to thrombosis and gangrene of the pancreas. Pancreatic destruction may be localized and confined to one area or may involve the entire organ.

Elastase is activated by trypsin and causes elastic fibers of the blood vessels and ducts to dissolve. The necrosis of blood vessels results in bleeding, ranging from minor bleeding to massive hemorrhage of pancreatic tissue. Another pancreatic

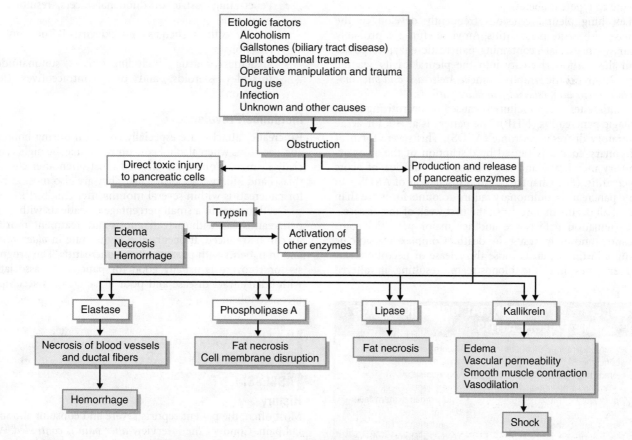

FIG. 62-2 The process of autodigestion in acute pancreatitis.

enzyme, kallikrein, causes the release of vasoactive peptides, bradykinin, and a plasma kinin known as *kallidin*. These substances contribute to vasodilation and increased vascular permeability, further compounding the hemorrhagic process. This massive destruction of blood vessels by necrosis may lead to generalized hemorrhage with blood escaping into the retroperitoneal tissues. *The patient with hemorrhagic pancreatitis is critically ill, and extensive pancreatic destruction and shock may lead to death. The majority of deaths in patients with acute pancreatitis result from irreversible shock.*

The *inflammatory stage* occurs when leukocytes cluster around the hemorrhagic and necrotic areas of the pancreas. A secondary bacterial process may lead to suppuration (pus formation) of the pancreatic parenchyma or the formation of an abscess. (See discussion of Pancreatic Abscess on p. 1328.) Mild infected lesions may be absorbed. When infected lesions are severe, calcification and fibrosis occur. If the infected fluid becomes walled off by fibrous tissue, a pancreatic pseudocyst is formed. (See discussion of Pancreatic Pseudocyst on p. 1329.)

Complications of Acute Pancreatitis

Acute pancreatitis may result in severe, life-threatening complications (Table 62-3). Jaundice occurs from swelling of the head of the pancreas, which slows bile flow through the common bile duct. The bile duct may also be compressed by calculi (stones) or a pancreatic pseudocyst. The resulting total bile flow obstruction causes severe jaundice. Intermittent hyperglycemia occurs from the release of glucagon, as well as the decreased release of insulin due to damage to the pancreatic islet cells. Total destruction of the pancreas may occur, leading to type 1 diabetes.

Left lung pleural effusions frequently develop in the patient with acute pancreatitis. Amylase effusions probably occur when exudate containing pancreatic enzymes passes from the peritoneal cavity into the pleural cavity via the transdiaphragmatic lymph channels. *Atelectasis and pneumonia may occur also, especially in older patients.*

Multi-system organ failure is caused by necrotizing hemorrhagic pancreatitis (NHP). The patient is at risk for acute respiratory distress syndrome (ARDS). This severe form of pulmonary edema is caused by disruption of the alveolar-capillary membrane and is a serious complication of acute pancreatitis. (See Chapter 34 for a discussion of ARDS.) In acute pancreatitis, pulmonary failure accounts for more than half of all deaths that occur in the first week of the disease.

Coagulation defects are another major potential complication and may result in death. Complex physiologic changes in the pancreas cause the release of necrotic tissue and enzymes into the bloodstream, resulting in altered coagulation. Disseminated intravascular coagulation (DIC) involves hypercoagulation of the blood, with consumption of clotting factors and the development of microthrombi.

Shock in acute pancreatitis results from peripheral vasodilation from the released vasoactive substances and the retroperitoneal loss of protein-rich fluid from proteolytic digestion. Hypovolemia may result in decreased renal perfusion and acute renal failure. Paralytic (adynamic) ileus results from peritoneal irritation and seepage of pancreatic enzymes into the abdominal cavity.

Etiology and Genetic Risk

In many cases, the cause of pancreatitis is not known, but many factors can injure the pancreas. The most common cause is biliary tract disease, with gallstones accounting for almost half of the cases of obstructive pancreatitis. Acute pancreatitis may occur as a result of trauma from surgical manipulation after biliary tract, pancreatic, gastric, and duodenal procedures, such as cholecystectomy, the Whipple procedure, and partial gastrectomy. The trauma may also occur as a complication of the diagnostic procedure *endoscopic retrograde cholangiopancreatography (ERCP), although this rarely occurs.*

Other causative factors include:
- Trauma: external (blunt trauma, stab wounds, gunshot wounds [GSWs])
- Pancreatic obstruction: tumors, cysts, or abscesses; abnormal organ structure
- Metabolic disturbances: hyperlipidemia, hyperparathyroidism, or hypercalcemia
- Renal disturbances: failure or transplantation
- Familial, inherited pancreatitis
- Penetrating gastric or duodenal ulcers, resulting in peritonitis
- Viral infections, such as coxsackievirus B infection
- Alcoholism
- Toxicities of drugs, including opiates, sulfonamides, thiazides, steroids, and oral contraceptives (less common)

Incidence/Prevalence

Pancreatic "attacks" are especially common during holidays and vacations when alcohol consumption may be high, especially in men. Women are affected most often after cholelithiasis and biliary tract problems. They are also most at risk for pancreatitis within several months after childbirth.

Death occurs in a small percentage of patients with acute pancreatitis, but with early diagnosis and treatment, mortality can be reduced. It occurs at a higher rate in *older adults* and in patients with postoperative pancreatitis. The prognosis for recovery is usually good for pancreatitis associated with biliary tract disease and poor if pancreatitis accompanies alcoholism.

PATIENT-CENTERED COLLABORATIVE CARE

ASSESSMENT

History

Most often, the patient reports severe and constant abdominal pain. Conduct the interview *after pain is controlled*. Ask whether the abdominal pain occurs when drinking alcohol or

---

TABLE 62-3 POTENTIAL COMPLICATIONS OF ACUTE PANCREATITIS	
• Pancreatic infection (causes septic shock)	• Acute respiratory distress syndrome (ARDS)
• Hemorrhage (necrotizing hemorrhagic pancreatitis [NHP])	• Atelectasis
• Acute kidney failure	• Pneumonia
• Paralytic ileus	• Multi-organ system failure
• Hypovolemic shock	• Disseminated intravascular coagulation (DIC)
• Pleural effusion	• Type 2 diabetes mellitus

eating a high-fat meal. Obtain information about alcohol usage, including the amount of alcohol consumed during what period of time (i.e., years of consumption, how much usually consumed over a particular period). Question the patient about a family or personal history of alcoholism, pancreatitis, trauma, or biliary tract disease. Ask whether any abdominal surgical interventions, such as cholecystectomy, or diagnostic procedures, such as ERCP, have been performed recently.

Ask about other medical problems known to cause pancreatitis, including peptic ulcer disease, renal failure, vascular disorders, hyperparathyroidism, and hyperlipidemia. Inquire about recent viral infections. Ask the patient or family member to list all prescription and over-the-counter (OTC) drugs taken recently, including nutritional and herbal supplements.

Physical Assessment/Clinical Manifestations

The diagnosis of pancreatitis is made based on the clinical presentation combined with the results of diagnostic studies—both laboratory and imaging assessments. Clinical manifestations of acute pancreatitis vary widely and depend on the severity of the inflammation. Typically, a patient is diagnosed after presenting with severe abdominal pain in the mid-epigastric area or left upper quadrant. Assess the intensity and quality of pain. The patient often states that the pain had a sudden onset and radiates to the back, left flank, or left shoulder. The pain is described as intense, boring (feeling that it is going through the body), and continuous and is worsened by lying in the supine position. Often the patient finds relief by assuming the fetal position (with the knees drawn up to the chest and the spine flexed) or by sitting upright and bending forward. He or she may report weight loss resulting from nausea and vomiting. Ask a nursing assistant or technician to weigh the patient.

When performing an abdominal assessment, inspect for:
- Generalized jaundice
- Gray-blue discoloration of the abdomen and periumbilical area
- Gray-blue discoloration of the flanks, caused by pancreatic enzyme leakage to cutaneous tissue from the peritoneal cavity

Listen for bowel sounds; absent or decreased bowel sounds usually indicate paralytic (adynamic) ileus. On light palpation, note abdominal tenderness, rigidity, and guarding as a result of peritonitis. A palpable mass may be found if a pancreatic pseudocyst is present. Pancreatic ascites creates a dull sound on percussion.

Monitor and record vital signs frequently to assess for elevated temperature, tachycardia, and decreased blood

---

❗ NURSING SAFETY PRIORITY

Critical Rescue

For the patient with acute pancreatitis, monitor for significant changes in vital signs that may indicate the life-threatening complication of shock. Hypotension and tachycardia may result from pancreatic hemorrhage, excessive fluid volume shifting, or the toxic effects of abdominal sepsis from enzyme damage. Observe the patient for changes in behavior and level of consciousness (LOC) that may be related to alcohol withdrawal, hypoxia, or impending sepsis with shock.

---

pressure, or delegate and supervise this activity. Respiratory problems, such as left lung pleural effusions, atelectasis, and pneumonia, are common in patients with acute pancreatitis. Auscultate the lung fields for adventitious sounds or diminished breath sounds, and observe for dyspnea or orthopnea.

Psychosocial Assessment

If excessive alcohol is a causative factor, tactfully explore the patient's alcohol intake history. Provide patient privacy and establish a trusting relationship. Discuss the intake of alcohol and the reasons for overindulging. Ask him or her when increased drinking episodes occur and, in particular, whether binges occur during holidays, vacations, or weekends or revolve around particular activities, such as television viewing. Question the patient about any recent traumatic or stressful event that may have contributed to increased alcohol consumption, such as the death of a family member or a job loss.

Laboratory Assessment

Diagnostic laboratory abnormalities are typical in patients with acute pancreatitis (Table 62-4). A variety of pancreatic and nonpancreatic disorders can cause increased serum amylase levels. In patients with pancreatitis, *amylase* levels usually increase within 12 to 24 hours and remain elevated for 2 to 3 days. Persistent elevations may be an indicator of pancreatic abscess or pseudocyst (Pagana & Pagana, 2010).

Lipase also helps determine the presence of acute pancreatitis. Serum levels may rise later than amylase and remain elevated for up to 2 weeks. Because these levels stay elevated for such a long time, the health care provider may find this test useful in diagnosing patients who are not examined until several days after the initial onset of symptoms. An increase in lipase and amylase in the urine is also expected (Pagana & Pagana, 2010).

If pancreatitis is accompanied by biliary dysfunction (biliary pancreatitis), serum *bilirubin* and *alkaline phosphatase* levels are usually elevated. A sensitive indicator of biliary

---

TABLE 62-4 **CAUSES OF DIAGNOSTIC LABORATORY ABNORMALITIES IN ACUTE PANCREATITIS**

ABNORMAL FINDING	CAUSE
Cardinal Diagnostic Tests	
Increased *serum* amylase	Pancreatic cell injury
Elevated *serum* lipase	Pancreatic cell injury
Elevated *serum* trypsin	Pancreatic cell injury
Elevated *serum* elastase	Pancreatic cell injury
Other Diagnostic Tests	
Elevated serum glucose	Pancreatic cell injury, resulting in impaired carbohydrate metabolism; decreased insulin release
Decreased serum calcium and magnesium	Fatty acids combined with calcium; seen in fat necrosis
Elevated bilirubin	Hepatobiliary obstructive process
Elevated alanine aminotransferase	Hepatobiliary involvement
Elevated leukocyte count	Inflammatory response

obstruction in acute pancreatitis is serum *alanine amino-transferase (ALT)*. A threefold or greater rise in concentration indicates that the diagnosis of acute biliary pancreatitis is valid. Elevated *white blood cell (WBC) count and differential, erythrocyte sedimentation rate (ESR),* and serum *glucose* levels are also common in acute pancreatitis. The levels often correlate with disease severity.

Decreased serum *calcium* and *magnesium* levels are seen with fat necrosis. Calcium levels may fall and remain decreased for 7 to 10 days. Those that consistently remain below 8 mg/dL are associated with a poor prognosis. Other tests include the basic metabolic panel (BMP), complete blood count (CBC), triglycerides, serum total protein, and albumin. The blood urea nitrogen (BUN), serum glucose, and triglycerides are usually elevated. Hemoconcentration is common as a result of third-space fluid loss. Leukocytosis (elevated WBCs) and thrombocytopenia (decreased platelets) are common (Holcomb, 2007). Albumin levels are decreased because cytokines (e.g., tumor necrosis factor [TNF]) released as part of the inflammatory response allow it to move from the bloodstream into the extravascular space. The presence of C-reactive protein suggests pancreatic inflammation and necrosis.

Imaging Assessment

Abdominal ultrasound is the most sensitive test to diagnose causes of pancreatitis like gallstones and can be performed at the bedside. However, it is not helpful in viewing the pancreas because of overlying bowel gas. Therefore *contrast-enhanced computed tomography (CT)* provides a more reliable image and diagnosis of acute pancreatitis. This noninvasive technique may also be used to rule out pancreatic pseudocyst or ductal calculi.

An abdominal x-ray may also reveal gallstones. A chest x-ray may show elevation of the left side of the diaphragm or pleural effusion. Pancreatic stones are best diagnosed through ERCP.

ANALYSIS

The priority problems for patients with acute pancreatitis are:
1. Acute Pain related to pancreatic inflammation and enzyme leakage
2. Inadequate nutrition related to the inability to ingest food and absorb nutrients

PLANNING AND IMPLEMENTATION

Managing Acute Pain

Planning: Expected Outcomes. The patient with acute pancreatitis is expected to state that he or she has a decrease in or absence of abdominal pain, as evidenced by a pain intensity scale measurement.

Interventions. The priorities for patient care are to provide supportive care by relieving symptoms, to decrease inflammation, and to anticipate or treat complications. As for any patient, continually assess for and support the ABCs (airway, breathing, and circulation). In collaboration with the respiratory therapist, if available, provide oxygen and other respiratory support as needed. The collaborative plan of care depends on the severity of the illness.

Abdominal pain is the most common symptom of pancreatitis. The main focus of nursing care is aimed at controlling pain by interventions that decrease GI tract activity, thus decreasing pancreatic stimulation. Pain assessment to measure

the effectiveness of these interventions is an essential part of nursing care.

Nonsurgical Management. Mild pancreatitis requires hydration with IV fluids, pain control, and drug therapy. The health care team initially attempts to relieve pain with nonsurgical interventions, which include fasting and rest, drug therapy, and comfort measures. If the patient has a life-threatening complication or requires frequent assessment, he or she is admitted to a critical care unit for invasive hemodynamic monitoring.

To rest the pancreas and reduce pancreatic enzyme secretion, withhold food and fluids during the acute period. The health care provider prescribes IV isotonic fluid administration to maintain hydration. IV replacement of calcium and magnesium may also be needed. Measure and document intake and output. Some patients have an indwelling urinary catheter to obtain accurate measurements.

Nasogastric drainage and suction are reserved for more *severely ill* patients who have continuous vomiting or biliary obstruction. Gastric decompression using a nasogastric tube (NGT) prevents gastric juices from flowing into the duodenum.

> ### ! NURSING SAFETY PRIORITY
> #### Action Alert
> Because paralytic (adynamic) ileus is a common complication of acute pancreatitis, prolonged nasogastric intubation may be necessary. Assess frequently for the return of peristalsis by asking the patient if he or she has passed flatus or had a stool. The return of bowel sounds is not reliable as an indicator of peristalsis return.

To decrease pain, the primary drug class used is opioid. Other drugs may also be prescribed. Pain management for acute pancreatitis typically begins with the administration of opioids by patient-controlled analgesia (PCA). Drugs such as morphine or hydromorphone (Dilaudid) are typically used because meperidine (Demerol) can cause seizures, especially in older adults. Other options that have been used successfully to manage acute pain include IV or transdermal fentanyl and epidural analgesia.

In *mild* pancreatitis, the pain usually subsides in 2 to 3 days. However, with *severe* acute pancreatitis, the abdominal pain and tenderness may persist for up to 2 weeks. The dosages and intervals of drug administration are individualized according to the severity of the disease and the symptoms.

Histamine receptor antagonists (e.g., ranitidine [Zantac]) and proton pump inhibitors (e.g., omeprazole [Prilosec]) help decrease gastric acid secretion. Antibiotics may be used, but they are indicated primarily for patients with acute necrotizing pancreatitis. Common drugs used include cefuroxime (Zinacef) and ceftazidime (Ceptaz).

Helping the patient assume a side-lying position (with the legs drawn up to the chest) may decrease the abdominal pain of pancreatitis. Sitting with the knees flexed toward the chest is also helpful.

If the patient is NPO or has an NGT, remind assistive nursing personnel to implement frequent oral hygiene measures to keep mucous membranes moist and free of inflammation or crusting. Because of the drying effect of drugs and the absence of oral fluids, the mouth and oral cavity may be extremely dry, resulting in considerable discomfort and possibly parotitis (inflammation of the parotid [salivary] glands).

> ## ! NURSING SAFETY PRIORITY
> ### Action Alert
>
> For the patient with acute pancreatitis, monitor his or her respiratory status every 8 hours or more often as needed, and provide oxygen to promote comfort in breathing. Respiratory complications such as pleural effusions increase patient discomfort. Fluid overload can be detected by assessing for weight gain, listening for crackles, and observing for dyspnea. Carefully monitor for signs of respiratory failure.
>
> Observe for signs and symptoms of hypocalcemia by assessing for Chvostek's and Trousseau's signs. These tests cause muscle spasms after stimulating the associated nerves. Chapter 13 discusses assessment and interventions for patients with hypocalcemia in more detail.

Lowering the patient's anxiety level may also substantially reduce pain. Explain all procedures and other aspects of patient care thoroughly. Provide reassurance, offer diversional activities such as music and reading material, and encourage visitors to direct attention away from the pain.

If pancreatitis was caused by gallstones, an ERCP with a sphincterotomy (opening of the sphincter of Oddi) may be performed on an urgent or emergent basis. If this procedure is not successful, surgery is required. ERCP is described in detail in Chapter 55.

Surgical Management. Surgical intervention for acute pancreatitis is usually not indicated. However, if an ERCP is not successful in removing gallstones, a laparoscopic cholecystectomy may be performed as described on p. 1319 in the discussion of Surgical Management in the Cholecystitis section.

Complications of pancreatitis, such as pancreatic pseudocyst and abscess, may also require surgical intervention. Laparoscopy (minimally invasive surgery [MIS]) may be done to drain an abscess or pseudocyst. For patients who are high surgical risks, pseudocysts or abscesses can be treated by percutaneous drainage under CT guidance.

Promoting Nutrition

Planning: Expected Outcomes. The patient with acute pancreatitis is expected to have adequate nutrition to meet his or her metabolic needs.

Interventions. The patient is maintained on NPO status in the early stages of pancreatitis. Antiemetics for nausea and vomiting are prescribed as needed. Patients who have severe pancreatitis and are unable to eat for 24 to 48 hours after illness onset may begin jejunal tube feeding unless paralytic ileus is present. *Early* nutritional intervention enhances immune system functioning and may prevent complications and worsening inflammation. Enteral feeding is preferred over total parenteral nutrition (TPN) because it causes fewer episodes of glucose elevation and other complications associated with TPN. Be sure that the patient is weighed every day. Collaborate with the health care provider, dietitian, and pharmacist to plan and implement the most appropriate nutritional intervention. Chapter 63 describes collaborative care of patients receiving enteral feeding and TPN.

When food is tolerated during the healing phase, the health care provider prescribes small, frequent, moderate- to high-carbohydrate, high-protein, low-fat meals. Foods should be bland with little spice. GI stimulants such as caffeine-containing foods (tea, coffee, cola, and chocolate), as well as alcohol, should be avoided. Monitor the patient beginning to resume oral food intake for nausea, vomiting, and diarrhea. *If any of these symptoms occur, notify the health care provider immediately.*

To boost caloric intake, commercial liquid nutritional preparations supplement the diet. The health care provider may also prescribe fat-soluble and other vitamin and mineral replacement supplements. Glutamine, omega-3 fatty acids, fiber, antioxidants, and/or nucleotides may be added to the patient's nutrition plan.

Community-Based Care

Home care preparation is individualized for each patient's circumstances. Some patients may be severely weakened from their acute illness and need to confine activity to one floor, limiting stair climbing and other strenuous activities until they regain their strength. Collaborate with the case manager to plan the best place for the patient to recover and resources that may be needed.

Education needs to be started early in the hospitalization period—as soon as the acute episodes of pain have subsided. Assess the patient's and family's knowledge of the disease.

The desired outcomes for discharge planning and education are to avoid further episodes of pancreatitis and prevent progression to a chronic disease. If the patient abuses alcohol, instruct him or her to abstain from drinking to prevent further pain attacks and extension of inflammation and pancreatic insufficiency. Tell the patient that if alcohol is consumed, acute pain will return and further autodigestion of the pancreas may lead to chronic pancreatitis.

Teach the patient to notify the health care provider after discharge to home if acute abdominal pain or biliary tract disease (as evidenced by jaundice, clay-colored stools, or darkened urine) occurs. These signs and symptoms are possible indicators of complications or disease progression.

Patients with acute pancreatitis may require several visits by a home care nurse if the hospital course was complicated. In these cases, home care may be needed for wound care and assistance with ADLs. The patient requires medical follow-up

> ## ? DECISION-MAKING CHALLENGE
> ### Patient-Centered Care; Evidence-Based Practice; Teamwork and Collaboration; Informatics
>
> A 78-year-old man is admitted from home to the medical unit with acute pancreatitis secondary to a history of gallstones, hypertension, osteoarthritis, and type 2 diabetes mellitus. He has lost 20 pounds (9.0 kg) in the past 2 months and reports severe boring-like abdominal pain, fatigue, and weakness. On physical assessment, he has decreased bowel sounds in all quadrants, crackles in the bases of his lungs, and signs of dehydration. Vital signs are: T, 100° F; P, 110; R, 36; and BP, 102/58.
>
> 1. What is the priority for this patient's care at this time? What current evidence supports your answer? Where would you look for current evidence that would help you answer this question? (Be specific in your answer.)
> 2. What laboratory findings would you expect him to have? Why?
> 3. With whom should you collaborate to meet the desired outcomes for his care?
> 4. What community support and health teaching is he going to require when he is discharged?

with the primary care physician or nurse practitioner to monitor the disease process. For those with alcoholism, provide information about groups such as Alcoholics Anonymous (AA). Family members may attend support groups such as Al-Anon and Alateen.

EVALUATION: OUTCOMES

Evaluate the care of the patient with acute pancreatitis based on the identified priority patient problems. The expected outcomes include that the patient will:

- Have control of abdominal pain, as indicated by self-report
- Have adequate nutrients available to meet metabolic needs

CHRONIC PANCREATITIS

Pathophysiology

Chronic pancreatitis is a progressive, destructive disease of the pancreas that has remissions and exacerbations ("flare-ups"). Inflammation and fibrosis of the tissue contribute to pancreatic insufficiency and diminished function of the organ.

Chronic pancreatitis can be classified into several categories. *Alcoholism* is the primary risk factor for chronic calcifying pancreatitis (CCP), the most common type. In the early stages of the disease, pancreatic secretions precipitate as insoluble proteins that plug the pancreatic ducts and flow of pancreatic juices. As the protein plugs become more widespread, the cellular lining of the ducts changes and ulcerates. This inflammatory process causes fibrosis of the pancreatic tissue. Intraductal calcification and marked pancreatic tissue destruction (necrosis) develop in the late stages. The organ becomes hard and firm as a result of cell atrophy and pancreatic insufficiency.

Chronic calcifying pancreatitis is found predominantly in men, but the incidence in women is increasing. In women, chronic pancreatitis occurs more commonly among those with biliary tract disease (cholecystitis and cholelithiasis).

Chronic obstructive pancreatitis develops from inflammation, spasm, and obstruction of the sphincter of Oddi, often from cholelithiasis (gallstones). Inflammatory and sclerotic lesions occur in the head of the pancreas and around the ducts, causing an obstruction and backflow of pancreatic secretions. (See Complications of Acute Pancreatitis, p. 1322.)

Autoimmune pancreatitis is a chronic inflammatory process in which immunoglobulins invade the pancreas. Other organs may also be infiltrated, including the lungs and liver. Whereas other types of chronic pancreatitis may predispose the patient to pancreatic cancer, there is no evidence that autoimmune pancreatitis is a risk factor (Novotny et al., 2010).

Idiopathic and hereditary chronic pancreatitis may be associated with *SPINK1* and *CFTR* gene mutations (Midha et al., 2010). The protein encoded by the *SPINK1* gene is a trypsin inhibitor. The *CFTR* gene is associated with cystic fibrosis. Research on these gene mutations can help develop targeted drug therapy for treatment of these diseases.

Pancreatic insufficiency in any type of chronic pancreatitis causes loss of *exocrine* function. Most patients with chronic pancreatitis have decreased pancreatic secretions and bicarbonate. Pancreatic enzyme secretion must be greatly reduced to produce steatorrhea resulting from severe malabsorption

of fats. These characteristic stools are pale, bulky, and frothy and have an offensive odor. The action of colonic bacteria on unabsorbed lipids and proteins is responsible for the extremely foul odor. On inspection of the stools, the fat content is visible. In severe chronic pancreatitis, stool fat output may be more than 40 g/day.

Fat malabsorption also contributes to weight loss and muscle wasting (a decrease in muscle mass) and leads to general debilitation. Protein malabsorption results in a "starvation" edema of the feet, legs, and hands caused by decreased levels of circulating albumin.

The loss of pancreatic *endocrine* function is responsible for the development of diabetes mellitus in patients with chronic pancreatic insufficiency. (See Chapter 67 for a complete discussion of diabetes mellitus.)

The patient with chronic pancreatitis may have pulmonary complications, such as pleuritic pain, pleural effusions, and pulmonary infiltrates. Pancreatic ascites may decrease diaphragmatic excursion and lung expansion, resulting in impaired ventilation. In the ill patient with chronic pancreatitis, acute respiratory distress syndrome (ARDS) may develop.

PATIENT-CENTERED COLLABORATIVE CARE

ASSESSMENT

Many of the clinical manifestations of chronic pancreatitis differ from those of an acute inflammation. Abdominal pain is the major clinical manifestation for most types of pancreatitis (Chart 62-2). For those with chronic pancreatitis, pain is typically describes as a continuous burning or gnawing dullness with periods of acute exacerbation (flare-ups). The pain is very intense and relentless. The frequency of acute exacerbations may increase as the pancreatic fibrosis develops.

Perform an abdominal assessment. Abdominal tenderness is less intense in patients with chronic pancreatitis than in those with acute pancreatitis. A mass may be palpated in the left upper quadrant, which may suggest a pancreatic pseudocyst or abscess. Massive pancreatic ascites may be present, producing dullness on abdominal percussion. Because respiratory complications can occur, auscultate the lung fields for adventitious sounds or decreased aeration and observe for dyspnea or orthopnea.

CHART 62-2 **KEY FEATURES**

Chronic Pancreatitis

- Intense abdominal pain (major clinical manifestation) that is continuous and burning or gnawing
- Abdominal tenderness
- Ascites
- Possible left upper quadrant mass (if pseudocyst or abscess is present)
- Respiratory compromise manifested by adventitious or diminished breath sounds, dyspnea, or orthopnea
- Steatorrhea; clay-colored stools
- Weight loss
- Jaundice
- Dark urine
- Polyuria, polydipsia, polyphagia (diabetes mellitus)

Ask the patient to collect a random stool specimen if able, or ask him or her to describe the stools. The specimen may show steatorrhea (foul-smelling fatty stools that may increase in volume as pancreatic insufficiency progresses and lipase production decreases). Assess for unintentional weight loss, muscle wasting, jaundice, dark urine, and the manifestations of diabetes mellitus, such as polyuria (increased urinary output), polydipsia (excessive thirst), and polyphagia (increased appetite).

Diagnosis is based on the patient's clinical manifestations and laboratory and imaging assessment. Endoscopic retrograde cholangiopancreatography (ERCP) is done to visualize the pancreatic and common bile ducts. Imaging studies such as computed tomography (CT) scanning, contrast-enhanced magnetic resonance imaging (MRI), abdominal ultrasound (US), and endoscopic ultrasound (EUS) are also useful in making the diagnosis. In chronic pancreatitis, laboratory findings include normal or moderately elevated serum amylase and lipase levels. Obstruction of the intrahepatic bile duct can cause elevated serum bilirubin and alkaline phosphatase levels. Intermittent elevations in serum glucose levels are common and can be detected by blood glucose monitoring, both fasting and non-fasting.

▌INTERVENTIONS

The focus of caring for the patient with chronic pancreatitis is to manage pain, assist in maintaining a sufficient nutritional intake, and prevent recurrence.

Nonsurgical Management

Nonsurgical interventions include primarily drug and nutrition therapy. The major intervention for the pain of chronic pancreatitis is drug therapy. Medicate the patient as prescribed according to the assessment of the intensity of pain. Evaluate the effectiveness of the drug intervention. Opioid analgesia is most frequently used initially, but dependency may occur. Non-opioid analgesics may be tried to relieve pain. (See Chapter 5 for other interventions for chronic pain.)

Pancreatic-enzyme replacement therapy (PERT) is the standard of care to prevent malnutrition, malabsorption, and excessive weight loss (Chart 62-3). Pancrelipase is usually prescribed in capsule or tablet form and contains varying amounts of amylase, lipase, and protease. Pancrelipase delayed-release capsules (Creon) or enteric tablets should not be crushed or chewed.

! NURSING SAFETY PRIORITY

Drug Alert

Teach the patient who is taking pancreatic-enzyme replacement therapy to take these drugs with meals and snacks and a glass of water. Instruct patients who have difficulty swallowing either to cover the capsules with applesauce or, if needed, open the capsules and spread their contents over applesauce, mashed fruit, or rice cereal. Enzyme preparations should not be mixed with foods containing proteins because the enzymatic action dissolves the food into a watery substance. Be sure that patients drink a full glass of water after taking the drug to ensure that none of the enzymes remain in the mouth. Advise patients to wipe their lips with a wet towel to prevent the skin irritation and breakdown that residual enzymes can cause.

The dosage of pancreatic enzymes depends on the severity of the malabsorption. Record the number and consistency of

---

CHART 62-3   PATIENT AND FAMILY EDUCATION: PREPARING FOR SELF-MANAGEMENT

Enzyme Replacement for the Patient with Chronic Pancreatitis

- Take pancreatic enzymes with meals and snacks and follow with a glass of water.
- Administer enzymes after antacid or H_2 blockers. (Decreased pH inactivates drug.)
- Swallow the tablets or capsules without chewing to minimize oral irritation and to allow the drug to be released slowly.
- If you cannot swallow the capsule, pierce the gelatin casing and place contents in applesauce.
- Do not mix enzyme preparations in protein-containing foods.
- Wipe your lips after taking enzymes to avoid skin irritation.
- Do not crush enteric-coated preparations.
- Follow up on all scheduled laboratory testing. (Pancrelipase can cause an increase in uric acid levels.)

---

stools per day to monitor the effectiveness of enzyme therapy. If pancreatic enzyme treatment is effective, the stools should become less frequent and less fatty.

If the patient has diabetes, the health care provider prescribes insulin or oral hypoglycemic agents for glucose control. Patients maintained on total parenteral nutrition (TPN) are particularly susceptible to elevated glucose levels and may require regular insulin additives to the solution. Closely monitor blood glucose so that hyperglycemia is controlled. Check finger-stick blood glucose (FSBG) or sugar (FSBS) levels every 2 to 4 hours. Chapter 63 describes in detail the care associated with TPN.

The health care provider may also prescribe drug therapy to decrease gastric acid. Gastric acid destroys the lipase needed to break down fats. Controlling the acidity of the stomach with H_2 blockers or proton pump inhibitors or neutralizing stomach acid with oral sodium bicarbonate may enhance the effectiveness of PERT.

Protein and fat malabsorption result in significant weight loss and decreased muscle mass in the patient with chronic pancreatitis. Therefore the nutritional interventions for acute pancreatitis are also used for chronic pancreatitis. The patient often limits food intake to avoid increased pain. For this reason, nutrition maintenance is often difficult to achieve. Patients receive either total parenteral nutrition (TPN) or total enteral nutrition (TEN), including vitamin and mineral replacement.

Collaborate with the dietitian to teach the patient about long-term dietary management. He or she needs an increased number of calories, up to 4000 to 6000 calories/day, to maintain weight. Those foods high in carbohydrates and protein also assist in the healing process. Foods high in fat are avoided because they cause or increase diarrhea. Teach all patients to avoid alcohol. Alcohol-cessation programs may be recommended.

Surgical Management

Surgery is not a primary intervention for the treatment of chronic pancreatitis. However, it may be indicated for ongoing abdominal pain, incapacitating relapses of pain, or complications such as abscesses and pseudocysts.

The underlying pathologic changes determine the procedure indicated. Using laparoscopy, the surgeon incises and drains an abscess or pseudocyst. Laparoscopic cholecystectomy or choledochotomy (incision of the common bile duct) may be indicated if biliary tract disease is an underlying cause of pancreatitis. If the pancreatic duct sphincter is fibrotic, the surgeon performs a sphincterotomy (incision of the sphincter) to enlarge it. Endoscopic sphincterotomy may be used for patients who are poor surgical candidates.

In some cases, laparoscopic distal pancreatectomy may be appropriate for resection of the distal pancreas or pancreas head. Endoscopic pancreatic necrosectomy and natural orifice transluminal endoscopic surgery (NOTES) are becoming more common for removing necrosed pancreatic tissue. Both procedures are performed through the GI wall without a visible skin incision. The NOTES procedure is discussed in Surgical Management on p. 1319 in the Cholecystitis section.

In a few cases, pancreas transplantation may be done. However, this procedure is performed most often for patients with severe, uncontrolled diabetes. Chapter 67 discusses pancreas transplantation.

Community-Based Care

Collaborate with the hospital-based case manager (CM) or discharge planner about home care or follow-up in another setting. A community-based CM may continue to follow the patient after hospital discharge. If the patient is discharged to home, the activity area should be limited to one floor until he or she regains strength and can increase activity. Teach patients and families that toilet facilities must be easily accessible because of chronic steatorrhea and frequent defecation. If they are not easily accessible, a bedside commode is obtained for the home.

Because there is no known cure for chronic pancreatitis, patient and family education is aimed at preventing acute episodes of the disease, providing long-term care, and promoting health maintenance (Chart 62-4). Teach the patient to avoid known irritating substances, such as caffeinated beverages (stimulates the GI system) and alcohol. Collaborate with the dietitian in diet teaching, which focuses on eating bland, low-fat, frequent meals and avoiding rich, fatty foods. Stress the importance of adhering to the nutritional recommendations. Written instructions are essential, with consideration of personal and cultural food preferences.

Remind the patient and family members or significant others of the importance of adhering to pancreatic enzyme replacement. The patient must take the prescribed enzymes with meals and snacks to aid in the digestion of food and promote the absorption of fats and proteins. Teach the patient to take the enzymes before or at the beginning of the meal. Instruct him or her to report any increase in abdominal distention, cramping, and foul-smelling, frothy, fatty stools to the health care provider so that these supplements may be increased as needed. Remind the patient to report any skin breakdown so that therapeutic interventions to promote skin integrity can be started. Abdominal fistulas are common and present a difficult challenge because pancreatic secretions irritate the skin.

The frequency of defecation (whether continent or incontinent) poses challenging skin care problems. Instruct the patient to keep the skin dry and free of the abrasive fatty stools, which damage the skin. The skin should be cleaned thoroughly after each stool and a moisture barrier applied to prevent breakdown and maintain skin integrity. Many products on the market actively repel stool from the skin.

If the patient develops diabetes mellitus as a result of chronic pancreatitis, management of elevated glucose levels after discharge from the hospital may require oral antidiabetic agents or insulin injections. If this is the case, collaborate with the certified diabetic educator (CDE) to provide in-depth teaching concerning diabetes, its signs and symptoms, medical management, drug therapy, nutrition therapy, blood glucose monitoring, and general care.

Chronic illnesses are devastating for families. The high costs of medical insurance, medical treatment, and drug therapy cause serious financial problems. Often the patient with chronic pancreatitis is unable to work. Collaborate with the CM about ways to assist the patient with resources for financial help.

The patient may require several home visits by nurses, depending on the severity of the chronic health problems and home maintenance and support needs. The nurse assesses the patient for pain management, adherence to the nutritional plan and alcohol abstinence, the effectiveness of pancreatic enzyme therapy, and psychosocial adaptation to a chronic illness. Refer him or her and the family to a counselor or a self-help group, such as Alcoholics Anonymous (www.aa.org) and Al-Anon (www.al-anon.org), if appropriate.

CHART 62-4 PATIENT AND FAMILY EDUCATION: PREPARING FOR SELF-MANAGEMENT

Prevention of Exacerbations of Chronic Pancreatitis

- Avoid things that make your symptoms worse, such as drinking caffeinated beverages.
- Avoid alcohol ingestion; refer to self-help group for assistance.
- Avoid nicotine.
- Eat bland, low-fat, high-protein, moderate-carbohydrate meals; avoid gastric stimulants, such as spices.
- Eat small meals and snacks high in calories.
- Take the pancreatic enzymes that have been prescribed for you with meals.
- Rest frequently; restrict your activity to one floor until you regain your strength.

❓ NCLEX EXAMINATION CHALLENGE
Physiological Integrity

The physician assistant prescribes pancreatic enzyme replacement capsules for a client with chronic pancreatitis. What health teaching will the nurse provide?
A. "Take the enzymes after meals to be most effective."
B. "Swallow the capsule whole or with applesauce."
C. "Drink a full glass of milk after taking the drug."
D. "Crush the capsules and tablets and mix with juice."

PANCREATIC ABSCESS

Pancreatic abscesses are the most serious complication of acute necrotizing pancreatitis. If untreated, they are always fatal. After surgery, the recurrence rate is high. The abscesses form from collections of purulent liquefaction of the necrotic pancreas.

Pancreatic abscesses occur after severe acute pancreatitis, episodes of chronic pancreatitis, or gallbladder surgery. The development of either a single abscess or multiple abscesses results from extensive inflammatory necrosis of the pancreas that is readily invaded by infectious organisms, such as enteric bacteria and *Candida*. They can erode through the retroperitoneum into the bowel mesentery, the mediastinum, the pleural space, or the pelvis.

Patients with pancreatic abscesses often appear more seriously ill than those with pseudocysts. Clinical manifestations are similar. However, the temperature in patients with abscesses may spike to as high as 104° F (40° C). Blood cultures are helpful in revealing the infective organism. Pleural effusions commonly accompany these abscesses if they enter the pleural space. Ultrasonography and contrast-enhanced computed tomography (CT) cannot differentiate between pancreatic pseudocysts and abscesses.

Drainage via the percutaneous method or laparoscopy should be performed as soon as possible to prevent sepsis. Antibiotic treatment alone does not resolve the abscess. Death rates remain high even after surgical drainage. Many patients require multiple drainage procedures for repeated abscesses.

PANCREATIC PSEUDOCYST

Pathophysiology

Pancreatic pseudocysts, or false cysts, are so named because, unlike true cysts, they do not have an epithelial lining. They are encapsulated, saclike structures that form on or surround the pancreas. The pseudocyst wall is inflamed, vascular, and fibrotic. It may contain up to several liters of straw-colored or dark brown viscous fluid, the enzymatic exudate of the pancreas (McCance et al., 2010). Risk factors for pseudocysts are acute pancreatitis, abdominal trauma, and chronic pancreatitis.

PATIENT-CENTERED COLLABORATIVE CARE

A pseudocyst can be palpated as an epigastric mass in about half of all cases. The primary presenting symptom is epigastric pain radiating to the back. Other common clinical manifestations include abdominal fullness, nausea, vomiting, and jaundice. Pseudocysts are diagnosed and their growth and resolution monitored by serial pancreatic diagnostic testing. Complications of pseudocyst formation include:

- Hemorrhage
- Infection
- Obstruction of the bowel, biliary tract, or splenic vein
- Abscess
- Fistula formation
- Pancreatic ascites

Pseudocysts may spontaneously resolve, or they may rupture and produce hemorrhage. Surgical intervention is necessary if the pseudocyst does not resolve within 6 to 8 weeks or if complications develop. Possible surgeries include:

- Percutaneous drainage using a needle, usually under CT scan guidance
- Endoscopic-assisted drainage using an endoscope to locate the pseudocyst
- Surgical drainage of the pseudocyst into the stomach or jejunum

To provide external drainage, the surgeon inserts a sump drainage tube to remove pancreatic secretions and exudate. Pancreatic fistulas are common after surgery, and skin breakdown from corrosive pancreatic enzymes in patients who have external drainage presents a major nursing care challenge.

PANCREATIC CANCER

Pathophysiology

Cancer of the pancreas is a leading cause of cancer deaths each year in the United States. It is difficult to diagnose early because the pancreas is hidden and surrounded by other organs. Treatment has limited results, and 5-year survival rates are low (American Cancer Society [ACS], 2010).

Pancreatic tumors usually originate from epithelial cells of the pancreatic ductal system. If the tumor is discovered in the early stages, the tumor cells may be localized within the glandular organ. However, this is highly unlikely. Most often, the tumor is discovered in the late stages of development and may be a well-defined mass or is diffusely spread throughout the pancreas.

The tumor may be a primary cancer, or it may result from metastasis from cancers of the lung, breast, thyroid, kidney, or skin. Primary tumors are generally adenocarcinomas and grow in well-differentiated glandular patterns. They grow rapidly and spread to surrounding organs (stomach, duodenum, gallbladder, and intestine) by direct extension and invasion of lymphatic and vascular systems. This highly metastatic lesion may eventually invade the lung, peritoneum, liver, spleen, and lymph nodes.

Clinical manifestations depend on the site of origin or metastasis. The head of the pancreas is the most common site. The tumors are usually small lesions with poorly defined margins. Jaundice results from tumor compression and obstruction of the common bile duct and from gallbladder dilation, causing the organ to enlarge.

Cancers of the body and tail of the pancreas are usually large and invade the entire tail and body. These tumors may be palpable abdominal masses, especially in the thin patient. Through metastatic spread via the splenic vein, metastasis to the liver may cause hepatomegaly (enlargement of the liver up to two to three times its normal size). Cancers of the body and tail spread more extensively than do pancreatic head carcinomas, with invasion of the retroperitoneum, vertebral column, spleen, adrenal glands, colon, or stomach. Regardless of where it originates, it spreads rapidly through the lymphatic and venous systems to other organs.

Venous thromboembolism is a common complication of pancreatic cancer. Necrotic products of the pancreatic tumor are believed to have thromboplastic properties resulting in the blood's hypercoagulable state. In addition, the patient is at high risk because of decreased mobility and extensive surgical manipulation.

GENETIC/GENOMIC CONSIDERATIONS

A small number of those with pancreatic cancer have an inherited risk. Mutations in certain oncogenes have been identified. Mutations have also been revealed in tumor suppressor genes, such as *p16* and *BRCA2*—the same mutation that makes some women susceptible to breast and ovarian cancer. Genes responsible for hereditary nonpolyposis colorectal cancer can also increase a person's risk for pancreatic cancer (ACS, 2010).

The exact cause of pancreatic cancer is unknown. High-risk populations are those in their sixth to eighth decades of life and those with a personal history of smoking.

Other risk factors associated with the disease include:
- Diabetes mellitus
- Chronic pancreatitis
- Cirrhosis
- High intake of red meat, especially processed meat like bacon
- Long-term exposure to chemicals such as gasoline and pesticides
- Obesity

PATIENT-CENTERED COLLABORATIVE CARE

ASSESSMENT

Pancreatic cancer often presents in a slow and vague manner. The presenting symptoms depend somewhat on the location of the tumor. The first sign may be jaundice, which suggests late, advanced disease (Chart 62-5). Jaundice occurs because the gallbladder and liver are commonly involved. As the tumor spreads, the green-gold skin color associated with obstructive jaundice progressively worsens. Ask the patient whether the color of the stool and urine has changed. As a result of the obstructive process, the stool is clay colored and the urine is dark and frothy. Inspect the skin for dryness and scratch marks, indicating pruritus from jaundice caused by bile salt collection. Assess the sclerae for icterus (yellowing) and the mucous membranes for signs of jaundice.

The enlarged gallbladder and liver may be palpable. In advanced cases of pancreatic carcinoma, the tumor may be felt as a firm, fixed mass in the left upper abdominal quadrant or epigastric region.

The most common concern is fatigue, which is described as a diminished energy level and an increased need for rest relative to the level of activity. The patient notices an inability to perform usual physical or intellectual activities.

Question the patient about abdominal pain, which is usually described as a vague, constant dullness in the upper abdomen and nonspecific in nature. Pain also indicates advanced stages of the disease and may be related to eating or activity. Ask whether the patient has pain in other areas of the body. Referred back pain may be caused by pressure on the nerve plexus. Some patients have leg or calf pain with swelling and redness as a result of deep vein thrombosis or thrombophlebitis.

CHART 62-5 **KEY FEATURES**

Pancreatic Cancer

- Jaundice
- Clay- (light) colored stools
- Dark urine
- Abdominal pain: usually vague, dull, or nonspecific that radiates into the back
- Weight loss
- Anorexia
- Nausea or vomiting
- Glucose intolerance
- Splenomegaly (enlarged spleen)
- Flatulence
- Gastrointestinal bleeding
- Ascites (abdominal fluid)
- Leg or calf pain (from thrombophlebitis)
- Weakness and fatigue

Weigh the patient to determine the extent of weight loss and whether it has occurred rapidly. Ask about food intake and intolerances. Anorexia accompanied by early satiety, nausea, flatulence (gas), and vomiting are common. GI bleeding may develop from esophageal or gastric varices caused by the tumor pressing on the portal vein. A new diagnosis of diabetes is found in some patients.

In addition to the focused history, perform a general abdominal assessment. In particular, observe for distention and swelling, which may be ascites (abdominal fluid). Percussion over the ascitic abdomen elicits dullness, seen in the advanced stages of the disease process.

No specific blood tests diagnose pancreatic cancer. Serum amylase and lipase levels, as well as alkaline phosphatase and bilirubin levels, are increased. The degree of elevation depends on the acuteness or chronicity of the pancreatic and biliary damage. Elevated carcinoembryonic antigen (CEA) levels occur in most patients with pancreatic cancer. This test may provide early information about the presence of tumor cells. Other tumor markers such as CA 19-9 and CA 242 have been found to be useful serologic tests for monitoring a proven diagnosis and for continuing surveillance for potential spread or recurrence (Pagana & Pagana, 2010).

Abdominal ultrasound and contrast-enhanced computed tomography (CT) are the most commonly used imaging techniques for confirming a tumor and can differentiate the tumor from a cyst. Endoscopic ultrasonography can also be performed to sample tissue for diagnosis and provide information on tumor type and size (Riehl, 2007). Contrast harmonic echo-endoscopic ultrasound increases the accuracy of diagnosing solid pancreatic masses (Fusaroli et al., 2010).

Endoscopic retrograde cholangiopancreatography (ERCP) also provides visual diagnostic data. An alternative to ERCP is a percutaneous transhepatic biliary cholangiogram with placement of a percutaneous transhepatic biliary drain (PTBD). This drain decompresses the blocked biliary system by draining bile, either internally, externally, or both. Aspiration of pancreatic ascitic fluid by abdominal paracentesis may reveal cancer cells and elevated amylase levels.

INTERVENTIONS

Management of the patient with pancreatic cancer is geared toward preventing tumor spread and decreasing pain. These measures are not curative, only palliative. The cancers are often metastatic and recur despite treatment.

Nonsurgical Management

As in other types of cancer, chemotherapy or radiation is used to relieve pain by shrinking the tumor. It may be used before, after, or instead of surgery. *Chemotherapy* has had limited success in increasing survival time. In most cases, combining agents has been more successful than single-agent chemotherapy. 5-Fluorouracil (5-FU), a commonly used drug, may be given alone or with gemcitabine (Gemzar) for locally advanced, or unresectable, pancreatic cancers. Gemcitabine may also be given with capecitabine (Xeloda), docetaxel (Taxotere), and/or erlotinib (Tarceva), a targeted agent for unresectable or metastatic tumors. Some patients receive three or four drugs and have had more tumor shrinkage as a result. Observe for adverse drug effects, such as fatigue, rash, anorexia, and diarrhea.

Other targeted therapies being investigated include growth factor inhibitors, anti-angiogenesis factors, and kinase inhibitors (also known as *tyrosine kinase inhibitors*). Kinase inhibitors are a newer group of drugs that focus on cancer cells with little or no effect on healthy cells. Chapter 24 describes general nursing interventions associated with chemotherapy.

To control pain, the patient takes high doses of opioid analgesics (usually morphine) as prescribed and uses other comfort measures before the pain escalates and peaks. Because of the poor prognosis, drug dependency is not a consideration. Chapter 5 describes in detail the care of the patient with chronic cancer pain.

Intensive external beam *radiation* therapy to the pancreas may offer pain relief by shrinking tumor cells, alleviating obstruction, and improving food absorption. It does not improve survival rates. Implantation of radioactive iodine (^{125}I) seeds, in combination with systemic or intra-arterial administration of floxuridine (FUDR), has also been used. The patient may experience discomfort during and after the radiation treatments. Chapter 24 describes radiation therapy in more detail.

For patients experiencing biliary obstruction who are high surgical risks, biliary stents placed percutaneously (through the skin) can ensure patency to relieve pain. These stents are devices made of plastic materials that keep the ducts of the biliary system open. Using another approach, self-expandable stents may be inserted endoscopically to relieve obstruction.

Surgical Management

Complete surgical resection of the pancreatic tumor offers the patient with pancreatic cancer the only effective treatment, but it is done only in patients with small tumors. *Partial pancreatectomy* is the preferred surgery for tumors smaller than 3 centimeters in diameter (Halls & Ward-Smith, 2007). Recent technologic advances have expanded the role of minimally invasive surgery (MIS) via laparoscopy in the staging, palliation, and removal of pancreatic cancers. The procedure selected depends on the purpose of the surgery and stage of the disease. For example, if the patient has a biliary obstruction, a laparoscopic procedure to relieve the obstruction is performed. This procedure diverts bile drainage into the jejunum.

For larger tumors, the surgeon may perform either a *radical pancreatectomy* or the *Whipple procedure (pancreaticoduodenectomy)*. These procedures have traditionally been done using an open surgical approach. Because of new advances in laparoscopic technology using a hand-assist device, this method is beginning to replace the conventional method. Some surgeons are not yet trained in how to perform this technique. Therefore the traditional open surgical approach remains the most common method of performing these surgeries.

Preoperative Care. The patient with pancreatic cancer may be a poor surgical risk because of malnutrition and debilitation. Specific care depends on the type of surgical approach being used.

Often, in the late stages of pancreatic cancer or before the Whipple procedure, the physician inserts a small catheter into the jejunum (jejunostomy) so that enteral feedings may be given. This feeding method is preferred to prevent reflux and to facilitate absorption. Feedings are started in low concentrations and volumes and are gradually increased as tolerated.

Provide feedings using a pump to maintain a constant volume, and assess for diarrhea frequency to determine tolerance. Chapter 63 provides additional information about enteral feeding.

For optimal nutrition, TPN may be necessary in addition to tube feedings or as a single measure to provide nutrition. When central venous access is required, a peripherally inserted central catheter (PICC) or other type of IV catheter may be necessary. Meticulous IV line care is an important nursing measure to prevent catheter sepsis. Sterile dressing changes and site observation are extremely important (see Chapter 15). Additional nursing care measures for the patient receiving TPN are given in Chapter 63. Monitor nutrition indicators such as serum prealbumin and albumin.

For the laparoscopic procedure, no bowel preparation is needed. However, either approach requires that the patient have nothing by mouth (NPO) for at least 6 to 8 hours before surgery. Surgeon preference and agency policy determine the preferred protocol for preoperative preparation.

Operative Procedures. The Whipple procedure (radical pancreaticoduodenectomy) involves extensive surgical manipulation and is used most often to treat cancer of the head of the pancreas. The procedure entails removal of the proximal head of the pancreas, the duodenum, a portion of the jejunum, the stomach (partial or total gastrectomy), and the gallbladder, with anastomosis of the pancreatic duct (pancreaticojejunostomy), the common bile duct (choledochojejunostomy), and the stomach (gastrojejunostomy) to the jejunum (Fig. 62-3). In addition, the surgeon may remove the spleen (splenectomy).

Postoperative Care. In addition to routine postoperative care measures, the patient who has undergone an open radical pancreaticoduodenectomy requires intensive nursing care

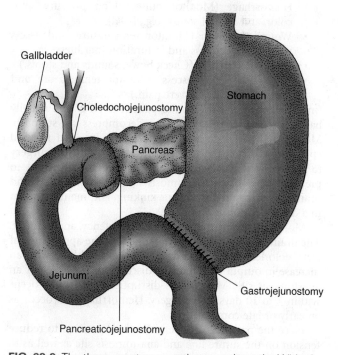

FIG. 62-3 The three anastomoses that constitute the Whipple procedure: choledochojejunostomy, pancreaticojejunostomy, and gastrojejunostomy.

TABLE 62-5 **POTENTIAL COMPLICATIONS OF THE WHIPPLE PROCEDURE**

Cardiovascular Complications
- Hemorrhage at anastomosis sites with hypovolemia
- Myocardial infarction
- Heart failure
- Thrombophlebitis

Pulmonary Complications
- Atelectasis
- Pneumonia
- Pulmonary embolism
- Acute respiratory distress syndrome
- Pulmonary edema

Gastrointestinal Complications
- Adynamic (paralytic) ileus
- Gastric retention
- Gastric ulceration
- Bowel obstruction from peritonitis
- Acute pancreatitis
- Hepatic failure
- Thrombosis to mesentery

Wound Complications
- Infection
- Dehiscence
- Fistulas: pancreatic, gastric, and biliary

Metabolic Complications
- Unstable diabetes mellitus
- Renal failure

---

and is usually admitted to a surgical critical care unit. Observe for multiple potential complications of the open Whipple procedure as listed in Table 62-5.

The primary benefit of MIS is the patient's fast postoperative recovery and less pain than with traditional open procedures. The patient having the laparoscopic Whipple surgery or radical pancreatectomy is also less at risk for severe complications. For patients having one of these procedures, observe for and implement preventive measures for these surgical complications:

- Diabetes (Check blood glucose often.)
- Hemorrhage (Monitor pulse, blood pressure, skin color, and mental status [e.g., LOC].)
- Wound infection (Monitor temperature, and assess wounds for redness and induration [hardness].)
- Bowel obstruction (Check bowel sounds and stools.)
- Intra-abdominal abscess (Monitor temperature and patient's report of severe pain.)

Immediately after surgery, the patient is NPO and usually has a nasogastric tube (NGT) to decompress the stomach. Monitor GI drainage and tube patency. In open surgical approaches, biliary drainage tubes are placed during surgery to remove drainage and secretions from the area and to prevent stress on the anastomosis sites. Assess the tubes and drainage devices for tension or kinking, and maintain them in a dependent position.

Monitor the drainage for color, consistency, and amount. The drainage should be serosanguineous. The appearance of clear, colorless, bile-tinged drainage or frank blood with an increase in output may indicate disruption or leakage of an anastomosis site. Most of the disruptions of the site occur within 7 to 10 days after surgery. Hemorrhage can occur as an early or late complication.

Place the patient in the semi-Fowler's position to reduce tension on the suture line and anastomosis site as well as to optimize lung expansion. Stress can be decreased by maintaining NGT drainage at a low or high intermittent suction level to keep the remaining stomach (if a partial gastrectomy

is done) or the jejunum (if a total gastrectomy is done) free of excessive fluid buildup and pressure. The NGT also reduces stimulation of the remaining pancreatic tissue.

The development of a fistula (an abnormal passageway) is the most common and most serious postoperative complication. Biliary, pancreatic, or gastric fistulas result from partial or total breakdown of an anastomosis site. The secretions that drain from the fistula contain bile, pancreatic enzymes, or gastric secretions, depending on which site is ruptured. *These secretions, particularly pancreatic fluid, are corrosive and irritating to the skin, and internal leakage causes chemical peritonitis.* Peritonitis (inflammation and infection of the peritoneum causing boardlike abdominal rigidity) requires treatment with multiple antibiotics. *If you suspect any postoperative complications resulting from MIS or open surgical approaches, call the surgeon immediately and provide assessment findings that support your concerns.*

Because the *open* Whipple procedure is extensive and can take many hours to complete, maintaining fluid and electrolyte balance can be difficult. Patients often have significant intraoperative blood loss and postoperative bleeding. The intestine is exposed to air for long periods, and fluid evaporates. Significant losses of fluid and electrolytes occur from the NGT and other drainage tubes. In addition, these patients may be malnourished and have low serum levels of protein and albumin, which maintain colloid osmotic pressure within the circulating system. Reduction in the serum osmotic pressure makes the patient likely to develop third spacing of body fluids, with fluid moving from the vascular to the interstitial space, resulting in shock. These problems are less likely to occur when MIS is used. Therefore, when possible, the trained surgeon prefers to perform laparoscopic Whipple procedures to shorten operating time and prevent the many complications that can occur.

Closely monitor vital signs for decreased blood pressure and increased heart rate, decreased vascular pressures with a pulmonary artery catheter (Swan-Ganz catheter) (in ICU setting), and decreased urine output to detect early signs of hypovolemia and prevent shock. Be alert for pitting edema of the extremities, dependent edema in the sacrum and back, and an intake that far exceeds output. Maintain sequential compression devices to prevent deep vein thrombosis.

Maintenance of prescribed IV isotonic fluid replacement with colloid replacements is important. Monitor hemoglobin and hematocrit values to assess for blood loss and the need for blood transfusions. Review electrolyte values for decreased serum levels of sodium, potassium, chloride, and calcium. IV fluid concentrations must be altered to correct these electrolyte imbalances. The physician prescribes replacement of electrolytes as needed.

Immediately after the Whipple procedure, the patient may have hyperglycemia or hypoglycemia as a result of stress and surgical manipulation of the pancreas. Most of the endocrine cells (responsible for insulin and glucagon secretion) are located in the body and tail of the pancreas. In some patients, up to half of the gland remains and diabetes does not develop. However, a large number of patients are diabetic before surgery. For patients having a radical pancreatectomy, administer insulin as prescribed because the entire pancreas is removed. Monitor glucose levels frequently during the early postoperative period, and administer insulin injections as prescribed.

? NCLEX EXAMINATION CHALLENGE

Physiological Integrity

A client has had an open Whipple procedure for pancreatic cancer. Which nursing interventions are appropriate for this client in the postoperative period? **Select all that apply.**
A. Maintain IV fluids, and monitor for fluid imbalance.
B. Assess for signs and symptoms of deep vein thrombosis.
C. Connect the nasogastric tube to high intermittent suction.
D. Start pancreatic enzyme replacements as soon as possible.
E. Check finger-stick blood glucose levels regularly.
F. Tell the client to lie flat to protect the incision.

Community-Based Care

The patient with pancreatic cancer is usually followed by a case manager (CM), both in the hospital and in the home or other community-based setting. Collaborate with the CM to ensure that the patient receives cost-effective treatment and that his or her needs are met.

Home Care Management

The stage of progression of pancreatic cancer and available home care resources determine whether the patient can be discharged to home or whether additional care is needed in a skilled nursing facility or with a hospice provider. Home care preparations depend on the patient's physical and activity limitations and should be tailored to his or her needs. Coordinate care with the patient, family, or whoever will be providing care after discharge from the hospital—home care provider, hospice care provider, or extended-care provider.

The patient and family need compassionate emotional support to deal with issues related to this illness. The diagnosis of pancreatic cancer can frighten and overwhelm the patient and family. Assist family members in looking realistically and objectively at the amount of physical care required. Tell family members that their own physical and emotional health are at risk during this stressful period and that supportive counseling may be needed. If the family does not have a religious affiliation or a spiritual leader (e.g., a minister or a rabbi) to provide support, suggest alternative counseling options. Refer patients and families to the certified hospital chaplain if desired. It is appropriate for the nurse to make the initial contact or appointment according to the patient's or family's wishes.

Teaching for Self-Management

When the patient is discharged to home, many interventions are palliative and aimed at managing symptoms such as pain. In many cases, the diagnosis of pancreatic cancer is made a few months before death occurs. The patient needs time to adjust to the diagnosis, which is usually made too late for cure or prolonged survival. Help the patient identify what needs to be done to prepare for death, including end-of-life care. For example, he or she may want to write a will or see family members and friends whom he or she has not seen recently. The patient needs to make known to family members or others his or her specific requests for the funeral or memorial service. These actions help prepare for death in a dignified manner. Chapter 9 discusses in detail anticipatory grieving and preparation for death, as well as symptom management during the end of life.

Health Care Resources

Regular home care nursing and assistive nursing personnel visits may be scheduled to assist the patient and family by providing physical, psychological, and supportive care. Supply information about local hospice care (see Chapter 9) and cancer support groups.

NURSING CONCEPT REVIEW

What might you NOTICE if the patient is experiencing inadequate digestion and nutrition as a result of gallbladder and pancreatic disorders?
- Report of intense abdominal pain
- Report of nausea, especially after food
- Report of anorexia
- Vomiting
- Jaundice
- Report of weight loss
- Dark urine
- Clay-colored stools

What should you INTERPRET and how should you RESPOND to a patient experiencing inadequate digestion and nutrition as a result of gallbladder and pancreatic disorders?

Perform and interpret physical assessment, including:
- Take vital signs to assess for hypovolemia and fever.
- Assess respiratory status, including breath sounds.
- Conduct a complete pain assessment if possible.
- Weigh the patient.

- Check laboratory values, especially enzyme levels like amylase and lipase, liver function studies, and CBC. Assess vomitus for quality and amount.

Respond by:
- Keeping the patient's head of the bed elevated and knees flexed
- Providing pain management by comfort measures and analgesia
- Providing oxygen if patient is having dyspnea or adventitious breath sounds
- Reassuring the patient who may be concerned about possible cancer

On what should you REFLECT?
- Observe patient for improvement in signs and symptoms, including pain control.
- Think about what could have caused the health problem.
- Think about what else you could do to help the patient meet desired outcomes.
- Plan health teaching for patient discharge.

GET READY FOR THE NCLEX® EXAMINATION!

KEY POINTS

Review these Key Points for each NCLEX Examination Client Needs Category.

Safe and Effective Care Environment
- When caring for a patient with a T-tube, do not place the drainage bag higher than the tube insertion site.
- Recognize that acute pain relief is the first priority for patients with acute pancreatitis.
- Be aware that patients with biliary and pancreatic disorders are at high risk for biliary obstruction, a serious and painful complication.

Health Promotion and Maintenance
- Recognize that obese, middle-aged women are most likely to have gallbladder disease.
- Teach patients to avoid losing weight too quickly and to keep weight under control to help prevent gallbladder disease.
- Instruct patients about ways to prevent exacerbations of chronic pancreatitis as outlined in Chart 62-4.

Psychosocial Integrity
- Provide pain relief measures for patients with acute pancreatitis to reduce anxiety.
- Refer patients with pancreatitis who use excessive alcohol to community resources such as Alcoholics Anonymous.

- Refer patients with pancreatic cancer for support services such as spiritual leaders and counselors.
- Help prepare the pancreatic cancer patient and family for the death and dying process.

Physiological Integrity
- Be aware that autodigestion of the pancreas causes severe pain in patients with acute pancreatitis (see Fig. 62-2).
- Monitor serum laboratory values, especially amylase and lipase (both elevated), in patients with pancreatitis (see Table 62-4).
- Assess for common clinical manifestations of cholecystitis as listed in Chart 62-1.
- For patients with acute pancreatitis, provide pain management including opioid analgesia.
- Assess for common clinical manifestations of chronic pancreatitis as listed in Chart 62-2.
- Teach patients about enzyme replacement therapy as described in Chart 62-3.
- Assess patients with presenting clinical manifestations of pancreatic cancer as described in Chart 62-5.
- Observe for and implement interventions to prevent life-threatening complications of the Whipple procedure as outlined in Table 62-5.

Care of Patients with Malnutrition and Obesity

Cherie R. Rebar and Donna D. Ignatavicius

LEARNING OUTCOMES

Safe and Effective Care Environment

1. Collaborate with members of the health care team when providing care for patients with malnutrition or obesity.
2. Protect bariatric patients from injury.
3. Select appropriate activities to delegate to unlicensed assistive personnel to promote a patient's nutrition.

Health Promotion and Maintenance

4. Provide care that meets the special nutrition needs of older adults.
5. Teach overweight and obese patients the importance of lifestyle changes to promote health.
6. Perform a nutrition screening for all patients to determine if they are at high risk for nutritional health problems.
7. Identify the key recommendations from the *Dietary Guidelines for Americans, 2010* document.

Psychosocial Integrity

8. Assess patient responses to being obese.

Physiological Integrity

9. Interpret findings of a nutrition screening and assessment.

10. Calculate body mass index (BMI), and interpret findings.
11. Describe the risk factors for malnutrition, especially for older adults.
12. Explain why serum visceral protein levels indicate change in nutritional status.
13. Identify the role of nutritional supplements in restoring or maintaining nutrition.
14. Describe complications of total enteral nutrition (TEN).
15. Explain how to prevent complications of total parenteral nutrition (TPN).
16. Explain how to maintain enteral tube patency.
17. Describe evidence-based practices to prevent aspiration for patients with nasoenteric tubes.
18. Explain the medical complications associated with obesity.
19. Identify the role of drug therapy in the management of obesity.
20. Prioritize nursing care for patients having bariatric surgery.
21. Develop a discharge teaching plan for patients having bariatric surgery.

Carbohydrates, protein, and fat are nutrients in food that supply the body with energy. In healthy people, most of this energy undergoes digestion and is absorbed from the GI tract. Food energy is used to maintain body temperature, respiration, cardiac output, muscle function, protein synthesis, and the storage and metabolism of food sources. Therefore proper *nutrition* plays a major role in promoting and maintaining health.

Energy balance refers to the relationship between energy used and energy stored. Weight loss occurs when energy

TABLE 63-1 EXAMPLES OF 2010 DIETARY GUIDELINES FOR AMERICANS

- Control total calorie intake to manage body weight.
- Consume less than 300 mg per day of dietary cholesterol.
- Increase intake of fat-free or low-fat milk and milk products, such as milk, yogurt, cheese, or fortified soy products.
- Choose a variety of protein foods, which include seafood, lean meat and poultry, eggs, beans and peas, soy products, and unsalted nuts and seeds.
- Reduce the intake of calories from solid fats and added sugars.
- Reduce daily sodium intake to less than 2300 mg and further reduce intake to 1500 mg among persons who are 51 years or older and those of any age who are African American or have hypertension, diabetes, or chronic kidney disease.
- Limit the consumption of foods that contain refined grains, especially refined grains that contain solid fats, added sugars, and sodium.
- Increase vegetable and fruit intake.

Source: Dietary Guidelines for Americans Council. (2010). Retrieved March 31, 2011, from www.cnpp.usda.gov/Publications/DietaryGuidelines/2010/DGAC/Report/A-ExecSummary.pdf.

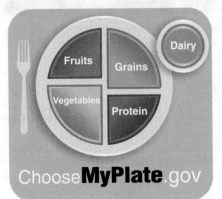

FIG. 63-1 The U.S. Department of Agriculture MyPlate.

used is more than intake. If food intake is more than energy used, weight is gained. Body proteins are used for energy when calorie intake is insufficient. The body attempts to meet its calorie requirements even if it is at the expense of protein needs.

NUTRITION STANDARDS FOR HEALTH PROMOTION AND MAINTENANCE

The role of nutrition in disease has been a subject of interest for many years. The current focus is on health promotion and the prevention of disease by healthy eating and exercise. In the United States, the Dietary Guidelines for Americans are revised by the U.S. Department of Agriculture (USDA) and the U.S. Department of Health and Human Services (DHHS) every 5 years. The most recent guidelines (2010) emphasize the need to include preferences of specific racial/ethnic groups, vegetarians, and other populations when selecting foods to maintain a healthful diet that is balanced with moderation and variety. If alcohol is consumed, it should be limited to one drink per day for women and two drinks for men (USDA, 2010). Examples of other guidelines are listed in Table 63-1.

The USDA also recently designed a picture to remind people about the good foods to increase and the foods that should be reduced in the daily diet. Fig. 63-1 illustrates the USDA's MyPlate to show that half of each meal should consist of fruits and vegetables. When grains are consumed, half of them should be whole grains rather than refined grain products.

An increasing number of people are adopting a variety of vegetarian diet patterns for health, environmental, or moral reasons. In general, vegetarians are leaner than those who consume meat. The lacto-vegetarian eats milk, cheese, and dairy foods but avoids meat, fish, poultry, and eggs. The lacto-ovo-vegetarian includes eggs in his or her diet. The vegan eats only foods of plant origin. Some people among these groups eat fish as well. Vegans can develop anemia as a result of vitamin B_{12} deficiency. Therefore they should include a daily source of vitamin B_{12} in their diets, such as a fortified

breakfast cereal, fortified soy beverage, or meat substitute. All vegetarians should ensure that they get adequate amounts of calcium, iron, zinc, and vitamins D and B_{12}. Well-planned vegetarian diets can provide adequate nutrition. The National Agriculture Library (2008) publishes a Vegetarian Nutrition Resource List that provides credible resources regarding vegetarian health.

⊕ CULTURAL AWARENESS

Many people have specific food preferences based on their ethnicity or race. For example, for people of Hispanic descent, tortillas, beans, and rice *may* be desired over pasta, risotto, and potatoes. *Never assume that a person's racial or ethnic background means that he or she eats only foods associated with his or her primary ethnicity.* Health teaching about nutrition should incorporate any cultural preferences (also see Chapter 4).

Some people have food allergies or intolerances. For instance, lactose intolerance (lactose is found in milk and milk products) is a common problem that occurs in a number of ethnic groups. It is found more often in Mexican Americans and black people as well as in some American Indian groups, Asian Americans, and Ashkenazi Jews. A small percentage of white people, particularly those of Mediterranean descent (e.g., Greek, Italian), are also lactose intolerant. The cause of lactose intolerance is an inadequate amount of the lactase enzyme, which converts lactose into absorbable glucose. Patients may benefit from learning more about the management of lactose intolerance from resources provided by organizations such as the American Dietetic Association.

CONSIDERATIONS FOR OLDER ADULTS

The USDA recommends that older adults drink eight glasses of water a day and eat plenty of fiber to prevent or manage constipation. It also suggests daily calcium and vitamins D and B_{12} supplements and a reduction in sodium and cholesterol-containing foods.

One of the most recent publications from Health Canada on nutrition is the Canada Food Guide. Compared with previous documents, it includes more culturally diverse foods, information on *trans* fats, customized individual recommendations, and exercise guidelines. Several booklets can be purchased to help people select the best foods and nutrients from the new Guide, such as *Eating Well with Canada's Food Guide.* In addition, Canada has published a separate booklet to address the special needs of some of its indigenous people. The *Eating Well with Canada's Food Guide—First Nations,*

Inuit, and Métis includes berries, wild plants, and wild game to reflect the values and traditions for aboriginal people living in Canada (Health Canada, 2007).

NUTRITIONAL ASSESSMENT

Malnutrition (also called *undernutrition*) and obesity are common nutritional health problems. These problems lead to deficits that cause many comorbidities and complications, including death.

Nutritional status reflects the balance between nutrient requirements and intake. Common factors that affect these requirements include age, gender, disease, infection, and psychological stress. Nutrient intake is influenced by eating behavior, economic factors, emotional stability, disease, drug therapy, and cultural factors.

Evaluation of nutritional status is an important part of total patient assessment and includes:

- Review of the nutritional history
- Food and fluid intake record
- Laboratory data
- Food-drug interactions
- Health history and physical assessment
- Anthropometric measurements
- Psychosocial assessment

Monitor the nutritional status of a patient during hospitalization as an important part of your initial assessment. Collaborate with the interdisciplinary health care team to identify patients at risk for nutritional problems.

Initial Nutritional Screening

Not every patient needs a complete nutritional assessment, but it is important to identify those at risk for problems through screening. An initial screening provides an inexpensive, quick way of determining which patients need more extensive nutritional assessment by the health care team. *The Joint Commission Patient Care Standards require that a nutritional screening occur within 24 hours of the patient's hospital admission. If indicated, an in-depth nutritional assessment should be performed.* When patients are in the hospital more than a week, nutritional assessment should be part of the daily plan of care.

The initial nutritional screening includes inspection, measured height and weight, weight history, usual eating habits, ability to chew and swallow, and any recent changes in appetite or food intake. Examples of questions that help identify patients at risk for nutritional problems are part of the history and physical assessment (Chart 63-1).

The Mini Nutritional Assessment (MNA), a two-part tool that has been tested worldwide, provides a reliable, rapid assessment for patients in the community and in any health care setting. The *first* part (A-F) is a screening section that takes 3 minutes to complete and asks about food intake, mobility, and body mass index (BMI) (described on p. 1339). It also screens for weight loss, acute illness, and psychological health problems. If the patient scores 11 points or less, the *second* part (G-R) of the MNA is completed, for an additional 12 questions. The entire assessment takes less than 15 minutes (Fig. 63-2) (DiMaria-Ghalili & Guenter, 2008). A new MNA® Short Form can be used as a stand-alone tool to evaluate whether the older patient is well-nourished, at risk for malnutrition, or malnourished. The alternative is to take the

---

CHART 63-1 BEST PRACTICE FOR PATIENT SAFETY & QUALITY CARE

Nutritional Screening Assessment

General
- Does the patient have any conditions that cause nutrient loss, such as malabsorption syndromes, draining abscesses, wounds, fistulas, or prolonged diarrhea?
- Does the patient have any conditions that increase the need for nutrients, such as fever, burn, injury, sepsis, or antineoplastic therapies?
- Has the patient been NPO for 3 days or more?
- Is the patient receiving a modified diet or a diet restricted in one or more nutrients?
- Is the patient being enterally or parenterally fed?
- Does the patient describe food allergies, lactose intolerance, or limited food preferences?
- Has the patient experienced a recent unexplained weight loss?
- Is the patient on drug therapy, either prescription, over-the-counter, or herbal/natural products?

Gastrointestinal
- Does the patient report nausea, indigestion, vomiting, diarrhea, or constipation?
- Does the patient exhibit glossitis (tongue inflammation), stomatitis (oral inflammation), or esophagitis?
- Does the patient have difficulty chewing or swallowing?
- Does the patient have a partial or total GI obstruction?
- What is the patient's state of dentition?

Cardiovascular
- Does the patient have ascites or edema?
- Is the patient able to perform ADLs?
- Does the patient have heart failure?

Genitourinary
- Is fluid intake about equal to fluid output?
- Does the patient have an ostomy?
- Is the patient hemodialyzed or peritoneally dialyzed?

Respiratory
- Is the patient receiving mechanical ventilatory support?
- Is the patient receiving oxygen via nasal prongs?
- Does the patient have chronic obstructive pulmonary disease (COPD) or asthma?

Integumentary
- Does the patient have abnormal nail or hair changes?
- Does the patient have rashes or dermatitis?
- Does the patient have dry or pale mucous membranes or decreased skin turgor?
- Does the patient have pressure areas on the sacrum, hips, heels, or ankles?

Extremities
- Does the patient have pedal edema?
- Does the patient have cachexia?

Modified with courtesy of Ross Products Division, Abbott Laboratories, Columbus, OH.

---

patient's calf circumference, which can be a reliable alternative if BMI is unavailable.

Anthropometric Measurements

Anthropometric measurements are noninvasive methods of evaluating nutritional status. These measurements include height and weight and assessment of body fat.

NESTLÉ NUTRITION SERVICES

Mini Nutritional Assessment (MNA)

Nestlé

Last name: _____ First name: _____ Sex: _____ Date: _____

Age: _____ Weight, kg: _____ Height, cm: _____ I.D. Number: _____

Complete the screen by filling in the boxes with the appropriate numbers.
Add the numbers for the screen. If score is 11 or less, continue with the assessment to gain a Malnutrition Indicator Score.

Screening

A Has food intake declined over the past 3 months due to loss of appetite, digestive problems, chewing or swallowing difficulties?
0 = severe loss of appetite
1 = moderate loss of appetite
2 = no loss of appetite ☐

B Weight loss during last 3 months
0 = weight loss greater than 3 kg (6.6 lbs)
1 = does not know
2 = weight loss between 1 and 3 kg (2.2 and 6.6 lbs)
3 = no weight loss ☐

C Mobility
0 = bed or chair bound
1 = able to get out of bed/chair but does not go out
2 = goes out ☐

D Has suffered psychological stress or acute disease in the past 3 months
0 = yes   2 = no ☐

E Neuropsychological problems
0 = severe dementia or depression
1 = mild dementia
2 = no psychological problems ☐

F Body Mass Index (BMI) (weight in kg) / (height in m)²
0 = BMI less than 19
1 = BMI 19 to less than 21
2 = BMI 21 to less than 23
3 = BMI 23 or greater ☐

Screening score (subtotal max. 14 points) ☐ ☐
12 points or greater Normal – not at risk – no need to complete assessment
11 points or below Possible malnutrition – continue assessment

Assessment

G Lives independently (not in a nursing home or hospital)
0 = no   1 = yes ☐

H Takes more than 3 prescription drugs per day
0 = yes   1 = no ☐

I Pressure sores or skin ulcers
0 = yes   1 = no ☐

J How many full meals does the patient eat daily?
0 = 1 meal
1 = 2 meals
2 = 3 meals ☐

K Selected consumption markers for protein intake
• At least one serving of dairy products (milk, cheese, yogurt) per day? yes ☐ no ☐
• Two or more servings of legumes or eggs per week? yes ☐ no ☐
• Meat, fish or poultry every day yes ☐ no ☐
0.0 = if 0 or 1 yes
0.5 = if 2 yes
1.0 = if 3 yes ☐.☐

L Consumes two or more servings of fruits or vegetables per day?
0 = no   1 = yes ☐

M How much fluid (water, juice, coffee, tea, milk…) is consumed per day?
0.0 = less than 3 cups
0.5 = 3 to 5 cups
1.0 = more than 5 cups ☐.☐

N Mode of feeding
0 = unable to eat without assistance
1 = self-fed with some difficulty
2 = self-fed without any problem ☐

O Self view of nutritional status
0 = views self as being malnourished
1 = is uncertain of nutritional state
2 = views self as having no nutritional problem ☐

P In comparison with other people of the same age, how does the patient consider his/her health status?
0.0 = not as good
0.5 = does not know
1.0 = as good
2.0 = better ☐.☐

Q Mid-arm circumference (MAC) in cm
0.0 = MAC less than 21
0.5 = MAC 21 to 22
1.0 = MAC 22 or greater ☐.☐

R Calf circumference (CC) in cm
0 = CC less than 31   1 = CC 31 or greater ☐

Assessment (max. 16 points) ☐ ☐.☐

Screening score ☐ ☐

Total Assessment (max. 30 points) ☐ ☐.☐

Malnutrition Indicator Score

17 to 23.5 points   at risk of malnutrition ☐

Less than 17 points   malnourished ☐

Ref.: Guigoz Y, Vellas B and Garry PJ. 1994. Mini Nutritional Assessment: A practical assessment tool for grading the nutritional state of elderly patients. *Facts and Research in Gerontology.* Supplement #2:15-59.
Rubenstein LZ, Harker J, Guigoz Y and Vellas B. Comprehensive Geriatric Assessment (CGA) and the MNA: An Overview of CGA, Nutritional Assessment, and Development of a Shortened Version of the MNA. In: "Mini Nutritional Assessment (MNA): Research and Practice in the Elderly". Vellas B, Garry PJ and Guigoz Y, editors. Nestlé Nutrition Workshop Series. Clinical & Performance Programme, vol. 1. Karger, Bâle, in press.

FIG. 63-2 The Mini Nutritional Assessment (MNA).

Obtain a current *height and weight* to provide a baseline. Be sure to obtain accurate measurements because patients tend to overestimate height and underestimate weight. Measurements taken days or weeks later may indicate an early change in nutritional status. *You may delegate this activity to unlicensed assistive personnel (UAP) under your supervision.*

Patients should be measured and weighed while wearing minimal clothing and no shoes. Determine the height in inches or centimeters using the measuring stick of a weight scale if the patient can stand. He or she should stand erect and look straight ahead, with the heels together and the arms at the sides. For patients who cannot stand or those who cannot stand erect (e.g., some older adults), use a sliding-blade knee height caliper, if available. This device uses the distance between the patient's patella and heel to estimate height. It is especially useful for patients who have knee or hip contractures.

UAP weigh ambulatory patients with an upright balance-beam scale. Non-ambulatory patients can be weighed with a movable wheelchair balance-beam scale or a bed scale.

! NURSING SAFETY PRIORITY

Action Alert

> Be sure that the manufacturer calibrates weight scales twice yearly for accurate readings. For daily or sequential weights, obtain the weight at the same time each day, if possible, preferably before breakfast. Conditions such as congestive heart failure and renal disease cause weight gain; dehydration and conditions such as cancer cause weight loss. *Weight is the most reliable indicator of fluid gain or loss, so accurate weights are essential!*

Normal weights for adult men and women are available from several reference standards, including the revised Metropolitan Life tables. Some health care professionals prefer these tables because they consider body-build differences by gender and body frame size.

Changes in body weight can be expressed by three different formulas:

1. Weight as a percentage of ideal body weight (IBW):

$$\%IBW = \frac{Current\ weight}{Ideal\ body\ weight} \times 100$$

2. Current weight as a percentage of usual body weight (UBW):

$$\%UBW = \frac{Current\ weight}{Usual\ body\ weight} \times 100$$

3. Change in weight:

$$Weight\ change = \frac{Usual\ weight - Current\ weight}{Usual\ weight} \times 100$$

An unintentional weight loss of 10% over a 6-month period at any time significantly affects nutritional status and should be evaluated. Depending on the patient's needs, weights may need to be taken daily, several times a week, or weekly for monitoring status and the effectiveness of nutritional support.

In the health care setting, *assessment of body fat* is usually calculated by the dietitian. For people who participate in a structured exercise program in the community, this assessment is typically performed by a fitness trainer or physical therapist.

The body mass index (BMI) is a measure of nutritional status that does not depend on frame size. It indirectly estimates total fat stores within the body by the relationship of weight to height. *Therefore an accurate height is as important as an accurate weight.*

A simple calculation for estimating BMI can be programmed into handheld computers or calculators using one of these two formulas:

$$BMI = \frac{Weight\ (lb)}{Height\ (in\ inches)^2} \times 703$$

$$BMI = \frac{Weight\ (kg)}{Height\ (in\ meters)^2}$$

BMI can also be determined using a table that is linked with height and weight. The least risk for malnutrition is associated with scores between 18.5 and 25. BMIs above and below these values are associated with increased health risks (Centers for Disease Control and Prevention [CDC], 2009).

CONSIDERATIONS FOR OLDER ADULTS

> Body weight and BMI usually increase throughout adulthood until about 60 years of age. As people get older, they become less hungry and eat less, even if they are healthy. Older adults should have a BMI between 23 and 27 (DiMaria-Ghalili & Amella, 2005).
>
> The average daily energy intake expended by this group tends to be more than the average energy intake. This physiologic change has been called the "anorexia of aging" (Conte et al., 2009). Many older adults are underweight, leading to undernutrition and increased risk for illness.

? NCLEX EXAMINATION CHALLENGE

Health Promotion and Maintenance

> An older adult is admitted to the hospital with pressure ulcers and septicemia. His height is 5 feet, 10 inches (1.78 meters), and he weighs 342 pounds (155 kg). His current body mass index (BMI) is _____. (Your answer should be rounded to the nearest tenth.)

Skinfold measurements estimate body fat and can be measured by either the nurse or the dietitian. The *triceps and subscapular* skinfolds are most commonly measured using a special caliper. Both are compared with standard measurements and recorded as percentiles.

The *midarm circumference (MAC) and calf circumference (CC)* can be obtained to measure muscle mass and subcutaneous fat. These measurements are needed if the Mini Nutritional Assessment tool is used. To measure MAC, place a flexible tape around the upper arm at the midpoint, taking care to hold the tape firmly but gently to avoid compressing the tissue. This measurement is usually recorded in centimeters. The midarm muscle mass (MAMM) measures the amount of muscle in the body and is a sensitive indicator of protein reserves. It can be computed from the MAC and the triceps skinfold measure. The CC is obtained using a similar procedure on the calf.

MALNUTRITION

Pathophysiology

Protein-energy malnutrition (PEM), also known as protein-calorie malnutrition (PCM), may present in three forms: marasmus, kwashiorkor, and marasmic-kwashiorkor. Marasmus is generally a calorie malnutrition in which body fat and protein are wasted. Serum proteins are often preserved. Kwashiorkor is a lack of protein quantity and quality in the presence of adequate calories. Body weight is more normal, and serum proteins are low. Marasmic-kwashiorkor is a combined protein and energy malnutrition. This problem often presents clinically when metabolic stress is imposed on a chronically starved patient. The outcome of unrecognized or untreated PEM is often dysfunction or disability and increased morbidity and mortality.

Malnutrition (also called *undernutrition*) is a multinutrient problem because foods that are good sources of calories and protein are also good sources of other nutrients. In the malnourished patient, protein catabolism exceeds protein intake and synthesis, resulting in negative nitrogen balance, weight loss, decreased muscle mass, and weakness.

The function of the liver, heart, lungs, GI tract, and immune system decreases in the patient with malnutrition. A decrease in serum proteins (hypoproteinemia) occurs as protein synthesis in the liver decreases. Vital capacity is also reduced as a result of respiratory muscle atrophy. Cardiac output diminishes. Malabsorption occurs because of atrophy of GI mucosa and the loss of intestinal villi.

Other common complications of severe malnutrition in adults include:

- Leanness and cachexia (muscle wasting with prolonged malnutrition)
- Decreased activity tolerance
- Lethargy
- Intolerance to cold
- Edema
- Dry, flaking skin and various types of dermatitis
- Poor wound healing
- Possible death
- Infection, particularly postoperative infection and sepsis

Malnutrition results from inadequate nutrient intake, increased nutrient losses, and increased nutrient requirements. Inadequate nutrient intake can be linked to poverty, lack of education, substance abuse, decreased appetite, and a decline in functional ability to eat independently, particularly in older adults. Infectious diseases, such as tuberculosis and human immune deficiency virus (HIV) infection, can also cause PEM. Diseases that produce diarrhea and infections leading to anorexia result in negative calorie and protein balance. Anorexia then leads to poor food intake. Vomiting causes decreased intestinal absorption with increased nutrient losses. Medical treatments such as chemotherapy can also cause malnutrition. In addition, catabolic processes, such as that caused by prolonged immobility, increase nutrient requirements and metabolic losses.

Inadequate nutrient intake can result also when a person is admitted to the hospital or long-term care facility. For example, decreased staffing may not allow time for patients who need to be fed, especially older adults, who may eat slowly. Many diagnostic tests, surgery, trauma, and unexpected medical complications require a period of NPO or cause anorexia (loss of appetite).

🌐 CULTURAL AWARENESS

In some cases, malnutrition results when the provided meals are different from what the patient usually eats. Be sure to identify specific food preferences that the patient can eat and enjoy that are in keeping with his or her cultural practices.

CONSIDERATIONS FOR OLDER ADULTS

Older adults in the community or in any health care setting are most at risk for poor nutrition, especially PEM. Risk factors include physiologic changes of aging, environmental factors, and health problems. Chart 63-2 lists some of these major factors. Chapter 3 discusses nutrition for older adults in more detail.

Acute PEM may develop in patients who were adequately nourished before hospitalization but experience starvation while in a catabolic state from infection, stress, or injury. *Chronic* PEM can occur in those who have cancer, end-stage kidney or liver disease, or chronic neurologic disease.

Eating disorders, such as anorexia nervosa and bulimia nervosa seen most often in teens and young adults, also lead to malnutrition. Anorexia nervosa is a self-induced starvation resulting from a fear of fatness, even though the patient is underweight. Bulimia nervosa is characterized by episodes of binge eating in which the patient ingests a large amount of food in a short time. The binge eating is followed by some form of purging behavior, such as self-induced vomiting or excessive use of laxatives and diuretics. If not treated, death can result from starvation, infection, or suicide. Information about eating disorders can be found in textbooks on mental/behavioral health nursing.

CHART 63-2 **NURSING FOCUS ON THE OLDER ADULT**

Risk Assessment for Malnutrition

Assess for:

- Decreased appetite
- Weight loss
- Poor-fitting or no dentures/poor dental health
- Poor eyesight
- Dry mouth
- Limited income
- Lack of transportation
- Inability to prepare meals because of functional decline or fatigue
- Loneliness and/or depression
- Chronic constipation (e.g., in patients with Alzheimer's disease)
- Decreased meal enjoyment
- Chronic physical illness
- "Failure to thrive" (a combination of three of five symptoms, including weakness, slow walking speed, low physical activity, unintentional weight loss, exhaustion)
- Prescription and OTC drugs (including herbs, vitamins, and minerals)
- Acute or chronic pain

PATIENT-CENTERED COLLABORATIVE CARE

ASSESSMENT

History

Review the medical history to determine the possibility of increased metabolic needs or nutritional losses, chronic disease, trauma, recent surgery of the GI tract, drug and alcohol abuse, and recent significant weight loss. Each of these conditions can contribute to malnutrition. For older adults, explore mental status changes and note poor eyesight, diseases affecting major organs, constipation or incontinence, and slowed reactions. Review prescription and over-the-counter (OTC) drugs, including vitamin, mineral, herbal, and other nutritional supplements.

For patients who live independently in the community, the nurse may assess their performance of instrumental activities of daily living (IADLs). Functional status can best be evaluated for institutionalized patients by assessing their ADL performance. Poor nutrition is a major contributing factor to decreased functional ability.

In collaboration with the dietitian, obtain information about the patient's usual daily food intake, eating behaviors, change in appetite, and recent weight changes. If the patient is able to communicate, ask him or her to describe the usual foods eaten daily, cultural food preferences, and the times of meals and snacks. If available, ask the family these questions if the patient cannot communicate. If the patient cannot understand the questions due to language differences, locate an interpreter to assist with communication. The dietitian can more thoroughly analyze the diet, if necessary, based on your initial nutritional screening.

Ask about changes in eating habits as a result of illness, and document any change in appetite, taste, and weight loss. *A weight loss of 5% or more in 30 days, a weight loss of 10% in 6 months, or a weight that is below ideal may indicate malnutrition.*

! NURSING SAFETY PRIORITY

Action Alert

When assessing for malnutrition, assess for difficulty or pain in chewing or swallowing. *Unrecognized dysphagia is a common problem among nursing home residents and can cause malnutrition, dehydration, and aspiration pneumonia.* Ask the patient whether any foods are avoided and why. Ask UAP to report any choking while the patient eats. Record the occurrence of nausea, vomiting, heartburn, or any other symptoms of discomfort with eating.

Ask the patient about dental health problems, including the presence of dentures. Dentures or partial plates that do not fit well interfere with food intake. Dental caries (decay) or missing teeth may also cause discomfort while eating.

Physical Assessment/Clinical Manifestations

Assess for manifestations of various nutrient deficiencies (Table 63-2). Inspect the patient's hair, eyes, oral cavity, nails, and musculoskeletal and neurologic systems. Examine the condition of the skin, including any reddened or open areas. The previously described anthropometric measurements

TABLE 63-2	MANIFESTATIONS OF NUTRIENT DEFICIENCIES
SIGN/SYMPTOM	**POTENTIAL NUTRIENT DEFICIENCY**
Hair	
Alopecia	Zinc
Easy to remove	Protein
Lackluster hair	Protein
"Corkscrew" hair	Vitamin C
Decreased pigmentation	Protein
Eyes	
Xerosis of conjunctiva	Vitamin A
Corneal vascularization	Riboflavin
Keratomalacia	Vitamin A
Bitot's spots	Vitamin A
Gastrointestinal Tract	
Nausea, vomiting	Pyridoxine
Diarrhea	Zinc, niacin
Stomatitis	Pyridoxine, riboflavin, iron
Cheilosis	Pyridoxine, iron
Glossitis	Pyridoxine, zinc, niacin, folic acid, vitamin B_{12}
Magenta tongue	Vitamin A, riboflavin
Swollen, bleeding gums	Vitamin C
Fissured tongue	Niacin
Hepatomegaly	Protein
Skin	
Dry and scaling	Vitamin A
Petechiae/ecchymoses	Vitamin C
Follicular hyperkeratosis	Vitamin A
Nasolabial seborrhea	Niacin
Bilateral dermatitis	Niacin
Extremities	
Subcutaneous fat loss	Calories
Muscle wastage	Calories, protein
Edema	Protein
Osteomalacia, bone pain, rickets	Vitamin D
Hematologic	
Anemia	Vitamin B_{12}, iron, folic acid, copper, vitamin E
Leukopenia, neutropenia	Copper
Low prothrombin time, prolonged clotting time	Vitamin K, manganese
Neurologic	
Disorientation	Niacin, thiamine
Confabulation	Thiamine
Neuropathy	Thiamine, pyridoxine, chromium
Paresthesia	Thiamine, pyridoxine, vitamin B_{12}
Cardiovascular	
Congestive heart failure, cardiomegaly, tachycardia	Thiamine
Cardiomyopathy	Selenium
Cardiac dysrhythmias	Magnesium

Courtesy of Ross Products Division, Abbott Laboratories, Columbus, OH.

may also be obtained. The nurse or UAP should monitor all food and fluid intake and note any mouth pain or difficulty in chewing or swallowing. A 3-day caloric intake may be collected and then calculated by the dietitian.

Psychosocial Assessment

The psychosocial history provides information about the patient's economic status, occupation, educational level, gender orientation, ethnicity/race, living and cooking arrangements, and mental status. Determine whether financial resources are adequate for providing the necessary food. If resources are inadequate, the social worker or case manager may refer the patient and family to available community services. Chapter 3 discusses nutrition in older adults in more detail.

Laboratory Assessment

Laboratory tests supply objective data that can support subjective data and identify preclinical deficiencies. However, they must be carefully interpreted with regard to the total patient; an isolated value may yield an inaccurate conclusion.

A low *hemoglobin* level may indicate anemia, recent hemorrhage, or hemodilution caused by fluid retention. Hemoglobin may also be low secondary to conditions such as low serum albumin, infection, catabolism, or chronic disease. High levels may indicate hemoconcentration or dehydration, or they may be secondary to liver disease.

Low *hematocrit* levels may reflect anemia, hemorrhage, excessive fluid, renal disease, or cirrhosis. High hematocrit levels may indicate dehydration or hemoconcentration.

Serum albumin, thyroxine-binding prealbumin, and transferrin are measures of visceral proteins. Serum *albumin* is a plasma protein that reflects the nutritional status of the patient a few weeks before testing and is therefore not the most sensitive test. In addition, patients who are dehydrated often have high levels of albumin and those with fluid excess have a lowered value. The normal serum albumin level for men and women is 3.5 to 5.0 g/dL or 35 to 50 g/L (SI units) (Pagana & Pagana, 2010).

Thyroxine-binding prealbumin (PAB) is a plasma protein that provides a more sensitive indicator of nutritional deficiency because of its short half-life of 2 days. Depending on the laboratory test used, the normal PAB range is 15 to 36 mg/dL or 150 to 360 mg/L (SI units) (Pagana & Pagana, 2010). PAB can also assess improvement in nutritional status with refeeding; levels can increase by 1 mg/dL daily with adequate nutritional support.

Although not used as commonly, serum transferrin, an iron-transport protein, can be measured directly or calculated as an indirect measurement of total iron-binding capacity (TIBC). It has a short half-life of 8 to 10 days and therefore is also a more sensitive indicator of protein status than albumin.

Cholesterol levels normally range between 160 and 200 mg/dL in adult men and women. Values are typically low with malabsorption, liver disease, pernicious anemia, end-stage cancer, or sepsis. A cholesterol level below 160 mg/dL has been identified as a possible indicator of malnutrition. Cholesterol testing is discussed in more detail in Chapter 35.

Total lymphocyte count (TLC) can be used to assess immune function. Malnutrition suppresses the immune system and leaves the patient more likely to get an infection. When a patient is malnourished, the TLC is usually decreased to below 1500/mm³.

ANALYSIS

The priority problem for the patient with malnutrition is:
1. Inadequate nutrition to meet body needs related to inability to ingest or digest food or absorb nutrients.

PLANNING AND IMPLEMENTATION

Improving Nutrition

Planning: Expected Outcomes. The patient with malnutrition is expected to have nutrients available to meet his or her metabolic needs as evidenced by normal serum proteins and adequate hydration.

Interventions. The preferred route for nutritional intake is through the GI tract because it enhances the immune system and is safer, easier, less expensive, and more enjoyable.

Nutrition Management. The dietitian calculates the nutrients required daily and plans the patient's diet. In collaboration with the health care provider and dietitian, provide high-calorie, nutrient-rich foods (e.g., milkshakes, cheese, supplement drinks like Boost or Ensure). Assess the patient's food likes and dislikes. A feeding schedule of six small meals may be tolerated better than three large ones. A pureed or

---

> **! NURSING SAFETY PRIORITY**
>
> **Action Alert**
>
> Malnourished ill patients often need to be encouraged to eat. Instruct UAP who are feeding patients to keep food at the appropriate temperature and to provide mouth care before feeding. Assess for other needs, such as pain management, and provide interventions to make the patient comfortable. Pain can prevent patients from enjoying their meals. Remove bedpans, urinals, and emesis basins from sight. Provide a quiet environment, which is conducive to eating. Soft music may calm those with advanced dementia or delirium. Appropriate time should be taken so that the patient does not feel rushed through a meal.

> **CONSIDERATIONS FOR OLDER ADULTS**
>
> Some patients, especially older adults, may take a long time to eat even small quantities of food because they tend to be less hungry than younger adults. If available, suggest that family members bring in favorite or ethnic foods that the patient might be more likely to eat. Teach them about ways to encourage the patient to increase food intake. Chart 63-3 describes additional interventions to promote nutritional intake in older adults.
>
> Restorative feeding programs help nursing home residents who need special assistance. These residents often eat in a separate dining area so that time and attention can be given to them. Some nursing homes have designated food and nutrition nursing assistants and/or trained volunteers who are primarily responsible for promoting and maintaining nutrition and hydration. Delegate and supervise these UAPs during resident mealtime.
>
> If the patient cannot take in enough nutrients in food, fortified medical nutritional supplements (MNSs) (e.g., Ensure, Sustacal, Carnation Instant Breakfast [also available as lactose-free supplement]) may be given, especially to older adults. Many commercial enteral products are available. For patients with medical diagnoses such as liver and renal disease or diabetes, special products that meet those needs are available.

dental soft diet may be easier for those who have problems chewing or are edentulous (toothless).

Nutritional supplements used in acute care, long-term care, and home care can be costly. In addition, patients may refuse them and the supplements are then wasted. In a classic study, Bender et al. (2000) found that a more successful alternative to having the MNS given by nursing assistant staff in the nursing home was to have the supplements delivered by nurses during their usual medication passes. In this study, the nurses gave 60 mL or more of the MNS at least four times a day with the residents' medications. As a result, the patients gained weight and had fewer pressure ulcers, thus making the program very cost-effective and providing positive clinical outcomes.

Nutritional supplements are supplied as liquid formulas, powders, soups, coffee, and puddings in a variety of flavors. They come in different degrees of sweetness and are also available as modular supplements that provide single nutrients. Examples of modular supplements are Polycose glucose polymers for carbohydrates and Resource Beneprotein for protein, both available in liquid and powder form.

Carbohydrate modulars are useful only if additional calories are needed. Protein modulars are indicated when metabolic stress causes a need for higher protein intake.

The dietitian may ask the nursing staff to keep a food and fluid intake record for at least 3 consecutive days to help assess the patient's nutritional status. Delegate this activity to UAP under your supervision. UAP also weigh the patient daily, every 3 days, or once a week, depending on the health care setting and severity of malnutrition.

Drug Therapy. Multivitamins, zinc, and an iron preparation are often prescribed to treat or prevent anemia. Monitor the patient's hemoglobin and hematocrit levels. Drug therapy can affect nutritional status. For example, iron can cause constipation and zinc can cause nausea and vomiting.

If the patient still does not receive enough nutrition by mouth using the interventions just mentioned, request specialized nutrition support (SNS). SNS consists of either total enteral nutrition (TEN) or total parenteral nutrition (TPN).

Total Enteral Nutrition. Patients often cannot meet the desired outcomes of nutritional therapy through their usual oral intake because of increased metabolic demands or a decreased ability to eat. Therefore TEN using enteral tube feeding may be necessary to supplement oral intake or to provide total nutritional support.

Patients likely to receive TEN can be divided into three groups:

- Those who can eat but cannot maintain adequate nutrition by oral intake of food alone
- Those who have permanent neuromuscular impairment and cannot swallow
- Those who do not have permanent neuromuscular impairment but are critically ill and cannot eat because of their condition

Patients in the first group are often older adults or patients receiving cancer treatment who cannot meet their calorie and protein needs. In some cases, this artificial nutrition and hydration may not be desired. For example, some patients have advance directives stating that they do not want to be kept alive by artificial nutrition and hydration if certain conditions exist. *However, legal and ethical questions arise when patients are not able to make their wishes known!*

For many years it was believed that withholding food and fluids would cause discomfort. Terminally or chronically ill patients who do not eat and drink may not suffer. In fact, they may be more comfortable if food and fluids are withheld. *The decision to feed is complex, and there is no clear right or wrong answer. To compound this legal and ethical dilemma, medical complications (e.g., aspiration, pressure ulcers) are common in older adults who are tube-fed.*

Decisions about these dilemmas are aided by the advice of interdisciplinary ethics committees in health care facilities. When clinicians are making decisions about the desirability of tube feedings in these cases, the focus should be on achieving consensus by:

- Reviewing what is known about tube feedings, especially their risks and benefits
- Reviewing the medical facts about the patient
- Investigating any available evidence that would help understand the patient's wishes
- Obtaining the opinions of all stakeholders in the situation
- Delaying any action until consensus is achieved

CHART 63-3 NURSING FOCUS ON THE OLDER ADULT

Promoting Nutritional Intake

- Be sure patient is toileted and receives mouth care before mealtime.
- Make sure that patient has glasses and hearing aids in place, if appropriate, during meals.
- Be sure that bedpans, urinals, and emesis basins are removed from sight.
- Give analgesics to control pain and/or antiemetics for nausea at least 1 hour before mealtime.
- Remind unlicensed assistive personnel (UAP) to have patient sit in chair, if possible, at mealtime.
- If needed, open cartons and packages and cut up food at the patient's and/or family's request.
- Observe the patient during meals for food intake.
- Ask the patient about food likes and dislikes and ethnic food preferences.
- Encourage self-feeding, or feed the patient slowly; *delegate* this activity to UAP if desired.
- If feeding patient, sit at eye-level if culturally appropriate.
- Create an environment that is conducive to eating and socialization and relaxation, if possible.
- Decrease distractions, such as environmental noise from television, music, or other people.
- Provide adequate, nonglaring lighting.
- Keep patient away from offensive or medicinal odors.
- Keep eye contact with the patient during the meal if culturally appropriate.
- Serve snacks with activities, especially in long-term care settings; *delegate* this activity to UAP if desired.
- Document the percentage of food eaten at each meal and snack; *delegate* this activity to UAP if appropriate.
- Ensure that meals are visually appealing, appetizing, appropriately warm or cold, and properly prepared.
- Do not interrupt patients during mealtimes for nonurgent procedures or rounds.
- Assess for need for supplements between meals and at bedtime.
- Review the patient's drug profile, and discuss with the health care provider the use of drugs that might be suppressing appetite.
- If the patient is depressed, be sure that the depression is treated by the health care provider.

Those in the second group of patients likely to receive TEN usually have permanent swallowing problems and require some type of feeding tube for delivery of the enteral product on a long-term basis. Examples of conditions that can cause permanent swallowing problems are strokes, severe head trauma, and advanced multiple sclerosis. Patients in the third group receive enteral nutrition for as long as their illness lasts. The feeding is discontinued when the patient's condition improves and he or she can eat again. TEN is contraindicated for patients in states of significant hemodynamic compromise, such as those with diffuse peritonitis, severe acute or chronic pancreatitis, intestinal obstruction, intractable vomiting or diarrhea, and paralytic ileus (Bankhead et al., 2009).

Many commercially prepared enteral products are available. A therapeutic combination of carbohydrates, fat, vitamins, minerals, and trace elements is available in liquid form. Differences among products allow the dietitian to select the right formula for each patient. A prescription from the health care provider is required for enteral nutrition, but the dietitian usually makes the recommendation and computes the amount and type of product needed for each patient.

❓ NCLEX EXAMINATION CHALLENGE

Health Promotion and Maintenance

An older client admitted to the hospital from the nursing home refuses to eat anything on her meal tray. What instructions will the nurse give to the nursing assistant who is attempting to feed the client? **Select all that apply.**

A. "Feed her the soft food because she has no teeth."
B. "Place the fork in her hand and leave the room."
C. "Sit at her level so that she can feel more comfortable."
D. "Take your time feeding her and don't rush her."
E. "Offer her the Ensure supplement instead of feeding her."
F. "Ask the client what foods she likes and dislikes."

Methods of Administering Total Enteral Nutrition. TEN is administered as "tube feedings" through one of the available GI tubes, either through a nasoenteric or enterostomal tube. It can be used in the patient's home or any health care setting.

A nasoenteric tube (NET) is any feeding tube inserted nasally and then advanced into the GI tract, such as a Keofeed, Entriflex, or Dobbhoff tube. Commonly used NETs include the nasogastric (NG) tube and the smaller (small-bore) nasoduodenal tube (NDT) (Fig. 63-3, *A*). A nasojejunal tube (NJT) is also available but is used less often than the other NETs.

The NDTs are used for delivering *short-term* enteral feedings (usually less than 4 weeks) because they are easy to use and are safer for the patient at risk for aspiration *if the tip of the tube is placed below the pyloric sphincter of the stomach and into the duodenum.* Small-bore polyurethane or silicone tubes from 8 to 12 Fr external diameter are preferred. The smaller tubes are more comfortable and are less likely to cause complications such as nasal irritation, sinusitis, tissue erosion, and pulmonary compromise.

Enterostomal feeding tubes are used for patients who need *long-term* enteral feeding. The most common types are gastrostomies and jejunostomies. The surgeon directly accesses the GI tract using various surgical, endoscopic, and laparoscopic techniques.

A gastrostomy is a stoma created from the abdominal wall into the stomach, through which a short feeding tube is inserted by the surgeon. It may require a small abdominal incision or may be placed endoscopically. This tube is called a percutaneous endoscopic gastrostomy (PEG) or dual-access gastrostomy-jejunostomy (PEG/J) tube. The PEG does not require general anesthesia for placement and is more secure and more durable than traditional gastrostomies. An alternative to either device is the low-profile gastrostomy device (LPGD) (Fig. 63-3, *B* and *C*). The LPGD is available

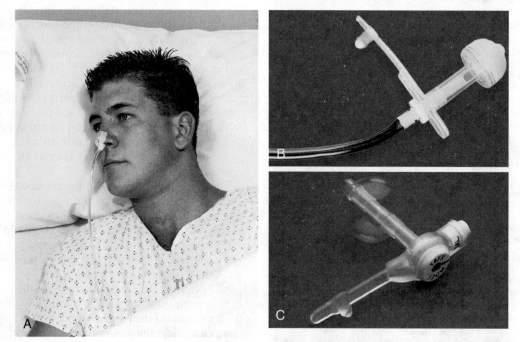

FIG. 63-3 Feeding tubes used for total enteral nutrition. **A,** Nasoduodenal tube. **B** and **C,** Gastrostomy tubes.

with a firm or balloon-style internal bumper or retention disk. An anti-reflux valve keeps GI contents from leaking onto the skin. This device is less irritating to the skin, longer lasting, and more cosmetically pleasing. It also allows greater patient independence. However, skin-level devices do not allow easy access for checking residuals (the amount of feeding that remains in the stomach).

Jejunostomies are used less often than gastrostomies. A jejunostomy is used for long-term feedings when it is desirable to bypass the stomach, such as with gastric disease, upper GI obstruction, and abnormal gastric or duodenal emptying.

Tube feedings are administered by bolus feeding, continuous feeding, and cyclic feeding. Bolus feeding is an intermittent feeding of a specified amount of enteral product at set intervals during a 24-hour period, typically every 4 hours. This method can be accomplished manually or by infusion through a mechanical pump or controller device. Another method of tube feeding is continuous enteral feeding. Continuous feeding is similar to IV therapy in that small amounts are continuously infused (by gravity drip or by a pump or controller device) over a specified time. The most commonly seen method, cyclic feeding, is the same as continuous feeding except the infusion is stopped for a specified time in each 24-hour period, usually 6 hours or longer ("down time"). Down time typically occurs in the morning to allow bathing, treatments, and other activities.

Infusion rates for cyclic feedings (and to some extent for intermittent bolus feeding) vary with the total amount of solution to be infused, the specific composition of the product, and the response of the patient to the feeding. The health care provider and dietitian usually decide the type, rate, and method of tube feeding, as well as the amount of additional water ("free water") needed. If the patient can swallow small amounts of food, he or she may also eat orally while the tube is in place.

The nurse is responsible for the care and maintenance of the feeding tube and the enteral feeding. Chart 63-4 lists best practices for the patient receiving TEN.

Complications of Total Enteral Nutrition. The nursing priority for care is patient safety, including preventing, assessing, and managing complications associated with tube feeding. Some complications of therapy result from the type of tube used to administer the feeding, and others result from the enteral product itself. The most common problem is the development of a clogged tube. Use the tips in Chart 63-5 to maintain tube patency.

Patients receiving TEN are at risk for several other complications, including refeeding syndrome, tube misplacement and dislodgement, abdominal distention and nausea/vomiting, and fluid and electrolyte imbalance, often associated with diarrhea. These problems can be prevented if the patient is carefully monitored and complications are detected early.

Refeeding Syndrome. Refeeding syndrome is a life-threatening metabolic complication that can occur when nutrition is restarted for a patient who is in a *starvation* state. When a patient is starved for nutrition, the body breaks down fat and protein, rather than carbohydrates, for energy. Protein catabolism leads to muscle and cell loss, often in major organs like the heart, liver, and lungs. The body's cells lose valuable electrolytes, including potassium and phosphate, into the plasma. Insulin secretion decreases in response to these changes. When *refeeding* begins, insulin production resumes and the cells take up glucose and electrolytes from the bloodstream, thus depleting serum levels.

❗ NURSING SAFETY PRIORITY

Critical Rescue

The electrolyte shift of refeeding syndrome can cause cardiovascular, respiratory, and neurologic problems, primarily as a result of hypophosphatemia (Mehanna et al., 2008). Observe for clinical manifestations of this electrolyte imbalance, including shallow respirations, weakness, acute confusion, seizures, and increased bleeding tendency. Report and document your findings immediately. More information on fluid and electrolyte imbalance can be found in Chapter 13.

CHART 63-4   BEST PRACTICE FOR PATIENT SAFETY & QUALITY CARE

Tube Feeding Care and Maintenance

- If nasogastric or nasoduodenal feeding is prescribed, use a soft, flexible, small-bore feeding tube (smaller than 12 Fr). *The initial placement of the tube should be confirmed by x-ray study.* Secure the tube with tape or a commercial attachment device after applying a skin protectant; change the tape regularly.
- Check tube placement by x-ray study when the correct position of the tube is in question; *an x-ray study is the most reliable method.*
- If a gastrostomy or jejunostomy tube is used, assess the insertion site for signs of infection or excoriation (e.g., excessive redness, drainage). Rotate the tube 360 degrees each day, and check for in-and-out play of about ¼ inch (0.6 cm). If the tube cannot be moved, notify the health care provider immediately because the retention disk may be embedded in the tissue. Cover the site with a dry, sterile dressing, and change the dressing at least once a day.
- Check and record the residual volume every 4 to 6 hours, or per facility policy, by aspirating stomach contents into a syringe. If residual feeding is obtained, check with the health care provider for the appropriate intervention (usually to slow or stop the feeding for a time) or use the American Society of Parenteral and Enteral Nutrition (ASPEN) best practice recommendations.
- Check the feeding pump to ensure proper mechanical operation.
- Ensure that the enteral product is infused at the prescribed rate (mL/hr).
- Change the feeding bag and tubing every 24 to 48 hours; label the bag with the date and time of the change with your initials. Use an irrigation set for no more than 24 hours.
- For continuous or cyclic feeding, add only 4 hours of product to the bag at a time to prevent bacterial growth. *A closed system is preferred, and each set should be used no longer than 24 hours.*
- Wear clean gloves when changing or opening the feeding system or adding product; wipe the lid of the formula can with clean gauze; wear sterile gloves for critically ill or immunocompromised patients.
- Label open cans with date and time opened; cover, and keep refrigerated. Discard any unused open cans after 24 hours.
- *Do not use blue (or any color) food dye in formula because it does not assess aspiration and can cause serious complications.*
- To prevent aspiration, keep the head of the bed elevated at least 30 degrees during the feeding and for at least 1 hour after the feeding for bolus feeding; continuously maintain semi-Fowler's position for patients receiving cyclic or continuous feeding.
- Monitor laboratory values, especially blood urea nitrogen (BUN), serum electrolytes, hematocrit, prealbumin, and glucose.
- Monitor for complications of tube feeding, especially diarrhea.
- Monitor and carefully record the patient's weight and intake and output as requested by the physician or dietitian.

Maintaining a Patent Feeding Tube

- Flush the tube with 20 to 30 mL of water (or the amount prescribed by the health care provider or dietitian):
  - At least every 4 hours during a continuous tube feeding
  - Before and after each intermittent tube feeding
  - Before and after drug administration (use warm water)
  - After checking residual volume
- If the tube becomes clogged, use 30 mL of water for flushing, applying gentle pressure with a 50-mL piston syringe.
- Avoid the use of carbonated beverage, except for existing clogs *when water is not effective.* Do not use cranberry juice.
- Whenever possible, use liquid medications instead of crushed tablets unless liquid forms cause diarrhea; make sure that the drug is compatible with the feeding solution.
- Do not mix drugs with the feeding product before giving. Crush tablets as finely as possible, and dissolve in warm water. *(Check to see which tablets are safe to crush. For example, do not crush slow-acting [SA] or slow-release [SR] drugs.)*
- Consider use of automatic flush feeding pump such as Flexiflo or Kangaroo.

Refeeding syndrome can be prevented if patients are carefully assessed and managed for nutritional needs. Interventions to supplement or replace nutrition should be implemented early before the patient is in a starvation state.

Tube Misplacement and Dislodgement. A less common but more serious complication is misplacement or dislodgement of the tube, *which can cause aspiration and possible death.* Lung intubation occurs in up to 27% of enteral tubes placed in hospitalized patients (Elpern et al., 2007). *Immediately remove any tube that you suspect is dislodged!* The Joint Commission's National Patient Safety Goals and the Centers for Medicare and Medicaid require all health care facilities to establish and implement procedures and systems to prevent patient harm from medical complications.

Several techniques should be used to confirm proper placement to prevent harm and to keep the patient safe. *An x-ray is the most accurate confirmation method and should always be done upon initial tube insertion.* After the initial placement is confirmed, check the placement before each intermittent feeding or at least every 4 to 8 hours during feeding. Also check placement before each drug administration.

The traditional auscultatory method for checking tube placement may not be reliable, especially for patients with small-bore tubes. In this method, the nurse instills 20 to 30 mL of air into the tube ("insufflation") while listening over the epigastric area (stomach) with a stethoscope. *The resulting whooshing sound does not guarantee correct tube placement!*

Although some patients have respiratory distress if the tube is misplaced into the lungs, some do not. Therefore better methods for patient safety are being researched. Several safer procedures have been recommended for checking tube placement *after the initial placement has been confirmed by x-ray.* These methods include:

- Testing aspirated contents for pH, bilirubin, trypsin, or pepsin
- Assessing for carbon dioxide using capnometry

Some hospitals and nursing homes support testing the *pH of GI contents* at the bedside. To perform this procedure, aspirate a sample of the GI content, observe its color, and test its pH. When aspirating fluid, wait at least 1 hour after drug administration and then flush the tube with 20 mL of air to clear it. Collect the aspirate, and test it with pH paper. The pH of gastric fluid ranges from 0 to 4.0. If the tube has moved down into the intestines, the pH will be between 7.0 and 8.0. If the tube is in the lungs, the pH will be greater than 6.0. The pH may also be as high as 6 if the patient takes certain drugs, such as H_2 blockers (e.g., ranitidine [Zantac] and famotidine [Pepcid]). Because these drugs affect pH, bilirubin testing or capnometry may be more reliable and valid methods for predicting tube location.

A newer method that has been researched is the use of *capnometry* to determine if carbon dioxide is emitted from the tube (Elpern et al., 2007). A device to measure the presence of the gas is attached to the end of the tube after placement. The test is positive for carbon dioxide if the tube is placed into the lungs, rather than the stomach. *The tube should be immediately removed if the gas is detected.*

> ! **NURSING SAFETY PRIORITY**
>
> ### Action Alert
>
> *If enteral tubes are misplaced or become dislodged, the patient is likely to aspirate. Aspiration pneumonia is a common, life-threatening complication associated with TEN, especially for older adults. Observe for increasing temperature and pulse, as well as for other signs of dehydration such as dry mucous membranes and decreased urinary output. Auscultate lungs every 4 to 8 hours to check for diminishing breath sounds, especially in lower lobes. Patients may become short of breath and report chest discomfort. A chest x-ray confirms this diagnosis, and treatment with antibiotics is started.*

Abdominal Distention and Nausea/Vomiting. Abdominal distention, nausea, and vomiting during tube feeding are often caused by overfeeding. To *prevent* overfeeding, check gastric residual volumes every 4 to 6 hours, depending on facility policy and the needs of the patient. The American Society of Parenteral and Enteral Nutrition (ASPEN) recommends holding a feeding if the gastric residual volumes are more than 200 mL on two consecutive assessments. In some facilities, feedings are temporarily held if the gastric residual is 100 mL or more, depending on the patient. After a period of rest, the feeding can be restarted at a lower flow rate.

A problem with frequent residual assessments is that the formula may clog the tube during aspiration, even if flushed with water. If the patient's residual volumes have been low or zero and he or she has no abdominal distention, nausea, or vomiting, consider discontinuing these assessments, depending on facility policy.

Fluid and Electrolyte Imbalances. Patients receiving enteral nutrition therapy are at an increased risk for fluid imbalances. They are often older or debilitated and may also have cardiac or renal problems. Fluid imbalances associated with enteral nutrition are usually related to the body's response to increased serum osmolarity, but *fluid overload* from too much tube feeding can also occur.

Osmolarity is the amount or concentration of particles dissolved in solution. This concentration exerts a specific osmotic pressure within the solution. Normal osmolarity of extracellular fluid (ECF) ranges between 270 and 300 mOsm. Enteral feeding products range in osmolarity from isotonic (about 300 mOsm) to extremely hypertonic (600 mOsm).

Electrolytes (including sodium) contribute to this hypertonicity, but more of the osmolarity is determined by the concentration of proteins and sugar molecules in the enteral product. Even when the product is isotonic, the ECF can become hyperosmolar unless some hypotonic fluids are also administered to the patient. This situation is most likely to develop in patients who are unconscious, unable to respond to the thirst reflex, on fluid restrictions, or receiving hyperosmotic enteral preparations.

Because increased plasma osmolarity is largely a result of extra glucose and proteins (which tend to remain in the plasma rather than move to interstitial spaces), the plasma osmotic pressure (water-pulling pressure) is increased. In this situation, intracellular and interstitial water move into and expand the plasma volume. This volume expansion results in an increased renal excretion of water (in patients with normal renal function) and leads to osmotic *dehydration*. If patients do *not* have normal renal and cardiac function, expansion of the plasma volume can lead to circulatory overload and pulmonary edema, especially in older adults. Assess for signs and symptoms of circulatory overload, such as peripheral edema, sudden weight gain, crackles, dyspnea, increased blood pressure, and bounding pulse. Collaborate with the dietitian and health care provider to plan the correct amount of fluid to be provided.

Excessive *diarrhea* may develop when hyperosmolar enteral preparations are delivered quickly. This situation can also lead to *dehydration* through excessive water loss. Collaborate with the health care provider and dietitian for recommendations to prevent diarrhea. The dietitian usually changes the feeding to a more iso-osmolar formula. Most of these formulas can be started full strength but slowly at 15 to 20 mL/hr. The rate is gradually increased as the patient tolerates and as the expected nutritional outcome is achieved.

If diarrhea continues, especially if it has a very foul odor, the patient should be evaluated for *Clostridium difficile* or other infectious organisms. Contamination can occur because of repeated and often faulty handling of the feeding solution and system. *Wear clean gloves when changing systems and adding product. Sterile gloves may help prevent infection in critically ill or immunocompromised patients. A closed feeding system is preferred over an open one because the chance of contamination is lessened* (see Chart 63-4). Tubes with ports also minimize contamination by eliminating the need to open the feeding system to administer drugs.

In some cases, diarrhea may be the result of multiple liquid medications, such as elixirs and suspensions that have a very high osmolarity. Examples include acetaminophen (Tylenol), furosemide (Lasix), and phenytoin (Dilantin). Patients receiving multiple liquid drugs should be evaluated by the health care provider to determine whether their drug regimen can be changed to prevent diarrhea. Diluting these liquids may also be an option.

Depending on the patient's state of health, some electrolyte imbalances can be avoided. This is achieved by the use of enteral preparations containing lower concentrations of the electrolytes that the patient cannot handle well. For example, renal patients with high potassium levels receive a special formula that is used for this imbalance.

The two most common electrolyte imbalances associated with enteral nutrition therapy are hyperkalemia and hyponatremia. Both of these conditions may be related to

hyperglycemia-induced hyperosmolarity of the plasma and the resultant osmotic diuresis. Fluid and electrolyte imbalances are discussed in detail in Chapter 13.

Parenteral Nutrition. When a patient cannot effectively use the GI tract for nutrition, either partial or total parenteral nutrition therapy may maintain or improve his or her nutritional status. This form of IV therapy differs from standard IV therapy in that any or all nutrients (carbohydrates, proteins, fats, vitamins, minerals, and trace elements) can be given. One liter of IV fluid containing 5% dextrose, which is often used as standard therapy, provides only 170 kcal. A hospitalized patient typically receives 3 to 4 L a day, for a total number of calories ranging between 500 and 700 a day. This calorie intake is not sufficient when the patient requires IV therapy for a prolonged period and cannot eat an adequate diet or has increased calorie needs for tissue repair and building.

Partial Parenteral Nutrition. Partial, or peripheral, parenteral nutrition (PPN) is usually given through a cannula or catheter in a large distal vein of the arm or through a peripherally inserted central catheter (PICC line). (See Chapter 15 for care of patients with PICC lines.) This nutritional alternative is used for some patients who can eat but are not able to take in enough nutrients to meet their needs. The patient must have adequate peripheral vein access and be able to tolerate large volumes of fluid to have PPN. Two types of solutions are commonly used in various combinations for PPN: IV fat (lipid) emulsions (IVFEs) and amino acid–dextrose solutions. IVFEs are usually given using a piggyback method.

> ## ! NURSING SAFETY PRIORITY
> ### *Critical Rescue*
>
> For patients receiving fat emulsions, monitor for manifestations of fat overload syndrome, especially in those who are critically ill. These manifestations include fever, increased triglycerides, clotting problems, and multi-system organ failure. Discontinue the IVFE infusion and report any of these changes to the health care provider immediately if this complication is suspected.

Most IVFEs (20% fat emulsion) are isotonic, but the tonicity of commercially prepared amino acid–dextrose solutions ranges from 300 mOsm to nearly 900 mOsm for PPN. Amino acid–dextrose solutions are considered more stable than IVFEs and therefore additives (e.g., vitamins, minerals, electrolytes, trace elements) tend to be mixed with them. These solutions must be delivered through an in-line filter and are administered by an infusion pump for an accurate and constant delivery rate.

Some PPN products are a *mixture* of lipids (10% or 20% fat emulsion) and an amino acid–dextrose (usually 10%) solution. This mixture of three types of nutrients is referred to as a *3:1, total nutrient admixture (TNA), or triple-mix solution.*

Total Parenteral Nutrition. When the patient requires intensive nutritional support for an extended time, the health care provider prescribes centrally administered total parenteral nutrition (TPN). TPN is delivered through access to central veins, usually through a PICC line or the subclavian or internal jugular veins. Central venous catheters and associated nursing care are described in detail in Chapter 15.

Total parenteral nutrition solutions contain higher concentrations of dextrose and proteins, usually in the form of synthetic amino acids or protein hydrolysates (3% to 5%). These solutions are hyperosmotic (three to six times the osmolarity of normal blood). The base solutions are available as commercially prepared solutions. The hospital or community pharmacist adds components (specific electrolytes, minerals, trace elements, and insulin) according to the patient's nutritional needs. This therapy provides needed calories and spares body proteins from catabolism for energy requirements.

The TPN solutions are administered with an infusion pump. The osmolarity of the fluid and the concentrations of the specific components make controlled delivery essential.

Patients receiving parenteral nutrition fluids are at risk for a wide variety of serious and potentially life-threatening complications. Complications may result from the solutions or from the peripheral or central venous catheter. The following discussion is limited to the complications that involve fluid or electrolyte balance. Complications of IV cannulas and central venous catheters are discussed in Chapter 15, including infection and sepsis.

Patients receiving parenteral nutrition therapy are at high risk for fluid imbalance. Not only is fluid delivered directly into the venous system, but also the extreme hyperosmolarity of the solutions stimulates fluid shifts between body fluid compartments. The hyperosmolarity is caused by their amino acid and dextrose concentrations. Increased dextrose causes hyperglycemia (increased blood glucose). As a result, some of the dextrose moves into the interstitial and intracellular spaces, where it is metabolized. However, dextrose remains in the plasma volume when the solutions are administered too rapidly, without enough insulin coverage, or in the presence of hyponatremia and hypokalemia. The result is a shift of water from the interstitial and intracellular spaces into the plasma. Expansion of the plasma volume together with hyperglycemia can cause osmotic diuresis and lead to serious dehydration and hypovolemic shock. If the patient also has cardiac or renal dysfunction, he or she may develop fluid overload, congestive heart failure, and pulmonary edema. Monitor the infusion rate of the parenteral fluid, and give insulin as prescribed.

Monitor for these complications by taking daily weights and by recording accurate intake and output while the patient is receiving parenteral nutrition. Serum glucose and electrolyte values are also monitored (Chart 63-6). Report any major changes or abnormalities to the health care provider, and document all assessments and interventions.

Patients receiving TPN are at an increased risk for many different electrolyte imbalances, depending on the composition of the solution and whether a fluid imbalance occurs. The health care provider usually requests frequent determinations of serum electrolyte levels to detect these imbalances. The risk for metabolic and electrolyte complications is reduced when the rate of administration is carefully controlled and patients are closely monitored for response to treatment. Potassium and sodium imbalances are common, especially when insulin is also administered as part of the therapy. Calcium imbalances, particularly hypercalcemia, are associated with TPN, although immobility may play more of a role than the actual therapy in developing this imbalance.

CHART 63-6   **BEST PRACTICE FOR PATIENT SAFETY & QUALITY CARE**

Care and Maintenance of Total Parenteral Nutrition

- Check each bag of total parenteral nutrition (TPN) solution for accuracy by comparing it with the physician's or pharmacist's prescription.
- Monitor the IV pump for accuracy in delivering the prescribed hourly rate.
- If the TPN solution is temporarily unavailable, give 10% dextrose/water (D/W) or 20% D/W until the TPN solution can be obtained.
- If the TPN administration is not on time ("behind"), do not attempt to "catch up" by increasing the rate.
- Monitor the patient's weight daily or according to facility protocol.
- Monitor serum electrolytes and glucose daily or per facility protocol. (Many facilities require finger-stick blood sugars [FSBSs] every 4 hours, especially if the patient is receiving insulin. Urine testing for ketones may also be requested.)
- Monitor for, report, and document complications, including fluid and electrolyte imbalances.
- Monitor and carefully record the patient's intake and output.
- Assess the patient's IV site for signs of infection or infiltration (see Chapter 15).
- Change the IV tubing every 24 hours or per facility protocol.
- Change the dressing around the IV site every 48 to 72 hours or per facility protocol.
- Before administering TPN, have a second nurse check the prescription and solution to prevent patient harm.

Community-Based Care

Malnourished patients can be cared for in a variety of settings, including the acute care hospital, transitional care unit, nursing home, or their own home. Malnutrition is often diagnosed when the patient is admitted to the acute care hospital or shortly after hospitalization if complications such as poor wound healing or sepsis occur. If the patient is severely compromised, he or she may require admission to a traditional nursing home for either transitional or long-term care. If adequate home support is available, he or she may be discharged to home in the care of a family member or other caregiver. Home care nurses may be needed to monitor and direct the care.

Home Care Management

The malnourished patient needs a variety of resources at home to continue aggressive nutrition support. If he or she can consume food by the oral route, the case manager or other discharge planner determines whether financial resources are available for the necessary nutrition supplements. If the hospital provides ambulatory nutrition counseling services, the patient is scheduled for follow-up after discharge for assessment of weight gain.

Teaching for Self-Management

The dietitian teaches the malnourished patient and family about high-calorie, high-protein diet and nutritional supplements. In collaboration with the pharmacist, review specific parenteral solutions with the patient and family or significant others.

Reinforce the importance of adhering to the prescribed diet, and review any drugs the patient may be taking. If using an iron preparation, teach the importance of taking the drug immediately before or during meals. Caution the patient that iron tends to cause constipation. For the older adult already susceptible to constipation, emphasize the importance of measures for prevention, including adequate fiber intake, adequate fluids, and exercise.

Some patients are discharged to home with enteral or parenteral nutrition. Teach the family or other caregiver how to continue these therapies. Remind caregivers to consider the psychosocial aspects of these alternative methods for nutrition. For example, the caregiver can bring the enteral product and napkin to the patient on a decorative tray to make the feeding experience more elegant and "normal." Moving the feeding equipment out of view of the patient when it is not in use is also helpful.

Health Care Resources

The malnourished patient discharged to home on enteral or parenteral nutrition support needs the specialized services of a home nutrition therapy team. This team generally consists of the physician, nurse, dietitian, pharmacist, and case manager or social worker. Several commercial companies supply these services to patients at home in addition to the feeding supplies and formulas and health teaching.

▌EVALUATION: OUTCOMES

Evaluate the care of the malnourished patient based on the identified priority patient problem. The primary expected outcome is that he or she has available nutrients to meet the metabolic demands for maintaining weight and total protein and has adequate hydration.

OBESITY

Pathophysiology

Obesity, like cancer, is not just one disease but, instead, many conditions with varying causes. The terms *obesity* and *overweight* are often used interchangeably, but they refer to different health problems. Overweight is an increase in body weight for height compared with a reference standard, or up to 10% greater than ideal body weight (IBW). However, this weight may not reflect excess body fat. It is possible for well-developed athletes to appear overweight because of increased muscle (lean) mass, in which the proportion of muscle to fat is greater than average.

Obesity refers to an excess amount of body fat when compared with lean body mass. The normal amount of body fat in *men* is between 15% and 20% of body weight. For *women*, the normal amount is 18% to 32%. An obese person weighs at least 20% above the upper limit of the normal range for ideal body weight. Morbid obesity, also called *extreme obesity*, refers to a weight that has a severely negative effect on health—usually more than 100% above IBW.

More than 72 million Americans are obese (Clancy, 2010), and another third of Americans are overweight. About 10% or more of adults are morbidly obese. *This problem is the second leading cause of preventable deaths in the United States, second only to smoking, and has become a national crisis. Obesity across the life span is considered an epidemic in the United States and Canada. Worldwide, it is recognized as a major global health problem, costing billions of dollars for health care and lost productivity.*

The pathophysiology of obesity is very complex. A number of chemicals in the body, including hormones known as *adipokines*, work together to affect appetite and fat metabolism:

- Leptin: a hormone released by fat cells and possibly by gastric cells; it also acts on the hypothalamus to control appetite
- Adiponectin: an anti-inflammatory and insulin sensitizing hormone
- Resistin: a hormone produced by fat cells that creates resistance to insulin activity
- Inflammatory cytokines: such as inflammatory interleukins and tumor necrosis factor–alpha
- Apolipoprotein E: one of several regulators of lipoprotein metabolism
- Cholecystokinin: a hormone that stimulates digestive juices and may work with leptin to increase or decrease appetite
- Ghrelin: the "hunger hormone" that is secreted in the stomach; increases in a fasting state and decreases after a meal

Some adipokines are neuropeptides, including orexins and anorexins, which play a role in body weight. Orexins are appetite stimulants; examples are ghrelin secreted by the stomach and peptide YY from the intestines. Anorexins decrease appetite and include leptin and insulin (McCance et al., 2010). Increased circulating plasma levels of orexins are associated with the development of obesity. However, in some people, high levels of leptin may not be effective in suppressing appetite—a condition known as *leptin resistance*. In this case, overeating and excessive weight gain can result. Hyperleptinemia also stimulates the autonomic nervous system and contributes to blood vessel inflammation and ventricular hypertrophy. These actions may help explain why obese patients are most at risk for hypertension, atherosclerosis, and heart disease (Kulie et al., 2011). Obesity is also associated with insulin resistance, which predisposes obese patients to type 2 diabetes mellitus (see Chapter 67).

Obesity is determined by weight compared with height, BMI, and waist circumference. To establish the percentage of IBW, the *height and weight* of the patient are compared with the midpoint of the desirable weight using an accepted reference standard. The *body mass index (BMI)*, as described previously, is a measure of heaviness and is only an indirect indicator of body fat. It reflects the combined effects of body build, proportions, lean body mass, and body fat. However, BMI has substantial correlations with fat mass for adult men and women and has been validated as a risk factor for cardiovascular disease. A BMI of 25 to 29.9 indicates that a person is overweight. A BMI of 30 or more indicates obesity. *People who are morbidly obese have a BMI of greater than 40 and are at a major risk for life-threatening health problems.*

The distribution of excess body fat rather than the degree of obesity has been used to predict increased health risks. For example, the waist circumference (WC) is a stronger predictor of coronary artery disease (CAD) than is the BMI. A WC greater than 35 inches (89 cm) in women, and a WC greater than 40 inches (102 cm) in men indicate central obesity (National Institute of Diabetes and Digestive and Kidney Diseases, 2008). Central obesity is a major risk factor for CAD, stroke, type 2 diabetes, some cancers (e.g., colon, breast), sleep apnea, and early death.

TABLE 63-3	COMMON COMPLICATIONS OF OBESITY
• Type 2 diabetes mellitus • Hypertension • Hyperlipidemia (increased serum lipids) • Coronary artery disease (CAD) • Stroke • Peripheral artery disease (PAD) • Metabolic syndrome • Obstructive sleep apnea	• Obesity hypoventilation syndrome • Depression and other mental health/behavioral health problems • Urinary incontinence • Cholelithiasis (gallstones) • Gout • Chronic back pain • Early osteoarthritis • Decreased wound healing

The waist-to-hip ratio (WHR) is also a predictor of CAD. This measure differentiates peripheral lower body obesity from central obesity. A WHR of 0.95 or greater in men (0.8 or greater in women) indicates android obesity with excess fat at the waist and abdomen.

Complications of Obesity

The major complications of obesity affect primarily the cardiovascular and respiratory systems. However, excess weight can also cause degeneration of the musculoskeletal system, especially the joints (osteoarthritis). Obese people are also more susceptible to infections and infectious diseases than are thinner people and tend to heal more slowly. Table 63-3 lists some of the most common complications of obesity.

Etiology and Genetic Risk

The causes of obesity involve complex interrelationships of many environmental, genetic, and behavioral factors. A number of causes of both human and animal obesity have been identified.

One of the most common causes of being overweight or obese is eating *high-fat and high-cholesterol diets.* Obesity is associated with diet when it contains a significant amount of *saturated* fat, which increases low-density lipoproteins (LDL-C). *Trans* fatty acids (TFAs), saturated fats, and cholesterol are linked to obesity and CAD (American Heart Association, 2010). By contrast, monounsaturated and polyunsaturated fats are healthy fats.

TFA is made when food manufacturers add hydrogen to vegetable oil, a process known as *hydrogenation.* This process increases the food's shelf life and flavor. Large amounts of TFA can be found in vegetable shortening, commercial baked goods, snack foods, and French fries. Food labels in the United States and Canada include amounts of total fat, subtypes of fat, and cholesterol content per serving.

Physical inactivity has been identified as another cause of overweight and obesity. The major barriers to increasing physical activity include a lack of time or decreased mobility associated with prolonged illness. Regular exercise is associated with lower death rates for adults of any age. It also increases lean muscle, decreases body fat, aids in weight control, and enhances psychological well-being. Regular exercise can also decrease the risk for falling in older adults (see Chapter 3).

Although some people think that regular exercise has to include joining a fitness program or exercising for long periods, simple forms of exercise like walking 20 minutes provide the same type of benefit. Older adults can engage in this type of exercise. It does not cost money (like joining a program) and provides health benefits such as strengthening joints and improving cardiovascular health.

Another cause of obesity is *drug therapy.* Some prescribed drugs contribute to weight gain when they are taken on a long-term basis. Examples include:

*   Corticosteroids
*   Estrogens and certain progestins
*   Nonsteroidal anti-inflammatory drugs (NSAIDs)
*   Antihypertensives
*   Antidepressants and other psychoactive drugs
*   Antiepileptic drugs
*   Certain oral antidiabetic agents

GENETIC/GENOMIC CONSIDERATIONS

Familial and genetic factors seem to play a very important role in obesity. When both parents are overweight, about 80% of their children will be overweight. If neither parent is overweight, fewer than 10% of the children will be overweight. In studies of identical twins, nonidentical twins, and parent-sibling relationships, about 50% of the difference in body fatness is transmitted to children and about 50% of this amount is genetically controlled (McCance et al., 2010).

Genetic composition may predispose some people, but not others, to obesity. Leptin, the hormone encoded by the *ob* gene, appears to send a message to the brain that the body has stored enough fat. This message serves as a signal to stop eating. In some obese people, other gene mutations have been identified, including an abnormality of the melanocortin-4 receptor that inhibits appetite in families with a history of obesity.

A small number of obese people have disorders of the neuroendocrine system. Examples include injury to the hypothalamus, Cushing's disease, polycystic ovary failure, hypogonadism, and growth hormone deficiency.

Health Promotion and Maintenance

Obesity is a major public health problem and is associated with many complications, including death. As a result of this increasing problem, the *Healthy People 2010* agenda addressed the need to reduce the proportion of children, adolescents, and adults who are obese. The new *Healthy People 2020 objectives for Nutrition and Weight Status* include specific population targets related to obesity and healthy nutritional habits (Table 63-4). In collaboration with the dietitian, teach the importance of weight management and exercise to improve health. Even a 5% weight loss can drastically decrease the risk for coronary artery disease (CAD) and diabetes mellitus.

PATIENT-CENTERED COLLABORATIVE CARE

■ ASSESSMENT

History

In addition to taking a complete history regarding present and past health problems, collect this information about the patient in collaboration with the dietitian:

*   Economic status
*   Usual food intake
*   Eating behavior
*   Cultural background
*   Attitude toward food

TABLE 63-4 **MEETING *HEALTHY PEOPLE 2020* SAMPLE OBJECTIVES AND TARGETS: NUTRITION AND WEIGHT STATUS**
• Reduce the proportion of adults who are obese (by 10%).
• Increase the proportion of adults who are at a healthy weight (by 10%).
• Increase the proportion of physician visits made by adult patients that include counseling about nutrition or diet (by 15.2%).
• Increase the proportion of primary care physicians who regularly assess body mass index (BMI) in their adult patients (by 10%).
• Increase the contribution of total vegetables to the diets of the population aged 2 years and older (to 1.1 cups per 1000 calories).
• Increase the contribution of fruits to the diets of the population aged 2 years and older (to 0.9 cups per 1000 calories).
• Reduce consumption of saturated fat in the population aged 2 years and older (by 9.5%).

- Appetite
- Chronic diseases
- Drugs (prescribed and OTC, including herbal preparations)
- Physical activity/functional ability
- Family history of obesity
- Developmental level

A nutritional history usually includes a 24-hour recall of food intake and the frequency with which foods are consumed. The adequacy of the diet can be evaluated by comparing the amount and types of foods consumed daily with the established standards. The dietitian then provides a more detailed analysis of nutritional intake.

Physical Assessment/Clinical Manifestations

Obtain an accurate height and weight. The dietitian calculates the percentage of ideal body weight (% IBW) and the body mass index (BMI). He or she may also:
- Measure the waist circumference
- Calculate the waist-to-hip ratio
- Determine arm and calf circumferences

Examine the skin of the obese patient for reddened or open areas. Lift skinfold areas, such as pendulous breasts and abdominal aprons (panniculus), to observe for *Candida* (yeast) (a condition called *intertrigo*) or other infections or lesions. Infection of the panniculus is referred to as panniculitis.

Psychosocial Assessment

Obtain a psychosocial history to determine the patient's circumstances and emotional factors that might prevent successful therapy or that might be worsened by therapy. Interview the patient to determine his or her perception of current weight and weight reduction. Some patients do not view weight as a problem, which affects treatment and outcome. Ask the patient questions about his or her health beliefs related to being overweight, such as:
- What does food mean to you?
- Do you want to lose weight?
- What prevents you from losing weight?
- What do you think will motivate you to lose weight?
- How do you think you might benefit from losing weight?

Many patients report that they have tried multiple diets to lose weight but either the diets have not worked or they regained the weight they had initially lost. People who attempt restrictive diets become easy targets for the billion-dollar weight-loss industry, yet most dieters regain lost weight. This problem can be even more concerning for the older adult who loses weight and then regains it. Recent studies have shown that this cycle may contribute to loss of lean muscle mass, especially in older men (Lee et al., 2010).

The results of dieting and other efforts can lead to a sense of failure and lowered self-esteem, which often stimulates more overeating. Many overweight and obese people eat in response to environmental and emotional stressors rather than because they are hungry. Ask patients to identify their perceived stressors and what triggers their need for food.

Lifestyle changes are difficult without adequate family and community support. Assess useful coping strategies and support systems that the patient can use during treatment for obesity.

Explore the patient's history to assess:
- Attempts at weight-reduction diets and outcomes
- Effects of obesity on lifestyle
- Effects of obesity on social interactions
- Mental health/behavioral health problems, such as depression
- Effects of obesity on intimate relationships, especially sexuality

Obese men often experience erectile dysfunction (ED), which can cause or worsen depression. Women often experience changes in their menstrual cycles and may have problems getting pregnant.

▌INTERVENTIONS

Weight is lost only when energy used is greater than intake. Weight loss may be accomplished by nutritional modification with or without the aid of drugs and in combination with a regular exercise program. Patients who may be candidates for surgical treatment include those who have:
- Repeated failure of nonsurgical interventions
- A BMI equal to or greater than 40
- Weight more than 100% above IBW (i.e., morbidly obese)

Nonsurgical Management

Various nutritional approaches and drug therapy have attempted to help obese patients achieve permanent weight loss.

Diet Programs. Diets for helping people lose weight include fasting, very-low-calorie diets, balanced and unbalanced low-energy diets, and novelty diets.

Short-term fasting programs have not been successful in treating morbidly obese patients, and prolonged fasting does not produce permanent benefits. Most patients regain the weight that was lost by this method. In addition, the risks associated with fasting (e.g., severe ketosis) require close medical supervision.

Very-low-calorie diets generally provide 200 to 800 calories/day. Two types of these diets are the *protein-sparing modified fast* and the *liquid formula diet*. The protein-sparing modified fast provides protein of high biologic value (1.5 g/kg of desirable body weight daily) within a limited number of calories. The diet produces rapid weight loss while preserving lean body mass. The liquid formula diet provides between 33 and 70 g of protein daily.

Both diets require an initial cardiac evaluation, supervision by an interdisciplinary health care team with monitoring by a physician, nutrition counseling by a dietitian, and supplementation with vitamins and minerals. These diets are only one part of a weight-reduction program. Patients who are on these diets should receive nutrition education, psychological counseling, exercise, and behavior therapy. Comparable weight losses have been achieved with both diets, but again, most patients regain the weight they lost.

Nutritionally *balanced diets* generally provide about 1200 calories/day with a conventional distribution of carbohydrate, protein, and fat. Vitamin and mineral supplements may be necessary if energy intakes fall below 1200 calories for women and 1800 calories for men. This diet provides conventional foods that are economical and easy to obtain. Thus the outcome of weight loss is facilitated, and it is hoped that loss is maintained. For example, Weight Watchers is an organization that provides education about nutritionally balanced diets based on a point system. They offer on-site weekly group support meetings or the option of an online community.

Unbalanced low-energy diets, such as the low-carbohydrate diet (e.g., Atkins or South Beach diet), restrict one or more nutrients. Protein and vegetables are encouraged, but certain carbohydrates and high-fat foods are not. Although they remain controversial in the medical community, these diets are extremely popular. Scientific outcome data have been conflicting.

Novelty diets, such as the grapefruit diet, the Cookie diet, and the Hollywood diet, are often nutritionally *inadequate*. This type of diet implies that a certain food or liquid increases metabolic rate or accelerates the oxidation of body fat. Weight loss is achieved because energy is restricted by food choice, but patients do not sustain weight loss after stopping the diet.

Nutrition Therapy. Nutritional recommendations for each patient should be developed through close interaction among the patient, family, physician, nurse, and dietitian. The diet should meet the patient's needs, habits, and lifestyle and should be realistic.

The dietitian develops a diet plan and instructs the patient. At a minimum, the diet should:
- Have a scientific rationale
- Be nutritionally adequate for all nutrients
- Have a low risk-benefit ratio
- Be practical and conducive to long-term success

Calorie estimates are easily calculated. Resting metabolic rate is determined using a gender-specific formula that incorporates the appropriate activity factor. This figure reflects the total calories needed daily for maintaining current weight. To encourage a weight loss of 1 pound (2.2 kg) a week, the dietitian subtracts 500 calories each day. To encourage a weight loss of 2 pounds (4.4 kg) a week, 1000 calories each day are subtracted. The amount of weight lost varies with the patient's food intake, level of physical activity, and water losses. A reasonable expected outcome of 5% to 10% loss of body weight has been shown to improve glycemic control and reduce cholesterol and blood pressure. These benefits continue if the weight loss is sustained.

Exercise Program. A major intervention to manage obesity is to increase the type and amount of daily exercise to burn calories along with change in eating habits. For most people, adding exercise to a nutritional intervention produces more weight loss than just dieting alone. More of the weight lost is fat, which preserves lean body mass. An increase in exercise can reduce the waist circumference and the waist-to-hip ratio.

Teach patients that increasing and maintaining physical activity levels are important in maintaining weight loss. Many overweight or obese patients are so unfit that it may take several months of conditioning before they can exercise sufficiently to lose weight.

The physical therapist or exercise physiologist or assistant first obtains a clinical exercise and health history. It is important to determine the patient's current exercise pattern, if any, and exercise habits over a lifetime. Teach about the importance of an exercise component in a weight-loss program. The patient's desire to participate in an exercise program and his or her preferred types of exercise are also identified.

The health care provider may evaluate the patient by an exercise stress test. Not all patients need one, but those with chronic disease may need the results to assist with an individual exercise plan. Patients are counseled about unusual signs and symptoms during exercise (e.g., chest pain) and what to do if they occur. The physical therapist or exercise physiologist first emphasizes the importance of exercising consistently and then stresses its duration, intensity, and frequency.

A minimum-level workout should be developed so that consistency can be achieved. The expected outcome is to maintain a lifetime of increased physical activity. The patient is likely to be less fatigued and discouraged with a low-intensity, short-duration program. Encourage sedentary (physically inactive) patients to increase their activity by walking 30 to 40 minutes at least 5 days each week. The activity may be performed all at once or divided over the course of the day. Remind the patient to exercise only under the supervision of the physician. All members of the interdisciplinary team should encourage and support any increase in physical activity. Structured national programs with support staff, such as Curves, may be helpful for some patients. The staff typically offer diet counseling as well as cardiovascular and muscle-toning activities.

Drug Therapy. A BMI of 30 or a BMI of 27 with comorbidities is one indicator for the use of drug therapy. Anorectic drugs suppress appetite, which reduces food intake and, over time, may result in weight loss. The Food and Drug Administration in the United States has pulled several drugs off the market and not approved other drugs due to concerns about cardiovascular complications associated with long-term use. The only *prescription* drug still available for the *long-term* treatment of obesity is orlistat (Xenical).

Orlistat inhibits lipase and leads to partial hydrolysis of triglycerides. Because fats are only partially digested and absorbed, calorie intake is decreased. The usual dosage is 120 mg three times daily. Most patients taking this drug have GI symptoms that include loose stools, abdominal cramps, and nausea unless they reduce their fat intake to less than 30% of their food intake each day. Therefore it should be used with caution and limited to adults between 18 and 75 years of age. Treatment is usually not extended beyond 12 months. A lower-dose 60-mg orlistat tablet (Alli) is the only *over-the-counter* weight loss aid product that has received FDA approval for long-term use.

Other sympathomimetic drugs suppress appetite for *short-term* use along with a structured weight-management and exercise program. These drugs act on the central nervous system, including suppressing the appetite center in the hypothalamus. Examples include phentermine (Adipex-P), diethylpropion (Tenuate, Tenuate Dospan), and phendimetrazine (Bontril).

> ### ! NURSING SAFETY PRIORITY
> #### *Drug Alert*
>
> Patients with hypertension, heart disease, and hyperthyroidism should not take anorectic drugs because they may worsen their symptoms. These drugs are not prescribed for any patient taking psychoactive agents because they cause similar side effects. Teach patients who are candidates for sympathomimetic drugs about side effects, which include:
> - Palpitations
> - Diarrhea or constipation
> - Restlessness
> - Insomnia
> - Dry mouth
> - Blurred vision (especially Bontril)
> - Change in sex drive or activity
> - Anxiety

Behavioral Management. Behavioral management of obesity helps the patient change daily eating habits to lose weight. This ongoing process should produce a change in behavior. Self-monitoring techniques include keeping a record of foods eaten (food diary), exercise patterns, and emotional and situational factors. Stimulus control involves controlling the external cues that promote overeating. Reinforcement techniques are used to self-reward the behavior change. Cognitive restructuring involves modifying negative beliefs by learning positive coping self-statements. Counseling by health care professionals must continue before, during, and after treatment. The 12-step program offered by Overeaters Anonymous (www.oa.org) has helped many people lose weight, especially those who are compulsive eaters.

Complementary and Alternative Therapies. Many complementary and alternative therapies have been tested and used for obesity. These modalities aim to suppress appetite and therefore limit food intake to lose weight:
- Acupuncture
- Acupressure
- Ayurvedic (a combination of holistic approaches)
- Hypnosis

Descriptions of most of these methods can be found in Chapter 2.

Surgical Management

At any weight, some patients seek to improve their appearance by having a variety of cosmetic procedures to reduce the amount of adipose tissue in selected areas of the body. A typical example of this type of surgery is liposuction, which can be done in a physician's office or ambulatory surgery center. Although the patient's appearance improves, if weight gain continues, the fatty tissue will return. This procedure is not a solution for people who are morbidly obese.

Morbidly obese people who do not respond to traditional interventions may be considered for a major surgical procedure aimed at producing permanent weight loss. Patients with a body mass index (BMI) of 40 or greater or a BMI of 35 or greater along with additional risk factors are considered for surgery. Surgery has been perceived as a last resort to address weight issues, but it *is the only method that has a long-term impact on morbid obesity.*

Bariatrics is a branch of medicine that manages obesity and its related diseases. Surgical procedures include these three types: gastric restrictive, malabsorption, or both. *Restrictive* surgeries decrease the volume capacity of the stomach to limit the amount of food that can be eaten at one time. As the name implies, *malabsorption* procedures interfere with the absorption of food and nutrients from the GI tract.

Every year, more than 100,000 people in the United States have these procedures, and that number is rapidly increasing. The surgeon may use a conventional open approach or minimally invasive surgery (MIS). Most patients have MIS by having either the laparoscopic adjustable gastric band (LAGB) or the laparoscopic sleeve gastrectomy (LSG). Both procedures are classified as restrictive surgeries (Kaser & Kukla, 2009). The decision of whether the patient is a candidate for the MIS is based on weight, body build, history of abdominal surgery, and co-existing medical complications. With any surgical approach, patients must agree to modify their lifestyle and follow stringent protocols to lose weight and keep the weight off. After bariatric surgery, many patients no longer have complications of obesity, such as diabetes mellitus, hypertension, depression, or sleep apnea.

Preoperative Care. Preoperative care is similar to that for any patient undergoing abdominal surgery or laparoscopy (see Chapter 16). However, obese patients are at increased surgical risks of pulmonary and thromboembolitic complications, as well as death. Some surgeons require limited weight loss before bariatric surgery to decrease these complications. Patients also have a thorough psychological assessment and testing to detect depression, substance abuse, or other mental health/behavioral health problem that could interfere with their success after surgery. Additional assessments to evaluate cognitive ability, coping skills, development, motivation, expectations, and support systems are also performed. Patients who are not alert and oriented or do not have sufficient strength and mobility are not considered for bariatric surgery. *The primary role of the nurse is to reinforce health teaching in preparation for surgery.* Most bariatric surgical centers provide education sessions for groups of patients who plan to have a bariatric procedure.

Operative Procedures. Gastric restriction surgeries allow for normal digestion without the risk for nutritional deficiencies. In the LAGB procedure, the surgeon places an adjustable band to create a small proximal stomach pouch through a laparoscope (Fig. 63-4, *A*). The band may or may not be inflatable. For example, the REALIZE® band requires that saline be injected into a balloon to control the tightness of the band. This type of procedure is considered to be restrictive; malabsorption complications do not usually occur (Pettit, 2009). For the LSG, the surgeon removes the portion of the stomach where ghrelin, the "hunger hormone," is secreted. Restrictive surgeries are the easiest to perform and can be reversed. However, weight lost is often regained after a period of time. By contrast, patients having the malabsorption procedures maintain 60% to 70% of their weight loss even after 20 years.

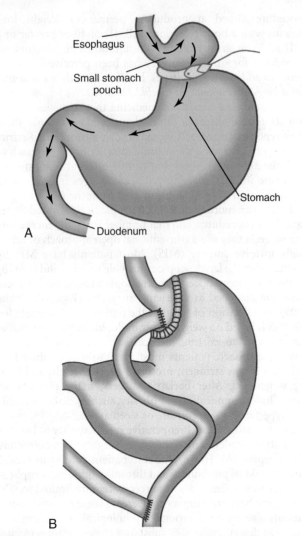

FIG. 63-4 Bariatric surgical procedures. **A,** Adjustable banded gastroplasty. **B,** Roux-en-Y gastric bypass (RNYGB).

The most common *malabsorption surgery* performed in the United States is the *Roux-en-Y gastric bypass (RNYGB)*, which is often done as a robotic surgical procedure. Other procedures less commonly done are the biliopancreatic diversion (rarely done) and the duodenal switch. All of these procedures result in quicker weight loss, but they are more invasive with a higher risk for postoperative complications. In RNYGB, most commonly just called a gastric bypass, gastric resection is combined with malabsorption surgery. The patient's stomach, duodenum, and part of the jejunum are bypassed so that fewer calories can be absorbed (see Fig. 63-4, *B*).

Postoperative Care. Postoperative care depends on the type of surgery—the conventional open approach or the minimally invasive technique. Although many patients have MIS, they are considered as having major abdominal surgery along with all its risks and are cared for accordingly. These patients may require less than 24 hours in the hospital; some may need 1 to 2 days. Patients with open procedures may need several days to recover.

Patients having one of the MIS procedures have less pain, scarring, and blood loss. They typically have a faster recovery time and a faster return to daily activities.

The priority for immediate care of postoperative bariatric surgery patients is airway management. Patients with short and thick necks often have compromised airways and need aggressive respiratory support, possibly mechanical ventilation in the critical care unit.

All patients experience some degree of pain, but it is usually less severe when MIS is done. Patients may use patient-controlled analgesia (PCA) with morphine for up to the first 24 hours. All patients receive oral opioid analgesic agents as prescribed after the PCA is discontinued. Liquid forms of drug therapy are preferred. Acute pain management is discussed in detail in Chapter 5.

Care of the bariatric surgical patient is similar to that of any patient having abdominal or laparoscopic surgery. *A major focus is patient and staff safety.* Special bariatric equipment and accommodations, including an extra-wide bed and additional personnel for moving the patient, are needed for both the surgical suite and postoperative care units. Weight-rated beds must be wide enough to allow the patient to turn. Bed rails should not be touching the body because they can cause pressure areas. Pressure between skinfolds, as well as tubes and catheters, can also cause skin breakdown. Monitor the skin in these areas, and keep it clean and dry.

> **❗ NURSING SAFETY PRIORITY**
>
> ***Action Alert***
>
> Some patients who have bariatric surgery have a nasogastric (NG) tube put in place, especially after open surgical procedures. In gastroplasty procedures, the NG tube drains both the proximal pouch and the distal stomach. Closely monitor the tube for patency. Never reposition the tube, because its movement can disrupt the suture line! The NG tube is removed on the second day if the patient is passing flatus.

Clear liquids are introduced slowly if the patient can tolerate water, and 1-ounce cups are used for each serving. Pureed foods, juice, and soups thinned with broth, water, or milk are added to the diet 24 to 48 hours after clear liquids are tolerated. Typically, the patient can increase the volume to 1 ounce over 5 minutes or until satisfied, but the diet is limited to liquids or pureed foods for 6 weeks. The patient then progresses to regular food, with an emphasis on nutrient-dense foods. Nausea, vomiting, or discomfort occurs if too much liquid is ingested.

> **❗ NURSING SAFETY PRIORITY**
>
> ***Critical Rescue***
>
> *Anastomotic leaks are the most common serious complication and cause of death after gastric bypass surgery. Monitor for manifestations of this life-threatening problem, including increasing back, shoulder, or abdominal pain; restlessness; and unexplained tachycardia and oliguria (scant urine). Report any of these findings to the surgeon immediately!*

In addition to the postoperative complications typically associated with abdominal and laparoscopic surgeries, bariatric patients have special needs and risks. Implement these measures to prevent complications:

- Apply an abdominal binder to prevent wound dehiscence for open surgical procedures.

- Place the patient in semi-Fowler's position or use bi-level or continuous positive airway pressure (BiPAP or CPAP) ventilation at night to improve breathing and decrease risk for sleep apnea or other pulmonary complications, such as pneumonia and atelectasis.
- Monitor oxygen saturation; provide oxygen at 2 L/min as prescribed.
- Apply sequential compression stockings and administer prophylactic anticoagulant (usually heparin) therapy as prescribed to help prevent thromboembolitic complications, including pulmonary embolism (PE).
- Observe skin areas and folds for redness, excoriation, or breakdown to treat these problems early.
- Use absorbent padding between folds to prevent pressure areas and skin breakdown; make sure that tubes and catheters are not causing pressure as well.
- Remove urinary catheter within 24 hours after surgery to prevent urinary tract infection.
- Assist the patient out of bed on the day of surgery; encourage and assist with turning every 2 hours using an appropriate weight-bearing overhead trapeze. Collaborate with the physical or occupational therapist if needed for transfers or ambulation assistive devices, such as walkers.
- Ambulate patient as soon as possible to prevent postoperative complications, such as deep vein thrombosis and pulmonary embolus.
- Measure and record abdominal girth daily, as requested.
- In collaboration with the dietitian, provide six small feedings and plenty of fluids to prevent dehydration.
- Observe for signs and symptoms of dumping syndrome (caused by food entering the small intestine instead of the stomach) after *gastric bypass*, such as tachycardia, nausea, diarrhea, and abdominal cramping.

❓ DECISION-MAKING CHALLENGE

Patient-Centered Care; Evidence-Based Practice; Teamwork and Collaboration; Informatics

A 34-year-old morbidly obese man had a laparoscopic adjustable gastric band procedure yesterday afternoon as part of a long-term plan for weight loss. He tells you that he is afraid he is going to die. He also tells you that he is scared that his two young children, ages 2 and 5, will become "fat like me." As he talks with you, his respiratory rate increases to over 40 breaths per minute. He is having diaphoresis and places his hand on his chest as he speaks.

1. What patient problems do you think he is having at this time? What data support your answer?
2. What health assessments will you perform at this time and why?
3. How will you respond to his problems at this time and why?
4. When he is ready for discharge, what health teaching will you provide related to the *Healthy People 2020* and *2010 Dietary Guidelines for Americans*? Find the complete evidence-based documents on the Internet and develop a teaching plan for this patient.
5. With whom will you collaborate as you prepare for his discharge to home?

Community-Based Care

Obese patients are cared for in a variety of settings, including the acute care hospital and transitional care unit (particularly after surgery) or in their own home. Obesity is a chronic,

---

CHART 63-7 PATIENT AND FAMILY EDUCATION: PREPARING FOR SELF-MANAGEMENT

Discharge Teaching for the Patient After Bariatric Surgery

Nutrition: Diet progression, nutrient (including vitamin and mineral) supplements, hydration guidelines

Drug therapy: Analgesics and antiemetic drugs, if needed; drugs for other health problems

Wound care: Clean procedure for open or laparoscopic wounds; cover during shower or bath

Activity level: Restrictions, such as avoiding lifting; activity progression; return to driving and work

Signs and symptoms to report: Fever; excessive nausea or vomiting; epigastric, back, or shoulder pain; red, hot, and/or draining wound(s); pain, redness, or swelling in legs; chest pain; difficulty breathing

Follow-up care: Health care provider office or clinic visits, support groups and other community resources, counseling for patient and family

Continuing education: Nutrition and exercise classes; follow-up visits with dietitian

---

lifelong problem. Diets, drug therapy, exercise, and behavior modification can produce short-term weight losses with reasonable safety. However, most patients who do lose weight often regain the weight. Treatment of obesity should focus on the long-term reduction of health risks and medical problems associated with obesity, improving quality of life, and promoting a health-oriented lifestyle. Interdisciplinary team members need to provide a nonjudgmental, supportive atmosphere that encourages the patient to:

- Increase physical activity
- Decrease fat intake and reliance on appetite-reducing drugs
- Establish a normal eating pattern in response to physiologic hunger
- Address psychological problems and concerns

Frequent, long-term ambulatory care follow-up coordinated by a case manager is essential for successful treatment.

Teach patients that bowel changes are common after surgery, including constipation. Vitamin and mineral supplements are often needed after surgery, especially vitamin D, B-complex vitamins, iron, and calcium.

The most important features of health teaching for any obese patient and family focus on health-related behavior patterns. In collaboration with the dietitian, counsel the patient on a healthful eating pattern. The physical therapist or exercise physiologist recommends an appropriate exercise program. A psychologist may recommend cognitive restructuring approaches that help alter dysfunctional eating patterns. For patients who have surgery, additional discharge teaching is needed. Chart 63-7 lists the important areas that should be reviewed.

Bariatric surgery results in a major lifestyle change and a variety of emotions. During weight loss, the patient may become depressed or anxious. Some experience a "hibernation phase" for about a month after surgery because of physical and emotional adjustments. Patients are usually followed closely by the surgeon and dietitian for several years.

Encourage them to keep all appointments and to adhere to the community-based treatment plan to ensure success. Plastic surgery, such as panniculectomy (removal of the abdominal apron, or panniculus), may be performed after weight is stabilized, usually in about 18 to 24 months.

Provide the patient with a list of available community resources, such as Overeaters Anonymous (www.oa.org) and the American Obesity Association (www.obesity.org). For surgical patients, the American Society for Metabolic and Bariatric Surgery (www.asmbs.org) may be helpful.

NURSING CONCEPT REVIEW

What might you NOTICE if the patient is experiencing inadequate nutrition as a result of malnutrition or obesity?

Malnutrition
- Weight below ideal body weight or report of unexplained weight loss of 10 pounds in 6 months
- Dry, flaky skin
- Brittle nails and hair
- Leanness
- Activity intolerance
- Report of lethargy or fatigue
- Weakness
- Complications, such as infections, pressure ulcers, poor healing

Obesity
- Weight at least 20% above ideal
- Excessive fat
- Shortness of breath during activity or at rest
- Slowed movement
- Change in gait or limping
- Complications, such as type 2 diabetes mellitus, hypertension, depression

What should you INTERPRET and how should you RESPOND to a patient experiencing inadequate nutrition as a result of malnutrition or obesity?

Perform and interpret assessments, including:
- Take and record height and weight.
- Calculate BMI based on height and weight.
- Check laboratory values for hematocrit and hemoglobin and visceral proteins.

- Take complete medical history to determine associated complications and cause of nutritional problem.
- Assess impact of nutritional status on daily life, including ADLs.
- Assess coping mechanisms, especially for patients who are morbidly obese.

Respond by:
- Teaching patients about their need for a healthy nutritional state
- Teaching patients how to either lose or gain weight, depending on their specific problem (e.g., nutritional supplements for malnutrition; restrictive diet and exercise for obesity)
- Teaching patients to weigh frequently
- Monitoring changes in serum visceral proteins (especially prealbumin) as an indicator of improved nutrition for malnourished patients
- Initiating total enteral or total parenteral nutrition as prescribed for malnutrition
- Informing morbidly obese patients about bariatric surgery options

On what should you REFLECT?
- Monitor patient for indicators of improved nutrition (e.g., increased prealbumin and weight for malnutrition; weight loss and decreased fat for obesity).
- Think about what may have caused these nutritional problems and how they can be prevented.
- Think about what else you can do to improve nutritional health of patients you care for.

GET READY FOR THE NCLEX® EXAMINATION!

KEY POINTS

Review these Key Points for each NCLEX Examination Client Needs Category.

Safe and Effective Care Environment
- Ensure that feeding tube placement is verified by x-ray; check placement every 4 to 8 hours by aspirating gastric contents and assessing pH for nasogastric tubes.
- Place patients receiving tube feeding in a semi-Fowler's position at all times to prevent aspiration; check residual contents every 4 hours or as designated per facility policy.

- Use gloves when changing feeding system tubing or adding product; use sterile gloves when working with critically ill or immunocompromised patients.
- Use a feeding pump when the patient receives continuous or cyclic tube feeding.
- Collaborate with the interdisciplinary health care team, especially the dietitian, health care provider, and case manager, when caring for patients with malnutrition or obesity.

- Be sure that bariatric furniture and equipment are available for the obese patient in the hospital or other health care setting; avoid pressure on skinfold areas.

Health Promotion and Maintenance

- Perform nutritional screening for all patients to determine if they are at risk (see Charts 63-1 and 63-2).
- For patients receiving enteral or parenteral nutrition at home, teach family members or other caregivers how to provide nutrition while avoiding complications.
- Teach patients who are undernourished to eat high-protein, high-calorie foods and nutritional supplements.
- Instruct obese patients about the importance of health care provider–approved exercise for weight reduction.

Psychosocial Integrity

- Be aware that some obese patients may not view their weight as a problem and are therefore unlikely to be part of a weight-reduction plan.
- Recognize that obesity can cause depression or anxiety, low self-esteem, and a disturbed body image.
- Be aware of legal and ethical issues related to tube-feeding older adults with chronic or terminal illness.

Physiological Integrity

- Review serum prealbumin, hemoglobin, and hematocrit levels to identify patients at nutritional risk.
- Older patients are at increased risk for malnutrition (see Chart 63-2).
- Assess patients with severe malnutrition for common complications, such as edema; lethargy; and dry, flaking skin.
- Implement interventions to promote nutritional intake in older adults as specified in Chart 63-3.
- Provide nursing interventions for managing total enteral nutrition as listed in Chart 63-4.

- Maintain feeding tube patency for patients receiving total enteral nutrition as described in Chart 63-5.
- Provide care for patients receiving total parenteral nutrition as specified in Chart 63-6.
- Recognize that many people are following low-carbohydrate rather than low-fat diets to lose weight.
- Recall that normal body mass index (BMI) for adults should be between 18.5 and 25; older adults should have a BMI between 23 and 27. A BMI of 27 to 30 indicates overweight, over 30 indicates obesity, and 40 and greater indicates morbid obesity.
- Recall that obesity causes early onset of many chronic illnesses, such as osteoarthritis, diabetes mellitus, hypertension, and coronary artery disease. Pulmonary problems, such as obstructive sleep apnea, delayed wound healing, and infections are also common.
- Remember that bariatric surgery includes gastric restriction procedures or gastric bypass; a panniculectomy may be performed to remove skinfolds once weight is stabilized.
- Be alert for signs and symptoms of anastomotic leak after bariatric surgery, including severe pain, restlessness, anxiety, and unexplained tachycardia.
- Provide postoperative care for patients having bariatric surgery to prevent complications such as wound dehiscence, respiratory distress, skin breakdown, and thromboembolitic complications, such as pulmonary embolism. Observe for complications, such as dumping syndrome in patients who have a gastric bypass. Tachycardia, nausea, diarrhea, and abdominal cramping are common manifestations of dumping syndrome.
- Provide discharge teaching for patients having bariatric surgery as described in Chart 63-7.

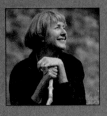

CHAPTER

64

Assessment of the Endocrine System

M. Linda Workman

 WEBSITE

LEARNING OUTCOMES

Safe and Effective Care Environment

1. Ensure that agency laboratory procedures for collecting and handling specimens for endocrine function studies are followed.

Health Promotion and Maintenance

2. Identify factors that place patients at risk for endocrine health problems.
3. Teach everyone about the dangers of misusing or abusing hormones or steroids.

Psychosocial Integrity

4. Encourage the patient to express concerns about a change in appearance, sexuality, or fertility.
5. Assess whether the patient has experienced recent changes in behavior or responses to stress.
6. Teach patients and family members about what to expect during tests and procedures to assess for endocrine problems.

Physiological Integrity

7. Describe the relationship between hormones and receptor sites.
8. Explain negative feedback as a control mechanism for hormone secretion.
9. Apply the principles of anatomy and physiology to understand the role of the endocrine system in homeostasis.
10. Identify adaptations in nursing assessment or interventions needed because of age-related changes in endocrine function.
11. Interpret laboratory test findings and clinical manifestations for patients with possible endocrine problems.

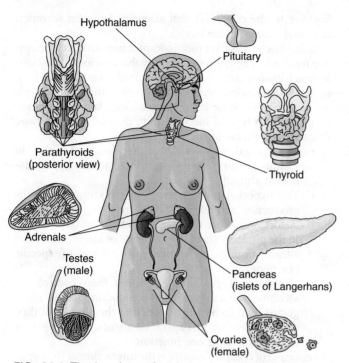

FIG. 64-1 The locations of various glands within the endocrine system.

TABLE 64-1	PRINCIPAL HORMONES OF THE ENDOCRINE GLANDS
GLAND	**HORMONES**
Hypothalamus	Corticotropin-releasing hormone (CRH)
	Thyrotropin-releasing hormone (TRH)
	Gonadotropin-releasing hormone (GnRH)
	Growth hormone–releasing hormone (GHRH)
	Growth hormone–inhibiting hormone (somatostatin GHIH)
	Prolactin-inhibiting hormone (PIH)
	Melanocyte-inhibiting hormone (MIH)
Anterior pituitary	Thyroid-stimulating hormone (TSH), also known as *thyrotropin*
	Adrenocorticotropic hormone (ACTH, corticotropin)
	Luteinizing hormone (LH), also known as *Leydig cell–stimulating hormone (LCSH)*
	Follicle-stimulating hormone (FSH)
	Prolactin (PRL)
	Growth hormone (GH)
	Melanocyte-stimulating hormone (MSH)
Posterior pituitary	Vasopressin (antidiuretic hormone [ADH])
	Oxytocin
Thyroid	Triiodothyronine (T_3)
	Thyroxine (T_4)
	Calcitonin
Parathyroid	Parathyroid hormone (PTH)
Adrenal cortex	Glucocorticoids (cortisol)
	Mineralocorticoids (aldosterone)
Ovary	Estrogen
	Progesterone
Testes	Testosterone
Pancreas	Insulin
	Glucagon
	Somatostatin

The endocrine system is made up of glands in many tissues and organs in a variety of body areas (Fig. 64-1). The purpose of all endocrine glands is to secrete hormones, which are natural chemicals that exert their effects on specific tissues known as target tissues. Target tissues are usually located some distance from the endocrine gland, with no direct physical connection between the endocrine gland and its target tissue. For this reason, endocrine glands are called "ductless" glands and must use the blood to transport secreted hormones to the target tissues (McCance et al., 2010). Endocrine glands include:
- Hypothalamus (a neuroendocrine gland)
- Pituitary gland
- Adrenal glands
- Thyroid gland
- Islet cells of the pancreas
- Parathyroid glands
- Gonads

The endocrine system works with the nervous system to control overall body function, known as neuroendocrine regulation. Many interactions must occur between the endocrine system and all other body systems to ensure that each system maintains a constant normal balance (homeostasis) in response to environmental changes. For example, neuroendocrine control of body systems keeps the internal body temperature at or near 98.6° F (37° C), even when environmental temperatures vary. Other actions keep the serum sodium level between 136 and 145 mEq/L (mmol/L), regardless of whether a person eats 2 g or 12 g of sodium per day.

Table 64-1 lists hormones secreted by various endocrine glands. Hormones travel through the blood to all body areas but exert their actions only on target tissues. They recognize their target tissues and exert their actions by binding to receptors on or within the target tissue cells. In general, each receptor site type is specific for only one hormone. Hormone-receptor actions work in a "lock and key" manner in that only the correct hormone (key) can bind to and activate the receptor site (lock) (Fig. 64-2). Binding a hormone to its receptor causes the target tissue to change its activity, producing specific responses.

Disorders of the endocrine system usually are related to:
- An excess of a specific hormone
- A deficiency of a specific hormone
- A receptor defect

ANATOMY AND PHYSIOLOGY REVIEW

The control of cellular function by any hormone depends on a series of reactions working through negative feedback control mechanisms. Hormone secretion usually depends on the need of the body for the final action of that hormone. When a body condition starts to move away from the normal range and a specific action or response is needed to correct this change, secretion of the hormone capable of starting the correcting action or response is stimulated until the need (demand) is met and the body condition returns to the normal range. As the correction occurs, hormone secretion decreases (and may halt). This type of control for hormone synthesis is "negative feedback" because the hormone causes the *opposite* action of the initial condition change.

An example of a simple negative feedback hormone response is the control of insulin secretion. When blood glucose levels start to rise above normal, the hormone *insulin* is secreted. Insulin increases glucose uptake by the cells, causing a *decrease* in blood glucose levels. Thus the action of insulin (decreasing blood glucose levels) is the opposite of or

negative to the condition that stimulated insulin secretion (elevated blood glucose levels).

Some hormones have more complex interactions for negative feedback. These interactions involve a series of reactions in which more than one endocrine gland, as well as the final target tissues, is stimulated. In this situation, the first hormone in the series may have another endocrine gland as its target tissue. For this type of mechanism to maintain homeostasis, this series of interactions must occur:

- The central nervous system receives and reacts to various sensory inputs transmitted to the hypothalamus as stimuli.
- The hypothalamus responds to the stimuli with the production and release of either releasing or inhibiting factors, which are transported to the pituitary.
- In the pituitary gland, the releasing or inhibiting factors either stimulate or inhibit the release of specific hormones.
- The anterior pituitary hormones then control the secretion of hormones in other endocrine glands. These glands then secrete hormones into the blood that then act on their target organs or tissues, resulting in a change of at least one function.

An example of complex control is the interaction of the hypothalamus and the anterior pituitary with the adrenal cortex (Fig. 64-3). Low blood levels of cortisol from the adrenal cortex stimulate the secretion of corticotropic-releasing hormone (CRH) in the hypothalamus. CRH stimulates the anterior pituitary gland to secrete adrenocorticotropic hormone (ACTH). ACTH then triggers the release of cortisol from the adrenal cortex. The rising blood levels of cortisol

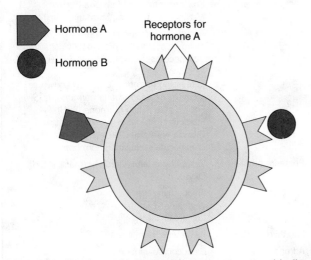

FIG. 64-2 "Lock and Key" hormone-receptor binding. *Hormone A* fits and binds to its receptors, causing a change in cell action. *Hormone B* does not fit or bind to receptors; no change in cell action results.

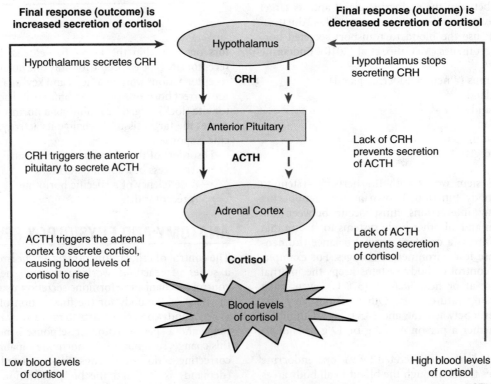

FIG. 64-3 Examples of positive and negative feedback control of hormone secretion. *ACTH,* Adrenocorticotropic hormone; *CRH,* corticotropic hormone.

inhibit CRH release from the hypothalamus. Without CRH, the anterior pituitary gland stops secretion of ACTH. In response, normal blood cortisol levels are maintained.

The normal blood level range of each hormone is well defined. Excesses or deficiencies of hormone secretion can lead to pathologic conditions.

Hypothalamus and Pituitary Glands

The hypothalamus is a small area of nerve and glandular tissue located beneath the thalamus in the brain. Nerve fibers connect the hypothalamus to the rest of the central nervous system. The hypothalamus shares a small, closed circulatory system with the anterior pituitary gland, known as the hypothalamic-hypophysial portal system. This system allows hormones produced in the hypothalamus to travel directly to the anterior pituitary gland so that only very small amounts are wasted in systemic circulation.

The endocrine function of the hypothalamus is to produce regulatory hormones (see Table 64-1). Some of these hormones are released into the blood and travel to the anterior pituitary, where they either stimulate or inhibit the release of anterior pituitary hormones.

The pituitary gland is located at the base of the brain in a protective pocket of the sphenoid bone (see Fig. 64-1). The pituitary gland is about 1 cm in diameter and is divided into the anterior lobe (adenohypophysis) and the posterior lobe (neurohypophysis). Nerve fibers in the hypophysial stalk connect the hypothalamus to the posterior pituitary (Fig. 64-4).

In response to the releasing hormones of the hypothalamus, the anterior pituitary secretes tropic hormones, which are hormones that stimulate other endocrine glands. Other pituitary hormones, such as prolactin, produce their effect directly on final target tissues (Table 64-2).

The hormones of the posterior pituitary, vasopressin (antidiuretic hormone [ADH]) and oxytocin, are produced in the hypothalamus and sent through the nerve tracts that connect the hypothalamus with the posterior pituitary. These hormones are stored in the nerve endings of the posterior pituitary and are released into the blood when needed.

Other factors can affect the release of hormones from the pituitary gland. Drugs, diet, lifestyle, and pathologic conditions can increase or decrease pituitary hormone secretion.

Gonads

The gonads are the male and female reproductive endocrine glands. Male gonads are the *testes,* and female gonads are the *ovaries.* Function of these glands begins at puberty.

During puberty in the male, the increased secretion of gonadotropins (luteinizing hormone [LH] and follicle-stimulating hormone [FSH]) from the anterior pituitary gland stimulates maturation of the testes, production of testosterone, and maturation of the external genitalia. During puberty in the female, increased secretion of the same gonadotropins stimulates ovarian maturation, estrogen production, ovulation, and maturation of the external genitalia.

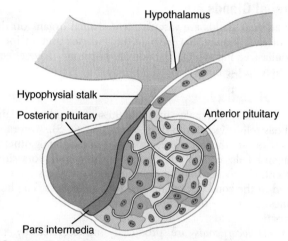

FIG. 64-4 The hypothalamus, hypophysial stalk, anterior pituitary gland, and posterior pituitary gland.

TABLE 64-2	PITUITARY HORMONES: TARGET TISSUES AND SUBSEQUENT ACTIONS	
HORMONE	**TARGET TISSUE**	**ACTIONS**
Anterior Pituitary		
TSH (thyroid-stimulating hormone or thyrotropin)	Thyroid	Stimulates synthesis and release of thyroid hormone
ACTH (adrenocorticotropic hormone, corticotropin)	Adrenal cortex	Stimulates synthesis and release of corticosteroids and adrenocortical growth
LH (luteinizing hormone [known as *Leydig cell–stimulating hormone* in males])	Ovary	Stimulates ovulation and progesterone secretion
	Testis	Stimulates testosterone secretion
FSH (follicle-stimulating hormone [known as *interstitial cell–* or *Sertoli cell–stimulating hormone* in males])	Ovary	Stimulates estrogen secretion and follicle maturation
	Testis	Stimulates spermatogenesis
PRL (prolactin)	Mammary glands	Stimulates breast milk production
GH (growth hormone)	Bone and soft tissue	Promotes growth through lipolysis, protein anabolism, and insulin antagonism
MSH (melanocyte-stimulating hormone)	Melanocytes	Promotes pigmentation
Posterior Pituitary*		
Vasopressin (antidiuretic hormone [ADH])	Kidney	Promotes water reabsorption
Oxytocin	Uterus and mammary glands	Stimulates uterine contractions and ejection of breast milk

*These hormones are synthesized in the hypothalamus and are stored in the posterior pituitary gland. They are transported from the hypothalamus down the hypothalamic stalk to the posterior pituitary while bound to proteins known as *neurophysins.*

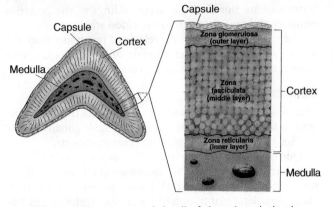

FIG. 64-5 The structural detail of the adrenal gland.

The function of the testes and ovaries is detailed in Chapter 72.

Adrenal Glands

The adrenal glands are vascular, tent-shaped organs on the top of each kidney that have an outer cortex and an inner medulla (see Fig. 64-1). The adrenal hormones have effects throughout the body.

Adrenal Cortex

The adrenal cortex makes up about 90% of the adrenal gland and has cells divided into three layers (Fig. 64-5). Mineralocorticoids are the hormones produced in the zona glomerulosa and help control the body's sodium and potassium content. Glucocorticoids, androgens, and estrogens are produced in the zona fasciculata and zona reticularis. The hormones secreted by the cortex are often called adrenal steroids or corticosteroids.

Mineralocorticoids are produced and secreted by the adrenal cortex to help control body fluids and electrolytes. Aldosterone is the major mineralocorticoid and maintains extracellular fluid volume. It promotes sodium and water reabsorption and potassium excretion in the kidney tubules. Aldosterone secretion is regulated by the renin-angiotensin system, serum potassium ion concentration, and adrenocorticotropic hormone (ACTH).

Renin is produced by specialized cells of the renal afferent arterioles. Its release is triggered by a decrease in extracellular fluid volume from blood loss, sodium loss, or posture changes. Renin converts renin substrate (formerly called *angiotensinogen*), a plasma protein, to angiotensin I. Angiotensin I is converted by a converting enzyme to form angiotensin II, the active form of angiotensin. In turn, angiotensin II stimulates the secretion of aldosterone. Chapter 13 (see Fig. 13-6) further explains the renin-angiotensin system. Aldosterone causes the kidney to reabsorb sodium and water to bring the plasma volume and osmolarity back to normal.

Serum potassium level also controls aldosterone secretion. The adrenal cortex secretes aldosterone when the serum potassium level increases above normal by as little as 0.1 mEq/L. Aldosterone then enhances kidney excretion of potassium to reduce the blood level back to normal.

Glucocorticoids are produced by the adrenal cortex and are essential for life. The main glucocorticoid produced by the adrenal cortex is cortisol. Cortisol affects:

TABLE 64-3	FUNCTIONS OF GLUCOCORTICOID HORMONES

- Prevent hypoglycemia by increasing liver gluconeogenesis and inhibiting peripheral glucose use
- Maintain excitability and responsiveness of cardiac muscle
- Increase lipolysis, releasing glycerol and free fatty acids
- Increase protein catabolism
- Degrade collagen and connective tissue
- Increase the number of mature neutrophils released from bone marrow
- Exert anti-inflammatory effects that decrease the migration of inflammatory cells to sites of injury
- Maintain behavior and cognitive functions

- Carbohydrate, protein, and fat metabolism
- The body's response to stress
- Emotional stability
- Immune function

Cortisol also influences other important body processes. For example, it must be present for catecholamine action and maintaining the normal excitability of the heart muscle cells. Glucocorticoid functions are listed in Table 64-3.

Glucocorticoid release is regulated directly by the anterior pituitary hormone *ACTH* and indirectly by the hypothalamic corticotropin-releasing hormone *(CRH)*. The release of CRH and ACTH is affected by the serum level of free cortisol, the normal sleep-wake cycle, and stress.

As described earlier and shown in Fig. 64-3, when blood cortisol levels are low, the hypothalamus secretes CRH, which triggers the pituitary to release ACTH. Then ACTH triggers the adrenal cortex to secrete cortisol. Adequate or elevated blood levels of cortisol *inhibit* the release of CRH and ACTH. This inhibitory effect is an example of a negative feedback system.

Glucocorticoid release peaks in the morning and reaches its lowest level 12 hours after each peak. Emotional, chemical, or physical stress increases the release of glucocorticoids.

Sex hormones (androgens and estrogens) are secreted in low levels by the adrenal cortex in both genders. Adrenal secretion of these hormones is usually not significant because the gonads (testes and ovaries) secrete much larger amounts of androgens and estrogens. In women, however, the adrenal gland is the major source of androgens. Women who have adrenal insufficiency or who have had surgical removal of the adrenals may need a small amount of testosterone replacement.

Adrenal Medulla

The adrenal medulla is a sympathetic nerve ganglion that has secretory cells. Stimulation of the sympathetic nervous system causes the release of adrenal medullary hormones, the catecholamines (which include epinephrine and norepinephrine). These hormones travel to all areas of the body through the blood and exert their effects on target cells. The adrenal medullary hormones are not essential for life because they also are secreted by other body tissues, but they do play a role in the physiologic stress response.

The adrenal medulla secretes about 15% norepinephrine (NE) and 85% epinephrine. Hormone effects vary with the specific receptor in the cell membranes of the target tissue.

TABLE 64-4 CATECHOLAMINE RECEPTORS AND EFFECTS OF ADRENAL MEDULLARY HORMONE STIMULATION ON SELECTED ORGANS AND TISSUES

ORGAN OR TISSUE	RECEPTORS	EFFECTS
Heart	Beta$_1$	Increased heart rate Increased contractility
Blood vessels	Alpha Beta$_2$	Vasoconstriction Vasodilation
Gastrointestinal tract	Alpha Beta	Increased sphincter tone Decreased motility
Kidneys	Beta$_2$	Increased renin release
Bronchioles	Beta$_2$	Relaxation; dilation
Bladder	Alpha Beta$_2$	Sphincter contractions Relaxation of detrusor muscle
Skin	Alpha	Increased sweating
Fat cells	Beta	Increased lipolysis
Liver	Alpha	Increased gluconeogenesis and glycogenolysis
Pancreas	Alpha	Decreased glucagon and insulin release
	Beta	Increased glucagon and insulin release
Eyes	Alpha	Dilation of pupils

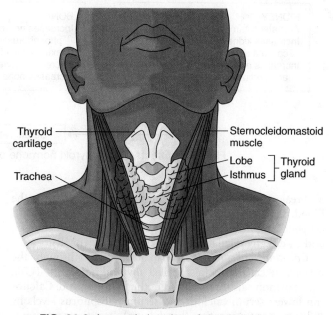

FIG. 64-6 Anatomic location of the thyroid gland.

TABLE 64-5 FUNCTIONS OF THYROID HORMONES IN ADULTS

- Control metabolic rate of all cells
- Promote sufficient pituitary secretion of growth hormone and gonadotropins
- Regulate protein, carbohydrate, and fat metabolism
- Exert effects on heart rate and contractility
- Increase red blood cell production
- Affect respiratory rate and drive
- Increase bone formation and decrease bone resorption of calcium
- Act as insulin antagonists

These receptors are of two types: alpha adrenergic and beta adrenergic. Both types of receptors are further classified as alpha$_1$ and alpha$_2$ receptors and beta$_1$, beta$_2$, and beta$_3$ receptors. NE acts mainly on alpha-adrenergic receptors, and epinephrine acts mainly on beta-adrenergic receptors.

Catecholamines exert their actions on many target organs (Table 64-4). Activation of the sympathetic nervous system, which then releases adrenal medullary catecholamines, is an important part of the body's response to stress. Catecholamines are secreted in small amounts at all times to maintain homeostasis. Stress triggers increased secretion of these hormones. This sympathetic activation results in the "fight-or-flight" response, a state of heightened physical and emotional awareness.

Thyroid Gland

The thyroid gland is in the anterior neck, directly below the cricoid cartilage (Fig. 64-6). It has two lobes joined by a thin strip of tissue *(isthmus)* in front of the trachea.

The thyroid gland has a rich blood supply and is composed of follicular and parafollicular cells. Follicular cells produce the thyroid hormones thyroxine (T$_4$) and triiodothyronine (T$_3$). Parafollicular cells produce thyrocalcitonin (TCT, or calcitonin), which helps regulate serum calcium levels.

Control of metabolism occurs through T$_3$ and T$_4$. Both hormones increase metabolism, which causes an increase in oxygen use and heat production in all tissues. The two hormones differ in structure, but their functions are the same. Most circulating T$_4$ and T$_3$ are bound to plasma proteins. The free hormone moves into the cell, where it binds to its receptor in the cell nucleus. Once in the cell, T$_4$ is converted to T$_3$, the most active thyroid hormone. The conversion of T$_4$ to T$_3$ is impaired by stress, starvation, dyes, beta blockers, amiodarone, corticosteroids, and propyl-thiouracil (PTU). Cold temperatures increase the conversion. Table 64-5 lists thyroid hormone functions.

Secretion of T$_3$ and T$_4$ is controlled by the hypothalamic-pituitary-thyroid gland axis negative feedback mechanism. The hypothalamus secretes thyrotropin-releasing hormone (TRH). TRH triggers the anterior pituitary gland to secrete thyroid-stimulating hormone (TSH), which then stimulates the thyroid gland to make and release thyroid hormones. If thyroid hormone levels are high, TRH and TSH release is inhibited. If thyroid hormone levels are low, TRH and TSH release is increased. Cold and stress are two factors that cause the hypothalamus to secrete TRH, which then stimulates the anterior pituitary to secrete TSH.

Thyroid hormone production involves a series of steps. Dietary intake of protein and iodine is needed to produce thyroid hormones. Iodine is absorbed from the intestinal tract as iodide. The thyroid gland withdraws iodide from the blood and concentrates it. After iodide is in the thyroid, it combines with the amino acid *tyrosine* to form T$_4$ and T$_3$. These hormones bind to thyroglobulin and are stored in the follicular cells of the thyroid gland. With stimulation, T$_4$ and

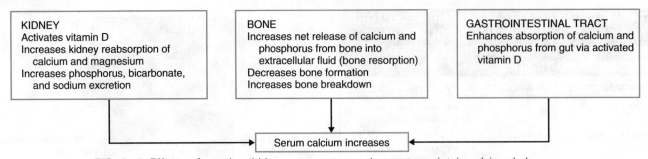

KIDNEY	BONE	GASTROINTESTINAL TRACT
Activates vitamin D Increases kidney reabsorption of calcium and magnesium Increases phosphorus, bicarbonate, and sodium excretion	Increases net release of calcium and phosphorus from bone into extracellular fluid (bone resorption) Decreases bone formation Increases bone breakdown	Enhances absorption of calcium and phosphorus from gut via activated vitamin D

Serum calcium increases

FIG. 64-7 Effects of parathyroid hormone on target tissues to maintain calcium balance.

T_3 break off from thyroglobulin and are released into the blood. They enter many cells, bind to the nucleus, and turn on genes important in metabolism. Thus the presence of T_4 and T_3 directly regulates basal metabolic rate (BMR).

Calcium and phosphorus balance occurs through the actions of calcitonin (also called *thyrocalcitonin,* or *TCT*). This hormone also is produced in the thyroid gland. Calcitonin lowers serum calcium and serum phosphorus levels by reducing bone resorption (breakdown). Its actions are opposite of parathyroid hormone.

The serum calcium level determines calcitonin secretion. Low serum calcium levels suppress the release of calcitonin. Elevated serum calcium levels increase its secretion.

Parathyroid Glands

The parathyroid glands consist of four small glands located close to or within the back surface of the thyroid gland (see Fig. 64-1). The chief cells of the parathyroid glands secrete parathyroid hormone (PTH).

Parathyroid hormone regulates calcium and phosphorus metabolism by acting on bones, the kidneys, and the GI tract (Fig. 64-7). Bone is the main storage site of calcium. PTH increases bone resorption (bone release of calcium into the blood from bone storage sites), thus increasing serum calcium. In the kidneys, PTH activates vitamin D, which then increases the absorption of calcium and phosphorus from the intestines. In the kidney tubules, PTH allows calcium to be reabsorbed and put back into the blood.

Serum calcium level determines PTH secretion. Secretion decreases when serum calcium levels are high, and it increases when serum calcium levels are low. Serum phosphorus levels also affect PTH secretion. PTH and calcitonin work together to maintain normal calcium levels in the blood and extracellular fluid.

Pancreas

The pancreas lies behind the stomach and has exocrine and endocrine functions. The exocrine function of the pancreas involves the secretion of digestive enzymes through ducts that empty into the duodenum. The cells in the islets of Langerhans perform the pancreatic endocrine functions (Fig. 64-8). About one million islet cells are found throughout the pancreas.

The islets have three distinct cell types: alpha cells, which secrete glucagon; beta cells, which secrete insulin; and delta cells, which secrete somatostatin. Glucagon and insulin affect carbohydrate, protein, and fat metabolism. Somatostatin, which is secreted not only in the pancreas but also in the intestinal tract and the brain, inhibits the release of glucagon

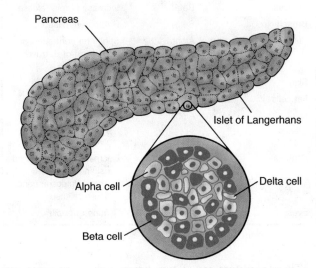

FIG. 64-8 The cells of the islets of Langerhans of the pancreas.

and insulin from the pancreas. It also inhibits the release of gastrin, secretin, and other GI peptides.

Glucagon is a hormone that increases blood glucose levels. It is triggered by decreased blood glucose levels and increased blood amino acid levels. Together with epinephrine, growth hormone (GH), and cortisol, glucagon prevents hypoglycemia. Chapter 67 discusses glucagon function in more detail.

Insulin promotes the movement and storage of carbohydrate (CHO), protein, and fat (Table 64-6). It lowers blood glucose levels by enhancing glucose movement across cell membranes and into the cells of many tissues. Basal levels of insulin are secreted continuously to control metabolism. Insulin secretion rises in response to an increase in blood

❓ NCLEX EXAMINATION CHALLENGE

Physiological Integrity

Which hormone levels should the nurse expect to change in response to a client receiving a continuous cortisol infusion over a 24-hour period when the endocrine negative feedback mechanism is functioning properly?

A. Lower-than-normal serum cortisol levels; lower-than-normal serum ACTH levels

B. Lower-than-normal serum cortisol levels; higher-than-normal serum ACTH levels

C. Higher-than-normal serum cortisol levels; lower-than-normal serum ACTH levels

D. Higher-than-normal serum cortisol levels; higher-than-normal serum ACTH levels

CHART 64-1   NURSING FOCUS ON THE OLDER ADULT

Changes in the Endocrine System Related to Aging

CHANGES	CLINICAL FINDINGS	NURSING ACTIONS/ADAPTATIONS
Decreased antidiuretic hormone (ADH) production	Urine is more dilute and may not concentrate when fluid intake is low.	The patient is at greater risk for dehydration as a result of urine loss. Assess the older patient more frequently for dehydration. If fluids are not restricted because of another health problem, teach unlicensed assistive personnel (UAP) to offer fluids at least every 2 hours while awake.
Decreased ovarian production of estrogen	Bone density decreases.	Teach the patient to engage in regular exercise and weight-bearing activity to maintain bone density. Handle the patient carefully to avoid injury from pathologic fractures.
	Skin is thinner, drier, and at greater risk for injury.	Avoid pulling or dragging the patient. Use minimal tape on the skin. Assist patients confined to bed or chairs to change positions at least every 2 hours. Teach patients to use moisturizers on the skin and to avoid agents that promote skin dryness.
	Perineal and vaginal tissues become drier, and the risk for cystitis increases.	Perform or assist the patient to perform perineal care at least twice daily. Unless another health problem requires fluid restriction, encourage all women to drink at least 2 liters of fluids daily. Teach sexually active women to urinate immediately after sexual intercourse. Teach sexually active women that using vaginal lubricants with sexual activity can reduce discomfort and the risk for tissue damage.
Decreased glucose tolerance	Weight becomes greater than ideal along with: • Elevated fasting blood glucose level • Elevated random blood glucose level • Slow wound healing • Frequent yeast infections • Polydipsia • Polyuria	Obtain a family history of obesity and type 2 diabetes. Encourage the patient to engage in regular exercise and to keep body weight within 10 lbs of ideal. Teach patients the clinical manifestations of diabetes, and instruct them to report any of these manifestations to the health care provider. Suggest diabetes testing for any patient with: • Persistent vaginal candidiasis • Failure of a foot or leg skin wound to heal in 2 weeks or less • Increased hunger and thirst • Noticeable decrease in energy level
Decreased general metabolism	Less tolerant of cold. Decreased appetite. Decreased heart rate & blood pressure (BP).	Can be difficult to distinguish from hypothyroidism. Check for additional manifestations of: • Lethargy • Constipation (as a change from usual bowel habits) • Decreased cognition • Slowed speech • Body temperature consistently below 97° F (36° C) • Heart rate below 60 beats/min Teach patients to dress warmly in cool or cold weather.

TABLE 64-6   ANABOLIC EFFECTS OF INSULIN

Effects on Liver
• Promotes glycogen synthesis and storage
• Inhibits glycogenolysis, gluconeogenesis, and ketogenesis
• Increases triglyceride synthesis

Effects on Muscle
• Promotes protein synthesis
• Increases amino acid transport
• Promotes glycogenesis

Effects on Fat
• Increases fatty acid synthesis
• Promotes triglyceride storage
• Decreases lipolysis

glucose levels. More information on insulin is presented in Chapter 67.

Endocrine Changes Associated with Aging

The effects of aging on the endocrine system vary widely. The three endocrine tissues that usually have reduced function with aging are the gonads, the thyroid gland, and the endocrine pancreas (Lamberts, 2008; Touhy & Jett, 2010). It is difficult to distinguish normal from abnormal endocrine activity because of these other age-related variables:

• Acute and chronic illnesses
• Alterations in diet, activity, and lean body mass–to-fat ratio
• Disturbances in sleep patterns
• Decreased metabolic clearance rate of hormones
• Increased use of multiple drugs that may affect hormone function

It is important to consider these factors when assessing the older adult with endocrine dysfunction.

Encourage the older adult to participate in regular screening examinations, including fasting and random blood glucose checks, calcium level determinations, and thyroid function testing. Chart 64-1 lists the endocrine changes that occur in the older adult.

ASSESSMENT METHODS

Patient History

Use a systems approach to obtain the history of patients with a possible endocrine problem. This approach can be difficult because of the variety and combination of clinical manifestations. Identify the patient's response to actual or perceived changes, and discuss the potential diagnostic and

---

CHART 64-2 ENDOCRINE ASSESSMENT

Using Gordon's Functional Health Patterns

Nutritional-Metabolic Pattern

- What is your typical daily food intake? Describe a day's meals, snacks, and vitamins.
- How much salt do you typically add to your food? Do you use salt substitutes?
- How is your appetite?
- Do you have any difficulty chewing or swallowing?
- What is your typical daily fluid intake? What types of fluids (water, juices, soft drinks, coffee, tea)? How much?
- Have you had any recent change in your weight? Weight gain? Weight loss? How much?
- Have you noticed a change in the tightness of your rings or shoes? Tighter? Looser?
- Have you noticed any change in thirst?

Elimination Pattern

- What is your usual bowel elimination pattern? Frequency? Character? Discomfort? Laxative use?
- What is your usual urinary elimination pattern? Frequency? Amount? Color? Odor? Control?
- Have you noticed a change in the amount of urine?
- Do you have any problem with excessive perspiration?
- Do you have any other type of drainage?

Sleep-Rest Pattern

- Do you have any difficulty falling asleep when you go to bed?
- Is there a change in the number of hours you sleep per night?
- Do you take any drugs to help you sleep?
- About how many times do you awaken during the night?
- Do you have any difficulty getting back to sleep?
- Are you bothered by nightmares or vivid dreams?
- Do you have difficulty awakening in the morning?
- Do you feel generally rested and ready for daily activities after sleep?
- Do you take scheduled naps or rest periods during the day?
- Do you find yourself falling asleep at work or at home while reading or watching television?
- Have you noticed any difficulty in your ability to concentrate?

Sexuality-Reproductive Pattern

- Are you sexually active?
- Are you satisfied with your level of sexual activity?

- Do you participate in sex as often as you would like?
- Do you participate in sex as often as your partner would like?
- Have you noticed a change in your interest in having sex over the past year?

Female:

- At what age did menstruation start?
- How regular are your periods?
- Do you have any pain, cramping, or clotting during your periods?
- Have you ever been pregnant? What was the outcome of the pregnancy(ies)?
- Do you use contraceptives? What type? Have you had any problems with your chosen method of contraception?
- Do you have any pain during intercourse?

Activity-Exercise Pattern

- Do you feel you have sufficient energy to perform tasks or routines that are required of you?
- Do you feel you have sufficient energy to do what you would like to do?
- Do you exercise? How often? For how long each time? What type(s) of exercise do you perform?
- What activities do you perform in your spare time?
- What is your ability to perform the following tasks?

Feeding _____	Grooming _____
Bathing _____	General Mobility _____
Toileting _____	Cooking _____
Bed Mobility _____	Home Maintenance _____
Dressing _____	Shopping _____

Functional Levels Code

Level 0: Full self-care
Level I: Requires use of equipment or device
Level II: Requires help from another person(s): assistance, supervision, teaching
Level III: Requires help from another person(s) and equipment or device
Level IV: Dependent; does not participate in self-care

Based on Gordon, M. (2011). *Manual of nursing diagnosis* (12th ed.). New York: Jones & Bartlett.

---

management plan. Chart 64-2 lists assessment questions based on Gordon's Functional Health Patterns (Gordon, 2011). Although endocrine problems can disturb any health pattern, the patterns most commonly affected are nutritional-metabolic, activity-exercise, elimination, sleep-rest, and sexuality-reproductive. These data are combined with physical, psychosocial, and laboratory findings for a complete assessment of endocrine function.

The age and gender of the patient provide baseline assessment data. Certain disorders are more common in older than in younger patients, such as diabetes mellitus, loss of ovarian function, and decreased thyroid function.

Manifestations of endocrine disorders can be gender related, such as the sexual effects of hyperpituitarism and hypopituitarism (see Chapter 65). Thyroid problems are more common in women (McCance et al., 2010). Assess for a history of endocrine dysfunction, manifestations that could indicate an endocrine disorder, and hospitalizations. Ask about past and current drugs, such as hydrocortisone, levothyroxine, oral contraceptives, and antihypertensive agents.

The use of exogenous hormone drugs, when not needed for hormone replacement, can cause serious dysfunction in many endocrine glands. Use the opportunity to warn patients about the dangers of misusing or abusing hormone-based drugs such as androgens and thyroid hormones.

Because the patient's socioeconomic status is a sensitive issue, explore whether his or her resources are adequate for a healthy diet, needed drugs, and consistent health care follow-up. It may be appropriate to involve social service and home care agencies at an early stage.

Nutrition History

Nutritional changes or GI tract disturbances may reflect many different endocrine problems. Ask about a history of nausea, vomiting, and abdominal pain. An increase or decrease in food or fluid intake may also indicate specific disorders. For example, diabetes insipidus triggers excessive thirst, and adrenal hypofunction triggers salt craving. Hunger and thirst also are associated with diabetes mellitus. Rapid changes in weight without diet changes are often associated with several endocrine disorders, including diabetes mellitus and thyroid problems.

Dietary deficiencies, especially of protein and iodide-containing foods (saltwater fish and seafood, iodized table salt), may be a cause of an endocrine disorder. Teach the patient about a well-balanced diet that includes at least 60 g of protein daily, less animal fat, and fewer concentrated simple sugars. Teach patients who do not eat saltwater fish on a regular basis to use iodized salt in food preparation.

Family History and Genetic Risk

Ask the patient about any family history of obesity, growth or development difficulties, diabetes mellitus, infertility, or thyroid disorders. These problems may have an autosomal dominant, recessive, or cluster pattern of inheritance.

Current Health Problems

Focus on the patient's reason for seeking health care, asking questions such as:

- Did the symptoms occur gradually, or was the onset sudden?
- Have you been treated for this problem in the past?
- How have the current problems affected your activities of daily living?

These questions can provide clues to specific endocrine disorders. Also explore changes in energy levels, elimination patterns, sexual and reproductive functions, and physical features.

Energy level changes occur with many endocrine problems, especially thyroid problems (see Chapter 66) and adrenal problems (see Chapter 65). Ask the patient about any change in ability to perform ADLs, and assess his or her current energy level. For instance, has he or she been sleeping longer, or are fatigue and generalized weakness present?

Elimination is also affected by the endocrine system. Identify the patient's past pattern of elimination to determine deviations from the normal routine. Ask about the amount and frequency of urination. Does he or she urinate frequently in large amounts? Does the patient wake during the night to urinate (nocturia), or is pain present with urination (dysuria)? Information about the frequency of bowel movements and their consistency and color may provide clues to problems in fluid balance or metabolic rate (i.e., thyroid function).

Sexual and reproductive functions are greatly affected by endocrine disturbances. Ask women about any changes in the menstrual cycle, such as increased flow, duration, and frequency of menses; pain or excessive cramping; or a recent change in the regularity of menses. Ask men whether they have experienced impotence. Question both men and women about a change in libido (sexual desire) or any fertility problems.

Physical appearance changes can reflect an endocrine problem. Discuss any changes that the patient perceives in physical features. Obvious changes are identified during the physical assessment, but patients may be able to describe some of the more subtle changes. Ask about changes in:

- Hair texture and distribution
- Facial contours and eye protrusion
- Voice quality
- Body proportions
- Secondary sexual characteristics

For example, you might ask a man whether he is shaving less often or a woman if she has noticed an increase in facial hair. These changes may be associated with pituitary, thyroid, parathyroid, or adrenal dysfunction.

NCLEX EXAMINATION CHALLENGE
Physiological Integrity

Which client assessment finding indicates to the nurse the need to assess further for a possible endocrine problem?
A. A history of taking oral contraceptives for more than 2 years
B. A weight loss of 15 lbs in the past 6 weeks without dieting
C. The client's father's diagnosis of prostate cancer
D. A recent need for corrective lenses

Physical Assessment
Inspection

An endocrine problem can change physical features because of its effect on growth and development, regulation of sex hormone levels, fluid and electrolyte balance, and the body's use of nutrients. Different clinical findings can occur with many endocrine disorders or with nonendocrine problems.

Use a head-to-toe approach to inspect the patient. Observe the patient's general appearance, and assess height, weight, fat distribution, and muscle mass in relation to age. It is important to remember that heredity and age rather than a health problem may be responsible for some physical features (e.g., short stature).

When examining the head, focus on abnormalities of facial structure, features, and expression, such as:

- Prominent forehead or jaw
- Round or puffy face
- Dull or flat expression
- Exophthalmos (protruding eyeballs and retracted upper lids)

Check the lower half of the neck for a visible enlargement of the thyroid gland. Normally the thyroid tissue cannot be observed. The isthmus may be noticeable when the patient swallows. Jugular vein distention may be seen on inspection of the neck and can indicate fluid overload.

Skin changes may reflect a specific endocrine dysfunction. Observe skin color, and look for areas of pigment loss (hypopigmentation) or hyperpigmentation. Fungal skin infections, slow wound healing, bruising, and petechiae are often seen in patients with adrenal hyperfunction. Skin infections, foot ulcers, and slow wound healing are common among patients with diabetes mellitus. In secondary hypofunction of the adrenal glands, the skin over the finger joints, elbows, and knees, as well as any scar tissue, may show increased pigmentation due to increased levels of adrenocorticotropic hormone (ACTH) and melanocyte-stimulating hormone.

Vitiligo (patchy areas of pigment loss with increased pigmentation at the edges) is seen with primary hypofunction of the adrenal glands and is caused by autoimmune destruction of melanocytes in the skin. Areas of pigment loss most often occur on the face, neck, and extremities. Mucous membranes may have large areas of uneven pigmentation. Document the location, color, distribution, and size of skin color changes and lesions.

Inspect the patient's fingernails for malformation, thickness, or brittleness, all of which may suggest thyroid gland problems. Examine the extremities and the base of the spine for edema, which suggests a fluid and electrolyte imbalance.

Inspection of the trunk can show signs of specific endocrine dysfunction. Check for any abnormalities in chest size and symmetry. Truncal obesity and the presence of a "buffalo hump" between the shoulders on the back may indicate adrenocortical excess. Hormonal imbalance may also change secondary sexual characteristics. Inspect the breasts of both men and women for size, symmetry, pigmentation, and discharge. Striae (reddish purple "stretch marks") on the breasts or abdomen are often seen with adrenocortical excess.

Assess the patient's hair distribution for indications of endocrine gland dysfunction. Changes can include hirsutism (excessive growth of body hair, especially on the face, chest, and the linea alba of the abdomen of women), excessive hair loss, or changes in hair texture.

Examination of the genitalia may reveal a dysfunction in hormone secretion. Observe the size of the scrotum and penis or of the labia and clitoris in relation to standards for the patient's age. The distribution and quantity of pubic hair are often affected in hypogonadism.

Palpation

The thyroid gland and the testes can be examined by palpation. Chapters 72 and 75 discuss examination of the testes. The thyroid gland is palpated for size, symmetry, general shape, and the presence of nodules or other irregularities.

Palpate the thyroid gland by standing either behind or in front of the patient (Fig. 64-9). The posterior approach may be easier (Jarvis, 2012). Having the patient swallow sips of water during the examination helps the clinician palpate the thyroid gland.

Ask the patient to sit and to lower the chin. Using the posterior approach, place the thumbs of both your hands on the back of the patient's neck, with the fingers curved around to the front of the neck on either side of the trachea. Ask the patient to swallow, and then locate the isthmus of the thyroid as you feel it rising. Identify the anterior surface of the thyroid lobe. To examine the thyroid, proceed in this way:
- Turn the patient's head to the right.
- Displace the thyroid cartilage to the right with the fingers of your left hand.
- Palpate the right lobe with your right hand.
- Reverse this procedure to examine the left lobe.

! NURSING SAFETY PRIORITY

Action Alert

Always palpate the thyroid gently because vigorous palpation can stimulate a thyroid storm in a person who has or is suspected to have hyperthyroidism.

Auscultation

Auscultate the chest to assess cardiac rate and rhythm. Document this information to use later as a means of assessing treatment effectiveness. Some endocrine problems induce dysrhythmias. Many endocrine disturbances can cause dehydration and volume depletion. Therefore document any

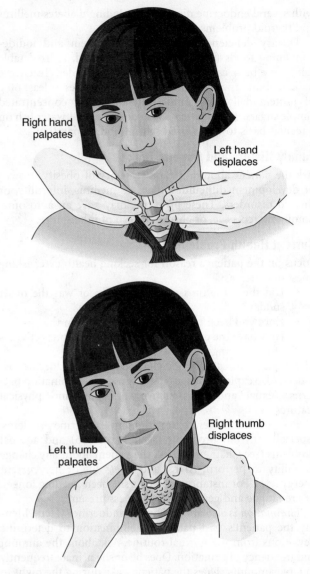

Right hand palpates

Left hand displaces

Left thumb palpates

Right thumb displaces

FIG. 64-9 Techniques for palpation of the thyroid gland.

difference in the patient's blood pressure and pulse in the lying, standing, or sitting positions (orthostatic vital signs).

If an enlarged thyroid gland is palpated, auscultate the area of enlargement for bruits. Hypertrophy of the thyroid gland causes an increase in vascular flow, which may result in bruits.

Psychosocial Assessment

Information obtained from the history and physical examination may help identify psychosocial problems. Assess the patient's coping skills, support systems, and health-related beliefs. Many endocrine problems can change a patient's behaviors, personality, and psychological responses. Ask the patient whether he or she has noticed a change in how stress is handled, frequency of crying, or degree of patience and anger expression. The patient may not recognize these changes in himself or herself. When possible, ask the family about changes in the patient's behaviors or personality.

A number of endocrine disorders affect the patient's perception of self. For example, body features can change significantly in disorders of the pituitary, adrenal, and thyroid

Endocrine Testing

For blood tests:
- Check your laboratory's method of handling hormone test samples for tube type, timing, drugs to be administered as part of the test, etc. For example, blood samples drawn for catecholamines must be placed on ice and taken to the laboratory immediately.
- Explain the procedure and any restrictions to the patient.
- If you are drawing blood samples from a line, clear the IV line thoroughly. Do not use a double- or triple-lumen line to obtain samples; contamination or dilution from another port is possible.
- Emphasize the importance of taking a drug prescribed for the test on *time*. Tell the patient to set an alarm if the drug is to be taken during the night.

For urine tests:
- Instruct the patient to begin the urine collection (whether for 2, 4, 8, 12, or 24 hours) by first emptying his or her bladder.
- Remind the patient to *not* save the urine specimen that begins the collection. The timing for the urine collection begins *after* this specimen.
- Tell the patient to note the time of the discarded specimen and to plan to collect all urine from this time until the end of the urine collection period.
- To end the collection, instruct the patient to empty his or her bladder at the end of the timed period and *add* that urine to the collection.
- Check with the laboratory to determine any special handling of the urine specimen (e.g., Is a preservative needed? Does the container need to be kept cold?).
- If needed, make sure that the preservative has been added to the collection container at the *beginning* of the collection.
- Tell the patient about any preservative and the need to avoid splashing urine from the container, because some preservatives make the urine caustic.
- If the specimen must be kept cool or cold, instruct the patient to place the container in an inexpensive cooler with ice. The specimen container should not be kept with food or drinks.

glands. Infertility, impotence, and other changes in sexual function may result from endocrine dysfunction. Encourage the patient to express his or her feelings and concerns about a change in appearance or in sexual function. Ask about any difficulty in coping with such changes.

Patients with endocrine problems may require lifelong drugs and follow-up care. Assess their readiness to learn and ability to carry out specific self-management skills. Patients may also face financial difficulties resulting from a prolonged medical regimen or loss of employment. A referral to social service agencies may be needed.

Diagnostic Assessment
Laboratory Assessment

For the patient with possible endocrine dysfunction, laboratory tests are an essential part of the diagnostic process. Body fluids commonly used for these tests include blood, urine, and saliva (Klee, 2008). Regardless of the test requested, check with the agency's laboratory to ensure proper collection and handling of the specimen for accurate results. The specialized testing for specific disorders is described in Chapters 65 to 67. Best practices for the collection of specimens for general endocrine testing are listed in Chart 64-3.

Stimulation/Suppression Tests. Measurement of specific hormone blood levels does not always distinguish between the normal and the abnormal. The wide normal range for some hormones makes it necessary to trigger responses by stimulation or suppression tests.

For the patient who might have an underactive endocrine gland, a stimulus may be provided to determine whether the gland is capable of normal hormone production. This method is called *stimulation testing.* Measured amounts of selected hormones are given to stimulate the target gland to maximum production. Hormone levels are then measured and compared with expected normal values. Failure of the hormone level to rise with stimulation indicates hypofunction. For example, insulin injection should stimulate increased release of growth hormone (GH) and adrenocorticotropic hormone (ACTH) from a normal anterior pituitary gland. When insulin injection does not result in increased release of these hormones, a problem with the anterior pituitary gland is likely, especially hypofunction.

Suppression tests are used when hormone levels are high or in the upper range of normal. Failure of suppression of hormone production during testing indicates hyperfunction. For example, when a bolus of glucose is given orally or intravenously, the normal anterior pituitary responds by suppressing the release of GH. A hyperfunctioning anterior pituitary gland fails to suppress GH release when blood glucose levels are elevated rapidly.

Assays. An assay measures the level of a specific hormone in blood or other body fluid. Some assays are indirect, such as the radioimmunoassay. Other hormone assay methods include immunometric assays, chromatographic assays, and mass spectrometry. An immunometric assay uses a large antibody with a component that "captures" the hormone and a second component that creates a signal when the antibody binds to the hormone (antigen). Chromatographic assays separate molecules in the serum by size, light absorption, and other properties. Each hormone has very specific properties that allow it to separate from other blood substances and form a unique bandwidth. Mass spectrometry methods also allow individual hormones to separate from other serum molecules based on the amount (mass) and charge of individual components. On a graph, these separate hormones each shows as a unique "spike" pattern. Many different hormone concentrations can be analyzed at the same time by this method.

Venous Sampling. In addition to general blood levels of hormones, another endocrine assessment test is venous sampling of blood from specific endocrine glands. Blood samples are taken directly from veins that drain a specific endocrine gland and hormone levels are measured. This test is used when a biopsy fails to identify a suspected mass. Unexpected blood hormone levels may indicate the location of a mass, a dysfunctional gland, or a dysfunctional part of a gland.

Urine Tests. Hormone levels and their metabolites in the urine are often measured to determine endocrine function. Because many of the endocrine hormones are secreted in a pulsatile fashion, measurement of a specific hormone in a 24-hour urine collection, rather than as a single blood or urine sample, better reflects the overall function of certain glands, such as the adrenal gland. Teach the patient how to collect a 24-hour urine sample (see also Chart 64-3).

Certain hormones require additives in the container at the beginning of the collection. Instruct the patient not to discard the preservative from the container and to use caution when handling it because some solutions are caustic. Remind him or her that this collection is timed for *exactly* 24 hours. Instruct the patient to avoid taking any unnecessary drugs during endocrine testing because some drugs can interfere with the laboratory assays.

Tests for Glucose. Tests for functions of the islet cells of the pancreas are indirect. They measure the *result* of pancreatic islet cell function. Blood glucose values and the oral glucose tolerance test help diagnose diabetes mellitus. The glycosylated hemoglobin (HbA_{1C}) value reveals the *average* blood glucose level over a period of 2 to 3 months. (See Chapter 67 for a full discussion of diabetes mellitus.)

Imaging Assessment

Anterior, posterior, and lateral skull x-rays may be used to view the sella turcica. Erosion of the sella turcica indicates invasion of the wall from an abnormal growth.

Magnetic resonance imaging (MRI) with contrast is the most sensitive method of imaging the pituitary gland, although computed tomography (CT) scans can also be used to evaluate it. The thyroid, parathyroid glands, ovaries, and testes are evaluated by ultrasound. In addition, CT scans are used to evaluate the adrenal glands, ovaries, and pancreas.

Other Diagnostic Assessment

Needle biopsy is a relatively safe and quick outpatient procedure used to indicate the composition of thyroid nodules. It is used to determine whether surgical intervention is needed.

? DECISION-MAKING CHALLENGE
Patient-Centered Care

The patient is a 50-year-old man who is being seen because he has been leaking clear fluid from both breasts for several weeks. Among the tests that have been requested to check for a pituitary tumor is a suppression test with IV glucose. He is very nervous over the possibility of having what he calls a "brain tumor" and of receiving the glucose intravenously. He tells you he does not need this test because he does not have diabetes, but his older brother does have the disease.
1. Is the patient correct in thinking that a pituitary tumor is a brain tumor? Why or why not?
2. How is the glucose suppression test related to diabetes?
3. Can this test be avoided or changed to reduce his apprehension? If so, in what way?

GET READY FOR THE NCLEX® EXAMINATION!

▍KEY POINTS

Review these Key Points for each NCLEX Examination Client Needs Category.

Safe and Effective Care Environment
- Follow the laboratory's procedures for collecting and handling specimens for endocrine function studies.

Health Promotion and Maintenance
- Teach all patients that abusing or misusing hormones or steroids can have an adverse effect on endocrine function.

Psychosocial Integrity
- Encourage the patient to express concerns about a change in appearance, sexual function, or fertility as a result of a possible endocrine problem.

- Explain all diagnostic procedures, restrictions, and follow-up care to the patient scheduled for endocrine tests.
- Ask family members about changes in the patient's personality or behavior.

Physiological Integrity
- The onset of endocrine problems can be slow and insidious or abrupt and life threatening.
- Ask the patient about other family members with endocrine disorders, because some problems have a genetic component.
- Ask the patient what prescribed and over-the-counter drugs are taken on a regular basis, because some drugs can alter endocrine function.

Care of Patients with Pituitary and Adrenal Gland Problems

M. Linda Workman

LEARNING OUTCOMES

Safe and Effective Care Environment

1. Protect the patient with antidiuretic hormone (ADH) deficiency from dehydration.
2. Use appropriate interventions to prevent injury in the patient who has hypercortisolism.
3. Modify the environment to reduce stimulation for the patient with pheochromocytoma.

Health Promotion and Maintenance

4. Teach patients how to avoid increasing intracranial pressure after pituitary surgery.
5. Identify the teaching priorities for the patient taking hormone replacement therapy for pituitary or adrenal hypofunction.
6. Teach patients how to monitor therapy effectiveness for diabetes insipidus or syndrome of inappropriate ADH (SIADH).

Psychosocial Integrity

7. Be accepting of patient behavior.

8. Encourage the patient and family to express concerns about a change in endocrine health.
9. Explain all disease management–related procedures to the patient and family.

Physiological Integrity

10. Compare the common clinical manifestations associated with pituitary hypofunction and pituitary hyperfunction.
11. Coordinate nursing care for the patient immediately after a transsphenoidal hypophysectomy.
12. Interpret clinical changes and laboratory data to determine the effectiveness of therapy for diabetes insipidus and for SIADH.
13. Compare the clinical manifestations of hypercortisolism and adrenal insufficiency.
14. Prioritize nursing care for the patient with acute adrenal insufficiency.
15. Coordinate nursing care for the patient with Cushing's disease or syndrome.

Hormones secreted from the pituitary gland and adrenal glands influence the function of many tissues and organs. When any of these glands secrete too much or too little of one or more hormones, the effects are widespread and may induce psychological, as well as physical, changes. The anterior pituitary gland regulates growth, metabolism, pigmentation, and sexual development. The posterior pituitary gland secretes vasopressin, also known as *antidiuretic hormone* or *ADH*. Posterior pituitary problems result in fluid and electrolyte imbalances. The adrenal gland produces and secretes hormones that influence homeostasis and are life sustaining. Nursing care for the patient with pituitary or adrenal gland disorders includes assessment, patient education, evaluation of patient response to therapy, and providing support.

A complete history and physical examination are performed to detect specific clinical findings. The patient also often undergoes many diagnostic tests and relies on the nurse for specific instructions and explanations. Surgical intervention may be indicated. The patient often needs lifelong hormone replacement therapy, and physical and emotional support are critical.

DISORDERS OF THE ANTERIOR PITUITARY GLAND

The anterior pituitary gland (adenohypophysis) controls growth, metabolic activity, and sexual development through the actions of these hormones:

- Growth hormone (GH; somatotropin)
- Thyrotropin (thyroid-stimulating hormone [TSH])
- Corticotropin (adrenocorticotropic hormone [ACTH])
- Follicle-stimulating hormone (FSH)
- Luteinizing hormone (LH)
- Melanocyte-stimulating hormone (MSH)
- Prolactin (PRL)

Hormone disorders of the anterior pituitary gland can result from problems arising within the anterior pituitary gland itself (*primary pituitary dysfunction*) or from problems in the hypothalamus that change anterior pituitary function (*secondary pituitary dysfunction*). In either case, one or more hormones may be undersecreted (*pituitary hypofunction*) or oversecreted (*pituitary hyperfunction*).

HYPOPITUITARISM

Pathophysiology

A person with hypopituitarism has a deficiency of one or more anterior pituitary hormones, resulting in metabolic problems and sexual dysfunction. If only one hormone is affected, the condition is known as *selective hypopituitarism*. Decreased production of *all* of the anterior pituitary hormones is an extremely rare condition known as panhypopituitarism.

More commonly, there is a decrease in the secretion of one hormone and a lesser decrease in the secretion of other hormones. Deficiencies of *adrenocorticotropic hormone (ACTH)* and *thyroid-stimulating hormone (TSH)* are the *most* life threatening because they cause a decrease in the secretion of vital hormones from the adrenal and thyroid glands. Adrenal gland hypofunction is discussed on pp. 1381-1384; hypothyroidism is discussed in Chapter 66.

Deficiency of the gonadotropins (luteinizing hormone [LH] and follicle-stimulating hormone [FSH]—hormones that stimulate the ovaries and testes to produce sex hormones) changes sexual function in both men and women. In men, gonadotropin deficiency results in testicular failure, with decreased testosterone production from the Leydig cells and decreased or absent sperm production. Decreased testosterone levels in men cause sterility. In women, gonadotropin deficiency results in ovarian failure, amenorrhea, and infertility.

Growth hormone (GH) deficiency changes tissue growth patterns indirectly. GH itself has little effect on tissues and cells; however, it stimulates the liver to produce somatomedins. These substances, especially somatomedin C, then enhance growth activities in cells and tissues. Somatomedin C is responsible for bone and cartilage growth and maintenance.

GH deficiency may be a result of decreased GH production, failure of the liver to produce somatomedins, or a failure of the cells or tissues to respond to the somatomedins. Deficiency in children leads to short stature and other manifestations of growth retardation. Deficiency in adults does not affect height but does increase the rate of bone destructive activity, leading to thinner, more fragile bones (osteoporosis) and an increased risk for fractures.

The cause of hypopituitarism varies. Benign or malignant pituitary tumors can compress and destroy pituitary tissue. Pituitary function can be impaired by severe malnutrition or rapid loss of body fat, such as in people with anorexia nervosa (a disorder in which people see themselves as overweight and eat so little that starvation results). Shock or severe hypotension reduces blood flow to the pituitary gland, leading to hypoxia and infarction. Other causes of hypopituitarism include head trauma, brain tumors or infection, radiation or surgery of the head and brain, and acquired immune deficiency syndrome (AIDS) (Melmed & Kleinberg, 2008). *Idiopathic hypopituitarism* is an isolated hormone deficiency with an unknown cause.

Postpartum hemorrhage is the most common cause of pituitary infarction, which results in decreased hormone secretion. This clinical problem is known as *Sheehan's syndrome*. The pituitary gland normally enlarges during pregnancy, and when hypotension results from hemorrhage, ischemia and necrosis of the gland occur. Usually this condition develops immediately after delivery, although some cases have occurred several years later.

PATIENT-CENTERED COLLABORATIVE CARE

ASSESSMENT

Changes in physical appearance and target organ function occur with deficiencies of specific pituitary hormones (Chart 65-1). Gonadotropin (LH and FSH) deficiency results in the loss of or change in secondary sex characteristics in men and women. While assessing the male patient, look for facial and body hair loss. Ask about episodes of impotence and decreased *libido* (sex drive). Women may report amenorrhea (absence of menstrual periods), dyspareunia (painful intercourse), infertility, and decreased libido. While examining the female patient, check for dry skin, breast atrophy, and a decreased amount or absence of axillary and pubic hair.

Neurologic manifestations of hypopituitarism as a result of tumor growth often first occur as changes in vision. Assess the patient's visual acuity, especially peripheral vision, for changes or loss. Temporal headaches are a common finding. Other manifestations may include diplopia (double vision) and ocular muscle paralysis, limiting eye movement.

Laboratory findings vary widely with hypopituitarism. Some pituitary hormone levels may be measured directly. Often, however, the *effects* of the hormones, rather than their actual levels, are assessed. Blood levels of triiodothyronine (T_3) and thyroxine (T_4) from the thyroid, as well as testosterone and estradiol from the gonads, are measured easily. If levels of one or all of these hormones are low or in the low-normal range, further evaluation is necessary. Levels of pituitary gonadotropins (LH and FSH) and TSH are sufficient if function of the target organ is apparent. Function of LH

CHART 65-1 KEY FEATURES

Pituitary Hypofunction

DEFICIENT HORMONE	CLINICAL MANIFESTATIONS
Anterior Pituitary Hormones	
Growth hormone (GH)	Decreased bone density Pathologic fractures Decreased muscle strength Increased serum cholesterol levels
Gonadotropins (luteinizing hormone [LH], follicle-stimulating hormone [FSH])	Women: • Amenorrhea • Anovulation • Low estrogen levels • Breast atrophy • Loss of bone density • Decreased axillary and pubic hair • Decreased libido Men: • Decreased facial hair • Decreased ejaculate volume • Reduced muscle mass • Loss of bone density • Decreased body hair • Decreased libido • Impotence
Thyroid-stimulating hormone (thyrotropin) (TSH)	Decreased thyroid hormone levels Weight gain Intolerance to cold Scalp alopecia Hirsutism Menstrual abnormalities Decreased libido Slowed cognition Lethargy
Adrenocorticotropic hormone (ACTH)	Decreased serum cortisol levels Pale, sallow complexion Malaise and lethargy Anorexia Postural hypotension Headache Hypoglycemia Hyponatremia Decreased axillary and pubic hair (women)
Posterior Pituitary Hormones	

Vasopressin (antidiuretic hormone [ADH])	Diabetes insipidus:
	• Greatly increased urine output
	• Low urine specific gravity (<1.005)
	• Hypovolemia:
	  Hypotension
	  Dehydration
	• Increased plasma osmolarity
	• Increased thirst
	• Output does not decrease when fluid intake decreases

and FSH is assessed by observing for the presence of secondary sexual characteristics. Function of TSH is assessed by measuring circulating levels of thyroid hormones. ACTH levels may be normal or low, and prolactin (PRL) levels are low to high.

Stimulation testing can be useful to evaluate pituitary function. For example, insulin injection in people with normal pituitary function causes an increased release of GH

and ACTH. With decreased pituitary function, levels of either of these hormones remain unchanged.

Pituitary problems may cause changes in the sella turcica (the bony nest where the pituitary gland rests) that can be seen with skull x-rays. Changes may include enlargement, erosion, and calcifications as a result of pituitary tumors. Computed tomography (CT) and magnetic resonance imaging (MRI) can more distinctly define bone or soft-tissue lesions. An angiogram may be used to rule out the presence of an aneurysm or other vascular problems in the area before surgery.

INTERVENTIONS

Management of the adult with hypopituitarism focuses on replacement of deficient hormones. Older patients or those with a chronic disease often require a lower amount of hormone replacement. Men who have gonadotropin deficiency receive sex steroid replacement therapy with androgens (testosterone). The most effective route of androgen replacement is IM, although use of transdermal testosterone patches is increasing. Instruct the patient in self-administration. Therapy begins with high-dose testosterone and is continued until virilization (presence of male secondary sex characteristics) is achieved. Maximal effects of treatment include increases in penis size, libido, muscle mass, bone size, and bone strength. Chest, facial, pubic, and axillary hair growth also increases, and the voice deepens. Patients usually report improved self-esteem and body image after therapy is initiated. The dose may then be decreased, but therapy continues throughout life.

Androgen therapy is avoided in men with prostate cancer. Side effects of testosterone therapy include gynecomastia (male breast tissue development), acne, baldness, and prostate enlargement.

Achieving fertility in these patients is difficult and requires additional parenteral testosterone therapy and injections of human chorionic gonadotropin (hCG). Teach the patient about the additional therapy, and provide emotional support because the outcome of fertility treatment is uncertain.

Women who have gonadotropin deficiency receive hormone replacement with a combination of estrogen and progesterone. The risk for hypertension or thrombosis (formation of blood clots in deep veins) is increased with estrogen therapy, especially among women who smoke. Emphasize measures to reduce risk and the need for regular health visits. For women who wish to become pregnant, clomiphene (Clomid) may be given to induce ovulation. Gonadotropin-releasing hormone (GnRH) and hCG are used to stimulate ovulation if therapy with clomiphene fails.

Adult patients with GH deficiency may be treated with injections of GH, although this treatment is rare.

NCLEX EXAMINATION CHALLENGE

Health Promotion and Maintenance

Which precaution is most important for the nurse to teach the female client undergoing drug therapy with estrogen and progesterone for hypopituitarism?
A. "Use a nonhormonal form of contraception to prevent an unplanned pregnancy."
B. "Wear a hat with a brim and use sunscreen when outdoors."
C. "Do not smoke or use nicotine in any form."
D. "Avoid drinking alcoholic beverages."

HYPERPITUITARISM

Pathophysiology

Hyperpituitarism is hormone oversecretion that occurs with pituitary tumors or tissue hyperplasia (tissue overgrowth). Tumors occur most often in the anterior pituitary cells that produce growth hormone (GH), prolactin (PRL), and adrenocorticotropic hormone (ACTH). Overproduction of PRL also may occur in response to tumors that overproduce GH and ACTH. Excess ACTH may occur with increased secretion of melanocyte-stimulating hormone (MSH).

GENETIC/GENOMIC CONSIDERATIONS

An uncommon cause of hyperpituitarism is multiple endocrine neoplasia, type 1 (MEN1), in which there is inactivation of the suppressor gene MENIN (Melmed & Kleinberg, 2008). This problem has an autosomal dominant inheritance pattern and is usually expressed as a benign tumor that affects the pituitary, parathyroid glands, and pancreas. In pituitary function, MEN1 leads to excessive production of growth hormone and acromegaly. Ask a patient suspected of having acromegaly whether either parent also has this problem or has had a tumor of the pancreas or parathyroid glands.

The most common cause of hyperpituitarism is a pituitary adenoma—a benign tumor of one or more tissues within the anterior pituitary. Adenomas are classified by size, invasiveness, and the hormone secreted. An invasive pituitary adenoma involves a portion or all of the sella turcica. When the sella turcica is not involved, the adenoma is "enclosed."

As an adenoma gets larger and compresses brain tissue, neurologic symptoms, as well as endocrine symptoms, may occur. Such symptoms may include visual changes, headache, and increased intracranial pressure (ICP).

Prolactin (PRL)-secreting tumors are the most common type of pituitary adenoma. Excessive PRL inhibits the secretion of gonadotropins and sex hormones in men and women, resulting in galactorrhea (breast milk production), amenorrhea, and infertility.

Overproduction of GH in adults results in acromegaly (Fig. 65-1). The onset may be gradual with slow progression, and changes may remain unnoticed for years before diagnosis of the disorder. Early detection and treatment are essential to prevent irreversible changes in the soft tissues, such as those of the face, hands, feet, and skin. Other changes include increased skeletal thickness, hypertrophy of the skin, and enlargement of many organs, such as the liver and heart. Some changes may be reversible after treatment, but skeletal changes are permanent.

Bone thinning and bone cell overgrowth occur slowly. Degeneration of joint cartilage and hypertrophy of ligaments, vocal cords, and eustachian tubes are common. Nerve entrapment occurs because of tissue overgrowth and myelin loss in peripheral nerves. Because GH blocks the action of insulin, hyperglycemia (elevated blood glucose levels) is also common.

Excess ACTH overstimulates the adrenal cortex. The result is excessive production of glucocorticoids, mineralocorticoids, and androgens, which leads to the development of Cushing's disease (see Hypercortisolism [Cushing's Disease], pp. 1384-1390).

Usually, hyperpituitarism is caused by hormone-secreting benign tumors (adenomas) arising from one pituitary cell type. It can also be caused by hypothalamic problems that lead to excessive production of releasing hormones, which then overstimulate the normal pituitary gland.

PATIENT-CENTERED COLLABORATIVE CARE

ASSESSMENT

The manifestations of hyperpituitarism vary, depending on which hormone is produced in excess. Obtain data about the patient's age, gender, and family history. Ask about any change in hat, glove, ring, or shoe size. Fatigue and lethargy are common. The patient with high GH levels may have backache and arthralgias (joint pain) from bone changes. Ask specifically about headaches and changes in vision.

The patient with hypersecretion of PRL often reports difficulties in sexual functioning. Ask women about menstrual changes (e.g., amenorrhea, irregular menses, and difficulty in becoming pregnant) and about decreased libido or dyspareunia (painful intercourse). Men may report decreased libido and impotence.

Changes in appearance and target organ function occur with excesses of specific anterior pituitary hormones (Chart 65-2). Initial manifestations of GH excess are increases in lip and nose sizes, a prominent brow ridge, and increases in head, hand, and foot sizes. The patient with hyperpituitarism often seeks health care because of dramatic changes in appearance. Assess the impact of these changes on self-image and personal relationships.

In hyperpituitarism, usually only one hormone is produced in excess because the cell types within the pituitary gland are so individually organized. The most common hormones produced in excess are PRL, ACTH, and GH. Tumors producing TSH, luteinizing hormone (LH), or follicle-stimulating hormone (FSH) are rare, and elevations of these hormones warrant evaluation. Elevations of LH and FSH are normal in the postmenopausal woman.

Imaging assessment for hyperpituitarism is the same as for hypopituitarism. Skull x-rays are used to identify abnormalities of the sella turcica. CT scans and MRI can define soft-tissue lesions, and angiography can rule out an aneurysm or vascular malformations.

Suppression testing can help diagnose hyperpituitarism and determine whether the normal negative feedback control mechanisms for hormonal regulation are intact. For example, high blood glucose levels suppress the release of GH. In a suppression test, 100 g of oral glucose or 0.5 g/kg of body weight is given IV. GH levels are measured serially for up to 120 minutes. GH levels that do not fall below 5 ng/mL indicate a positive (abnormal) result.

INTERVENTIONS

The expected outcomes of management for the patient who has hyperpituitarism are to return hormone levels to normal or near normal, reduce or eliminate headache and visual disturbances, prevent complications, and reverse as many of the body changes as possible.

Nonsurgical Management

Encourage the patient to express concerns about his or her altered physical appearance. Help him or her identify personal strengths and positive characteristics, reinforcing each

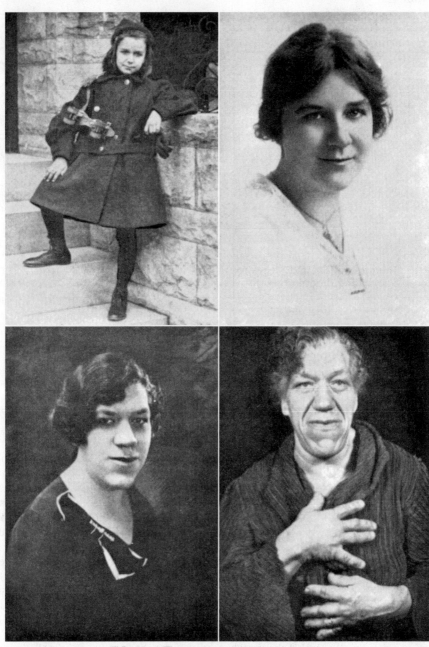

FIG. 65-1 The progression of acromegaly.

patient's uniqueness and importance. Galactorrhea, gynecomastia, and reduced sexual functioning can disturb self-image and personal identity. Reassure the patient that treatment may reverse some of these problems. Encourage the patient to discuss his or her feelings.

Drug therapy may be used alone or in combination with surgery and/or radiation. The most common drugs used are dopamine agonists, including bromocriptine mesylate (Parlodel), cabergoline (Dostinex), and pergolide (Permax) (Melmed & Kleinberg, 2008). These drugs stimulate dopamine receptors in the brain and inhibit the release of GH and PRL. In most cases, small tumors decrease until the pituitary gland is of normal size. Large pituitary tumors usually decrease to some extent. In patients with acromegaly, bromocriptine reduces GH levels and decreases tumor size,

especially when GH levels remain high after surgery or before the full effect of radiation therapy has occurred.

Side effects of bromocriptine include orthostatic (postural) hypotension, gastric irritation, nausea, headaches, abdominal cramps, and constipation. Give bromocriptine with a meal or a snack to reduce some of these side effects. Treatment starts with a low dose and is gradually increased until the desired level (usually 7.5 mg/day) is reached. *If pregnancy occurs, the drug is stopped immediately.*

Other agents used for acromegaly are the somatostatin analogs, especially octreotide (Sandostatin), and a growth hormone receptor blocker, pegvisomant (Somavert). Octreotide inhibits GH release through negative feedback. Pegvisomant blocks growth hormone (GH) receptor activity and production of insulin-like growth factor (IGF). Although

CHART 65-2   **KEY FEATURES**

Anterior Pituitary Hyperfunction

Prolactin (PRL)
- Hypogonadism (loss of secondary sexual characteristics)
- Decreased gonadotropin levels
- Galactorrhea
- Increased body fat
- Increased serum prolactin levels

Growth Hormone (GH)
Acromegaly
- Folding of the scalp skin
- Thickened lips
- Coarse facial features
- Increasing head size
- Protrusion of the lower jaw
- Deepening of the voice
- Tufting of the fingertips
- Enlarged hands and feet
- Joint enlargement and pain
- Kyphosis and backache
- Barrel-shaped chest
- Excessive sweating
- Hyperglycemia
- Airway narrowing, sleep apnea
- Enlarged heart, lungs, and liver

Adrenocorticotropic Hormone (ACTH)
Cushing's Disease (Pituitary)
- Elevated plasma cortisol levels
- Weight gain
- Truncal obesity
- "Moon face"
- Extremity muscle wasting
- Loss of bone density
- Hypertension
- Hyperglycemia
- Purple striae
- Acne
- Thin, easily damaged skin
- Hyperpigmentation

Thyrotropin (Thyroid-Stimulating Hormone [TSH])
- Elevated plasma TSH levels
- Elevated plasma thyroid hormone levels
- Weight loss
- Tachycardia and dysrhythmias
- Heat intolerance
- Increased GI motility
- Fine tremors

Gonadotropins (Luteinizing Hormone [LH], Follicle-Stimulating Hormone [FSH])
Men:
- Elevated LH and FSH levels
- Hypogonadism or hypergonadism

Women:
- Normal LH and FSH levels
(The most common clinical manifestations in men and women are related to the physical presence of a tumor rather than to excessive hormone secretion.)

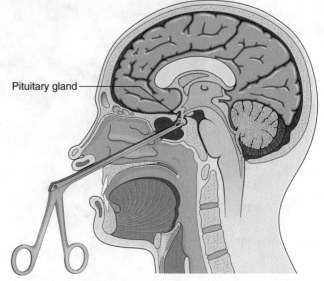

FIG. 65-2 The transsphenoidal surgical approach to the pituitary gland. Selective adenomectomy leaves normal pituitary tissue undisturbed.

and vision problems. Use of the gamma knife procedure is increasing the accuracy of radiation therapy.

Surgical Management

Surgical removal of the pituitary gland and tumor (hypophysectomy) is the most common treatment for hyperpituitarism.

Preoperative Care. Explain that hypophysectomy decreases hormone levels, relieves headaches, and may reverse changes in sexual functioning. Body changes, organ enlargement, and visual changes are not usually reversible. Explain that because nasal packing is present for 2 to 3 days after surgery, it will be necessary to breathe through the mouth, and a "mustache" dressing ("drip" pad) will be placed under the nose. Instruct the patient not to brush teeth, cough, sneeze, blow the nose, or bend forward after surgery. These activities can increase intracranial pressure (ICP) and delay healing.

Operative Procedures. Depending on tumor size and other patient factors, a minimally invasive endoscopic transnasal approach may be used instead of the more traditional transsphenoidal approach (Fig. 65-2). Although both procedures are less invasive than a craniotomy, the endoscopic approach uses smaller diameter instruments and results in less damage to nasal structures (Graham et al., 2009). Both procedures are performed with the patient in a semi-sitting position. For the transsphenoidal approach, the surgeon makes an incision just above the upper lip and reaches the pituitary gland through the sphenoid sinus. After the gland is removed, a muscle graft is taken, often from the thigh, to support the area and prevent leakage of cerebrospinal fluid (CSF). Nasal packing is inserted after the incision is closed, and a mustache dressing is applied. If the tumor cannot be reached by either the endoscopic transnasal approach or the transsphenoidal approach, a craniotomy may be indicated (see Chapter 47).

Postoperative Care. Monitor the patient's neurologic response, and document any changes in vision or mental

these therapies are effective, a disadvantage is that they must be given as an injection on a daily or weekly schedule. A major side effect is gallbladder disease. Pegvisomant may cause an increase in tumor size.

! NURSING SAFETY PRIORITY

Drug Alert

Teach patients taking bromocriptine to seek medical care immediately if chest pain, dizziness, or watery nasal discharge occurs because of the possibility of serious side effects, including cardiac dysrhythmias, coronary artery spasms, and cerebrospinal fluid leakage.

Radiation therapy is not useful in the immediate management of acute hyperpituitarism. These therapy regimens take a long time to complete, and several years may pass before a therapeutic effect can be seen. Side effects of radiation therapy include hypopituitarism, optic nerve damage, and other eye

status, altered level of consciousness, or decreased strength of the extremities. Observe the patient for complications such as transient diabetes insipidus (discussed on pp. 1378-1380), CSF leakage, infection, and increased ICP.

Teach the patient to report any postnasal drip or increased swallowing, which might indicate leakage of CSF. Keep the head of the bed elevated after surgery. Assess nasal drainage for quantity, quality, and the presence of glucose (which indicates that the fluid is CSF). A light yellow color at the edge of the clear drainage on the dressing is called the "halo sign" and indicates CSF. If the patient has persistent, severe headaches, CSF fluid may have leaked into the sinus area. Most CSF leaks resolve with bedrest. If the CSF leak persists, the physician may perform a spinal tap to reduce CSF pressure. Surgical intervention is rarely necessary.

Teach the patient to avoid coughing early after surgery because it increases pressure in the incision area and may lead to a CSF leak. Remind the patient to perform deep-breathing exercises hourly while awake to prevent pulmonary problems. Patients may have mouth dryness from mouth breathing. Perform frequent oral rinses, and apply a lubricating jelly to dry lips.

Infection can occur after surgery. Specifically assess for manifestations of meningitis, such as headache, fever, and nuchal (neck) rigidity. The surgeon may prescribe antibiotics, analgesics, and antipyretics.

If the entire pituitary gland has been removed, replacement of thyroid hormones and glucocorticoids is lifelong. Best practices for care after surgery are listed in Chart 65-3.

After surgery, the patient needs daily self-management regimens and frequent checkups. He or she may need strategies to reduce stress. The home care nurse performs a focused assessment during any home visit to a patient who has undergone a hypophysectomy (Chart 65-4). Review drug regimens and manifestations of infection and cerebral edema with the family.

After a transsphenoidal hypophysectomy, advise the patient to avoid activities that might interfere with healing. Teach him or her to avoid bending over from the waist to pick

up objects or tie shoes because this position increases ICP. Teach the patient to bend the knees and then lower the body to pick up fallen objects. ICP also increases when the patient strains to have a bowel movement. Suggest techniques to prevent constipation, such as eating high-fiber foods, drinking plenty of fluids, and using stool softeners or laxatives. Activities that increase ICP should be avoided for up to 2 months after surgery.

Teach the patient to avoid toothbrushing for about 2 weeks after surgery until the incision has healed. Frequent mouth care (every 4 to 6 hours) with mouthwash and daily flossing provide adequate oral hygiene. Numbness in the area of the incision and a decreased sense of smell are expected after surgery and usually last 3 to 4 months. Advise the patient to use a mirror to check the gums for bleeding, because reduced sensation increases the risk for injury.

After a hypophysectomy, hormone replacement with vasopressin may be needed to maintain fluid balance. (See discussion of Interventions on pp. 1378-1380 in the Diabetes Insipidus section.) If the anterior portion of the pituitary gland is removed, instruct the patient in cortisol, thyroid, and gonadal hormone replacement. Teach the patient to report the return of any symptoms of hyperpituitarism immediately to the primary health care provider.

NCLEX EXAMINATION CHALLENGE

Safe and Effective Care Environment

The nurse notes that the mustache dressing of a client who is 12 hours postoperative from a transsphenoidal hypophysectomy is wet. What is the nurse's best action?

A. Reapply a dry dressing and document this expected response.
B. Ask the client whether other symptoms of a cold are present.
C. Notify the surgeon or the Rapid Response Team.
D. Test the drainage for the presence of glucose.

DISORDERS OF THE POSTERIOR PITUITARY GLAND

Disorders of the posterior pituitary gland (neurohypophysis) are related to a deficiency or excess of the hormone *vasopressin* (antidiuretic hormone [ADH]) and usually occur independently from anterior pituitary problems. Diabetes insipidus occurs with ADH deficiency, and the syndrome of inappropriate antidiuretic hormone (SIADH) occurs with ADH excess.

DIABETES INSIPIDUS

Pathophysiology

Diabetes insipidus (DI) is a water metabolism problem caused by an ADH deficiency (either a decrease in ADH synthesis or an inability of the kidneys to respond to ADH). ADH deficiency results in the excretion of large volumes of dilute urine. Without ADH, distal kidney tubules and collecting ducts do not reabsorb water, leading to polyuria (excessive water loss through urination) and dehydration.

Dehydration caused by this massive water loss increases plasma osmolarity, which stimulates the osmoreceptors to relay a sensation of thirst to the cerebral cortex. Thirst promotes increased fluid intake and aids in maintaining water homeostasis. *If the thirst mechanism is poor or absent or if the person is unable to obtain water, dehydration becomes more severe and can lead to death.*

NURSING SAFETY PRIORITY

Critical Rescue

Ensure that no patient suspected of having DI is deprived of fluids for more than 4 hours, because he or she cannot reduce urine output and severe dehydration can result.

ADH deficiency is classified as nephrogenic, drug-related, primary, or secondary, depending on whether the problem is caused by insufficient production of ADH or an inability of the kidney to respond to the presence of ADH (Simmons, 2010).

Nephrogenic diabetes insipidus is an inherited disorder. The kidney tubules do not respond to the actions of ADH, which results in poor water reabsorption by the kidney. The actual amount of hormone produced is not deficient.

Primary diabetes insipidus is caused by a defect in the hypothalamus or pituitary gland, resulting in a lack of ADH production or release. *Secondary diabetes insipidus* can result from tumors in or near the hypothalamus or pituitary gland, head trauma, infectious processes, surgical procedures (hypophysectomy), or metastatic tumors. Less often, it is caused by brain hemorrhage, brain disease, or cerebral aneurysm, which reduces ADH production.

Drug-related diabetes insipidus is usually caused by lithium carbonate (Eskalith, Lithobid, Carbolith ♣) and demeclocycline (Declomycin). These drugs can interfere with the response of the kidneys to ADH.

CHART 65-5 KEY FEATURES

Diabetes Insipidus

Cardiovascular Manifestations
- Hypotension
- Decreased pulse pressure
- Tachycardia
- Peripheral pulses weak, easily blocked
- Hemoconcentration:
  - Increased hemoglobin
  - Increased hematocrit
  - Increased BUN

Kidney/Urinary Manifestations
- Increased urine output:
  - Dilute, low specific gravity
  - Hypo-osmolar

Skin Manifestations
- Poor turgor
- Dry mucous membranes

Neurologic Manifestations
- Increased sensation of thirst
- Irritability*
- Decreased cognition*
- Hyperthermia*
- Lethargy to coma*
- Ataxia*

BUN, Blood urea nitrogen.
*Occurs when access to water is limited and rapid dehydration results.

PATIENT-CENTERED COLLABORATIVE CARE

ASSESSMENT

Most manifestations of DI are related to dehydration (Chart 65-5) (Simmons, 2010). The key manifestations are an increase in the frequency of urination and excessive thirst. Ask about a history of any known causative factors, such as recent surgery, head trauma, or drug use (e.g., lithium). Although increased fluid intake prevents serious volume depletion, the patient who is deprived of fluids or who cannot increase oral fluid intake may develop shock from fluid loss. Manifestations of dehydration, such as poor skin turgor and dry or cracked mucous membranes or skin, may be present. (See Chapter 13 for further discussion of dehydration.)

Water loss produces changes in blood and urine tests. The first step in diagnosis is to measure a 24-hour fluid intake and output without restricting food or fluid intake. DI is considered if urine output is more than 4 L during this period and is greater than the volume ingested. *The amount of urine excreted in 24 hours may vary from 4 to 30 L/day.* Urine is dilute with a low specific gravity (less than 1.005) and low osmolarity (50 to 200 mOsm/kg).

INTERVENTIONS

Management focuses on controlling manifestations with drug therapy (Chart 65-6). If only a partial deficit of ADH is present, effective control can be achieved with oral chlorpropamide (Diabinese, Novo-Propamide ♣). This drug increases the action of existing ADH and possibly has a stimulating effect on the production of ADH in the hypothalamus.

CHART 65-6 COMMON EXAMPLES OF DRUG THERAPY

Diabetes Insipidus

DRUG/DOSAGE	PURPOSE/ACTION	NURSING INTERVENTIONS	RATIONALES
Desmopressin (DDAVP, Rhinal Tube, Minirin, Stimate) Tablets: 0.1-0.2 mg orally twice daily Nasal spray: 10-20 mcg every 8-12 hr Parenteral: 1-2 mcg IV or subcutaneously every 12 hr	The drug is a synthetic type of ADH that serves as a replacement. It binds to kidney receptors and enhances the reabsorption of water, thus reducing urine output.	Teach the patient using the inhaled form of the drug to blow the nose before taking the drug. Teach the patient using the inhaled form to sit upright and hold his or her breath when spraying or using the rhinal tube. Warn the patient not to drink more than 3 L of fluids daily while on this drug. Teach the patient to weigh himself or herself daily and to notify the health care provider if 2 lbs or more is gained in 24 hours. Tell the patient to notify the health care provider if he or she experiences a persistent headache or acute confusion.	Drug is absorbed through the nasal mucosa. Nasal secretions can dilute the drug and inhibit its absorption. Sitting upright and holding the breath keeps the drug in contact with the nasal mucosa, rather than going down the throat, enhancing drug absorption. Drug promotes fluid retention and can lead to fluid overload. A rapid increase in weight is an indicator of excessive fluid retention and may require a change in drug dosage. These are manifestations of water toxicity, which must be treated before seizure activity occurs.
Vasopressin (Pitressin) 5-10 units parenterally two to four times daily	The drug is an exogenous form of ADH that serves as a replacement. It binds to kidney receptors and enhances the reabsorption of water, thus reducing urine output.	For the hospitalized patient, monitor for signs of water intoxication, such as listlessness, drowsiness, confusion, headache, anuria, and weight gain. Warn the patient not to drink more than 3 L of fluids daily while on this drug. Teach the patient to weigh himself or herself daily and to notify the health care provider if 2 lbs or more is gained in 24 hours. Tell the patient to notify the health care provider if he or she experiences a persistent headache or acute confusion.	Vasopressin-induced water intoxication can also lead to seizures, coma, and death. Drug promotes fluid retention and can lead to fluid overload. A rapid increase in weight is an indicator of excessive fluid retention and may require a change in drug dosage. These are manifestations of water toxicity, which must be treated before seizure activity occurs.
Chlorpropamide (Diabinese, Insulase) 250-500 mg orally daily	The drug is an antidiabetic agent that also has some antidiuretic activity through an unknown mechanism. It decreases urine output.	Ask whether the patient has any allergies to sulfa-based drugs. Teach patients the manifestations of hypoglycemia and to always carry candy or concentrated sugar with them.	Drug contains sulfa, and a person who is hypersensitive to sulfa drugs is likely to also be hypersensitive to this drug. The main action of the drug is to lower blood glucose levels. When taken by a person whose blood glucose level is normal, hypoglycemia can result.

ADH, Antidiuretic hormone.

! NURSING SAFETY PRIORITY
Drug Alert

Diabinese and Diamox are sound-alike, look-alike drugs. Do not confuse them. Diamox is a type of diuretic, which could increase urine output and the risk for dehydration.

! NURSING SAFETY PRIORITY
Drug Alert

The parenteral form of desmopressin is 10 times stronger than the oral form, and the dosage must be reduced.

When ADH deficiency is severe, ADH is replaced in amounts sufficient to maintain water balance. Desmopressin acetate (DDAVP) is a synthetic form of vasopressin given orally or intranasally in a metered spray and is the drug of choice (Robinson & Verbalis, 2008). The frequency of dosing varies with patient responses. Teach patients that each metered spray delivers 10 mcg, and those with mild DI may need only one or two doses in 24 hours. For more severe DI, one or two metered doses two or three times daily may be needed. During severe dehydration, ADH may be given IV or IM. Ulceration of the mucous membranes, allergy, a sensation of chest tightness, and lung inhalation of the spray may occur with use of the intranasal preparations. If side effects occur or if the patient has an upper respiratory infection, oral or subcutaneous vasopressin is used.

For the hospitalized patient with DI, nursing management focuses on early detection of dehydration and maintaining adequate hydration. Interventions include accurately measuring fluid intake and output, checking urine specific gravity, and recording the patient's weight daily.

Urge the patient to drink fluids in an amount equal to urine output. If fluids are given IV, ensure the patency of the access catheter and accurately monitor the amount infused hourly.

The patient with permanent DI requires lifelong desmopressin or vasopressin therapy. Assess his or her ability to follow instructions and participate in health care. Teach that polyuria and polydipsia are signals for the need for another dose.

Drugs for DI induce water retention and can cause fluid overload (see Chapter 13). *Teach all patients taking these drugs to weigh themselves daily to identify weight gain.* Stress the importance of using the same scale and weighing at the same time of day while wearing a similar amount of clothing. If weight gain or other signs of water toxicity occur (e.g., persistent headache, acute confusion), instruct the patient or family that the patient must go to the emergency department or call 911. Instruct the patient to wear a medical alert bracelet identifying the disorder and drugs.

❓ NCLEX EXAMINATION CHALLENGE

Physiological Integrity

Which response in a client with diabetes insipidus indicates to the nurse that another dose of desmopressin acetate (DDAVP) is needed?
A. Urine output and specific gravity are increased.
B. Urine output is increased and urine specific gravity is decreased.
C. Urine output and specific gravity are decreased.
D. Urine output is decreased and urine specific gravity is increased.

SYNDROME OF INAPPROPRIATE ANTIDIURETIC HORMONE

Pathophysiology

The syndrome of inappropriate antidiuretic hormone (SIADH) is a problem in which vasopressin (antidiuretic hormone [ADH]) is secreted even when plasma osmolarity is low or normal. A decrease in plasma osmolarity normally inhibits ADH production and secretion. SIADH is also known as the *Schwartz-Bartter syndrome.* SIADH occurs with many pathologic conditions (e.g., cancer therapy) and with specific drugs, including selective serotonin reuptake inhibitors (Fitzgerald, 2008). Table 65-1 lists specific drugs and other common causes of SIADH.

In SIADH, ADH continues to be released even when plasma is hypo-osmolar. Water is *retained,* which results in dilutional hyponatremia (a decreased serum sodium level) and fluid overload. The increase in plasma volume increases the glomerular filtration rate and inhibits the release of renin

and aldosterone. The combined effect is an increased sodium loss in urine, leading to greater hyponatremia.

PATIENT-CENTERED COLLABORATIVE CARE

ASSESSMENT

Ask the patient about his or her medical history, which may reveal conditions that occur with the development of SIADH. Information about these conditions should be obtained:
- Recent head trauma
- Cerebrovascular disease
- Tuberculosis or other pulmonary disease
- Cancer
- All past and current drug use

The early manifestations of SIADH are related to water retention. GI disturbances, such as loss of appetite, nausea, and vomiting, may occur first. Weigh the patient, and document any recent weight gain. Use this information to monitor responses to therapy. In SIADH, free water (not salt) is retained and dependent edema is not usually present, even though water is retained.

Water retention, hyponatremia, and fluid shifts affect central nervous system function, especially when the serum sodium level drops below 115 mEq/L. The patient may have lethargy, headaches, hostility, disorientation, and a change in level of consciousness. Manifestations can progress from lethargy and headaches to decreased responsiveness, seizures, and coma. Assess deep tendon reflexes, which are usually decreased.

Vital sign changes include a full and bounding pulse (caused by the increased fluid volume) and hypothermia (caused by central nervous system disturbance). Chapter 13 presents other findings that occur with hyponatremia.

Water retention changes both plasma and urine osmolarity. Urine volume decreases, and urine osmolarity increases. Plasma volume increases, and plasma osmolarity decreases. Elevated urine sodium levels and specific gravity reflect increased urine concentration. Serum sodium levels are decreased, often as low as 110 mEq/L, because of fluid retention and sodium loss.

Radioimmunoassay of ADH can diagnose SIADH when ADH levels are inappropriately elevated when plasma osmolarity is normal or decreased.

INTERVENTIONS

Medical interventions for SIADH focus on restricting fluid intake, promoting the excretion of water, replacing any lost sodium, and interfering with the action of ADH. Nursing interventions focus on monitoring response to therapy, preventing complications, teaching the patient and family about fluid restrictions and drug therapy, and preventing injury.

Fluid restriction is essential because fluid intake further dilutes plasma sodium levels. In some cases, fluid intake may be kept as low as 500 to 600 mL/24 hr. Dilute tube feedings with saline rather than plain water, and use saline to irrigate GI tubes. Mix drugs to be given by GI tube with saline.

Measure intake, output, and daily weights to assess the degree of fluid restriction needed. A weight gain of 2 pounds or more per day or a gradual increase over several days is

TABLE 65-1	CONDITIONS CAUSING THE SYNDROME OF INAPPROPRIATE ANTIDIURETIC HORMONE
Malignancies	**CNS Disorders**
• Small cell lung cancer	• Trauma
• Pancreatic, duodenal, and GU carcinomas	• Infection
	• Tumors (primary or metastatic)
• Thymoma	• Strokes
• Hodgkin's lymphoma	• Porphyria
• Non-Hodgkin's lymphoma	• Systemic lupus erythematosus
Pulmonary Disorders	**Drugs**
• Viral and bacterial pneumonia	• Exogenous ADH
	• Chlorpropamide
• Lung abscesses	• Vincristine
• Active tuberculosis	• Cyclophosphamide
• Pneumothorax	• Carbamazepine
• Chronic lung diseases	• Opioids
• Mycoses	• Tricyclic antidepressants
• Positive-pressure ventilation	• General anesthetics

ADH, Antidiuretic hormone; *CNS,* central nervous system; *GU,* genitourinary.

cause for concern. A 1-kg weight increase is equal to a 1000-mL fluid retention (1 kg = 1 L). The patient may be uncomfortable during fluid restriction. Keep mucous membranes moist by offering frequent oral rinsing (remind the patient not to swallow the rinses).

Drug therapy with tolvaptan (Samsca) or conivaptan (Vaprisol) is used to treat SIADH when hyponatremia is present in hospitalized patients. These drugs are vasopressin antagonists that promote water excretion without causing sodium loss (Belavic, 2010). Tolvaptan is an oral drug, and conivaptan is given IV. Tolvaptan has a black box warning that rapid increases in serum sodium levels (those greater than a 12 mEq/L increase in 24 hours) have been associated with central nervous system demyelination that can lead to serious complications and death.

! NURSING SAFETY PRIORITY

Drug Alert

Administer tolvaptan or conivaptan only in the hospital setting so that serum sodium levels can be monitored closely for the development of hypernatremia.

Diuretics may be used to manage SIADH when sodium levels are near normal and heart failure is present. Be aware of the diuretic effects on sodium loss. Sodium loss can be potentiated, further contributing to the problems caused by SIADH. For milder SIADH, demeclocycline (Declomycin), an oral antibiotic, may help correct the fluid imbalance, although the drug is not approved for this problem.

Hypertonic saline (i.e., 3% sodium chloride [3% NaCl]) may be used to treat SIADH when the serum sodium level is very low. Give IV saline cautiously because it may add to existing fluid overload and promote heart failure. If the patient needs routine IV fluids, a saline solution rather than a water solution is prescribed.

Monitor the patient's response to therapy to prevent the fluid overload from SIADH from becoming worse, leading to pulmonary edema and heart failure. Any patient with SIADH, regardless of age, is at risk for these complications. The older adult or one who has coexisting cardiac problems, kidney problems, pulmonary problems, or liver problems is at greater risk.

Monitor for increased fluid overload (bounding pulse, increasing neck vein distention, crackles in lungs, increasing peripheral edema, reduced urine output) at least every 2 hours. *Pulmonary edema can occur very quickly and can lead to death.* Notify the health care provider of any change that indicates the fluid overload from SIADH either is not responding to therapy or is becoming worse.

Providing a safe environment is needed when the serum sodium level falls below 120 mEq/L. Possible neurologic changes and the risk for seizures increase as a result of osmotic fluid shifts into brain tissue. Observe for and document changes in the patient's neurologic status. Assess for subtle changes, such as muscle twitching, before they progress to seizures or coma. Check orientation to time, place, and person every 2 hours because disorientation or confusion may be present. Reduce environmental noise and lighting to prevent overstimulation.

Flow sheets with continuing information about the level of consciousness, motor and sensory neurologic assessments, and laboratory data are helpful in detecting neurologic trends. The frequency of neurologic checks depends on the patient's status. For the patient with SIADH who is hyponatremic but alert, awake, and oriented, neurologic checks every 4 hours are sufficient. For the patient who has had a change in level of consciousness, perform neurologic checks at least every hour. Inspect the environment every shift, making sure that basic safety measures, such as siderails being securely in place, are observed.

? NCLEX EXAMINATION CHALLENGE

Safe and Effective Care Environment

The serum electrolyte values for a client with syndrome of inappropriate antidiuretic hormone being treated with tolvaptan (Samsca) indicate the following changes within the past 12 hours. Which change does the nurse report immediately to the health care provider?
A. Serum potassium decrease from 4.2 mEq/L to 3.8 mEq/L
B. Serum sodium increase from 122 mEq/L to 140 mEq/L
C. Serum calcium increase from 9.5 mg/dL to 10.2 mg/dL
D. Serum chloride decrease from 109 mEq/L to 99 mEq/L

DISORDERS OF THE ADRENAL GLAND

ADRENAL GLAND HYPOFUNCTION

Pathophysiology

Production of adrenocortical steroids may decrease as a result of inadequate secretion of adrenocorticotropic hormone (ACTH), dysfunction of the hypothalamic-pituitary control mechanism, or direct dysfunction of adrenal gland tissue. Manifestations may develop gradually or occur quickly with stress. In acute adrenocortical insufficiency (adrenal crisis), life-threatening manifestations may appear without warning.

Insufficiency of adrenocortical steroids causes problems through the loss of aldosterone and cortisol action. Impaired secretion of cortisol results in decreased gluconeogenesis (making glucose from proteins) along with depletion of liver and muscle glycogen, leading to hypoglycemia (low blood glucose levels). Glomerular filtration and gastric acid production decrease, leading to reduced urea nitrogen excretion, causing anorexia and weight loss.

Reduced aldosterone secretion causes potassium, sodium, and water imbalances. Potassium excretion is decreased, causing hyperkalemia. Sodium and water excretion are increased, causing hyponatremia and hypovolemia. Potassium retention also promotes reabsorption of hydrogen ions, which can lead to acidosis.

Low adrenal androgen levels decrease the body, axillary, and pubic hair, especially in women, because the adrenals produce most of the androgens in females. The severity of symptoms is related to the degree of hormone deficiency.

Acute adrenal insufficiency, or addisonian crisis, is a life-threatening event in which the need for cortisol and aldosterone is greater than the available supply. Often, it occurs in response to a stressful event (e.g., surgery, trauma, severe infection), especially when the adrenal hormone output is already reduced. The problems of acute adrenal insufficiency are the same as those of chronic insufficiency but are more severe. *Unless intervention is initiated promptly, however, sodium levels fall and potassium levels rise rapidly. Severe hypotension results from the blood volume depletion that occurs with the loss of aldosterone.* Best practices for emergency care of patients with acute adrenal insufficiency are listed in Chart 65-7.

Adrenal insufficiency (Addison's disease) is classified as primary or secondary. Causes of primary and secondary adrenal insufficiency are listed in Table 65-2. A common cause of secondary adrenal insufficiency is the sudden cessation of long-term glucocorticoid therapy. This therapy suppresses production of glucocorticoids through negative feedback by causing atrophy of the adrenal cortex. Glucocorticoid drugs must be withdrawn gradually to allow for pituitary production of ACTH and activation of adrenal cells to produce cortisol.

CHART 65-7 BEST PRACTICE FOR PATIENT SAFETY & QUALITY CARE

Emergency Care of the Patient with Acute Adrenal Insufficiency

Hormone Replacement
- Start rapid infusion of normal saline or dextrose 5% in normal saline.
- Initial dose of hydrocortisone sodium succinate (Solu-Cortef) is 100 to 300 mg or dexamethasone 4 to 12 mg as an IV bolus.
- Infuse additional 100 mg of hydrocortisone sodium succinate by continuous IV drip over the next 8 hours.
- Give hydrocortisone 50 mg IM concomitantly every 12 hours.
- Initiate an H_2 histamine blocker (e.g., ranitidine) IV for ulcer prevention.

Hyperkalemia Management
- Administer insulin (20 to 50 units) with dextrose (20 to 50 mg) in normal saline to shift potassium into cells.
- Administer potassium binding and excreting resin (e.g., Kayexalate).
- Give loop or thiazide diuretics.
- Avoid potassium-sparing diuretics, as prescribed.
- Initiate potassium restriction.
- Monitor intake and output.
- Monitor heart rate, rhythm, and ECG for manifestations of hyperkalemia (slow heart rate; heart block; tall, peaked T waves; fibrillation; asystole).

Hypoglycemia Management
- Administer IV glucose, as prescribed.
- Administer glucagon, as needed and prescribed.
- Maintain IV access.
- Monitor blood glucose level hourly.

ECG, Electrocardiogram.

TABLE 65-2 CAUSES OF PRIMARY AND SECONDARY ADRENAL INSUFFICIENCY

Primary Causes	Secondary Causes
• Idiopathic (autoimmune) disease*	• Pituitary tumors
• Tuberculosis	• Postpartum pituitary necrosis (Sheehan's syndrome)
• Metastatic cancer	• Hypophysectomy
• Fungal lesions	• High-dose pituitary radiation
• AIDS	• High-dose whole-brain radiation
• Hemorrhage	
• Gram-negative sepsis (Waterhouse-Friderichsen syndrome)	
• Adrenalectomy	
• Abdominal radiation therapy	
• Drugs (mitotane) and toxins	

AIDS, Acquired immune deficiency syndrome.
*Most common cause.

PATIENT-CENTERED COLLABORATIVE CARE

ASSESSMENT

History

When possible, take the history from the patient. If he or she is confused, ask the family about manifestations and factors that cause adrenal hypofunction. Ask about any change in activity level, because lethargy, fatigue, and muscle weakness are often present. Include questions about salt intake because salt craving often occurs with adrenal hypofunction.

GI problems, such as anorexia, nausea, vomiting, diarrhea, and abdominal pain, often occur. Ask about weight loss during the past months. Women may have menstrual changes related to weight loss, and men may report impotence.

Ask whether the patient has had radiation to the abdomen or head. Document medical problems (e.g., tuberculosis or previous brain surgery) and all past and current drugs, especially steroids, anticoagulants, opioids, or cytotoxic drugs.

Physical Assessment/Clinical Manifestations

The manifestations of adrenal insufficiency vary, and the severity is related to the degree of hormone deficiency (Chart 65-8). In patients with primary insufficiency, plasma ACTH and melanocyte-stimulating hormone (MSH) levels are in response to the adrenal-hypothalamic-pituitary feedback system. Elevated MSH levels result in areas of increased pigmentation (Fig. 65-3). In primary autoimmune disease, patchy areas of decreased pigmentation may occur because of destruction of skin melanocytes. Body hair may also be decreased. In secondary disease, skin pigmentation is not changed.

Assess for signs of hypoglycemia (e.g., sweating, headaches, tachycardia, and tremors) and fluid depletion (postural hypotension and dehydration). Hyperkalemia (elevated blood potassium levels) can cause dysrhythmias with an irregular heart rate and result in cardiac arrest.

CHART 65-8 KEY FEATURES

Adrenal Insufficiency

Neuromuscular Manifestations
- Muscle weakness
- Fatigue
- Joint/muscle pain

Gastrointestinal Manifestations
- Anorexia
- Nausea, vomiting
- Abdominal pain
- Bowel changes (constipation/diarrhea)
- Weight loss
- Salt craving

Skin Manifestations
- Vitiligo
- Hyperpigmentation

Cardiovascular Manifestations
- Anemia
- Hypotension
- Hyponatremia
- Hyperkalemia
- Hypercalcemia

Psychosocial Assessment

Depending on the degree of imbalance, patients may appear lethargic, depressed, confused, and even psychotic or fearful. Observe the patient, and check his or her orientation to person, place, and time. Families may report that the patient has a decreased energy level, experiences wide mood swings, and is forgetful.

Diagnostic Assessment

Laboratory findings include low serum cortisol, low fasting blood glucose, low sodium, elevated potassium, and increased blood urea nitrogen (BUN) levels (Chart 65-9). In primary disease, the eosinophil count and ACTH level are elevated. Plasma cortisol levels do not rise during stimulation tests.

Urinary 17-hydroxycorticosteroids are the glucocorticoid metabolites, and 17-ketosteroid levels reflect the adrenal

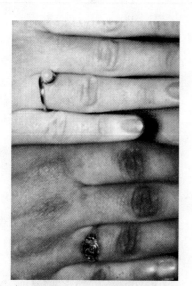

FIG. 65-3 The increased pigmentation seen in primary adrenocortical insufficiency.

androgen metabolites. Both levels are in the low or low-normal range in adrenal hypofunction.

An ACTH stimulation test is the most definitive test for adrenal insufficiency (Stewart, 2008). ACTH 0.25 to 1 mg is given IV, and plasma cortisol levels are obtained at 30-minute and 1-hour intervals. In primary insufficiency, the cortisol response is absent or very decreased. In secondary insufficiency, it is increased. When acute adrenal insufficiency is suspected, treatment is started without stimulation testing.

Imaging Assessment

Skull x-rays, CT, MRI, and arteriography may help determine the cause of pituitary problems leading to adrenal insufficiency. CT scans may show adrenal gland atrophy.

INTERVENTIONS

Nursing interventions focus on promoting fluid balance, monitoring for fluid deficit, and preventing hypoglycemia. Weigh the patient daily, and record intake and output. Assess vital signs every 1 to 4 hours, depending on the patient's condition and the presence of dysrhythmias or postural hypotension. Monitor laboratory values to identify hemoconcentration (e.g., increased hematocrit or BUN). Chapter 13 discusses fluid volume deficit in detail.

Cortisol and aldosterone deficiencies are corrected by replacement therapy. Hydrocortisone corrects glucocorticoid deficiency (Chart 65-10). Oral cortisol replacement regimens vary. The most common drug used for this purpose is prednisone. Generally, divided doses are given, with two-thirds given in the morning and one-third in the late afternoon to mimic the normal release of this hormone. Although most patients do well on this regimen, some may not tolerate the dosage or may need more.

An additional mineralocorticoid hormone, such as fludrocortisone (Florinef), may be needed to maintain electrolyte balance (especially sodium and potassium). Dosage adjustment may be needed, especially in hot weather when more sodium is lost because of excessive perspiration. *Salt*

CHART 65-9	**LABORATORY PROFILE**		
Adrenal Gland Assessment			
		SIGNIFICANCE OF ABNORMAL FINDINGS	
TEST	**NORMAL RANGE FOR ADULTS**	**HYPOFUNCTION OF THE ADRENAL GLAND**	**HYPERFUNCTION OF THE ADRENAL GLAND**
Sodium	136-145 mEq/L	Decreased	Increased
Potassium	3.5-5.0 mEq/L	Increased	Decreased
Glucose	70-115 mg/dL *Older adults:* slightly increased	Normal to decreased	Normal to increased
Calcium	9-10.5 mg/dL (total) 4.5-5.6 mg/dL (ionized) *Older adults:* slightly decreased	Increased	Decreased
Bicarbonate	23-30 mEq/L	Increased	Decreased
BUN	10-20 mg/dL *Older adults:* may be slightly higher	Increased	Normal
Cortisol	6 AM to 8 AM: 5-23 mcg/dL or 138-635 SI units (nmol/L) 4 PM to 6 PM: 3-13 mcg/dL or 83-359 SI units (nmol/L)	Decreased	Increased

BUN, Blood urea nitrogen; *SI,* International System of Units.

CHART 65-10	COMMON EXAMPLES OF DRUG THERAPY		
Hypofunction of the Adrenal Gland			
DRUG	**USUAL DOSAGE**	**NURSING INTERVENTIONS**	**RATIONALES**
Cortisone	25-50 mg orally either once daily in AM or daily in divided doses	Instruct the patient to take the drug with meals or a snack.	GI irritation can occur.
Hydrocortisone (Cortef, Hycort ✦)	20-50 mg orally either once daily in AM or daily in divided doses	Instruct the patient to report these signs or symptoms of excessive drug therapy: • Rapid weight gain • Round face • Fluid retention	Cushing's syndrome, which indicates a need for dosage adjustment, can occur.
Prednisone (Winpred ✦)	5-10 mg orally either once daily in AM or daily in divided doses	Instruct the patient to report illness, such as: • Severe diarrhea • Vomiting • Fever	Other conditions may indicate a need for dosage change. The usual daily dosage may not be adequate during periods of illness or severe stress.
Fludrocortisone (Florinef)	0.05-0.2 mg orally daily	Monitor the patient's blood pressure. Instruct the patient to report weight gain or edema.	Hypertension is a potential side effect. Sodium-related fluid retention is possible.

! NURSING SAFETY PRIORITY

Drug Alert

Prednisone and prednisolone are sound-alike drugs, and care is needed not to confuse them. Although they are both corticosteroids, they are not interchangeable because prednisolone is several times more potent than prednisone and dosages are not the same.

restriction or diuretic therapy should not be started without considering whether it might lead to an adrenal crisis.

ADRENAL GLAND HYPERFUNCTION

The adrenal gland may oversecrete just one hormone or all adrenal hormones. Hypersecretion by the adrenal cortex results in hypercortisolism (e.g., Cushing's disease or Cushing's syndrome), hyperaldosteronism (excessive mineralocorticoid production), or excessive androgen production. Hyperstimulation of the adrenal medulla caused by a tumor (pheochromocytoma) results in excessive secretion of catecholamines (epinephrine and norepinephrine).

HYPERCORTISOLISM (CUSHING'S DISEASE)

Pathophysiology

Cushing's disease is the exaggerated secretion of cortisol from the adrenal cortex, causing widespread problems. It is caused by either a problem in the adrenal cortex itself, a problem in the anterior pituitary gland, or a problem in the hypothalamus. In addition, glucocorticoid therapy can also lead to problems of hypercortisolism.

The presence of excess glucocorticoids, regardless of the cause, affects metabolism and all body systems. An increase in total body fat results from slow turnover of plasma fatty acids. This fat is redistributed, producing truncal obesity, "buffalo hump," and "moon face" (Fig. 65-4). Increases in the breakdown of tissue protein and an increase in urine nitrogen excretion also occur, resulting in decreased muscle mass and muscle strength, thin skin, and fragile capillaries. The effects on minerals lead to bone density loss.

High levels of corticosteroids kill lymphocytes and shrink organs containing lymphocytes, such as the spleen and the

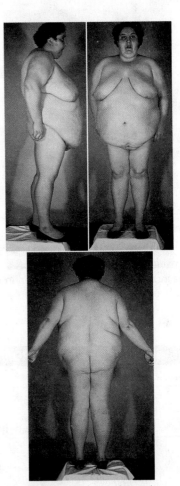

FIG. 65-4 The typical appearance of a patient with Cushing's disease or syndrome. Note truncal obesity, moon face, buffalo hump, thinner arms and legs, and abdominal striae.

lymph nodes. Eosinophils and macrophages are reduced. Although the number of neutrophils may be increased, the reduction of cytokines makes these cells less active. Thus inflammatory and immune response protections are reduced.

TABLE 65-3	CONDITIONS CAUSING INCREASED CORTISOL SECRETION
Endogenous Secretion (Cushing's Disease)	**Exogenous Administration (Cushing's Syndrome)**
• Bilateral adrenal hyperplasia*	• Therapeutic use of ACTH or glucocorticoids—most commonly for treatment of:
• Pituitary adenoma increasing the production of ACTH (pituitary Cushing's disease)	• Asthma
• Malignancies: carcinomas of the lung, GI tract, pancreas	• Autoimmune disorders
	• Organ transplantation
• Adrenal adenomas or carcinomas	• Cancer chemotherapy
	• Allergic responses
	• Chronic fibrosis

ACTH, Adrenocorticotropic hormone.
*Most common cause.

In most cases, increased androgen production also occurs and causes acne, hirsutism (increased hair growth), and occasionally clitoral hypertrophy. Increased androgen production disrupts the normal ovarian hormone feedback mechanism, decreasing the ovary's production of estrogens and progesterone. Oligomenorrhea (scant or infrequent menses) occurs as a result.

Etiology

Cushing's disease or syndrome is a group of clinical problems caused by an excess of cortisol. Table 65-3 lists causes of cortisol excess. When the anterior pituitary gland oversecretes adrenocorticotropic hormone (ACTH), this hormone causes hyperplasia of the adrenal cortex in both adrenal glands and an excess of most hormones secreted by the adrenal cortex. (See Fig. 64-3 in Chapter 64.) This problem is known as pituitary Cushing's disease because the tissue causing the problem is the pituitary. When the excess glucocorticoids are caused by a problem in the actual adrenal cortex, usually a benign tumor (adrenal adenoma), the problem is called adrenal Cushing's disease and usually occurs in only one adrenal gland. When glucocorticoid excess results from drug therapy for another health problem, it is known as Cushing's syndrome.

Incidence/Prevalence

The most common cause of Cushing's disease is a pituitary adenoma. Adrenal adenomas account for only about 15% of the disease (Stewart, 2008). Women are more likely than men to develop Cushing's disease. The actual incidence of Cushing's syndrome from chronic use of exogenous corticosteroids is not known. However, because these drugs are commonly used to control serious chronic inflammatory conditions such as asthma, other respiratory problems, and rheumatoid arthritis, Cushing's syndrome is more common than Cushing's disease and affects both genders equally.

PATIENT-CENTERED COLLABORATIVE CARE

ASSESSMENT

History

Ask about the patient's other health problems and drug therapies, because glucocorticoid therapy is a common cause of hypercortisolism. Regardless of cause, the patient has many

CHART 65-11	KEY FEATURES

Hypercortisolism (Cushing's Disease/Syndrome)

General Appearance
• Fat redistribution:
  • Moon face
  • Buffalo hump
  • Truncal obesity
• Weight gain

Cardiovascular Manifestations
• Hypertension
• Increased risk for thromboembolic events
• Frequent dependent edema
• Capillary fragility:
  • Bruising
  • Petechiae

Musculoskeletal Manifestations
• Muscle atrophy (most apparent in extremities)
• Osteoporosis (bone density loss)
  • Pathologic fractures
  • Decreased height with vertebral collapse
  • Aseptic necrosis of the femur head
  • Slow or poor healing of bone fractures

Skin Manifestations
• Thinning skin ("paper-like" appearance, especially on the back of the hands)
• Striae
• Increased pigmentation (with ectopic or pituitary production of ACTH)

Immune System Manifestations
• Increased risk for infection
• Decreased immune function:
  • Decreased circulating lymphocytes
  • Decreased production of immunoglobulins (antibodies)
• Decreased inflammatory responses:
  • Decreased eosinophil count
  • Slight increase in neutrophil count but activity is reduced
• Decreased production of pro-inflammatory cytokines, histamine, and prostaglandins
• Manifestations of infection/inflammation may be masked

ACTH, Adrenocorticotropic hormone.

changes because of the widespread effect of excessive cortisol levels. Record age, gender, and usual weight. He or she may report a significant weight gain and an increased appetite. Ask about changes in activity or sleep patterns, fatigue, and muscle weakness. Ask about bone pain or a history of fractures because osteoporosis is common in hypercortisolism. Ask about a history of frequent infections and easy bruising, which suggest hypercortisolism. Women often stop menstruating. GI problems include ulcer formation from increased hydrochloric acid secretion and decreased production of protective gastric mucus.

Physical Assessment/Clinical Manifestations

The patient with hypercortisolism has specific physical changes, although all body systems are affected (see Fig. 65-4 and Chart 65-11). Observe the patient's general appearance. Changes in fat distribution may result in fat pads on the neck, back, and shoulders ("buffalo hump"); an enlarged trunk with thin arms and legs; and a round face ("moon face"). Other changes include muscle wasting and weakness. Assess and document changes, and use these findings to prioritize patient problems and interventions.

Skin changes result from increased blood vessel fragility and include bruises, thin or translucent skin, and wounds that have not healed. Reddish purple striae ("stretch marks") occur on the abdomen, thighs, and upper arms because of the destructive effect of cortisol on collagen.

Excessive cortisol secretion causes acne and a fine coating of hair over the face and body. In women, look for the presence of hirsutism, clitoral hypertrophy, and male pattern balding related to androgen excess.

Cardiac changes occur as a result of altered water and mineral metabolism. Both sodium and water are reabsorbed and retained, leading to hypervolemia and edema formation. Blood pressure is elevated and pulses are full and bounding.

Musculoskeletal changes occur as a result of nitrogen depletion and mineral loss. Muscle mass decreases, especially in arms and legs, which look too small in proportion to the trunk (see Fig. 65-4). Muscle weakness increases the risk for falls. Bone is thinner as a result of mineral loss, and osteoporosis is common, increasing the risk for pathologic fractures.

Glucose metabolism is profoundly affected by hypercortisolism. Fasting blood glucose levels are high because the liver is stimulated to convert more glycogen to glucose and the insulin receptors are less sensitive, so blood glucose does not move as easily into the tissues. In addition, muscle mass loss reduces glucose uptake.

Immune changes caused by excess cortisol result in immunosuppression and an increased risk for infection. Excess cortisol reduces the number of circulating lymphocytes, inhibits macrophage activity, reduces antibody synthesis, and inhibits production of cytokines and inflammatory chemicals (e.g., histamine). These patients not only are at greater risk for infection but also may not have the expected inflammatory manifestations (fever, purulent exudate, redness in the affected area) when an infection is present.

Psychosocial Assessment

Hypercortisolism can result in emotional instability, and patients often say that they do not feel like themselves anymore. Ask about mood swings, irritability, confusion, or depression. Ask the patient whether he or she has been crying or laughing inappropriately or has had difficulty concentrating. Family members often report changes in the patient's mental or emotional status. The patient may have neurotic or psychotic behavior as a result of high blood cortisol levels. In addition, the hormones stimulate the central nervous system, heightening the awareness of and responses to sensory stimulation. The patient often reports sleep difficulties and fatigue.

Laboratory Assessment

Laboratory tests include blood, salivary, and urine cortisol levels. These are high in patients with hypercortisolism regardless of the origin of the disorder. Plasma ACTH levels vary, depending on the cause of the problem. In pituitary Cushing's disease, ACTH levels are elevated. In adrenal Cushing's disease or when Cushing's syndrome results from chronic steroid use, ACTH levels are very low.

Salivary cortisol levels may be used to detect hypercortisolism. This test is accurate in assessing cortisol levels because cortisol-binding proteins are not present in saliva. Usually, salivary cortisol levels are obtained at midnight (Stewart, 2008). Saliva, not spit, is needed for the assay. Saliva is easily and painlessly collected with the use of a salivary specimen cushion placed in the cheek next to the salivary gland. A normal salivary cortisol level is lower than 2.0 ng/mL. Higher levels indicate hypercortisolism.

Urine is tested to measure levels of free cortisol and the metabolites of cortisol and androgens (17-hydroxycorticosteroids and 17-ketosteroids). In Cushing's disease, levels of urine cortisol and androgens are all elevated in a 24-hour specimen, as are urine calcium, potassium, and glucose levels (Fraser & Van Uum, 2010).

Dexamethasone suppression testing can screen for hypercortisolism and may take place overnight or over a 3-day period. Set doses of dexamethasone are given. A 24-hour urine collection follows drug administration. When urinary 17-hydroxycorticosteroid excretion and cortisol levels are suppressed by dexamethasone, Cushing's disease is not present.

Additional laboratory findings that accompany hypercortisolism include:

- Increased blood glucose level
- Decreased lymphocyte count
- Increased sodium level
- Decreased serum calcium level
- Decreased serum potassium level

Imaging Assessment

Imaging for hypercortisolism includes x-rays, CT scans, MRI, and arteriography. These images can identify lesions of the adrenal or pituitary glands, lung, GI tract, or pancreas.

ANALYSIS

The priority problems for patients with Cushing's disease or Cushing's syndrome are:

1. Fluid overload
2. Risk for Injury related to skin thinning, poor wound healing, and bone density loss
3. Potential for infection
4. Potential for acute adrenal insufficiency

PLANNING AND IMPLEMENTATION

Expected outcomes of hypercortisolism management are the reduction of plasma cortisol levels, removal of tumors, and restoration of normal or acceptable body appearance. When the disorder is caused by pituitary or adrenal problems, cure is possible. When caused by drug therapy for another health problem, the focus is to prevent complications from hypercortisolism.

Restoring Fluid Volume Balance

Planning: Expected Outcomes. The patient with hypercortisolism is expected to achieve and maintain an acceptable fluid balance. Indicators include that these parameters are within or close to the normal range:

- Blood pressure
- Stable body weight
- Serum electrolytes

Interventions. Interventions for patients with fluid overload from hypercortisolism focus on ensuring patient safety, restoring fluid balance, and providing supportive care. Depending on the cause, surgical management may be used to reduce cortisol production.

Nonsurgical Management. Patient safety, drug therapy, nutrition therapy, and monitoring are the basis of nonsurgical interventions for hypercortisolism and fluid overload.

Patient safety includes preventing fluid overload from becoming worse, leading to pulmonary edema and heart failure. Any patient with fluid overload, regardless of age, is at risk for these complications. The older adult or one who has coexisting cardiac problems, kidney problems, pulmonary problems, or liver problems is at greater risk.

Monitor for indicators of increased fluid overload (bounding pulse, increasing neck vein distention, lung crackles, increasing peripheral edema, reduced urine output) at least every 2 hours. *Pulmonary edema can occur very quickly and can lead to death.* Notify the health care provider of any change that indicates fluid overload either is not responding to therapy or is becoming worse.

The patient with fluid overload and dependent edema is at risk for skin breakdown. Use a pressure-reducing or pressure-relieving overlay on the mattress. Assess skin pressure areas, especially the coccyx, elbows, hips, and heels, daily for redness or open areas. Many patients with fluid overload may be receiving oxygen by mask or nasal cannula. Check the skin around the mask, nares, and ears and under the elastic band. Assist the patient to change positions every 2 hours, or ensure that others delegated to perform this intervention are diligent in this action.

Drug therapy involves the use of drugs that interfere with adrenocorticotropic hormone (ACTH) production or adrenal hormone synthesis for temporary relief. Aminoglutethimide (Elipten, Cytadren) and metyrapone (Metopirone) use different pathways to decrease cortisol production. For patients with hypercortisolism from increased ACTH production, cyproheptadine (Periactin) may be used because it interferes with ACTH production. Mitotane (Lysodren) is an adrenal cytotoxic agent used for inoperable tumors causing hypercortisolism.

Monitor the patient for response to drug therapy, especially weight loss and increased urine output. Observe for manifestations of electrolyte imbalance, especially changes in electrocardiogram (ECG) patterns. Assess laboratory findings, especially sodium and potassium values, every 8 hours or whenever they are drawn.

Nutrition therapy for the patient with hypercortisolism may involve restrictions of both fluid and sodium intake to control fluid volume. Review the patient's serum sodium levels whenever fluid overload is present. Often sodium restriction involves only "no added salt" to ordinary table foods when fluid overload is mild. For more pronounced fluid overload, the patient may be restricted to anywhere from 2 g/day to 4 g/day of sodium. When sodium restriction is ongoing, teach the patient and family how to check food labels for sodium content and how to keep a daily record of sodium ingested. Explain to the patient and family the reason for any fluid restriction and the importance of adhering to the prescribed restriction.

Monitoring intake and output, as well as weight, provides information on therapy effectiveness. Ensure that unlicensed assistive personnel (UAP) understand that these measurements need to be accurate, not just estimated, because treatment decisions are based on these findings. In addition to regulating the total amount of fluid ingested in a 24-hour period, schedule fluid offerings throughout the 24 hours. Teach UAP to check urine for color and character and to report these findings. Check the urine specific gravity (a specific gravity below 1.005 may indicate fluid overload). If IV therapy is used, infuse the exact amount prescribed.

Fluid retention may not be visible. Remember that rapid weight gain is the best indicator of fluid retention and overload. Metabolism can account for no more than a half pound of weight gain in one day. Each pound of weight gained (after the first half pound) equates to 500 mL of retained

water. Weigh the patient at the same time every day (before breakfast), using the same scale. Whenever possible, have the patient wear the same type of clothing for each weigh-in.

Radiation therapy may be used to treat hypercortisolism caused by pituitary adenomas. However, radiation is not always effective and often destroys normal tissue. Observe for any changes in the patient's neurologic status, such as headache, elevated blood pressure or pulse, disorientation, or changes in pupil size or reaction. The patient may have skin dryness, redness, flushing, or alopecia at the radiation site. Review these possible side effects with the patient. Chapter 47 discusses radiation therapy to the head.

Surgical Management. The surgical treatment of adrenocortical hypersecretion depends on the cause of the disease. When adrenal hyperfunction is due to increased pituitary secretion of ACTH, removal of a pituitary adenoma may be attempted. In many instances, a total hypophysectomy (surgical removal of the pituitary gland) is needed. Hypophysectomy is performed via the transsphenoidal or transfrontal craniotomy route. (See earlier discussion of hypophysectomy on pp. 1376-1377; see also Chapter 47 for nursing care of patients undergoing a craniotomy.) If hypercortisolism is caused by adrenal tumors, a partial or complete adrenalectomy (removal of the adrenal gland) may be needed.

Preoperative Care. Electrolyte imbalances are corrected before surgery. Continue to monitor blood potassium, sodium, and chloride levels. Dysrhythmias from potassium imbalance may occur, and cardiac monitoring is needed. Hyperglycemia is controlled before surgery, and blood glucose levels are monitored.

The patient with hypercortisolism is at risk for complications such as infections and fractures. Prevent infection with handwashing and aseptic technique. Decrease the risk for falls by raising top siderails and encouraging the patient to ask for assistance when getting out of bed. A high-calorie, high-protein diet is prescribed before surgery.

Glucocorticoid preparations are given before surgery. The patient continues to receive glucocorticoids during surgery to prevent adrenal crisis because the removal of the tumor results in a sudden drop in cortisol levels. Before surgery, discuss the care needs for after surgery and the need for long-term drug therapy.

Operative Procedures. A unilateral adrenalectomy is performed when one gland is involved. A bilateral adrenalectomy is needed when ACTH-producing tumors cannot be treated by other means or when both adrenal glands are diseased. Surgery can be abdominal or through the lateral flank. The flank approach is preferred because the abdominal cavity is not entered and complications are reduced. A laparoscopic adrenalectomy, a minimally invasive surgical approach, is increasingly being used and reduces some complications after surgery.

Postoperative Care. After an adrenalectomy, the patient is usually sent to a critical care unit. Immediately after surgery, assess the patient every 15 minutes for shock (e.g., hypotension; a rapid, weak pulse; and a decreasing urine output) due to possible insufficient glucocorticoid replacement. Monitor ongoing vital signs and other hemodynamic variables (central venous pressure, pulmonary wedge pressure), intake and output, daily weights, and serum electrolyte levels.

After a bilateral adrenalectomy, patients require lifelong glucocorticoid and mineralocorticoid replacement, starting immediately after surgery. In unilateral adrenalectomy, hormone replacement continues until the remaining adrenal gland increases hormone production. This therapy may be needed for up to 2 years after surgery.

NCLEX EXAMINATION CHALLENGE

Health Promotion and Maintenance

Which precaution is most important for the nurse to teach a client who is prescribed oral corticosteroids for hormone replacement therapy after a unilateral adrenalectomy?
A. "Do not stop taking this drug without consulting your prescriber."
B. "Avoid crowds and people who are ill."
C. "Be sure to take this drug with food."
D. "Reduce your salt intake."

Preventing Injury

The patient who has hypercortisolism is at risk for injury from skin breakdown, bone fractures, and GI bleeding. Prevention of these injuries is a major nursing care focus.

Planning: Expected Outcomes. The patient with hypercortisolism is expected to avoid injury. Indicators include:

- Skin is intact.
- Minimal or no bruising is present.
- Bones are intact.
- Stools, vomitus, and other GI secretions contain no gross or occult blood.

Interventions. Priority nursing interventions for prevention of injury focus on skin assessment and protection, coordinating care to ensure gentle handling, and patient teaching regarding drug therapy for prevention of GI ulcers.

Skin injury is a continuing risk for any patient who has hypercortisolism. Even when surgery has corrected the cortisol excess, the changes induced in the skin and blood vessels remain for weeks to months. Assess the skin for reddened areas, excoriation, breakdown, and edema. If mobility is decreased, turn the patient every 2 hours and pad bony prominences.

Instruct the patient to avoid activities that can result in skin trauma. To reduce tissue injury, teach him or her to use a soft toothbrush and an electric shaver. Instruct patients to keep the skin clean and to dry it thoroughly after washing. Excessive dryness can be prevented by using a moisturizing lotion.

Adhesive tape often causes skin breakdown. Use tape sparingly, and use caution when removing it. After venipuncture or arterial puncture, the patient may have increased bleeding because of blood vessel fragility. Exert pressure over the site for longer than normal to prevent bleeding and bruising.

Pathologic fractures from bone density loss and osteoporosis are possible for months to years after cortisol levels return to normal. Teach the patient about safety issues and dietary needs. When helping the patient move in bed, use a lift sheet instead of grasping him or her. Remind the patient to call for help when ambulating. Review the use of walkers or canes, if needed. Keep rooms free of objects that might cause a fall. Teach UAP to use a gait belt when walking with a patient who has bone density loss.

Coordinate with a dietitian to teach the patient about nutrition therapy. A high-calorie diet is prescribed that includes items from all of the major food groups and increased amounts of calcium and vitamin D. Generous amounts of milk, cheese, yogurt, and green leafy and root vegetables add calcium to promote bone density. Advise the patient to avoid caffeine and alcohol, which increase the risk for GI ulcers and may promote bone density loss.

GI bleeding is common with hypercortisolism as a result of systemic changes. Cortisol inhibits production of the thick, gel-like mucus that protects the stomach lining, decreases blood flow to the area, and triggers the release of excess hydrochloric acid. Although surgery reduces the hypercortisolism, the normal protective mucus and increased blood flow may take days to weeks to return. Interventions focus on reducing gastric irritation, usually through drug therapy to protect the GI mucosa and decrease the secretion of hydrochloric acid.

Antacids buffer stomach acids and protect the GI mucosa. Teach the patient that these drugs should be taken on a regular schedule rather than on an as-needed basis.

Some agents block the H_2 receptors in the gastric mucosa. When histamine binds to these receptors, a series of actions release hydrochloric acid. Drugs that block the H_2-receptor site include cimetidine (Tagamet, Peptol ✦, Novo-Cimetine ✦), ranitidine (Zantac, Apo-Ranitidine ✦), famotidine (Pepcid), and nizatidine (Axid). Omeprazole (Losec ✦, Prilosec) and esomeprazole (Nexium) inhibit the gastric proton pump and prevent the formation of hydrochloric acid.

Encourage the patient to reduce or eliminate habits that contribute to gastric irritation, such as consuming alcohol or caffeine, smoking, and fasting. Discuss other prescribed and over-the-counter drugs that he or she may be taking. NSAIDs and drugs that contain aspirin or other salicylates can cause gastritis and intensify GI bleeding.

Preventing Infection

Glucocorticoids reduce both inflammation and the immune responses, increasing the risk for infection. For the patient who is taking glucocorticoid replacement therapy, the risk is ongoing. For the patient who is recovering from surgery to prevent hypercortisolism, the infection risk continues for weeks after surgery.

Planning: Expected Outcomes. The patient with hypercortisolism is expected to remain free from infection and avoid situations that increase the risk for infection. Indicators include these manifestations and behaviors:

- Absence of fever and foul-smelling or purulent drainage
- Absence of cough, chest pain, and dyspnea
- Absence of urinary frequency, urgency, or pain and burning
- Avoids crowds and large gatherings
- Obtains appropriate vaccinations
- Washes hands frequently

Interventions. A major focus in caring for the patient with hypercortisolism is protection from infection. All personnel must use extreme care during all nursing procedures. Thorough handwashing is of the utmost importance. Anyone with an upper respiratory tract infection who must enter the patient's room must wear a mask. Observe strict procedures when performing dressing changes or any invasive procedure.

Continually assess the patient for possible infection. Manifestations may not be obvious because hypercortisolism suppresses manifestations of infection. Fever and the formation of pus (indicators of infection) depend on the presence of white blood cells (WBCs). The immunosuppressed patient may have a severe infection without pus and with only a low-grade fever.

Monitor the patient's daily complete blood count (CBC) with differential WBC count and absolute neutrophil count (ANC). Inspect the mouth during every shift for lesions and mucosa breakdown. Assess the lungs every 8 hours for crackles, wheezes, or reduced breath sounds. Assess all urine for odor and cloudiness. Ask about any urgency, burning, or pain on urination.

Take vital signs at least every 4 hours to assess for fever. A temperature elevation of even 1° F (or 0.5° C) above baseline is significant for a patient who is immunosuppressed and indicates infection until it has been proved otherwise.

Skin care is important for preventing infection because the skin may be the patient's only intact defense. Teach him or her about hygiene, and urge daily bathing. If the patient is immobile, turn him or her every hour and apply skin lubricants.

Perform pulmonary hygiene every 2 to 4 hours. Listen to the lungs for crackles, wheezes, or reduced breath sounds. Urge the patient to cough and deep breathe or to perform sustained maximum inhalations every hour while awake.

Preventing Acute Adrenal Insufficiency

The patient most at risk for acute adrenal insufficiency is the one who has Cushing's syndrome as a result of glucocorticoid drug therapy. The exogenous drug inhibits the feedback control pathway (see Fig. 64-3 in Chapter 64), preventing the hypothalamus from secreting corticotropin-releasing hormone (CRH). The lack of CRH inhibits secretion of ACTH from the anterior pituitary gland. Without normal levels of ACTH, the adrenal glands atrophy and completely stop production of any of the corticosteroids. As a result, the patient completely depends on the exogenous drug. If the drug is stopped, even for a day or two, the atrophied adrenal glands cannot produce the glucocorticoids and the patient develops acute adrenal insufficiency, a life-threatening condition. Management of this problem is described on p. 1382.

Community-Based Care
Home Care Management

The patient with hypercortisolism usually has muscle weakness and fatigue for some weeks after surgery and remains at risk for falls and other injury. These problems may necessitate one-floor living for a short time, and a home health aide may be needed to assist with hygiene, meal preparation, and maintenance.

Teaching for Self-Management

The patient taking exogenous glucocorticoids who is discharged to home remains at continuing risk for fluid volume excess. Teach him or her and the family to monitor the patient's weight at home. Verify that the patient understands the relationship between body weight and fluid balance. Suggest that a record of these daily weights be kept to show the health care provider at any checkups. Also, instruct the patient to call the health care provider if he or she gains more than 3 lbs in a week or more than 1 to 2 lbs in a 24-hour period.

Lifelong hormone replacement is needed after bilateral adrenalectomy. Teach the patient and family about adherence to the drug regimen and its side effects (Chart 65-12).

Protecting the patient from infection at home is just as important as it was during hospitalization. Urge him or her to use proper hygiene and to avoid crowds or others with infections. Encourage the patient and all people living in the same home with him or her to have yearly influenza vaccinations. Stress that the patient should immediately notify the

---

⍰ DECISION-MAKING CHALLENGE

Patient-Centered Care; Evidence-Based Practice

The patient is a 45-year-old woman who has recently been diagnosed with a chronic lung inflammation with pulmonary fibrosis. She has been prescribed 45 mg of prednisone daily to slow the progression of this disease and has been adherent to this therapy for the past 12 weeks. She now has a moon face, buffalo hump, acne, thinning scalp hair, and muscle weakness. Today, her blood pressure is elevated and she is being started on an antihypertensive drug, along with an H₂ histamine blocker. Since her last visit, she has gained 18 lbs. She tells you that she feels as though she has aged 20 years in 2 months, and that her appearance changes are "devastating." She is concerned about now having to take two more drugs on a daily basis. She also reveals to you that she did not take her prednisone for 3 days last week hoping that she would lose weight.

1. In what ways does prednisone induce the changes she shows and has described?
2. How should you address the issue of her not taking the prednisone as prescribed?
3. Is her weight gain irreversible while she is taking prednisone? Why or why not?
4. What should you tell her about the newly prescribed drugs?
5. What resources can you suggest to improve her appearance?

CHART 65-12 PATIENT AND FAMILY EDUCATION: PREPARING FOR SELF-MANAGEMENT

Cortisol Replacement Therapy

- Take your medication in divided doses—the first dose in the morning and the second dose between 4 and 6 PM.
- Take your medication with meals or snacks.
- Weigh yourself daily.
- Increase your dosage as directed for increased physical stress or severe emotional stress, including surgery, dental work, influenza, fever, pregnancy, and family problems.
- Never skip a dose of medication. If you have persistent vomiting or severe diarrhea and cannot take your medication by mouth for 24 to 36 hours, call your physician. If you cannot reach your physician, go to the nearest emergency department. You may need an injection to take the place of your usual oral medication.
- Always wear your medical alert bracelet or necklace.
- Make regular visits for health care follow-up.
- Learn how to give yourself an intramuscular injection of hydrocortisone.

health care provider if he or she has a fever or any other sign of infection. Chart 42-11 in Chapter 42 lists guidelines for patients for infection prevention.

Health Care Resources

Immediately after returning home, the patient may need a support person to stay and provide more attention than could be given by a visiting nurse or home care aide. Contact with the health care team is needed for follow-up and identification of potential problems. The patient taking corticosteroid therapy may have manifestations of adrenal insufficiency if the dosage is inadequate. Suggest that the patient obtain and wear a medical alert bracelet listing the condition and the drug replacement therapy.

EVALUATION: OUTCOMES

Evaluate the care of the patient with hypercortisolism based on the identified priority patient problems. The expected outcomes are that the patient should:

- Have an acceptable fluid balance
- Remain free from injury
- Remain free from infection
- Not experience acute adrenal insufficiency

Specific indicators for these outcomes are listed for each priority patient problem under the Planning and Implementation section (see earlier).

HYPERALDOSTERONISM

Pathophysiology

Hyperaldosteronism is an increased secretion of aldosterone with mineralocorticoid excess. Primary hyperaldosteronism (Conn's syndrome) results from excessive secretion of aldosterone from one or both adrenal glands, usually caused by a benign adrenal adenoma. In secondary hyperaldosteronism, excessive secretion of aldosterone is caused by high levels of angiotensin II that are stimulated by high plasma renin levels. Causes of high renin levels include kidney hypoxemia and the use of thiazide diuretics.

Increased aldosterone levels affect the kidney tubules and cause sodium retention with potassium and hydrogen ion excretion. Hypernatremia, hypokalemia, and metabolic alkalosis result. Sodium retention increases blood volume, which raises blood pressure but usually does not cause peripheral edema. The elevated blood pressure may cause strokes, heart attacks, and kidney damage. (See Chapter 13 for discussion of electrolyte imbalances.)

PATIENT-CENTERED COLLABORATIVE CARE

ASSESSMENT

Hypokalemia and elevated blood pressure are the most common problems of the patient with hyperaldosteronism. He or she may have headache, fatigue, muscle weakness, nocturia (excessive urination at night), and loss of stamina. Polydipsia (excessive fluid intake) and polyuria (excessive urine output) occur less frequently. Paresthesias (sensations of numbness and tingling) may occur if potassium depletion is severe (Crawford, & Harris, 2011).

Hyperaldosteronism is diagnosed on the basis of laboratory studies, x-rays, and imaging with CT or MRI. Serum

potassium levels are decreased, and sodium levels are elevated. Plasma renin levels are low, and aldosterone levels are high. Hydrogen ion loss leads to metabolic alkalemia (elevated blood pH). Urine has a low specific gravity and high aldosterone levels.

INTERVENTIONS

Surgery is the most common treatment for early-stage hyperaldosteronism. One or both adrenal glands may be removed. Surgery is not performed, however, until the patient's potassium levels are normal. Drugs used to increase potassium levels include spironolactone (Aldactone, Spirono, Sincomen ✦), a potassium-sparing diuretic and aldosterone antagonist. Potassium supplements may be prescribed to increase potassium levels before surgery. The patient may also benefit from a low-sodium diet before surgery, but sodium restriction is not needed after surgery because aldosterone levels return to normal.

The patient who has undergone a unilateral adrenalectomy may need temporary glucocorticoid replacement. Replacement is lifelong if both adrenal glands are removed. Glucocorticoids are given before surgery to prevent adrenal crisis. The patient receiving long-term replacement therapy should wear a medical alert bracelet. (See the discussion of adrenalectomy on pp. 1387-1389 in the Hypercortisolism [Cushing's Disease] section for more discussion of care after surgery and patient education.)

When surgery cannot be performed, spironolactone therapy is continued to control hypokalemia and hypertension. Because spironolactone is a potassium-sparing diuretic, hyperkalemia can occur in patients who have impaired kidney function or excessive potassium intake. Advise the patient to avoid potassium supplements and foods rich in potassium. Hyponatremia can occur with spironolactone therapy, and the patient may need increased dietary sodium. Instruct the patient to report symptoms of hyponatremia, such as dryness of the mouth, thirst, lethargy, or drowsiness. Teach patients to report any additional side effects of spironolactone therapy, including gynecomastia, diarrhea, drowsiness, headache, rash, urticaria (hives), confusion, erectile dysfunction, hirsutism, and amenorrhea.

PHEOCHROMOCYTOMA

Pathophysiology

Pheochromocytoma is a catecholamine-producing tumor that arises in the adrenal medulla. These tumors usually occur as a single lesion in one adrenal gland, although they can be bilateral or in the abdomen. Pheochromocytomas are usually benign, but at least 10% are malignant (Young, 2008).

The tumors produce, store, and release epinephrine and norepinephrine (NE). Excessive epinephrine and NE stimulate adrenergic receptors and can have wide-ranging adverse effects mimicking the action of the sympathetic division of the autonomic nervous system.

The cause is unknown, but some pheochromocytomas occur with inherited disorders such as neurofibromatosis (type 1), multiple endocrine neoplasia (MEN-2), Von Hippel-Lindau disease, and pheochromocytoma-paraganglioma syndrome (Cook, 2009). These tumors are rare and occur slightly more often in women. They can occur at any age but appear most commonly in patients between 40 and 60 years of age.

PATIENT-CENTERED COLLABORATIVE CARE

ASSESSMENT

The patient often has intermittent episodes of hypertension or attacks that range from a few minutes to several hours. During these episodes, the patient has severe headaches, palpitations, profuse diaphoresis, flushing, apprehension, or a sense of impending doom. Pain in the chest or abdomen, with nausea and vomiting, can also occur. Increased abdominal pressure, defecation, and vigorous abdominal palpation can provoke a hypertensive crisis. Drugs such as tricyclic antidepressants, droperidol, glucagon, metoclopramide, phenothiazines, and naloxone can induce a hypertensive crisis in the patient with pheochromocytoma. Foods or beverages high in tyramine (e.g., aged cheese, red wine) also induce hypertension. The patient may also report heat intolerance, weight loss, and tremors.

The most common diagnostic test is a 24-hour urine collection for vanillylmandelic acid (VMA) (a product of catecholamine metabolism), metanephrine, and catecholamines, all of which are elevated in the presence of a pheochromocytoma. Other tests that may be conducted when catecholamine levels are not consistent include the clonidine suppression test and, rarely, stimulation testing. MRI or CT scans can precisely locate tumors in the adrenal gland. After diagnosis, CT scans of the chest and abdomen may be used to locate any other tumors.

INTERVENTIONS

Surgery is the main treatment for a pheochromocytoma. One or both adrenal glands are removed (depending on whether the tumor is bilateral). After surgery, nursing interventions focus on promoting adequate tissue perfusion, nutritional needs, and comfort measures.

Hypertension is the hallmark of the disease and the most common serious complication after surgery (Daub, 2008). Monitor the blood pressure regularly, and place the cuff consistently on the same arm, with the patient in lying and standing positions. Identify stressors that may lead to a hypertensive crisis, and attempt to reduce them. Teach the patient to not smoke, drink caffeine-containing beverages, or change position suddenly. Provide a diet rich in calories, vitamins, and minerals.

! NURSING SAFETY PRIORITY

Action Alert

> Do not palpate the abdomen of a patient with a pheochromocytoma, because this action could stimulate a sudden release of catecholamines and trigger severe hypertension.

The patient often benefits from hydration before surgery because decreased blood volume increases the risk for hypotension during and after surgery. Assess the patient's hydration status, and report manifestations of dehydration or fluid overload.

Provide a calm, restful environment for the patient who has a severe headache. Instruct the patient to limit activity. A private, darkened room helps promote rest. If the patient is sleeping, avoid interruptions if possible.

The patient's blood pressure is stabilized with adrenergic blocking agents such as phenoxybenzamine (Dibenzyline) starting several weeks before surgery because of the increased risk for severe hypertension during surgery (Tsegay et al., 2008). The drug dosages are adjusted for 2 to 3 weeks before surgery until blood pressure is controlled and hypertensive attacks do not occur. The blood volume expands, and blood pressure in the supine position returns to normal.

Anesthetic agents and touching of the tumor during surgery can cause a catecholamine release. Short-acting alpha-adrenergic blockers are given by IV bolus or continuous infusion for a hypertensive crisis.

Nursing care after surgery is similar to that for the patient who has undergone an adrenalectomy (see Hypercortisolism [Cushing's Disease], pp. 1387-1389). Closely monitor the patient for hypertension and for hypotension (from the sudden decrease in catecholamine levels) and for hypovolemia. Hemorrhage and shock are possible, and plasma expanders or fluids may be needed. Monitor vital signs, as well as fluid intake and output. If opioids are given, check for their effect on blood pressure.

Tumors may be inoperable because of the patient's other medical conditions. Management then is medical, with alpha-adrenergic and beta-adrenergic blocking agents, because the tumors do not respond well to chemotherapy or radiation therapy. For these patients, self-measurement of blood pressure with home monitoring equipment is essential. (See Chapter 38 for teaching priorities and community-based care of the patient with chronic hypertension.)

GET READY FOR THE NCLEX® EXAMINATION!

KEY POINTS

Review these Key Points for each NCLEX Examination Client Needs Category.

Safe and Effective Care Environment

- Handle all patients with bone density loss carefully, using lift sheets whenever possible.
- Use good handwashing techniques before providing any care to a patient who is immunosuppressed.

Health Promotion and Maintenance

- Instruct the patient with adrenal insufficiency to wear a medical alert bracelet and to carry simple carbohydrates with them at all times.
- Teach the patient and family about the clinical manifestations of infection and when to seek medical advice.

GET READY FOR THE NCLEX® EXAMINATION!—cont'd

- Teach patients who have permanent endocrine hypofunction the proper techniques and timing of hormone replacement therapy.
- Teach patients with diabetes insipidus the proper way to self-administer desmopressin orally or by nasal spray.

Psychosocial Integrity

- Encourage the patient and family to express concerns about a change in health status.
- Explain all treatment procedures, restrictions, and follow-up care to the patient.
- Allow patients who experience a change in physical appearance to mourn this change.

Physiological Integrity

- Ensure that hormone replacement drugs are given as close to the prescribed times as possible.

- Use Infection Precautions for patients who are immunosuppressed.
- During the immediate period after a transsphenoidal or an endoscopic nasal hypophysectomy, teach the patient to avoid activities that increase intracranial pressure (e.g., bending at the waist, straining to have a bowel movement, coughing).
- Measure intake and output accurately on patients who have either diabetes insipidus or syndrome of inappropriate antidiuretic hormone (SIADH).
- Teach the patient with diabetes insipidus the manifestations of dehydration.
- Do not palpate the abdomen of a patient who has a pheochromocytoma.

Care of Patients with Problems of the Thyroid and Parathyroid Glands

M. Linda Workman

LEARNING OUTCOMES

Safe and Effective Care Environment

1. Adjust the environment for the patient with severe hypothyroidism or thyrotoxicosis.
2. Ensure the availability of suction and emergency intubation equipment for anyone who has thyroid or parathyroid surgery.
3. Prevent injury in the patient who has bone density loss or hypocalcemia.

Health Promotion and Maintenance

4. Teach patients taking thyroid hormone inhibitors the correct timing of therapy, side effects, adverse effects, and when to seek medical assistance.

Psychosocial Integrity

5. Be accepting of patient behavior and changes in appearance.

6. Inform patients and family members that changes in cognition and behavior resulting from thyroid problems are usually temporary.

Physiological Integrity

7. Compare the clinical manifestations of hyperthyroidism with those of hypothyroidism.
8. Interpret clinical changes and laboratory data to determine the effectiveness of interventions for thyroid problems.
9. Coordinate nursing care for the patient during the first 24 hours after thyroid or parathyroid surgery.
10. Identify teaching priorities for the patient taking thyroid hormone replacement therapy.
11. Compare the clinical manifestations of hyperparathyroidism with those of hypoparathyroidism.

The thyroid and parathyroid glands secrete hormones that affect overall metabolism, electrolyte balance, and excitable membrane activity. Thus problems of either gland usually have widespread effects and manifestations. Mild disturbances produce subtle problems. More severe disturbances may produce life-threatening problems.

THYROID DISORDERS

HYPERTHYROIDISM

Pathophysiology

Hyperthyroidism is excessive thyroid hormone secretion from the thyroid gland. The manifestations of hyper-

thyroidism are called thyrotoxicosis, regardless of the origin of the thyroid hormones (Davies & Larsen, 2008). (For example, a person who takes a large amount of synthetic thyroid hormones can have thyrotoxicosis but does not have hyperthyroidism.) Thyroid hormones increase metabolism in all body organs, and excesses produce many different manifestations. Hyperthyroidism can be temporary or permanent, depending on the cause.

In hyperthyroidism the excessive thyroid hormones stimulate most body systems, causing hypermetabolism and increased sympathetic nervous system activity. Many of the manifestations are caused by the body's response to the demands of hypermetabolism (Chart 66-1).

Thyroid hormones stimulate the heart, increasing both heart rate and stroke volume. These responses increase

CHART 66-1 KEY FEATURES

Hyperthyroidism

Skin Manifestations
- Diaphoresis (excessive sweating)
- Fine, soft, silky body hair
- Smooth, warm, moist skin
- Thinning of scalp hair

Pulmonary Manifestations
- Shortness of breath with or without exertion
- Rapid, shallow respirations
- Decreased vital capacity

Cardiovascular Manifestations
- Palpitations
- Chest pain
- Increased systolic blood pressure
- Widened pulse pressure
- Tachycardia
- Dysrhythmias

Gastrointestinal Manifestations
- Weight loss
- Increased appetite
- Increased stools
- Hypoproteinemia

Musculoskeletal Manifestations
- Muscle weakness
- Muscle wasting

Neurologic Manifestations
- Blurred or double vision
- Eye fatigue
- Corneal ulcers or infections
- Increased tears
- Injected (red) conjunctiva
- Photophobia
- Eyelid retraction, eyelid lag*
- Globe lag*
- Hyperactive deep tendon reflexes
- Tremors
- Insomnia

Metabolic Manifestations
- Increased basal metabolic rate
- Heat intolerance
- Low-grade fever
- Fatigue

Psychological/Emotional Manifestations
- Decreased attention span
- Restlessness
- Irritability
- Emotional lability
- Manic behavior

Reproductive Manifestations
- Amenorrhea
- Decreased menstrual flow
- Increased libido

Other Manifestations
- Goiter
- Wide-eyed or startled appearance (exophthalmos)*
- Decreased total white blood cell count
- Enlarged spleen

*Present in Graves' disease only.

cardiac output, systolic blood pressure, and blood flow (Burton, 2011).

Elevated thyroid hormone levels affect protein, lipid, and carbohydrate metabolism. Protein synthesis (buildup) and degradation (breakdown) are increased, but breakdown exceeds buildup, causing a net loss of body protein known as a negative nitrogen balance. Glucose tolerance is decreased, and the patient has hyperglycemia (elevated blood glucose levels). Fat metabolism is increased, and body fat decreases. Although the patient has an increased appetite, the increased metabolism causes weight loss and nutritional deficiency.

Thyroid hormones are produced in response to the stimulation hormones secreted by the hypothalamus and anterior pituitary glands. Thus oversecretion of thyroid hormones changes the secretion of hormones from the hypothalamus and anterior pituitary gland through negative feedback (see Chapter 64). Thyroid hormones also have some influence over sex hormone production in both men and women. Women have menstrual problems and decreased fertility.

Both men and women with hyperthyroidism have an increased libido (sexual urge or interest).

Etiology and Genetic Risk

Hyperthyroidism has many causes, the most common of which is Graves' disease, also called *toxic diffuse goiter*. Graves' disease is an autoimmune disorder in which antibodies (thyroid-stimulating immunoglobulins [TSIs]) are made and attach to the thyroid-stimulating hormone (TSH) receptors on the thyroid tissue. The thyroid gland responds by increasing the number and size of glandular cells, which enlarges the gland, forming a goiter, and overproduces thyroid hormones (thyrotoxicosis). Other manifestations specific to Graves' disease include exophthalmos (abnormal protrusion of the eyes) and pretibial myxedema (dry, waxy swelling of the front surfaces of the lower legs). *Not all patients with a goiter have hyperthyroidism.*

Hyperthyroidism caused by multiple thyroid nodules is termed toxic multinodular goiter. The nodules may be enlarged thyroid tissues or benign tumors (adenomas). These patients usually have had a goiter for years. The overproduction of thyroid hormones is milder than that seen in Graves' disease, and the patient does not have exophthalmos or pretibial edema.

Hyperthyroidism also can be caused by excessive use of thyroid replacement hormones. This type of problem is called exogenous hyperthyroidism.

GENETIC/GENOMIC CONSIDERATIONS

Graves' disease has a strong association with other autoimmune disorders, such as diabetes mellitus, vitiligo, and rheumatoid arthritis. It often occurs in both members of identical twins, with an inheritance pattern of familial clustering or complex, which suggests a polygenic gene-environmental interaction (Nussbaum et al., 2007).

Incidence/Prevalence

Hyperthyroidism is a common endocrine disorder. Graves' disease can occur at any age but is diagnosed most often in women between 20 and 40 years of age, affecting women about ten times more often than men (Davies & Larsen, 2008). Toxic multinodular goiter usually occurs after the age of 50 and affects women four times more often than men (McCance et al, 2010).

PATIENT-CENTERED COLLABORATIVE CARE

ASSESSMENT

History

The patient may have noticed many changes and problems because hyperthyroidism affects all body systems, although changes may occur over such a long period that not all patients are aware of them. Record age, gender, and usual weight. The patient may report a recent unplanned weight loss, an increased appetite, and an increase in the number of bowel movements per day.

A hallmark of hyperthyroidism is heat intolerance. The patient may have diaphoresis (increased sweating) even when environmental temperatures are comfortable for others. He or she often wears lighter clothing in cold weather. The patient

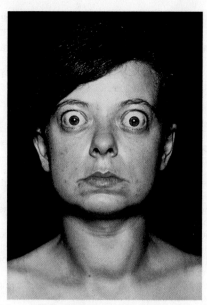

FIG. 66-1 Exophthalmos.

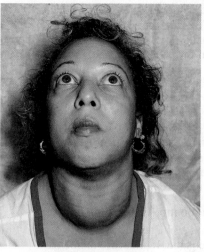

FIG. 66-2 Goiter.

TABLE 66-1	GOITER CLASSIFICATION
GOITER GRADE	DESCRIPTION
0	No palpable or visible goiter.
1	Mass is not visible with neck in the normal position. Goiter can be palpated and moves up when the patient swallows.
2	Mass is visible as swelling when the neck is in the normal position. Goiter is easily palpated and is usually asymmetric.

may also report palpitations or chest pain as a result of the cardiovascular effects. Ask about changes in breathing patterns, because dyspnea (with or without exertion) is common.

Visual changes may be the earliest problem the patient notices, especially exophthalmos with Graves' disease (Fig. 66-1). Ask about changes in vision, such as blurring or double vision and tiring of the eyes.

Ask whether he or she has noticed a change in energy level or in the ability to perform ADLs. Fatigue, weakness, and insomnia are common. Family and friends may report that the patient has become irritable or depressed.

Ask women about changes in menses, because amenorrhea or a decreased menstrual flow is common. Initially, both men and women may have an increase in libido, but this changes as the patient becomes more fatigued.

Explore the patient's medical history. Information about previous thyroid surgery or radiation therapy to the neck is important to obtain because some people remain hyperthyroid after surgery or are resistant to radiation therapy. Ask about past and current drugs, especially the use of thyroid hormone replacement or antithyroid drugs.

Physical Assessment/Clinical Manifestations

Exophthalmos is common in patients with Graves' disease. The wide-eyed or "startled" look is due to edema in the extraocular muscles and increased fatty tissue behind the eye, which pushes the eyeball forward. Pressure on the optic nerve may impair vision. Swelling and shortening of the muscles may cause problems with focusing. If the eyelid fails to close completely and the eye is unprotected, the eye may become overly dry and develop corneal ulcers or infection. Observe the patient's eyes for excessive tearing and a bloodshot appearance, and ask about sensitivity to light (photophobia).

Observe the patient's general appearance. In addition to the exophthalmos of Graves' disease, two other eye problems are common in all types of hyperthyroidism: eyelid retraction (eyelid lag) and globe (eyeball) lag. In eyelid lag, the upper eyelid fails to descend when the patient gazes slowly downward. In globe lag, the upper eyelid pulls back faster than the eyeball when the patient gazes upward. During assessment, ask the patient to look down and then up, and document the response.

Observe the size and symmetry of the thyroid gland. Palpate the thyroid gland to assess the presence of a mass or general enlargement. In goiter, a generalized thyroid enlargement, the thyroid gland may increase to four times its normal size (Fig. 66-2). Goiters are common in Graves's disease and are classified by size (Table 66-1). Bruits (turbulence from increased blood flow) may be heard in the neck with a stethoscope. (See Chapter 64 for thyroid palpation and auscultation.)

The cardiovascular problems of hyperthyroidism include increased systolic blood pressure, tachycardia, and dysrhythmias. Usually the diastolic pressure is decreased, causing a widened pulse pressure.

Inspect the hair and skin. Fine, soft, silky hair and smooth, warm, moist skin are common. Muscle weakness and hyperactive deep tendon reflexes are common. Observe motor movements of the hands for tremors. The patient may appear restless, irritable, and fatigued.

Psychosocial Assessment

The patient with hyperthyroidism often has wide mood swings, irritability, decreased attention span, and manic behavior. Hyperactivity often leads to fatigue because of the inability to sleep well. Some patients describe their activity as having two modes—either "full speed ahead" or "completely stopped." Ask whether he or she cries or laughs without cause or has difficulty concentrating. Family members often report a change in the patient's mental or emotional status.

Laboratory Assessment

Testing for hyperthyroidism involves measurement of blood values for triiodothyronine (T_3), thyroxine (T_4), T_3 resin uptake (T_3RU), and thyroid-stimulating hormone (TSH). Antibodies to TSH (TSH-RAb) are measured to diagnose Graves' disease. The most common changes in laboratory tests for Graves' disease and other forms of hyperthyroidism are listed in Chart 66-2.

Other Diagnostic Assessment

Thyroid scan evaluates the position, size, and functioning of the thyroid gland. Radioactive iodine (RAI [^{123}I]) is given by mouth, and the uptake of iodine by the thyroid gland (radioactive iodine uptake [RAIU]) is measured. The half-life of ^{123}I is short, and radiation precautions are not needed. Pregnancy should be ruled out before the scan is performed. The normal thyroid gland has an uptake of 5% to 35% of the given dose at 24 hours. RAIU is increased in hyperthyroidism.

Assess whether the patient has undergone procedures or has taken drugs that might affect the results of the scan. Procedures that use iodine-containing dye (e.g., renography) should not be performed for at least 4 weeks before a thyroid scan is done. Any drug that contains iodine should be discontinued for 1 week before the scan.

Ultrasonography of the thyroid gland can determine its size and the general composition of any masses or nodules. This procedure takes about 30 minutes to perform and is painless.

Electrocardiography (ECG) usually shows tachycardia. Other ECG changes with hyperthyroidism include atrial fibrillation, dysrhythmias, and changes in P and T waveforms.

? NCLEX EXAMINATION CHALLENGE

Physiological Integrity

Why is a goiter often present in clients who have Graves' disease?
A. The low circulating levels of thyroid hormones stimulate the feedback system and trigger the anterior pituitary gland to secrete more thyroid-stimulating hormone, which increases the numbers and size of glandular cells in the thyroid gland.
B. The autoantibodies stimulate the inflammatory and immune responses to increase the number of white blood cells circulating in the thyroid gland, which increases tissue size without increasing the number of glandular cells.
C. The excessive autoantibodies bind to the thyroid hormone receptor sites, which increases the number and size of glandular cells in the thyroid gland.
D. The autoantibodies stimulate blood vessel growth and blood storage within the thyroid gland, increasing its overall size.

▌ INTERVENTIONS

Because Graves' disease is the most common form of hyperthyroidism, the interventions discussed in the following sections include those specific for the problems that occur with Graves' disease. The purposes of medical management are to decrease the effect of thyroid hormone on cardiac function

---

CHART 66-2   LABORATORY PROFILE

Thyroid Function

TEST	NORMAL RANGE FOR ADULTS	SIGNIFICANCE OF ABNORMAL FINDINGS	
		HYPERTHYROIDISM	HYPOTHYROIDISM
Serum T_3	70-205 ng/dL, or 1.2-3.4 SI units	Increased	Decreased
Serum T_4	4-12 mcg/dL, or 51-154 SI units	Increased	Decreased
Free T_4 index	0.8-2.4 ng/dL, or 10-31 SI units	Increased	Decreased
T_3 resin uptake	24%-34% (varies with different laboratories)	Increased	Decreased
TRH stimulation test	Doubling of baseline TSH 30 min after IV injection of 500 mcg TRH (women have greater response)	Little or no TSH response	Delayed or poor TSH response in secondary hypothyroidism (pituitary failure) Elevated two or more times the normal in primary hypothyroidism (thyroid gland failure)
Thyroid suppression test	N/A	Fails to suppress RAIU or T_4 levels	No change in RAIU or T_4 levels
TSH stimulation test (thyroid stimulation test)	>10% in RAIU or >1.5 mcg/dL	N/A (test differentiates primary from secondary hypothyroidism)	No response in primary hypothyroidism Normal response in secondary hypothyroidism
Thyroid antibodies (antithyroglobulin antibody)	Titer <1:100	High titer of antithyroglobulin antibodies	Increased titers
Thyrotropin receptor antibodies (TSH-RAb)	Titer <130% of basal activity	High titers indicate Graves' disease	No response
TSH	0.3-5.0 μU/mL or 0.3-5.0 SI units.	Low in Graves' disease High in secondary or tertiary hyperthyroidism	High in primary disease Low in secondary or tertiary disease

N/A, Not applicable; *RAIU*, radioactive iodine uptake; *SI*, International System of Units; *T_3*, triiodothyronine; *T_4*, thyroxine; *TRH*, thyrotropin-releasing hormone; *TSH*, thyroid-stimulating hormone.

and to reduce thyroid hormone secretion. The priorities for nursing care focus on monitoring for complications, reducing stimulation, promoting comfort, and teaching the patient and family about therapeutic drugs and procedures.

Nonsurgical Management

Monitoring includes measuring the patient's apical pulse, blood pressure (BP), and temperature at least every 4 hours. Instruct the patient to report immediately any palpitations, dyspnea, vertigo, or chest pain. Increases in temperature may indicate a rapid worsening of the patient's condition and the onset of thyroid storm, a life-threatening event that occurs with uncontrolled hyperthyroidism and is characterized by high fever and severe hypertension. *Immediately report a temperature increase of even one degree Fahrenheit.* If this task is delegated to unlicensed assistive personnel (UAP), instruct them to report the patient's temperature to you as soon as it has been obtained. If a temperature elevation is reported, immediately assess the patient's cardiac status. If the patient has a cardiac monitor, check for dysrhythmias.

Reducing stimulation is important because a noisy or stressful environment can increase the manifestations of hyperthyroidism and increase the risk for cardiac complications. Encourage the patient to rest. Keep the environment as quiet as possible by closing the door to his or her room, limiting visitors, and eliminating or postponing nonessential care or treatments.

Promoting comfort can be accomplished through actions such as reducing the room temperature to decrease discomfort caused by heat intolerance. Instruct UAP to ensure the patient always has a fresh pitcher of ice water and to change the bed linen whenever it becomes damp from diaphoresis. Suggest that the patient take a cool shower several times each day. If showering is not possible, cool sponge baths may increase comfort. Prevent eye dryness in patients with exophthalmos by encouraging the use of artificial tears and by taping the eyelids closed for sleep.

Drug therapy with antithyroid drugs is the initial treatment of hyperthyroidism. Chart 66-3 lists teaching priorities for the patient receiving drug therapy for hyperthyroidism. The preferred drugs are the thionamides, which include propylthiouracil (PTU) and methimazole (Tapazole). These drugs block thyroid hormone production by preventing iodide binding in the thyroid gland (see Chart 66-3). In addition, PTU also prevents T_4 from being converted to the more powerful T_3 in the tissues. Methimazole doses are lower than PTU doses. The response to these drugs is delayed because the patient may have large amounts of stored thyroid hormones that continue to be released.

> **! NURSING SAFETY PRIORITY**
>
> *Drug Alert*
>
> Both propylthiouracil and methimazole are effective but dangerous drugs. Propylthiouracil now has a black box warning because it is associated with an incidence of serious liver injury and liver failure. Methimazole can cause birth defects. The Food and Drug Administration recommends that unless a patient is pregnant or is allergic to methimazole, propylthiouracil should be avoided. Assess any patient taking propylthiouracil for manifestations of liver problems (e.g., yellowing of the sclera and skin, dark urine, clay-colored stools, elevated liver enzymes) (Aschenbrenner, 2009).

Iodine preparations may be used for short-term therapy before surgery. They decrease blood flow through the thyroid gland, reducing the production and release of thyroid hormone. Improvement usually occurs within 2 weeks, but it may be weeks before metabolism returns to normal. This treatment can result in hypothyroidism, and the patient is monitored closely for the need to adjust the drug regimen.

Lithium also inhibits thyroid hormone release. However, its use is limited because of side effects such as depression, diabetes insipidus, tremors, nausea, and vomiting. Lithium may be used for a patient who cannot tolerate other antithyroid drugs.

Beta-adrenergic blocking drugs, such as propranolol (Inderal, Detensol ✦) may be used as supportive therapy. These drugs relieve diaphoresis, anxiety, tachycardia, and palpitations but do not inhibit thyroid hormone production. See Chapters 36 and 40 for a discussion of the actions and nursing implications of these agents.

Radioactive iodine (RAI) therapy is not used in pregnant women because ^{131}I crosses the placenta and can damage the fetal thyroid gland. The patient with hyperthyroidism may receive RAI in the form of oral ^{131}I. The dosage depends on the thyroid gland's size and sensitivity to radiation. The thyroid gland picks up the RAI, and some of the cells that produce thyroid hormone are destroyed by the local radiation. Because the thyroid gland stores thyroid hormones to some degree, the patient may not have complete symptom relief until 6 to 8 weeks after RAI therapy. Additional drug therapy for hyperthyroidism is still needed during the first few weeks after RAI treatment.

RAI therapy is performed on an outpatient basis. One dose may be sufficient, although some patients need a second or third dose. The radiation dose is low and is usually completely eliminated within a month; however, the source is unsealed, and some radioactivity is present in the patient's body fluids and stool for a few weeks after therapy (Al-Shakhrah, 2008). Radiation precautions are needed to prevent exposure to family members and other people. Chart 66-4 lists precautions to teach the patient during the first few weeks after receiving ^{131}I.

The degree of thyroid destruction varies. Some patients become hypothyroid as a result of treatment. This problem may occur within a few weeks, or it may take several years to develop. The patient then needs lifelong thyroid hormone replacement. All patients who have undergone RAI therapy should be monitored regularly for changes in thyroid function.

Surgical Management

Antithyroid drugs and RAI therapy are now the most common treatments for patients with hyperthyroidism. Surgery to remove all or part of the thyroid gland may be needed for patients who have a large goiter causing tracheal or esophageal compression or who do not have a good response to antithyroid drugs. Removal of all (total thyroidectomy) or part (subtotal thyroidectomy) of the thyroid tissue decreases the production of thyroid hormones. After a total thyroidectomy, patients must take lifelong thyroid hormone replacement.

Preoperative Care. If possible, the patient is treated with drug therapy first to have near-normal thyroid function (euthyroid) before thyroid surgery. This state is achieved

CHART 66-3   COMMON EXAMPLES OF DRUG THERAPY

Hyperthyroidism

DRUG/USUAL DOSAGE	PURPOSE/ACTION	NURSING INTERVENTION	RATIONALE
For Treatment of Mild to Moderate Hyperthyroidism			
Propylthiouracil (PTU, Propyl-Thyracil ✦) Initial dose 100-150 mg orally every 8 hr Maintenance dose 50-150 mg orally every 8 hr	Reduces manifestations of hyperthyroidism by preventing the new formation of thyroid hormones by inhibiting thyroid binding of iodide and by preventing the conversion of T_4 to T_3 in the tissues.	Teach patient to take the drug every 8 hr. Teach patient to avoid crowds and people who are ill. Teach patient to report darkening of the urine, a yellow appearance to the skin or whites of the eyes, and an increased tendency to bruise or bleed. Teach patient to check for weight gain, slow heart rate, and cold intolerance.	Taking the drug evenly throughout the day results in better drug action. Drug reduces blood cell counts and the immune response, increasing the risk for infection. These manifestations may indicate liver toxicity or failure, a possible side effect of the drug. These indicate hypothyroidism and may require a lower drug dose.
Methimazole (Northyx, Tapazole) Initial dose 5-20 mg orally every 8 hr Maintenance dose 1-4 mg orally every 8 hr	Reduces manifestations of hyperthyroidism by preventing the new formation of thyroid hormones by inhibiting thyroid binding of iodide.	Teach patient to take the drug every 8 hr. Remind women to notify their health care providers if they become pregnant. Teach patient to avoid crowds and people who are ill. Teach patient to check for weight gain, slow heart rate, and cold intolerance. Teach patient about the possibility of muscle and joint pain.	Taking the drug evenly throughout the day results in better drug action. This drug causes birth defects and should not be used during pregnancy. Drug reduces blood cell counts and the immune response, increasing the risk for infection. These indicate hypothyroidism and may require a lower drug dose. Knowing the side effects to expect reduces anxiety.
Lithium carbonate (Eskalith, Lithobid, Lithonate) 300 mg orally every 8 hr	Reduces the manifestations of hyperthyroidism by inhibiting the release of thyroid hormones (temporarily). Used only when the patient cannot take a thionamide.	Teach patient to take the drug every 8 hr. Teach patient to drink at least 3 to 4 quarts of fluids daily. Teach patient to check for weight gain, slow heart rate, and cold intolerance.	Taking the drug evenly throughout the day results in better drug action. Drug increases urine output and can cause dehydration. These indicate hypothyroidism and may require a lower drug dose.
For Initial Treatment of Severe Hyperthyroidism or Thyrotoxicosis			
Iodine and iodine-containing agents: Lugol's solution Saturated solution of potassium iodide (SSKI) Dosages vary depending on the agent, how the drug is administered, and the severity of the manifestations	The sudden excess of iodine rapidly inhibits thyroid hormone release and dramatically (but temporarily) resolves the cardiac and other manifestations of hyperthyroidism. These agents are not recommended for long-term therapy.	Administer these drugs 1 hour *after* a thionamide has been given. Check patient for a fever or rash, and ask about a metallic taste, mouth sores, sore throat, or GI distress.	Initially, the iodine agents can cause an increase in the production of thyroid hormones. Giving a thionamide first prevents this initial increase in thyroid hormone production. These are manifestations of *iodism*, a toxic effect of the drugs, and may require that the drug be discontinued.

Safety Precautions for the Patient Receiving an Unsealed Radioactive Isotope

- Use a toilet that is not used by others for least 2 weeks after receiving the radioactive iodine.
- Sit to urinate (males and females) to avoid splashing the seat, walls, and floor.
- Flush the toilet three times after each use.
- If urine is spilled on the toilet seat or floor, use paper tissues or towels to clean it up, bag them in sealable plastic bags, and take them to the hospital's radiation therapy department.
- Men with urinary incontinence should use condom catheters and a drainage bag rather than absorbent gel-filled briefs or pads.
- Women with urinary incontinence should use facial tissue layers in their clothing to catch the urine rather than absorbent gel-filled briefs or pads.
- Using a laxative on the second and third days after receiving the radioactive drug helps you excrete the contaminated stool faster (this also decreases the exposure of your abdominal organs to radiation).
- Wear only machine-washable clothing, and wash these items separate from others in your household.
- After washing your clothing, run the washing machine for a full cycle on empty before it is used to wash the clothing of others.
- Avoid close contact with pregnant women, infants, and young children for the first week after therapy. Remain at least 3 feet (about 1 meter) away from these people, and limit your exposure to them to no more than 1 hour daily.
- Some radioactivity will be in your saliva during the first week after therapy. Precautions to avoid exposing others to this contamination (both household members and trash collectors) include:
- Not sharing toothbrushes or toothpaste tubes
- Using disposable tissues, rather than cloth handkerchiefs, and either flushing used ones down the toilet or keeping them in a plastic bag and turning them in to the radiation department of the hospital for disposal
- Use disposable utensils, plates, and cups
- Selecting foods that can be eaten completely and do not result in a saliva-coated remnant (Foods to avoid are fruit with a core that can be contaminated, meat with a bone [e.g., chicken wings or legs, ribs])

Al-Shakhrah, I. (2008). Radioprotection using iodine-131 for thyroid cancer and hyperthyroidism: A review. *Clinical Journal of Oncology Nursing, 12*(6), 905-912.

with antithyroid drugs that decrease the secretion of thyroid hormones. In addition, iodine preparations are used to decrease thyroid size and vascularity, thereby reducing the risk for hemorrhage and the potential for thyroid storm during surgery.

Hypertension, dysrhythmias, and tachycardia must be controlled before surgery. The patient with hyperthyroidism is often not at an optimal weight and may need to follow a high-protein, high-carbohydrate diet for days or weeks before surgery.

Teach the patient to perform coughing and deep-breathing exercises. Stress the importance of supporting the neck when coughing or moving by placing both hands behind the neck. This action reduces the strain on the suture line. Explain that hoarseness may be present for a few days as a result of endotracheal tube placement during surgery.

Patients often fear thyroid surgery, perhaps because the incision is on the neck. Reassure the patient by calmly explaining the surgery and the care after surgery. Remind him or her that a drain as well as a dressing may be in place after surgery. Answer any questions the patient and family have.

Operative Procedures. A thyroidectomy is performed with the patient under general anesthesia. In the traditional open approach, the patient's neck is extended and the surgeon makes a "collar" incision just above the clavicle. The surgeon attempts to avoid the parathyroid glands and recurrent laryngeal nerves to reduce the risk for complications and injury. Minimally invasive video-assisted thyroidectomy is being used for some patients (Snissarenko et al., 2009).

With a subtotal thyroidectomy, the remaining thyroid tissues are sutured to the trachea. With a total thyroidectomy, the entire thyroid gland is removed but the parathyroid glands are left with an intact blood supply to prevent causing hypoparathyroidism.

Postoperative Care. *Monitoring the patient for complications is the most important nursing action after thyroid surgery.* Monitor vital signs every 15 minutes until the patient is stable and then every 30 minutes for 24 hours. Increase or decrease the monitoring of vital signs based on changes in the patient's condition.

Assess the patient's level of discomfort. Use sandbags or pillows to support the head and neck. Place the patient, while he or she is awake, in a semi-Fowler's position. When positioning the patient, decrease tension on the suture line by avoiding neck extension. Give prescribed drugs for pain control as needed.

Humidifying the air promotes easier respiration and thins respiratory secretions. Assist the patient to cough and deep-breathe every 30 minutes to 1 hour. Suction oral and tracheal secretions when necessary.

Thyroid surgery can cause hemorrhage, respiratory distress, parathyroid gland injury (resulting in hypocalcemia [low serum calcium levels] and tetany [hyperexcitability of nerves and muscles]), damage to the laryngeal nerves, and thyroid storm. Remain alert to the potential for complications, and identify manifestations early.

Hemorrhage is most likely to occur during the first 24 hours after surgery. Inspect the neck dressing and behind the patient's neck for blood. A drain may be present, and a moderate amount of serosanguineous drainage is normal. Hemorrhage may be seen as bleeding at the incision site or as respiratory distress caused by tracheal compression.

Respiratory distress can result from swelling, tetany, or damage to the laryngeal nerve resulting in spasms. Laryngeal stridor (harsh, high-pitched respiratory sounds) is heard in acute respiratory obstruction. Keep emergency tracheostomy equipment in the patient's room. Check that oxygen and suctioning equipment are nearby and in working order.

> **! NURSING SAFETY PRIORITY**
> *Critical Rescue*
>
> When stridor, dyspnea, or other symptoms of obstruction appear after thyroid surgery, notify the Rapid Response Team. In some agencies, nurses can remove clips or sutures when medical assistance is not immediately available and swelling at the surgical site is obstructing the airway.

Hypocalcemia and tetany may occur if the parathyroid glands are removed, damaged or their blood supply is impaired during thyroid surgery, resulting in decreased parathyroid hormone (PTH) levels. Ask the patient hourly about tingling around the mouth or of the toes and fingers. Assess for muscle twitching as a sign of calcium deficiency. Calcium gluconate or calcium chloride for IV use should be available in an emergency situation. (For information on the later signs of hypocalcemia, see the discussion of postoperative care on p. 1407 in the Hyperparathyroidism section, and p. 1408 in the Assessment discussion in the Hypoparathyroidism section. The care of patients with hypocalcemia is also discussed in Chapter 13.)

Laryngeal nerve damage may occur during surgery. This problem results in hoarseness and a weak voice. Assess the patient's voice at 2-hour intervals, and document any changes. Reassure the patient that hoarseness is usually temporary.

Thyroid storm, or thyroid crisis, is a life-threatening event that occurs in patients with uncontrolled hyperthyroidism and occurs most often with Graves' disease (McAdams-Jones, 2008). Manifestations of crisis develop quickly. It is often triggered by stressors such as trauma, infection, diabetic ketoacidosis, and pregnancy. Other conditions that can lead to thyroid storm include vigorous palpation of the goiter, exposure to iodine, and radioactive iodine (RAI) therapy. Although thyroid storm after surgery is less common because patients receive antithyroid drugs, beta blockers, and iodides before thyroid surgery, it can still occur.

The manifestations of thyroid storm are caused by excessive thyroid hormone release, which dramatically increases metabolic rate. *Key manifestations include fever, tachycardia, and systolic hypertension.* The patient may have GI problems such as abdominal pain, nausea, vomiting, and diarrhea. Often he or she is very anxious and has tremors. As the crisis progresses, the patient may become restless, confused, or psychotic and may have seizures, leading to coma. *Even with treatment, thyroid storm may lead to death.*

> **! NURSING SAFETY PRIORITY**
> *Critical Rescue*
>
> When caring for a patient with hyperthyroidism, even after a partial thyroidectomy, immediately report a temperature increase of even 1° F because it may indicate an impending thyroid crisis.

CHART 66-5 BEST PRACTICE FOR PATIENT SAFETY & QUALITY CARE

Emergency Care of the Patient During Thyroid Storm

- Maintain a patent airway and adequate ventilation.
- Give antithyroid drugs as prescribed: methimazole (Tapazole), up to 60 mg daily; propylthiouracil (PTU, Propyl-Thyracil ✦), 300 to 900 mg daily.
- Administer sodium iodide solution, 2 g IV daily as prescribed.
- Give propranolol (Inderal, Detensol ✦), 1 to 3 mg IV as prescribed. Give slowly over 3 minutes. The patient should be connected to a cardiac monitor, and a central venous pressure catheter should be in place.
- Give glucocorticoids as prescribed: hydrocortisone, 100 to 500 mg IV daily; prednisone, 4 to 60 mg IV daily; or dexamethasone, 2 mg IM every 6 hours.
- Monitor continually for cardiac dysrhythmias.
- Monitor vital signs every 30 minutes.
- Provide comfort measures, including a cooling blanket.
- Give non-salicylate antipyretics as prescribed.
- Correct dehydration with normal saline infusions.
- Apply cooling blanket or ice packs to reduce fever.

Emergency measures to prevent death vary with the intensity and type of specific symptoms. After the cause has been identified, interventions focus on maintaining airway patency, providing adequate ventilation, reducing fever, and stabilizing the hemodynamic status. Chart 66-5 outlines the best practices for emergency management of thyroid storm.

Eye and vision problems of Graves' disease are not corrected by treatment for hyperthyroidism. Treatment of infiltrative ophthalmopathy is symptomatic. Teach the patient with mild symptoms to elevate the head of the bed at night and to use artificial tears. If photophobia (sensitivity to light) is present, dark glasses or eye patches are often helpful. For those who cannot close the eyelids completely, recommend gently taping the lids closed with nonallergenic tape at bedtime. These actions prevent irritation and injury. If pressure behind the eye continues and forces the eye forward, blood supply to the eye can be compromised, leading to ischemia and blindness.

In severe cases, short-term steroid therapy is prescribed to reduce swelling and halt the infiltrative process. Prednisone (Deltasone, Winpred ✦) is given in high doses (often 120 mg daily) at first and then is tapered down according to the patient's response. Explain the need to reduce the prednisone gradually, and review its side effects with the patient.

Diuretics may be prescribed to decrease edema around the eye. Surgical intervention (orbital decompression) may be needed if loss of sight or damage to the eyeball is possible. However, it is not usually performed for cosmetic reasons alone (Leung et al., 2009).

Health teaching includes reviewing with the patient and family the manifestations of hyperthyroidism and instructing the patient to report an increase or recurrence of symptoms. Also teach about the manifestations of hypothyroidism (discussed in the next section) and the need for thyroid hormone replacement. Reinforce the need for regular follow-up because hypothyroidism can occur several years after radioactive iodine therapy.

If the patient has had surgery, the surgeon usually removes the sutures on the third or fourth postoperative day. Teach the patient to inspect the incision area and to report redness, tenderness, drainage, or swelling to the surgeon.

The discharged patient may continue to have mood changes as a result of hyperthyroidism. Explain the reason for mood swings to the patient and family, and reassure them that these will decrease with continued treatment.

? DECISION-MAKING CHALLENGE

Patient-Centered Care; Evidence-Based Practice

You are preparing the patient who is 2 days postoperative from a total thyroidectomy for Graves' disease to be discharged to home. She is relieved the surgery is over and tells you that she is so happy that drugs are no longer needed and that her appearance, especially the goiter and the protruding eyes, will return to normal. However, she is concerned that her voice is still hoarse today, although less so than yesterday.

1. Is she correct in thinking that drugs are no longer needed? Why or why not?
2. What will you teach her about her appearance?
3. What will you teach her about the hoarseness?
4. What are the additional teaching priorities for this patient?

HYPOTHYROIDISM

Pathophysiology

The manifestations of hypothyroidism (Chart 66-6) are the result of decreased metabolism from low levels of thyroid hormones. Thyroid cells may fail to produce sufficient levels of thyroid hormones (THs) for several reasons. Sometimes the cells themselves are damaged and no longer function normally. At other times, the thyroid cells are functional but the person does not ingest enough of the substances needed to make thyroid hormones, especially iodide and tyrosine. When the production of thyroid hormones is too low or absent, the blood levels of TH are very low and the patient has a decreased metabolic rate. This lowered metabolism causes the hypothalamus and anterior pituitary gland to make stimulatory hormones, especially thyroid-stimulating hormone (TSH), in an attempt to trigger hormone release from the poorly responsive thyroid gland. The TSH binds to thyroid cells and causes the thyroid gland to enlarge, forming a goiter, although thyroid hormone production does not increase.

Most tissues and organs are affected by the low metabolic rate caused by hypothyroidism. Cellular energy is decreased, and metabolites that are compounds of proteins and sugars called *glycosaminoglycans* build up inside cells; this buildup increases the mucus and water, forms cellular edema, and changes organ texture. The edema is mucinous (called myxedema), rather than edema caused by water alone, and changes the patient's appearance (Fig. 66-3). Nonpitting edema forms everywhere, especially around the eyes, in the hands and feet, and between the shoulder blades. The tongue thickens, and edema forms in the larynx, making the voice husky. All general physiologic function is decreased.

Myxedema coma is a rare, serious complication of untreated or poorly treated hypothyroidism. The decreased metabolism causes the heart muscle to become flabby and the

CHART 66-6 KEY FEATURES

Hypothyroidism

Skin Manifestations
- Cool, pale or yellowish, dry, coarse, scaly skin
- Thick, brittle nails
- Dry, coarse, brittle hair
- Decreased hair growth, with loss of eyebrow hair
- Poor wound healing

Pulmonary Manifestations
- Hypoventilation
- Pleural effusion
- Dyspnea

Cardiovascular Manifestations
- Bradycardia
- Dysrhythmias
- Enlarged heart
- Decreased activity tolerance
- Hypotension

Metabolic Manifestations
- Decreased basal metabolic rate
- Decreased body temperature
- Cold intolerance

Musculoskeletal Manifestations
- Muscle aches and pains
- Delayed contraction and relaxation of muscles

Neurologic Manifestations
- Slowing of intellectual functions:
  - Slowness or slurring of speech
  - Impaired memory
  - Inattentiveness
- Lethargy or somnolence
- Confusion
- Hearing loss
- Paresthesia (numbness and tingling) of the extremities
- Decreased tendon reflexes

Psychological/Emotional Manifestations
- Apathy
- Depression
- Paranoia
- Withdrawal

Gastrointestinal Manifestations
- Anorexia
- Weight gain
- Constipation
- Abdominal distention

Reproductive Manifestations
Women
- Changes in menses (amenorrhea or prolonged menstrual periods)
- Anovulation
- Decreased libido

Men
- Decreased libido
- Impotence

Other Manifestations
- Periorbital edema
- Facial puffiness
- Nonpitting edema of the hands and feet
- Hoarseness
- Goiter (enlarged thyroid gland)
- Thick tongue
- Increased sensitivity to opioids and tranquilizers
- Weakness, fatigue
- Decreased urine output
- Anemia
- Easy bruising
- Iron deficiency
- Folate deficiency
- Vitamin B_{12} deficiency

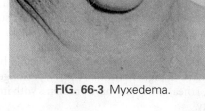

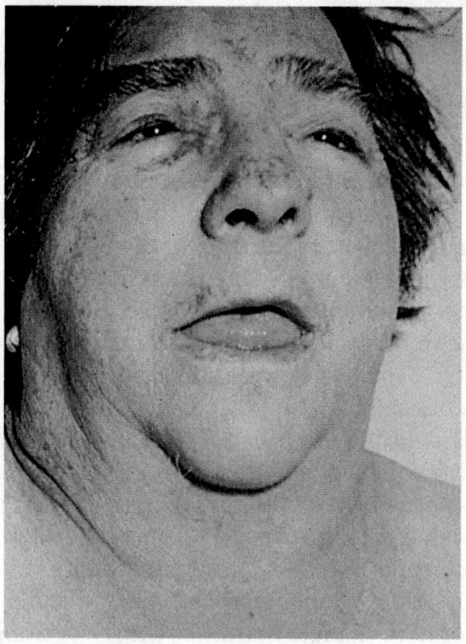

FIG. 66-3 Myxedema.

TABLE 66-2 CAUSES OF HYPOTHYROIDISM

Primary Causes
Decreased Thyroid Tissue
- Surgical removal of the thyroid
- Radiation-induced thyroid destruction
- Autoimmune thyroid destruction
- Congenital thyroid agenesis
- Congenital thyroid hypoplasia
- Congenital thyroid dysgenesis
- Cancer (thyroidal or metastatic)

Decreased Synthesis of Thyroid Hormone
- Endemic iodine deficiency
- Excessive exposure to iodine
- Drugs
  - Lithium
  - Phenylbutazone
  - Propylthiouracil
  - Sodium or potassium perchlorate
  - Aminoglutethimide

Secondary Causes
Inadequate Production of Thyroid-Stimulating Hormone
- Pituitary tumors, trauma, infections, or infarcts
- Congenital pituitary defects
- Hypothalamic tumors, trauma, infections, or infarcts

chamber size to increase. The result is decreased cardiac output and decreased perfusion to the brain and other vital organs. The decreased perfusion makes the already slowed cellular metabolism worse, resulting in tissue and organ failure. *The mortality rate for myxedema coma is extremely high, and this condition is considered a life-threatening emergency.* Myxedema coma can be caused by a variety of events, drugs, or conditions.

Etiology

Most cases of hypothyroidism in the United States occur as a result of thyroid surgery and radioactive iodine (RAI) treatment of hyperthyroidism. Worldwide, hypothyroidism is common in areas where the soil and water have little natural iodide, causing endemic goiter. (This problem was common in the midwest region of the United States before iodide was added to table salt and before saltwater fish was widely available.) Hypothyroidism is also caused by a variety of other conditions (Table 66-2).

Incidence/Prevalence

Hypothyroidism occurs most often in women between 30 and 60 years of age. Women are affected 7 to 10 times more often than men (McCance et al., 2010). An association exists between the development of hypothyroidism and diabetes mellitus. Incidence increases with age.

PATIENT-CENTERED COLLABORATIVE CARE

ASSESSMENT

History

A decrease in thyroid hormones produces many manifestations related to decreased metabolism. However, changes may have occurred slowly, often over weeks or months, and the patient may not have noticed them. Ask him or her to compare activity now with that of a year ago. The patient often reports an increase in time spent sleeping, sometimes up to 14 to 16 hours daily. Generalized weakness, anorexia, muscle aches, and paresthesias may also be present. Constipation is common, as is cold intolerance. Ask whether more blankets at night or sweaters and extra clothing, even in warm weather, have been needed. Some of these changes may be subtle and missed because they are considered part of the aging process.

Both men and women with hypothyroidism may report a decrease in libido. Women may have had difficulty becoming pregnant or have changes in menses (heavy, prolonged bleeding or amenorrhea). Men may have problems with impotence and infertility.

Ask the patient about current or previous use of drugs, such as lithium, thiocyanates, aminoglutethimide, sodium or potassium perchlorate, or cobalt. All these drugs can impair thyroid hormone production. In particular, the cardiac drug *amiodarone* (Cordarone) often has damaging effects on the thyroid gland (Kessenich & Higgs, 2010). Also determine whether the patient has ever been treated for hyperthyroidism and what specific treatment was used.

Physical Assessment/Clinical Manifestations

Observe the patient's overall appearance. Fig. 66-3 shows the typical appearance of an adult with hypothyroidism. Common changes include coarse features, edema around the eyes and face, a blank expression, and a thick tongue. The patient's overall muscle movement is slow. He or she may not speak clearly and may take a longer time to respond to questions.

Cardiac and respiratory functions are decreased. Heart rate may be below 60 beats per minute, and respiratory rate may be slower than normal. The patient's body temperature is often lower than 97° F.

Weight gain is very common, even when the person is ingesting an appropriate number of calories for size, age, and gender. Weigh the patient, and ask whether the result is the same or different from his or her weight a year ago.

Depending on the cause of hypothyroidism, the patient may have a goiter. However, some types of hypothyroidism do not induce a goiter and some types of hyperthyroidism do. Therefore the presence of a goiter suggests a thyroid problem but does not indicate whether the problem is excessive hormone secretion or too little hormone secretion.

Psychosocial Assessment

Hypothyroidism causes many problems in psychosocial functioning. Depression is the most common reason for seeking medical attention. Family members often bring the patient for the initial evaluation. The patient may be too lethargic, apathetic, or drowsy to recognize changes in his or her condition. Families may report that the patient is withdrawn and has reduced mental function. Assess his or her attention span and memory, both of which can be impaired by hypothyroidism. Weight gain may have a negative affect on body image. The mental slowness can contribute to social isolation.

Laboratory Assessment

Laboratory findings for hypothyroidism are the opposite of those for hyperthyroidism. Triiodothyronine (T_3) and thyroxine (T_4) serum levels are decreased. TSH levels are high in primary hypothyroidism but can be decreased or near normal in patients with secondary hypothyroidism (see Chart 66-2). Patients older than 80 years may have lower-than-normal levels of thyroid hormones without manifestations of hypothyroidism, and hormone replacement is not used until other manifestations are present (Touhy & Jett, 2010).

ANALYSIS

The priority problems for patients who have hypothyroidism are:

1. Decreased oxygenation related to decreased energy, obesity, muscle weakness, and fatigue
2. Hypotension related to altered heart rate and rhythm as a result of decreased myocardial metabolism
3. Altered cognitive functioning related to impaired brain metabolism and edema
4. Potential for myxedema coma

PLANNING AND IMPLEMENTATION

Both cardiac and respiratory problems are serious, and their management is a priority. However, the most common cause of death among patients with myxedema coma is respiratory failure.

Improving Oxygenation

Planning: Expected Outcomes. The patient with hypothyroidism is expected to have improved respiratory function and oxygenation. Indicators include:

- Maintenance of Spo_2 of at least 90%
- Absence of cyanosis
- Maintenance of cognitive orientation

Interventions. Observe and record the rate and depth of respirations. Measure oxygen saturation by pulse oximetry, and apply oxygen if the patient has hypoxemia. Auscultate the lungs for any problems, such as a decrease in breath sounds. If hypothyroidism is severe, the patient may have such severe respiratory distress that ventilatory support is required. Severe respiratory distress often occurs with myxedema coma.

Sedating a patient with hypothyroidism can make respiratory difficulties worse and is avoided, if possible. When sedation is needed, the dosage is reduced because hypothyroidism increases sensitivity to these drugs. Assess the patient receiving sedation for respiratory adequacy.

Preventing Hypotension

Planning: Expected Outcomes. The patient with hypothyroidism is expected to have adequate cardiovascular function and tissue perfusion. Indicators include that the patient:

- Maintains heart rate above 60 beats/min
- Maintains blood pressure within normal limits for his or her age and general health
- Has no dysrhythmias, peripheral edema, or neck vein distention

Interventions. The patient with hypothyroidism can have decreased blood pressure, bradycardia, and dysrhythmias. Priority nursing actions are focused on monitoring for condition changes and preventing complications. Monitor blood pressure and heart rate and rhythm, and observe closely for signs of shock, such as hypotension, decreasing urine output, and changes in mental status.

If hypothyroidism has been chronic, the patient may have cardiovascular disease. Instruct the patient to report episodes of chest pain or chest discomfort immediately.

The patient with hypothyroidism requires lifelong thyroid hormone replacement. Synthetic hormone preparations are usually prescribed. The most common is levothyroxine sodium (Synthroid, T_4, Eltroxin ✦). Therapy is started with low doses and gradually increased over a period of weeks. The patient with more severe symptoms of hypothyroidism is started on the lowest dose of thyroid hormone replacement. This caution is especially important when the patient has known cardiac problems. Starting at too high a dose or increasing the dose too rapidly can cause severe hypertension, heart failure, and myocardial infarction (Brent et al., 2008). *Teach patients, as well as their families, who are beginning thyroid replacement hormone therapy to take the drug exactly as prescribed and not to change the dose or schedule without consulting the health care provider. In addition, teach them not to switch brands because the response to different drug brands can vary.*

Assess the patient for chest pain and dyspnea during initiation of therapy. The final dosage is determined by blood levels of TSH and the patient's physical responses. The dosage and time required for symptom relief vary with each patient. Monitor for and teach the patient and family about the manifestations of hyperthyroidism (see Chart 66-1), which can occur with replacement therapy.

> ### ? NCLEX EXAMINATION CHALLENGE
> #### Safe and Effective Care Environment
> Which is the nurse's most important assessment before giving the client prescribed levothyroxine (Synthroid) the first oral dose of the drug?
> A. Measuring heart rate and rhythm
> B. Checking core body temperature
> C. Asking about an allergy to "sulfa" drugs
> D. Determining the level of gastric motility

Supporting Cognition

Planning: Expected Outcomes. The patient with hypothyroidism is expected to have cognitive function that is at a level that was present before the thyroid problem started. Indicators include that the patient:
- Demonstrates immediate memory
- Communicates clearly and appropriately for age and ability
- Is attentive during conversations

Interventions. Observe for and record the presence and severity of lethargy, drowsiness, memory deficit, poor attention span, and difficulty communicating. These problems should decrease with thyroid hormone treatment, and mental awareness usually returns to the patient's normal level within 2 weeks. Orient the patient to person, place, and time, and explain all procedures slowly and carefully. Provide a safe environment.

Family members may have difficulty coping with the patient's behavior. Encourage them to accept the mood changes and mental slowness as manifestations of the disease. Remind the family that these problems should improve with therapy.

Preventing Myxedema Coma

Any patient with hypothyroidism who has any other health problem or who is newly diagnosed is at risk for myxedema coma. Factors leading to myxedema coma include acute illness, surgery, chemotherapy, discontinuing thyroid replacement therapy, and the use of sedatives or opioids. Problems that often occur with this condition include:
- Coma
- Respiratory failure
- Hypotension
- Hyponatremia
- Hypothermia
- Hypoglycemia

> ### ! NURSING SAFETY PRIORITY
> #### Action Alert
> Myxedema coma can lead to shock, organ damage, and death. Assess the patient with hypothyroidism at least every 8 hours for changes that indicate increasing severity, especially changes in mental status, and report these promptly to the health care provider (Simmons, 2010).

Treatment is instituted quickly according to the patient's manifestations and without waiting for laboratory confirmation. Best practices for emergency care of the patient with myxedema coma are listed in Chart 66-7.

Community-Based Care

Hypothyroidism is usually a chronic condition. Patients with hypothyroidism are managed on an outpatient basis and may reside anywhere. Patients in acute care settings, subacute care settings, and rehabilitation centers may have long-standing hypothyroidism in addition to other acute or chronic health

> ### CHART 66-7 BEST PRACTICE FOR PATIENT SAFETY & QUALITY CARE
> #### Emergency Care of the Patient During Myxedema Coma
> - Maintain a patent airway.
> - Replace fluids with IV normal or hypertonic saline, as prescribed.
> - Give levothyroxine sodium IV as prescribed.
> - Give glucose IV as prescribed.
> - Give corticosteroids as prescribed.
> - Check the patient's temperature hourly.
> - Monitor blood pressure hourly.
> - Cover the patient with warm blankets.
> - Monitor for changes in mental status.
> - Turn every 2 hours.
> - Institute Aspiration Precautions.

problems. Ensure that whoever is responsible for overseeing the patient's daily care is aware of the condition and understands its treatment.

Home Care Management

The patient with hypothyroidism does not usually require changes in the home unless cognition has decreased to the point that he or she poses a danger to himself or herself. Activity intolerance and fatigue may necessitate one-floor living for a short time. If manifestations have not improved before discharge, discuss the need for extra heat or clothing because of cold intolerance. The patient who has a decreased attention span may need help with the drug regimen. Discuss this issue with the family and patient, and develop a plan for drug therapy. One person should be clearly designated as responsible for drug preparation and delivery so that doses are neither missed nor duplicated.

Teaching for Self-Management

The most important educational need for the patient with hypothyroidism is about hormone replacement therapy and its side effects. Emphasize the need for lifelong drugs, and review the manifestations of both hyperthyroidism and hypothyroidism. Teach the patient to wear a medical alert bracelet. Teach the patient and family when to seek medical interventions for dosage adjustment and the need for periodic blood tests of hormone levels. Instruct the patient to not take any over-the-counter (OTC) drugs because thyroid hormone preparations interact with many other drugs. Older patients may need additional information about the effects of aging on the thyroid gland (Chart 66-8).

Advise the patient to eat a well-balanced diet with adequate fiber and fluid intake to prevent constipation. Caution him or her that use of fiber supplements may interfere with the absorption of thyroid hormone. Thyroid hormones should be taken on an empty stomach. Remind the patient about the importance of adequate rest. Encourage family members to voice their concerns to the health care provider.

Assist the family in understanding that the time required for resolution of hypothyroidism varies. During this time, the patient may continue to have mental dullness or slowness. Teach the family to orient the patient often and to explain everything clearly, simply, and as often as needed.

Teach the patient to monitor himself or herself for therapy effectiveness. The two easiest parameters to check are need for sleep and bowel elimination. When the patient requires more sleep and is constipated, the dose of replacement hormone may need to be increased. When the patient has difficulty getting to sleep and has more bowel movements than normal for him or her, the dose may need to be decreased.

Health Care Resources

Immediately after returning home, the patient may need a support person to stay and provide more attention than could be given by a visiting nurse or home care aide. Contact with the health care team is needed for follow-up and identification of potential problems. The patient taking thyroid drugs may have manifestations of hypothyroidism if the dosage is inadequate or may have manifestations of hyperthyroidism if the dose is too high. A home care nurse performs a focused assessment at every home visit to the patient with thyroid dysfunction (Chart 66-9).

▌EVALUATION: OUTCOMES

Evaluate the care of the patient with hypothyroidism based on the identified priority patient problems. The expected outcomes are that the patient should:
- Maintain normal cardiovascular function
- Maintain adequate respiratory function
- Experience improvement in thought processes

Specific indicators for these outcomes are listed for each patient problem in the Planning and Implementation section (see earlier).

❓ NCLEX EXAMINATION CHALLENGE

Physiological Integrity

The client who has been taking levothyroxine (Synthroid) for 3 months reports all of the following conditions. Which condition indicates to the nurse that the drug dosage may need to be adjusted?
A. Difficulty sleeping
B. Increased urine output
C. Decreased sense of smell
D. Difficulty remembering to take the drug

THYROIDITIS

Pathophysiology

Thyroiditis is an inflammation of the thyroid gland. There are three types: acute, subacute, and chronic. Chronic thyroiditis (Hashimoto's disease) is the most common type.

Acute thyroiditis is caused by bacterial invasion of the thyroid gland. Manifestations include pain, neck tenderness, malaise, fever, and dysphagia (difficulty swallowing). It usually resolves with antibiotic therapy.

Subacute or granulomatous thyroiditis results from a viral infection of the thyroid gland after a cold or other upper respiratory infection. Manifestations include fever, chills, dysphagia, and muscle and joint pain. Pain can radiate to the ears and the jaw. The thyroid gland feels hard and enlarged on palpation. Thyroid function can remain normal, although hyperthyroidism or hypothyroidism may develop.

Chronic thyroiditis (Hashimoto's disease) is a common type of hypothyroidism that affects women more often than

The Patient with Thyroid Dysfunction

Assess cardiovascular status:
- Vital signs, including apical pulse, pulse pressure, presence or absence of orthostatic hypotension, and the quality and rhythm of peripheral pulses
- Presence or absence of peripheral edema
- Weight gain or loss

Assess cognition and mental status:
- Level of consciousness
- Orientation to time, place, and person
- Accurately reading a seven-word sentence containing no words greater than three syllables
- Can the patient count backward from 100 by threes?

Assess condition of skin and mucous membranes:
- Moistness of skin, most reliable on chest and back
- Skin temperature and color

Assess neuromuscular status:
- Reactivity of patellar and biceps reflexes
- Oral temperature
- Handgrip strength
- Steadiness of gait
- Presence or absence of fine tremors in the hand

Ask about:
- Sleep in the past 24 hours
- Patient warm enough or too warm indoors
- 24-hour diet recall
- 24-hour activity recall
- Over-the-counter and prescribed drugs taken
- Last bowel movement

Assess patient's understanding of illness and adherence with therapy:
- Manifestations to report to health care provider
- Drug therapy plan (correct timing and dose)

men, usually when patients are in their 30s to 50s (Brent et al., 2008). Hashimoto's disease is an autoimmune disorder that is usually triggered by a bacterial or viral infection. The thyroid is invaded by antithyroid antibodies and lymphocytes, causing thyroid tissue destruction. When large amounts of the gland are destroyed, serum thyroid hormone levels are low and secretion of thyroid-stimulating hormone (TSH) is increased.

PATIENT-CENTERED COLLABORATIVE CARE

The manifestations of Hashimoto's disease are dysphagia and painless enlargement of the gland. Diagnosis is based on circulating antithyroid antibodies and needle biopsy of the thyroid gland. Serum thyroid hormone levels, TSH levels, and radioactive iodine uptake (RAIU) vary with disease stage.

The patient is given thyroid hormone to prevent hypothyroidism and to suppress TSH secretion, which decreases the size of the thyroid gland. Surgery (subtotal thyroidectomy) is needed if the goiter does not respond to thyroid hormone, is disfiguring, or compresses other structures.

Nursing interventions focus on promoting comfort and teaching the patient about hypothyroidism, drugs, and surgery. (See discussion of Postoperative Care on pp. 1399-1400 in the Hyperthyroidism section.)

THYROID CANCER

Pathophysiology

The four distinct types of thyroid cancer are papillary, follicular, medullary, and anaplastic (American Cancer Society, 2011). The initial manifestation of thyroid cancer is a single, painless lump or nodule in the thyroid gland. Additional manifestations depend on the presence and location of metastasis (spread of cancer cells).

Papillary carcinoma, the most common type of thyroid cancer, occurs most often in younger women. It is a slow-growing tumor that can be present for years before spreading to nearby lymph nodes. When the tumor is confined to the thyroid gland, the chance for cure is good with a partial or total thyroidectomy.

Follicular carcinoma occurs most often in older patients. The cancer invades blood vessels and spreads to bone and lung tissue. It can adhere to the trachea, neck muscles, great vessels, and skin, resulting in dyspnea (difficulty breathing) and dysphagia (difficulty swallowing). When the tumor involves the recurrent laryngeal nerves, the patient may have a hoarse voice.

Medullary carcinoma is most common in patients older than 50 years. This tumor often occurs as part of multiple endocrine neoplasia (MEN) type II, a familial endocrine disorder. The tumor usually secretes calcitonin, adrenocorticotropic hormone (ACTH), prostaglandins, and serotonin.

Anaplastic carcinoma is a rapid-growing, aggressive tumor that directly invades nearby structures. Manifestations include stridor (harsh, high-pitched respiratory sounds), hoarseness, and dysphagia.

PATIENT-CENTERED COLLABORATIVE CARE

Radiation therapy is used most often for anaplastic carcinoma because this cancer has usually metastasized (spread) at diagnosis. Surgery is the treatment of choice for papillary, follicular, and medullary carcinomas. A total thyroidectomy is usually performed with a nodal neck dissection if regional lymph nodes are involved. (See the postoperative care discussion in the Surgical Management section for Hyperthyroidism on pp. 1399-1400.) Suppressive doses of thyroid hormone are usually taken for 3 months after surgery. A radioactive iodine uptake (RAIU) study is performed after

? NCLEX EXAMINATION CHALLENGE
Health Promotion and Maintenance

The client scheduled to receive a radioablative dose of ^{131}I for thyroid cancer asks how long he will need to use radiation precautions after receiving the treatment. What is the nurse's best response?
A. "Because the isotope collects in the tumor cells, precautions are needed until the cancer is completely gone."
B. "The dose of radiation is low, and most of it is excreted in the first week. Precautions are needed for only 2 weeks."
C. "You will need to use radiation precautions until the radiologist removes the radiation source from your thyroid gland."
D. "The radiation used is taken up by your thyroid gland, so only your thyroid is considered radioactive. Because the thyroid does not excrete to the outside of the body, precautions are needed only on the days you actually receive the treatment."

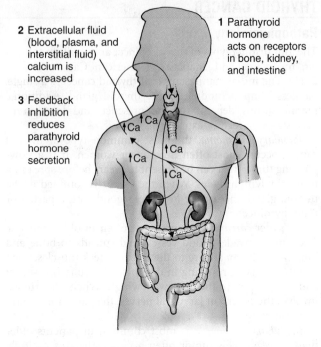

2 Extracellular fluid (blood, plasma, and interstitial fluid) calcium is increased

3 Feedback inhibition reduces parathyroid hormone secretion

1 Parathyroid hormone acts on receptors in bone, kidney, and intestine

FIG. 66-4 The physiologic actions of parathyroid hormone.

TABLE 66-3	CAUSES OF PARATHYROID DYSFUNCTION
Causes of Hyperparathyroidism	**Causes of Hypoparathyroidism**
• Parathyroid adenoma • Parathyroid carcinoma • Congenital hyperplasia • Neck trauma or radiation • Vitamin D deficiency • Chronic kidney disease with hypocalcemia • Parathyroid hormone–secreting carcinomas of the lung, kidney, or GI tract	• Surgical or radiation-induced thyroid ablation • Parathyroidectomy • Congenital dysgenesis • Idiopathic (autoimmune) hypoparathyroidism • Hypomagnesemia

drugs are withdrawn. If there is RAI uptake, the patient is treated with ablative (enough to destroy the tissue) amounts of RAI. (See Chart 66-4 for precautions to teach the patient receiving unsealed RAI therapy.) If thyroid cancer does not respond to RAI, chemotherapy is initiated.

Usually the patient is hypothyroid after treatment for thyroid cancer. Nursing interventions then focus on teaching the patient about hypothyroidism and its management. (See discussion of Patient-Centered Collaborative Care on pp. 1402-1404 in the Hypothyroidism section.)

PARATHYROID DISORDERS

HYPERPARATHYROIDISM

Pathophysiology

The parathyroid glands maintain calcium and phosphate balance (Fig. 66-4). Serum calcium level is normally maintained within a narrow range. Phosphate levels vary more widely. Increased levels of parathyroid hormone (PTH) act directly on the kidney, causing increased kidney reabsorption of calcium and increased phosphate excretion. These processes cause hypercalcemia (excessive calcium) and hypophosphatemia (inadequate phosphate) in the patient with hyperparathyroidism.

In bone, excessive PTH levels increase bone resorption (bone loss of calcium) by decreasing osteoblastic (bone production) activity and increasing osteoclastic (bone destruction) activity. This process releases calcium and phosphate into the blood and reduces bone density. With chronic calcium excess and hypercalcemia, calcium is deposited in soft tissues.

Although the exact triggering mechanisms are unknown, primary hyperparathyroidism results when one or more

parathyroid glands do not respond to the normal feedback of serum calcium. The most common cause is a benign tumor in one parathyroid gland. Table 66-3 lists other causes of hyperparathyroidism.

PATIENT-CENTERED COLLABORATIVE CARE

ASSESSMENT

Manifestations of hyperparathyroidism may be related either to the effects of excessive PTH or to the effects of the accompanying hypercalcemia.

Ask the patient about any bone fractures, recent weight loss, arthritis, or psychological distress. Determine whether the patient has received radiation treatment to the head or neck. The patient with long-standing disease may have a waxy pallor of the skin and bone deformities in the extremities and back.

High levels of PTH cause renal calculi (kidney stones) and deposits of calcium in the soft tissue of the kidney. Bone lesions are due to an increased rate of bone destruction and may result in pathologic fractures, bone cysts, and osteoporosis.

GI problems (e.g., anorexia, nausea, vomiting, epigastric pain, constipation, weight loss) are common, particularly when serum calcium levels are high. Elevated serum gastrin levels are caused by hypercalcemia and lead to peptic ulcer disease. Fatigue and lethargy may be present and become more severe as the serum calcium levels increase. When serum calcium levels are greater than 12 mg/dL, the patient may have psychosis with mental confusion, which leads to coma and death if left untreated. (See Chapter 13 for more information about hypercalcemia.)

Serum PTH, calcium, and phosphate levels and urine cyclic adenosine monophosphate (cAMP) are the most commonly used laboratory tests to detect hyperparathyroidism (Chart 66-10). X-rays may show kidney stones, calcium deposits, and bone lesions (e.g., cysts or fractures). Loss of bone density occurs in the patient with chronic hyperparathyroidism. Other diagnostic tests include arteriography, computed tomography (CT) scans, venous sampling of the thyroid for blood PTH levels, and ultrasonography. Explain the procedures and care for the patient undergoing diagnostic tests.

CHART 66-10 **LABORATORY PROFILE**

Parathyroid Function

TEST	NORMAL RANGE FOR ADULTS	SIGNIFICANCE OF ABNORMAL FINDINGS	
		HYPERPARATHYROIDISM	HYPOPARATHYROIDISM
Serum calcium	Total: 9.0-10.5 mg/dL or 2.25-2.75 SI units Ionized (active): 4.64-5.28 mg/dL or 1.16-1.32 SI units	Increased in primary hyperparathyroidism	Decreased
Serum phosphate	3.0-4.5 mg/dL or 0.97-1.45 SI units *Older adults:* May be slightly lower	Decreased	Increased
Serum magnesium	1.3-2.1 mEq/L	Increased	Decreased
Serum parathyroid hormone	C-terminal 50-330 pg/mL	Increased	Decreased
Vitamin D (calciferol)	14-60 ng/mL	Variable	Decreased
Urine cAMP	18.3-45.4 nmol/L in a 24-hour urine collection specimen	Increased	Decreased

SI, International System of Units; *cAMP,* cyclic adenosine monophosphate.

INTERVENTIONS

Nonsurgical Management

Diuretic and hydration therapies are used for reducing serum calcium levels in patients who are not candidates for surgery. Usually furosemide (Lasix, Uritol ✦), a diuretic that increases kidney excretion of calcium, is used together with IV saline in large volumes to promote calcium excretion. Priority nursing interventions focus on monitoring and preventing injury.

Monitor cardiac function and intake and output every 2 to 4 hours during hydration therapy. Continuous cardiac monitoring may be needed. Compare recent electrocardiogram (ECG) tracings with the patient's baseline tracings. Especially look for changes in the T waves and the QT interval, as well as changes in rate and rhythm. Closely monitor serum calcium levels, and immediately report any sudden drop to the health care provider. Sudden drops in calcium levels may cause tingling and numbness in the muscles.

Preventing injury is important because the patient with chronic hyperparathyroidism often has significant bone density loss and is at risk for pathologic fractures. Teach all members of the health care team to handle the patient carefully. Use a lift sheet to reposition the patient rather than pulling him or her. Ensure that the hospitalized patient is accompanied when ambulating to prevent falls.

Drug therapy is used when hydration and furosemide cannot reduce hypercalcemia or if it is necessary to discontinue IV fluids. Other drugs can help reduce the manifestations of hyperparathyroidism, especially those related to hypercalcemia.

Oral phosphates inhibit bone resorption and interfere with calcium absorption. IV phosphates are used only when serum calcium levels must be lowered rapidly. Calcitonin decreases the release of skeletal calcium and increases the kidney excretion of calcium. It is not effective when used alone because of its short duration of action. The therapeutic effects are greatly enhanced if calcitonin is given along with glucocorticoids.

Some drugs known as *calcium chelators* lower calcium levels by binding *(chelating)* calcium, which reduces the levels of free calcium. Mithramycin, a cytotoxic agent, is the most effective and potent calcium chelator used to lower serum calcium levels. In most patients, a single IV dose of 10 to 15 mg/kg of body weight by slow infusion can lower serum calcium levels within 48 hours. However, the toxic effects limit its use to two or three doses. *Thrombocytopenia* (decreased circulating platelets) and kidney and liver toxicity can result after only one dose. Liver function test, blood urea nitrogen and creatinine, complete blood count (CBC), and serum calcium levels are closely monitored in the patient receiving mithramycin. Another calcium chelator is penicillamine (Cuprimine, Pendramine).

Surgical Management

Surgical management of hyperparathyroidism is a parathyroidectomy. Before surgery, the patient is stabilized and calcium levels are decreased to near normal. If mithramycin has been used to lower serum calcium levels, studies to determine bleeding and clotting times are needed, as is a CBC to determine bone marrow function.

The operative procedure involves a transverse incision in the lower neck. All four parathyroid glands are examined for enlargement. If a tumor is present on one side but the other side is normal, the surgeon removes the glands containing tumor and leaves the remaining glands on the opposite side intact. If all four glands are diseased, they are all removed.

Nursing care before and after surgical removal of the parathyroid glands is the same as that for thyroidectomy. See the Preoperative Care section on pp. 1397-1399 and the Postoperative Care section on pp. 1399-1400 for specific nursing interventions.

The remaining glands, which may have atrophied as a result of PTH overproduction, require several days to several weeks to return to normal function. A hypocalcemic crisis can occur during this critical period. Usually, the surgeon requests the serum calcium to be assessed frequently after surgery. Check serum calcium levels immediately after surgery and every 4 hours thereafter until calcium levels stabilize. Monitor for manifestations of hypocalcemia, such as tingling and twitching in the extremities and face. Check for Trousseau's and Chvostek's signs, either of which indicates potential tetany (see Chapter 13).

The recurrent laryngeal nerve can be damaged. Assess the patient for changes in voice patterns and hoarseness.

When hyperparathyroidism is due to hyperplasia (tissue overgrowth), three glands plus half of the fourth gland are usually removed. If all four glands are removed, a small portion of a gland may be implanted in the forearm, where it produces PTH and maintains calcium homeostasis. If all these maneuvers fail, the patient will need lifelong treatment with calcium and vitamin D because the resulting hypoparathyroidism is permanent (see next section).

HYPOPARATHYROIDISM

Pathophysiology

Hypoparathyroidism is a rare endocrine disorder in which parathyroid function is decreased. Problems are directly related to a lack of parathyroid hormone (PTH) secretion or to decreased effectiveness of PTH on target tissue. Whether the problem is a lack of PTH secretion or an ineffectiveness of PTH on tissues, the result is the same: *hypocalcemia*.

Iatrogenic hypoparathyroidism, the most common form, is caused by the removal of all parathyroid tissue during total thyroidectomy or by deliberate surgical removal of the parathyroid glands.

Idiopathic hypoparathyroidism can occur spontaneously. The exact cause is unknown, but an autoimmune basis is suspected. It may occur with other autoimmune disorders such as adrenal insufficiency, hypothyroidism, diabetes mellitus, pernicious anemia, and vitiligo.

Hypomagnesemia (decreased serum magnesium levels) may also cause hypoparathyroidism. Hypomagnesemia is seen in alcoholics and in patients with malabsorption syndromes, chronic kidney disease, and malnutrition. It causes impairment of PTH secretion and may interfere with the effects of PTH on the bones, kidneys, and calcium regulation.

PATIENT-CENTERED COLLABORATIVE CARE

ASSESSMENT

Ask about any head or neck surgery or radiation therapy because these treatments may damage the parathyroid glands and cause hypoparathyroidism. Also determine whether the neck has ever sustained a serious injury in a car crash or by strangulation. Assess whether the patient has any manifestations of hypoparathyroidism, which may range from mild tingling and numbness to muscle tetany. Tingling and numbness around the mouth or in the hands and feet reflect mild to moderate hypocalcemia. Severe muscle cramps, spasms of the hands and feet, and seizures (with no loss of consciousness or incontinence) reflect a more severe hypocalcemia. The patient or family may notice mental changes ranging from irritability to psychosis.

The physical assessment may show excessive or inappropriate muscle contractions that cause finger, hand, and elbow flexion. This can signal an impending attack of tetany. Check for Chvostek's sign and Trousseau's sign; positive responses indicate potential tetany (see Chapter 13). Bands or pits may encircle the crowns of the teeth, which indicates a loss of calcium from the teeth with enamel loss.

Diagnostic tests for hypoparathyroidism include electroencephalography (EEG), blood tests, and CT scans. EEG changes revert to normal with correction of hypocalcemia. Serum calcium, phosphate, magnesium, vitamin D, and urine cyclic adenosine monophosphate (cAMP) levels may be used in the diagnostic workup for hypoparathyroidism (see Chart 66-10). The CT scan can show brain calcifications, which indicate chronic hypocalcemia.

INTERVENTIONS

Nonsurgical management of hypoparathyroidism focuses on correcting hypocalcemia, vitamin D deficiency, and hypomagnesemia. For patients with acute and severe hypocalcemia, IV calcium is given as a 10% solution of calcium chloride or calcium gluconate over 10 to 15 minutes. Acute vitamin D deficiency is treated with calcitriol (Rocaltrol), 0.5 to 2 mg daily. Acute hypomagnesemia is corrected with 50% magnesium sulfate in 2-mL doses (up to 4 g daily) either IM or IV. Long-term oral therapy for hypocalcemia involves the intake of calcium, 0.5 to 2 g daily, in divided doses.

Long-term therapy for vitamin D deficiency is 50,000 to 400,000 units of ergocalciferol daily. The dosage is adjusted to keep the patient's calcium level in the low-normal range (slightly hypocalcemic), enough to prevent symptoms of hypocalcemia. It must also be low enough to prevent increased urine calcium levels, which can lead to stone formation.

Nursing management includes teaching about the drug regimen and interventions to reduce anxiety. Teach the patient to eat foods high in calcium but low in phosphorus. Milk, yogurt, and processed cheeses are avoided because of their high phosphorus content. *Stress that therapy for hypocalcemia is lifelong.* Advise the patient to wear a medical alert bracelet. With adherence to the prescribed drug and diet regimen, the calcium level usually remains high enough to prevent a hypocalcemic crisis.

GET READY FOR THE NCLEX® EXAMINATION!

KEY POINTS

Review these Key Points for each NCLEX Examination Client Needs Category.

Safe and Effective Care Environment

• Keep the environment of a patient at risk for thyroid storm cool, dark, and quiet.

• Keep emergency suctioning and tracheostomy equipment in the room of a patient who has had thyroid or parathyroid surgery.

• Use a lift sheet to move or reposition a patient with hypocalcemia.

GET READY FOR THE NCLEX® EXAMINATION!—cont'd

Health Promotion and Maintenance

- Teach all patients to take antithyroid drugs or thyroid hormone replacement therapy as prescribed.
- Include the person who prepares the patient's meals when teaching about dietary electrolyte restrictions.
- Collaborate with the dietitian to teach patients about diets that are restricted in calcium or phosphate.

Psychosocial Integrity

- Be accepting of patient behavior.
- Remind patients and family members that changes in cognition and behavior related to thyroid problems are usually temporary.

- Encourage the patient who has a permanent change in appearance (e.g., exophthalmia) to mourn the change.

Physiological Integrity

- Monitor the hydration status of patients who have hypercalcemia.
- Teach patients that hormone replacement therapy for hypothyroidism is lifelong.
- Teach patients to use clinical manifestations (e.g., the number of bowel movements per day, the ability to sleep) as indicators of therapy effectiveness and when the dose of thyroid hormone replacement may need to be adjusted.

67

Care of Patients with Diabetes Mellitus

Margaret Elaine McLeod

℮volve WEBSITE

http://evolve.elsevier.com/Iggy/

Animation: Insulin Function
Answer Keys for NCLEX Examination Challenges and
   Decision-Making Challenges
Audio Glossary

Concept Map Creator
Concept Map: Diabetes Mellitus—Type 2
Key Points
Review Questions for the NCLEX® Examination

LEARNING OUTCOMES

Safe and Effective Care Environment

1. Assess the person who has diabetes for specific current and ongoing factors that pose threats to safety.
2. Administer insulin and other antidiabetic agents in a safe and accurate manner.
3. Apply the principles of infection control in the care of patients with diabetes.
4. Individualize patient teaching methods for diabetes management.
5. Teach patients and families the safe use of insulin injection equipment and glucose monitoring equipment.
6. Teach patients with peripheral neuropathy how to avoid injury.

Health Promotion and Maintenance

7. Encourage everyone to prevent type 2 diabetes by achieving and maintaining ideal weight and participating in regular exercise.
8. Teach all patients with diabetes how to self-manage their disease.
9. Teach the patient and family about the manifestations and emergency treatment of hypoglycemia and hyperglycemia.

Psychosocial Integrity

10. Allow the patient the opportunity to express concerns regarding the diagnosis of diabetes or the treatment regimen.
11. Explain all procedures, restrictions, drugs, and follow-up care to the patient and family.
12. Refer patients newly diagnosed with diabetes to local resources and support groups.

Physiological Integrity

13. Compare the risk factors, age of onset, manifestations, and pathologic mechanisms of type 1 and type 2 diabetes mellitus.
14. Explain the effects of insulin on carbohydrate, protein, and fat metabolism.
15. Explain how to mix different kinds of insulin together.
16. Evaluate laboratory data to determine effectiveness of the prescribed dietary, drug, and exercise therapies for diabetes.
17. Explain how to perform foot assessment and foot care for the patient with diabetes.
18. Collaborate with members of the health care team to provide care for patients with diabetic ketoacidosis (DKA) or hyperglycemic-hyperosmolar state (HHS).

Diabetes mellitus (DM) is a chronic metabolic disease that requires lifelong behavioral and lifestyle changes. A collaborative approach helps the patient successfully manage the disease. As part of the team, you will plan, organize, and coordinate care with other health care team members to provide care and education and promote the patient's health and well-being.

Diabetes is a major public health problem, and its complications, especially hypertension and hyperlipidemia (high blood lipid levels), cause many serious health problems. In the United States, diabetes mellitus (DM) is a leading cause of blindness, end-stage kidney disease, and foot or leg amputations. Many people have undiagnosed diabetes and, among those who are diagnosed, many have continuous high blood glucose levels. The complications of DM can be greatly reduced with glycemic (blood glucose) control along with management of hypertension and hyperlipidemia. Thus nursing priorities focus on helping the patient with diabetes achieve and maintain lifestyle changes that prevent long-term complications by keeping blood glucose levels and cholesterol levels as close to normal as possible (Young, 2011).

PATHOPHYSIOLOGY

Classification of Diabetes

For all types of diabetes mellitus (DM), the main feature is chronic hyperglycemia (high blood glucose level) resulting from problems with insulin secretion, insulin action, or both. The disease is classified by the underlying problem causing a lack of insulin and the severity of the insulin deficiency. Table 67-1 outlines the types of DM.

The Endocrine Pancreas

The pancreas has mostly exocrine functions that are related to digestion and endocrine functions that are related to blood glucose control. The endocrine portion of the pancreas has about 1 million small glands, the *islets of Langerhans*, scattered through the organ. The two types of islet cells important to glucose control are the *alpha cells*, which secrete glucagon, and the *beta cells*, which produce insulin and amylin. Glucagon is a "counterregulatory" hormone that has actions opposite those of insulin. It prevents *hypoglycemia* (low blood glucose levels) by triggering the release of glucose from cell storage sites. Insulin prevents hyperglycemia by allowing body cells to take up, use, and store carbohydrate, fat, and protein.

Active insulin is a protein made up of 51 amino acids. It is initially produced as inactive *proinsulin*, a prohormone that contains an additional amino acid chain (the C-peptide chain). Proinsulin is converted into active insulin by removal of the C-peptide (Fig. 67-1).

About 40 to 50 units of insulin is secreted daily directly into liver circulation in a two-step manner. It is secreted at low levels during fasting (basal insulin secretion) and at increased levels after eating (prandial). An early burst of insulin secretion occurs within 10 minutes of eating. This is followed by an increasing release that lasts until the blood glucose level is normal.

Glucose Homeostasis

Glucose is the main fuel for central nervous system (CNS) cells. Because the brain cannot produce or store much glucose, it needs a continuous supply from circulation to prevent

TABLE 67-1	CLASSIFICATION OF DIABETES MELLITUS

Type 1 Diabetes
- Beta-cell destruction leading to absolute insulin deficiency
- Autoimmune
- Idiopathic

Type 2 Diabetes
- Ranges from insulin resistance with relative insulin deficiency to secretory deficit with insulin resistance

Other Specific Conditions Resulting in Hyperglycemia
- Genetic defects of beta-cell function
- Genetic defects in insulin action
- Diseases of the exocrine pancreas: pancreatitis, trauma, neoplasia, cystic fibrosis, hemochromatosis
- Endocrinopathies: acromegaly, Cushing's disease, glucagonoma, pheochromocytoma, hyperthyroidism, aldosteronism
- Drug or chemical-induced conditions (from use of pentamidine, nicotinic acid, glucocorticoids, thyroid hormone, diazoxide, beta-adrenergic agents, thiazides, phenytoin, interferon-alpha, other drugs)
- Infections: congenital rubella, cytomegalovirus, human immune deficiency virus
- Uncommon forms of immune-related diabetes
- Other genetic syndromes associated with diabetes: Down syndrome, Klinefelter syndrome, Turner's syndrome, Huntington disease, and others

Gestational Diabetes Mellitus (GDM)
- Glucose intolerance with onset or first recognition during pregnancy

Data from American Diabetes Association (ADA). (2010a). Position statement: Diagnosis and classification of diabetes mellitus, *Diabetes Care, 33*(Suppl. 1), 62-69.

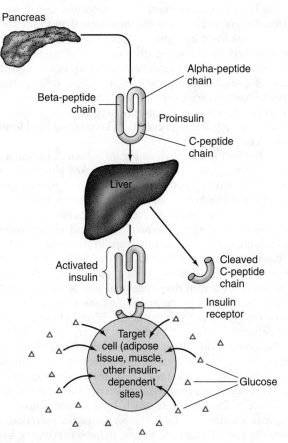

FIG. 67-1 Proinsulin, secreted by and stored in the beta cells of the islets of Langerhans in the pancreas, is transformed by the liver into active insulin. Insulin attaches to receptors on target cells, where it promotes glucose transport into the cells through the cell membranes.

neuronal dysfunction and cell death. Other organs can use both glucose and fatty acids to generate energy. Glucose is stored inside cells as glycogen in the liver and muscles, and free fatty acids are stored as triglyceride in fat cells. Fat is the most efficient means of storing energy. Fat has 9 calories of stored energy per gram. Protein and carbohydrate have only 4 calories per gram. During a prolonged fast or after illness or injury, proteins are broken down and some of the amino acids are converted into glucose.

Several organs and hormones play a role in maintaining glucose homeostasis. During the fasting state, when the stomach is empty, blood glucose is maintained between 60 and 150 mg/dL (3.3 and 8.3 mmol/L) by a balance between glucose uptake by cells and glucose production by the liver. Insulin plays a pivotal role in this process.

Movement of glucose into some cells requires the presence of specific carrier proteins, glucose transport (GLUT) proteins and insulin. Insulin is like a "key" that opens "locked" membranes to glucose, allowing glucose in the blood to move into cells to generate energy. Insulin starts this action by binding to insulin receptors on the cell membranes, which changes membrane permeability to glucose.

Insulin exerts many effects on metabolism and cellular processes in different body tissues and organs. The main metabolic effects of insulin are to stimulate glucose uptake in skeletal muscle and heart muscle and to suppress liver production of glucose and very-low-density lipoprotein (VLDL). In the liver, insulin promotes the production and storage of glycogen (glycogenesis) at the same time that it inhibits glycogen breakdown into glucose (glycogenolysis). It increases protein and lipid (fat) synthesis and inhibits ketogenesis (conversion of fats to acids) and gluconeogenesis (conversion of proteins to glucose). In muscle, insulin promotes protein and glycogen synthesis. In fat cells, it promotes triglyceride storage. Overall, insulin keeps blood glucose levels from becoming too high and helps keep blood lipid levels in the normal range.

In the *fasting state* (not eating for 8 hours), insulin secretion is suppressed, which leads to increased gluconeogenesis in the liver and kidneys, along with increased glucose generation by the breakdown of liver glycogen. In the fed state, insulin released from pancreatic beta cells reverses this process. Instead, glycogen breakdown and gluconeogenesis are inhibited. At the same time, insulin also enhances glucose uptake and use by cells and reduces both fat breakdown (lipolysis) and protein breakdown (proteolysis). When more glucose is present in liver cells than can be metabolized for energy or stored as glycogen, insulin causes the excess glucose to be converted to free fatty acids (FFAs). These extra FFAs are deposited as fat in fat cells.

Glucose in the blood after a meal is controlled by the emptying rate of the stomach and delivery of nutrients to the small intestine where they are absorbed into circulation. Incretin hormones (e.g., GLP-1), secreted in response to the presence of food in the stomach, have several actions. They increase insulin secretion, inhibit glucagon secretion, and slow the rate of gastric emptying, thereby preventing hyperglycemia after meals.

Counterregulatory hormones increase blood glucose by actions opposite those of insulin when more energy is needed. Glucagon is the main counterregulatory hormone. Other hormones that increase blood glucose levels are epinephrine,

TABLE 67-2	**PHYSIOLOGIC RESPONSE TO INSUFFICIENT INSULIN**

- Decreased glycogenesis (conversion of glucose to glycogen)
- Increased glycogenolysis (conversion of glycogen to glucose)
- Increased gluconeogenesis (formation of glucose from non-carbohydrate sources, such as amino acids and lactate)
- Increased lipolysis (breakdown of triglycerides to glycerol and free fatty acids)
- Increased ketogenesis (formation of ketones from free fatty acids)
- Proteolysis (breakdown of protein with amino acid release in muscles)

norepinephrine, growth hormone, and cortisol. The combined actions of insulin and counterregulatory hormones (discussed in the next section) keep blood glucose levels in the range of 60 to 100 mg/dL (3.3 to 5.6 mmol/L) to support brain functions. When glucose levels fall, insulin secretion stops and glucagon is released. Glucagon causes the release of glucose from the liver. Liver glucose is made through breakdown of glycogen to glucose (glycogenolysis) and conversion of amino acids into glucose (gluconeogenesis). When liver glucose is unavailable, the breakdown of fat (lipolysis) and the breakdown of proteins (proteolysis) provide fuel for energy.

Absence of Insulin

Insulin is needed to move glucose into most body tissues. The lack of insulin in diabetes, from either a lack of production or a problem with insulin use at its cell receptor, prevents some cells from using glucose for energy. The body then breaks down fat and protein in an attempt to provide energy and also increases the levels of counterregulatory hormones in an attempt to make glucose from other sources. Table 67-2 outlines the body's response to insufficient insulin.

Without insulin, glucose builds up in the blood, causing hyperglycemia, which is high blood glucose levels. Hyperglycemia causes fluid and electrolyte imbalances, leading to the classic symptoms of diabetes: polyuria, polydipsia, and polyphagia.

Polyuria is frequent and excessive urination and results from an osmotic diuresis caused by excess glucose in the urine. As a result of diuresis, sodium, chloride, and potassium are excreted in the urine and water loss is severe. Dehydration results, and polydipsia (excessive thirst) occurs. Because the cells receive no glucose, cell starvation triggers polyphagia (excessive eating). Despite eating vast amounts of food, the person remains in starvation until insulin is available to move glucose into the cells.

With insulin deficiency, fats break down, releasing free fatty acids. Conversion of fatty acids to ketone bodies (small acids) provides a backup energy source. Because ketone bodies, or "ketones," are abnormal breakdown products of fatty acids, they collect in the blood when insulin is not available, leading to metabolic acidosis.

The dehydration that occurs with diabetes leads to hemoconcentration (an increased blood concentration), hypovolemia (a decreased blood volume), hyperviscosity (thick, concentrated blood), poor tissue perfusion, and hypoxia (poor tissue oxygenation), especially to the brain. Hypoxic cells do not metabolize glucose efficiently, the Krebs' cycle is blocked, and lactic acid increases, causing more acidosis.

The excess acids caused by absence of insulin increase hydrogen ion (H^+) and carbon dioxide (CO_2) levels in the blood, causing metabolic acidosis. These products trigger the respiratory centers of the brain to increase the rate and depth of respiration in an attempt to excrete more carbon dioxide and acid. This type of breathing is known as Kussmaul respiration. Acetone is exhaled, giving the breath a "fruity" odor. When the lungs can no longer offset acidosis, the blood pH drops. Arterial blood gas studies show a metabolic acidosis (decreased pH with decreased arterial bicarbonate [HCO_3^-] levels) and compensatory respiratory alkalosis (decreased partial pressure of arterial carbon dioxide [$Paco_2$]).

Insulin lack initially causes potassium depletion. With the increased fluid loss from hyperglycemia, excessive potassium is excreted in the urine, leading to low serum potassium levels. High serum potassium levels may occur in acidosis because of the shift of potassium from inside the cells to the blood. Serum potassium levels in DM, then, may be low (hypokalemia), high (hyperkalemia), or normal, depending on hydration, the severity of acidosis, and the patient's response to treatment. Chapter 14 discusses acid-base balance and acidosis in more detail.

❓ NCLEX EXAMINATION CHALLENGE

Health Promotion and Maintenance

The client newly diagnosed with diabetes asks why he is always so thirsty. What is the nurse's best response?

A. "The extra glucose in the blood increases the blood sodium level, which increases your sense of thirst."

B. "Without insulin, glucose is excreted rather than used in the cells. The loss of glucose directly triggers thirst, especially for sugared drinks."

C. "The extra glucose in the blood makes the blood thicker, which then triggers thirst so that the water you drink will dilute the blood glucose level."

D. "Without insulin, glucose combines with blood cholesterol, which damages the kidneys, making you feel thirsty even when no water has been lost."

Acute Complications of Diabetes

Three glucose-related emergencies can occur in patients with diabetes:

- Diabetic ketoacidosis (DKA) caused by lack of insulin and ketosis
- Hyperglycemic-hyperosmolar state (HHS) caused by insulin deficiency and profound dehydration
- Hypoglycemia from too much insulin or too little glucose

All three problems require emergency treatment and can be fatal if treatment is delayed or incorrect. These problems and their interventions are described later.

Chronic Complications of Diabetes

Diabetes mellitus (DM) can lead to health problems and early death because of changes in large blood vessels (macrovascular) and small blood vessels (microvascular) in tissues and organs. Complications result from poor tissue circulation and cell death. Macrovascular complications, including coronary heart disease, cerebrovascular disease, and peripheral

vascular disease, lead to increased early death. Microvascular complications of blood vessel structure and function lead to nephropathy (kidney dysfunction), neuropathy (nerve dysfunction), and retinopathy (vision problems). Explanations for these diabetic vascular complications include:

- Chronic hyperglycemia thickens basement membranes, which causes organ damage.
- Glucose toxicity directly or indirectly affects functional cell integrity.
- Chronic ischemia in small blood vessels causes connective tissue hypoxia and microischemia.

Chronic high blood glucose levels are the main cause of microvascular complications and allow premature development of macrovascular complications. Additional risk factors that contribute to poor health outcomes for people with DM include smoking, physical inactivity, increased body weight, hypertension, and excessive blood levels of cholesterol and other fats. Many of these factors can be modified to reduced complications related to DM.

The Diabetes Control and Complications Trial (DCCT) showed that hyperglycemia is a critical factor for long-term complications in patients with type 1 DM. Intensive therapy aiming for blood glucose levels as close to normal as possible delays the onset and progression of retinopathy, nephropathy, neuropathy, and macrovascular disease. Additional studies show that intensive therapy with lowered blood glucose levels delays the onset of retinopathy, nephropathy, and neuropathy in patients with type 2 DM. A strong relationship exists between microvascular complications and blood glucose levels. For every percentage point decrease in HbA_{1c} (hemoglobin A_{1c}), a 35% reduction in the risk for kidney and eye complications has been shown.

Macrovascular Complications

Cardiovascular Disease. Diabetes mellitus (DM) is associated with a reduced life span, largely as a result of cardiovascular disease (CVD). Most patients with DM die as a result of a thrombotic event, usually myocardial infarction (MI). DM also affects the heart muscle, causing both systolic and diastolic heart failure. Left ventricular dysfunction with heart failure and fatal cardiac dysrhythmias are more common after MI in patients with DM.

Patients with diabetes, those with prediabetes, and those with metabolic syndrome are at increased risk for CVD. This excess risk affects women to a greater degree than men and is influenced by the patient's ethnic group. The Adult Treatment Panel III of the National Cholesterol Education Program recommends that diabetes be considered a "coronary heart disease risk equivalent" and a target for aggressive reduction of risk factors.

Patients with DM often also have the traditional cardiovascular risk factors of obesity, hypertension, dyslipidemia, and sedentary lifestyle. Cigarette smoking and a positive family history greatly increase risk for CVD. Kidney disease, indicated by albuminuria (presence of albumin in the urine), increases the risk for coronary heart disease and mortality from MI. Patients with DM often have higher levels of C-reactive protein (CRP), an acute-phase inflammatory marker associated with increased risk for cardiovascular problems and death.

Cardiovascular complication rates can be reduced through aggressive management of hyperglycemia, hypertension, and hyperlipidemia. The American Diabetes Association (ADA) recommends that blood pressure be maintained below 130/80 mm Hg and that low-density lipoprotein (LDL) cholesterol remain below 100 mg/dL (2.60 mmol/L) for patients without manifestations of CVD and to less than 70 mg/dL (1.8 mmol/L) for patients with manifestations of CVD (ADA, 2010b). Diets high in saturated fat raise total cholesterol and LDL cholesterol levels, which increase the risk for coronary artery disease. Lifestyle modifications that focus on reducing saturated fat, *trans* fat, and cholesterol intake; increasing intake of omega-3 fatty acids, fiber, and plant sterols; weight loss (if indicated); and increasing physical activity are recommended to improve the lipid profile for patients with DM (ADA, 2010b).

Priority nursing actions focus on interventions to reduce modifiable risk factors associated with CVD, such as smoking cessation, diet, exercise, blood pressure control, maintenance of prescribed aspirin use, and maintenance of prescribed lipid-lowering drug therapy.

Cerebrovascular Disease. The risk for stroke is 2 to 4 times higher in people with DM compared with those who do not have the disease. Diabetes also increases the likelihood of severe carotid atherosclerosis. Hypertension, hyperlipidemia, nephropathy, peripheral vascular disease, and alcohol and tobacco use further increase the risk for stroke in people with DM.

DM affects stroke outcomes as well. Patients with DM are likely to suffer irreversible brain damage with carotid emboli that produce only transient ischemic attacks in people without DM. Elevated blood glucose levels at the time of the stroke may lead to greater brain injury and higher mortality.

In addition, chronic hyperglycemia with microvascular disease may contribute to neuronal damage, brain atrophy, and cognitive impairment. These problems are more frequent and more severe in patients who have longer-duration DM and an increase in the complications of neuropathy and retinopathy (Roberts et al., 2008).

Microvascular Complications

Eye and Vision Complications. Legal blindness (a corrected visual acuity of 20/200 or less) is 25 times more common in patients with diabetes. Diabetic retinopathy (DR) is strongly related to the duration of diabetes. After 20 years of DM, nearly all patients with type 1 disease and most with type 2 disease have some degree of retinopathy. Unfortunately, DR has few manifestations until vision loss occurs.

The cause and progression of DR are related to problems that block retinal blood vessels and cause them to leak, leading to retinal hypoxia. Nonproliferative diabetic retinopathy (Fig. 67-2) causes structural problems in retinal vessels, including areas of poor retinal circulation, edema, hard fatty deposits in the eye, and retinal hemorrhages. Microaneurysms are small capillary wall dilations in retinal vessels that form throughout the eye and leak fluid and blood into the retina. This leakage causes retinal edema and hard exudates.

Other retinal problems include retinal hemorrhages, optic nerve atrophy from hypoxia, and venous beading. Venous beading is the abnormal appearance of retinal veins in which areas of swelling and constriction along a segment of vein resemble links of sausage. It occurs in areas of retinal ischemia. Nonproliferative diabetic retinopathies develop slowly and rarely cause reduced vision to the point of blindness.

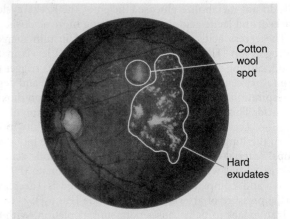

FIG. 67-2 Select ophthalmic changes seen in nonproliferative diabetic retinopathy.

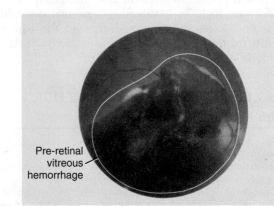

FIG. 67-3 Ophthalmic hemorrhage that is possible with proliferative diabetic retinopathy.

Proliferative diabetic retinopathy is the growth of new retinal blood vessels, also known as *neovascularization*. When retinal blood flow is poor and hypoxia develops, retinal cells secrete growth factors that stimulate formation of new blood vessels in the eye. These new vessels are thin, fragile, and bleed easily, leading to eye hemorrhage and vision loss (Fig. 67-3).

Vision loss from DR has several mechanisms. Central vision may be impaired by macular edema, which can occur at any stage of DR. Diabetic macular edema is characterized by increased blood vessel permeability and deposits of hard exudates at the center of the retina. This problem is the main cause of vision loss in the person with DM. Vision loss also occurs from macular degeneration, corneal scarring, and changes in lens shape or clarity.

Hyperglycemia may cause blurred vision, even with eyeglasses. Hypoglycemia may cause double vision. Cataracts occur at a younger age and progress faster among patients with DM. Open-angle glaucoma also is more common in patients with DM. The management of cataracts and glaucoma is the same as for patients who do not have diabetes (see Chapter 49).

Control of blood glucose, blood pressure, and blood lipid level is important in preventing DR. Thus patients with DM

TABLE 67-3	FEATURES OF DIABETIC NEUROPATHY	
	COMPLICATION	**MANIFESTATION**
Diffuse Neuropathies		
Distal symmetric polyneuropathy	Sensory alterations	Paresthesias: burning/tingling sensations, starting in toes and moving up legs
		Dysesthesias: burning, stinging, or stabbing pain
		Anesthesia: loss of sensation
	Motor alterations in intrinsic muscles of foot	Foot deformities: high arch, claw toes, hammertoes; shift of weight-bearing to metatarsal heads and tips of toes
Autonomic neuropathy	Anhidrosis	Drying, cracking of skin
	Gastrointestinal	Delayed gastric emptying, gastric retention, early satiety, bloating, nausea, vomiting, anorexia, constipation, diarrhea
	Neurogenic bladder	Atonic bladder, urinary retention
	Impotence	Erectile dysfunction
	Cardiovascular autonomic neuropathy	Early fatigue, weakness with exercise, orthostatic hypotension
	Defective counterregulation	Loss of warning signs of hypoglycemia
Focal Neuropathies		
Focal ischemia	Thoracolumbar radiculopathy with sensory and reflex loss	Pain radiating across back, side, and front of chest or abdomen
	Cranial nerve palsies, third and sixth nerves	Sudden diplopia or ptosis; eye pain
	Amyotrophy	Pain; asymmetric weakness; wasting of iliopsoas, quadriceps, and adductor muscles
Entrapment neuropathies	Median nerve	Carpal tunnel syndrome
	Popliteal nerve/knee	Footdrop
	Posterior tibial nerve at tarsal tunnel	Tarsal tunnel syndrome: sensory impairment in sole of foot; weakness of intrinsic muscles of foot; burning pain and paresthesias at ankle and plantar surface

should have routine ophthalmic evaluations to detect vision problems early before vision loss occurs.

CONSIDERATIONS FOR OLDER ADULTS

The older patient with diabetic retinopathy also has visual changes from aging. As a result, the patient's ability to perform self-care may be seriously affected. The patient with retinopathy may have blurred vision, distorted central vision, fluctuating vision, loss of color perception, and mobility problems resulting from loss of depth perception. It is especially important to assess the patient's ability to measure and inject insulin and to monitor blood glucose levels to determine if adaptive devices are needed to assist in self-management activities.

Diabetic Neuropathy. Neuropathy is a progressive deterioration of nerves that results in loss of nerve function. It is a common complication of DM and often involves all parts of the body. Damage to sensory nerve fibers results in either pain or loss of sensation. Damage to motor nerve fibers results in muscle weakness. Damage to nerve fibers in the autonomic nervous system can cause dysfunction in every part of the body. This combination of factors leads to the nerve damage in diabetic neuropathy (Bedlack, 2009):

- Metabolic factors of hyperglycemia, long duration of DM, hyperlipidemia, low insulin levels
- Damaged blood vessels leading to reduced neuronal oxygen and other nutrients
- Autoimmune neuronal inflammation
- Increased genetic susceptibility to nerve damage
- Smoking and alcohol use

Hyperglycemia leads to neuropathy through blood vessel changes that cause nerve hypoxia. Both the axon and its myelin sheath are damaged by reduced blood flow, resulting in blocked nerve impulse transmission. Excessive glucose is converted to sorbitol, which collects in nerves. The increased sorbitol also impairs motor nerve conduction. Common diabetic neuropathies are listed in Table 67-3. Autonomic nervous system neuropathy leads to problems in cardiovascular, GI, and urinary function. Keeping blood glucose levels in the normal range can slow the development and progression of diabetic neuropathies.

Diabetic neuropathy can be focal or diffuse, each with different causes and rates of progression. *Diffuse neuropathies* are the most common neuropathies in DM and involve widespread nerve function loss. They have a slow onset, affect both sides of the body, involve motor and sensory nerves, progress slowly, are permanent, and include autonomic nerve dysfunction. Late complications include foot ulcers and deformities.

Focal neuropathies affect a single nerve or nerve group and usually are caused by an acute ischemic event or by nerve trapping. Both problems lead to nerve damage or nerve death. Ischemic neuropathies occur when the blood supply to a nerve or nerve group is disrupted. The symptoms begin suddenly, affect only one side of the body area, and are self-limiting. Recovery time varies. The most common neuropathies affect the nerves that control the eye muscles. Manifestations begin with pain on one side of the face near the affected eye. The eye muscles become paralyzed, resulting in double vision. The problem usually resolves in 2 to 3 months.

Entrapment neuropathies stem from trapping and compressing a nerve in a body compartment or between tissues. Symptoms begin gradually and can occur anywhere. They may be bilateral, having a waxing and waning course without spontaneous recovery. An example of focal entrapment neuropathy is carpal tunnel syndrome.

Cardiovascular autonomic neuropathy (CAN) affects sympathetic and parasympathetic nerves of the heart and blood vessels. This problem contributes to left ventricular dysfunction, painless myocardial infarctions, and exercise intolerance. Most often, CAN leads to orthostatic (postural) hypotension and syncope (brief loss of consciousness on standing). These problems are due to failure of the heart and arteries to adjust to position changes by increasing heart rate and vascular tone. As a result, blood flow to the brain is interrupted briefly. Orthostatic hypotension and syncope increase the risk for falls, especially among older adults.

Autonomic neuropathy can affect the entire GI system. Common GI problems from diabetic neuropathy include gastroesophageal reflex, delayed gastric emptying and gastric retention, early satiety, heartburn, nausea, vomiting, and anorexia. Sluggish movement of the small intestine can lead to bacterial overgrowth, which causes bloating, gas, and diarrhea. Diarrhea caused by diabetes is chronic, may be severe, and often occurs at night. Constipation, the most common GI problem with DM, is intermittent and may alternate with bouts of diarrhea. Gastroparesis (delay in gastric emptying) is a cause of hypoglycemia.

Urinary problems from neuropathy results in incomplete emptying and urine retention, which leads to urinary infection and kidney problems. Manifestations include frequency, urgency, and incontinence.

Diabetic Nephropathy. Nephropathy is a pathologic change in the kidney that reduces kidney function and leads to kidney failure. Diabetes is the leading cause of end-stage kidney disease (ESKD) and kidney failure in the United States. Risk factors for nephropathy include a 10- to 15-year history of DM, diabetic retinopathy, poor blood glucose control, uncontrolled hypertension, and genetic predisposition. Studies have shown that the onset of diabetic kidney disease may be prevented and the progression to ESKD can be delayed by maintaining optimum blood glucose control, keeping blood pressure within the normal ranges, and using drug therapy to protect the kidneys (American Association of Diabetic Educators [AADE], 2009a). Drugs that protect the kidneys are the angiotensin-converting enzyme (ACE) inhibitors and the angiotensin receptor blockers (ARBs).

Kidney disease causes progressive albumin excretion and a declining glomerular filtration rate (GFR). The earliest manifestation of nephropathy is microalbuminuria (small amounts of albumin in the urine). Annual testing for microalbuminuria is recommended for patients who have had type 1 DM for at least 5 years and in everyone with type 2 DM (ADA, 2010b).

Chronic high blood glucose levels cause hypertension in kidney blood vessels and excess kidney perfusion. The increased pressure damages the kidney in many ways. The blood vessels become leakier, especially in the glomerulus. This leakiness allows filtration of larger particles (including albumin and other proteins), which then form deposits in the kidney tissue and blood vessels. Blood vessels narrow, decreasing kidney oxygenation and leading to kidney cell hypoxia and cell death. These processes worsen over time, with scarring of glomerular blood vessels and loss of urine filtration ability, leading to kidney failure.

Kidney damage is also related to hypertension for patients with DM and cardiovascular disease. Both systolic and diastolic hypertension speed the progression of diabetic nephropathy.

Male Erectile Dysfunction. Erectile dysfunction (ED) is the inability to achieve or maintain a penile erection sufficient for satisfactory sexual performance. ED occurs at a higher rate (about 50%) and an earlier age among men with DM as compared with the general population. This occurs 10 to 15 years earlier than in the general population and increases with age. It is related to poor blood glucose control, obesity, hypertension, heavy cigarette smoking, and the presence of other chronic vascular complications. Chapter 75 discusses erectile function problems in depth.

? NCLEX EXAMINATION CHALLENGE

Physiological Integrity

Why is controlling blood glucose levels important?
A. High blood glucose levels increase the risk for heart disease, strokes, blindness, and kidney failure.
B. High blood glucose levels increase the risk for seizure disorders, arthritis, osteoporosis, and bone fractures.
C. Low blood glucose levels increase the risk for peripheral neuropathy, Alzheimer's disease, and premature aging.
D. Low blood glucose levels increase the risk for obesity, pancreatitis, dehydration, and certain types of cancer.

Etiology and Genetic Risk

Type 1 Diabetes

Type 1 diabetes mellitus (DM) is an autoimmune disorder in which beta cells are destroyed in a genetically susceptible person (Table 67-4). The immune system fails to recognize normal body cells as "self" and takes destructive actions against them. In type 1 DM, immune system cells, mediators, and antibodies attack and destroy insulin-secreting cells in the islets. Although the exact cause of why normal cells are attacked by immune system cells is not known, people with certain tissue types are more likely to develop autoimmune diseases, including type 1 DM. Specifically, patients who have the tissue types *HLA-DR* or *HLA-DQ* are at an increased risk for type 1 DM. Certain viral infections, such as mumps and coxsackievirus infection, appear to trigger autoimmune destruction of pancreatic beta cells (McCance et al., 2010).

Indicators or markers of immune damage to insulin-producing cells (a key feature of type 1 DM) are the presence of blood antibodies directed against the beta cells themselves or against substances made by beta cells. Most patients with type 1 diabetes have islet cell antibodies (ICAs), insulin

---

GENETIC/GENOMIC CONSIDERATIONS

Risk for type 1 diabetes is determined by inheritance of genes coding for the *HLA-DR* and *HLA-DQ* tissue types. However, although inheritance of these genes increases the risk, most people with these genes do not develop type 1 diabetes. Development of the disease is an interactive effect of genetic predisposition and exposure to certain environmental factors. The risk for type 1 diabetes in the general population ranges from 1 in 400 to 1 in 1000. The risk greatly increases for those who have at least one parent with diabetes (from 1 in 20 to 1 in 50) (Nussbaum et al., 2007). It is unclear why some genetically susceptible people develop diabetes and others do not.

TABLE 67-4   DIFFERENTIATION OF TYPE 1 AND TYPE 2 DIABETES

FEATURES	TYPE 1	TYPE 2
Former names	Juvenile-onset diabetes	Adult-onset diabetes
	Ketosis-prone diabetes	Ketosis-resistant diabetes
	Insulin-dependent diabetes mellitus (IDDM)	Non–insulin-dependent diabetes mellitus (NIDDM)
Age at onset	Usually younger than 30 yr, occurs at any age	Peaks in 50s; may occur earlier
Symptoms	Abrupt onset, thirst, hunger, increased urine output, weight loss	Frequently none; thirst, fatigue, blurred vision, vascular or neural complications
Etiology	Viral infection	Not known
Pathology	Pancreatic beta-cell destruction	Insulin resistance Dysfunctional pancreatic beta cell
Antigen patterns	*HLA-DR, HLA-DQ*	None
Antibodies	ICAs present at diagnosis	None
Endogenous insulin and C-peptide	None	Low, normal, or high
Inheritance	Complex	Dominant, multifactorial
Nutritional status	Usually nonobese	60% to 80% obese
Insulin	All dependent on insulin	Required for 20% to 30%
Medical nutrition therapy	Mandatory	Mandatory

ICAs, Islet cell antibodies.

autoantibodies (IAAs), autoantibodies to glutamic acid decarboxylase (GAD), or autoantibodies to tyrosine phosphates. Circulating ICA and IAA may be present before manifestations of type 1 DM develop.

Type 2 Diabetes and Metabolic Syndrome

Type 2 DM is a progressive disorder in which the person has a combination of insulin resistance and decreased secretion of insulin by pancreatic beta cells. Insulin resistance (a reduced ability of cells to respond to insulin) develops from obesity and physical inactivity in a genetically susceptible person. Insulin resistance occurs before the onset of type 2 DM and often is accompanied by other cardiovascular risk factors of hyperlipidemia, hypertension, and increased clot formation. Most patients with type 2 DM are obese. With the increased rate of obesity occurring in younger people, the age of onset for type 2 DM is also decreasing. The specific causes of type 2 DM are not known, although insulin resistance and beta-cell failure have many genetic and nongenetic causes. Heredity plays a major role in the development of type 2 DM. Offspring of patients with type 2 DM have a 15% chance for developing the disease and a 30% risk for having impaired glucose tolerance. Specific gene defects have been identified in certain groups with high incidence rates of type 2 DM (Nussbaum et al., 2007).

Metabolic syndrome, also called *syndrome X,* is the simultaneous presence of metabolic factors known to increase risk for developing type 2 DM and cardiovascular disease. Features of the syndrome include:

- Abdominal obesity: waist circumference of 40 inches (100 cm) or more for men and 35 inches (88 cm) or more for women
- Hyperglycemia: fasting blood glucose level of 100 mg/dL or more or on drug treatment for elevated glucose
- Hypertension: systolic BP of 130 mm Hg or more or diastolic BP of 85 mg Hg or more or on drug treatment for hypertension
- Hyperlipidemia: triglyceride level of 150 mg/dL or more or on drug treatment for elevated triglycerides; high-density lipoprotein (HDL) cholesterol less than 40 mg/dL for men or less than 50 mg/dL for women

Any one of these health problems increases the rate of atherosclerosis and the risk for stroke, coronary heart disease, and early death. Teach patients about the lifestyle changes that can improve health. Reducing weight to within 20% of ideal or body mass index to less than 25 kg/m² by modifying diet and exercising more will reduce cardiovascular risk. Drug therapy may be required to achieve desired lipid and blood pressure outcomes.

Incidence/Prevalence

More than 57 million American adults have prediabetes, defined as impaired fasting glucose (IFG) or impaired glucose tolerance (IGT). IFG (fasting plasma glucose levels of 100 mg/dL [5.6 mmol/L] to 125 mg/dL [6.9 mmol/L]) and IGT (2-hr oral glucose tolerance values of 140 mg/dL [7.8 mmol/L] to 199 mg/dL [11.0 mmol/L]) are considered risk factors for diabetes and for cardiovascular disease. Over a 3- to 5-year period, people with prediabetes have a fivefold to fifteenfold higher risk for developing type 2 DM than do those with normal blood glucose levels. IFG and IGT are associated with obesity (especially abdominal or central obesity), dyslipidemia with high triglycerides and/or low HDL cholesterol, and hypertension (AADE, 2009b).

The Diabetes Prevention Trial demonstrated that changes in physical activity and eating habits (primarily reduced calories from fat) resulting in weight loss were associated with reduced diabetes risk. Encourage the person with prediabetes to adopt healthy eating habits that limit caloric and fat intake sufficient for weight reduction and to participate in physical activity in order to sustain weight loss.

Diabetes is the seventh leading cause of death in the United States, where it affects 25.8 million people, or 8.3% of the population. An additional 7.0 million people are unaware they have the disease (ADA, 2011).

About 90% of people with diabetes have type 2 DM. It is diagnosed most often among middle-aged and older adults, affecting about 9.6% of patients ages 20 to 59 years and 20.9% of patients ages 60 years or older. The prevalence of diabetes is higher for men than for women (ADA, 2011).

Although type 2 diabetes is a disease of middle-aged and older adults, recent surveys show an increase of the disorder in childhood and adolescence as a result of obesity. Because the prevalence of obesity is rising in North America, diabetes will become even more common. Obesity and a higher-than-normal body mass index (BMI) greatly increase the risk for diabetes.

HEALTH PROMOTION AND MAINTENANCE

Diabetes is a common disorder causing many preventable but devastating complications and is a major public health problem. Control of diabetes and its complications is a major focus for health promotion activities. No interventions are successful in preventing type 1 DM. Health promotion for patients with type 1 DM focuses on controlling hyperglycemia to reduce its long-term complications.

Adopting a low-calorie diet that results in weight loss and increasing physical activity have been shown to improve metabolic and cardiac risk factors. These improvements include reducing hypertension, increasing heart rate variability between resting rate and exercise rate, lowering triglyceride levels, increasing high-density lipoprotein cholesterol (the "good" cholesterol) levels, and reducing low-density lipoprotein cholesterol (the "bad" cholesterol) levels. These changes reduce the incidence of type 2 DM in older adults by 58% (Mozaffarian et al., 2009).

Teach all patients with DM that tight control of blood glucose levels can prevent many complications. Urge all patients with DM to regularly follow up with their health care provider or endocrinologist, to have their eyes and vision tested yearly by an ophthalmologist, and to have urine microalbumin levels assessed yearly. Early detection of changes in the eye or kidney permits adjustments in treatment regimens that can slow or halt progression of retinopathy and

---

🌐 CULTURAL AWARENESS

Diabetes is a significant health problem for African Americans, American Indians, and Mexican Americans. The increase in obesity and sedentary lifestyles in the U.S. population is the probable cause of this growing problem. The ADA has identified patients who should be tested for diabetes in Table 67-5.

Racial and ethnic differences affect clinical outcomes for patients with diabetes. The prevalence of hypertension in patients with diabetes is at least twice the rate of patients who do not have diabetes, with non-Hispanic whites and African Americans having the highest prevalence. Microvascular complications of the eyes, nerves, and kidneys are more common in African Americans and American Indians with diabetes than in non-Hispanic whites with diabetes. Possible factors for these differences include lack of access to health care, lifestyle issues, mistrust of the health care system, reduced financial resources, and lack of knowledge about the relationship between glucose control and complications.

❓ NCLEX EXAMINATION CHALLENGE

Health Promotion and Maintenance

The client newly diagnosed with type 2 diabetes asks how diabetes type 1 and diabetes type 2 are different. What is the nurse's best response?
A. "Diabetes type 1 develops in people younger than 40 years and diabetes type 2 develops only in older people."
B. "Diabetes type 2 develops in people younger than 40 years and diabetes type 1 develops only in older people."
C. "Patients with type 1 diabetes are at higher risk for obesity and heart disease, whereas patients with type 2 diabetes are at higher risk for strokes."
D. "Patients with type 1 diabetes produce no insulin and patients with type 2 diabetes produce insulin but their insulin receptors are not very sensitive to it."

TABLE 67-5   INDICATIONS FOR TESTING INDIVIDUALS FOR TYPE 2 DIABETES

- Testing for diabetes should be considered in people 45 years of age and older, particularly in those with a BMI greater than 25 kg/m². If normal, it should be repeated at 3-year intervals.
- Testing should be considered at a younger age or be carried out more frequently in people who are overweight (BMI >25 kg/m²) and have these additional associated factors:
  - Have a first-degree relative with diabetes
  - Are habitually physically inactive
  - Are members of a high-risk ethnic population (e.g., African American, Hispanic American, American Indian, Asian American, or Pacific Islander)
  - Deliver a baby weighing more than 9 pounds or have been diagnosed with GDM
  - Are hypertensive (>140/90 mm Hg)
  - Have a high-density lipoprotein (HDL) cholesterol level less than 35 mg/dL (0.90 mmol/L) and/or a triglyceride level greater than 250 mg/dL (2.82 mmol/L)
  - Have polycystic ovary syndrome
  - Have IFG or IGT on previous testing
  - Have a history of vascular disease

Data from American Diabetes Association (ADA). (2010a). Position statement: Diagnosis and classification of diabetes mellitus. *Diabetes Care, 33*(Suppl. 1), 14. *BMI*, Body mass index; *GDM*, gestational diabetes mellitus; *IFG*, impaired fasting glucose; *IGT*, impaired glucose tolerance.

---

nephropathy. Encourage all people to maintain weight within an appropriate range for height and body build and to engage in physical activity at least three times per week.

PATIENT-CENTERED COLLABORATIVE CARE

ASSESSMENT

History

Ask questions about risk factors and symptoms related to diabetes. Age is important because type 2 diabetes mellitus (DM) is more common in older patients, especially among African Americans and Mexican Americans. Ask women how large their children were at birth, because many women who develop type 2 DM had gestational diabetes or were glucose intolerant during pregnancy. These women often have given birth to infants weighing 9 pounds or more.

Assessing weight and weight change is important, because excess weight and obesity are risk factors for type 2 DM. The patient with type 1 DM often has weight loss with increased appetite during the weeks before diagnosis. For both types of DM, patients usually have fatigue, polyuria, and polydipsia. Ask about recent major or minor infections. In particular, ask women about frequent vaginal yeast infections. Ask all patients whether they have noticed that small skin injuries become infected more easily or take longer to heal. Also ask whether they have noticed any changes in vision or in the sense of touch.

Laboratory Assessment

Diagnosis of Diabetes. Diabetes can be diagnosed by assessing blood glucose levels. The ADA defines normal blood glucose values in Chart 67-1. ADA criteria for the diagnosis of type 2 DM are outlined in Table 67-6. A test result

CHART 67-1 LABORATORY PROFILE

Blood Glucose Values

TEST	NORMAL RANGE FOR ADULTS	SIGNIFICANCE OF ABNORMAL RESULTS
Fasting blood glucose test	<100 mg/dL (5.6 mmol/L) Older adults: Levels rise 1 mg/dL per decade of age	Levels >100 mg/dL (5.6 mmol/L) but <126 mg/dL (7.0 mmol/L) indicate impaired fasting glucose (IFG). Levels >126 mg/dL (7.0 mmol/L) obtained on at least two occasions are diagnostic of diabetes, even in older adults.
Glucose tolerance test (2-hr post-load result)	<140 mg/dL (7.8 mmol/L)	Levels >140 mg/dL (7.8 mmol/L) and <200 mg/dL (11.1 mmol/L) indicate impaired glucose tolerance (IGT). Levels >200 mg/dL (11.1 mmol/L) indicate provisional diagnosis of diabetes.
Glycosylated hemoglobin (hemoglobin A$_{1c}$ [HbA$_{1c}$]) test	4%-6%	Levels >8% indicate poor diabetic control and need for adherence to regimen or changes in therapy.

Data from American Diabetes Association (ADA). (2010a). Position statement: Diagnosis and classification of diabetes mellitus. *Diabetes Care, 33*(Suppl. 1), 42-47; American Diabetes Association (ADA). (2010b). Position statement: Standards of medical care in diabetes—2010. *Diabetes Care, 33*(Suppl. 1), 11-61.

TABLE 67-6 CRITERIA FOR THE DIAGNOSIS OF TYPE 2 DIABETES

A$_{1c}$ 6.5%. The test should be performed in a laboratory using a method that is NGSP certified and standardized to the DCCT assay.
Or
Fasting plasma glucose greater than 126 mg/dL (7.0 mmol/L). *Fasting* is defined as no caloric intake for at least 8 hr.
Or
2-hr plasma glucose greater than 200 mg/dL (11.1 mmol/L) during an oral glucose tolerance test. The test should be performed using a glucose load containing the equivalent of 75 g anhydrous glucose dissolved in water.
Or
In a patient with classic manifestations of hyperglycemia or hyperglycemic crisis, a casual blood glucose concentration greater than 200 mg/dL (11.1 mmol/L). *Casual* is defined as any time of the day without regard to time since last meal. The classic manifestations of diabetes include polyuria, polydipsia, and unexplained weight loss.

NOTE: In the absence of unequivocal hyperglycemia, the first three criteria should be confirmed by repeat testing.

Data from American Diabetes Association (ADA). (2010a). Position statement: Diagnosis and classification of diabetes mellitus. *Diabetes Care, 33*(Suppl. 1), 14. *NGSP,* National Glycohemoglobin Standardization Program; *DCCT,* Diabetes Control and Complications Trial.

CHART 67-2 PATIENT AND FAMILY EDUCATION: PREPARING FOR SELF-MANAGEMENT

Blood Glucose Testing

Fasting Blood Glucose
- Do not eat any food or drink any liquid except water for at least 8 hours before the test.

Oral Glucose Tolerance Test
- Eat a balanced diet with carbohydrate intake of at least 150 g for a minimum of 3 days before the test while maintaining normal physical activity.
- Carbohydrate restriction, bedrest, acute illness, and certain drugs interfere with the test. Phenytoin (Dilantin), anovulatory drugs, diuretics, nicotinic acid, and glucocorticoids adversely affect results.
- The test is performed in the morning after a 10- to 12-hour fast.
- A fasting blood sample is obtained.
- You will be asked to drink 300 mL of a flavored beverage containing 75 g of glucose within 5 minutes of the fasting blood sample.
- Blood samples are drawn at 30-minute intervals for 2 hours.
- During the test, you will remain at rest and not be able to smoke or drink liquids.

diagnostic of DM should be repeated to rule out laboratory error unless classic manifestations of hyperglycemia or hyperglycemic crisis are also present.

The diagnosis of diabetes mellitus has recently changed to include elevated glycosylated hemoglobin levels. This test was not previously recommended for diagnosing diabetes because of a lack of assay standardization. Glycosylated hemoglobin A$_{1c}$ (HbA$_{1c}$) is a test that measures how much glucose permanently attaches to a specific area of the hemoglobin molecule. Because glucose binds to a variety of proteins (including hemoglobin) through a process called *glycosylation,* the higher the blood glucose level is over time, the more glycosylated hemoglobin becomes. HbA$_{1c}$ testing is now highly standardized for accuracy and precision. The ADA defines HbA$_{1c}$ levels greater than 6.5% as diagnostic of DM (ADA, 2009).

Fasting plasma glucose (FPG) is used to diagnose diabetes in nonpregnant adults. The patient should have no caloric intake for at least 8 hours (water is permitted). The blood sample needs to be obtained before insulin or oral antidiabetic agents have been taken. A diagnosis of diabetes is made with two separate test results greater than 126 mg/dL (7 mmol/L) (ADA, 2010a). Patient and family education about blood glucose testing is presented in Chart 67-2. *Random* or *casual plasma* glucose greater than 200 mg/dL (7.0 mmol/L) is used to diagnose diabetes in patients with severe classic hyperglycemia or hyperglycemic crisis.

Oral glucose tolerance testing (OGTT) is the most sensitive test for the diagnosis of DM. However, it is not routinely used in the diagnosis because it is inconvenient to patients, costly, and time consuming compared with fasting blood glucose measures. The diagnosis of gestational diabetes mellitus (GDM) is based on the oral glucose tolerance test (75-g glucose load, 2-hr test or 100-g glucose load, 3-hr test). Before the test, review instructions from Chart 67-2 with the patient. He or she drinks a beverage containing a glucose load, and blood samples are collected at hourly intervals. Two or more of the plasma levels must be met or exceeded for a diagnosis of DM (ADA, 2010a).

Other blood tests for diabetes can help determine whether a patient has type 1 or type 2 DM, although they are not commonly used. Type 1 DM is an autoimmune disease with the presence of autoantibodies to proteins. The presence of islet cell antibodies (ICAs) is an indicator for type 1 DM. Measurement of C-peptide levels indicates beta secretory function of the pancreas. C-peptide levels correlate well with insulin levels and are used to diagnose type 1 DM.

Screening for Diabetes. Evidence from type 1 DM prevention studies suggests that measurement of islet cell antibodies identifies people who are at risk for developing type 1 DM. Testing to detect prediabetes and type 2 DM should be considered in patients older than 45 years and those defined as overweight (BMI greater than 25 kg/m²). Testing is considered for patients who are younger than 45 years and are overweight if they have additional risk factors for diabetes or have other health problems associated with diabetes. Screening for diabetes is done with hemoglobin A_{1c} levels or either fasting plasma glucose levels or the 2-hour OGTT (75-g glucose load) (ADA, 2010a; ADA, 2010b).

Ongoing Assessment. Glucose can bind to a variety of structures, including proteins, through a process called *glycosylation. Glycosylated hemoglobin assays* are useful because blood glucose permanently attaches to hemoglobin. The higher the blood glucose level is over time, the more glycosylated hemoglobin becomes. Thus glycosylated HbA_{1c} is a good indicator of the average blood glucose levels. Measurement of A_{1c} shows the average blood glucose level during the previous 120 days—the life span of red blood cells. HbA_{1c} testing is used to assess long-term glycemic control, as well as to predict the risk for complications. *Unlike the fasting blood glucose test, HbA_{1c} test results are not altered by eating habits the day before the test.* This testing is performed at diagnosis and at specific intervals to evaluate the treatment plan. Hemolysis, blood loss, and pregnancy all increase red blood cell turnover and reduce HbA_{1c} levels. Triglycerides and bilirubin interfere with the assay, leading to overestimation of A_{1c} levels in patients with hypertriglyceridemia. HbA_{1c} testing is recommended at least twice yearly in patients who are meeting expected treatment outcomes and have stable blood glucose control. Quarterly assessment is recommended for patients whose therapy has changed or who are not meeting prescribed glycemic levels (ADA, 2010a). Table 67-7 shows the correlation between HbA_{1c} and mean blood glucose levels.

When glucose binds to amino groups on serum proteins, especially albumin, the glycosylated protein product is called *fructosamine.* This product increases with elevated blood glucose levels in the same way as hemoglobin does. However, because serum proteins and albumin turn over in 14 days, compared with 120 days for red blood cells, these proteins can indicate blood glucose control over a shorter period. These measures are useful when tight control of blood glucose is necessary (e.g., pregnancy), in short-term follow-up of treatment changes, or in patients with hemoglobin abnormalities in which HbA_{1c} is not an accurate reflection of glucose control. Available tests are called *glycosylated serum albumin (GSA), glycosylated serum protein (GSP),* and *fructosamine.*

Urine Tests. Ketone bodies are a product of fat metabolism. The presence of moderate to high urine ketones (hyperketonuria) indicates a severe lack of insulin. Hyperketonuria

TABLE 67-7	CORRELATION BETWEEN HBA₁c LEVEL AND MEAN PLASMA GLUCOSE LEVELS	
	MEAN PLASMA GLUCOSE	
HBA₁c (%)	**MG/DL**	**MMOL/L**
6	126	7.0
7	154	8.6
8	183	10.2
9	212	11.8
10	240	13.4
11	269	14.9
12	298	16.5

Data from American Diabetes Association (ADA). (2010b). Position statement: Standards of medical care in diabetes—2010. *Diabetes Care, 33*(Suppl. 1), 19. *HbA₁c,* Hemoglobin A₁c.

in the presence of hyperglycemia is a medical emergency that, when detected early, can be treated with insulin and careful monitoring. Urine testing for ketones should be performed during acute illness or stress, when blood glucose levels consistently exceed 300 mg/dL (16.7 mmol/L), during pregnancy, or when any symptoms of ketoacidosis are present. Ketone testing also is recommended for patients with diabetes participating in a weight-loss program. Hyperketonuria without hyperglycemia suggests that weight loss is occurring without disrupting blood glucose control.

Ketone bodies include beta-hydroxybutyric acid, acetoacetic acid, and acetone. They appear in urine in the same proportion as they do in blood but are affected by urine volume and concentration. Ketones are variably reabsorbed by the kidney tubules and may be present in urine long after blood levels have returned to normal. For these reasons, urine ketone bodies are not used to evaluate the effectiveness of treatment for ketoacidosis.

Tests for kidney function are important because the presence of urine protein without kidney symptoms may indicate microvascular changes in the kidney. Urine albumin excretion rates of 20 to 200 g/min (30 to 300 mg/hr) indicate microalbuminuria. Even minor elevations of albumin are associated with increased mortality.

Once clinical proteinuria has been detected, kidney function (e.g., glomerular filtration rate) is assessed by creatinine clearance tests (see Chapter 68). In patients with nephropathy, a rise in serum creatinine level is related to both poor blood glucose control and hypertension.

Urine glucose testing is an indirect measurement of blood glucose and is much less precise than blood glucose testing. Fluid intake, urine elimination patterns, and certain drugs affect the results. This test may be appropriate for a quick screening but should not be used for monitoring diabetes management.

ANALYSIS

Priority problems for patients with diabetes are:
1. Potential for injury related to hyperglycemia
2. Potential for impaired wound healing related to endocrine and vascular effects of diabetes
3. Potential for injury related to diabetic neuropathy
4. Pain related to diabetic neuropathy

5. Potential for injury related to diabetic retinopathy–induced reduced vision
6. Potential for kidney disease related to impaired renal circulation
7. Potential for hypoglycemia
8. Potential for diabetic ketoacidosis
9. Potential for hyperglycemic-hyperosmolar state and coma

PLANNING AND IMPLEMENTATION

The management of diabetes mellitus (DM) is complex and involves extensive patient education. The Concept Map on p. 1422 highlights care issues for the patient with type 2 DM.

Preventing Injury from Hyperglycemia

Planning: Expected Outcomes. The patient with diabetes is expected to manage DM and prevent disease progression by maintaining blood glucose levels in the expected range. Indicators are that the patient consistently demonstrates these behaviors:

- Performs treatment regimen as prescribed
- Follows recommended diet
- Monitors blood glucose using correct testing procedures
- Manages symptoms of hyperglycemia
- Seeks health care if blood glucose levels fluctuate outside of recommended parameters
- Meets recommended activity levels
- Uses drugs as prescribed
- Maintains optimum weight
- Problem-solves about barriers to self-management

Interventions

Nonsurgical Management. Nonsurgical management of diabetes mellitus (DM) involves nutritional interventions, blood glucose monitoring, a planned exercise program, and in some instances, drugs to lower blood glucose levels. The nurse, together with the patient, physician, dietitian, pharmacist, case manager, and in some cases, physical therapist, plans, coordinates, and delivers care.

The American Diabetes Association (ADA) has proposed these treatment outcomes for glycosylated hemoglobin (HbA$_{1c}$) and blood glucose levels (ADA, 2010a):

- HbA$_{1c}$ levels are maintained at 7% or below.
- The majority of premeal (preprandial) blood glucose levels are 70 to 130 mg/dL (3.9 to 7.2 mmol/L).
- Peak after-meal (postprandial) blood glucose levels are less than 180 mg/dL (<10.0 mmol/L).

Drug Therapy. Drug therapy is indicated when a patient with type 2 DM does not achieve blood glucose control with diet changes, regular exercise, and stress management. Several categories of drugs are available to lower blood glucose levels. Patients with type 1 DM require insulin therapy for blood glucose control.

Drugs are started at the lowest effective dose and increased every 1 to 2 weeks until the patient reaches desired blood glucose control or the maximum dosage. If the maximum dosage of one agent does not control blood glucose levels, a second agent with a different mechanism of action may be added. Insulin therapy is indicated for the patient with type 2 DM when blood glucose cannot be controlled with the use of two or three different antidiabetic agents.

Antidiabetic drugs are not a substitute for dietary modification and exercise. Teach the patient about the need for continuing dietary restrictions and regular exercise while taking antidiabetic drugs.

Drug Selection. The choice of antidiabetic drug is based on cost, the patient's ability to manage multiple drug dosages, age, and response to the drugs. Shorter-acting drugs (e.g., glipizide) are preferred for older patients, those with irregular eating schedules, and those with liver, kidney, or cardiac function problems. Longer-acting drugs (e.g., glyburide, glimepiride) with once-daily dosing are better for adherence. Beta-cell function in type 2 DM often declines over time, reducing the effectiveness of some drugs. The treatment regimen for a patient with type 2 DM may eventually require insulin therapy either alone or with oral drugs.

Antidiabetic Drugs. Drug therapy is prescribed when dietary control has proven insufficient or if the patient is highly symptomatic. Some antidiabetic drugs are oral agents and others require subcutaneous injection.

Insulin Secretagogues. Insulin secretagogues stimulate insulin release from pancreatic beta cells and are used for patients who are still able to produce insulin. These drugs work by blocking potassium in pancreatic beta cells, which increases the time the beta cells spend in the calcium-release stage of cell signaling. This extra time allows for a higher intracellular calcium level, which then signals each beta cell to release more insulin.

Sulfonylurea Agents. Sulfonylurea agents lower fasting plasma glucose levels by triggering the release of insulin from beta cells. Drugs in this class differ in strength, overall effects, metabolism, and risk for complications (Chart 67-3). First-generation sulfonylurea drugs are seldom used.

Side effects of sulfonylurea agents include weight gain and hypoglycemia. Underweight older adults with cardiovascular, liver, or kidney impairment are more susceptible to hypoglycemia. Many drugs interact with sulfonylureas (Table 67-8).

Meglitinide Analogs. *Meglitinide analogs* are classified as insulin secretagogues and have actions and adverse effects similar to those of sulfonylureas. Repaglinide (Prandin) and Nateglinide (Starlix) were designed to increase meal-related insulin secretion. They are rapidly absorbed and have a short duration of action. Meglitinide analogs lower HbA$_{1c}$ levels by an average of 1.5 percentage points.

Repaglinide (Prandin) is taken before meals, has a rapid onset with a limited duration of action, and is used to treat both fasting and after-meal hyperglycemia. Adverse effects include hypoglycemia, GI disturbances, upper respiratory infections, joint and back pain, and headache.

Nateglinide (Starlix) is rapidly absorbed and stimulates insulin secretion within 20 minutes of ingestion. It is taken just before meals to control mealtime hyperglycemia and improves overall glycemic control in patients with type 2 DM. The major adverse effect is hypoglycemia. Teach patients who skip meals to also skip their scheduled dose of Starlix to reduce the risk for hypoglycemia.

Text continued on page 1428.

Concept Map: Diabetes Mellitus — Type 2

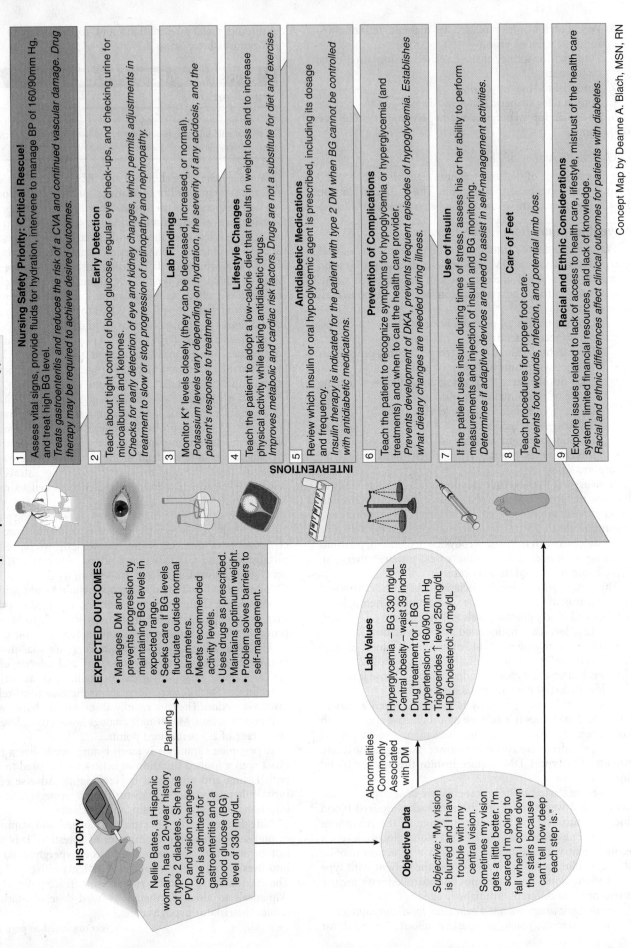

INTERVENTIONS

1 **Nursing Safety Priority: Critical Rescue!**
Assess vital signs, provide fluids for hydration, intervene to manage BP of 160/90mm Hg, and treat high BG level.
Treats gastroenteritis and reduces the risk of a CVA and continued vascular damage. Drug therapy may be required to achieve desired outcomes.

2 **Early Detection**
Teach about tight control of blood glucose, regular eye check-ups, and checking urine for microalbumin and ketones.
Checks for early detection of eye and kidney changes, which permits adjustments in treatment to slow or stop progression of retinopathy and nephropathy.

3 **Lab Findings**
Monitor K+ levels closely (they can be decreased, increased, or normal).
Potassium levels vary depending on hydration, the severity of any acidosis, and the patient's response to treatment.

4 **Lifestyle Changes**
Teach the patient to adopt a low-calorie diet that results in weight loss and to increase physical activity while taking antidiabetic drugs.
Improves metabolic and cardiac risk factors. Drugs are not a substitute for diet and exercise.

5 **Antidiabetic Medications**
Review which insulin or oral hypoglycemic agent is prescribed, including its dosage and frequency.
Insulin therapy is indicated for the patient with type 2 DM when BG cannot be controlled with antidiabetic medications.

6 **Prevention of Complications**
Teach the patient to recognize symptoms for hypoglycemia or hyperglycemia (and treatments) and when to call the health care provider.
Prevents development of DKA, prevents frequent episodes of hypoglycemia. Establishes what dietary changes are needed during illness.

7 **Use of Insulin**
If the patient uses insulin during times of stress, assess his or her ability to perform measurements and injection of insulin and BG monitoring.
Determines if adaptive devices are need to assist in self-management activities.

8 **Care of Feet**
Teach procedures for proper foot care.
Prevents foot wounds, infection, and potential limb loss.

9 **Racial and Ethnic Considerations**
Explore issues related to lack of access to health care, lifestyle, mistrust of the health care system, limited financial resources, and lack of knowledge.
Racial and ethnic differences affect clinical outcomes for patients with diabetes.

Concept Map by Deanne A. Blach, MSN, RN

EXPECTED OUTCOMES
- Manages DM and prevents progression by maintaining BG levels in expected range.
- Seeks care if BG levels fluctuate outside normal parameters.
- Meets recommended activity levels.
- Uses drugs as prescribed.
- Maintains optimum weight.
- Problem solves barriers to self-management.

Planning

HISTORY

Nellie Bates, a Hispanic woman, has a 20-year history of type 2 diabetes. She has PVD and vision changes. She is admitted for gastroenteritis and a blood glucose (BG) level of 330 mg/dL.

Lab Values
- Hyperglycemia – BG 330 mg/dL
- Central obesity – waist 39 inches
- Drug treatment for ↑ BG
- Hypertension: 160/90 mm Hg
- Triglycerides ↑ level 250 mg/dL
- HDL cholesterol: 40 mg/dL

Abnormalities Commonly Associated with DM

Objective Data

Subjective: "My vision is blurred and I have trouble with my central vision. Sometimes my vision gets a little better. I'm scared I'm going to fall when I come down the stairs because I can't tell how deep each step is."

CHART 67-3 COMMON EXAMPLES OF DRUG THERAPY

Diabetes Mellitus

	USE IN DIABETES	NURSING INTERVENTIONS	RATIONALES
Secretagogues			
Second-Generation Sulfonylurea Agents			
Glipizide (Glucotrol) Usual dose: 5-10 mg every 12 hr Glucotrol XL (Extended-release form) 5-20 mg orally once daily	Increase insulin secretion in the treatment of type 2 diabetes.	Teach patients to take the drug 30 min before meals.	Taking the drug 30 min before a meal achieves the best after-meal blood glucose concentration.
		Teach patients how to prevent and treat hypoglycemia.	Because the drug induces insulin secretion, hypoglycemia is possible.
		Monitor patients with impaired kidney function carefully for hypoglycemia.	The drug is eliminated by the kidney. Patients with impaired kidney function have higher blood levels of the drug and are at risk for hypoglycemia.
		Instruct patients to swallow the extended-release form of the drug whole and not divided, chewed, or crushed.	Damaging the extended-release form of the drug causes the rapid release of the entire dose and can cause hypoglycemia.
Glimepiride (Amaryl) Initial dose: 1-2 mg orally once daily Maintenance dose: 1-4 mg orally once daily Maximum dose: 8 mg daily	Used as single therapy or in combination with metformin or insulin in treatment of type 2 diabetes.	Teach patients to take the drug as a single daily dose with the first main meal of the day. Teach patients how to prevent and treat hypoglycemia.	Debilitated or malnourished patients or those with impaired kidney or liver function are more sensitive to blood glucose–lowering effects of glimepiride.
Meglitinide Analogs			
Repaglinide (Prandin) Usual dose: 0.5-4 mg orally daily	Increase insulin secretion in the treatment of type 2 diabetes. Short-acting agent used to prevent postmeal blood glucose elevation.	Teach patients to take the drug 1-30 min before meals.	Drug is most effective when administered with or just before eating a meal.
		Teach patients to omit the drug when skipping a meal, and instruct them to add a dose if an extra meal is eaten.	Hypoglycemia may occur shortly after dosing when the meal is delayed or omitted.
Nateglinide (Starlix) Usual dose: 60-120 mg orally before meals	Increase insulin secretion in the treatment of type 2 diabetes. Short-acting agent used to prevent postmeal blood glucose elevation.	Teach patients to take the drug 3 times daily, 1-30 min before meals.	Drug is most effective when administered with or just before eating a meal.
		Teach patients to omit the drug when skipping a meal, and instruct them to add a dose if an extra meal is eaten.	Hypoglycemia may occur shortly after dosing when the meal is delayed or omitted.
Biguanides			
Metformin (Glucophage) Usual dose: 850 mg orally twice daily with the morning and evening meals (Glucophage XL) Usual dose: 500-2000 mg orally daily before breakfast	Lowers both basal and postmeal blood glucose levels in patients with type 2 diabetes by reducing hepatic glucose production and increasing tissue sensitivity to insulin.	Teach patients to take the drug with food.	Adverse GI side effects such as diarrhea, nausea, vomiting, flatulence, indigestion, and abdominal discomfort are common. Taking the drug with food reduces these effects.
		Monitor liver and kidney function before starting metformin and periodically thereafter.	Metformin should be used with caution in older patients since aging is associated with reduced kidney function. Metformin is contraindicated in people with serum creatinine in males >1.5 mg/dL (132.6 μmol/L), and in females >1.4 mg/dL (123.8 μmol/L).
		Monitor cardiopulmonary status throughout therapy.	Metformin should not be used in patients with congestive heart failure requiring drug therapy. These patients are at risk for hypoperfusion and hypoxemia, conditions which increase the risk for lactic acidosis.
		Monitor for conditions that increase risk for lactic acidosis.	Metformin is contraindicated in people with risk factors for lactic acidosis: reduced kidney function, liver impairment, respiratory insufficiency, severe infection, alcohol abuse.
		Instruct patients taking metformin to report symptoms of lactic acidosis: malaise, unusual muscle pain, respiratory distress, increasing somnolence, and abdominal distress.	Onset of lactic acidosis is subtle and accompanied by nonspecific symptoms.

Continued

CHART 67-3 COMMON EXAMPLES OF DRUG THERAPY

Diabetes Mellitus—cont'd

	USE IN DIABETES	NURSING INTERVENTIONS	RATIONALES
Metformin—cont'd		Instruct patients taking metformin to report any illness that causes severe vomiting, diarrhea, or fever.	Precipitating events for lactic acidosis include hypoxemia, dehydration, and sepsis.
		Withhold metformin for 48 hr before use of iodinated contrast materials used in certain radiographic studies.	Iodinated contrast materials can alter kidney function and increase the risk for lactic acidosis. Metformin therapy is restarted when kidney function has returned to normal.
		Instruct patients taking Glucophage XL that tablets must be swallowed whole and never crushed or chewed.	Damaging the extended-release form of the drug causes the rapid release of the entire dose and can cause hypoglycemia.
Alpha-Glucosidase Inhibitors			
Acarbose (Precose) Usual dose: 50-100 mg orally three times daily	Used to prevent postmeal blood glucose elevation in the treatment of type 2 diabetes.	Teach patients to take with the first bite of each main meal.	Acarbose must be taken at the beginning of a meal to be fully effective.
		Instruct patients to take the missed dose at the next meal and to avoid taking a double dose of the drug.	Acarbose works only when taken at the beginning of a meal. If it is not taken at that time, it should not be taken until the next meal.
		Monitor for abdominal pain, diarrhea, and flatulence.	GI side effects are very common. Symptoms can be reduced by slow titration of dose.
		Teach patients about dietary habits to decrease GI discomfort.	Avoiding foods that will increase GI discomfort such as rich foods, sauces, beverages including beer and carbonated soft drinks, gas-producing foods such as beans, nuts, bran cereals, broccoli, and cabbage reduce the GI side effects of the drug. Meals and snacks should be low in fat. Drinking plenty of water, especially in the early part of the day, and avoiding overeating also reduce symptoms.
		Monitor kidney function.	Drug may accumulate in patients with kidney dysfunction; drug not recommended for patients with serum creatinine >2 mg/dL (176.8 µmol/L).
		Monitor liver function tests. Emphasize the need to report symptoms of unexplained nausea, vomiting, abdominal pain, fatigue, anorexia, or dark urine.	Acarbose is associated with elevation in serum transaminase levels. Doses >150 mg/day associated with increases in ALT and AST (SGOT). ALT should be checked every 3 months for first year and periodically thereafter.
		Instruct patients receiving acarbose to treat hypoglycemia with glucose tablets, glucose gel, or low-fat milk.	Acarbose does not cause hypoglycemia when given alone. Hypoglycemia caused by other agents should be treated with oral dextrose. Sucrose (table sugar or candy bars) will not reverse symptoms of hypoglycemia due to acarbose.
		Teach patients to store the drug according to manufacturer's directions.	Remove from wrapper immediately before taking the drug to prevent deterioration of acarbose.
Miglitol (Glyset) Usual dose: 50 mg orally three times daily	Used to prevent postmeal blood glucose elevation in the treatment of type 2 diabetes.	Instruct patients to take the drug with the first bite of each main meal.	Miglitol must be taken at the beginning of a meal to be fully effective.
		Monitor kidney function.	Drug may accumulate in patients with kidney dysfunction; drug not recommended for patients with serum creatinine >2 mg/dL.
		Monitor for abdominal pain, diarrhea, and flatulence.	GI side effects are very common. Symptoms can be reduced by slow titration of dose.
		Monitor liver function tests.	Miglitol is associated with elevation in serum transaminase levels.
		Emphasize the need to report symptoms of unexplained nausea, vomiting, abdominal pain, fatigue, anorexia, or dark urine.	These manifestations are associated with reduced liver function.

Drug	Nursing Interventions	Rationales
	Teach patients taking miglitol to treat hypoglycemia with glucose tablets, glucose gel, or low-fat milk.	Miglitol does not cause hypoglycemia when given alone. Hypoglycemia caused by other agents should be treated with oral dextrose. Sucrose (table sugar or candy bars) will not reverse symptoms of hypoglycemia due to acarbose.
Thiazolidinediones		
Pioglitazone (Actos) Usual dose: 15 mg or 30 mg once orally daily without regard to meals	Emphasize the need for liver function tests as recommended. Instruct patients to report symptoms of unexplained nausea, vomiting, abdominal pain, fatigue, anorexia, or dark urine.	Rare cases of liver failure have occurred with pioglitazone. Liver function tests are measured at the start of therapy and at regular intervals thereafter. Not recommended for moderate to severe liver impairment (ALT >2.5 upper limit of normal or active liver disease) or in patients with jaundice.
	Advise women of the need for effective contraception during therapy.	Administration of pioglitazone with certain oral contraceptives may reduce the plasma concentration of the oral contraceptive. Postmenopausal women with insulin resistance may resume ovulation during therapy.
	Monitor weight; assess for edema and shortness of breath.	Fluid retention can lead to weight gain and can cause or exacerbate congestive heart failure.
	Stress importance of continuing therapy even if a response is not evident within 2 weeks.	Full therapeutic response may not be evident for 8-12 weeks after initiation of therapy.
Rosiglitazone (Avandia) Usual dose: 4 mg orally daily in the morning, or 2 mg twice daily in the morning and evening without regard to food	Emphasize the need for liver function tests as recommended. Instruct the patient to report symptoms of unexplained nausea, vomiting, abdominal pain, fatigue, anorexia, or dark urine.	Rare cases of liver failure have occurred with rosiglitazone. Liver function tests are measured at the start of therapy and at regular intervals thereafter. Not recommended for moderate to severe liver impairment (ALT >2.5 upper limit of normal or active liver disease) or in patients with jaundice.
	Advise women of the need for effective contraception during therapy.	Administration of rosiglitazone with certain oral contraceptives may reduce the plasma concentration of the oral contraceptive. Postmenopausal women with insulin resistance may resume ovulation during therapy.
	Monitor weight; assess for edema and shortness of breath.	Fluid retention can lead to weight gain and can cause or exacerbate congestive heart failure.
	Stress importance of continuing therapy even if a response is not evident within 2 weeks.	Full therapeutic response may not be evident for 2-3 months after initiation of therapy.
Fixed Combinations		
Actoplus Met (pioglitazone/ metformin) Usual doses: 15 mg/500 mg or 15 mg/850 mg orally once or twice daily	Instruct patients in measures to prevent and treat hypoglycemia.	Hypoglycemia may occur when metformin is given in combination with thiazolidinedione agent. Refer to Nursing Interventions and Rationales listed for pioglitazone and metformin.
Avandamet (rosiglitazone/ metformin) Usual oral doses: 1 mg/500 mg 2 mg/500 mg 4 mg/500 mg Maximum dose: 8 mg/2000 mg daily	Teach patients to take the drug in divided doses with meals. Teach patients how to prevent and treat hypoglycemia.	Hypoglycemia may occur when metformin is given in combination with thiazolidinedione agent. Refer to Nursing Interventions and Rationales listed for metformin and rosiglitazone.

Continued

CHART 67-3 COMMON EXAMPLES OF DRUG THERAPY

Diabetes Mellitus—cont'd

	USE IN DIABETES	NURSING INTERVENTIONS	RATIONALES
Avandaryl (glimepiride/rosiglitazone) Usual oral doses: 1 mg/4 mg 2 mg/4 mg 4 mg/4 mg Maximum dose: 4 mg/8 mg daily	Rosiglitazone added to regimen when blood glucose is inadequately controlled on glimepiride therapy alone.	Teach patients how to prevent and treat hypoglycemia.	Hypoglycemia may occur when glimepiride is given in combination with thiazolidinedione agent. Refer to Nursing Interventions and Rationales listed for rosiglitazone and glimepiride.
Duetact (glimepiride/pioglitazone) Usual once daily doses: 2 mg/30 mg 4 mg/30 mg	Pioglitazone added to regimen when blood glucose is inadequately controlled on glimepiride therapy alone.	Teach patients how to prevent and treat hypoglycemia.	Hypoglycemia may occur when glimepiride is given in combination with thiazolidinedione agent. Refer to Nursing Interventions and Rationales listed for pioglitazone and glimepiride.
Glucovance (glyburide/metformin) Usual oral twice-daily doses: 1.25 mg/250 mg 2.5 mg/500 mg 5 mg/500 mg	Metformin added to regimen when blood glucose is inadequately controlled on glyburide therapy alone.	Teach patients how to prevent and treat hypoglycemia.	Hypoglycemia may occur when metformin is given in combination with sulfonylurea agent. Refer to Nursing Interventions and Rationales listed for metformin and glyburide.
Janumet (sitagliptin/metformin) Usual oral twice-daily doses: 100 mg/1000 mg 100 mg/2000 mg Maximum dose: 100 mg/2000 mg	Sitagliptin added to regimen when blood glucose is inadequately controlled on metformin therapy alone.	Teach patients to take the drug twice daily with meals.	Refer to Nursing Interventions and Rationales listed for sitagliptin and metformin.
Metaglip (glipizide/metformin) Usual oral twice-daily doses: 2.5 mg/250 mg 2.5 mg/500 mg 5 mg/500 mg	Metformin added to regimen when blood glucose is inadequately controlled on glipizide therapy alone.	Teach patients to take the drug with meals. Teach patients how to prevent and treat hypoglycemia.	Hypoglycemia may occur when metformin is given in combination with sulfonylurea agent. Refer to Nursing Interventions and Rationales listed for metformin and glipizide.
PrandiMet (repaglinide/metformin) Usual oral doses taken two or three times daily: 1 mg/500 mg 2 mg/500 mg Maximum dose: 10 mg/2500 mg	Repaglinide added to regimen when blood glucose is inadequately controlled on metformin therapy alone.	Instruct patients in measures to prevent and treat hypoglycemia.	Hypoglycemia may occur when metformin is given in combination with repaglinide. Refer to Nursing Interventions and Rationales listed for repaglinide and metformin.
Amylin Analog **Pramlintide (Symlin)** Initial subcutaneous dose immediately before each meal: 15 mcg Maintenance dose: 30 mcg or 60 mcg	Used for people with type 1 or type 2 diabetes who have not received desired glucose control with optimal insulin therapy.	Teach the patient to prepare and self-administer pramlintide. Instruct the patient in measures to prevent and treat hypoglycemia. Instruct the patient to eat at least 250 calories or 30 g of	A U-100 insulin syringe is used to administer pramlintide. It is necessary to convert the microgram dosage to insulin syringe unit increments. Pramlintide carries a Black Box Warning for severe insulin-induced hypoglycemia. The risk for hypoglycemia is greatest within 3 hours of injection.

Drug / Dose	Usage	Nursing Interventions	Rationale
		Instruct the patient in measures to avoid drug incompatibilities: Do not mix pramlintide and insulin together in the same syringe. Inject pramlintide into an anatomical site distant from the insulin injection site.	Pramlintide and insulin are not compatible when mixed together.
Incretin Mimetics (GLP-1 agonist) Exenatide (Byetta) Initial subcutaneous dose: 5 mcg twice daily Maintenance dose: 10 mcg twice daily	Exenatide is used as monotherapy or as part of 2- or 3-drug regimen for patients with type 2 diabetes.	Teach the patient to prepare and self-administer exenatide. Instruct patients to administer as subcutaneous injection within 60 minutes before morning and evening meals (or two main meals of the day). Teach patients the actions to take for missed doses of the drug. Instruct the patient in measures to prevent and treat hypoglycemia. Instruct patient to discontinue use of the drug and to report symptoms of unexplained persistent severe abdominal pain with or without nausea and vomiting. Teach patients to discontinue use of the drug and to report symptoms of hypersensitive reactions to their provider.	Exenatide is available in a prefilled pen containing 60 doses for 30 days of use. Patient education in use of the pen is necessary to ensure that the patient receives the correct dose of the drug. Instruct patients to take the missed dose at the next meal. Exenatide is not given after a meal. Hypoglycemia has been reported when exenatide is given in combination with a sulfonylurea agent. Acute pancreatitis, including both fatal and nonfatal hemorrhagic or necrotizing pancreatitis, has been reported in patients taking exenatide. Hypersensitive reactions including exfoliative dermatitis, urticaria, skin rash, and Stevens-Johnson syndrome have been reported in patients taking exenatide.
Liraglutide (Victoza) Initiate at 0.6 mg per day for 1 week Increase to 1.2 mg after 1 week Maximum once daily subcutaneous dose: 1.8 mg	Liraglutide is used as single drug therapy or as part of 2- or 3-drug regimen for patients with type 2 diabetes.	Instruct patients to administer once daily, at any time of the day, independent of meals. Inject subcutaneously in abdomen, thigh, or upper arm. Monitor for nausea, vomiting, diarrhea, dyspepsia, and constipation. Instruct patients in measures to prevent and treat hypoglycemia. Observe and report symptoms of pancreatitis: persistent severe abdominal pain with or without nausea and vomiting.	Liraglutide is available in a prefilled multi-dose pen. Patient education in use of the pen is necessary to ensure that the patient receives the correct dose of the drug. Side effects tend to be dose-related and lessen over time. Hypoglycemia may occur when liraglutide is given in combination with a sulfonylurea agent. Pancreatitis has been reported in patients taking liraglutide.
DPP-4 Inhibitors Sitagliptin (Januvia) Recommended dose: 100 mg orally once daily	Sitagliptin is used as single drug therapy or as part of 2- or 3-drug regimen for patients with type 2 diabetes.	Instruct patients to administer once daily, with or without food. Instruct patient to discontinue use of the drug and to report symptoms of unexplained persistent severe abdominal pain with or without nausea and vomiting.	Drug is effective with or without food and does not increase the risk for hypoglycemia. Acute pancreatitis, including both fatal and nonfatal hemorrhagic or necrotizing pancreatitis, has been reported in patients taking sitagliptin.
Saxagliptin (Onglyza) Recommended dose: 2.5 mg or 5 mg orally once daily	Saxagliptin is used as single drug therapy or as part of 2- or 3-drug regimen for patients with type 2 diabetes.	Instruct patients to administer once daily, with or without food. Instruct patients in measures to prevent and treat hypoglycemia.	Drug is effective with or without food and does not increase the risk for hypoglycemia. Hypoglycemia may occur when saxagliptin is given in combination with glyburide.

ALT, Alanine aminotransferase; AST, aspartate aminotransferase; SGOT, serum glutamate oxaloacetate transaminase.

TABLE 67-8   DRUG INTERACTIONS WITH SULFONYLUREA AGENTS

POTENTIATE HYPOGLYCEMIA	WORSEN HYPERGLYCEMIA
Angiotensin-converting agents (captopril [Capoten], enalapril [Vasotec])	Adrenalin
Alcohol	Calcium channel blocking agents (diltiazem [Cardizem], nifedipine [Procardia])
Allopurinol (Zyloprim)	Corticosteroids (prednisone)
Analgesics (azapropazone, phenylbutazone, salicylates)	Diazoxide (Proglycem [oral], Hyperstat [IV])
Antifungal azoles (fluconazole [Diflucan], ketoconazole [Nizoral], miconazole [Monistat])	Estrogen (Estrace, Premarin)
Beta-adrenergic blocking agents (atenolol, [Tenormin], propranolol [Inderal])	Estrogen-progesterone–containing oral contraceptives (Brevicon, Depo-Provera, Estrostep)
Chloramphenicol (Chloromycetin)	Furosemide (Lasix)
Clofibrate (Atromid-S)	Isoniazid (INH)
Warfarin (Coumadin)	Nicotinic acid (Nicolar)
Fluoroquinolones (ciprofloxacin [Cipro], gatifloxacin [Tequin], levofloxacin [Levaquin])	Phenothiazines (chlorpromazine [Thorazine], prochlorperazine [Compazine], trifluoperazine [Stelazine])
Heparin	Phenytoin (Dilantin)
Histamine H_2 antagonists (cimetidine [Tagamet], ranitidine [Zantac])	Rifampin (Rifadin)
	Sympathomimetics
Monoamine oxidase (MAO) inhibitors (phenelzine [Nardil])	Thiazide diuretics (hydrochlorothiazide [HydroDIURIL], chlorothiazide [Diuril])
NSAIDs (indomethacin [Indocin], ibuprofen [Advil])	
Octreotide (Sandostatin)	
Probenecid (Benemid, Probalan)	
Sulfinpyrazone (Anturane)	
Sulfonamides (trimethoprim/sulfamethoxazole [Bactrim], sulfisoxazole [Gantrisin])	
Tricyclic antidepressants (amitriptyline hydrochloride, desipramine hydrochloride [Norpramin], doxepin hydrochloride [Sinequan])	

Data from *AHFS Drug Information*. (2009). Bethesda, MD: American Society of Health-System Pharmacists.

Insulin Sensitizers. Insulin sensitizers include biguanides (metformin) and thiazolidinediones (TZDs). Metformin (Glucophage) does not increase insulin secretion. It decreases liver glucose production, thereby reducing fasting plasma glucose release, and improves insulin receptor sensitivity. TZDs bind to a regulatory protein, peroxisome proliferator–activated receptor (PPAR)), that controls expression of genes that regulate glucose and fat metabolism. TZDs increase cellular utilization of glucose, which lowers blood glucose levels.

The ADA recommends metformin as initial therapy for type 2 DM because the drug does not induce weight gain or hypoglycemia and has a relatively low cost and few adverse effects. It should not be given to anyone with kidney disease and elevated blood creatinine levels. The drug should be withheld for 48 hours before and after using contrast material and surgical procedures requiring anesthesia. Metformin lowers HbA_{1c} levels by an average of 1.5 percentage points.

The most common side effects are abdominal discomfort and diarrhea. Metformin can cause lactic acidosis in patients with kidney problems and should not be used in conditions that decrease drug clearance, such as liver disease, alcoholism, or severe congestive heart failure or in patients older than 80 years. Hypoxemia, dehydration, and sepsis also increase the risk for lactic acidosis. Symptoms of lactic acidosis can be subtle. Teach the patient to report symptoms of fatigue, unusual muscle pain, difficulty breathing, unusual or unexpected stomach discomfort, dizziness, lightheadedness, or irregular heartbeats to the primary care provider. Instruct patients to take metformin with meals to reduce GI effects. Caution against excessive alcohol intake because alcohol increases the risk for lactic acidosis.

! NURSING SAFETY PRIORITY

Drug Alert

> Metformin can cause lactic acidosis in patients with renal insufficiency and should not be used by anyone with kidney disease. To prevent kidney damage, the drug should be withheld after using contrast material or any surgical procedure requiring anesthesia until adequate kidney function is established.

Thiazolidinediones (TZDs) improve insulin sensitivity and reduce liver glucose production. TZDs also improve insulin action in muscle, fat, and liver tissue. The two drugs in this class are rosiglitazone (Avandia) and pioglitazone (Actos).

! NURSING SAFETY PRIORITY

Drug Alert

> Do not confuse Actos with Actonel. Actos is an oral antidiabetic drug from the thiazolidinedione class, and Actonel is a drug that prevents calcium loss from bones.

All drugs in this class reduce blood lipid levels. Major side effects of TZD treatment are an increase in adipose tissue and fluid retention. Some patients taking these drugs gain weight. Edema, with development of congestive heart failure, is possible but rare. Other side effects include infection, headache, peripheral edema, and pain. Patients taking these drugs should have periodic liver function studies because of the potential for liver damage. There is an increased incidence of fractures of the upper arms, hands, and feet in women using rosiglitazone and pioglitazone. TZDs lower HbA_{1c} levels by an average of 0.5 to 1.4 percentage points.

Rosiglitazone has been associated with an increased risk for heart-related deaths, bone fracture, and macular edema. In May 2011, the FDA issued prescribing information, which includes this black box warning:

- Prescription of rosiglitazone, either as a single drug or combined with other drugs, is limited to only those patients who are already using the drug and whose disease cannot be adequately controlled by other drugs or a combination of drugs. It is absolutely contraindicated in patients with any symptomatic heart failure.

- Rosiglitazone causes or exacerbates congestive heart failure in some patients. Monitor for signs and symptoms of heart failure (excessive rapid weight gain, difficulty breathing and/or swelling) after starting treatment or after increases in dosage of rosiglitazone. If heart failure signs and symptoms occur, the heart failure should be managed appropriately and discontinuation of rosiglitazone must be considered.
- Rosiglitazone is available only through pharmacies that are certified by the Avandia-Rosiglitazone Medicines Access Programs.

(A Black Box Warning is a government designation indicating that a drug has at least one serious side effect and must be used with caution.)

Alpha-Glucosidase Inhibitors. Alpha-glucosidase inhibitors prevent after-meal hyperglycemia by delaying absorption of carbohydrate from the small intestine. These drugs inhibit enzymes in the intestinal tract, reducing the rate of digestion of starches and the absorption of glucose. This action prevents a sudden blood glucose surge after meals. Acarbose *delays* rather than prevents glucose absorption and does not cause weight loss. Alpha-glucosidase inhibitors lower HbA_{1c} levels by an average of 0.5 to 0.8 percentage points.

The most common side effects are flatulence, diarrhea, and abdominal discomfort. There are two drugs in this class. Acarbose (Precose, Prandase ♣) is well tolerated when started at a low dose (25 mg once daily to three times daily with meals) and increased slowly. At higher doses, poor carbohydrate absorption occurs. Miglitol (Glyset) should be taken three times daily with the first bite of each main meal.

These drugs do not cause hypoglycemia unless given with sulfonylureas or insulin. Because alpha-glucosidase inhibitors delay carbohydrate absorption and interfere with the conversion of complex sugars to glucose, many of the standard products used to manage hypoglycemia have a slower onset of action. These drugs do not inhibit absorption of glucose or lactose. Teach patients to use oral glucose tablets, glucose gel, or low-fat milk to manage hypoglycemia. Severe hypoglycemia may require glucose infusion or glucagon injection.

Incretin Mimetics. Incretin mimetics are natural "gut" hormones that, along with insulin, also lower plasma glucose levels. These agents include glucagon-like peptide-1 (GLP-1) and glucose-dependent insulinotropic polypeptide (GIP) that are released by the intestine throughout the day in response to food intake (Appel, 2011). GLP-1 has effects on the stomach, liver, pancreas, and brain to work together to regulate blood glucose. It lowers glucagon secretion from the pancreas, leading to reduced liver glucose production. It also delays gastric emptying, slows the rate of nutrient absorption into the blood, and reduces food intake, all of which lower blood glucose levels. GLP and GIP are rapidly metabolized by an enzyme known as *DPP-4,* which inactivates their effects. Patients with type 2 DM have a reduced incretin effect, indicating that they have either a decreased level of incretin hormones or a resistance to their effects. Two incretin agents are approved for use in patients with type 2 DM—exenatide (Byetta) and liraglutide (Victoza). Incretin

agents lower HbA_{1c} levels by an average of 0.5 to 1.0 percentage points.

Exenatide (Byetta) is a GLP-1 agonist. It mimics the actions of GLP-1, stimulating insulin secretion only when blood glucose is high. This action restores "first phase" insulin release and improves blood glucose control by lowering both after-meal and fasting blood glucose levels. The drug is approved for use as a single agent or in combination with a sulfonylurea, metformin, or thiazolidinedione in patients with type 2 DM.

The main side effect of exenatide is nausea. Most patients lose weight as a result of the anorexic effect of the drug. It stimulates insulin secretion and may cause hypoglycemia when given with sulfonylurea drugs (which also stimulate insulin secretion) but not with metformin alone. Exenatide should not be used for patients with end-stage kidney disease or those with kidney impairment that reduces glomerular filtration to less than 30 mL/min.

Exenatide is available as a fixed-dose prefilled pen injector delivering either 5 mcg or 10 mcg of drug per dose. It is injected subcutaneously in thigh, abdomen, or upper arm within 60 minutes *before* the morning and evening meals or before the two main meals of the day. Teach patients not to administer exenatide *after* a meal. Unopened prefilled pens are stored in a refrigerator between 36° F and 46° F (2° C and 8° C). Opened pen injectors can be stored for up to 30 days at room temperature in a closed container protected from heat and light. Instruct the patient to discard an open pen after 30 days even if it is not empty.

Liraglutide (Victoza) is a glucagon-like peptide-1 (GLP-1) agonist approved as an addition to diet and exercise to improve glycemic control in adults with type 2 DM. It enhances glucose-dependent insulin secretion from the pancreas, suppresses excess glucagon secretion, delays gastric emptying, reduces appetite, and preserves beta-cell mass and function.

The most common adverse effects are GI related and included nausea, vomiting, diarrhea, dyspepsia and constipation. The frequency of effects tends to be dose-related and decreased over time. Hypoglycemia is uncommon, and occurs more often in combination with a sulfonylurea agent. Liraglutide carries a black box warning for thyroid tumors and is not to be used by patients with a history of medullary thyroid carcinoma (Appel, 2011).

Liraglutide is available as a solution for subcutaneous injection in a prefilled multi-dose pen. It is administered once daily at any time of the day, independent of meals. Each pen delivers doses of 0.6 mg, 1.2 mg, or 1.8 mg. Unopened prefilled pens should be stored under refrigeration between 36° F and 46° F (2° C and 8° C). Opened pens can be stored for up to 30 days at controlled room temperature between 59° F and 86° F (15° C and 30° C) or in a refrigerator. Pens need to be protected from excessive heat and sunlight. Therapy with liraglutide begins at 0.6 daily mg for 1 week. This dose is intended to reduce GI symptoms during initial titration. After 1 week, the dose is increased to 1.2 mg daily and to 1.8 mg daily, if needed.

Monitor patients taking incretin mimetics for symptoms of pancreatitis. Teach patients to discontinue use of the drug and to report symptoms of unexplained, persistent severe abdominal pain with or without nausea and vomiting to their primary care provider as soon as possible.

DPP-4 Inhibitors. DPP-4 inhibitors work by inhibiting the enzyme that inactivates the incretin hormones (Martin, 2010). As a result, more natural incretin hormones (GLP-1 and GIP) are available to regulate blood glucose. Glucagon levels are decreased, and insulin secretion from pancreatic beta cells is increased. The two DPP-4 inhibitors approved for use in patients with type 2 DM are sitagliptin (Januvia) and saxagliptin (Onglyza). DPP-4 inhibitors lower HbA$_{1c}$ levels by an average of 0.6 to 0.9 percentage points.

Sitagliptin increases the body's active incretin hormone levels, reducing both before-meal and after-meal blood glucose levels. It works only when blood glucose is elevated. Sitagliptin is approved as single agent therapy for patients with type 2 DM unable to manage the disease with diet and exercise alone and as add-on therapy for those patients with inadequate blood glucose control who are also taking a sulfonylurea, metformin, or thiazolidinediones. The recommended dose is 100 mg orally, once daily, with or without food. Dosage adjustment is needed for patients with moderate to severe kidney impairment.

Side effects include stuffy or runny nose, sore throat, upper respiratory infection, and GI effects of abdominal pain, nausea, and diarrhea. Monitor for symptoms of kidney impairment. Hypersensitivity reactions including exfoliative dermatitis, urticaria, skin rash, and Stevens-Johnson syndrome have been reported. Teach patients to discontinue use of the drug and to report symptoms of hypersensitive reactions to their health care provider.

Patients taking sitagliptin (Januvia) should be monitored for symptoms of pancreatitis. Acute pancreatitis, including both fatal and nonfatal hemorrhagic or necrotizing pancreatitis, has been reported in patients who received sitagliptin therapy. Teach patients to discontinue use of the drug and to report symptoms of unexplained, persistent severe abdominal pain with or without nausea and vomiting to their health care provider as soon as possible.

Saxagliptin (Onglyza) lowers HbA$_{1c}$ levels in patients with type 2 diabetes when used alone or in combination with metformin, sulfonylurea, or thiazolidinediones (TZDs). Common adverse effects include nasopharyngitis, headache, diarrhea, upper respiratory infection, urinary tract infection, and peripheral edema. Hypoglycemia was reported, particularly when saxagliptin was given in combination with glyburide.

Amylin Analogs. Amylin analogs are drugs similar to amylin, a naturally occurring hormone produced by beta cells in the pancreas that works with and is co-secreted with insulin in response to blood glucose elevation. Amylin levels are deficient in patients with type 1 DM who are also deficient in insulin. Pramlintide (Symlin), an analog of amylin, is approved for patients with either type 1 or type 2 DM treated with insulin. It is indicated as adjunct therapy for patients who use mealtime insulin delivery and have not achieved desirable glucose control despite optimum insulin therapy.

Pramlintide works by three mechanisms: delayed gastric emptying, reducing after-meal blood glucose levels, and triggering satiety (in the brain). (Satiety leads to decreased caloric intake and eventual weight loss.) The initial dose of pramlintide is 15 mcg subcutaneously before meals with at least 250 calories or 30 g of carbohydrate. It can be given up to 4 times per day. Dosage is increased in 15-mcg increments to a target dose of 30 mcg or 60 mcg. Pramlintide alters gastric

uptake. Therefore instruct patients to take oral drugs in which rapid onset of action is important (e.g., analgesics) either 1 hour before or 2 hours after eating.

Teach the patient to prepare and self-administer pramlintide. A U-100 syringe is used to administer the drug. However, it is necessary to convert the microgram dosage to insulin syringe unit increments (e.g., 15 mcg is equal to 2.5 units on a U-100 insulin syringe). Teach the patient to inject pramlintide into a site different from where insulin is injected.

! NURSING SAFETY PRIORITY
Drug Alert

> Do not mix pramlintide and insulin in the same syringe because the pH of the two drugs is not compatible.

Nausea, vomiting, and anorexia are common side effects of pramlintide therapy. It should not be used for patients with symptomatic gastroparesis. Pramlintide carries a black box warning for insulin-induced severe hypoglycemia. The hypoglycemic risk is higher in patients with type 1 DM and usually occurs within 3 hours of injection. The black box also warns about the risk for hypoglycemia during driving or operating heavy equipment.

Combination Agents. Combination agents combine drugs with different mechanisms of action. Glucovance, for example, combines glyburide with metformin. Combining drugs with different mechanisms of action may be highly effective in maintaining desired blood glucose control. Some patients may need a combination of oral agents and insulin to control blood glucose levels.

? NCLEX EXAMINATION CHALLENGE
Safe and Effective Care Environment

> A client with type 2 diabetes who also has heart failure is prescribed metformin extended-release (Glucophage XR) once daily. On assessment, the nurse finds that the client now has muscle aches, drowsiness, low blood pressure, and a slow, irregular heartbeat. What is the nurse's best action?
> A. Assess the client's blood glucose level and prepare to administer IV glucose.
> B. Reassure the client that these symptoms are normal effects of this drug.
> C. Hold the dose and notify the prescriber immediately.
> D. Administer the drug at bedtime to prevent falls.

Insulin Therapy. Insulin therapy is needed for type 1 DM and also may be used for type 2 DM. The safety of insulin therapy in older patients may be affected by reduced vision, mobility and coordination problems, and decreased memory. There are many types of insulin and regimens that have the purpose of achieving normal blood glucose levels. Because insulin is a small protein that is quickly digested and inactivated in the GI tract, it must be administered as an injection or by another route that bypasses the GI tract.

Types of Insulin. Insulin is manufactured using DNA technology to synthesize pure human insulin. Insulin analogs are synthetic human insulins in which the structure of the insulin molecule is altered to change the rate of absorption and duration of action within the body. One example is Lispro insulin, a rapid-acting insulin analog that is created by switching the

TABLE 67-9	TIME ACTIVITY OF PHARMACEUTICAL INSULIN				
PREPARATION	**BRAND**	**ONSET (HR)**	**PEAK (HR)**	**DURATION (HR)**
Rapid-Acting Insulin				
Insulin aspart	NovoLog	0.25	1-3	3-5
Insulin glulisine	Apidra	0.3	0.5-1.5	3-4
Human lispro injection	Humalog	0.25	0.5-1.5	5
Short-Acting Insulin				
Regular human insulin injection	Humulin R	0.5	2-4	5-7
	Novolin R	0.5	2.5-5	8
	ReliOn R			
Humulin R (Concentrated U-500)	Humulin R (U-500)	1.5	4-12	24
Intermediate-Acting Insulin				
Isophane Insulin NPH injection	Humulin N	1.5	4-12	16-24+
	Novolin N			
	ReliOn N			
70% human insulin isophane suspension/30% human insulin injection	Humulin 70/30	0.5	2-12	24
	Novolin 70/30			
	ReliOn 70/30			
50% human insulin isophane suspension/50% human insulin injection	Humulin 50/50	0.5	3-5	24
70% insulin aspart protamine suspension/30% insulin aspart injection	NovoLog Mix 70/30	0.25	1-4	24
75% insulin lispro protamine suspension/25% insulin lispro injection	Humalog Mix 75/25	0.25	1-2	24
Long-Acting Insulin				
Insulin glargine injection	Lantus	2-4	None	24
Insulin detemir injection	Levemir	1	6-8	5.7-24

positions of lysine and proline in one area of the insulin molecule.

Rapid-, short-, intermediate-, and long-acting forms of insulin can be injected separately, and some can be mixed in the same syringe. Insulin is available in concentrations of 100 units/mL (U-100) or 500 units/mL (U-500). U-500 is used only in rare cases of insulin resistance.

Teach the patient that the insulin types, the injection technique, the site of injection, and the patient response can all affect the absorption, onset, degree, and duration of insulin activity. Reinforce that changing insulins may affect blood glucose control and should be done only under supervision of the health care provider. Table 67-9 outlines the time activity of human insulin.

❓ NCLEX EXAMINATION CHALLENGE

Health Promotion and Maintenance

The client newly diagnosed with type 1 diabetes asks why insulin is given only by injection and not as an oral drug. What is the nurse's best response?
A. "Injected insulin works faster than oral drugs to lower blood glucose levels."
B. "Oral insulin is so weak that it would require very high dosages to be effective."
C. "Insulin is a small protein that is destroyed by stomach acids and intestinal enzymes."
D. "Insulin is a "high alert drug" and could more easily be abused if it were available as an oral agent."

Insulin Regimens. Insulin regimens try to duplicate the normal insulin release pattern from the pancreas. The pancreas produces a constant *(basal)* amount of insulin that balances liver glucose production with glucose use and maintains normal blood glucose levels between meals. The pancreas also produces additional *(prandial)* insulin to prevent blood glucose elevation after meals. The insulin dose required for blood glucose control varies among patients. A usual starting dose is between 0.5 and 1 unit/kg of body weight per day. For multiple-dose regimens or continuous subcutaneous insulin infusion (CSII), basal insulin makes up about 40% to 50% of the total daily dosage, with the remainder divided into premeal doses of rapid-acting insulin analogs or regular insulin. Basal insulin coverage is provided by NPH insulin or by intermediate-acting and long-acting insulin analogs, insulin glargine (Lantus) or insulin detemir (Levemir). Because the rate of absorption is slowed by increasing the dosage, adjustments in dosage should be made no more than every 3 to 4 days. Dosage adjustments are based on the results of blood glucose monitoring.

Single daily injection protocols require insulin injection only once daily. This protocol may include one injection of intermediate- or long-acting insulin or a combination of short- and intermediate-acting insulin. Many patients with type 2 diabetes combine once-daily insulin injection with oral agent therapy.

Multiple-component insulin therapy combines short- and intermediate-acting insulin injected twice daily. Two thirds of the daily dose is given before breakfast and one third before the evening meal. Ratios of intermediate-acting and regular insulin are based on results of blood glucose monitoring.

Intensified regimens include a basal dose of intermediate- or long-acting insulin and a bolus dose of short- or rapid-acting insulin designed to bring the next blood glucose value into the target range. Blood glucose elevations above the target range are treated with "correction" doses of short- or rapid-acting insulin. The patient's blood glucose patterns determine insulin dosage. Frequency of blood glucose monitoring is based on the timed action of short- and intermediate- or long-acting insulins and may occur as often as eight times daily. Blood glucose testing 1 to 2 hours after meals and within 10 minutes before the next meal helps determine the adequacy of the bolus dose. The patient determines the effects of basal insulin by monitoring blood glucose levels before breakfast (fasting) and before the evening meal.

Patients on intensified insulin regimens need extensive education to achieve target blood glucose values. They need to know how to adjust insulin doses and understand nutrition therapy to maintain dietary flexibility and target blood glucose values. Patients must also be able to accurately monitor blood glucose levels so that therapy decisions can be based on accurate data.

Regardless of the specific insulin regimen, adherence to insulin injection schedules is critical in achieving glycemic control and maintaining HbA_{1c} levels below the 7% needed to reduce long-term complications. At times, skipping an occasional insulin dose may be related to an unusual meal pattern for a day or a change in exercise. However, many patients continue to "skip" insulin doses regularly, which increases their overall risk for serious health problems and early death. Determining what factors are associated with this behavior can help nurses and other health care professionals provide an individualized approach to assisting the patient with DM to understand the benefits of insulin therapy adherence (Peyrot et al., 2010). (See the Evidence-Based Practice box at right.)

Factors Influencing Insulin Absorption. Many factors affect insulin absorption and availability, including injection site; timing, type, or dose of insulin used; and physical activity.

Injection site area affects the speed of insulin absorption. Fig. 67-4 shows common insulin injection areas. Absorption is fastest in the abdomen, followed by the deltoid, thigh, and buttocks. Rotating injection site areas prevents lipohypertrophy (increased fat deposits in the skin) and lipoatrophy (loss of fatty tissue, leaving an uneven appearance). Rotation *within* one anatomic site is preferred to rotation from one area to another to prevent day-to-day changes in absorption. The abdomen (except for a 2-inch radius around the navel) is the preferred injection site area because it provides the most rapid insulin absorption.

Absorption rate is determined by insulin properties. The longer the duration of action, the more unpredictable is absorption. Larger doses of insulin also prolong the absorption. Factors that increase blood flow from the injection site, such as local application of heat, massage of the area, and exercise of the injected area, increase insulin absorption. Scarred sites often become favorite injection sites because they are less sensitive to pain, but these areas usually slow the rate of insulin absorption.

Injection depth changes insulin absorption. Usually, injections are made into the subcutaneous tissue. Most patients

EVIDENCE-BASED PRACTICE

Why Do Adults with Diabetes Omit Prescribed Insulin Doses?

Peyrot, M., Rubin, R., Kruger, D., & Travis, L. (2010). Correlates of insulin injection omission. *Diabetes Care, 33*(2), 240-245.

Both type 1 and type 2 diabetes mellitus (DM) result in severe and life-shortening complications when blood glucose levels are not controlled. Extensive research has shown that maintaining hemoglobin A_{1c} levels below 7% dramatically reduces or delays these complications. For people with type 1 DM, insulin therapy is required for blood glucose control. For many people with type 2 DM, insulin therapy is needed when other drug therapies are no longer effective. Intentional omission of insulin has been identified as a relatively common behavior in adolescents with DM. This study sought to determine to what degree intentional insulin omission occurs in adults with DM and what personal factors are associated with this behavior.

A total of 502 adults with diabetes were recruited into this online survey-based descriptive study, all of whom were prescribed insulin therapy. The majority, 77%, had type 2 DM and 23% had type 1 DM. Of these 502 subjects, 57% reported having intentionally omitted an insulin dose on occasion; however, 20% reported intentionally omitting insulin doses regularly. The incidence was highest among those with type 2 DM. Other variables that correlated with the behavior of regularly omitting insulin doses were lower socioeconomic level, not having followed a healthy diet, and having a prescribed insulin regimen that required more frequent daily injections. Insulin injection factors that correlated with omitting insulin doses included the perception that injections were painful and embarrassing and that insulin scheduling interfered with the life activities of eating, exercising, and working. Some of the factors that either did not correlate with omitting insulin doses or had only minimal influence were race/ethnicity, education level, and the presence of depressive symptoms.

Level of Evidence: 4

Although very large, the study was descriptive in nature without randomization of subject selection or assignment. The information collected relied on subject self-report. The methods of statistical analysis were appropriate for the research questions posed.

Commentary: Implications for Practice and Research

The results of this study indicate that insulin omission is more common among people with type 2 DM. The researchers postulated that perhaps this group may view their disease as less serious than type 1 DM, especially if they retain any beta-cell function. These subjects also viewed the use of insulin to be more burdensome, painful, and embarrassing than did those with type 1 DM.

Because the overall damage caused by hyperglycemia is the same regardless of the category of DM, it is imperative that patients with type 2 DM understand the relationship between poor blood glucose control and development of complications. Nurses and other members of the health care team must convey the benefits of tight glycemic control that insulin therapy provides, as well as the benefits of a healthy diet. One factor possibly contributing to this problem is a lack of continuing access to support from health care professionals, especially diabetes educators. Assisting the patient to access local and online information and support services may help increase understanding about the disease and its effective therapy.

Some of the issues regarding the "pain" of injections can be reduced by teaching patients about the use of smaller needles, as well as injection into body areas with less sensitivity. Nurses can help patients identify ways and means to self-inject insulin without drawing undo attention and to disguise injection site bruising.

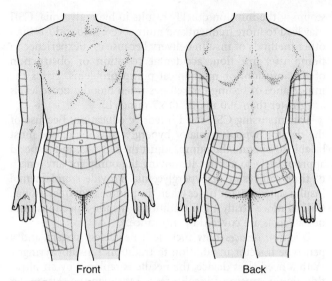

FIG. 67-4 Common insulin injection areas and sites.

Front   Back

TABLE 67-10	AMERICAN DIABETES ASSOCIATION GUIDELINES FOR THE MIXING OF INSULINS

- Patients whose condition is well controlled on a particular mixed-insulin regimen should maintain their standard procedure for preparing insulin doses.
- No other drug or diluents should be mixed with any insulin product unless approved by the prescribing health care provider.
- Insulin glargine should not be mixed with any other forms of insulin because of the low pH of its diluent.
- Currently available NPH and short-acting insulin formulations when mixed may be used immediately or stored for future use.
- Rapid-acting insulin can be mixed with NPH insulin.
- When rapid-acting insulin is mixed with either an intermediate-acting or a long-acting insulin, the mixture should be injected within 15 minutes before a meal.
- Insulin formulations may change; therefore manufacturers should be consulted when their recommendations appear to conflict with the American Diabetes Association guidelines.

Data from American Diabetes Association (ADA). (2004). Insulin administration. *Diabetes Care, 27*(Suppl. 1), 106-109.

lightly grasp a fold of skin and inject at a 90-degree angle. Aspiration for blood is not needed. A thin patient may need to pinch the skin and inject at a 45-degree angle to avoid IM injection. IM injection has a faster absorption and is not used for routine insulin use. Assess the older patient's ability to inject insulin, and arrange for assistance when self-care is no longer possible.

Timing of injection affects blood glucose levels. The interval between premeal injections and eating, known as "lag time," affects blood glucose levels after meals. Insulin lispro, insulin aspart, and insulin glulisine have rapid onsets of action and should be given within 10 minutes before mealtime when blood glucose is in the target range. If hyperglycemia or hypoglycemia is not present, these insulins can be given at any time from 10 minutes before mealtime to just before eating or even immediately after eating. Regular insulin should be given at least 20 to 30 minutes before eating when glucose levels are within the target range. When blood glucose levels are above the target range, the lag time should be increased to permit insulin to begin to have an effect sooner. Rapid-acting insulin analogs can be given 15 minutes before and regular insulin 30 to 60 minutes before eating a meal. When blood glucose levels are below the target range, injection of regular insulin should be delayed until immediately before eating and injection of rapid-acting insulin should be delayed until sometime after eating the meal.

Mixing insulins can change the time of peak action. Mixtures of short- and intermediate-acting insulins produce a more normal blood glucose response in some patients than does a single dose. The patient's response to mixed insulin may differ from the response to the same insulins given separately.

When rapid-acting (Humalog or NovoLog) or short-acting (regular) insulin is mixed with a longer-acting insulin, draw the shorter-acting dose into the syringe first. This action prevents contamination of the shorter-acting insulin vial with the longer-acting insulin. Short-acting and NPH insulins may be used immediately when mixed, or they may be stored. Mixing clouds the solution and makes the onset of action and peak effect time less predictable. Follow American

Diabetes Association (ADA) guidelines for mixing insulins (Table 67-10).

! NURSING SAFETY PRIORITY
Drug Alert

Do not mix any other insulin type with insulin glargine, insulin detemir, or with any of the premixed insulin formulations, such as Humalog Mix 75/25.

Complications of Insulin Therapy. Hypoglycemia from insulin excess has many causes. Its effects and treatment are discussed on pp. 1451-1454 in the Preventing Hypoglycemia section.

Lipoatrophy is a loss of fat tissue in areas of repeated injection that results from an immune reaction to impurities in insulin. Treatment consists of injection of insulin at the edge of the atrophied area. Lipohypertrophy is an increased swelling of fat that occurs at the site of repeated insulin injections. The overlying skin has decreased sensitivity, and the area can become large and unsightly. Treatment consists of rotating the injection site among different body areas. Teach patients who take insulin to rotate injection sites to prevent lipohypertrophy.

Two conditions of fasting hyperglycemia can occur (Fig. 67-5). *Dawn phenomenon* results from a nighttime release of growth hormone that causes blood glucose elevations at about 5 to 6 AM. It is managed by providing more insulin for the overnight period (e.g., giving the evening dose of intermediate-acting insulin at 10 PM). *Somogyi phenomenon* is morning hyperglycemia from the counterregulatory response to nighttime hypoglycemia. It is managed by ensuring adequate dietary intake at bedtime and evaluating the insulin dose and exercise programs to prevent conditions that lead to hypoglycemia. Both problems are diagnosed by blood glucose monitoring during the night. Help identify these problems, and teach the patient and family about management.

Alternative Methods of Insulin Administration. Many methods of insulin delivery are available in addition to traditional subcutaneous injections.

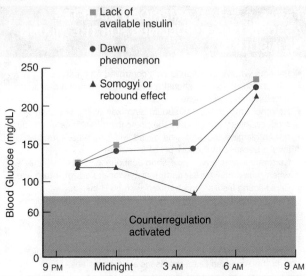

FIG. 67-5 Three blood glucose phenomena in patients with diabetes.

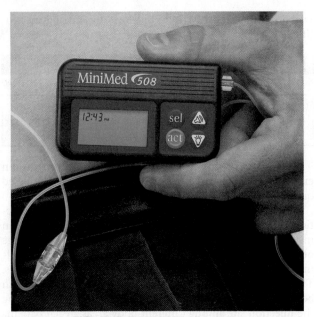

FIG. 67-6 External insulin pump.

Continuous subcutaneous infusion of a basal dose of insulin (CSII) with increases in insulin at mealtimes is more effective in controlling blood glucose levels than a multiple-injection schedule. CSII allows flexibility in meal timing, because if a meal is skipped, the additional mealtime dose of insulin is not given. It is given by an externally worn pump containing a syringe and reservoir with rapid-acting insulin and is connected to the patient by an infusion set. Teach him or her to adjust the amount of insulin based on data from blood glucose monitoring. Rapid-acting insulin analogs are used with insulin infusion pumps (Fig. 67-6).

Problems with CSII include skin infections that can occur when the infusion site is not cleaned or the needle is not changed every 2 to 3 days. When the patient is receiving rapid-acting insulin and has normal blood glucose levels, stopping the infusion quickly results in hyperglycemia. CSII may lead to more frequent and more severe ketoacidosis than other methods of insulin delivery because of inexperience in pump use, infection, accidental cessation or obstruction of the infusion, or mechanical pump problems. Stress the importance of testing for ketones when blood glucose levels are greater than 300 mg/dL (16.7 mmol/L).

Patients using CSII need intensive education. Because of the risk for hypoglycemia or hyperglycemia, he or she must be able to operate the pump, adjust the settings, and respond appropriately to alarms. Removing the pump for any length of time can result in hyperglycemia. Provide supplemental insulin schedules for times when the pump is not operational. CSII is more costly than traditional insulin injections, and not all costs are covered by insurance.

Injection devices now include a needleless system and a pen-type injector in addition to traditional insulin syringes. With a needleless device, the needle is replaced by an ultra-thin liquid stream of insulin forced through the skin under high pressure. Insulin given by jet injection is absorbed at a faster rate and has a shorter duration of action. Cost is a drawback to this system.

Patient Education: Drugs. Provide specific instructions about insulin therapy, new drug therapies, and self-monitoring of blood glucose levels.

Insulin storage varies by use. Teach patients to refrigerate insulin that is not in use to maintain potency, prevent exposure to sunlight, and inhibit bacterial growth. Insulin in use may be kept at room temperature for up to 28 days to reduce irritation at the injection site caused by cold insulin.

To prevent loss of drug potency, teach the patient to avoid exposing insulin to temperatures below 36° F (2.2° C) or above 86° F (30° C), to avoid excessive shaking, and to protect insulin from direct heat and light. Insulin should not be allowed to freeze. Insulin glargine (Lantus) should be stored in a refrigerator (36° to 46° F [2.2° to 7.8° C]) even when in use. Teach patients to discard any unused insulin after 28 days.

Teach patients to always have a spare bottle of each type of insulin used. A slight loss in potency may occur after the bottle has been in use for more than 30 days, even when the expiration date has not passed. Prefilled syringes are stable up to 30 days when refrigerated. If possible, store prefilled syringes in the upright position, with the needle pointing upward, so that insulin particles do not clog it. Teach patients to roll prefilled syringes between the hands before using. The effect of premixing insulins on blood glucose control is assessed by examining blood glucose levels.

Dose preparation is critical for insulin effectiveness and patient safety. Teach patients that the person giving the insulin needs to inspect the insulin before each use for changes (e.g., clumping, frosting, precipitation, or change in clarity or color) that may indicate loss in potency. Rapid-acting, short-acting, and glargine insulins should be clear, and all other types of insulin should be uniformly cloudy after gently rolling the vial between the hands. If potency is questionable, another vial of the same type of insulin should be used.

Syringes are the most commonly used method to administer insulin. The standard insulin syringes are marked in insulin units. They are available in 1-mL (100-U), ½-mL (50-U), and ³⁄₁₀-mL (30-U) sizes. The unit scale on the barrel of the syringe differs with the syringe size and manufacturer.

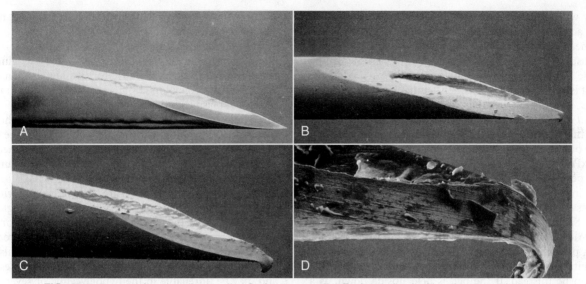

FIG. 67-7 Reuse of an insulin needle. **A,** A new needle. **B,** A needle that has been used once. **C,** A needle that has been used twice. **D,** A needle that has been used six times.

CHART 67-4 PATIENT AND FAMILY EDUCATION: PREPARING FOR SELF-MANAGEMENT

Subcutaneous Insulin Administration

- Wash your hands.
- Inspect the bottle for the type of insulin and the expiration date.
- Gently roll the bottle of intermediate-acting insulin in the palms of your hands to mix the insulin.
- Clean the rubber stopper with an alcohol swab.
- Remove the needle cover, and pull back the plunger to draw air into the syringe. The amount of air should be equal to the insulin dose. Push the needle through the rubber stopper, and inject the air into the insulin bottle.
- Turn the bottle upside down, and draw the insulin dose into the syringe.
- Remove air bubbles in the syringe by tapping on the syringe or injecting air back into the bottle. Redraw the correct amount.
- Make certain the tip of the plunger is on the line for your dose of insulin. Magnifiers are available to assist in measuring accurate doses of insulin.
- Remove the needle from the bottle. Recap the needle if the insulin is not to be given immediately.
- Select a site within your injection area that has not been used in the past month.
- Clean your skin with an alcohol swab. Lightly grasp an area of skin, and insert the needle at a 90-degree angle.
- Push the plunger all the way down. This will push the insulin into your body. Release the pinched skin.
- Pull the needle straight out quickly. Do not rub the place where you gave the shot.
- Dispose of the syringe and needle without recapping in a puncture-proof container.

CHART 67-5 PATIENT AND FAMILY EDUCATION: PREPARING FOR SELF-MANAGMENT

How to Mix a Prescribed Dose of 10 Units of Regular Insulin and 20 Units of NPH Insulin

- Wash your hands.
- Inspect the bottle for the type of insulin and the expiration date.
- Gently roll the bottle of intermediate-acting (NPH) insulin in the palms of your hands to mix the insulin.
- Clean the rubber stopper with an alcohol swab.
- Inject 20 units of air into the NPH insulin bottle. The amount of air should be equal to the dose of insulin needed. Always inject air into the intermediate-acting insulin first. Withdraw the needle.
- Inject 10 units of air into the regular insulin bottle. The amount of air is equal to the dose of insulin desired.
- Withdraw 10 units of regular insulin. Be sure that the syringe is free of air bubbles. Always withdraw the shorter-acting insulin first.
- Withdraw 20 units of NPH insulin with the same syringe, being careful not to inject any short-acting insulin into the bottle. (A total of 30 units should be in the syringe.)

Manufacturers recommend that disposable needles be used only once. Reuse of an insulin syringe and needle can compromise insulin sterility. Most insulins contain products that inhibit growth of bacteria commonly found on the skin; however, most patients with diabetes are at an increased risk for infection. Another reason to not reuse smaller (30- and 31-gauge) needles is that even with one injection, the needle tip can become bent to form a hook, which can lacerate tissue or break off to leave needle fragments in the skin (Fig. 67-7). Teach the patient to discard the syringe and needle after one use by participating in a community program, such as a drop-off center for household hazardous waste, or in a national disposal program, such as a "sharps" mail-back program (in accordance with The Joint Commission's National Patient Safety Goals). Information on needle disposal can be obtained at www.safeneedledisposal.org.

Pen-type injectors hold small, lightweight, prefilled insulin cartridges. The injectors are easy to carry and make intensive

Insulin syringe needles are measured in 28-, 29-, 30-, and 31-gauge and in lengths of ½-inch and ⁵⁄₁₆-inch. Short needles are not used for obese patients because of poor insulin absorption. To ensure accurate insulin measurement, instruct the patient to always buy the same type of syringe. Charts 67-4 and 67-5 review instructions for drawing up a single insulin injection and for mixing regular and NPH insulin in the same syringe.

therapy with multiple injections easier. These devices allow greater accuracy than traditional insulin syringes, especially when measuring small doses. Discuss proper storage for pre-filled insulin pens or cartridges. More drugs are becoming available in a prefilled syringe or cartridge. Ensure that the product is appropriate to the patient's unique needs. *Pen-type injectors are not designed for independent use by visually impaired patients or by those with cognitive impairment.* Ensure that the patient has received education on its use. Each syringe or cartridge has specific requirements. Patients using the FlexPen (Novo Nordisk) must be able to attach a needle and to perform an air shot of 2 units to ensure that a dose of insulin is administered. The Institute for Safe Medication Practices (ISMP) and The Joint Commission's National Patient Safety Goals identify insulin as a *High-Alert* drug. (High-Alert drugs are those that have an increased risk for causing patient harm if given in error.) The ISMP cautions that digital displays on some of the newer insulin formulations can be misread. If the pen is held upside down, as a left-handed person might do, a dose of 52 units actually appears to be a dose of 25 units, and a dose of 12 units looks like a dose of 21 units.

ⓘ DECISION-MAKING CHALLENGE

Patient-Centered Care

You are teaching a 22-year-old woman newly diagnosed with type 1 diabetes how to self-administer insulin. This is the second teaching session, and she can draw up the correct amount and maintain sterility. She has not been able to actually inject the needle into her skin, saying "It doesn't hurt but I just can't stand to push that needle in." She has not had any difficulty when her sister or the nurse has injected the insulin.

1. What should your immediate response be?
2. What modifications in your teaching technique can you make?
3. Is it critical that the patient learn to inject herself at this session? Why or why not?
4. Is there any type of adaptation that can help with this problem?

Patient Education: Blood Glucose Monitoring. Self-monitoring of blood glucose (SMBG) levels provides information to assess effectiveness of the management plan. SMBG allows patients and providers to evaluate patient response to therapy and assess whether glycemic targets are being reached. Results of SMBG are useful in preventing hypoglycemia and adjusting drug therapy, nutrition therapy, and physical activity. Assessment of blood glucose levels is very important for these situations:

- Symptoms of hypoglycemia/hyperglycemia
- Hypoglycemic unawareness
- Periods of illness
- Before and after exercise
- Gastroparesis
- Adjustment of diabetes medications
- Evaluation of other drug therapies (e.g., steroids)
- Preconception planning
- Pregnancy

Technique for SMBG follows principles that are the same for most self-monitoring systems. The finger is pricked, a drop of blood flows over or is drawn into a testing strip or disc impregnated with chemicals, and the glucose value is displayed in mg/dL or mmol/L. Most meters display blood glucose results on a screen. For vision-impaired patients, "talking meters" are available to allow independence in blood glucose monitoring.

Home blood glucose meters measure glucose in whole blood, whereas most laboratory tests measure glucose in plasma, which is generally 10% to 15% higher than glucose measured in whole blood. Many meters currently in use give results as "plasma equivalents" even though they are measuring whole blood. This value is calculated from the whole blood glucose reading using a formula built into the glucose meter. This conversion allows patients to compare their home glucose monitoring results with laboratory measurements of glucose.

Data obtained from SMBG are evaluated along with other measures of blood glucose (e.g., glycosylated hemoglobin, or hemoglobin A_{1c} [HbA_{1c}], values) or periodic laboratory blood glucose tests. Even when SMBG is performed correctly, the results are affected by hematocrit values (anemia falsely elevates glucose values; polycythemia falsely depresses them) and may be unreliable in the hypoglycemic or severe hyperglycemic ranges.

Blood glucose meters must meet the accuracy standards set by the International Organization for Standardization (IOS). According to the IOS, blood glucose meters must provide results that are within 20% of a laboratory standard 90% of the time. The performance of SMBG systems depends on accuracy of the specific blood glucose meter, operator proficiency, and test strip quality. Results are influenced by the size and quality of the blood sample; the meter's calibration to the strip in use; environmental conditions of altitude, temperature, and moisture; and patient-specific conditions of hematocrit level, triglyceride level, high levels of substances such as ascorbic acid in blood, and the presence of hypotension or hypoxia.

Accuracy of the blood glucose monitor is ensured when the manufacturer's directions are followed. The most significant source of error in blood glucose measurement is related to the skill of the user and not to errors of the instrument. Common errors in SMBG involve failure to obtain a sufficient blood drop, poor storage of test strips, using expired strips, and not changing the code number on the meter to match the strip bottle code. Help the patient select a meter based on cost of the meter and strips, ease of use, and availability of repair and servicing. Provide training, explain and demonstrate procedures, assess visual acuity, and check the patient's ability to perform the procedure through a return demonstration. Glucose meters are designed to reduce user error as much as possible. Newer meters no longer require wiping the blood from the strip in timed sequence, include error signals for inadequate sample size, "lock out" if control solutions are not tested, and store hundreds of SMBG results. (See the Consumer Guide published yearly in the January edition of Diabetes Forecast [forecast.diabetes.org] for information to help patients determine which blood glucose meter best meets their needs.)

Even when highly trained personnel tested meters under optimal conditions, accuracy and precision varied widely among capillary blood glucose monitoring devices. Teach patients to properly calibrate the machine. Instruct them to re-check the calibration and re-test if they obtain a test result that is unusual for them and whenever they are in doubt about test accuracy. Continued retraining of patients performing SMBG helps ensure accurate results because performance accuracy deteriorates over time. Laboratory glucose determinations are more accurate than SMBG.

Frequency of testing varies with the complexity of the drug schedules and the patient's prescribed therapy target outcomes. The ADA recommends that patients taking multiple insulin injections or using insulin pump therapy monitor glucose levels three or more times daily. For patients taking less-frequent injections of insulin, non-insulin therapy, or nutrition therapy alone, SMBG is useful for evaluation of therapy.

Blood glucose therapy target goals are set individually for each patient. The entire health care team works with him or her to reach target blood glucose levels. The ADA recommends that patients with type 1 diabetes aim for HbA1c values less than 7%, premeal glucose levels of 70 to 130 mg/dL (3.9 to 7.2 mmol/L), and postmeal glucose levels less than 180 mg/dL (10.0 mmol/L) (ADA, 2010b).

Infection control measures are needed for SMBG. Teach the patient to follow Centers for Disease Control and Prevention (CDC) guidelines for infection control during SMBG. The chance of becoming infected from blood glucose monitoring processes is reduced by handwashing before monitoring and by not reusing lancets. *Instruct patients to not share their blood glucose monitoring equipment.* Hepatitis B virus can survive in a dried state for at least 1 week. Infection can be spread by the lancet holder even when the lancet itself has been changed. Small particles of blood can stick to the device and infect multiple users. Regular cleaning of the meter is critical for infection control. Remind health care staff who perform blood glucose testing and family members who help with testing to wear gloves.

Many meters have sophisticated data-handling capabilities. Many can be downloaded by a cable or by infrared technology to a computer that has diabetes management software. Some meters allow entry of additional data such as insulin dose, amounts of carbohydrate eaten, or exercise. A radio link to an insulin pump allows automatic transfer of glucose readings to a calculator that assists the patient in deciding on an appropriate insulin dose.

! NURSING SAFETY PRIORITY

Action Alert

> Prevent hypoglycemia by ensuring that appropriate blood glucose testing products are used for patients receiving parenteral maltose, parenteral galactose, and oral xylose products.

The U.S. Food and Drug Administration issued an Important Safety Information Notice about blood glucose measurement following use of parenteral maltose, parenteral galactose, and oral xylose-containing products.

When patients receive icodextrin (EXTRANEAL) peritoneal dialysis solution, blood glucose values obtained using point-of-care blood glucose monitors may be falsely elevated. Icodextrin is metabolized to maltose, and the presence of maltose in blood can cause readings to be falsely elevated when using some, but not all, portable glucose monitors. Insulin therapy based on falsely elevated blood glucose values has caused hypoglycemia, coma, and death. Products containing maltose, galactose, and xylose also cause blood glucose readings to be falsely elevated. Maltose is found in immune globulin intravenous (Octagam 5%, Gamimune N 5%),

rho(D) immune globulin (WinRho SDF), and vaccinia immune globulin (VIG-IV). Galactose and xylose are found in some foods, herbs, and dietary supplements; they are also used in diagnostic tests.

Portable glucose monitors using test strips with glucose dehydrogenase pyrroloquinoline quinone (GDH-PQQ) or glucose-dye-oxidoreductase (GDO) reagents cannot distinguish between glucose, maltose, and other sugars and will provide falsely elevated "glucose" readings in the presence of these sugars. The GDH-PQQ and GDO reagent-based glucose monitors are widely available and commonly used in hospital settings to provide point-of-care blood glucose testing. Various manufacturers, including Abbott, Bayer, Roche, CH Diagnostics, and Home Diagnostics, have glucose strips that use GDH-PQQ technology.

It is important that staff understand the potential for hypoglycemia when patients are admitted to the hospital. In that instance, it is safest to monitor blood glucose patterns by laboratory methods. Blood glucose monitoring needs to be performed with a system whose tests strips use a different enzyme technology. The best resource for guidance in selecting a glucose monitoring system that is not reactive to maltose interference is the manufacturer of the test strip. Some manufacturers produce test strips that use more than one type of enzyme technology.

Alternate site testing allows patients to obtain blood from sites other than the fingertip and is available on many meters. However, use caution when interpreting results obtained from alternate sites. These results are not necessarily the same as those from the fingertip when tested at the same time. Comparison studies have shown wide variation between fingertip and alternate sites, and the variation is most evident during times when blood glucose levels are rapidly changing. Teach patients that there is a lag time for blood glucose levels between the fingertip and other sites when blood glucose levels are changing rapidly and that the fingertip reading is the only safe choice at those times.

! NURSING SAFETY PRIORITY

Critical Rescue

> Teach patients with a history of hypoglycemic unawareness not to test at alternative sites.

Continuous blood glucose monitoring (CGM) systems monitor glucose levels in interstitial fluid. The system consists of three parts: a disposable sensor that measures glucose levels, a transmitter that is attached to the sensor, and a receiver that displays and stores glucose information. A thin plastic sensor is inserted into subcutaneous tissue. Electrodes measure interstitial glucose concentrations and convert these values to blood glucose levels. The transmitter attached to the sensor uses radiofrequency communication to send information to the receiver, which provides real-time glucose information to the user. After an initiation or warm-up period, the sensor gives glucose values every 1 to 5 minutes. Sensors are approved for 3- to 7-day use, depending on the manufacturer. CGM provides information about the current blood glucose level, provides short-term feedback about results of treatment, and provides warnings when glucose readings become dangerously high or low. Most available sensors require at least two capillary glucose readings per day for calibration of

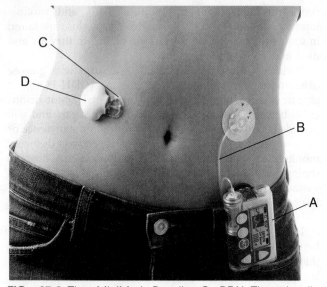

FIG. 67-8 The MiniMed Paradigm® REAL-Time Insulin Pump and Continuous Glucose Monitoring System. **A,** Pump. **B,** Injection cannula. **C,** Glucose sensor. **D,** Data transmitter.

the sensor. Sensor accuracy depends on these calibrations. There may be a lag time between the capillary glucose measurement and the glucose sensor value. If the blood glucose value is changing rapidly, the time between capillary and interstitial glucose values may be as long as 30 minutes. For this reason, capillary glucose readings need to be checked on all extreme values and before any corrective treatment is given.

Fig. 67-8 shows this type of system. The costs for CGM systems are substantial. The initial device varies from $400 to more than $2000. An additional monthly charge of at least $300 includes the cost of disposable sensors, which last between 3 to 7 days, and additional glucose test strips used to calibrate the sensors and perform FDA-required capillary glucose testing before treatment decisions are made.

Continuous glucose monitoring is meant to supplement, not replace, finger stick tests. Insulin should be given only after confirming the results of any of the continuous glucose monitoring systems.

Nutrition Therapy. Effective self-management of diabetes requires that the meal plan, education, and counseling programs be "patientized" for each patient. A dietitian should be a member of the treatment team. The nurse, dietitian, patient, and family work together on all aspects of the meal plan, which must be realistic and as flexible as possible. Plans that consider the patient's cultural background, financial status, and lifestyle are more likely to be successful.

Desired Outcomes of Nutrition Therapy. The ADA (2008) advocates that nutrition therapy focuses on these outcomes:
- Achieving and maintaining blood glucose levels in the normal range or as close to normal as is safely possible
- Achieving and maintaining a blood lipid profile that reduces the risk for vascular disease
- Achieving blood pressure levels in the normal range or as close to normal as is safely possible
- Preventing or slowing the rate of development of the chronic complications of diabetes by modifying nutrient intake and lifestyle

- Addressing patient nutrition needs taking into account personal and cultural preferences and willingness to change
- Maintaining the pleasure of eating by limiting food choices only when indicated by scientific evidence
- Meeting the nutritional needs of unique times of the life cycle, particularly for pregnant and lactating women and for older adults with diabetes
- Providing self-management training for patients treated with insulin or insulin secretagogues for exercising safely, including the prevention and treatment of hypoglycemia, and managing diabetes during acute illness

Principles of Nutrition in Diabetes. The dietitian develops a meal plan based on the patient's usual food intake, weight-management expectations, and lipid and blood glucose patterns. Day-to-day consistency in the timing and amount of food eaten helps control blood glucose. Patients receiving insulin therapy need to eat at times that are coordinated with the timed action of insulin. Teach patients using intense insulin therapy to adjust premeal insulin to allow for timing and quantity changes in their meal plan.

Carbohydrate recommendation for the patient with diabetes is a diet containing 45% to 65% of calories from carbohydrate, with a minimum intake of 130 g carbohydrate/day. The diet should include carbohydrate from fruit, vegetables, whole grains, legumes, and low-fat milk. Diets restricting total carbohydrate to less than 130 g/day are not recommended in the management of diabetes (ADA, 2008).

Food choices that prevent after-meal (*postprandial*) blood glucose elevation are important in achieving blood glucose control. The amount and types of carbohydrate consumed have the greatest impact on after-meal blood glucose levels.

The percentage of calories from carbohydrates is determined for each patient. Various starches have different blood glucose responses. Place the emphasis on the *total amount* of carbohydrate consumed each day rather than the source of the carbohydrate. Little evidence supports the assumption that sugars are more rapidly absorbed than starches and cause blood glucose values to increase more rapidly.

Dietary fat and cholesterol intake for people with diabetes focuses on limiting saturated fatty acids, *trans* fatty acids, and cholesterol to reduce the risk for cardiovascular disease. Current recommendations from the ADA (2008, 2010b) for patients with diabetes are:
- Limiting saturated fatty intake to less than 7% of total calories
- Minimizing intake of *trans* fat
- Limiting dietary cholesterol to less than 200 mg/day
- Having two or more servings of fish per week (with the exception of commercially fried fish) to provide n-3 polyunsaturated fatty acids

Trans fatty acids raise low-density lipoprotein (LDL) cholesterol and lower high-density lipoprotein (HDL) cholesterol; both actions increase the risk for cardiovascular disease. *Trans* fatty acids are found in hard margarine and in foods prepared with or fried in hydrogenated and partly hydrogenated oils. Teach the patient to restrict intake of *trans* fatty acids by limiting the amount of commercially fried foods and bakery goods eaten.

Further dietary fat restrictions for patients with diabetes are determined by a dietitian based on specific lipid levels.

Adults with diabetes should be tested annually for abnormalities of fasting serum cholesterol, triglyceride, HDL cholesterol, and calculated LDL cholesterol levels (ADA, 2008).

Protein intake of 15% to 20% of total daily calories is appropriate for patients with diabetes and normal kidney function. In patients with microalbuminuria, reducing protein intake to 10% of calories (0.8-1.0 g/kg) may slow progression of kidney failure. Reducing protein intake to not more than 0.8 g/kg body weight in later stages of chronic kidney disease may improve function (ADA, 2008).

Fiber improves carbohydrate metabolism and lowers cholesterol levels. Taste and texture, limited food choices, and GI side effects make it difficult to achieve a high-fiber intake. Assist the patient to first reach the target of 14 g per 1000 calories. The American Heart Association recommends a fiber intake of 25 g each day. Teach the patient to select a variety of fiber-containing foods such as legumes, fiber-rich cereals (more than 5 g fiber/serving), fruits, vegetables, and whole-grain products because they provide vitamins, minerals, and other substances important for good health.

Teach the patient that adding high-fiber foods to the diet gradually can reduce abdominal cramping, loose stools, and flatulence. An increase in fluid intake should accompany increased fiber intake. The nurse and the patient should pay careful attention to blood glucose levels because hypoglycemia can result when dietary fiber intake increases significantly.

Sweeteners include sucrose and a variety of nonnutritive substances. Dietary sucrose does not increase blood glucose more than equal amounts of other starches. Intake of sucrose and sucrose-containing foods by patients with diabetes does not need to be restricted out of a concern for causing hyperglycemia. Sucrose can be included in the meal plan as long as it is adequately covered with insulin or other glucose-lowering agents.

The use of products to enhance the taste of food while not disturbing blood glucose control is desirable. The FDA has approved five nonnutritive sweeteners: saccharin, aspartame, acesulfame, neotame, and sucralose.

Alcohol consumption can affect blood glucose levels. Levels are not affected by *moderate* use of alcohol when diabetes is well controlled. Teach patients with diabetes that two alcoholic beverages for men and one for women can be ingested with, and in addition to, the usual meal plan. (One alcoholic beverage equals 12 ounces of beer, 5 ounces of wine, or 1 and ½ ounces of distilled spirits.) Alcohol raises plasma triglycerides. Thus reducing or abstaining from alcohol is important for patients with hyperlipidemia. One alcoholic beverage is substituted for two fat exchanges when calculating caloric intake (ADA, 2008).

> ### ! NURSING SAFETY PRIORITY
> **Action Alert**
>
> Because of the potential for alcohol-induced hypoglycemia, instruct the patient with diabetes to ingest alcohol only with or shortly after meals.

Patient Education: Prescribed Nutrition Plan. No one meal plan is right for all patients with diabetes. Each patient's nutrition recommendations are based on blood glucose monitoring results, total blood lipid levels, and glycosylated hemoglobin (HbA_{1c}). These tests help determine whether current meal and exercise patterns need adjustment or whether present habits need reinforcement. A specific nutritional prescription is developed for each patient.

Reinforce information provided by the dietitian. The patient with DM needs to understand how to adjust food intake during illness, planned exercise, and social occasions (e.g., restaurant meals) when the usual time of eating is delayed. He or she may be unable to follow the prescribed plan because of an inability to see, read, or understand printed materials. Share dietary information with the person who prepares the meals. The dietitian sees each patient at least yearly to identify changes in lifestyle and make appropriate nutrition therapy changes. Some patients, such as those with weight control problems or low incomes, may need more frequent evaluation and counseling.

> ### ? NCLEX EXAMINATION CHALLENGE
> **Health Promotion and Maintenance**
>
> Which statement made by the client during nutritional counseling indicates to the nurse that the client with diabetes type 1 correctly understands his or her nutritional needs?
> A. "If I completely eliminate carbohydrates from my diet, I will not need to take insulin."
> B. "I will make certain that I eat at least 130 g of carbohydrate each day regardless of my activity level."
> C. "My intake of protein in terms of grams and calories should be the same as my intake of carbohydrate."
> D. "My intake of unsaturated fats in terms of grams and calories should be the same as my intake of protein."

Meal Planning Strategies. Many meal planning approaches are available. Each approach emphasizes different aspects of nutrition.

Exchange systems are based on three food groups: carbohydrates, meat and meat substitutes, and fat. The exchange list for meal planning assumes that foods with similar nutrient content affect blood glucose levels similarly. Plans based on the exchange system produce predictable blood glucose responses. The patient's prescription identifies how many items from each food group are to be eaten at a meal or snack. Information can be obtained from the American Dietetic Association at www.eatright.org.

Carbohydrate (CHO) counting is a simple approach to meal planning that uses label information of the nutritional content of packaged food items. Because fat and protein have little effect on after-meal blood glucose levels, CHO counting focuses on the nutrient that has the greatest impact on these levels. It uses total grams of carbohydrate, regardless of the food source. The dietitian determines the number of grams of carbohydrate to be eaten at each meal and snack and helps the patient make appropriate food choices. This method is effective in achieving overall blood glucose control when carbohydrate intake is consistent from day to day.

Patients using intensive insulin or pump therapies can use CHO counting to determine insulin coverage. After the amount of insulin needed to cover the usual meal is determined, insulin may be added or subtracted for changes in carbohydrate intake. An initial formula of 1 unit of rapid-acting insulin for each 15 g of carbohydrate provides flexibility to meal plans. The patient determines the grams of carbohydrate in a specific meal or snack by reading labels or

TABLE 67-11	CARBOHYDRATE COUNTING			
MEAL	FOOD SOURCE	GRAMS OF CARBOHYDRATES	TOTAL	INSULIN DOSE* (1:15 RATIO)
Breakfast	2 slices honey grain bread	32		
	¼ cup egg substitute	0		
	½ cup orange juice	15		
	1 tablespoon lower-fat margarine	0	47	3
Lunch	2 oz tuna, canned in water	0		
	1 hamburger bun	30		
	Fat-free Pringles (#15)	15		
	1 tablespoon reduced-fat mayonnaise	0		
	1 tomato and 1 lettuce slice	0		
	1 medium dill pickle	0		
	Sugar-free pudding made with fat-free milk	15	60	4
Supper	3 oz chicken breast, grilled	0		
	1 small (3 oz) baked potato	15		
	1 cup steamed broccoli	10		
	1 French roll	25		
	1 tablespoon lower-fat margarine	0		
	2 tablespoons reduced-fat sour cream	0		
	½ cup canned pineapple (in own juice)	15	65	4

*Insulin dose has been rounded off to the nearest whole unit.

weighing and measuring each item. The total grams of carbohydrate are used to calculate the bolus dose of insulin based on his or her prescribed insulin-to-carbohydrate ratio. See Table 67-11 for an example of carbohydrate counting.

People at high risk for type 2 diabetes are encouraged to achieve moderate weight loss (7% total body weight), participate in regular physical activity (150 minutes per week), and reduce caloric and dietary fat intake. These at-risk people are also encouraged to increase fiber intake to at least 14 g per 1000 calories consumed and to eat foods containing whole grains.

Special considerations for type 1 diabetes include developing insulin regimens that conform to the patient's preferred meal routines, food preferences, and exercise patterns. Patients using rapid-acting insulin by injection or an insulin pump should adjust insulin doses based on the carbohydrate content of the meals and snacks. Insulin-to-carbohydrate ratios are developed and are used to provide mealtime insulin doses. Blood glucose monitoring before and 2 hours after meals determines whether the insulin-to-carbohydrate ratio is correct. For patients who are on fixed insulin regimens and do not adjust premeal insulin dosages, consistency of timing of meals and the amount of CHO eaten at each meal is important to prevent hypoglycemia.

Physical exercise can cause hypoglycemia if insulin is not decreased before activity. For planned exercise, reduction in insulin dosage is the preferred method for hypoglycemia prevention. For unplanned exercise, intake of additional CHO is usually needed. Moderate exercise increases glucose utilization by 2 to 3 mg/kg/min. A 70-kg person would need about 10 to 15 g additional CHO per hour of moderate-intensity physical activity. More CHO is needed for intense activity (ADA, 2008).

It is important for patients with type 1 diabetes to avoid gaining weight. Hyperinsulinemia (chronic high blood insulin levels) can occur with intensive treatment schedules and may result in weight gain. These patients may need to manage hyperglycemia by restricting calories rather than increasing insulin. Weight gain can be minimized by following the prescribed meal plan, getting regular exercise, and avoiding overtreatment of hypoglycemia.

Special considerations for type 2 diabetes focus on lifestyle changes. Many patients with type 2 diabetes are overweight and insulin resistant. Nutrition therapy stresses lifestyle changes that reduce calories eaten and increase calories expended through physical activity. Many patients also have abnormal blood fat levels and hypertension (metabolic syndrome), making reductions of saturated fat, cholesterol, and sodium desirable. A moderate caloric restriction (250 to 500 calories less than average daily intake) and an increase in physical activity improve diabetic control and weight control. Decreases of more than 10% of body weight can result in

CONSIDERATIONS FOR OLDER ADULTS

Older patients are at increased risk for malnutrition, hypoglycemia, and especially dehydration, a factor in the development of hyperglycemic-hyperosmolar state (HHS). Many factors contribute to malnutrition. Nutritional needs of the older adult change as the person's taste, smell, and appetite diminish and his or her ability to obtain and prepare food decreases. Older patients who prepare their own food or have tooth loss or poorly fitting dentures may not eat enough food. Neuropathy with gastric retention or diarrhea compounds poor food intake. Impaired cognition and depression may disrupt self-care. Older patients may have a marginal food supply because of inadequate income, may have poor understanding of meal-planning needs, or may live alone and have reduced incentive to prepare or eat proper meals. They may eat in restaurants or live in situations in which they have little control over meal preparation. Regular visits by home health nurses can assist older patients in following a diabetic meal plan.

A realistic approach to nutrition therapy is essential for the older patient with diabetes. Changing the eating habits of 60 to 70 years is very difficult. The nurse, dietitian, and patient assess the patient's usual eating patterns. Teach the older patient taking antidiabetic drugs about the importance of eating meals and snacks at the same time every day, eating the same amount of food from day to day, and eating all food allowed on the diet.

significant improvement in HbA_{1c}. Decreasing intake of cholesterol-raising fatty acids helps reduce the risk for cardiovascular disease.

When patients with type 2 diabetes need insulin, consistency in timing and carbohydrate content of meals is important. Division of the total daily calories into three meals or into smaller meals and snacks is based on patient preference.

Exercise Therapy. Regular exercise is an essential part of diabetic management. It has beneficial effects on carbohydrate metabolism and insulin sensitivity. Programs of increased physical activity and weight loss reduce the incidence of type 2 diabetes in patients with impaired glucose tolerance (AADE, 2008).

Plasma glucose levels remain stable in physically active patients without diabetes because of the balance between glucose use by exercising muscles and glucose production by the liver. Exercise does not result in hyperglycemia or hypoglycemia. The patient with type 1 DM cannot make the hormonal changes needed to maintain stable blood glucose levels during exercise. Without an adequate insulin supply, cells cannot use glucose. Low insulin levels trigger release of glucagon and epinephrine (counterregulatory hormones) to increase liver glucose production, further raising blood glucose levels. In the absence of insulin, free fatty acids become the source of energy. Exercise in the patient with uncontrolled diabetes results in further hyperglycemia and the formation of ketone bodies. He or she may have prolonged elevated blood glucose levels after vigorous exercise.

Exercise in the person with diabetes can cause hypoglycemia because of increased muscle glucose uptake and inhibited glucose release from the liver. It can occur during exercise and for up to 24 hours after exercise. Replacement of muscle and liver glycogen stores, along with increased insulin sensitivity after exercise, causes insulin requirements to drop.

Benefits of Exercise. Appropriate exercise results in better regulation of blood glucose levels and lowering of insulin requirements for patients with type 1 DM. Exercise also increases insulin sensitivity, which enhances cell uptake of glucose and promotes weight loss.

Regular exercise decreases risk for cardiovascular disease. It decreases most blood lipid levels and increases high-density lipoproteins (HDLs). Exercise decreases blood pressure and improves cardiovascular function. Regular vigorous physical activity prevents or delays type 2 DM by reducing body weight, insulin resistance, and glucose intolerance.

Adjustments for Diabetes Complications. Exercise in the presence of long-term complications of diabetes often requires some adjustment. Vigorous aerobic or resistance exercise may be contraindicated in the presence of proliferative diabetic retinopathy or severe nonproliferative diabetic retinopathy. Teach the patient with retinopathy to avoid the Valsalva maneuver (breath holding while bearing down) and activities that increase blood pressure. Heavy lifting, rapid head motion, or jarring activities can cause vitreous hemorrhage or retinal detachment. Decreased pain sensation in the extremities increases the risk for skin breakdown and infection and for joint destruction. Teach patients with peripheral neuropathy to wear proper footwear and to examine their feet daily for lesions. Teach anyone with a foot injury or open sore to engage in non–weight-bearing activities such as swimming, bicycling, or arm exercises. Those with autonomic neuropathy are at increased risk for exercise-induced injury from impaired temperature control, postural hypotension, and impaired thirst with risk for dehydration. Physical activity also can increase urine protein excretion. Encourage high-risk patients to start with short periods of low-intensity exercise and to increase the intensity and duration slowly (ADA, 2010b).

Safety Assessment. Assessment before initiating an exercise program is necessary to ensure patient safety. Although current ADA guidelines do not recommend routine screening for patients with diabetes who have no manifestations of cardiovascular disease, be alert to conditions that might predispose the patient to injury or that contraindicate certain types of exercise. Regular physical activity increases the risk for both musculoskeletal injury and life-threatening cardiovascular events. The ADA recommends screening when any of these conditions exist (Roelker, 2008):

- Typical or atypical chest pain
- Abnormal electrocardiogram (ECG) suggestive of ischemia or infarction
- Peripheral or carotid occlusive disease
- Age older than 35 years with sedentary lifestyle in a patient who plans a vigorous exercise program
- Two or more risk factors in addition to diabetes, such as dyslipidemia, hypertension, tobacco use
- Family history for premature coronary artery disease, or microalbuminuria or macroalbuminuria of more than 10 years' duration
- Age older than 25 years and type 1 diabetes of more than 15 years' duration
- Severe autonomic neuropathy, severe peripheral neuropathy, history of foot lesions, and unstable proliferative retinopathy

Screening for coronary artery disease before an exercise program is started is recommended for patients with cardiovascular risk factors. The purpose of exercise treadmill testing (ETT) is to determine if a person can exercise to 85% of their predicted heart rate without having ischemic changes. Also, ETT provides information about exercise capacity and functional status. Failure to achieve 85% of the predicted heart rate is associated with increased death from all causes.

Imaging studies provide information regarding the risk for exercise-induced ischemia. Medical stress tests with vasodilator therapy are recommended for patients who are not able to exercise or who have abnormal ECG. Stress echocardiography provides information about left ventricular systolic, left ventricular diastolic, and valvular function, and it assesses for evidence of exercise-induced ischemia. Additional tests may be performed to determine the presence of obstructive lesions in coronary arteries.

The positive benefits of exercise are short term (i.e., triglyceride reduction lasts for up to 72 hours). Advise people with DM to perform at least 150 min/week of moderate-intensive aerobic physical activity, or 75 min/week of vigorous aerobic physical activity or an equivalent combination of the two. In the absence of contraindications, patients with type 2 diabetes are urged to perform resistance exercise 3 times a week, targeting all major muscle groups (ADA 2010b). The effect of a single bout of aerobic exercise on insulin sensitivity lasts 24 to 72 hours, depending on the duration and intensity of the activity. The ADA recommends that there be no more than 2 consecutive days without aerobic physical activity.

A 5- to 10-minute warm-up period with stretching and low-intensity exercise before exercise prepares the skeletal muscles, heart, and lungs for a progressive increase in exercise intensity. After the activity session, a cool-down should be performed similarly to the warm-up. The cool-down should last 5 to 10 minutes and gradually bring the heart rate down to pre-exercise level.

Guidelines for exercise are based on blood glucose levels and urine ketone levels. Recommend that the patient test blood glucose before exercise, at intervals during exercise, and after exercise to determine if it is safe to exercise and to evaluate the effects of exercise. The absence of urine ketones indicates that enough insulin is available for glucose transport and that exercise should be effective in lowering blood glucose levels. *When urine ketones are present, the patient should* NOT *exercise.* Ketones indicate that current insulin levels are not adequate and that exercise would elevate blood glucose levels. Carbohydrate foods should be ingested to raise blood glucose levels above 100 mg/dL (5.6 mmol/L) before engaging in exercise.

! NURSING SAFETY PRIORITY

Critical Rescue

Teach patients with type 1 diabetes to perform vigorous exercise only when blood glucose levels are 100 to 250 mg/dL (5.6 to 13.8 mmol/L) and no ketones are present in the urine.

Patient Education: Exercise Promotion. Chart 67-6 lists tips to teach the patient and family about self-management and exercise. Instruct the patient to wear shoes with good traction and cushioning and to examine the feet daily and after

CHART 67-6 PATIENT AND FAMILY EDUCATION: PREPARING FOR SELF-MANAGEMENT

Exercise

* Teach the patient about the relationship between regularly scheduled exercise and blood glucose levels, blood lipid levels, and complications of diabetes.
* Reinforce the level of exercise recommended for the patient based on his or her physical health.
* Instruct the patient to wear appropriate footwear designed for exercise.
* Remind the patient to examine his or her feet daily and after exercising.
* Warn the patient not to exercise within 1 hour of insulin injection or near the time of peak insulin action.
* Teach patients how to prevent hypoglycemia during exercise:
  * Do not exercise unless blood glucose level is at least 80 and less than 250 mg/dL.
  * Have a carbohydrate snack before exercising if 1 hour has passed since the last meal or if the planned exercise is high intensity.
  * Carry a simple sugar to eat during exercise if symptoms of hypoglycemia occur.
  * Ensure that identification information about diabetes is carried during exercise.
* Remind the patient to check blood glucose levels more frequently on days in which exercise is performed and that extra carbohydrate and less insulin may be needed during the 24-hour period after extensive exercise.

exercise. Warn him or her to not exercise in extreme heat or cold or during periods of poor blood glucose control. Teach the patient to stay hydrated, especially during and after exercise in a warm environment.

Teach patients not to exercise within 1 hour of insulin injection or at the peak time of insulin action. Exercise can increase absorption of insulin from the injection site, increasing blood insulin levels. The risk for hypoglycemia increases when insulin is injected into an area that is exercised.

Teach patients about the risk for hypoglycemia and its preventive measures. Those taking insulin secretagogues or insulin should monitor blood glucose levels to determine the effects of exercise. Reinforce that snacks containing rapidly absorbable carbohydrate may be eaten before and during exercise to maintain normal blood glucose levels. Extra carbohydrate may be needed for up to 24 hours after exercise to prevent hypoglycemia. The amount of additional carbohydrate is directed by the results of blood glucose monitoring. Teach the patient to decrease insulin dosage before planned exercise as directed.

Advise the nonobese patient who is taking insulin secretagogues or insulin to have a carbohydrate-containing snack before exercise if at least 1 hour has passed since the last food was eaten or if high-intensity exercise is planned. Additional carbohydrate intake is not needed when the blood glucose level exceeds 100 mg/dL (5.6 mmol/L) before exercise and the planned activity is of low intensity and short duration. When vigorous activity of long duration is planned, teach the patient to eat an additional 15 to 30 g of carbohydrate for every 30 to 60 minutes of exercise. Snacks such as fruit, fruit juice, bread products, and whole milk can prevent hypoglycemia. Teach patients to carry a simple sugar (hard candy) to eat if symptoms of hypoglycemia occur. Also instruct them to carry identifying information about having diabetes.

CONSIDERATIONS FOR OLDER ADULTS

With age, the ability of the heart and lungs to deliver oxygen to tissues and organs declines. These changes may be due more to decline in muscle mass than to changes in cardiac output. Aerobic activities are important in maintaining muscle mass. Healthy older adults are able to maintain cardiac output by increasing stroke volume during exercise.

The emphasis for any activity program is on changing sedentary behavior to active behavior at any level. Encourage sedentary older adults to begin with low-intensity physical activity. Start low-intensity activities in short sessions (less than 10 minutes); include warm-up and cool-down components with active stretching. Changes in activity levels should be gradual. Formal evaluation by a physical therapist and/or occupational therapist may be needed.

In the absence of retinopathy-related restrictions, strength (resistance) training for major muscles of the legs, arms, stomach, and trunk, performed two or three times weekly, helps preserve muscle mass and minimizes general functional decline. Examples of specific exercise can be found at www.geri.com.

Blood Glucose Control in Hospitalized Patients. Hyperglycemia in hospitalized patients occurs for many reasons and is associated with poor outcomes. In patients without a previous diagnosis of diabetes, elevated blood glucose may be due to "stress hyperglycemia." Hyperglycemia may result from decline in basic level of glucose control caused by illness, decreased physical activity, withholding of antidiabetic drugs, administration of drugs that cause hyperglycemia such as corticosteroids, and initiation of tube feedings or parenteral nutrition.

Hyperglycemia among general medical-surgical patients is linked with higher infection rates, longer hospital stays, increased need for intensive care, and greater mortality. Serum glucose levels greater than 200 mg/mL (11.0 mmol/L) after cardiothoracic surgical procedures are associated with higher rates of wound infection. Admission glucose levels greater than 198 mg/dL (10.9 mmol/L) are associated with greater risk for mortality and complications. Hypoglycemia, defined as blood glucose values lower than 40 mg/dL (2.2 mmol/L), is considered an independent risk factor for mortality.

Current American Association of Clinical Endocrinologists (AACE) and ADA guidelines recommend treatment protocols that maintain blood glucose levels between 140 and 180 mg/dL (7.8 and 10.0 mmol/L) for critically ill patients. For the majority of non–critically ill patients, premeal glucose targets should be lower than 140 mg/dL (7.8 mmol/L) in conjunction with random blood glucose values less than 180 mg/dL (10.0 mmol/L). To prevent hypoglycemia, insulin regimens should be reviewed if blood glucose levels fall below 100 mg/dL (5.6 mmol/L) and should be modified when blood glucose levels are less than 70 mg/dL (3.9 mmol/L) (ADA, 2010b).

Continuous IV insulin solutions are the most effective method for achieving glycemic targets in the intensive care setting. Scheduled subcutaneous injection with basal, meal, and correction elements is the preferred method for achieving and maintaining glucose control in non–critically ill patients. Using correction dose or "supplemental insulin" to correct premeal hyperglycemia in addition to scheduled prandial and basal insulin is recommended. The correction dose is determined by the patient's insulin sensitivity and current blood glucose level. The health care provider calculates sensitivity by adding up the patient's total daily insulin requirement and dividing that amount into 1500 (for type 2 DM) or 1700 (for type 1 DM).

Prevention of hypoglycemia is also part of managing blood glucose levels. Causes of inpatient hypoglycemia include an inappropriate insulin type, mismatch between insulin type and/or timing of nutritional intake, and altered nutritional intake without insulin dosage adjustment. Many facilities have protocols for hypoglycemia treatment that direct staff to provide carbohydrate replacement if the patient is alert and able to swallow, or to administer 50% dextrose intravenously or glucagon by subcutaneous injection if the patient cannot swallow.

There is confusion about whether to give or to hold insulin from a patient who is NPO. Administration of rapid-acting or short-acting insulin, as well as amylin and incretin mimetics, will cause hypoglycemia if a patient is not eating. Basal insulin should be administered when the patient is NPO because it treats baseline glucose levels. Insulin mixtures are not administered because they contain some short-acting or rapid-acting insulin and will cause hypoglycemia.

Surgical Management. Surgical interventions for diabetes include transplantation of the pancreas. Successful transplantation improves quality of life by eliminating the need for insulin injections, blood glucose monitoring, and many dietary restrictions. It can eliminate the acute complications related to blood glucose control but is only partially successful in reversing long-term diabetes complications. Pancreatic transplant is successful when the patient no longer needs insulin therapy and all blood measures of glucose are normal.

Transplantation requires lifelong drug therapy to prevent graft rejection. These drug regimens have toxic side effects that restrict their use to patients who have serious progressive complications of diabetes. In addition, some anti-rejection drugs have the effect of increasing blood glucose levels. Pancreas-alone transplants are considered for patients with severe metabolic complications, clinical and emotional problems with insulin that are so severe as to be incapacitating, and consistent failure of insulin-based therapy to prevent acute complications.

Pancreas transplantation is considered in patients with diabetes and end-stage kidney disease who have had or plan to have a kidney transplant. Normal blood glucose levels after pancreas transplantation improve kidney graft survival. Pancreas graft survival is better when performed at the time of the kidney transplant.

Whole-Pancreas Transplantation. Improved surgical techniques and newer anti-rejection drugs have improved transplantation outcomes. The 1-year survival rate for patients is above 95%, with more than 83% of patients remaining free of insulin injection and diet restrictions after 1 year. The degree of *HLA* tissue-type matching affects the results.

Pancreatic transplantation is performed in one of three ways: pancreas alone (PTA), pancreas after kidney transplant (PAK), and simultaneous pancreas and kidney transplant (SPK). SPK is the ideal procedure for patients with DM and uremia.

Operative Procedure. Most pancreatic transplants are from cadaver donors using a total pancreas still attached to the exit of the pancreatic duct. Because the pancreas performs important digestive functions, the recipient's pancreas is left in place and the donated pancreas is placed in the pelvis. The insulin released by the pancreas graft is secreted into the bloodstream. The new pancreas also produces about 800 to 1000 mL of fluid daily, which is diverted to either the bladder or the bowel.

Chronic loss of pancreatic secretions can cause dehydration and electrolyte imbalance, and drainage of these fluids into the urinary bladder causes irritation. When the pancreas is attached to the bladder, the loss of fluid rich in bicarbonate may cause acidosis. Some techniques allow intestinal drainage of pancreatic fluids.

Rejection Management. A combination of drugs and antibodies are used to reverse rejection. (See Chapter 19 for a listing of agents used to prevent or treat transplant rejection.) Patients undergoing anti-rejection therapy first receive drugs to prevent viral, bacterial, and fungal infection because of the risk for opportunistic infections.

In most episodes of rejections, kidney problems occur before pancreatic problems. An increase in serum creatinine indicates rejection of both the transplanted kidney and the pancreas. In patients with bladder drainage of pancreatic hormones, a decrease in the urine amylase level by 25% is an indication to treat rejection. High blood glucose levels are a later marker of rejection and usually indicate irreversible graft failure.

Long-Term Effects. Long-term anti-rejection therapy increases the risk for infection, cancer, and atherosclerosis.

The transplanted pancreas does not duplicate all the functions of a normal pancreas. When insulin drains into systemic rather than portal (liver) circulation, blood insulin levels rise (*hyperinsulinemia*) and increase the risk for hypertension and macrovascular disease.

Complications. Complications are common in patients taking long-term anti-rejection therapy. Monitor laboratory values, fluid and electrolyte status, physical changes, and changes in vital signs to identify possible complications. Early removal of IV and intra-arterial lines, use of sterile technique with dressing changes and catheter irrigations, strict handwashing by all health care personnel, and good pulmonary hygiene help prevent infection.

Complications immediately after surgery include thrombosis, pancreatitis, anastomosis leak with infection, and rejection of the transplanted pancreas. Pancreatic blood vessel thrombosis occurs in about 30% of patients after transplantation. Observe for and report any sudden drop in urine amylase levels, rapid increases in blood glucose, gross hematuria (bloody urine), and tenderness or pain in the graft area (iliac fossa). Pancreatitis in the transplanted organ occurs to some degree in all patients after surgery. Report elevations in serum amylase that persist after 48 to 96 hours.

The most serious complication of enteric-drained pancreas transplantation is leaking and intra-abdominal abscess. Observe for and report elevation in temperature, abdominal discomfort, and elevation in white blood cell (WBC) count. Bladder-drained pancreas transplantation has a lower rate of intra-abdominal abscess formation. However, drainage of bicarbonate-rich fluid with pancreatic enzymes into the urinary bladder can cause urinary tract infections, cystitis, urethritis, and balanitis. Metabolic acidosis occurs from the loss of large amounts of alkaline pancreatic secretions.

Assess for and document manifestations of rejection. In acute rejection, decreased kidney function is indicated by increased serum creatinine, decreased urine output, hypertension, increased weight, graft tenderness, and fever. Proteinuria is often the first indicator of chronic graft rejection. Check for increased blood amylase, lipase, or glucose; decreased urine amylase; graft tenderness; hyperglycemia; and fever. *It is especially important to assess for signs of infection and start appropriate therapy. Fever can indicate both infection and rejection.*

Monitor for side effects of the anti-rejection drugs. Cyclosporine (Neoral) is toxic to the kidney. Signs of toxicity are elevated creatinine and decreased urine output. Monitor WBC counts daily, because azathioprine (Imuran) can suppress bone marrow function. Prednisone has many side effects, including elevated blood glucose levels. Common side effects of tacrolimus (Prograf) are hypertension, kidney toxicity, neurotoxicity, GI toxicity, and glucose intolerance.

The patient's quality of life improves as a result of freedom from the need for insulin, a less restricted lifestyle, and a return to a normal diet. Stress, however, the potential need for insulin injections to treat hyperglycemia caused by anti-rejection drugs.

Islet Cell Transplantation. Islet cell transplantation eliminates the need for insulin and protects against the complications of diabetes. Wider use of this procedure is hindered by the limited supply of beta cells available for transplantation and by issues related to rejection. Islet cells from tissue-typed (*HLA*-matched) cadaver pancreas glands are injected into the portal vein. The new cells lodge in the liver and begin to function, secreting insulin and maintaining near-perfect blood glucose control.

Islet cell transplantation may successfully restore long-term endogenous insulin production and glycemic control in patients with type 1 diabetes and unstable baseline control. Currently, most patients undergoing this procedure eventually have a progressive loss of islet cell function over time. Very few islet cell transplant recipients have remained insulin-free for more than 4 years. The reasons for this gradual loss of function are not known and make this procedure a long-term but temporary intervention. It is considered an experimental procedure.

Enhancing Surgical Recovery

Planning: Expected Outcomes. The patient with diabetes undergoing a surgical procedure is expected to recover completely without complications. Indicators include:

- Wound healing
- Absence of infection
- Maintenance of blood glucose levels within expected range
- Discharge readiness

Interventions. Surgery is a physical and emotional stressor, and the patient with diabetes has a higher risk for complications. Anesthesia and surgery cause a stress response with release of counterregulatory hormones that elevate blood glucose. Stress hormones suppress insulin action, increasing the risk for ketoacidosis and metabolic acidosis. Hyperglycemic-hyperosmolar state (HHS) (previously known as *hyperglycemic-hyperosmolar nonketotic syndrome [HHNS]*) is a common complication after major surgery and is associated with increased mortality. Diuresis from hyperglycemia can cause severe dehydration and increase the risk for kidney failure.

Complications of diabetes increase the risk for surgical complications. Patients with DM are at higher risk for hypertension, ischemic heart disease, cerebrovascular disease, MI, and cardiomyopathy. Heart failure is a serious risk factor and must be improved before surgery. Damage to nerves controlling the heart and blood vessels (autonomic neuropathy) may result in sudden tachycardia, bradycardia, or postural hypotension. The patient with DM is at risk for acute kidney injury and urinary retention after surgery, especially if he or she has albumin in the urine (indicator of kidney damage). Nerves to the intestinal wall and sphincters can be impaired, leading to delayed gastric emptying and reflux of gastric acid, which increases the risk for aspiration with anesthesia. Autonomic neuropathy may cause paralytic ileus after surgery.

Preoperative Care. Patients undergoing major surgery should be admitted to the hospital 2 to 3 days before surgery to optimize blood glucose control. Second-generation sulfonylureas are discontinued 1 day before surgery. Metformin (Glucophage) is stopped 48 hours before surgery and restarted only after kidney function is normal. All other oral drugs are stopped the day of surgery. Patients taking long-acting insulin may need to be switched to intermediate-acting insulin forms 1 to 2 days before surgery.

Preoperative blood glucose levels should be less than 200 mg/dL (11.1 mmol/L). Higher levels can cause neutrophil dysfunction and increased infection rates. They also impair wound healing by altering collagen formation, which decreases wound strength.

Plan ahead for pain control after surgery. Pain, a stressor, triggers the release of counterregulatory hormones, increasing blood glucose levels and insulin needs. Opioid analgesics slow GI motility and alter blood glucose levels. The older patient who receives opioids is more at risk for confusion, paralytic ileus, hypoventilation, hypotension, and urinary retention. Patient-controlled analgesia (PCA) systems reduce respiratory complications and confusion. (See Chapter 5 for pain interventions and Chapter 16 for general preoperative care.)

Intraoperative Care. IV infusion of insulin, glucose, and potassium is standard therapy for perioperative management of diabetes. The purpose is to keep the glucose level between 140 and 180 mg/dL (7.8 and 10.0 mmol/L) during surgery to prevent hypoglycemia and reduce risks from hyperglycemia. Levels below 180 mg/dL (10.0 mmol/L) reduce the risk for wound infection. Insulin/glucose infusion rates are based on hourly capillary glucose tests. Higher insulin doses may be needed because stress releases glucagon and epinephrine. Patients with DM should receive about 5 g of glucose per hour during surgery to prevent hypoglycemia, ketosis, and protein breakdown.

Monitor the patient's temperature—it may be lowered deliberately in some surgical procedures and inadvertently in others. Low operating room temperatures and large incisions also lower body temperature. Hypothermia decreases metabolic needs, depresses heart rate and contractility, causes vasoconstriction, and impairs insulin release, resulting in high blood glucose levels. Monitor arterial blood gas values for acidosis.

Postoperative Care. Hyperglycemia is associated with increased mortality and morbidity after surgical procedures. Current AACE and ADA guidelines recommend insulin protocols that maintain blood glucose levels between 140 and 180 mg/dL (7.8 and 10.0 mmol/L) for critically ill patients. Targets less than 110 mg/dL (6.1 mmol/L) are avoided (Moghissi et al., 2009).

Protocols and computer-based programs can be used to determine the insulin infusion rate required to maintain blood glucose levels within a defined target range. Many insulin infusion algorithms are implemented by nursing staff. Continue glucose and insulin infusions as prescribed until the patient is stable and can tolerate oral feedings. Short-term insulin therapy may be needed after surgery for the patient who usually uses oral agents. For those receiving insulin therapy, dosage adjustments may be required until the stress of surgery subsides.

Monitoring. Patients with autonomic neuropathy or vascular disease need close monitoring to avoid hypotension or respiratory arrest. Those who take beta blockers for hypertension need close monitoring for hypoglycemia because these drugs mask symptoms of hypoglycemia. Patients with azotemia (increased protein or nitrogen waste products in the blood) may have problems with fluid management. Check central venous pressure or pulmonary artery pressure as needed.

! NURSING SAFETY PRIORITY

Critical Rescue

When a patient who has had reasonably controlled blood glucose levels in the hospital develops an unexpected rise in blood glucose values, check for wound infection.

Glucose levels are a sensitive marker of counterregulatory hormones, which are often activated before patients become febrile. Hyperglycemia often occurs before a fever.

Hyperkalemia (high blood potassium level) is common in patients with mild to moderate kidney failure and can lead to cardiac dysrhythmia. In other patients, hypokalemia (low blood potassium level) may occur and be made worse by insulin and glucose given during surgery. Monitor the cardiac rhythm and serum potassium values.

Cardiovascular monitoring using serial electrocardiograms (ECGs) is recommended for older patients with diabetes, those with long-standing type 1 DM, and those with heart disease. Patients with diabetes are at higher risk for MI after surgery with a higher mortality rate. Changes in ECG or in potassium level may indicate a silent MI.

Kidney monitoring, especially observing fluid balance, helps detect acute kidney injury. Diagnosis of kidney impairment may require the use of x-ray studies using dyes, which may be nephrotoxic. Management of infections may require the use of nephrotoxic antibiotics. Ensure adequate hydration when these drugs are used. Check for impending kidney failure by assessing fluid and electrolyte status.

Nutritional Care. Patients requiring clear or full liquid diets should receive about 200 g of carbohydrate daily in equally divided amounts at meals and snack times. Liquids should not be sugar-free. For tube feedings, either a standard formula (50% carbohydrate) or a lower-carbohydrate formula (33%-40% carbohydrate) may be used. Most patients require 25 to 35 calories per kg of body weight every 24 hours. After surgery, food intake is initiated as quickly as possible, and progression from clear liquids to solid foods should be accomplished as rapidly as tolerated (ADA, 2008).

Use of total parenteral nutrition (TPN) in patients with diabetes can cause severe metabolic changes. Anticipate that hyperglycemia will occur with TPN therapy. Monitor blood glucose often to determine the need for supplemental short-acting insulin. Insulin can be added to the TPN infusion or given as a separate IV infusion.

Returning to a normal meal plan as soon as possible after surgery promotes healing and metabolic balance. When oral foods are tolerated, make sure the patient takes at least 150 to 200 g of carbohydrate daily to prevent hypoglycemia.

Preventing Injury from Peripheral Neuropathy

Planning: Expected Outcomes. The patient with diabetes is expected to identify factors that increase the risk for injury, practice proper foot care, and maintain intact skin on the feet. Indicators include that the patient consistently demonstrates these behaviors:

- Follows preventive foot care practices
- Cleanses and inspects the feet daily
- Wears properly fitting shoes
- Avoids walking in bare feet
- Trims toenails properly
- Reports nonhealing breaks in the skin of the feet to the health care provider

Interventions. Patients with DM need intensive teaching about foot care. *Foot injury is the most common complication of diabetes leading to hospitalization.* Studies have shown that patients with DM have up to a 25% lifetime risk for developing a foot ulcer. Once an ulcer has developed, there is an increased risk for wound progression that will eventually lead to amputation. Almost all lower extremity amputations are

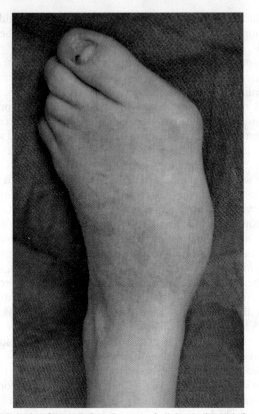

FIG. 67-9 A "Charcot foot" type of diabetic foot deformity.

preceded by foot ulcers. The 5-year mortality rate after leg or foot amputation ranges from 39% to 67% (National Institute of Diabetes and Digestive and Kidney Diseases [NIDDK], 2011). Diabetic foot ulcers are the result of a combination of factors. The major causes of diabetic foot ulcers are peripheral neuropathy and ischemia from peripheral vascular disease.

Motor neuropathy results in damage to the nerves of the intrinsic foot muscles that lead to imbalance between flexion and extension of the foot. This imbalance leads to anatomic foot deformities that create abnormal bony prominences and pressure points that gradually cause skin breakdown and ulceration. In claw toe deformity, toes are hyperextended and increase pressure on the metatarsal heads ("ball" of the foot), resulting in ulceration. Thinning or shifting of the fat pad under the metatarsal heads decreases cushioning and increases areas of pressure. These changes predispose the patient to callus formation, ulceration, and infection. The Charcot foot is a type of diabetic foot deformity with multiple anatomic abnormalities, often including a hallux valgus (turning inward of the great toe) (Fig. 67-9). The foot is warm, swollen, and painful. Walking collapses the arch, shortens the foot, and gives the foot a "rocker bottom" shape.

Autonomic neuropathy causes loss of normal sweating and skin temperature regulation, resulting in dry, thinning skin. Skin cracks and fissures increase the risk for infection. Sensory neuropathy may cause tingling or burning, but more often it produces numbness and reduced sensation. Without sensation, the patient does not notice injuries to the foot and does not treat them. Peripheral arterial disease commonly affects the tibial and peroneal arteries of the calf, resulting in reduced blood supply to the foot. This problem increases the risk for ulcer formation and reduces ulcer healing (McCance et al., 2010).

Foot injuries can be caused by walking barefoot, wearing ill-fitting shoes, sustaining thermal injuries from heat (e.g., hot water bottles, heating pads, baths), or receiving caustic burns from over-the-counter corn treatments. Because the blood supply to the diabetic foot is poor, these injuries can lead to amputation.

Ulcers result from continued pressure. Plantar ulcers (on the sole, usually the ball) are from standing or walking. Those on the top or sides of the foot usually are from shoes. The increased pressure causes calluses. Ulcers usually form over or around the great toe, under the metatarsal heads, and on the tops of claw toes.

Broken skin increases the risk for infection. Skin tends to break in areas of pressure. Infection is common in diabetic foot ulcers and, once present, is difficult to treat. Infection also impairs glucose control, leading to higher blood glucose levels and reduced immune defenses, which further increases the risk for infection.

Prevention of High-Risk Conditions. Neuropathy of the feet and legs can be delayed by keeping blood glucose levels as near normal as possible. Poor blood glucose control increases the risk for neuropathy and amputation. Intensive therapy reduces the risk for peripheral sensory neuropathy by 60%. Urge smoking cessation to reduce the risk for vascular complications.

The risk for ulcers or amputation increases with duration of diabetes. Other risk factors are male gender; poor glucose control; and cardiovascular, retinal, or kidney complications. Foot-related risks include poor gait and stepping mechanics, peripheral neuropathy, increased pressure (callus, erythema, hemorrhage under a callus, limited joint mobility, foot deformities, or severe nail pathology), peripheral vascular disease, and a history of ulcers or amputation.

Peripheral Neuropathy Management. The feet should be evaluated closely at least annually. Chart 67-7 lists self-management activities for prevention of injury from peripheral neuropathy, and Table 67-12 lists foot risk categories.

Complete a full foot assessment as outlined in Chart 67-8. Sensory examination with Semmes-Weinstein monofilaments is the most practical measure of the risk for foot ulcers. The nylon monofilament is mounted on a holder standardized to exert a 10-g force. There is no agreement on the exact number of sites to test. A person who cannot feel the 10-g pressure at any point is at increased risk for ulcers. To perform the examination:

- Provide a quiet and relaxed setting. Ask the patient to close his or her eyes during the test.
- Test the monofilament on the patient's cheek so he or she knows what to expect.
- Test the sites noted in Fig. 67-10.
- Apply the monofilament at a right angle to the skin surface.
- Apply enough force to bend the filament using a smooth, not jabbing, motion (Fig. 67-11).
- The approach, contact, and removal of the filament at each site should take 1 to 2 seconds.
- Apply the filament along the perimeter and **not** on an ulcer site, callus, scar, or necrotic tissue. Do not slide

Peripheral Neuropathy and Safety

- Protect feet and other body areas where sensation is reduced (e.g., do not walk around in bare feet or stocking feet; always wear shoes with a protective sole).
- Be sure shoes are long enough and wide enough to prevent creating sores or blisters.
- Provide a long break-in period for new shoes; do not wear new shoes for longer than 2 hours at a time.
- Avoid pointed-toe shoes and shoes with heels higher than 2 inches.
- Inspect your feet daily (with a mirror) for open areas or redness.
- Avoid extremes of temperature; wear warm clothing in the winter, especially over hands, feet, and ears.
- Test water temperature with a thermometer when washing dishes or bathing. Use warm water rather than hot water (less than 110° F).
- Use potholders when cooking.
- Use gloves when washing dishes or gardening.
- Do not eat foods that are "steaming hot," allow them to cool before placing them in your mouth.
- Eat foods that are high in fiber (e.g., fruit, whole grain cereals, vegetables).
- Drink two to three liters of fluid (nonalcoholic) daily unless your health care provider has told you to restrict fluid intake.
- Get up from a lying or sitting position slowly. If you feel dizzy, sit back down until the dizziness fades before standing and then stand in place for a few seconds before walking or using the stairs.
- Look at your feet and the floor or ground where you are walking to assess how the ground, floor, or step changes to prevent tripping or falling.
- Avoid using area rugs, especially those that slide easily.
- Use handrails when going up or down steps.

TABLE 67-12   FOOT RISK CATEGORIES

Risk Categories	Management Categories
Risk Category 0	**Management Category 0**
• Has disease that leads to insensitivity	• Examine feet at each visit, at least four times per year
• Has protective sensation	• Foot clinic visit once a year
• Has not had a plantar ulcer	• Patient education
Risk Category 1	**Management Category 1**
• Does not have protective sensation	• Examine feet at each visit, at least four times per year
• Has not had a plantar ulcer	• Foot clinic visit every 6 months
• Does not have a foot deformity	• Soft insoles
	• Patient education
Risk Category 2	**Management Category 2**
• Does not have protective sensation	• Examine feet at each visit, at least 4 times per year
• Has not had a plantar ulcer	• Foot clinic visit every 3-4 months
• Does have a foot deformity	• Custom-molded insoles
	• Prescription footwear
	• Patient education
Risk Category 3	**Management Category 3**
• Does not have protective sensation	• Examine feet at each visit, at least four times per year
• Has history of plantar ulcer	• Foot clinic visit every 1-2 months
	• Custom-molded insoles
	• Prescription footwear
	• Patient education

From Gillis W. Long Hansen's Disease Center Rehabilitation Branch. (1992). *Foot screening: Care of the foot in diabetes—The Carville approach.* Carville, LA: Department of Health and Human Services.

the filament across the skin or make repeated contact at the test site.

Randomize the sequence of applying the filament throughout the examination. Have the patient identify where the filament touched rather than asking "Do you feel this?"

Footwear. All patients with any degree of peripheral neuropathy need to wear protective shoes. They should be fitted by an experienced shoe fitter, such as a certified podiatrist. The shoe should be $\frac{1}{2}$ to $\frac{5}{8}$ inch longer than the longest toe. Heels should be less than 2 inches high. Shoes that are too tight damage tissue when worn for 4 hours or longer. Teach the patient to change shoes by midday and again in the evening. Socks or stockings need to fit properly and be appropriate for the planned activity. Socks should feel soft and have no thick seams, creases, or holes. They should pad the foot and absorb excess moisture. Teach patients to avoid tight stockings or those that have constricting bands. Patients with toe deformities should buy custom shoes with high, wide toe boxes and extra depth. Those with severely deformed feet, such as Charcot feet, need specially molded shoes. All new shoes need a long break-in period with frequent inspection for irritation or blistering.

Foot Care. Teach patients about preventive foot care and the need for examination of the feet and legs at each visit to a health care provider. Identify patients with high-risk foot conditions, and teach them about foot care. Explain problems caused by loss of protective sensation, the importance of

CHART 67-8   FOCUSED ASSESSMENT

The Diabetic Foot

Assess the patient for risk for diabetic foot problems:
- History of previous ulcer
- History of previous amputation

Assess the foot for abnormal skin and nail conditions:
- Dry, cracked, fissured skin
- Ulcers
- Toenails: thickened, long nails; ingrown nails
- Tinea pedis; onychomycosis (mycotic nails)

Assess the foot for status of circulation:
- Symptoms of claudication
- Presence or absence of dorsalis pedis or posterior tibial pulse
- Prolonged capillary filling time (greater than 25 seconds)
- Presence or absence of hair growth on the top of the foot

Assess the foot for evidence of deformity:
- Calluses, corns
- Prominent metatarsal heads (metatarsal head is easily felt under the skin)
- Toe contractures: clawed toes, hammertoes
- Hallux valgus or bunions
- Charcot foot ("rocker bottom")

Assess the foot for loss of strength:
- Limited ankle joint range of motion
- Limited motion of great toe

Assess the foot for loss of protective sensation:
- Numbness, burning, tingling
- Semmes-Weinstein monofilament testing at 10 points on each foot

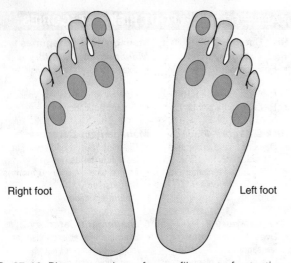

FIG. 67-10 Placement sites of monofilaments for testing of protective sensation.

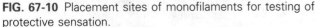

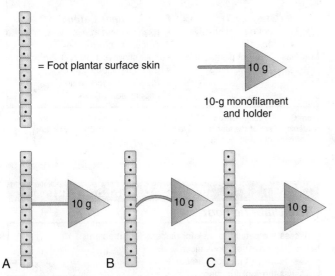

FIG. 67-11 Correct technique for sensation testing with 10-g monofilament. **A,** Apply monofilament to designated areas of the foot sole (intact skin only, see Fig. 67-10). **B,** Apply pressure to the filament until either the patient states he or she can feel the pressure or until the filament bends (see pp. 1446-1447). **C,** Quickly remove the filament without sliding it or touching other areas of the foot.

monitoring the feet daily, proper care of the feet (including nail and skin care), and how to select appropriate footwear. Advise patients with neuropathy to break in new shoes slowly to reduce the risk for blisters.

Teach patients to inspect their feet daily. Assess their ability to inspect all areas of the foot and to perform foot care. Teach family members how to inspect and care for the patient's feet if the patient cannot. Chart 67-9 lists foot care instructions for self-management.

Wound Care. The standards of care for diabetic ulcers are a moist wound environment, débridement of necrotic tissue, and elimination of pressure (*offloading*).

Wound environment is influenced by the dressing. Dressings reduce or prevent infection, allow débridement, reduce

---

CHART 67-9   PATIENT AND FAMILY EDUCATION: PREPARING FOR SELF MANAGEMENT

Foot Care Instructions

- Inspect your feet daily, especially the area between the toes.
- Wash your feet daily with lukewarm water and soap. Dry thoroughly.
- Apply moisturizing cream to your feet after bathing. Do not apply to the area between your toes.
- Change into clean cotton socks every day.
- Do not wear the same pair of shoes 2 days in a row, and wear only shoes made of breathable materials, such as leather or cloth.
- Check your shoes for foreign objects (nails, pebbles) before putting them on. Check inside the shoes for cracks or tears in the lining.
- Purchase shoes that have plenty of room for your toes. Buy shoes later in the day, when feet are normally larger. Break in new shoes gradually.
- Wear socks to keep your feet warm.
- Trim your nails straight across with a nail clipper. Smooth the nails with an emery board.
- See your physician or nurse immediately if you have blisters, sores, or infections. Protect the area with a dry, sterile dressing. Do not use adhesive tape to secure dressing.
- Do not treat blisters, sores, or infections with home remedies.
- Do not smoke.
- Do not step into the bathtub without checking the temperature of the water with your wrist or thermometer. Optimal temperature is 95° F (35° C). Maximum temperature is 110° F (43° C).
- Do not use very hot or cold water. Never use hot water bottles, heating pads, or portable heaters to warm your feet.
- Do not treat corns, blisters, bunions, calluses, or ingrown toenails yourself.
- Do not go barefooted.
- Do not wear sandals with open toes or straps between the toes.
- Do not cross your legs or wear garters or tight stockings that constrict blood flow.
- Do not soak your feet.

wound pain, and stimulate granulation tissue. Many commercial products are available. Antiseptics such as povidone iodine, hydrogen peroxide, and chlorhexidine interfere with wound healing. Dressings that keep the wound moist are essential.

Débridement removes dead tissues that support bacterial growth. Proper débridement is needed to reduce the risk for infection and to reduce pressure around the wound. It is accomplished with surgery, topical débriding agents, and dressings. Mechanical débridement, although helpful, can delay healing by removing newly formed tissue.

Eliminating pressure on an infected area is essential to wound healing. Teach patients with foot ulcers to not wear a shoe on the affected foot while the ulcer is healing. Those with poor sensation may keep walking on an ulcer because it does not hurt. This results in pressure necrosis that delays healing and increases ulcer size. Pressure is reduced by specialized orthotic devices, custom-molded shoe inserts, or shoe adjustments that redistribute weight.

The purpose of offloading is to redistribute force away from ulcer sites and pressure points to wider areas of the foot. Several products are available for offloading, including total-contact casting, half shoes, removable cast walkers, wheelchairs, and crutches. Total-contact casts redistribute pressure over the bottom of the foot. Casting material is molded to the foot and leg so pressure is spread along the entire surface of contact, thereby reducing vertical force. The almost complete elimination of motion of the total-contact cast reduces plantar shear forces. The cast is removed 24 to 48 hours after application to inspect the foot and the cast fit. The cast is replaced and then removed and reapplied weekly thereafter until the ulcer is healed. *Teach the patient that foot ulcers will recur unless weight is permanently redistributed.*

Growth factors applied to wounds increase healing by stimulating new tissue and enhancing cell growth. This treatment has helped heal foot ulcers present for many months or even years. Because it is costly, this therapy is usually performed in specialized treatment centers.

❓ DECISION-MAKING CHALLENGE

Patient-Centered Care; Teamwork and Collaboration

The patient, Angelina Lopez, is a 44-year-old woman who was diagnosed with type 2 diabetes on admission for a wound infection of her right foot. She stepped on a piece of a small toy while walking in her bare feet at home. The toy broke the skin of the foot and lodged there, leading to infection. She was unaware of the presence of the toy and sought medical help only when her foot began to drain purulent fluid and smell. Examination of her retinas shows damage indicating she has had diabetes for at least 10 years. She is overweight and hypertensive (for which she has just been prescribed an antihypertensive). She is crying and tells you that her grandmother in Mexico died after an amputation because of diabetes. She says she just doesn't understand how she "caught" diabetes and is worried that she too will die young.

1. What specific risk factors led to the wound infection?
2. What will you tell her about "catching" diabetes?
3. Is she or is she not at risk for dying young? Why or why not?
4. What will you say immediately to address her worry?
5. What are the teaching priorities for this patient?

Managing Pain

Planning: Expected Outcomes. The patient with neuropathic pain is expected to experience relief of pain. Indicators include these consistent behaviors:

- Uses preventive measures
- Uses available resources to increase comfort
- Reports pain controlled

Interventions. Neuropathic pain results from damage anywhere along the nerve. The mechanism for neuropathic pain in the patient with diabetes is unclear. Many patients with diabetes suffer from the painful neuropathy. Common symptoms of diabetic neuropathy include:

- Burning
- Muscle cramps
- Piercing, stabbing, or darting pain
- Metatarsalgia (feeling as if you are walking on marbles)
- Hyperalgesia (exaggerated pain response)
- Allodynia (pain in response to normally nonpainful stimuli)
- Tingling, numbness, and loss of proprioception in lower extremities

Maintaining normal blood glucose levels and avoiding extreme fluctuations prevent neuropathy and relieve symptoms of acute nerve dysfunction. Rapid improvement in blood glucose control may actually trigger acute peripheral neuropathy.

Several pharmacologic agents are used to manage neuropathic pain. The anticonvulsants *gabapentin* (Neurontin) and *pregabalin* (Lyrica) and the serotonin-norepinephrine reuptake inhibitor (SNRI) *duloxetine* (Cymbalta) are approved for management of peripheral neuropathic pain. Tricyclic antidepressants such as amitriptyline hydrochloride (Elavil, Levate ✦) and nortriptyline (Pamelor) are widely used for neuropathic pain but are not approved for this purpose and have some significant side effects. Their use is contraindicated for older adults and those with cardiovascular disease.

The burning of neuropathy may respond to capsaicin cream 0.075% (Axsain ✦, Zostrix-HP). This drug reduces amounts of substance P, which is involved in pain transmission (see Chapter 5). Teach the patient to apply it four times daily for several weeks. Neuropathic pain may worsen for several days after therapy is started before improving.

Unpleasant symptoms are noted with abrupt discontinuation of many of these drugs. Teach the patient about possible side effects of the drug before its initiation, and warn him or her to avoid abrupt discontinuation. A gradual reduction in the dose rather than abrupt cessation is recommended to prevent side effects.

Provide support and practical information on measures to reduce pain. Simple measures such as a bed cradle to lift bed clothes off hypersensitive skin can be beneficial. Assist the patient to maintain stable glucose control. *All patients with neuropathy are at increased risk for foot ulcers and require more frequent assessment and education in routine foot management.*

Preventing Injury from Reduced Vision

Planning: Expected Outcomes. The patient with diabetes is expected to be free of injury related to reduced vision and to maintain current level of vision. Indicators include:

- No further reduction of visual fields
- No double vision

Interventions

Blood Glucose Control. Poor blood glucose control, proteinuria, diastolic hypertension, and long duration of diabetes are risk factors for diabetic retinopathy and vision loss. Surgical intervention for retinal hemorrhage or new retinal blood vessel growth can reduce vision loss.

Besides regular eye examinations to evaluate retinopathy, urge the patient with impaired vision to have an optometrist or ophthalmologist assess the remaining vision and prescribe appropriate eyewear. A functional vision assessment, performed by a low-vision technician, rehabilitation teacher, or diabetes educator, determines the patient's use of lighting, contrast, non-optical and low-vision devices, large-print options, and use of central or peripheral vision. Low-vision reading aids include products or devices such as closed circuit television systems, handheld magnifiers, desktop systems, portable low-vision aids, talking calculators, talking and large-print books, check-writing guides, and telescopic lenses. The American Foundation for the Blind maintains a list of services for visually impaired people that is organized by type of service and geographic area. More information is available at (800) 232-5463 and www.afb.org.

Environmental Management. Not all visually impaired patients need special devices. Adjustments in lighting, contrast, color, distance, type size of printed materials, and eye movement often improve visual abilities. Instruct the patient to supplement overhead fluorescent lighting with an incandescent lamp directed toward the workspace. Placing dark equipment against a white or yellow background (or vice versa) provides contrast to enhance vision. Coding objects such as vials of insulin with bright colors or with felt-tipped markers helps identify the correct bottle. Bringing the blood glucose lancet or insulin syringe close to the eye makes it easier to see. Suggest large type or bold print to ease reading. Teach the patient to use peripheral vision.

Prefilled insulin pens are not approved for use by people with severe visual impairment unless they are assisted by a person with good vision who is trained to use the pen correctly. Adaptive devices can help the patient self-administer insulin independently. Some syringes may have a magnifier attached to the syringe. Other devices include preset dose gauges (which measure the space between the end of the syringe barrel and the plunger) to help the patient draw up the correct amount of insulin by feeling this distance. The blind patient can accurately measure insulin by using products such as the Count-A-Dose Insulin Measuring Device. This device is designed to be used with the BD Lo-Dose syringe. It holds two insulin vials and has a slot to direct the syringe needle into the vials' rubber stoppers. The patient draws insulin into the syringe by turning a thumb-wheel, which clicks for each unit (clicks can be both heard and felt). (See the Consumer Guide published yearly in the January edition of Diabetes Forecast [forecast.diabetes.org] for information to help patients determine which adaptive devices best meet their needs.) When teaching the patient to use an adaptive device, stress:

- Differentiating between bottles of fast-acting and slower-acting insulin by wrapping a rubber band around the fast-acting insulin bottle
- Ensuring proper placement of the device on the syringe
- Holding the insulin bottle upright when measuring insulin
- Avoiding air bubbles in the syringe by pulling a small amount of insulin into the syringe, moving the plunger in and out three times, and measuring insulin on the fourth draw

Design a system to determine how many doses can be drawn from a bottle so the patient does not inject air from an empty bottle instead of insulin.

Specialized adaptive equipment also is available to assist with blood glucose monitoring techniques. Assist the patient to select a blood glucose monitoring device best suited to his or her level of visual impairment. For patients with reliable low vision, monitors with large display screens and easy-to-use features may be used. The Prodigy Voice (Diagnostic Devices) is fully audio for patients who are visually impaired. The monitor uses no coding, has automatic turn-on with test strip insertion, and has a button for repeating the last message. Assess the ability of the patient to obtain an adequate blood sample and to apply it to the test strip. Commercially made blood drop guides can assist with this task.

Reducing the Risk for Kidney Disease

Planning: Expected Outcomes. The patient with diabetes is expected to maintain a normal urine elimination pattern. Indicators include:

- Urine protein levels within normal limits
- 24-hour intake and output balance

- Blood urea nitrogen (BUN) and serum creatinine within the normal ranges
- Serum electrolytes within the normal ranges

Interventions

Prevention. Tight control of blood glucose levels may slow kidney disease in patients with type 1 diabetes. Diabetic kidney disease is more likely to develop in those with poor blood glucose control. Progression to end-stage kidney disease can be delayed or prevented by normalizing blood pressure, correcting hyperlipidemia, and restricting dietary protein. Control of hypertension is essential for the reduction of diabetic nephropathy (ADA, 2010c). Both systolic and diastolic hypertension greatly accelerate the progression of diabetic kidney disease.

Stress the need for evaluation of kidney function according to the ADA Standards of Care. Glomerular filtration rate (GFR) is the best overall measure of kidney function. Serum creatinine should be measured at least annually for an estimation of GFR in all patients with diabetes (ADA, 2010b). An annual test for microalbuminuria is performed for patients who have had type 1 DM for over 5 years and in all those with type 2 DM starting at diagnosis and during pregnancy.

After 5 or more years of DM, the earliest change signaling diabetic kidney disease is an excretion of 30 to 299 mg of albumin per day *(microalbuminuria)*. When albumin excretion rises above 300 mg per day, it is termed *albuminuria*. Screening for microalbuminuria is performed by three methods: (1) random spot urine collection to measure the albumin-creatinine ratio, (2) 24-hour urine collection to measure creatinine clearance, and (3) timed urine collection (e.g., 4 hours or overnight). Timed urine collections are not reliable in patients with neuropathy and incomplete bladder emptying. The preferred method of screening for microalbuminuria is by measuring the albumin-to-creatinine ratio in a random spot urine collection (ADA, 2010c).

Aggressive control of blood glucose and hypertension in patients without microalbuminuria can avoid nephropathy. Once microalbuminuria develops, management focuses on controlling blood pressure and blood glucose, restricting dietary protein, avoiding nephrotoxic agents, promptly treating urinary tract infections, and preventing dehydration.

Control of blood pressure and blood glucose levels requires the patient's participation and effort. Prescribed drugs must be taken according to schedules, and dietary restriction must be maintained. Teach patients about the roles of blood pressure and blood glucose levels in kidney disease. Help them maintain normal blood glucose levels and blood pressure levels below 130/80 mm Hg. Stress the need for yearly screening for microalbuminuria.

Smoking cessation is important in halting the progression of diabetic kidney disease. Smoking increases the risk for development of microalbuminuria, increases the rate of advancement to proteinuria, and accelerates the rate of progression of kidney disease in patients with either type 1 or type 2 DM. Teach the patient about the risks of smoking, and refer him or her to appropriate resources for assistance in smoking cessation.

Any urinary tract infection (UTI) can lead to kidney infection and further reduce kidney function. Explain the manifestations of UTI. Urge the patient to take antibiotics exactly as prescribed, completing the entire course of treatment.

Reinforce the need for follow-up urine cultures to reduce the risk for kidney damage. Avoid indwelling urinary catheters when possible.

Drugs can affect kidney function either through toxic effects on the kidney or by an acute but reversible reduction in function. The most common nephrotoxic drugs are antifungal agents (amphotericin B) and aminoglycoside antibiotics such as amikacin (Amikin), streptomycin, kanamycin (Kantrex), gentamicin (Garamycin), and tobramycin (Tobrex). Outside the hospital, the leading nephrotoxic agents are NSAIDs such as ibuprofen (Advil) or naproxen (Aleve). To prevent accidental ingestion of nephrotoxic drugs, teach the patient to check with a health care provider before taking over-the-counter drugs or herbal remedies.

Radiocontrast dyes can also affect kidney function, especially in patients with preexisting kidney problems. Monitor IV hydration before and after contrast is used to prevent contrast-induced nephropathy in patients with diabetes.

Drug Therapy. Use of angiotensin-converting enzyme (ACE) inhibitors (ACEIs) or angiotensin receptor blockers (ARBs) is recommended for all patients with microalbuminuria or advanced stages of nephropathy (ADA, 2010c). ACE inhibitors reduce the level of albuminuria and the rate of progression of kidney disease. These drugs have not shown to be effective in primary prevention of microalbuminuria. Monitor serum potassium levels for development of hyperkalemia.

Nutrition Therapy. Patients with nephropathy should restrict dietary protein to 0.8 g/kg of body weight per day. Once the glomerular filtration rate (GFR) starts falling, further reducing protein may slow the decline in kidney function (ADA, 2010c). Because lifelong dietary restrictions are difficult, provide ongoing teaching to encourage adherence.

Fluid and Electrolyte Management. Fluid and electrolyte management can prevent more loss of kidney function. Avoiding dehydration is important for kidney perfusion and function. Assess fluid balance, and use measures to prevent dehydration. The most common cause of dehydration in patients with diabetes is overuse of diuretics. Teach patients to report edema or symptoms of orthostatic hypotension, and provide ongoing education to promote nutrition therapy.

Dialysis for patients with DM and kidney failure is the same as for patients without diabetes (see Chapter 71). The dosage of insulin needs to be adjusted when dialysis starts.

Preventing Hypoglycemia

Hypoglycemia is defined as the presence of Whipple's triad: manifestations consistent with low blood glucose, a low plasma glucose concentration, and resolution of symptoms or signs after plasma glucose concentration is raised. Hypoglycemic symptoms are mediated through both the central and peripheral nervous systems. Once plasma glucose levels fall below 70 mg/dL (3.88 mmol/L), a sequence of events begins with release of counterregulatory hormones, stimulation of the autonomic nervous system, and production of *neurogenic* and *neuroglycopenic* symptoms. Peripheral autonomic symptoms (adrenergic), including sweating, irritability, tremulousness, anxiety, tachycardia, and hunger, serve as an early warning system and occur before the central neuroglycopenic symptoms (confusion, paralysis, seizure, and coma) due to central glucose deprivation. *Neuroglycopenic symptoms* occur when brain glucose *gradually declines* to a

TABLE 67-13	SYMPTOMS OF HYPOGLYCEMIA
Neuroglycopenic Symptoms	**Neurogenic Symptoms**
• Weakness	• Adrenergic:
• Fatigue	• Shaky/tremulous
• Difficulty thinking	• Heart pounding
• Confusion	• Nervous/anxious
• Behavior changes	• Cholinergic:
• Emotional instability	• Sweaty
• Seizures	• Hungry
• Loss of consciousness	• Tingling
• Brain damage	
• Death	

low level. *Neurologic symptoms* result from autonomic nervous activity triggered by a *rapid decline* in blood glucose (Table 67-13).

Central nervous system (CNS) function depends on a continuous supply of glucose in the blood. The brain cannot make glucose and stores only a few minutes' supply as glycogen. This needed supply is not maintained when the blood glucose level falls below critical levels.

The first defense against falling blood glucose levels in a person who does not have diabetes is decreased insulin secretion, decreased glucose use, and increased glucose production. Normally, insulin secretion decreases when blood glucose levels drop to about 83 mg/dL (4.5 mmol/L). Counterregulatory hormones are activated at about 67 mg/dL (3.7 mmol/L), a level well above the threshold for symptoms of hypoglycemia. The main counterregulatory hormone is glucagon. Epinephrine also becomes important in patients with DM who are deficient in glucagon. Both glucagon and epinephrine raise blood glucose levels by stimulating liver glycogen breakdown and conversion of protein to glucose. Epinephrine also limits insulin secretion. Growth hormone and cortisol also are important during prolonged hypoglycemia. Their effects do not become evident until 4 hours after the onset of hypoglycemia.

Type 1 DM disrupts the body's response to hypoglycemia, a change that occurs within 1 to 5 years of diagnosis. Regulation of circulating insulin levels is lost because insulin comes from an injection rather than from the pancreas. As blood glucose levels fall, insulin levels do not decrease. Over time, the pancreas loses it ability to secrete glucagon in response to hypoglycemia. After a few more years of type 1 DM, the response of epinephrine to falling blood glucose levels is also reduced. It does respond, but it takes a lower blood glucose level to become active. These problems greatly increase the risk for severe hypoglycemia.

A second problem with long-standing type 1 DM is *hypoglycemic unawareness,* in which patients no longer have the warning symptoms of impending hypoglycemia that should prompt them to take preventive action. This problem occurs most often in patients who have had type 1 DM for 30 years or longer.

The blood glucose level at which symptoms of hypoglycemia occur varies among patients. Many have symptoms when blood glucose levels are well above 50 mg/dL (2.8 mmol/L), especially if the level dropped rapidly or they are used to chronic hyperglycemia. Thus clinical criteria used to

TABLE 67-14　DIFFERENTIATION OF HYPOGLYCEMIA AND HYPERGLYCEMIA

FEATURE	HYPOGLYCEMIA	HYPERGLYCEMIA
Skin	Cool, clammy	Warm, moist
Dehydration	Absent	Present
Respirations	No particular or consistent change	Rapid, deep*; Kussmaul type; acetone odor ("fruity" odor) to breath
Mental status	Anxious, nervous,* irritable, mental confusion,* seizures, coma	Varies from alert to stuporous, obtunded, or frank coma
Symptoms	Weakness,* double vision, blurred vision, hunger, tachycardia, palpitations	No specific symptoms for DKA Acidosis; hypercapnia; abdominal cramps, nausea and vomiting Dehydration: decreased neck vein filling, orthostatic hypotension, tachycardia, poor skin turgor
Glucose	<70 mg/dL (3.9 mmol/L)	>250 mg/dL (13.8 mmol/L)
Ketones	Negative	Positive

DKA, Diabetic ketoacidosis.
*Classic symptoms.

categorize hypoglycemia are based on severity rather than blood glucose levels. In mild hypoglycemia, the patient remains alert and able to self-manage symptoms. In severe hypoglycemia, neurologic function is so impaired that he or she needs another person's help to increase blood glucose levels.

Planning: Expected Outcomes. The patient with DM is expected to have decreased episodes of hypoglycemia and remain oriented to person, place, and time, as indicated by a Glasgow Coma Scale score above 7.

Interventions. A blood glucose level below 70 mg/dL (3.9 mmol/L) alerts you to assess for manifestations of hypoglycemia (Table 67-13; see also Table 67-14).

Blood Glucose Management. Monitor blood glucose levels before giving antidiabetic drugs, before meals, before bedtime, and when the patient is symptomatic. All patients who take insulin, those taking long-acting insulin secretagogues (glyburide [glibenclamide]), and those taking metformin in combination with glyburide (Glucovance) are at risk for hypoglycemia. This risk is increased if they are older, have liver or kidney impairment, or are taking drugs that enhance the effects of antidiabetic drugs. Proper patient selection, drug dosage, and instructions are important factors in avoiding severe hypoglycemia. Hypoglycemia may be difficult to recognize in those who take beta-blocking drugs. Symptoms become less intense and less obvious. Manifestations of hypoglycemia in older patients may be mistaken for other conditions.

The most common causes of hypoglycemia are:
- Too much insulin as it relates to food intake and physical activity
- Insulin injected at the wrong time relative to food intake and physical activity
- The wrong type of insulin injected at the wrong time

- Decreased food intake resulting from missed or delayed meals
- Delayed gastric emptying from gastroparesis
- Decrease liver glucose production after alcohol ingestion
- Increased insulin sensitivity as a result of regular exercise and weight loss
- Decreased insulin clearance from progressive kidney failure

Nutrition Therapy. When the patient is hypoglycemic, start carbohydrate replacement per physician prescription or standing protocols. Ingestion of 15 to 20 g of glucose is the preferred treatment for hypoglycemia. If the patient can swallow, give a liquid form of carbohydrate, although any source of carbohydrate can be used to treat hypoglycemia. Ingestion of 15 to 20 g of glucose is the preferred treatment for blood glucose levels less than 70 mg/dL (3.9 mmol/L), repeated in about 15 minutes if manifestations have not improved or if blood glucose levels are still less than 70. The amount of carbohydrate should be increased to 30 g when treating glucose levels less than 50 mg/dL (2.8 mmol/L).

Ten grams of oral glucose raises plasma glucose levels by about 40 mg/dL over 30 minutes, and 20 g of oral glucose raises plasma glucose levels by about 60 mg/dL over 45 minutes. Glucose levels often begin to fall about 60 minutes after glucose ingestion. Specific recommendations are listed in Chart 67-10.

The blood glucose level determines the form and amount of glucose used. The response to treatment of hypoglycemia should be apparent in 10 to 20 minutes; however, test plasma glucose again in about 60 minutes because additional treatment may be needed. Fluid is absorbed much more quickly from the GI tract than are solids. Concentrated sweet fluids, such as juice with sugar added or a soft drink, may slow absorption.

Management of hypoglycemia requires ingestion of glucose or glucose-containing foods. The blood glucose response correlates better with the glucose content rather than the carbohydrate content of the food. Adding protein to carbohydrate does not improve blood glucose response and does not prevent subsequent hypoglycemia. Adding fat may retard and then prolong the blood glucose response, resulting in post-treatment hyperglycemia. Commercially available products provide predictable glucose absorption.

Drug Therapy. Glucagon given subcutaneously or IM and 50% dextrose given IV is used for patients who cannot swallow. Glucagon is the main counterregulatory hormone and is used as therapy for severe hypoglycemia in DM. It converts liver glycogen to glucose but is not effective in starved patients who have little liver glycogen. Take care to prevent aspiration in patients receiving glucagon, because it often causes vomiting. Give 50% dextrose carefully to avoid extravasation because it is hyperosmolar and can damage tissue. The effects of glucagon and dextrose are temporary. After the patient responds and is no longer nauseated, give a simple sugar followed by a small snack or meal. IV glucose is used to maintain mild hyperglycemia. Diazoxide (Proglycem) or octreotide (Sandostatin) may be required to treat sulfonylurea-induced hypoglycemia. Evaluate response by monitoring blood glucose levels for several hours. Symptoms may persist for an hour or more after treatment. A target blood glucose level is 70 to 110 mg/dL (3.9 to 6.2 mmol/L).

CHART 67-10 PATIENT AND FAMILY EDUCATION: PREPARING FOR SELF-MANAGEMENT

Treatment of Hypoglycemia at Home

For *mild* hypoglycemia (hungry, irritable, shaky, weak, headache, fully conscious; blood glucose usually less than 60 mg/dL [3.4 mmol/L]):
- Treat the symptoms of hypoglycemia with 10 to 15 g of carbohydrate. You may use one of the following:
  - Glucose tablets or glucose gel (dosage is printed on the package)
  - ½ cup of fruit juice
  - ½ cup of regular (nondiet) soft drink
  - 8 ounces of skim milk
  - 6 to 10 hard candies
  - 4 cubes of sugar
  - 4 teaspoons of sugar
  - 6 saltines
  - 3 graham crackers
  - 1 tablespoon of honey or syrup
- Re-test blood glucose in 15 minutes.
- Repeat this treatment if symptoms do not resolve.
- Eat a small snack of carbohydrate and protein if your next meal is more than an hour away.

For *moderate* hypoglycemia (cold, clammy skin; pale; rapid pulse; rapid, shallow respirations; marked change in mood; drowsiness; blood glucose usually less than 40 mg/dL [2.2 mmol/L]):
- Treat the symptoms of hypoglycemia with 15 to 30 g of rapidly absorbed carbohydrate.
- Take additional food, such as low-fat milk or cheese, after 10 to 15 minutes.

For *severe* hypoglycemia (unable to swallow; unconsciousness or convulsions; blood glucose usually less than 20 mg/dL [1.0 mmol/L]):
- Treatment administered by family members:
  - Administer 1 mg of glucagon as intramuscular or subcutaneous injection.
  - Administer a second dose in 10 minutes if the person remains unconscious.
  - Notify a primary care provider immediately, and follow instructions.
  - If still unconscious, transport the person to the emergency department.
  - Give a small meal when the person wakes up and is no longer nauseated.

! NURSING SAFETY PRIORITY

Critical Rescue

For the patient with *severe* hypoglycemia (unable to swallow, unconscious or convulsing, blood glucose usually less than 20 mg/dL [1.0 mmol/L]), treat by:
1. Giving glucagon 1 mg subcutaneously or IM
2. Repeating the dose in 10 minutes if the patient remains unconscious
3. Notifying the primary health care provider immediately, and following instructions

Prevention Strategies. Teach the patient how to prevent hypoglycemia by avoiding the four common causes of hypoglycemia. These are (1) excess insulin, (2) deficient intake or absorption of food, (3) exercise, and (4) alcohol intake.

Insulin excess from variable absorption of insulin can cause hypoglycemia even when insulin is injected correctly. This excess also can be caused by lowered insulin resistance, which occurs with termination of pregnancy or resolution of an infection. Increased insulin sensitivity can occur with weight loss or exercise programs. Differences in insulin formulation can result in hypoglycemia. Teach the patient to not change insulin brands without medical supervision.

Deficient food intake from inadequate or incorrectly timed meals can result in hypoglycemia. Changes in gastric absorption may cause hypoglycemia in patients with delayed gastric emptying. This problem is more common in those with DM of long duration, is more severe with solid than with liquid meals, and is made worse by illness or poor glucose control. Teach the patient about the importance of regularity in timing and quantity of food eaten.

Exercise usually causes blood glucose levels to fall in a patient with type 1 DM. Prolonged exercise increases cellular glucose uptake for several hours after exercise. Teach the patient about blood glucose monitoring and carbohydrate consumption before and during exercise.

Alcohol inhibits liver glucose production and leads to hypoglycemia. It interferes with the counterregulatory response to hypoglycemia and impairs glycogen breakdown, making exercise-induced hypoglycemia more severe. Alcohol is more likely to cause hypoglycemia when the patient does not eat for long periods, when basic nutrition is poor, and when glycogen stores are depleted. Teach him or her to ingest alcohol only with or shortly *after* eating a meal with enough carbohydrate to prevent hypoglycemia. Warn patients to avoid excess alcohol at bedtime to prevent nighttime hypoglycemia.

Patient and Family Education. The cause of hypoglycemia may be subtle. At the onset of menses, a fall in hormone levels decreases insulin needs and contributes to hypoglycemia. When patients switch to a new bottle of insulin, hypoglycemia may occur because the fresh insulin has greater potency. Some patients have hypoglycemia when they change injection sites. Drugs such as propranolol (Inderal, Detensol ✦) or other beta blockers mask warning signs and thus predispose patients to severe hypoglycemia. Some episodes of hypoglycemia occur without an obvious cause and are due to the erratic absorption of insulin, which can occur in any patient.

Many patients who have been treated in the emergency department for hypoglycemia do not receive adequate instruction on how to prevent another episode and are at continuing risk. Help each patient develop a personal treatment plan for hypoglycemia. Routinely taking 10 to 15 g of carbohydrate results in overtreatment of hypoglycemia in some patients and undertreatment in others. The exact glucose rise from a set amount of carbohydrate varies; however, using the estimate that each 5 g of carbohydrate raises blood glucose about 20 mg/dL is a good starting plan. For example, the patient may be directed to take:
- 20 to 30 g of carbohydrate if the blood glucose level is 50 mg/dL (2.8 mmol/L) or less
- 10 to 15 g of carbohydrate if the blood glucose level is 51 to 70 mg/dL (2.9 to 3.9 mmol/L)

Use blood glucose monitoring results to revise or reinforce this plan.

Encourage the patient to wear a medical alert bracelet, and help him or her obtain one. This bracelet is helpful if the patient becomes hypoglycemic and is unable to provide self-care.

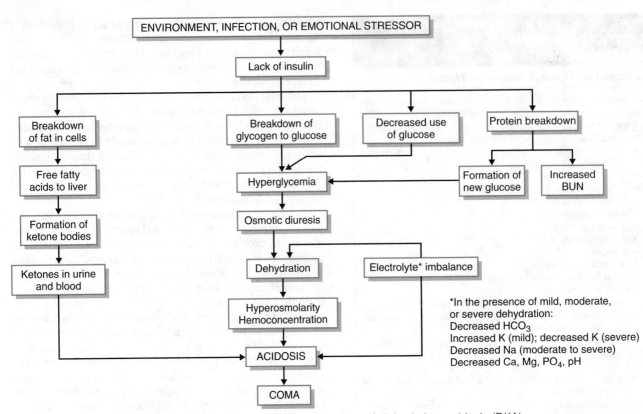

FIG. 67-12 The pathophysiologic mechanism of diabetic ketoacidosis (DKA).

Teach the patient and family about the manifestations of hypoglycemia. Emphasize that delaying a meal for more than 30 minutes raises the risk for hypoglycemia when using some insulin regimens. Instruct him or her to keep a carbohydrate source nearby at all times. Teach the patient and family how to administer glucagon.

Hypoglycemia is a major risk for patients receiving intensive insulin protocols who engage in exercise programs. Explain that nightmares or headaches on days after prolonged or severe exercise occur with hypoglycemia.

Establishing Treatment Plans. Blood glucose monitoring directs hypoglycemia treatment. Treatment continues until blood glucose levels reach and stay in the target range. Once blood glucose control is regained, the specific cause of each hypoglycemic episode should be determined and measures taken to prevent recurrence.

Preventing Diabetic Ketoacidosis

Diabetic ketoacidosis (DKA) is characterized by uncontrolled hyperglycemia, metabolic acidosis, and increased production of ketones. This condition results from the combination of insulin deficiency and an increase in counterregulatory hormone release (Fig. 67-12). Laboratory diagnosis of DKA is shown in Table 67-15. Hormonal changes lead to increased liver and kidney glucose production and decreased glucose use in peripheral tissues. Increased production of counterregulatory hormones leads to the production of ketoacids with resultant ketonemia and metabolic acidosis.

DKA occurs most often in patients with type 1 DM but also can occur in those with type 2 DM who are under severe stress (e.g., trauma, surgery, infection). The most common precipitating factor for development of DKA is infection. *Death occurs in up to 10% of these cases even with appropriate treatment.* Mortality is highest for older patients who also have infection, stroke, MI, vascular thrombosis, intestinal obstruction, or pneumonia.

Hyperglycemia leads to osmotic diuresis with dehydration and electrolyte loss. Classic symptoms of DKA include

TABLE 67-15	DIFFERENCES BETWEEN DIABETIC KETOACIDOSIS AND HYPERGLYCEMIC-HYPEROSMOLAR STATE	
	DIABETIC KETOACIDOSIS (DKA)	**HYPERGLYCEMIC-HYPEROSMOLAR STATE (HHS)**
Onset	Sudden	Gradual
Precipitating factors	Infection Other stressors Inadequate insulin dose	Infection Other stressors Poor fluid intake
Manifestations	Ketosis: Kussmaul respiration, "fruity" breath, nausea, abdominal pain	Altered central nervous system function with neurologic symptoms
	Dehydration or electrolyte loss: polyuria, polydipsia, weight loss, dry skin, sunken eyes, soft eyeballs, lethargy, coma	Dehydration or electrolyte loss: same as for DKA
Laboratory Findings		
Serum glucose	>300 mg/dL (16.7 mmol/L)	>600 mg/dL (33.3 mmol/L)
Osmolarity	Variable	>320 mOsm/L
Serum ketones	Positive at 1:2 dilutions	Negative
Serum pH	<7.35	>7.4
Serum HCO_3^-	<15 mEq/L	>20 mEq/L
Serum Na+	Low, normal, or high	Normal or low
BUN	>30 mg/dL; elevated because of dehydration	Elevated
Creatinine	>1.5 mg/dL; elevated because of dehydration	Elevated
Urine ketones	Positive	Negative

BUN, Blood urea nitrogen; *HCO_3^-,* bicarbonate; *Na+,* sodium.

polyuria, polydipsia, polyphagia, weight loss, vomiting, abdominal pain, dehydration, weakness, altered mental status, shock, and coma. Mental status can vary from total alertness to profound coma. As ketone levels rise, the buffering capacity of the body is exceeded, the pH of the blood decreases, and acidosis occurs. Kussmaul respirations (very deep and rapid respirations) cause respiratory alkalosis in an attempt to correct metabolic acidosis by exhaling carbon dioxide. Initial serum sodium levels may be low or normal. Initial potassium levels depend on how long DKA lasts before treatment. After therapy starts, serum potassium levels drop quickly.

Planning: Expected Outcomes. The patient is expected to have few episodes of hyperglycemia and avoid diabetic keto-acidosis. Indicators include that the patient consistently demonstrates these behaviors:

- Maintains blood glucose levels within the prescribed target range
- Adjusts insulin doses to match eating patterns and blood glucose levels during illness
- Maintains easily digestible liquid diet containing carbohydrate and salt when nauseated
- Describes correct procedure for urine ketone testing
- Describes when to seek help from health care professional

Interventions

Blood Glucose Management. Monitor for manifestations of DKA (see Table 67-15 and Fig. 67-12). Document and use these findings to determine therapy effectiveness. *First assess the airway, level of consciousness, hydration status, electrolytes, and blood glucose level.* Check the patient's blood pressure, pulse, and respirations every 15 minutes until stable. Record urine output, temperature, and mental status every hour. When a central venous catheter is present, assess central venous pressure every 30 minutes or as prescribed. After treatment starts and these values are stable, monitor and record vital signs every 4 hours. Use blood glucose values to assess therapy effectiveness and determine when to switch from saline to dextrose-containing solutions.

Fluid and Electrolyte Management. *Closely assess the patient's fluid status.* The kidneys are less able to respond to changes in pH or fluid and electrolyte balance, to concentrate urine, or to regulate blood osmolarity. The risk for kidney failure rises with age. Impaired bicarbonate reabsorption and acid excretion in poorly functioning kidney tubules can lead to acidosis. Cardiovascular disease can cause fluid retention. The dehydrated patient's lips and mouth may be dry and the tongue furrowed. Temperature may be elevated. Age-related skin changes, such as loss of elasticity and dryness, make skin turgor an unreliable sign of dehydration in the older patient. In patients with poor kidney function and excess fluid volume, assess for edema around the eyes and in the limbs, increasing abdominal girth, increasing blood pressure and pulse volume, jugular venous distention, and orthostatic hypotension. Edema occurs with excess interstitial fluid and often is not apparent until interstitial volume increases by 2 to 3 L. Daily weights are good indicators of fluid status because 1 kg of body weight equals 1 L of fluid.

Check the clinical indicators of fluid imbalance. Fluid overload can cause hypertension, especially in patients with kidney failure. Jugular venous pressure increases with volume overload. Orthostatic hypotension may indicate volume depletion. In that case, jugular venous pulsation may not be visible at a 45-degree angle. In severe volume depletion, the jugular venous pulsation may not be visible even with the patient lying flat.

The first outcome of fluid therapy is to restore volume and maintain perfusion to the brain, heart, and kidneys. Typically, initial infusion rates are 15 to 20 mL/kg/hr during the first hour (Fowler, 2009).

The second outcome of fluid therapy, replacing total body fluid losses, is achieved more slowly. The choice for fluid replacement depends on hemodynamics (status of blood pressure), the state of hydration, serum electrolyte levels, and urine output. In general, hypotonic fluids are infused at 4 to 14 mL/kg/hr after the initial fluid bolus. When blood glucose levels reach 250 mg/dL (13.8 mmol/L), give 5% dextrose in 0.45% saline. This solution prevents hypoglycemia and cerebral edema, which can occur when serum osmolarity declines too rapidly.

During the first 24 hours of treatment, the patient needs enough fluids to replace the actual volume deficit and ongoing losses. This may be as much as 6 to 10 L. Assess cardiac, kidney, and mental status to avoid fluid overload. Watch for signs of congestive heart failure and pulmonary edema. Central venous pressure may be monitored for older patients and those with myocardial disease. Assess the status of fluid replacement by monitoring blood pressure and intake and output.

Drug Therapy. The outcome of insulin therapy is to lower serum glucose by about 50 to 75 mg/dL/hr. Unless the episode of DKA is mild, regular insulin by continuous IV infusion is the treatment of choice. Effective blood insulin levels are reached quickly when an IV bolus dose is given at the start of the infusion. An initial IV bolus dose of 0.1 unit/kg is followed by an IV infusion of 0.1 unit/kg/hr. Continuous insulin infusion is used because of the 4-minute half-life of IV insulin and because of the delayed onset of action and prolonged half-life of subcutaneous regular insulin. Subcutaneous insulin is started when the patient can take oral fluids and ketosis has stopped. Criteria for resolution of DKA include blood glucose less than 200 mg/mL along with a serum bicarbonate level higher than 18 mEq/L, venous pH higher than 7.3, and a calculated ion gap of less than 12 mEq/L. Assess therapy effectiveness by hourly blood glucose measurements.

Acidosis Management. The key diagnostic feature of DKA is elevation in circulating total body ketone concentration. The severity of DKA is best assessed by measurements of serum β-hydroxybutyrate. Accumulation of ketoacids results in an increased anion gap metabolic acidosis. The anion gap is calculated by subtracting the sum of chloride and bicarbonate concentration from the sodium concentration. A normal anion gap is between 7 and 9 mEq/L; an anion gap greater than 10 to 12 mEq/L indicates metabolic acidosis.

Despite total-body potassium depletion, mild to moderate hyperkalemia is common in patients with hyperglycemia. Insulin therapy, correction of acidosis, and volume expansion decrease serum potassium concentration. To prevent hypokalemia, potassium replacement is initiated after serum levels fall below normal. *Assess for signs of hypokalemia, including fatigue, malaise, confusion, muscle weakness, shallow respirations, abdominal distention or paralytic ileus, hypotension, and weak pulse.* An ECG shows cardiac conduction changes related to potassium. Hypokalemia is a common cause of death in the treatment of DKA.

! NURSING SAFETY PRIORITY

Critical Rescue

Before giving IV potassium, make sure the patient produces at least 30 mL/hr of urine.

Bicarbonate is used only for severe acidosis because it may reverse acidosis too rapidly and lead to severe hypokalemia, which can cause fatal cardiac dysrhythmias. Rapid correction can worsen the patient's mental status. Acidosis is corrected with fluid replacement and insulin therapy. Sodium bicarbonate, given by slow IV infusion over several hours, is indicated when the arterial pH is 7.0 or less or the serum bicarbonate level is less than 5 mEq/L (5 mmol/L).

After acid-base disturbances are corrected, efforts are directed toward determining the cause of DKA. Infection is the most common cause (see Table 67-15).

Patient and Family Education. Exploring the factors leading to DKA helps in planning specific educational efforts. Teach the patient and family to check blood glucose levels every 4 to 6 hours as long as symptoms such as anorexia,

---

CHART 67-11   PATIENT AND FAMILY EDUCATION: PREPARING FOR SELF-MANAGEMENT

Sick-Day Rules

- Notify your health care provider that you are ill.
- Monitor your blood glucose at least every 4 hours.
- Test your urine for ketones when your blood glucose level is greater than 240 mg/dL (13.8 mmol/L).
- Continue to take insulin or oral antidiabetic agents.
- To prevent dehydration, drink 8 to 12 ounces of sugar-free liquids every hour that you are awake. If your blood glucose level is below your target range, drink fluids that contain sugar.
- Continue to eat meals at regular times.
- If unable to tolerate solid food because of nausea, consume more easily tolerated foods or liquids equal to the carbohydrate content of your usual meal.
- Call your primary care provider for any of these danger signals:
  - Persistent nausea and vomiting
  - Moderate or large ketones
  - Blood glucose elevation after two supplemental doses of insulin
  - High (101.5° F [38.6° C]) temperature or increasing fever; fever for more than 24 hours
- Treat symptoms (e.g., diarrhea, nausea, vomiting, fever) as directed by your primary care provider.
- Get plenty of rest.

---

nausea, and vomiting are present and as long as glucose levels exceed 250 mg/dL (13.8 mmol/L). Teach them to check urine ketone levels when blood glucose levels exceed 300 mg/dL (16.7 mmol/L).

Teach the patient to reduce the risk for dehydration by maintaining food and fluid intake. Unless another health problem is present that requires fluid restriction, suggest that he or she drink at least 3 L of fluid daily and increase this amount when infection is present. When nausea is present, instruct the patient to take liquids containing both glucose and electrolytes (e.g., soda pop, diluted fruit juice, and sports drinks [Gatorade]). Small amounts of fluid may be tolerated even when vomiting is present. When blood glucose levels are normal or elevated, the patient should take 8 to 12 ounces (240 to 360 mL) of calorie-free and caffeine-free liquids every hour while awake to prevent dehydration.

Liquids containing carbohydrate can be taken if the patient with diabetes cannot eat solid food. Ingesting at least 150 g of carbohydrate daily reduces the risk for starvation ketosis. After consulting a primary care provider, urge the patient to take additional rapid-acting (lispro) or short-acting (regular) insulin based on blood glucose levels.

Instruct the patient and family to consult the primary care provider when these problems occur:

- Blood glucose exceeds 250 mg/dL (13.8 mmol/L).
- Ketonuria lasts for more than 24 hours.
- The patient cannot take food or fluids.
- Illness lasts more than 1 to 2 days.

Also instruct them to detect hyperglycemia by monitoring blood glucose whenever the patient is ill. Illness can result in dehydration with DKA, hyperglycemic-hyperosmolar state, or both. The sooner the patient seeks treatment, the less severe the metabolic alteration. He or she should not omit insulin therapy during illness. Chart 67-11 lists guidelines for the ill patient.

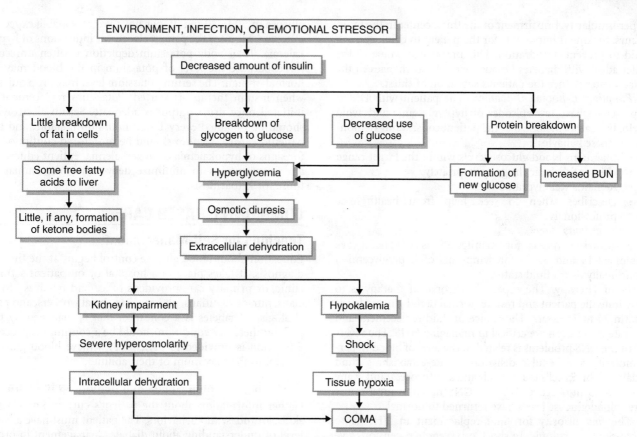

FIG. 67-13 The pathophysiologic mechanism of hyperglycemic-hyperosmolar state (HHS). *BUN,* Blood urea nitrogen.

Preventing Hyperglycemic-Hyperosmolar State

Hyperglycemic-hyperosmolar state (HHS), formerly known as *hyperglycemic-hyperosmolar nonketotic syndrome (HHNS),* is a hyperosmolar (increased blood osmolarity) state caused by hyperglycemia. The processes of HHS are outlined in Fig. 67-13. Both HHS and diabetic ketoacidosis (DKA) are caused by hyperglycemia and dehydration. HHS differs from DKA in that ketone levels are low or absent and blood glucose levels are much higher. Blood glucose levels may exceed 600 mg/dL (33.3 mmol/L), and blood osmolarity may exceed 320 mOsm/L. Other biochemical problems with HHS also are more severe than those with DKA. Table 67-15 lists the differences between DKA and HHS.

HHS is the end result of a sustained osmotic diuresis. Kidney impairment in HHS allows for extremely high blood glucose levels. Glucose impairs the concentrating ability of the kidney. Normally, kidneys act as a safety valve to eliminate glucose above levels around 180 mg/dL (10.0 mmol/L). As serum concentrations of glucose exceed the renal threshold, the kidney's capacity to reabsorb glucose is exceeded.

Decreased blood volume, caused by osmotic diuresis, or underlying kidney disease, common in many older patients with diabetes, results in further deterioration of kidney function. The decreased volume further reduces glomerular filtration rate, causing the glucose level to increase. Decreased kidney perfusion from hypovolemia further impairs kidney function.

Myocardial infarction, sepsis, pancreatitis, stroke, and some drugs (glucocorticoids, diuretics, phenytoin [Dilantin], propranolol [Inderal], and calcium channel blockers) also

CONSIDERATIONS FOR OLDER ADULTS

HHS occurs most often in older patients with type 2 diabetes mellitus, many of whom did not know that they had diabetes. Mortality rates in older patients are as high as 40% to 70%. The onset of HHS is slow and may not be recognized. The older patient often seeks medical attention later and is sicker than the younger patient. HHS does not occur in adequately hydrated patients. Older patients are at greater risk for dehydration and HHS because of age-related changes in thirst perception and poor urine-concentrating abilities.

Many older adults take diuretics, which contributes to dehydration. In the long-term care settings and for home-bound older adults who depend on others for oral intake, many patients do not ingest enough fluids and can more easily become dehydrated. Ensure that older adults with diabetes are weighed every 3 days or weekly to monitor trends and detect dehydration early.

may cause HHS. Central nervous system (CNS) changes range from confusion to complete coma. Unlike DKA, patients with HHS may have seizures, myoclonic jerking, and reversible paralysis. The degree of neurologic impairment is related to serum osmolarity, with coma occurring once serum osmolarity is greater than 350 mOsm/L (350 mmol/L).

The development of HHS rather than DKA is related to residual insulin secretion. In HHS, the patient secretes just enough insulin to prevent ketosis but not enough to prevent hyperglycemia. The hyperglycemia of HHS is more severe than that of DKA, greatly increasing the blood osmolarity and causing profound diuresis. Severe dehydration and electrolyte loss occur, and the patient may lose 15% to 25% of body fluid. When dehydration is severe, glucose is not filtered into the urine, causing even greater hyperglycemia and hyperosmolarity. Impairment of the thirst center in the brain occurs, making it impossible for the patient to drink enough fluid to prevent dehydration. This problem is worse in the older adult with diabetes because age-related changes in the thirst center reduce the patient's sensation of thirst.

Planning: Expected Outcomes. The patient with DM is expected to have few episodes of hyperglycemia and avoid HHS. Indicators include that the patient consistently demonstrates these behaviors:

- Maintains blood glucose levels within the target range
- Uses antidiabetic drugs appropriately
- Remains well hydrated
- Describes when to seek help from health care professionals

Interventions

Monitoring. Assess for manifestations of HHS. (See Tables 67-14 and 67-15 for symptoms of hyperglycemia.) Continually assess fluid status.

Fluid Therapy. The expected outcome of therapy is to rehydrate the patient and restore normal blood glucose levels within 36 to 72 hours. The choice of fluid replacement and the rate of infusion are critical in managing HHS. The severity of the CNS problems is related to the level of blood hyperosmolarity and cellular dehydration. Re-establishing fluid balance in brain cells is a difficult and slow process, and many patients do not recover baseline CNS function until hours after blood glucose levels have returned to normal.

The *first* priority for fluid replacement in HHS is to increase blood volume. In shock or severe hypotension, give normal saline. Otherwise, use half-normal saline because it more rapidly corrects the water deficit. Infuse fluids at 1 L/hr until central venous pressure or pulmonary capillary wedge pressure begins to rise or until blood pressure and urine output are adequate. The rate is then reduced to 100 to 200 mL/hr. Half of the estimated water deficit is replaced in the first 12 hours, and the rest is given over the next 36 hours. Body weight, urine output, kidney function, and the presence or absence of pulmonary congestion and jugular venous distention determine the rate of fluid infusion. In patients with congestive heart failure, kidney disease, or acute kidney injury (failure), monitor central venous pressure. *Assess the patient hourly for signs of cerebral edema—abrupt changes in mental status, abnormal neurologic signs, and coma.* Lack of improvement in level of consciousness may indicate inadequate rates of fluid replacement or reduction in plasma osmolarity. Regression after initial improvement may indicate a too-rapid reduction in plasma osmolarity. A slow but steady improvement in CNS function is the best evidence that fluid management is satisfactory.

> **! NURSING SAFETY PRIORITY**
>
> **Critical Rescue**
>
> For patients being managed for a hyperglycemic-hyperosmolar state, immediately report changes in the level of consciousness; changes in pupil size, shape, or reaction; or seizures.

Continuing Therapy. IV insulin is administered after adequate fluids have been replaced. The typical intervention is an initial bolus dose of 0.15 unit per kg IV followed by an infusion of 0.1 unit per kg per hour until blood glucose levels fall to 250 mg/dL (13.9 mmol/L). A reduction of blood glucose of 50 to 70 mg/dL per hour is a reasonable expected outcome. Monitor the patient closely for indications of hypokalemia. Total body potassium depletion is often unrecognized because the level of potassium in the blood may be normal or high. The serum potassium level may drop quickly when insulin therapy is started. Potassium replacement is initiated once urine output is adequate. Serum electrolytes should be obtained every 1 to 2 hours until stable, and the patient's cardiac rhythm should be monitored continuously for signs of hypokalemia or hyperkalemia. Patient education and interventions to minimize dehydration are similar to those for ketoacidosis.

COMMUNITY-BASED CARE

Teaching for Self-Management

Education about blood glucose control begins at the time of diagnosis. It takes place in a hospital or outpatient setting, clinic, or primary care provider's office and involves physicians, nurses, dietitians, pharmacists, social workers, and psychologists. Diabetes is a condition that is managed by the patient; therefore education should be a continuous process. Education is provided to patients to achieve blood glucose control to the maximum of their abilities.

Assessing Learning Needs and Readiness to Learn

Gather information about the patient's current knowledge, skills, attitudes, and behaviors. The patient must have a basic level of understanding about diabetes management in order to reach target blood glucose levels. Assess his or her awareness of diabetes and the needs of both patient and family before teaching. This assessment includes:

- Health and medical history
- Nutrition history and practices
- Physical activity and exercise behaviors
- Prescription and over-the-counter medications, and complementary and alternative therapies and practices
- Factors that influence learning such as education and literacy levels, perceived learning needs, motivation to learn, and health beliefs
- Diabetes self-management behaviors, including experience with self-adjusting the treatment plan
- Previous diabetes self-management training, actual knowledge, and skills
- Physical factors including age, mobility, visual acuity, hearing, manual dexterity, alertness, attention span, and ability to concentrate or special needs or limitations requiring adaptive support and use of alternative skills
- Psychosocial concerns, factors, or issues including family and social support
- Current mental health status
- History of substance abuse including alcohol, tobacco, and recreational drugs
- Occupation, vocation, education level, financial status, and social, cultural, and religious practices
- Access to and use of health care resources

Adult learners want information that applies directly to them. Find out what concerns the patient most about having diabetes, and ask what he or she wants to learn. Learning is enhanced when it is related to what the learner already knows. Start with what the patient already knows, and build on that base. Because they will be managing their own care after discharge, patients tend to focus on issues most important to them. Treatment measures that need to start soon after diagnosis may be of more interest to the patient than long-term control. Learning is reinforced and retained when it can be applied immediately and repeatedly.

The patient's physical condition dictates the timing of teaching. He or she does not have the energy to learn complex information when blood glucose levels are fluctuating. Explaining that well-controlled blood glucose levels improve the sense of well-being can help the patient accept the therapy plan. Pace your teaching to match the patient's energy level. Use an informal teaching process until he or she feels able to attend a formal class.

Each patient learns in his or her own way. A successful diabetes education program combines several teaching methods. Some patients learn better when they read pamphlets. Others learn better when they watch videos. Learning improves when the equipment is handled, techniques are practiced, success is rewarded, and errors are corrected immediately.

Assessing Physical, Cognitive, and Emotional Limitations

Assess the patient's education and reading level to determine what level of information to present. He or she must be able to understand the printed material. It is important to match the literacy level of printed material provided to the literacy level of the patient. Even highly educated patients do not want to read complicated information when they are sick. Develop creative teaching strategies for the patient who cannot read.

Assess the patient's ability to read printed information, insulin labels, and markings on syringes and equipment. Many with type 2 diabetes have presbyopia (age-related farsightedness) and other visual problems made worse by blurred vision caused by fluctuating blood glucose levels.

Assess the patient's ability to reason with numbers and other mathematical concepts. Adjusting insulin dosage based on blood glucose monitoring is a difficult concept and may not be appropriate for patients who cannot understand it. Managing drugs, exercise, and diet requires complex interpretation and behavior.

Assess manual dexterity for any physical limitations that may alter the teaching plan. A hand injury, tremors, or severe arthritis may require a change in insulin preparation.

Information is best learned when the patient is ready. Those with newly diagnosed diabetes are facing a life crisis. Some are motivated to learn information and are willing to change lifelong behaviors. Others may grieve the loss of their previous lifestyle and use denial to cope. In this instance, the patient may not be able to learn needed information right away.

Survival Skills Information

The initial phase of diabetes education involves teaching information necessary for the survival of anyone diagnosed with diabetes. Survival information includes:
- Simple information on pathophysiology of diabetes
- Learning how to prepare and administer insulin or how to take oral drugs for diabetes
- Basic diet information
- Monitoring of blood glucose and ketones

- Recognition, treatment, and prevention of hypoglycemia and hyperglycemia
- Sick-day management
- Where to buy diabetes supplies and how to store them
- When and how to notify the primary care provider

A dietitian provides the initial diet instruction. The patient needs to understand what to eat, how much to eat, and when to eat. Stress the importance of eating on time and the dangers of skipping meals. He or she must know how to maintain food intake during illness. Reinforce dietary instruction, answer questions, and refer questions to the dietitian or primary care provider as indicated.

After being taught, the patient should be able to identify the drugs needed to control blood glucose levels. If insulin is used, he or she must be able to prepare and give the dose accurately using sterile technique. The patient must also be able to state when insulin is to be injected, where insulin is injected, and how insulin is stored. Stress the dangers of skipping doses. Carefully review drug interactions, especially with older patients taking oral antidiabetic drugs.

Patients should be able to state their plan for regular physical activity. They must be able to describe the relationship between exercise and blood glucose control and identify situations in which activity should not be performed. Provide guidelines for additional carbohydrate intake to prevent hypoglycemia from excessive exercise.

The patient also must be able to state the plan for monitoring blood glucose. The person doing the monitoring must be able to do the procedure accurately and understand the results. Explain when blood glucose should be monitored, acceptable ranges, and actions to take when results are out of these ranges. If the patient cannot perform self-monitoring of blood glucose (SMBG) because of illness, ensure that a resource (e.g., home care agency, health clinic, or primary care provider's office) will be available to do the monitoring.

The most important part of survival-level education is to ensure that the patient understands the significance, symptoms, causes, and treatment of hypoglycemia. He or she must be able to state the causes of hypoglycemia and the activities needed to prevent it. The patient must be able to describe appropriate carbohydrates to have available and the need to notify the physician of hypoglycemic episodes. Teach a family member how and when to inject glucagon.

The patient also must understand the significance of hyperglycemia and its relationship to illness. Instruct him or her on actions to take during illness and when to communicate with the primary care provider.

Most of this information is best retained when the patient is ready to learn. Education is a challenge because patients tend to be hospitalized for shorter periods. All diabetes education may be provided in an outpatient setting, where contact with the patient is limited. Important information must be squeezed into the time available. Many patients do not progress in self-management beyond the survival level because of psychological barriers.

In-Depth Education

In-depth education and counseling involve teaching more detailed information related to survival skills, as well as helping the patient learn preventive measures for avoiding long-term complications. Educational sessions with patient and family are needed to "patientize" the diabetes regimen for their needs and abilities. Education is often provided by a team of a physician, nurse educator, dietitian, social worker, pharmacist, psychologist, case manager, and other health care professionals as needed. It may occur in various outpatient settings.

Besides knowledge gained at the survival level, the patient should be able to discuss the action of insulin in the body and the effects of insulin deficiency. He or she should also be able to explain the effects of diet, drugs, and activity on blood glucose. The patient should be able to relate maintaining normal blood glucose levels to preventing complications. This includes relating changes in glucose level to the possible need for a change in insulin dosage.

The patient must be able to describe the meal plan and explain the adjustments needed to meet diabetic diet requirements. He or she should state how food intake should be altered when eating out or increasing exercise. *The patient must be able to list specific foods to be eaten to prevent and treat hypoglycemia, as well as adjustments to make when ill.* Include in this teaching the family member usually responsible for buying groceries and preparing meals.

The patient with diabetes must be able to prepare and give insulin accurately and must be able to discuss the onset, peak, and duration of the insulin used. Review formulas for self-adjustment in insulin (when permitted by the physician), and explain blood glucose monitoring requirements needed to evaluate the effects of additional insulin. If the patient takes an oral antidiabetic drug, ask him or her to identify the drug and describe its prescribed schedule. The patient must identify over-the-counter drugs with the potential to cause adverse interactions and the need to inform all care providers of the drug regimen.

Review how to perform desired physical activities safely. The patient must state blood glucose levels that are safe for exercise, the frequency of SMBG during exercise, drug adjustments before exercise, food required before exercise, and what food to have available during exercise. He or she should be aware of the risk for injury during exercise and explain the importance of protective footwear.

The purposes of in-depth education are to help the patient solve problems of blood glucose fluctuation through the use of SMBG. He or she should be able to identify practices, such as travel (Chart 67-12), that cause blood glucose to fluctuate and to treat these problems with supplemental insulin, changes in activity, or changes in diet. Ask him or her to demonstrate urine ketone testing and to describe when urine ketones should be measured.

The patient must be able to describe a plan for periodic evaluation of blood glucose control by the primary care provider, as well as periodic dental and eye examinations. He or she must be able to perform foot care, wear properly fitting shoes, and describe hazards related to foot care. The patient must be able to describe ways to reduce specific risk factors, such as cigarette smoking and hypertension.

The patient must state that diabetes is a lifelong disease that requires lifestyle changes, describe the changes being made, and indicate those that need to be made. He or she should be able to identify stress-producing situations and discuss ways to reduce stress.

Psychosocial Preparation

The diagnosis of diabetes may represent a loss of control. All but a few patients lose flexibility. Life becomes ordered, and routines must be followed. Certain events surrounding

---

CHART 67-12   PATIENT AND FAMILY EDUCATION: PREPARING FOR SELF-MANAGEMENT

Travel Tips for Patients with Diabetes

Before traveling, visit your primary care provider and diabetes educator.
- See your physician to make certain you do not have any other health problems.
- Obtain a letter from your physician (typed on office letterhead) that indicates you have diabetes and lists the drugs you are taking.
- Obtain any needed immunizations or inoculations.
- Obtain prescriptions from your physician for your drugs, including glucagon if you take insulin, and prescriptions for motion sickness, nausea and vomiting, and traveler's diarrhea.
- Develop a plan for changing strengths of insulin if you are traveling to a country that does not carry the type of insulin you use. Learn how to use a U-100 syringe to draw up U-40 insulin.
- Develop a plan for meal and drug adjustment across time zones. Eastbound travel will shorten the day, requiring a reduction in the amount of drug needed. Westbound travel may add an extra meal to the day and require additional drug.
- Obtain a list of foods from your diabetes educator that you can substitute for food served in restaurants or airplanes.

If you are traveling by air, train, or boat, call ahead and request special meals for those with diabetes.
- Plan for delays in eating.
- Eat something every 4 hours.
- Drink a glass of water every 2 hours to prevent dehydration.
- Do not assume that special meals will be available; substitute items you cannot eat with foods you have in your travel kit.

Notify airline and hotel personnel that you have diabetes.
- Always wear medical alert identification and keep your medical alert card in your wallet.

While traveling:
- Check your blood glucose level frequently.
- Do not engage in activities when blood glucose levels are lower than 65 mg/dL.
- Stretch and walk around every 2 hours to help your circulation.
- Check your feet frequently for blisters and sores. You may be doing more walking than usual.
- Take extra shoes with you, and plan to change shoes often when walking more than normal.
- Protect your skin against exposure to the sun. Drug-induced photosensitivity can occur with some oral hypoglycemic agents.

Always have your travel kit with you; do not check your kit along with the rest of your luggage. Include these items in your travel kit:
- Insulin bottles in boxes with prescription labels
- Twice as much drug and twice as many supplies as you think you will need (pack drugs separately from checked luggage)
- Insulin stored in an insulated carrying case that will maintain temperatures according to the manufacturer's directions
- The letter from your physician (typed on office letterhead) that indicates you have diabetes and lists the drugs you are taking
- A supply of fast-acting sugar (e.g., glucose tablets or gel, hard candy, sugar cubes), as well as longer-acting foods (e.g., cheese and crackers, peanut butter and crackers)
- A self-monitoring diary

---

diabetes are predictable. Taking an insulin injection and not eating for several hours causes hypoglycemia. Poorly controlled diabetes leads to complications and premature death. Tight control of blood glucose levels prevents complications.

The stress of diabetes is in addition to the demands of normal daily life. The patient must be able to integrate the demands of diabetes into daily and recreational schedules while keeping blood glucose stable.

Assist in healthy psychological adaptation to diabetes by providing successful educational experiences. Mastery of blood glucose monitoring helps the patient feel that he or she has control over the disease. Knowing the effects of extra activities, extra food, or extra insulin is helpful in learning to adjust the regimen.

Feeling a sense of control over the condition does much to promote a positive attitude about diabetes. Success in injecting insulin provides concrete evidence that he or she can master the disease. Teach by breaking a task into small, achievable units to ensure mastery. For example, a patient may begin learning how to inject insulin by first obtaining an accurate dose.

Devote as much teaching time as possible to insulin injection and blood glucose monitoring. Patients with newly diagnosed diabetes are often fearful of giving themselves injections. After this technique has been mastered, they become less anxious and are able to attend to other tasks.

Recognize that not everyone will have a healthy adaptation to diabetes. Major depression affects many patients with diabetes and severely impacts quality of life and all aspects of functioning, including self-management behaviors. Clinical anxiety disorder is another problem common in patients with diabetes. Refer those who have significant problems coping with the day-to-day demands of diabetes to mental health counseling for appropriate treatment.

Home Care Management

Patients with diabetes self-manage their disease. Each day they decide what to eat, whether to exercise, and whether to take prescribed drugs. Maintaining blood glucose control depends on the accuracy of self-management skills. The main role of the health care professional is to provide support and education and to empower the patient to make informed decisions. Self-management education allows patients to identify their problems and provides techniques to help them make decisions, take appropriate actions, and alter these actions as needed.

Provide information about resources. The patient must know whom to contact in case of emergency. Older adults who live alone need to have daily telephone contact with a friend or neighbor. The patient may also need help shopping and preparing meals. He or she may have limited access to transportation and may not have sufficient supplies of food, particularly in bad weather. Because of the likelihood of visual problems in older patients, they may need assistance in preparing insulin syringes for injection or in monitoring blood glucose. Make referrals to home care or public health agencies as needed. Chart 67-13 identifies areas for assessment during a home or clinic visit.

▌EVALUATION: OUTCOMES

Evaluate the care of the patient with diabetes based on the identified priority patient problems. Outcome success for diabetes education is the ability of the patient to maintain blood glucose levels within their established target range. General outcome criteria are listed below and in Table 67-16. More specific outcomes are listed with each priority patient problem. The expected outcomes include that the patient should:

- Achieve blood glucose control
- Avoid acute and chronic complications of diabetes

CHART 67-13   FOCUSED ASSESSMENT

The Insulin-Dependent Patient with Diabetes During a Home or Clinic Visit

- Assess overall mental status, wakefulness, ability to converse.
- Take vital signs and weight:
  - Fever could indicate infection.
  - Are blood pressure and weight within target range? If not, why?
- Question patient regarding any change in visual acuity; check current visual acuity.
- Inspect oral mucous membranes, gums, and teeth.
- Question patient about injection areas used; inspect areas being used; assess whether patient is using areas and sites appropriately.
- Inspect skin for intactness, wounds that have not healed, new sores, ulcers, bruises, or burns; assess any previously known wounds for infection, progression of healing.
- Question patient regarding foot care.
- Assess lower extremities and feet for peripheral pulses, lack of or decreased sensation, abnormal sensations, breaks in skin integrity, condition of toes and nails.
- Question patient regarding color and consistency of stools and frequency of bowel movements; assess abdomen for bowel sounds.
- Review patient's home health diary:
  - Is blood glucose within targeted range? If not, why?
  - Is glucose monitoring being recorded often enough?
  - Is the patient's food intake adequate and appropriate? If not, why?
  - Is exercise occurring regularly? If not, why?
- Assess patient's ability to perform self-monitoring of blood glucose.
- Assess patient's procedures for obtaining and storing insulin and syringes, cleaning equipment, disposing of syringes and needles.
- Assess patient's insulin preparation and injection technique.

TABLE 67-16   OUTCOME CRITERIA FOR DIABETES TEACHING

Before being discharged to home, the patient with diabetes or the significant other should be able to:

- Tell why insulin or an oral hypoglycemic agent is being prescribed.
- Name which insulin or oral hypoglycemic agent is being prescribed, and name the dosage and frequency of administration.
- Discuss the relationship between mealtime and the action of insulin or the oral hypoglycemic agent.
- Discuss plans to follow diabetic diet instructions.
- Prepare and administer insulin accurately.
- Test blood for glucose, or state plans for having blood glucose levels monitored.
- Test urine for ketones, and state when this test should be done.
- Verbalize how to store insulin.
- List symptoms that indicate a hypoglycemic reaction.
- Tell what carbohydrate sources are used to treat hypoglycemic reactions.
- Tell what symptoms indicate hyperglycemia.
- Tell what dietary changes are needed during illness.
- Verbalize when to call the physician or the nurse (frequent episodes of hypoglycemia, symptoms of hyperglycemia).
- Verbalize the procedures for proper foot care.

- Have a satisfactory and complete postoperative recovery without complications
- Avoid injury
- Experience relief of pain
- Maintain optimal vision
- Maintain a urine output in the expected range

- Have an optimal level of mental status functioning
- Have decreased episodes of hypoglycemia
- Have decreased episodes of hyperglycemia

Specific indicators for these outcomes are listed for each priority patient problem under the Planning and Implementation section (see earlier).

GET READY FOR THE NCLEX® EXAMINATION!

KEY POINTS

Review these Key Points for each NCLEX Examination Client Needs Category.

Safe and Effective Care Environment

- Use aseptic technique during any invasive procedure when caring for a patient with diabetes.
- Administer antidiabetic drugs and insulin in a safe manner.
- Use good handwashing techniques before providing any care to a patient who has diabetes.
- Wash your hands before and after testing the patient's blood glucose levels.

Health Promotion and Maintenance

- Encourage all patients to maintain weight within an appropriate range.
- Encourage all patients, including patients with diabetes, to participate regularly in exercise or physical activity appropriate to their health status.
- Teach the patient and family about the manifestations of infection and when to seek medical advice.
- Instruct patients with diabetes to wear a medical alert bracelet.
- Instruct patients to not share blood glucose monitoring equipment.
- Reinforce to all patients with diabetes that tight control over blood glucose levels reduces the risk for the vascular complications of diabetes.
- Remind patients with diabetes to have yearly eye examinations by an ophthalmologist.
- Teach patients with peripheral neuropathy to use a bath thermometer to test water for bathing, to avoid walking barefoot, and to inspect their feet daily.

Psychosocial Integrity

- Explore with the patient what the diagnosis of diabetes means to him or her.
- Allow the patient the opportunity to express concerns about the diagnosis of diabetes or the treatment regimen.
- Explain all procedures, restrictions, drugs, and follow-up care to the patient and family.
- Pace your education sessions to match the learning needs and style of the patient.
- Use return demonstration strategies when teaching the patient about drug regimen, insulin injection, blood glucose monitoring, and foot assessment.

- Refer patients newly diagnosed with diabetes to local resources and support groups.
- Assess patients' visual acuity and peripheral tactile sensation to determine needed adjustments in teaching self-medication and self-monitoring of blood glucose levels.

Physiological Integrity

- Teach the patient about any drugs to be continued after discharge from the hospital.
- Instruct the patient and family on the manifestations of complications and when to seek assistance.
- Instruct all patients with diabetes to avoid becoming dehydrated and to drink at least 3 L of water each day unless another medical condition requires fluid restriction.
- Instruct patients who are taking sulfonylurea drugs about an increased risk for hypoglycemic reactions.
- Teach patients who are taking metformin the clinical manifestations of lactic acidosis (fatigue, dizziness, difficulty breathing, stomach discomfort, irregular heartbeat).
- Warn patients to not take over-the-counter drugs with their oral antidiabetic drugs without consulting their primary care provider.
- When mixing different kinds of insulin together, draw the shorter-acting insulin into the syringe before drawing up the longer-acting insulin.
- Never dilute or mix insulin glargine with any other insulin or solution.
- Teach patients to rotate insulin injection sites within one area rather than to another area to prevent changes in absorption.
- Avoid injecting insulin within a 2-inch radius of the umbilicus.
- Avoid IM insulin injection.
- Teach patients to administer an accurate dose of insulin using a prefilled or disposable insulin pen.
- Teach patients who experience Somogyi phenomenon (early morning hyperglycemia) to ensure an adequate dietary intake at bedtime.
- Instruct patients to always carry a glucose source.
- Teach patients who exercise to test urine for ketone bodies if blood glucose levels are greater than 250 mg/dL before engaging in strenuous exercise.
- Instruct patients in foot care as outlined in Chart 67-9.

CONCEPT OVERVIEW

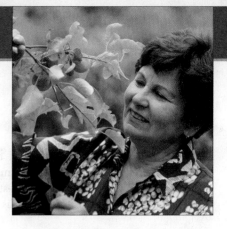

Urinary Elimination

The need for urinary elimination is really the need for homeostasis—the ability of the body to maintain its internal environment at a "steady state" and within very narrow ranges of normal, regardless of external changes. The body works best when blood and other extracellular fluids have a serum sodium concentration of 135 to 145 mEq/L (mmol/L) and a serum potassium level of 3.5 to 5.0 mEq/L (mmol/L). Serious health problems and death occur when these electrolytes are much higher or lower than these normal ranges. Keeping the amount of total body water, especially blood volume, within the normal range is also important to proper function and health. When blood volume is too high, hypertension develops and damages vital organs. When blood volume is too low, hypotension can be so severe that vital organs are not perfused with oxygen and become hypoxic. In addition, protein waste products containing nitrogen, such as urea, act as a poison and must be prevented from getting too high. Humans ingest many foods and liquids that contain water, electrolytes, and substances that will be converted to waste products. Without control mechanisms to balance the intake of these substances with their elimination, we would rapidly accumulate too much of everything and die.

As part of the renal/urinary system, the kidneys are responsible for maintaining this balance of what is taken into the body, what is allowed to remain in the body, and what is eliminated from the body. Although some products are eliminated in the stool, there is no discrimination or adjustment in bowel elimination. Urinary elimination, however, allows a person to eat and drink almost anything (except poisons and infectious organisms) in almost any amount without upsetting the homeostatic balance for body water, electrolytes, waste products, and blood pressure. For example, on one day a person may drink 2 L of fluids and eat food that contains 2 g of sodium and 5 g of potassium. The next day this same person may drink 3 L of fluids and eat food that contains 12 g of sodium and 10 g of potassium. Yet because the kidneys selectively adjust to change the amount of each substance that gets eliminated, the blood pressure, serum sodium, and serum potassium levels remain the same and within the normal ranges on both days. A "steady-state" or homeostatic balance of these substances is maintained because the kidneys adjust the output to match the intake (Fig. 1).

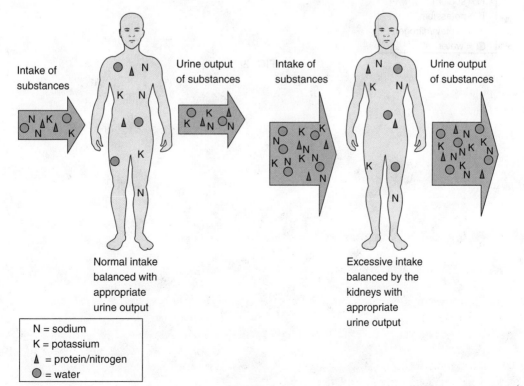

FIG. 1

When kidney function is impaired to any degree as a result of renal/urinary problems, the human need for urinary elimination is not met and the steady-state homeostasis of water, electrolyte, and waste products is disrupted (Fig. 2).

Without intervention, this lack of steady state leads to excesses of body water, electrolytes, and nitrogenous waste products that interfere with normal organ function and can cause death.

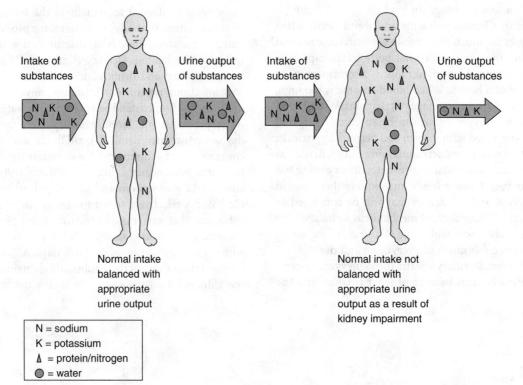

FIG. 2

CHAPTER

68

Assessment of the Renal/Urinary System

Chris Winkelman

⊖volve WEBSITE

http://evolve.elsevier.com/Iggy/

Animation: Filtration
Animation: Nephrons
Answer Key for NCLEX Examination Challenges and
   Decision-Making Challenges

Audio Glossary
Key Points
Review Questions for the NCLEX® Examination

LEARNING OUTCOMES

Safe and Effective Care Environment

1. Use Standard Precautions when handling urine specimens or examining the patient's genitalia.
2. Determine whether the patient has risks for an allergic reaction to contrast dyes or a drug–contrast dye adverse interaction before testing procedures.
3. Verify that informed consent has been obtained and that the patient has a clear understanding of the potential risks before he or she undergoes invasive procedures to assess the kidneys and urinary function.
4. Examine individual patient factors contributing to safety risks.

Health Promotion and Maintenance

5. Teach all people about the importance of maintaining an adequate oral fluid intake.

6. Teach about or assist with cleansing of the perineum or urinary meatus after using the toilet and during daily bathing or showering.

Psychosocial Integrity

7. Use language comfortable for the patient during assessment of the kidneys and urinary system.
8. Encourage the patient to express feelings or concerns about a change in kidney or bladder function.
9. Respect the patient's dignity when performing kidney and urinary assessment.
10. Explain all diagnostic procedures, restrictions, and follow-up care to the patient scheduled for tests.

Physiological Integrity

11. Briefly review the relevant anatomy and physiology of the kidney and urinary system.

LEARNING OUTCOMES—cont'd

12. Describe age-related changes in the kidney and urinary system.
13. Describe the correct techniques to use in physically assessing the kidney and urinary system.
14. Use laboratory data to distinguish between dehydration and kidney impairment.

15. Describe how to obtain a sterile urine specimen from a urinary catheter.
16. Coordinate nursing care for the patient during the first 24 hours after IV urography.
17. Coordinate nursing care for the patient during the first 24 hours after a kidney biopsy.

The kidneys help maintain health in many ways. Most important for urinary elimination, they maintain body fluid volume and composition and filter waste products for elimination. The kidneys also help regulate blood pressure and acid-base balance, produce erythropoietin for red blood cell (RBC) synthesis, and convert vitamin D to an active form.

The renal system includes the kidneys and the entire urinary tract. The ureters, bladder, and urethra are the drainage route for the excretion of urine. Structural or functional problems in the kidney or urinary tract may alter fluid, electrolyte, and acid-base balance.

Assessment of the patient at risk for or with actual problems of the kidney or urinary system begins with a history and physical assessment. Understanding the anatomy, physiology, and diagnostic tests of the renal system helps you in problem-solving about kidney function in the clinical setting. It also assists you in teaching the patient about the purpose of procedures and in physically and emotionally preparing the patient for assessment.

ANATOMY AND PHYSIOLOGY REVIEW

Kidneys

Structure

Gross Anatomy. Normally, two kidneys are located behind the peritoneum, not really in the abdominal cavity, one on either side of the spine (Fig. 68-1). The adult kidney is 4 to 5

inches (10 to 13 cm) long, 2 to 3 inches (5 to 7 cm) wide, and about 1 inch (2.5 to 3 cm) thick. It weighs about 8 ounces (250 g). The left kidney is slightly longer and narrower than the right kidney. Larger-than-usual kidneys may indicate obstruction or polycystic disease. Smaller-than-usual kidneys may indicate chronic kidney disease (CKD).

Variation in kidney shape and number is not uncommon and does not necessarily mean there is also a problem in kidney function. Some people have more than two kidneys or may have only one, large, horseshoe-shaped kidney. As long as tests of kidney function are normal, these variations are of no significance.

Several layers of tissue surround the kidney, providing protection and support. On the outer surface of the kidney is a layer of fibrous tissue called the capsule (Fig. 68-2). This capsule covers most of the kidney except the hilum, which is the area where the renal artery and nerve plexus enter and the renal vein and ureter exit. The renal capsule is surrounded by layers of fat and connective tissue.

Lying beneath the renal capsule are the two layers of functional kidney tissue—the cortex and the medulla. The renal cortex is the outer tissue layer and is covered by the renal capsule. The medulla is the medullary tissue lying below the cortex in the shape of many fans. Each "fan" is called a pyramid, and there are 12 to 18 pyramids per kidney. The renal columns are cortical tissue that dips down into the interior of the kidney and separates the pyramids.

The tip, or end, of each pyramid is called a papilla. The papillae drain urine into the collecting system. A cuplike structure called a calyx collects the urine at the end of each papilla. The calices join together to form the renal pelvis, which narrows to become the ureter.

The kidneys have a rich blood supply and receive 20% to 25% of the total cardiac output. Blood flow to the kidneys varies from about 600 to 1300 mL/min. The blood supply to each kidney comes from the renal artery, which branches from the abdominal aorta. The renal artery divides into progressively smaller arteries, supplying all blood to areas of the kidney tissue (parenchyma) and the nephrons. The smallest arteries (afferent arterioles) feed the nephrons directly to form urine.

Venous blood from the kidneys starts with the capillaries surrounding each nephron. These capillaries drain into progressively larger veins, with blood eventually returned to the inferior vena cava through the renal vein.

Microscopic Anatomy. The nephron is the "working" or functional unit of the kidney, and it is here that urine is actually formed from blood. There are about 1 million nephrons per kidney, and each nephron separately makes urine from blood.

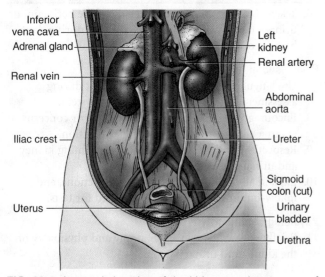

FIG. 68-1 Anatomic location of the kidneys and structures of the urinary system.

Inferior vena cava
Adrenal gland
Renal vein
Iliac crest
Uterus
Left kidney
Renal artery
Abdominal aorta
Ureter
Sigmoid colon (cut)
Urinary bladder
Urethra

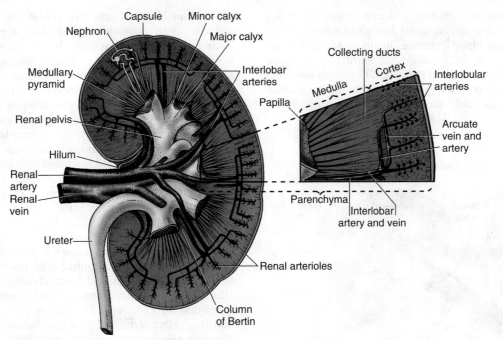

FIG. 68-2 Bisection of the kidney showing the major structures of the kidney.

There are two types of nephrons: cortical nephrons and juxtamedullary nephrons. The cortical nephrons are short, with all parts located in the renal cortex. The juxtamedullary nephrons (about 20% of all nephrons) are longer, and their tubes and blood vessels dip deeply into the medulla. The purpose of the juxtamedullary nephrons is to concentrate urine during times of low fluid intake. The ability to concentrate urine allows for continued excretion of body wastes with less fluid loss.

Blood supply to the nephron is delivered through the afferent arteriole—the smallest, most distal portion of the renal arterial system. From the afferent arteriole, blood flows into the glomerulus, which is a series of specialized capillary loops. It is through these capillaries that water and small particles are filtered from the blood to make urine. The remaining blood leaves the glomerulus through the efferent arteriole, which is the first vessel in the venous system of the kidney. From the efferent arteriole, blood exits into one of two additional capillary systems:

- The *peritubular capillaries* around the tubular part of the cortical nephrons
- The *vasa recta* around the tubular part of juxtamedullary nephrons

Each nephron is a tubelike structure with distinct parts (Fig. 68-3). The tube begins with Bowman's capsule, a saclike structure that surrounds the glomerulus. The tubular tissue of Bowman's capsule narrows into the *proximal convoluted tubule (PCT)*. The PCT twists and turns, finally straightening into the descending limb of the *loop of Henle*. The descending loop of Henle dips in the direction of the medulla but forms a hairpin loop and comes back up into the cortex as the ascending loop of Henle.

There are two segments of the ascending limb of the loop of Henle: the thin segment and the thick segment. The *distal convoluted tubule (DCT)* forms from the thick segment of the ascending limb of the loop of Henle. The DCT ends in one

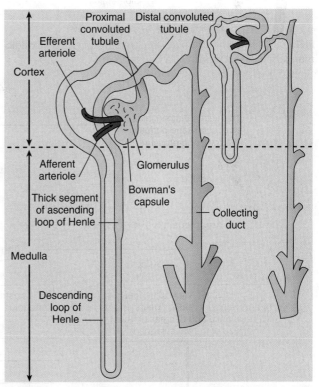

FIG. 68-3 Anatomy of the nephron, the functional unit of the kidney. Note that the particular nephron labeled here is a juxtamedullary nephron.

of many collecting ducts located in the kidney tissue. The urine in the collecting ducts passes through the papillae and empties into the renal pelvis.

Special cells in the afferent arteriole, efferent arteriole, and DCT are known as the juxtaglomerular complex (Fig. 68-4).

These specialized cells produce and store renin. Renin is a hormone that helps regulate blood flow, glomerular filtration rate (GFR), and blood pressure. Renin is secreted when sensing cells in the DCT (called the *macula densa*) sense changes in blood volume and pressure. The macula densa lies next to the renin-producing cells. Renin is produced when the macula densa cells sense that blood volume, blood

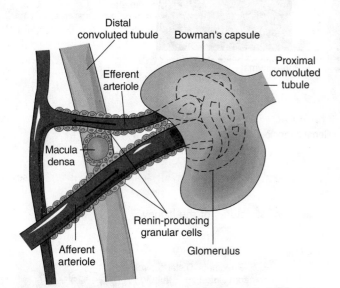

FIG. 68-4 The juxtaglomerular complex showing juxtaglomerular cells and the macula densa.

pressure, or blood sodium level is low. Renin then converts renin substrate (angiotensinogen) into angiotensin I. This leads to a series of reactions that cause secretion of the hormone *aldosterone* (Fig. 68-5). Aldosterone increases kidney reabsorption of sodium and water, restoring blood pressure, blood volume, and blood sodium levels. It also promotes excretion of potassium. (See Chapter 13 for more discussion of the renin-angiotensin-aldosterone pathway.)

The glomerular capillary wall has three layers (Fig. 68-6): the endothelium, the basement membrane, and the epithelium. The endothelial and epithelial cells lining these capillaries are separated by pores that filter water and small particles from the blood into Bowman's capsule. This fluid is called the "filtrate" or "early urine."

Function

The kidneys have both regulatory and hormonal functions. The regulatory functions control fluid, electrolyte, and acid-base balance. The hormonal functions control red blood cell (RBC) formation, blood pressure, and vitamin D activation.

Regulatory Functions. The kidney processes that maintain fluid, electrolyte, and acid-base balance are glomerular filtration, tubular reabsorption, and tubular secretion. These processes use filtration, diffusion, active transport, and osmosis. (See Chapter 13 for a review of these actions.) Table 68-1 lists the functions of nephron tubules and blood vessels.

Glomerular filtration is the first process in urine formation. As blood passes from the afferent arteriole into the glomerulus, water, electrolytes, and other small particles (e.g., creatinine, urea nitrogen, glucose) are filtered across the glomerular

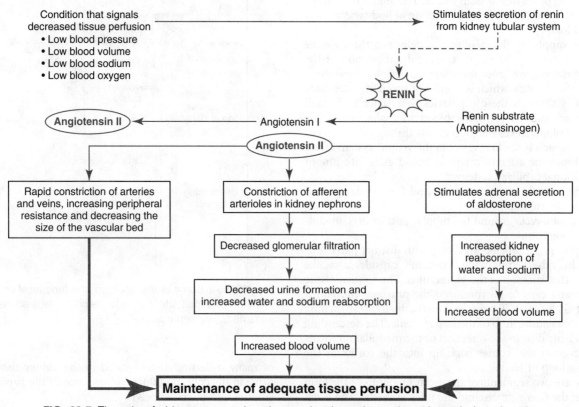

FIG. 68-5 The role of aldosterone, renin substrate (angiotensinogen), angiotensin I, and angiotensin II in the renal regulation of water and sodium.

membrane into the Bowman's capsule to form *glomerular filtrate*. As the filtrate enters the proximal convoluted tubule (PCT), it is called *tubular filtrate*.

Large particles, such as blood cells, albumin, and other proteins, are too large to filter through the glomerular capillary walls. *Therefore these substances are not normally present in the filtrate or in the final urine.*

About 180 L of glomerular filtrate is formed from the blood each day. The rate of filtration is expressed in milliliters per minute. Normal glomerular filtration rate (GFR) averages 125 mL/min. If the entire amount of filtrate were excreted as urine, death would occur quickly from dehydration. Actually, only about 1 to 3 L is excreted each day as urine. The rest is reabsorbed back into the circulatory system.

The GFR is controlled by blood pressure and blood flow. The ability of the kidneys to self-regulate renal blood pressure and renal blood flow keeps GFR constant. GFR is controlled by selectively constricting and dilating the afferent and efferent arterioles. When the afferent arteriole is constricted or the efferent arteriole is dilated, pressure in the glomerular capillaries falls and filtration decreases. When the afferent arteriole is dilated or the efferent arteriole is constricted, pressure in the glomerular capillaries rises and filtration increases. Through this process, the kidney can maintain a constant GFR, even when systemic blood pressure changes. When systolic pressure drops below about 70 mm Hg, these processes cannot compensate and GFR stops.

Tubular reabsorption is the second process involved in urine formation. This reabsorption of most of the filtrate keeps normal urine output at 1 to 3 L/day and prevents

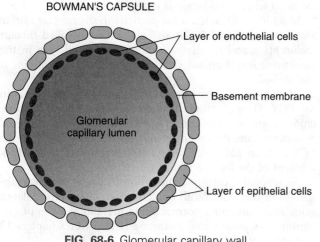

BOWMAN'S CAPSULE

Layer of endothelial cells

Basement membrane

Glomerular capillary lumen

Layer of epithelial cells

FIG. 68-6 Glomerular capillary wall.

TABLE 68-1   VASCULAR AND TUBULAR COMPONENTS OF THE NEPHRON

STRUCTURE	ANATOMIC FEATURES	PHYSIOLOGIC ASPECTS	STRUCTURE	ANATOMIC FEATURES	PHYSIOLOGIC ASPECTS
Vascular Components			Proximal convoluted tubule (PCT)	Evolves from and is continuous with Bowman's capsule Specialized cellular lining facilitates tubular reabsorption	Site for reabsorption of sodium, chloride, water, glucose, amino acids, potassium, calcium, bicarbonate, phosphate, and urea
Afferent arteriole	Delivers arterial blood from the branches of the renal artery into the glomerulus	Autoregulation of renal blood flow via vasoconstriction or vasodilation Renin-producing granular cells			
			Loop of Henle	Continues from PCT Juxtamedullary nephrons dip deep into the medulla Permeable to water, urea, and sodium chloride	Regulation of water balance
Glomerulus	Capillary loops with thin, semipermeable membrane	Site of glomerular filtration Glomerular filtration occurs when hydrostatic pressure (blood pressure) is greater than opposing forces (tubular filtrate and oncotic pressure)	Descending limb (DL)	Continues from the loop of Henle Permeable to water, urea, and sodium chloride	Regulation of water balance
Efferent arteriole	Delivers arterial blood from the glomerulus into the peritubular capillaries or the vasa recta	Autoregulation of renal blood flow via vasoconstriction or vasodilation Renin-producing granular cells	Ascending limb (AL)	Emerges from DL as it turns and is redirected up toward the renal cortex	Potassium and magnesium reabsorption in the thick segment Thin segment is impermeable to water
Peritubular capillaries (PTCs) and vasa recta (VR)	PTCs: surround tubular components of cortical nephrons VR: surround tubular components of juxtamedullary nephrons	Tubular reabsorption and tubular secretion allow movement of water and solutes to or from the tubules, interstitium, and blood	Distal convoluted tubule (DCT)	Evolves from AL and twists so the macula densa cells lie adjacent to the juxtaglomerular cells of afferent arteriole	Site of additional water and electrolyte reabsorption, including bicarbonate Potassium and hydrogen secretion
Tubular Components			Collecting ducts	Collect formed urine from several tubules and deliver it into the renal pelvis	Receptor sites for antidiuretic hormone regulation of water balance
Bowman's capsule (BC)	Thin membranous sac surrounding 7/8 of the glomerulus	Collects glomerular filtrate (GF) and funnels it into the tubule			

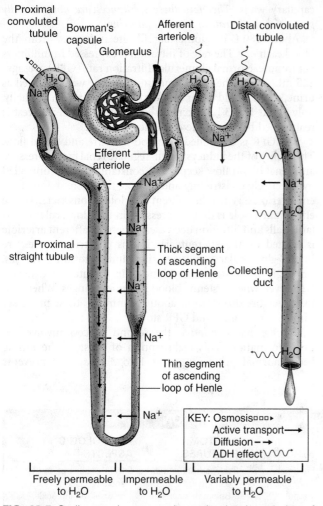

FIG. 68-7 Sodium and water reabsorption by the tubules of a cortical nephron. *ADH,* Antidiuretic hormone; *Na⁺,* sodium.

dehydration. As the filtrate passes through the tubular parts of the nephron, most of the water and electrolytes is reabsorbed. Reabsorption returns particles (solutes) and water to the blood. Reabsorption occurs *from the filtrate* across the tubular lumen of the nephron and into the blood of the peritubular capillaries. The PCT reabsorbs about 65% of the total glomerular filtrate.

The tubules return about 99% of all filtered water back into the body (Fig. 68-7). Most water reabsorption occurs as the filtrate passes through the PCT. Water reabsorption continues as the filtrate flows down the descending loop of Henle. The thin and thick segments of the ascending loop of Henle are *not* permeable to water, and water reabsorption does not occur here.

The distal convoluted tubule (DCT) can be permeable to water, and some water reabsorption can occur as the filtrate continues to flow through the tubule. The membrane of the DCT may be made more permeable to water through the action of antidiuretic hormone (ADH) and aldosterone. ADH increases tubular permeability to water, allowing water to leave the tube and be reabsorbed into the capillaries. ADH is also known as *vasopressin* and affects arteriole constriction. Arteriole constriction alters blood pressure, which, in turn,

affects the amount of fluid and solutes that exit glomeruli capillaries. Aldosterone promotes the reabsorption of sodium in the DCT. Water reabsorption occurs as a result of the movement of sodium (where sodium goes, water follows).

The ability of the kidneys to vary the volume or concentration of urine helps regulate water balance regardless of fluid intake. In this way, the healthy kidney can prevent dehydration when fluid intake is low and can prevent circulatory overload when fluid intake is excessive.

In addition to water, some particles in the tubular filtrate also *are returned to the blood.* This process is called *tubular reabsorption* and is selective. About 50% of all urea in the early urine is reabsorbed. On the other hand, no creatinine is reabsorbed.

Most sodium, chloride, and water reabsorption occurs in the PCT. The collecting ducts are the other site of sodium, chloride, and water reabsorption. Here reabsorption is caused by aldosterone. Potassium is also mostly reabsorbed in the PCT, with an additional 20% to 40% reabsorbed in the thick segment of the loop of Henle.

Bicarbonate, calcium, and phosphate are mostly reabsorbed in the PCT. Bicarbonate reabsorption helps balance acids and maintain a normal blood pH. Blood levels of calcitonin and parathyroid hormone (PTH) (see Chapters 13 and 66) control calcium balance.

The kidney reabsorbs some of the glucose filtered from the blood. However, there is a limit to how much glucose the kidney can reabsorb. This limit is called the renal threshold for glucose reabsorption or the transport maximum for glucose reabsorption. The usual renal threshold for glucose is about 220 mg/dL. This means that at a blood glucose level of 220 mg/dL or less, all glucose is reabsorbed and returned to the blood, with no glucose present in final urine. When blood glucose levels are greater than 220 mg/dL, some glucose stays in the filtrate and is present in the urine. Normally, almost all glucose and any amino acids or proteins are reabsorbed and are not present in the urine.

> **! NURSING SAFETY PRIORITY**
> *Action Alert*
>
> Report the presence of glucose or proteins in the urine of a patient undergoing a screening examination to the health care provider because this is an abnormal finding and requires further assessment.

Tubular secretion is the third process involved in urine formation. Like glomerular filtration, it allows substances to move from the blood into the early urine. During tubular secretion, substances move from the peritubular capillaries in reverse, across capillary membranes, and into the cells that line the tubules. From the cells, these substances are moved into the urine and are excreted from the body. Potassium (K⁺) and hydrogen (H⁺) ions are some of the substances moved in this way to maintain homeostasis of electrolytes and pH.

Hormonal Functions. The kidneys produce renin, prostaglandins, bradykinin, erythropoietin, and activated vitamin D (Table 68-2). Other kidney products, such as the kinins, change kidney blood flow and capillary permeability. The kidneys also help break down and excrete insulin.

Renin, as discussed on p. 1468 in the Microscopic Anatomy section, assists in blood pressure control. It is formed and

TABLE 68-2 RENAL HORMONE PRODUCTION AND HORMONES INFLUENCING RENAL FUNCTION

	SITE	ACTION
Renal Hormone Production		
Renin	Renin-producing granular cells	Raises blood pressure as result of angiotensin (local vasoconstriction) and aldosterone (volume expansion) secretion
Prostaglandins	Kidney tissues	Regulate intrarenal blood flow by vasodilation or vasoconstriction
Bradykinins	Juxtaglomerular cells of the arterioles	Increase blood flow (vasodilation) and vascular permeability
Erythropoietin	Kidney parenchyma	Stimulates bone marrow to make red blood cells
Activated vitamin D	Kidney parenchyma	Promotes absorption of calcium in the GI tract
Hormones Influencing Kidney Function		
Antidiuretic hormone (ADH, vasopressin)	Released from posterior pituitary	Makes DCT and CD permeable to water to maximize reabsorption and produce a concentrated urine
Aldosterone	Released from adrenal cortex	Promotes sodium reabsorption and potassium secretion in DCT and CD; water and chloride follow sodium movement
Natriuretic hormones	Cardiac atria, cardiac ventricle, brain	Cause tubular secretion of sodium

CD, Collecting duct; *DCT,* distal convoluted tubule.

released when there is a decrease in blood flow, blood volume, or blood pressure through the renal arterioles or when too little sodium is present in kidney blood. These conditions are detected through the receptors of the juxtaglomerular complex.

Renin release causes the production of *angiotensin II* through a series of steps (see Fig. 68-5). Angiotensin II increases systemic blood pressure through powerful blood vessel constricting effects and triggers the release of aldosterone from the adrenal glands. Aldosterone increases the reabsorption of sodium in the distal tubule of the nephron. Therefore more water is reabsorbed and blood pressure is increased because of increases in blood volume. When blood flow to the kidney is reduced, this system also regulates pressures in the nephron to prevent fluid loss and maintain circulating blood volume (see also Chapter 13).

Prostaglandins are produced in the kidney and many other tissues. Those produced specifically in the kidney are prostaglandin E_2 (PGE_2) and prostacyclin (PGI_2). These substances help regulate glomerular filtration, kidney vascular resistance, and renin production. PGE_2 acts on the distal tubule and collecting duct to increase sodium and water excretion.

Bradykinin is released by the kidney in response to the presence of angiotensin II, prostaglandins, and ADH. It is a small hormone that dilates the afferent arteriole and increases capillary membrane permeability to some solutes. These actions maintain kidney blood flow and reabsorption even when other conditions cause systemic blood vessel constriction.

Erythropoietin is produced and released in response to decreased oxygen tension in the kidney's blood supply. It triggers red blood cell (RBC) production in the bone marrow. When kidney function is poor, erythropoietin production decreases and the person becomes anemic.

Vitamin D activation occurs through a series of steps. Some of these steps take place in the skin when it is exposed to sunlight, and then more processing occurs in the liver. From there, vitamin D is converted to its active form (1,25-dihydroxy-cholecalciferol) in the kidney. It is needed to absorb calcium in the intestinal tract and to regulate calcium balance.

Ureters

Each kidney has a single ureter—a hollow tube that connects the renal pelvis with the urinary bladder. The ureter is about ½ inch (1.25 cm) in diameter and about 12 to 18 inches (30 to 45 cm) in length. The diameter of the ureter narrows in three areas:

- In the upper third of the ureter, at the point at which the renal pelvis becomes the ureter, is a narrowing known as the ureteropelvic junction (UPJ).
- The ureter also narrows as it bends toward the abdominal wall (aortoiliac bend).
- Each ureter narrows at the point it enters the bladder; this point is called the ureterovesical junction (UVJ).

The ureter tunnels through bladder tissue for a short distance and then opens into the bladder at the trigone (Fig. 68-8).

The ureter has three layers: an inner lining of mucous membrane (*urothelium*), a middle layer of smooth muscle fibers, and an outer layer of fibrous tissue. The outer layer contains the blood supply. The middle layer of muscle fibers is controlled by several nerve pathways from the lower spinal cord.

Contractions of the smooth muscle in the ureter move urine from the renal pelvis of the kidney to the bladder. Stretch receptors in the renal pelvis regulate this movement. For example, a large volume of urine in the renal pelvis triggers the stretch receptors, which respond by increasing ureteral contractions and ureter peristalsis.

Urinary Bladder
Structure

The urinary bladder is a muscular sac (see Fig. 68-8). The upper surface lies next to the peritoneal cavity. In men, the bladder is in front of the rectum. In women, it is in front of the vagina. The bladder lies directly behind the pubic bone.

The bladder is composed of the *body* (the rounded sac portion) and the *bladder neck* (posterior urethra), which connects to the bladder body. The bladder has three linings—an inner lining of epithelial cells (*urothelium*), middle layers of smooth muscle (*detrusor muscle*), and an outer lining. The *trigone* is an area on the posterior wall between the points of ureteral entry (ureterovesical junctions [UVJs]) and the urethra.

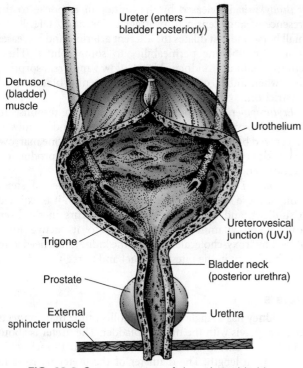

FIG. 68-8 Gross anatomy of the urinary bladder.

The internal urethral sphincter is the smooth detrusor muscle of the bladder neck and elastic tissue. The external urethral sphincter is skeletal muscle that surrounds the urethra. In men, the external sphincter surrounds the urethra at the base of the prostate gland. In women, the external sphincter is at the base of the bladder. The pudendal nerve from the spinal cord controls the external sphincter.

Function

The bladder is a temporary urine storage site. The bladder also provides continence and enables voiding. The secretions of the bladder lining resist bacteria.

Continence is the ability to voluntarily control bladder emptying. Bladder continence occurs during bladder filling through the combination of detrusor muscle relaxation, internal sphincter muscle tone, and external sphincter contraction. As the bladder fills with urine, stretch sensations are transmitted to spinal sacral nerves S2 and S3.

Maintaining continence occurs by the interaction of the nerves that control the muscles of the bladder, bladder neck, urethra, and pelvic floor, as well as by factors that close the urethra. During bladder filling, the sympathetic nervous system fibers prevent detrusor muscle contraction. These control centers are located in the cerebral cortex, the brainstem, and the sacral part of the spinal cord. For urethral closure to be adequate for continence, the mucosal surfaces must be in contact and must be adhesive. Contact depends on the presence and proper function of the involved nerves and muscles. Adhesion depends on the adequate secretion of mucus-like substances.

Micturition (voiding) is a reflex of autonomic control that triggers contraction of the detrusor muscle at the same time as relaxation of the external sphincter and the muscles of the pelvic floor. With detrusor muscle contraction, the UVJ of the ureter closes and the normally round bladder assumes the shape of a funnel. Voiding is a voluntary act as the result of a learned response and is controlled by the cerebral cortex and the brainstem. Contraction of the external sphincter inhibits the micturition reflex and prevents voiding.

Urethra

The urethra is a narrow tube lined with mucous membranes and epithelial cells. Its purpose is to eliminate urine from the bladder. The urethral meatus, or opening, is the endpoint of the urethra. In men, the urethra is about 6 to 8 inches (15 to 20 cm) long, with the meatus located at the tip of the penis. The male urethra has three sections:

- The prostatic urethra, which extends from the bladder to the prostate gland
- The membranous urethra, which extends to the wall of the pelvic floor
- The cavernous urethra, which is external and extends through the length of the penis

In women, the urethra is about 1 to 1.5 inches (2.5 to 3.75 cm) long and exits the bladder through the pelvic floor. The meatus lies slightly below the clitoris and directly in front of the vagina and rectum.

Kidney and Urinary System Changes Associated with Aging

Kidney Changes

Structural and functional changes occur in the kidney as a result of the aging process. These changes often affect health. The kidney loses cortical tissue and gets smaller by 80 years of age. This cortical loss is caused by reduced blood flow to the kidney. The medulla is not affected by aging, and the juxtamedullary nephron functions are preserved. However, the glomerular and tubular linings thicken. Both the number of glomeruli and their surface areas decrease with aging. Tubule length also decreases. These changes reduce the ability of the older adult to filter blood and excrete waste products.

Kidney size and function decrease with aging (Chart 68-1). Blood flow to the kidney declines by about 10% per decade as blood vessels thicken. This means that blood flow to the kidney is not as adaptive in older adults compared with younger adults, leaving nephrons more vulnerable to damage during episodes of either hypotension or hypertension.

Glomerular filtration rate (GFR) decreases with age, especially after 45 years of age. By age 65, the GFR is about 65 mL/min (half the rate of a young adult). This decline is more rapid in patients with diabetes, hypertension, or heart failure. As a result, the older patient is at greater risk for fluid overload. The combination of reduced kidney mass, reduced blood flow, and decreased GFR contributes to reduced drug clearance and a greater risk for drug reactions and kidney damage from drugs and contrast dyes in older adults.

Tubular changes with aging decrease the ability to concentrate urine, resulting in urgency (a sense of a nearly uncontrollable need to urinate) and nocturnal polyuria (increased urination at night). The regulation of sodium, acids, and bicarbonate remains effective but is less efficient. Along with an age-related impairment in the thirst mechanism, these changes increase the risk for dehydration and hypernatremia (increased blood sodium levels) in the older adult. Hormonal changes include a decrease in renin secretion, aldosterone levels, and activation of vitamin D.

CHART 68-1	NURSING FOCUS ON THE OLDER ADULT

Changes in the Renal/Urinary System Related to Aging

PHYSIOLOGIC CHANGE	NURSING INTERVENTIONS	RATIONALES
Decreased glomerular filtration rate (GFR)	Monitor hydration status. Ensure adequate fluid intake. Administer potentially nephrotoxic agents or drugs carefully.	With aging, the ability of the kidneys to regulate water balance is decreased. The kidneys are less able to conserve water when necessary. Dehydration results in decreased renal blood flow and increases the nephrotoxic potential of many agents. Acute or chronic kidney failure may result.
Nocturia	Ensure adequate nighttime lighting and a hazard-free environment. Ensure the availability of a toilet, bedpan, or urinal. Discourage excessive fluid intake for 2-4 hr before the patient retires for the evening. Evaluate drugs and timing.	Nocturia may occur from decreased renal concentrating ability associated with aging. The desire to maintain continence prompts people to seek the bathroom. Falls and injuries are common among older patients seeking bathroom facilities. Excessive fluid intake at night may increase nocturia. Some drugs increase urine output.
Decreased bladder capacity	Encourage the patient to use the toilet, bedpan, or urinal at least every 2 hr. Respond as soon as possible to the patient's indication of the need to void.	By emptying the bladder on a regular basis, urinary incontinence from overflow may be avoided. A quick response may alleviate episodes of urinary stress incontinence.
Weakened urinary sphincter muscles and shortened urethra in women	Provide thorough perineal care after each voiding.	The shortened urethra increases the potential for bladder infections. Good perineal hygiene may prevent skin irritations and urinary tract infection (UTI).
Tendency to retain urine	Observe the patient for urinary retention (e.g., bladder distention) or urinary tract infection (e.g., dysuria, foul odor, confusion). Provide privacy, assistance, and voiding stimulants such as warm water over the perineum as needed. Evaluate drugs for possible contribution to retention.	Urinary stasis may result in a UTI. UTIs may become bloodstream infections, resulting in urosepsis or septic shock. Nursing interventions can help initiate voiding. Anticholinergic drugs promote urinary retention.

Urinary Changes

Changes in the detrusor muscle elasticity lead to decreased bladder capacity and reduced ability to retain urine. The urge to void may cause immediate bladder emptying because the urinary sphincters lose tone and often become weaker with age. In women, weakened muscles shorten the urethra and promote incontinence. In men, an enlarged prostate gland makes starting the urine stream difficult and may cause urinary retention.

CULTURAL AWARENESS

African Americans have more rapid age-related decreases in GFR than do white people (Brenner, 2008). Kidney excretion of sodium is less effective in hypertensive African Americans who have high sodium intake, and the kidneys have about 20% less blood flow as a result of anatomic changes in small renal vessels and intrarenal responses to renin. Thus African-American patients are at greater risk for kidney failure than are white patients. Yearly health examinations should include urinalysis and checking for the presence of microalbuminuria.

ASSESSMENT METHODS

Patient History

One way to assess kidney and urologic function is to use Gordon's Functional Health Patterns (Gordon, 2011). The patterns most related to the renal system are Nutritional/Metabolic and Elimination (Chart 68-2).

Demographic information, such as age, gender, race, and ethnicity, is important to consider as nonmodifiable risk factors in the patient with any kidney or urinary problem. A sudden onset of hypertension in patients older than 50 years suggests possible kidney disease. Clinical changes with adult polycystic kidney disease typically occur in patients in their 40s or 50s. In men older than 50 years, altered urinary patterns accompany prostate disease.

Anatomic gender differences make some disorders worse or more common. For example, men rarely have urinary tract infections unless there are abnormalities, such as ureteral reflux or prostatic enlargement. Women have a shorter urethra and more commonly develop cystitis (bladder infection) because bacteria pass more readily into the bladder.

Ask the patient about any previous kidney or urologic problems, including tumors, infections, stones, or urologic surgery. A history of any chronic health problems, especially diabetes mellitus or hypertension, increases the risk for development of kidney disease because these disorders damage kidney blood vessels.

Ask the patient about chemical exposures at the workplace or with hobbies. Exposure to hydrocarbons (e.g., gasoline, oil), heavy metals (especially mercury and lead), and some gases (e.g., chlorine, toluene) can impair kidney function. Use this opportunity to teach patients who come into contact with chemicals at work or during leisure time activities to avoid direct skin or mucous membrane contact with these chemicals. Use of heroin, cocaine, methamphetamine, ecstasy,

---

CHART 68-2 RENAL/URINARY ASSESSMENT

Using Gordon's Functional Health Patterns

Nutritional/Metabolic Pattern

- What is your typical daily food intake? Describe a day's meals, snacks, and vitamins.
- How much salt do you typically add to your food? Do you use salt substitutes?
- How is your appetite?
- Have you experienced any nausea or vomiting?
- What is your typical daily fluid intake?
- What types of fluids do you drink (water, juices, soft drinks, coffee, tea)?
- How much fluid do you drink each day?
- Have you had any recent change in your weight? Weight gain? Weight loss? How much?
- Have you noticed a change in the tightness of your rings or shoes? Tighter? Looser?
- Have you noticed any skin changes lately? More dry? Less dry? Itchy?

Elimination Pattern

- What is your usual bowel elimination pattern? Frequency? Character? Discomfort? Laxatives?
- What is your usual urinary elimination pattern? Frequency? Amount? Color? Odor? Control?
- Have you noticed a change in the amount of urine?
- Do you have any problem with excessive perspiration?
- Do you have any other type of drainage?

Based on Gordon, M. (2011). *Manual of nursing diagnosis* (12th ed.). New York: Jones & Bartlett.

TABLE 68-3 COMMONLY USED RENAL AND URINARY TERMS

anuria Total urine output of less than 100 mL in 24 hours

azotemia Increased blood urea nitrogen and serum creatinine levels suggestive of kidney impairment but without outward symptoms of kidney failure

dysuria Discomfort or pain associated with micturition

frequency Feeling the need to void often, usually voiding small amounts of urine each time; may void every hour or even more frequently

hesitancy Difficulty in initiating the flow of urine, even when the bladder has sufficient urine to initiate a void and the sensation of the need to void is present

micturition The act of voiding

nocturia Awakening prematurely from sleep because of the need to empty the bladder

oliguria Decreased urine output; total urine output between 100 and 400 mL in 24 hours

polyuria Increased urine output; total urine output usually greater than 2000 mL in 24 hours

uremia Full-blown manifestations of kidney failure; sometimes referred to as the *uremic syndrome,* especially if the cause of the renal failure is unknown

urgency A sudden onset of the feeling of the need to void immediately; may result in incontinence if the patient is unable to get to toileting facilities quickly

---

and volatile solvents (inhalants) has also been associated with kidney damage.

Specifically ask the patient whether he or she has ever been told about the presence of protein or albumin in the urine. The question "Have you ever been told that your blood pressure is high?" may prompt a response different from the one to the question "Do you have high blood pressure?" Ask women about health problems during pregnancy (e.g., proteinuria, high blood pressure, gestational diabetes, urinary tract infections). Obtain information about:

- Chemical or environmental toxin exposure in occupational or other settings
- Recent travel to geographic regions that pose infectious disease risks
- Recent physical injuries
- Trauma
- Sexual contacts
- A history of altered patterns of urinary elimination

Socioeconomic status may influence health care practices. Prevention, early detection, and treatment of kidney or urinary problems may be limited by lack of insurance or access to health care, lack of transportation, and reduced income. Low income may also result in difficulty following medical advice, having prescriptions filled, and keeping follow-up appointments.

Educational level may affect health-seeking practices and the patient's understanding of a disease or its symptoms. Recurring urinary tract infections often result from inadequate or incomplete treatment, including lack of follow-up to ensure the infection is cleared. The lack of money to pay for antibiotics or nutritious foods may inhibit or delay recovery.

The patient's health beliefs affect the approach to health and illness. Cultural background or religious affiliation may influence the belief system.

The language used by patients may be different from that used by the health care professional. Anatomic or medical terms may have no meaning for the patient (Table 68-3). When obtaining a history, listen to and explore the terms used by the patient. By using the patient's own terms, you may help him or her provide a more complete description of the problem. This technique may increase the amount of information obtained and decrease the patient's discomfort when discussing bodily functions.

Nutrition History

Ask the patient with known or suspected kidney or urologic disorders about his or her usual diet and any recent changes in the diet. Note any excessive intake or omission of certain food categories. Ask about food and fluid intake. Assess how much and what types of fluids the patient drinks daily, especially fluids with a high calorie or caffeine content. Use this opportunity to teach the patient the importance of drinking about 3 L of fluid daily (if another medical problem does not require fluid restriction) to prevent dehydration and cystitis. If the patient has followed a diet for weight reduction, the details of the diet plan are important and collaboration with a dietitian may be needed. A high-protein intake can result in temporary kidney problems. For example, a patient at risk for calculi (stone) formation who ingests large amounts of protein or has a poor fluid intake may form new stones.

Ask about any change in appetite or in the ability to discriminate tastes. These symptoms can occur with the buildup of nitrogenous waste products from kidney failure. Changes in thirst or fluid intake may also cause changes in urine output. Endocrine disorders may also cause changes in thirst, fluid intake, and urine output (see Chapter 64 for a discussion of endocrine influences on fluid balance).

Medication History

Identify all of the patient's prescription drugs because many can impair kidney function. Ask about the duration of drug use and whether there have been any recent changes in prescribed drugs. Drugs for diabetes mellitus, hypertension, cardiac disorders, hormonal disorders, cancer, arthritis, and psychiatric disorders are potential causes of kidney dysfunction. Antibiotics, such as gentamicin (Garamycin, Cidomycin ✦), may also cause acute kidney injury. Drug-drug interactions and drug–contrast dye interactions also are potential causes of kidney dysfunction.

Explore the past and current use of over-the-counter (OTC) drugs or agents, including dietary supplements, vitamins and minerals, herbal agents, laxatives, analgesics, acetaminophen, and NSAIDs. Many of these agents affect kidney function. For example, dietary supplementation with synthetic creatine, used to increase muscle mass, has been associated with compromised kidney function. High-dose or long-term use of NSAIDs or acetaminophen can seriously reduce kidney function. Some agents are associated with hypertension, hematuria, or proteinuria, which may occur before kidney dysfunction.

Family History and Genetic Risk

The family history of the patient with a suspected kidney or urologic problem is important because some disorders have a familial inheritance pattern. Ask whether his or her siblings, parents, or grandparents have had kidney problems. Past terms used for kidney disease include *Bright's disease, nephritis,* and *nephrosis*. Patients may use these terms to describe kidney disease as it was known by their parents or grandparents years ago. Adult polycystic kidney disease can occur in either gender. Exposure to gadolinium-enhanced magnetic resonance imaging (MRI) can result in nephrogenic systemic fibrosis.

Current Health Problems

The effects of kidney failure result in changes in all body systems. Therefore document all of the patient's current health problems. Ask him or her to describe all health concerns, because some kidney disorders cause systemic problems or problems in other body systems. Recent upper respiratory problems, achy muscles or joints, chronic disease, or GI problems may be related to problems of kidney function.

Assess the kidney and urologic system specifically by asking about any changes in the appearance (color, odor, clarity) of the urine, pattern of urination, ability to initiate or control voiding, and other unusual symptoms. For example, urine that is reddish, dark brown or black, greenish, or different from the usual yellowish color usually prompts the patient to seek health care assistance. Urine typically has a mild but distinct odor of ammonia. An increase in the intensity of color, a change in odor quality, or a decrease in urine clarity may suggest infection.

Ask about changes in urination patterns, such as incontinence (involuntary bladder emptying), nocturia (urination at night), frequency, or an increase or decrease in the amount

of urine. The normal urine output for adults is about 1500 to 2000 mL/day, or within 500 mL of the volume of fluid ingested daily. Ask about how closely the urine output is to the volume of fluid ingested. The patient usually does not know the exact amount of urine produced. A bladder diary may provide useful data. Also ask whether:
- Initiating urine flow is difficult
- A burning sensation or other discomfort occurs with urination
- The force of the urine stream is decreased (in men)
- Persistent dribbling of urine is present

The onset of pain in the flank, in the lower abdomen or pelvic region, or in the perineal area triggers concern and usually prompts the patient to seek assistance. Ask about the onset, intensity, and duration of the pain, its location, and its association with any activity or event.

Pain associated with kidney or ureteral irritation is often severe and spasmodic. Pain that radiates into the perineal area, groin, scrotum, or labia is described as *renal colic*. This pain occurs with distention or spasm of the ureter, such as in an obstruction or the passing of a stone. Renal colic pain may be intermittent or continuous and may occur with pallor, diaphoresis, and hypotension. These general symptoms occur because of the location of the nerve tracts near or in the kidneys and ureters.

Because the kidneys are close to the GI organs and the nerve pathways are similar, GI manifestations may occur with kidney problems. These renointestinal reflexes often complicate the description of the kidney problem.

Uremia is the buildup of nitrogenous waste products in the blood as a result of kidney failure. Manifestations include anorexia, nausea and vomiting, muscle cramps, pruritus (itching), fatigue, and lethargy.

Physical Assessment

The physical assessment of the patient with a known or suspected kidney or urologic disorder includes general appearance, a review of body systems, and specific structure and functions of the kidney and urinary system.

Assess the patient's general appearance, and check the skin for the presence of any rashes, bruising, or yellowish discoloration. The skin and tissues may show edema, especially in the pedal (foot), pretibial (shin), and sacral tissues and around the eyes, which is associated with kidney disease. Use a stethoscope to listen to the lungs to determine whether fluid is present. Weigh the patient and measure blood pressure as a baseline for later comparisons.

Assess the level of consciousness and level of alertness. Record any deficits in memory, concentration, or thought processes. Family members may report subtle changes. Cognitive changes may be the result of the buildup of waste products when kidney disease is present.

Assessment of the Kidneys, Ureters, and Bladder

Assess the kidneys, ureters, and bladder during an abdominal assessment. Auscultate before percussion and palpation because these activities can enhance bowel sounds and obscure abdominal vascular sounds.

Inspect the abdomen and the flank regions with the patient in both the supine and the sitting positions. Observe the patient for asymmetry (e.g., swelling) or discoloration (e.g., bruising or redness) in the flank region, especially in the area

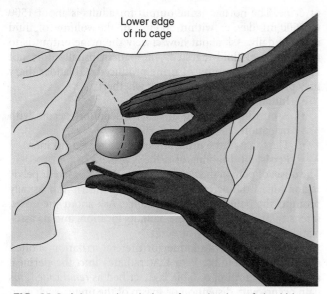

Lower edge of rib cage

FIG. 68-9 Advanced technique for palpation of the kidney.

of the costovertebral angle (CVA). The CVA is located between the lower portion of the twelfth rib and the vertebral column.

Listen for a bruit by placing a stethoscope over each renal artery on the midclavicular line. A **bruit** is an audible swishing sound produced when the volume of blood or the diameter of the blood vessel changes. It often occurs with blood flow through a narrowed vessel, as in renal artery stenosis.

Kidney palpation is usually performed by a physician or advanced practice nurse. It can help locate masses and areas of tenderness in or around the kidney. Lightly palpate the abdomen in all quadrants. Ask about areas of tenderness or pain, and examine nontender areas first. The outline of the bladder may be seen as high as the umbilicus in patients with severe bladder distention. *If tumor or aneurysm is suspected, palpation may harm the patient.*

Because the kidneys are located deep and posterior, palpation is easier in thin patients who have little abdominal musculature. For palpation of the right kidney, the patient is in a supine position while the examiner places one hand under the right flank and the other hand over the abdomen below the lower right part of the rib cage. The lower hand is used to raise the flank, and the upper hand depresses the abdomen as the patient takes a deep breath (Fig. 68-9). The left kidney is deeper and often cannot be palpated. A transplanted kidney is readily palpated in either the lower right or left abdominal quadrant. The normal kidney is smooth, firm, and nontender.

A distended bladder sounds dull when percussed. After gently palpating to determine the outline of the distended bladder, begin percussion on the lower abdomen and continue in the direction of the umbilicus until dull sounds are no longer produced. If you suspect bladder distention, use a portable bladder scanner to determine the amount of retained urine.

If the patient reports flank pain or tenderness, percuss the nontender flank first. Have the patient assume a sitting, side-lying, or supine position, and then form one of your hands into a clenched fist. Place your other hand flat over the CVA of the patient. Then quickly deliver a firm thump to your hand over the CVA area. Costovertebral tenderness often occurs with kidney infection or inflammation. Patients with inflammation or infection in the kidney or nearby structures may describe their pain as severe or as a constant, dull ache.

Assessment of the Urethra

Using a good light source and wearing gloves, inspect the urethra by examining the meatus and the tissues around it. Record any unusual discharge such as blood, mucus, or pus. Inspect the skin and mucous membranes of surrounding tissues. Record the presence of lesions, rashes, or other abnormalities of the penis or scrotum or of the labia or vaginal opening. Urethral irritation is suspected when the patient reports discomfort with urination. Use this opportunity to remind women to clean the perineum by wiping from front to back, never from back to front. Teach them that the front-to-back technique keeps organisms in stool from coming close to the urethra, which could increase the risk for infection.

Women from other cultures may have undergone female circumcision. This procedure alters the anatomic appearance of the vulvar-perineal area and increases the risk for urinary tract infections. It also makes urethral inspection or catheterization difficult. Document any noted anatomic changes and ask the patient to describe her hygiene practices for this area.

Psychosocial Assessment

Concerns about the urologic system may evoke fear, anger, embarrassment, anxiety, guilt, or sadness in the patient. Childhood learning often includes privacy with regard to toilet habits. Urologic disorders may bring up forgotten memories of difficult toilet training and bedwetting or of childhood experiences of exploring one's body. The patient may ignore symptoms or delay seeking health care because of emotional responses or cultural taboos about the urogenital area.

❓ NCLEX EXAMINATION CHALLENGE

Psychosocial Integrity

A 67-year-old client who had an abdominal x-ray as part of pre-admission testing for a gastrointestinal problem has just been told that he has a horseshoe-shaped kidney. He is very upset, telling the nurse that he has never had any health problems until the past month and now feels that he is "falling apart." What is the nurse's best response?
A. Remind him that it was lucky that he was being x-rayed anyway and that the problem was found at an early stage.
B. Reassure him that it is unlikely that the kidney shape is important since he has not had other kidney problems.
C. Ask him whether anyone else in his family has ever been diagnosed with a horseshoe-shaped kidney.
D. Reassure him that his health care provider will request a consultation with a kidney specialist.

Diagnostic Assessment
Laboratory Assessment

Blood Tests. Serum creatinine is produced when protein or muscle breaks down. Creatinine is filtered by the kidneys and excreted in the urine. Because muscle mass and protein breakdown are usually constant, the serum creatinine level is a good indicator of kidney function. Normal serum creatinine levels vary with age, gender, and body muscle mass.

LABORATORY PROFILE

Renal Function Blood Studies

TEST	NORMAL RANGE FOR ADULTS	SIGNIFICANCE OF ABNORMAL FINDINGS
Serum creatinine	*Males:* 0.6-1.2 mg/dL (53-106 mmol/L) *Females:* 0.5-1.1 mg/dL (44-97 mmol/L) *Older adults:* may be decreased	An *increased level* indicates kidney impairment. A *decreased level* may be caused by a decreased muscle mass.
Blood urea nitrogen (BUN)	10-20 mg/dL (3.6-7.1 mmol/L) *Older adults:* 60-90 yr: 8-23 mg/dL (2.9-8.2 mmol/L) Older than 90 yr: 10-31 mg/dL (3.6-11.1 mmol/L)	An *increased level* may indicate hepatic or renal disease, dehydration or decreased kidney perfusion, a high-protein diet, infection, stress, steroid use, GI bleeding, or other situations in which blood is in body tissues. A *decreased level* may indicate malnutrition, fluid volume excess, or severe hepatic damage.
BUN/creatinine ratio	Mass ratio: 12:1 to 20:1 Mole ratio: 48.5:1 to 80.8:1	An *increased ratio* may indicate fluid volume deficit, obstructive uropathy, catabolic state, or a high-protein diet. A *decreased ratio* may indicate fluid volume excess or acute renal tubular acidosis. *No change* in the ratio with increases in both the BUN and creatinine levels indicates renal impairment.

Data from Pagana, K.D., & Pagana, T.J. (2010). *Mosby's manual of diagnostic and laboratory tests* (4th ed.). St. Louis: Mosby.

Levels are slightly higher in men than in women because men tend to have a larger muscle mass than do women, but there are exceptions (Chart 68-3). Creatinine levels in bodybuilders tend to be higher than normal without reflecting a kidney function problem. Muscle mass and the amount of creatinine produced decrease with age. Because of decreased rates of creatinine clearance, however, the serum creatinine level remains relatively constant in older adults unless kidney disease is present.

No common pathologic condition other than kidney disease increases the serum creatinine level. The serum creatinine level does not increase until at least 50% of the kidney function is lost, and therefore *any* elevation of serum creatinine values is important and should be assessed further.

! NURSING SAFETY PRIORITY

Action Alert

An increase of serum creatinine 1.5 times above baseline or a decrease of urine output to <0.5 mL/kg/hr for 6 or more hours places a patient at risk for acute kidney injury. Monitor both baseline and trend values to determine risk for and actual kidney damage, especially among patients exposed to agents that can cause kidney dysfunction. Inform the health care provider of increased serum creatinine and decreased urine output values promptly.

Blood urea nitrogen (BUN) measures the kidney excretion of urea nitrogen, a by-product of protein breakdown in the liver. Urea nitrogen is produced mostly from liver metabolism of food sources of protein. The kidneys filter urea nitrogen from the blood and excrete the waste in urine. BUN levels indicate the extent of kidney clearance of this nitrogen waste product.

Other factors influence the BUN level, and an elevation does not always mean kidney disease is present (see Chart 68-3). For example, rapid cell destruction from infection, cancer treatment, or steroid therapy may elevate BUN level. In addition, blood is a protein. Blood in the tissues rather than in the blood vessels is reabsorbed as if it were a general protein. Thus reabsorbed blood protein is processed by the liver and increases BUN levels. This means that injured tissues can result in increased BUN levels even when kidney function is normal. Also, BUN is increased by protein turnover in exercising muscle and is elevated as a result of concentration during dehydration.

The liver must function properly to produce urea nitrogen. When liver and kidney dysfunction are present, urea nitrogen levels are actually *decreased* because the liver failure limits urea production. The BUN level is not always elevated with kidney disease and is not the best indicator of kidney function. However, an elevated BUN level is highly *suggestive* of kidney dysfunction.

Blood urea nitrogen to serum creatinine ratio can help determine whether non–kidney-related factors, such as low cardiac output or red blood cell destruction, are causing the elevated BUN level. When blood volume is deficient (e.g., dehydration) or cardiac output is low, the BUN level rises more rapidly than the serum creatinine level. As a result, the ratio of BUN to creatinine is *increased.*

When both the BUN and serum creatinine levels increase at the same rate, the BUN/creatinine ratio remains normal. However, the elevated serum creatinine and BUN levels suggest kidney dysfunction that is not related to dehydration or poor perfusion.

Blood osmolarity is a measure of the overall concentration of particles in the blood and is a good indicator of hydration status. The kidneys excrete or reabsorb water to keep blood osmolarity in the range of 285 to 295 mOsm/L. Osmolarity is slightly higher in older adults (285 to 301 mOsm/L). When blood osmolarity is decreased, the release of antidiuretic hormone (ADH) is inhibited. Without ADH, the distal tubule and collecting ducts are *not* permeable to water. As a result, water is *excreted,* not reabsorbed, and blood osmolarity increases. When blood osmolarity increases, ADH is released. ADH increases the permeability of the distal tubule to water. Then water is reabsorbed and blood osmolarity decreases.

Urine Tests

Urinalysis. Urinalysis is a part of any complete physical examination and is especially useful for patients with suspected kidney or urologic disorders (Chart 68-4). Ideally, the urine specimen is collected at the morning's first voiding. Specimens obtained at other times may be too dilute. The specimen may be collected by several techniques (Table 68-4).

Urine color comes from urochrome pigment. Color variations may result from increased levels of urochrome or other pigments, changes in the concentration or dilution of the urine, and the presence of drug metabolites in the urine. Urine smells faintly like ammonia and is normally clear without turbidity (cloudiness) or haziness.

CHART 68-4   LABORATORY PROFILE

Urinalysis

TEST	NORMAL RANGE FOR ADULTS	SIGNIFICANCE OF ABNORMAL FINDINGS
Color	Pale yellow	*Dark amber* indicates concentrated urine. *Very pale* yellow indicates dilute urine. *Dark red* or brown indicates blood in the urine. Brown also may indicate increased urinary bilirubin level. Red also may indicate the presence of myoglobin. *Other color* changes may result from diet or drugs.
Odor	Specific aroma, similar to ammonia	*Foul smell* indicates possible infection, dehydration, or ingestion of certain foods or drugs.
Turbidity	Clear	*Cloudy urine* indicates infection, sediment, or high levels of urinary protein.
Specific gravity	Usually 1.005-1.030; possible range 1.000-1.040 (after 12-hr fluid restriction, >1.025) *Older adult:* Decreased because of decreased concentrating ability	*Increased* in decreased kidney perfusion, inappropriate antidiuretic hormone secretion, or congestive heart failure. *Decreased* in chronic kidney disease, diabetes insipidus, malignant hypertension, diuretic administration, and lithium toxicity.
pH	Average: 6; possible range: 4.6-8	*Changes* are caused by diet, the administration of drugs, infection, freshness of the specimen, acid-base imbalance, and altered renal function.
Glucose	<0.5 g/day (<2.78 mmol/L)	*Presence* reflects hyperglycemia or a decrease in the renal threshold for glucose.
Ketones	None	*Presence* reflects incomplete metabolism of fatty acids, as in diabetic ketoacidosis, prolonged fasting, anorexia nervosa.
Protein	0.8 mg/dL	*Increased* amounts may indicate stress, infection, recent strenuous exercise, or glomerular disorders.
Bilirubin (urobilinogen)	None	*Presence* suggests liver or biliary disease or obstruction.
Red blood cells (RBCs)	0-2 per high-power field	*Increased* amounts are normal with indwelling or intermittent catheterization or menses but may reflect tumor, stones, trauma, glomerular disorders, cystitis, or bleeding disorders.
White blood cells (WBCs)	*Males:* 0-3 per high-power field *Females:* 0-5 per high-power field	*Increased* amounts may indicate an infectious or inflammatory process anywhere in the renal/urinary tract, renal transplant rejection, fever, or exercise.
Casts	A few or none, composed of RBC, WBC, protein, or tubular cell casts	*Increased* amounts indicate the presence of bacteria or protein, which is seen in severe kidney disease and could also indicate urinary calculi.
Crystals	None	*Presence* of normal or abnormal crystals may indicate that the specimen has been allowed to stand.
Bacteria	<1000 colonies/mL	*Increased* amounts indicate the need for urine culture to determine the presence of urinary tract infection.
Parasites	None	*Presence* of *Trichomonas vaginalis* indicates infection, usually of the urethra, prostate, or vagina.
Leukoesterase	None	*Presence* suggests urinary tract infection.
Nitrites	None	*Presence* suggests urinary *Escherichia coli.*

Specific gravity is the density of urine compared with water, which has a specific gravity of 1.000. Density is related to the number of particles in a specific volume of urine. The normal specific gravity of urine ranges from 1.005 to about 1.030. In kidney disease, changes in specific gravity do not reflect systemic fluid volume. For example, dilute urine with a low specific gravity may occur in a dehydrated patient who is deficient in antidiuretic hormone (ADH).

An *increase* in specific gravity occurs with dehydration, decreased kidney blood flow, or the presence of ADH. (ADH production is normally increased with stress, surgery, anesthetic agents, and certain drugs such as morphine and commonly used oral antidiabetic drugs.) In these situations, the normal kidney response is to reabsorb water and decrease urine output. As a result, the urine produced is more concentrated.

A *decrease* in specific gravity occurs with increased fluid intake, diuretic drugs, and diabetes insipidus. In these conditions, the normal kidney response is to excrete more water; thus urine output is increased. In kidney disease, the specific gravity decreases because the damaged kidneys reabsorb less water. The specific gravity does not vary with changes in plasma osmolarity (i.e., it becomes fixed).

pH is a measure of urine acidity or alkalinity. A pH value less than 7 is acidic, and a value greater than 7 is alkaline. Many factors influence urine acidity or alkalinity. A diet high in certain fruits and vegetables results in a more alkaline urine. A high-protein diet produces a more acidic urine. The presence of *Escherichia coli* in the urine also results in an acidic urine.

Urine specimens become more alkaline when left standing unrefrigerated for more than 1 hour, when bacteria are present, or when a specimen is left uncovered. Alkaline urine increases cell breakdown; thus the presence of red blood cells may be missed on analysis. Ensure that urine specimens are covered and delivered to the laboratory promptly or

TABLE 68-4 COLLECTION OF URINE SPECIMENS

NURSING INTERVENTIONS	RATIONALES
Voided Urine	
Collect the first specimen voided in the morning.	Urine is more concentrated in the early morning.
Send the specimen to the laboratory as soon as possible.	After urine is collected, cellular breakdown results in more alkaline urine.
Refrigerate the specimen if a delay is unavoidable.	Refrigeration delays the alkalinization of urine. Bacteria are more likely to multiply in an alkaline environment.
Clean-Catch Specimen	
Explain the purpose of the procedure to the patient.	Correct technique is needed to obtain a valid specimen.
Instruct the patient to self-clean before voiding:	Surface cleaning is necessary to remove secretions or bacteria from the urethral meatus.
Instruct the female patient to separate the labia and use the sponges and solution provided to wipe with three strokes over the urethra. The first two wiping strokes are over each side of the urethra; the third wiping stroke is centered over the urethra (from front to back).	
Instruct the male patient to retract the foreskin of the penis and to similarly clean the urethra, using three wiping strokes with the sponge and solution provided (from the head of the penis downward).	
Instruct the patient to initiate voiding after cleaning. The patient then stops and resumes voiding into the container. Only 1 ounce (30 mL) is needed; the remainder of the urine may be discarded into the commode.	A midstream collection further removes secretions and bacteria because urine flushes the distal portion of the internal urethra.
Ensure that the patient understands the procedure.	An improperly collected specimen may result in inappropriate or incomplete treatment.
Assist the patient as needed.	The patient's understanding and the nurse's assistance ensure proper collection.
Catheterized Specimen	
For non-indwelling (straight) catheters:	The one-time passage of a urinary catheter may be necessary to obtain an uncontaminated specimen for analysis or to measure the volume of residual urine.
Avoid routine use.	
Follow the facility's procedures for catheterization technique.	These procedures minimize bacterial entry.
For indwelling catheters:	Urine is collected from an indwelling catheter or tubing when patients have catheters for continence or long-term urinary drainage.
Apply a clamp to the drainage tubing, distal to the injection port.	Clamping allows urine to collect in the tubing at the location where the specimen is obtained.
Clean the injection port cap of the catheter drainage tubing with an appropriate antiseptic. Povidone-iodine solution or alcohol is acceptable.	Surface contamination is prevented by following the cleaning procedures.
Attach a sterile 5-mL syringe into the port and aspirate the quantity of urine required.	A minimum of 5 mL is needed for culture and sensitivity (C&S) testing.
Inject the urine sample into a sterile specimen container.	A sterile container is used for C&S specimens.
Remove the clamp to resume drainage.	
Properly dispose of the syringe.	
24-Hour Urine Collection	
Instruct the patient thoroughly.	A 24-hr collection of urine is necessary to quantify or calculate the rate of clearance of a particular substance.
Provide written materials to assist in instruction.	Instructional materials for patients, signs, etc. remind patients and staff to ensure that the total collection is completed.
Place signs appropriately.	
Inform all personnel or family caregivers of test in progress.	
Check laboratory or procedure manual on proper technique for maintaining the collection (e.g., on ice, in a refrigerator, or with a preservative).	Proper technique prevents breakdown of elements to be measured.
On initiation of the collection, ask the patient to void, discard the urine, and note the time. If a Foley catheter is in use, empty the tubing and drainage bag at the start time and discard the urine.	Proper techniques ensure that *all* urine formed within the 24-hr period is collected.
Collect all urine of the next 24 hr.	
Twenty-four hours after initiation, ask the patient to empty the bladder and add that urine to the container.	
Do not remove urine from the collection container for other specimens.	Urine in the container is not considered a "fresh" specimen and may be mixed with preservative.

refrigerated. During acidosis or alkalosis, the kidneys, along with blood buffers and the lungs, normally respond to keep serum pH normal. Chapter 14 discusses acid-base balance and imbalance.

Glucose is filtered by the glomerulus and is reabsorbed in the proximal tubule of the nephron. When the blood glucose level rises above 220 mg/dL, the renal threshold for reabsorption is exceeded and some glucose is present in the urine. Changes in the renal threshold for glucose occur in many patients, such as those with infection or those with long-standing diabetes mellitus. It is possible that their serum glucose level may be high (e.g., greater than 400 mg/dL) and glucose may still not be present in the urine. More often, these patients show glucose in the urine even when blood glucose levels are normal or only slightly elevated.

Ketone bodies are formed from the incomplete metabolism of fatty acids. Three types of ketone bodies are acetone, acetoacetic acid, and beta-hydroxybutyric acid. *Normally there are no ketones in urine.* Ketone bodies are produced when fat is used instead of glucose for cellular energy. Ketones present in the blood are partially excreted in the urine.

Protein, such as albumin, is not normally present in the urine. Levels greater than 300 mg/24 hr, or 200 mcg/min, are abnormal. Protein molecules are too large to pass through intact glomerular membranes. When glomerular membranes are not intact, protein molecules pass through and are excreted in the urine. Increased membrane permeability is caused by infection, inflammation, or immunologic problems. Some systemic problems cause production of abnormal proteins, such as globulin. These proteins are not detected by routine urinalysis and require electrophoresis or other tests for detection.

A random finding of proteinuria (protein in the urine) followed by a series of negative (normal) findings does not imply kidney disease. If infection is the cause of the proteinuria, urinalyses after elimination of the infection should be negative for protein. Persistent proteinuria needs further investigation.

Microalbuminuria is the presence of albumin in the urine that is not measurable by a urine dipstick or usual urinalysis procedures. Specialized assays are used to quickly analyze a freshly voided urine specimen for microscopic levels of albumin. The normal microalbumin levels in a freshly voided specimen should range between 2.0 and 20 mg/mmol for men and between 2.8 and 28 mg/mmol for women. Higher levels indicate microalbuminuria and could mean very early kidney disease, especially in patients with diabetes mellitus. In 24-hour urine specimens, levels of 30 to 300 mg/24 hr, or 20 to 200 mcg/min, indicate microalbuminuria.

Leukoesterase is an enzyme found in some white blood cells, especially neutrophils. When the number of these cells increases in the urine or they are broken *(lysed),* the urine then contains leukoesterase. The presence of leukoesterase and nitrites in the urine is a sensitive screen for assessing urinary tract infections. A normal reading is no leukoesterase in the urine. A positive test (+ sign) indicates increasing leukocytes in the urine.

Nitrites are not usually present in urine. Many types of bacteria, when present in the urine, convert nitrates (normally found in urine) into nitrites. A positive finding indicates urinary tract infection.

Sediment is precipitated particles in the urine. These particles include cells, casts, crystals, and bacteria. Normally, urine contains few, if any, cells. Types of cells abnormally present in the urine include tubular cells (from the tubule of the nephron), epithelial cells (from the lining of the urinary tract), red blood cells (RBCs), and white blood cells (WBCs).

Casts are structures formed around other particles. There may be casts of cells, bacteria, or protein. When cells, bacteria, or proteins are present in the urine, minerals and sticky materials clump around them and form a cast. Casts are described by the type of particle they have surrounded (e.g., RBC cast, WBC cast, tubular epithelial cast) or the stage of cast breakdown. Casts are described as "granular" (coarse or fine) and "waxy."

Urine crystals come from mineral salts as a result of diet, drugs, or disease. Common salt crystals are formed from calcium, oxalate, urea, phosphate, magnesium, or other substances. Some drugs, such as the sulfates, can also form crystals.

Bacteria multiply quickly, so the urine specimen must be analyzed promptly to avoid falsely elevated counts of bacterial colonization. Normally urine is sterile, but it is easily contaminated by perineal bacteria during collection.

Recent advances in technology and molecular biology are leading to new diagnostic tests using urine, including identification of biomarkers of disease and profiling for specific proteins. Markers are being used in investigation to identify early-onset kidney dysfunction, target therapy, and predict responsiveness to intervention. Markers for angiogenesis and kidney cell adhesion, regulation, and apoptosis will likely contribute to clinical diagnostics in the future.

Urine for Culture and Sensitivity. Urine is analyzed for the number and types of organisms present. Manifestations of infection and unexplained bacteria in a urine specimen are indications for urine culture and sensitivity testing. Bacteria from urine are placed in a medium with different antibiotics. In this way, we can know which antibiotics are effective in killing or stopping the growth of the organisms (organisms are "sensitive") and which are not effective (organisms are "resistant"). A clean-catch or catheter-derived specimen is best for culture and sensitivity testing.

Composite Urine Collections. Some urine collections are made for a specified number of hours (e.g., 24 hours) for more precise analysis of one or more substances. These collections are often used to measure urine levels of creatinine or urea nitrogen, sodium, chloride, calcium, catecholamines, or other components (Chart 68-5). For a composite urine specimen, *all* urine within the designated time frame must be collected (see Table 68-4). If other urine must be obtained while the collection is in progress, measure and record the amount collected but not added to the timed collection.

The urine collection may need to be refrigerated or stored on ice to prevent changes in the urine during the collection time. Follow the procedure from the laboratory for urine storage. The urine collection must be free from fecal contamination. Menstrual blood and toilet tissue also contaminate the specimen and can invalidate the results.

The collection of urine for a 24-hour period is often more difficult than it seems. With hospitalized patients, the cooperation of staff personnel, the patient, family members, and visitors is essential. Placing signs in the bathroom, instructing

CHART 68-5   LABORATORY PROFILE

24-Hour Urine Collections

COMPONENT	NORMAL RANGE FOR ADULTS	SIGNIFICANCE OF ABNORMAL FINDINGS
Creatinine	0.8-2 g/24 hr *Males:* 1-2 g/24 hr or 14-26 mg/kg/24 hr (124-230 μmol/kg/24 hr or 7.1-17.7 mmol/24 hr) *Females:* 0.6-1.8 g/24 hr or 11-20 mg/kg/24 hr (97-177 μmol/kg/24 hr or 5.3-15.9 mmol/24 hr) *Older adults:* 10 mg/kg/24 hr (88.4 μmol/kg/24 hr) at 90 yr	*Decreased amounts* indicate a deterioration in kidney function caused by kidney disease. *Increased amounts* occur with infections, exercise, diabetes mellitus, and meat meals.
Urea nitrogen	12-20 g/24 hr (0.43-0.71 mmol/24 hr)	*Decreased amounts* occur when kidney damage or liver disease is present. *Increased amounts* commonly result from a high-protein diet, dehydration, trauma, or sepsis.
Sodium	40-220 mEq/24 hr (40-220 mmol/24 hr)	*Decreased amounts* are seen in hemorrhage, shock, hyperaldosteronism, and prerenal acute kidney injury. *Increased amounts* are common with diuretic therapy, excessive salt intake, hypokalemia, and acute tubular necrosis.
Chloride	110-250 mEq/24 hr (110-250 mmol/24 hr) *Older adults:* 95-195 mEq/24 hr (95-195 mmol/24 hr)	*Decreased amounts* are seen in certain kidney diseases, malabsorption syndrome, pyloric obstruction, prolonged nasogastric tube drainage, diarrhea, diaphoresis, heart failure, and emphysema. *Increased amounts* are seen with hypokalemia, adrenal insufficiency, and massive diuresis.
Calcium	100-400 mg/24 hr (2.50-7.50 mmol/kg/24 hr)	*Decreased amounts* are often associated with hypocalcemia, hypoparathyroidism, nephrosis, and nephritis. *Increased amounts* are commonly seen with calcium kidney stones, hyperparathyroidism, sarcoidosis, certain cancers, immobilization, and hypercalcemia.
Total catecholamines*	<100 mcg/24 hr (<591 mmol/24 hr)	*Increased amounts* occur with pheochromocytoma, neuroblastomas, stress, or strenuous exercise.
Protein	1-14 mg/dL (10-140 mg/L) or 50-80 mg/24 hr at rest	*Increased amounts* indicate glomerular disease, nephrotic syndrome, diabetic nephropathy, urinary tract malignancies, and irritations.

*Epinephrine and norepinephrine only; dopamine is not measured.

the patient and family, and emphasizing the need to save the urine are helpful.

Creatinine Clearance. Creatinine clearance is a calculated measure of glomerular filtration rate. It is the best indication of overall kidney function. The amount of creatinine cleared from the blood (e.g., filtered into the urine) is measured in the total volume of urine excreted in a defined period. The optimal calculation for glomerular filtration rate (GFR) is based on a 24-hour urine collection, but urine can be collected for shorter periods (e.g., 8 or 12 hours). The analysis compares the urine creatinine level with the blood creatinine level, and therefore a blood specimen for creatinine must also be collected.

The laboratory or care provider calculates the creatinine clearance. The patient's age, gender, height, weight, diet, and activity level influence the expected amount of creatinine to be excreted. Thus these factors are considered when interpreting creatinine clearance test results. Although creatinine clearance can be calculated based on age, weight, serum creatinine, and other non-urine measures, a 24-hour collection and direct measurement is preferred for patients with high risk for or actual kidney dysfunction.

The rate of creatinine clearance is expressed as milliliters per minute per square meter of body surface area. The range for normal creatinine clearance is 90 to 139 mL/min/m^2 for men and 80 to 125 mL/min/m^2 for women.

Creatinine clearance values are used to determine the patient's current kidney function. Decreases in the creatinine clearance rate may require reducing drug doses and often signifies the need to further explore the cause of kidney deterioration.

Urine Electrolytes. Urine samples can be analyzed for electrolyte levels (e.g., sodium, chloride). Normally the amount of sodium excreted in the urine is nearly equal to that consumed. Urine sodium levels of less than 10 mEq/L indicate that the tubules are able to conserve (reabsorb) sodium.

Urine Osmolarity. Osmolarity measures the concentration of particles in solution. The particles in urine contributing to osmolarity include electrolytes, glucose, urea, and creatinine. Urine osmolarity can vary from 50 to 1400 mOsm/L, depending on the patient's hydration status and kidney function. With average fluid intake, the range for urine osmolarity is 300 to 900 mOsm/L. Electrolytes, acids, and other wastes of normal metabolism are continually produced. These particles are the solute load that must be excreted in the urine on a regular basis. This is referred to as *obligatory solute excretion.* If the patient loses excessive fluids, the kidney response is to save water while excreting wastes by excreting small amounts of highly concentrated urine. Diet, drugs, and activity can change urine osmolarity. Thus urine with an increased osmolarity is concentrated urine with less water and more

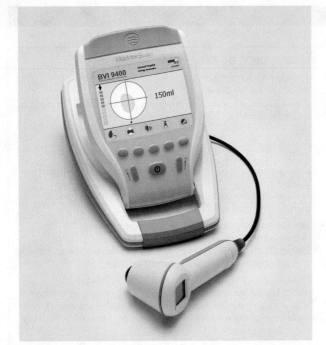

FIG. 68-10 The "BladderScan" BVI 9400, a handheld portable bladder scanner.

solutes. Urine with a decreased osmolarity is dilute urine with more water and fewer solutes.

? NCLEX EXAMINATION CHALLENGE

Physiological Integrity

A client's urinalysis shows all of the following results. Which result does the nurse report to the health care provider?
A. pH 5.8
B. Osmolarity 450
C. Nitrites present
D. Sodium 5 mEq/L

Bedside Sonography/Bladder Scanners. The use of portable ultrasound scanners in the hospital and rehabilitation setting by nurses is a noninvasive method of estimating bladder volume (Fig. 68-10). Bladder scanners are used to screen for post-void residual volumes and to determine the need for intermittent catheterization based on the amount of urine in the bladder rather than the time between catheterizations. There is no discomfort with the scan, and no patient preparation beyond an explanation of what to expect is required.

Explain why the procedure is being done and what sensations the patient might experience during the procedure. For example, "This test will measure the amount of urine in your bladder. I will place a gel pad just above your pubic area and then place the probe, which is a little bigger and heavier than a stethoscope, on the gel."

Before scanning, select the male or female icon on the bladder scanner. Using the female icon allows the scanner software to subtract the volume of the uterus from any measurement. Use the male icon on all men and on women who have undergone a hysterectomy.

Place an ultrasound gel pad right above the symphysis pubis (pubic bone), or moisten the round dome of the scan head area with 5 mL of conducting gel to improve ultrasound conduction. Use gel on the scanner head for obese patients and those with heavy body hair in the area to be scanned. Place the probe midline over the abdomen about 1.5 inches (4 cm) above the pubic bone. Aim the scan head so the ultrasound is projected toward the expected location of the bladder, typically toward the patient's coccyx. Press and release the scan button. The scan is complete with the sound of a beep, and a volume is displayed. Two readings are recommended for best accuracy. An aiming icon on the portable bladder scanner indicates whether the bladder image is centered on the crosshairs of the scan head. If the crosshairs on the aiming icon are not centered on the bladder, the measured volume may not be accurate.

Imaging Assessment

Many imaging procedures are used to diagnose abnormalities within the urinary system (Table 68-5). Explain the procedures thoroughly to the patient, prepare him or her, and provide follow-up care. Patient education materials for many urologic tests have been developed by professional organizations such as the Society for Urologic Nurses and Associates (www.suna.org/for patients) and are freely available.

Kidney, Ureter, and Bladder X-rays. An x-ray of the kidneys, ureters, and bladder (KUB) is a plain film of the abdomen obtained without any specific patient preparation. The KUB study shows gross anatomic features and obvious stones, strictures, calcifications, or obstructions in the urinary tract. This test identifies the shape, size, and relationship of the organs to other parts of the urinary tract. Other tests are needed to diagnose functional or structural problems.

There is no discomfort or risk from this procedure. Tell the patient that the x-ray will be taken while he or she is in a supine position. No specific follow-up care is needed.

Intravenous Urography. Other names for IV urography include *excretory urography* and (the older term) *IV pyelography (IVP)*.

Patient Preparation. Before urography, assess the patient (Chart 68-6) and explain the need for a bowel preparation. Report allergy information to the physician. Contrast reactions can be minor (nausea and vomiting, urticaria, itching, sneezing), moderate (nephrotoxic effects, congestive heart failure, pulmonary edema), or severe (bronchospasm, anaphylaxis). If the diagnostic test must be performed in a patient with a minor allergy to the contrast dye, drugs such as a steroid (prednisone or methylprednisolone) and an antihistamine (diphenhydramine hydrochloride [Benadryl, Allerdryl ✦]) are prescribed before the procedure to reduce the risk for an allergic response. Explain the rationale for the procedure to the patient.

Some preparations may be needed to ensure that urinary structures are not obscured by bowel contents. Some radiologists recommend a light evening meal or clear liquids and then fasting (NPO status) from midnight on the night before the procedure. Others recommend increased fluid intake to prevent dehydration up until the time of the procedure. Because some patients may vomit as a reaction to the IV contrast, some physicians prefer the patient to remain on NPO status for a few hours before the procedure. Hydration with IV fluids may be prescribed.

A bowel preparation is prescribed to remove fecal contents, fluid, and air from the gut, any of which could obscure part of the outline of the kidneys, ureters, and bladder. Bowel

TABLE 68-5   COMMON RADIOLOGIC AND SPECIAL DIAGNOSTIC TESTS FOR PATIENTS WITH DISORDERS OF THE KIDNEY AND URINARY SYSTEM

TEST	PURPOSE	COMMENTS
Radiography of kidneys, ureters, and bladder (KUB) (plain film of abdomen)	To screen for the presence of two kidneys To measure kidney size To detect gross obstruction	
Excretory urography	To measure kidney size To detect obstruction To assess parenchymal mass	Radiopaque contrast medium may cause an allergic (hypersensitivity) reaction in iodine-sensitive patients. Contrast agent is also hypertonic and increases the risk for acute kidney injury in adults with serum creatinine levels greater than 1.5 mg/dL. Nephrotoxic complications can be prevented by parenteral fluid administration.
Nephrotomography	To assess various planes of kidney tissue for cysts, tumors, or calculi	Same as for excretory urography.
Computed tomography (CT)	To measure kidney size To evaluate contour to assess for masses or obstruction	Contrast medium may provoke acute kidney injury. See comments with excretory urography for high-risk patients and preventive measures related to contrast. May be performed without contrast medium and still obtain adequate visualization.
Cystography and cystoscopy	To identify abnormalities of the bladder wall and urethral and ureteral occlusions To treat small obstructions or lesions via fulguration, lithotripsy, or removal with a stone basket	Instrumentation of the urinary tract increases the risk for infection. Monitor for infection for 48-72 hr after the procedure.
Voiding cystourethrography (VCUG)	To outline bladder's contour and detect urinary reflux from vesicourethral junctions	The risk for infection is similar to that in cystography because urinary catheterization is necessary. Monitor for postprocedure infection.
Ultrasonography (US)	To identify the size of the kidneys or obstruction in the kidneys or the lower urinary tract May detect tumors or cysts	Ultrasonography entails minimal risk to the patient. Ultrasonography is a good alternative to excretory urography.
MAG3 study 99m	To assess kidney function, structural abnormalities, kidney injury or impairment, obstruction, and kidney stones	Radioactive material (technetium Tc mertiatide) is used for this test.
Intravenous pyelography (IVP) (fluoroscopy)	To assess kidney function, identify anomalies To image kidney/urinary stones (size, location, radiodensity) To screen for kidney injury after trauma	Contraindicated during pregnancy (ionizing radiation is a risk to the fetus). Contrast dye can cause renal dysfunction. Colonic cleaning improves quality of image.
Magnetic resonance imaging (MRI)	Staging of cancers, similar to CT	Patient must be able to lie still (motion can interfere with imaging).
Renal scan	Evaluation of kidney blood flow Estimation of glomerular filtration rate Provides functional information without exposing the patient to iodinated contrast dye	ACE inhibitors should be held for 48 hours before the test. ACE inhibitors may be given during the test, placing the patient at risk for episodes of hypotension. Ensure adequate hydration for best results.

ACE, Angiotensin-converting enzyme.

preparation procedures vary but usually include the use of laxatives the day before the procedure. Enemas also may be prescribed, but their use is controversial because some air and fluid can be retained.

CONSIDERATIONS FOR OLDER ADULTS

Bowel preparation procedures increase the risk for dehydration, especially in older adult patients. To help prevent dehydration, contact the testing department and ask that urograms be scheduled early in the day for older patients.

The contrast dye is potentially kidney-damaging (nephrotoxic). The risk for *contrast-induced kidney failure* is greatest in patients who are older or dehydrated, who have some renal insufficiency (e.g., serum creatinine levels greater than 1.5 mg/dL), or who are also taking other nephrotoxic drugs.

In addition, patients taking metformin are at risk for lactic acidosis when they receive iodinated contrast media. Metformin should be discontinued 24 hours before the time of a procedure and for at least 48 hours after the procedure. Kidney function should be re-evaluated before the patient resumes metformin therapy.

All patients at risk for contrast-induced nephrotoxicity need additional IV fluids before the procedure to maintain hydration and decrease the risk for kidney damage. Acetylcysteine (an antioxidant) may be used to prevent contrast-induced nephrotoxic effects in radiologic procedures, although its benefits have not been proven. Diuretics may be given immediately after the dye is injected to enhance dye excretion in patients who are well hydrated.

Instruct the patient in the preparation procedures for the urogram, and explain the procedure so that he or she knows

CHART 68-6   BEST PRACTICE FOR PATIENT SAFETY & QUALITY CARE

Assessing the Patient About to Undergo a Diagnostic Test or Interventional Procedure Using Contrast Medium

Before the procedure:
- Ask the patient if he or she has ever had a reaction to contrast media. (Such a patient has the highest risk for having another reaction.)
- Ask the patient about a history of asthma. (Patients with asthma have been shown to be at greater risk for contrast reactions than the general public. When reactions do occur, they are more likely to be severe.)
- Ask the patient about known hay fever or food or drug allergies, especially to seafood, eggs, milk, or chocolate. (Contrast reactions have been reported to be as high as 15% in these patients.)
- Ask the patient to describe any specific allergic reactions (e.g., hives, facial edema, difficulty breathing, bronchospasm).
- Assess for a history of kidney impairment and for conditions that have been implicated in increasing the chance of developing kidney failure after contrast media (e.g., diabetic nephropathy, class IV heart failure, dehydration, concomitant use of potentially nephrotoxic drugs such as the aminoglycosides or NSAIDs, and cirrhosis).
- Ask the patient if he or she is taking metformin (Glucophage). (Metformin must be discontinued at least 24 hours before any study using contrast media because the life-threatening complication of lactic acidosis, although rare, could occur.)
- Assess hydration status by checking blood pressure, heart and respiratory rates, mucous membranes, skin turgor, and urine concentration.
- Ask the patient when he or she last ate or drank anything.

From Cohan, R.H., & Ellis, J.H. (1997). Iodinated contrast material in uroradiology: Choice of agent and management of complications. *Urologic Clinics of North America, 24*(3), 471-491.

! NURSING SAFETY PRIORITY

Drug Alert

Ensure that the patient who is prescribed metformin does not receive the drug after a procedure requiring IV contrast material until adequate kidney function has been determined.

---

what to expect (Chart 68-7). Intervene on behalf of the patient to ensure that questions are answered *before* the procedure.

Procedure. The dye is injected IV with the patient in a supine position. As blood (with the dye) rapidly circulates into the kidney blood vessels and is filtered by the glomeruli, the dye is excreted in the urine. A series of x-rays are taken at various times after injection. Nephrotomograms may be taken at the same time as the urogram. Tomograms take images of different planes of tissue and show any abnormalities present at varying depths. The technologist then asks the patient to empty the bladder and return for a few more x-rays. An outline of the kidneys, ureters, and bladder results as urine containing the dye is excreted.

The urogram provides information about:
- The number, size, shape, and location of the kidneys
- The adequacy of filling and the rate of excretion of contrast medium

CHART 68-7   PATIENT AND FAMILY EDUCATION: PREPARING FOR SELF-MANAGEMENT

Excretory Urogram

- The urogram outlines your urinary tract and helps determine any problems there.
- Notify your nurse or physician if you have had any reactions (allergic or otherwise) to any food or drugs, especially shellfish (e.g., shrimp, scallops, crab, lobster) or iodine, or to x-ray "dyes" such as contrast media; if you have a history of asthma; or if you are taking metformin (Glucophage) or Glucovance.
- The day before the test, follow the instructions about changes in your diet and fluid intake to be sure that as much information as possible is gained from the test.
- After you start the bowel preparation, you may need to be close to toileting facilities. The preparation drugs usually work quickly.
- You will be lying on an x-ray table with the x-ray machine above you for most of the procedure.
- A pressure band, similar to a large blood pressure cuff, may be placed around your stomach or abdomen to help obtain better x-rays.
- If you do not already have an IV access site, one will be started to give you the contrast agent.
- After the contrast is injected, you may feel a sense of warmth or heat as it travels throughout your body. You also may have a taste in your mouth that is sometimes described as metallic. These sensations last only a few seconds or minutes.
- When the pressure band is inflated, you may feel some tightness around your abdomen. The sensation is similar to the feeling on your arm when you have your blood pressure taken.
- A series of x-rays will be taken. You may be asked to empty your bladder and return to the table for more films. You also may be asked to have a standing film taken.
- After the test is completed, you are usually able to resume your normal activities and diet.
- You will not notice any change in the color or characteristics of your urine.
- Please do not hesitate to ask your nurse, physician, or x-ray technologist any question, no matter how slight the question may seem to you. It is important that you have as much understanding as possible.

- The number, size, location, appearance, and patency of the calices, pelves, and ureters
- The size, location, and nature of the urinary bladder

Follow-up Care. After the urogram, monitor the patient for altered kidney function and other effects from the dye. Ensure adequate hydration by urging the patient to take oral fluid or by giving IV fluids. Hydration reduces the risk for kidney damage. Monitor blood creatinine levels to assess ongoing kidney function.

Computed Tomography. Inform the patient that a computed tomography (CT) scan provides three-dimensional information about the kidneys, ureters, bladder, and surrounding tissues. The CT scan is performed in a special room, usually in the radiology department. It is usually performed after other diagnostic procedures and can provide information about tumors, cysts, abscesses, other masses, and obstruction. CT can also be used to image the kidney's vascular system (i.e., CT angiography). Some hospitals require patients having CT scans to be NPO for some period before the scan, although there is no specific evidence guiding this practice.

Determine whether the scan requires administration of a dye. Oral or injected contrast dye is usually given before starting the imaging procedure. Dye use may be omitted in patients at risk for contrast–induced acute kidney injury (AKI), but the images produced are less distinct.

When a dye is used, the follow-up care is the same as for IV urography. When no contrast or dye is used, there is no special postprocedural care.

Cystography and Cystourethrography. Explain the procedure to the patient. A urinary catheter is temporarily needed to instill contrast dye. The dye is needed to enhance x-ray visibility of the lower urinary tract.

In both cystography and cystourethrography, dye is instilled into the bladder via a urethral catheter. After bladder filling, x-rays are taken from the front, back, and side positions. For the voiding cystourethrogram (VCUG), the patient is requested to void and x-rays are taken during the voiding. A VCUG is obtained to determine whether urine refluxes into the ureter. The cystogram is often used in cases of trauma when urethral or bladder injury is suspected.

Monitor for infection as a result of catheter placement. In this test, the dye is not nephrotoxic because it does not enter the bloodstream and does not reach the kidney. Encourage fluid intake to dilute the urine and reduce the burning sensation from catheter irritation after removal. Monitor for changes in urine output because pelvic or urethral trauma may be present.

Renography (Kidney Scan). Explain that a kidney scan is performed to provide general information about blood flow to and in the kidneys. A small amount of radioactive material, a radionuclide, is used. Reassure the patient that there is no danger from the small amount of radioactive material present in the agent. Radionucleotides are not associated with nephrotoxicity.

For a kidney scan, the radionuclide is injected IV. After injection, the agent is absorbed into kidney tissue and gives off low-level radioactive emissions (scintillations). The amount of emission is measured by a scintillation counter. A special camera records the emissions and produces an image. At the same time, the rate and location of the emissions are recorded by computer and information about blood flow, or glomerular filtration, is provided.

In some cases, captopril (Capoten), an antihypertensive drug, is given at the start of the procedure to change blood flow in the kidney. This procedure is a "captopril renal scan." The drug can cause severe hypotension during and after the procedure.

When the patient can urinate, urination into a commode does not place anyone at risk from the small amount of radioactive material excreted. If he or she is incontinent, change the bed linens promptly and wear gloves for Standard Precautions. If captopril was used during the procedure, assess the patient's blood pressure frequently. Warn him or her to avoid rapid position changes and about the risk for falling as a result of orthostatic (positional) hypotension.

Ultrasonography. Inform the patient that ultrasonography does not cause discomfort and is without risk. This test usually requires a full bladder. Ask the patient to drink water, if needed, to help fill the bladder. This test applies sound waves to structures of different densities to produce images of the kidneys, ureters, and bladder and surrounding tissues. Ultrasonography allows assessment of kidney size, cortical thickness, and status of the calices. The test can identify obstruction in the urinary tract, tumors, cysts, and other masses without the use of contrast dye.

The patient undergoing kidney ultrasound is usually placed in the prone position. Sonographic gel is applied to the skin over the back and flank areas to enhance sound-wave conduction. A transducer in contact with and moving across the skin delivers sound waves and measures the echoes. Images of the internal structures are produced. Skin care to remove the gel is all that is needed after ultrasonography.

Renal Arteriography (Angiography). Renal arteriography allows dye to enter the renal blood vessels and generates images to determine blood vessel size and abnormalities. This test has largely been replaced by other imaging techniques (e.g., nuclear renal scans, ultrasonography, computed tomography) and is seldom used as a stand-alone diagnostic procedure. The most common use of renal arteriography is at the time of a renal angioplasty or other intervention.

Cystoscopy and Cystourethroscopy

Patient Preparation. Cystoscopy and cystourethroscopy are operative procedures and require completion of a preoperative checklist and a signed informed consent statement. The physician provides a complete description of and reasons for the procedure, and the nurse reinforces this information. Cystoscopy may be performed for diagnosis or treatment. This test is used to examine for bladder trauma (cystoscopy) or urethral trauma (cystourethroscopy) and to identify causes of urinary tract obstruction. Cystoscopy may be used to remove bladder tumors or an enlarged prostate gland.

Cystoscopy may be performed under general or local anesthesia with sedation. The patient's age and general health and the expected duration of the procedure are considered in the decision about anesthesia. A light evening meal may be eaten. Usually the patient is NPO after midnight on the night before the cystoscopy. A bowel preparation with laxatives or enemas is performed the evening before the procedure.

Procedure. The cystoscopy is performed in a designated cystoscopic examination room. If the procedure is performed in a surgical suite under general anesthesia, the usual surgical support personnel are present (see Chapter 17). This procedure is often performed in clinics, ambulatory surgery or short-procedure units, or urologist's office.

Assist the patient onto a table, and after sedation, place him or her in the lithotomy position. After the anesthesia is given and the area cleansed and draped, the urologist inserts a cystoscope through the urethra into the urinary bladder. This examination commonly includes the use of both the cystoscope and the urethroscope.

Follow-up Care. After this procedure with general anesthesia, the patient is returned to a postanesthesia care unit (PACU) or area. If local anesthesia and sedation were used, he or she may be returned directly to the hospital room. Patients undergoing cystoscopic examinations as outpatients are transferred to an area for monitoring before discharge to home. Monitor for airway patency and breathing, changes in vital signs (including temperature), and changes in urine output. Also observe for the complications of bleeding and infection.

A catheter may or may not be present after cystoscopy. The patient without a catheter has urinary frequency as a result of irritation from the procedure. The urine may be pink tinged, but gross bleeding is not expected. Bleeding or the presence of clots may obstruct the catheter and decrease urine output. Monitor urine output, and notify the physician of obvious blood clots or a decreased or absent urine output. Irrigate the Foley catheter with sterile saline, if prescribed. Notify the physician if the patient has a fever (with or without chills) or an elevated white blood cell (WBC) count, which suggests infection. Urge the patient to take oral fluids to increase urine output (which helps prevent clotting) and to reduce the burning sensation on urination.

Retrograde Procedures. Retrograde means going against the normal flow of urine. A retrograde examination of the ureters and pelves (*pyelogram*), the bladder (*cystogram*), and the urethra (*urethrogram*) involves instilling dye into the lower urinary tract. Because the dye is instilled directly to obtain an outline of the structures desired, the dye does not enter the bloodstream. Therefore the patient is not at risk for dye-induced acute kidney injury or a systemic allergic response.

The patient is prepared for retrograde procedures (retrograde pyelography, retrograde cystography, and retrograde urethrography) in the same way as for cystoscopy. Retrograde x-rays are obtained during the cystoscopy. After placement of the cystoscope by the urologist, catheters are placed into each ureter and contrast dye is instilled into each ureter and renal pelvis. The catheters are removed by the urologist, and x-rays are taken to outline these structures as the dye is excreted. The procedure identifies obstruction or structural abnormalities.

For patients undergoing retrograde cystoscopy or urethrography, contrast dye is instilled similarly into the bladder or urethra. Cystography and urethrography identify structural problems, such as fistulas, diverticula, and tumors.

After retrograde procedures, monitor the patient for infection caused by placing instruments in the urinary tract. Because these procedures are performed during cystoscopic examination, follow-up care is the same as that for cystoscopy.

Other Diagnostic Assessments

Urodynamic Studies. Urodynamic studies examine the processes of voiding and include:
- Tests of bladder capacity, pressure, and tone
- Studies of urethral pressure and urine flow
- Tests of perineal voluntary muscle function

These tests are often used along with voiding urographic or cystoscopic procedures to evaluate problems with urine flow.

Cystometrography (CMG) can determine how well the bladder wall (detrusor) muscle functions and how sensitive it is to stretching as the bladder fills. This test provides information about bladder capacity, bladder pressure, and voiding reflexes.

Explain the procedure, and inform the patient that a urinary catheter may be needed temporarily during the procedure. Ask the patient to void normally. Record the amount, rate of flow, and time of voiding. Insert a urinary catheter to measure the residual urine volume. The cystometer is attached to the catheter, and fluid is instilled via the catheter into the bladder. The point at which the patient first notes a feeling of the urge to void and the point at which he or she notes a strong urge to void are recorded. Bladder capacity and bladder pressure readings are recorded graphically. The patient is asked to void when the bladder instillation is complete (about

500 mL). The residual urine after voiding is recorded, and the catheter is removed. Electromyography of the perineal muscles may be performed during this examination.

For any procedure that involves inserting instruments into the urinary tract, monitor for infection. Record the patient's temperature, the character of the urine, and urine output volume.

Urethral pressure profile (also called a *urethral pressure profilometry [UPP]*) can provide information about the nature of urinary incontinence or urinary retention.

Explain the procedure, and inform the patient that a urinary catheter may be needed temporarily during the procedure. A special catheter with pressure-sensing capabilities is inserted into the bladder. Variations in the pressure of the smooth muscle of the urethra are recorded as the catheter is slowly withdrawn.

As with any study involving inserting instruments into the urinary tract, monitor the patient for manifestations of infection.

Urine stream testing is used to evaluate pelvic muscle strength and the effectiveness of pelvic muscles in stopping the flow of urine. It is useful in assessing urinary incontinence.

Explain the procedure, and reassure the patient that efforts will be made to ensure privacy. The patient is asked to begin urinating. Three to five seconds after urination begins, the examiner gives the patient a signal to stop urine flow. The length of time required to stop the flow of urine is recorded.

Cleaning the perineal area, as after any voiding, is all that is necessary after the urine stream test.

Electromyography (EMG) of the perineal muscles tests the strength of the muscles used in voiding. This information may help identify methods of improving continence. Inform the patient that some mild, temporary discomfort may accompany placement of the electrodes. In EMG of the perineal muscles, electrodes are placed in either the rectum or the urethra to measure muscle contraction and relaxation. After the completion of EMG, administer analgesics as prescribed to promote the patient's comfort.

❓ NCLEX EXAMINATION CHALLENGE
Safe and Effective Care Environment

Which assessments are most important for the nurse to perform when monitoring a client after a retrograde cystogram?
A. Temperature and urine character
B. Kidney tenderness and flank pain
C. 24-hour urine volume, BUN and creatinine levels
D. Angioedema and other indicators of systemic allergic response

Kidney Biopsy

Patient Preparation. Explain that a kidney biopsy can help determine a cause of unexplained kidney problems and can help direct or change therapy. Most kidney biopsies are performed percutaneously (through the skin and other tissues) using ultrasound or CT guidance. The patient signs an informed consent. Patients are NPO for 4 to 6 hours before the procedure.

Because of the risk for bleeding after the biopsy, coagulation studies such as platelet count, activated partial thromboplastin time (aPTT), prothrombin time (PT), and bleeding time are performed before surgery. A blood transfusion may be needed to correct anemia before biopsy. Hypertension and uremia increase the risk for bleeding, and antihypertensive drugs or dialysis may be prescribed before a biopsy.

Procedure. In a percutaneous biopsy, the nephrologist or radiologist obtains tissue samples without an incision. Patients receive sedation and are monitored throughout the procedure. The patient is placed in the prone position on the procedure table. The entry site is selected after taking preliminary images. The area is prepped and sterilely draped. A local anesthetic is injected, and the physician then inserts the biopsy device into the tissues toward the kidney. Needle depth and placement are confirmed by ultrasound or CT. While the patient holds his or her breath, the needle is advanced into the renal cortex. Samples are then taken with a spring-loaded coring biopsy needle and sent for pathologic study.

Follow-up Care. After a percutaneous biopsy, the major risk is bleeding from the biopsy site. For 24 hours after the biopsy, monitor the dressing site, vital signs, urine output, hemoglobin level, and hematocrit. Even if the dressing is dry and there is no hematoma, the patient could be bleeding from the site. An internal bleed is not readily visible but is suspected with flank pain, decreasing blood pressure, decreasing urine output, or other signs of hypovolemia or shock.

The patient follows a plan of strict bedrest, lying in a supine position with a back roll for additional support for 2 to 6 hours after the biopsy. The head of the bed may be elevated, and the patient may resume oral intake of food and fluids. After bedrest, the patient may have limited bathroom privileges if there is no evidence of bleeding.

Monitor for hematuria, the most common complication of kidney biopsy. Hematuria occurs microscopically in most patients, but 5% to 9% have gross hematuria. This problem usually resolves without treatment in 48 to 72 hours after the biopsy but can persist for 2 to 3 weeks. In rare cases, transfusions and surgery are required. There should be no obvious blood clots in the urine.

The patient may have some local pain after the biopsy. If aching originates at the biopsy site and begins to radiate to the flank and around the front of the abdomen, bleeding may have started or a hematoma is forming around the kidney. This pattern of discomfort with bleeding occurs because blood in the tissues around the kidney increases pressure on local nerve tracts.

If bleeding occurs, IV fluid, packed red blood cells, or both may be needed to prevent shock. In general, a small amount of bleeding creates enough pressure to compress bleeding sites. This is called a "tamponade effect." If tamponade does not occur and bleeding is extensive, surgery for hemostasis or even nephrectomy may be needed. A hematoma in, on, or around the kidney may become infected, requiring treatment with antibiotics and surgical drainage.

If no bleeding occurs, the patient can resume general activities after 24 hours. Instruct him or her to avoid lifting heavy objects, exercising, or performing other strenuous activities for 1 to 2 weeks after the biopsy procedure. Driving may also be restricted. Refer to Chapter 18 for general postoperative care for the patient undergoing an open kidney biopsy.

❓ DECISION-MAKING CHALLENGE
Safety; Patient-Centered Care

At the start of the shift, you are assessing a 36-year-old patient 12 hours after a percutaneous biopsy of the left kidney. You observe that the bruising around the site extends about 2 inches past the dressing (a total diameter of 4 inches) and is swollen. The patient rates his pain at a 5 on a 0-to-10 pain-rating scale, which is up from the 3 he reported several hours ago. When you empty the urinal, the urine is pink-tinged. The patient has been lying on his right side for the past several hours and asks if he can change positions.
1. What assessment information will you document in the chart?
2. What additional information should you ask the patient and assess directly?
3. How could you accurately monitor changes in the size of the bruising at the surgical site?
4. What would be the best position for this patient for the next 2 hours?
5. Should you notify the surgeon at this time? Why or why not?

NURSING CONCEPT REVIEW

What should you expect to NOTICE in a patient with adequate urinary elimination?

Vital signs
- Body temperature is within normal range.
- Blood pressure is within normal range.

Physical assessment
- Daily urine output is within 500 mL of daily fluid intake.
- Skin texture is normal (no edema or superficial crystals present).
- Skin color is appropriate for race with no excessive yellowing, bruising, or petechiae.
- Urine is clear and some variation of yellow in color.
- Patient voids 300 to 500 mL per voiding.
- Patient does not report pain or burning on urination.
- Patient has no difficulty starting or stopping the stream of urine.
- Patient is continent of urine and can maintain continence without sensation of urgency.
- Patient is alert and oriented.

Psychological assessment
- Patient is able to communicate concerns about the urinary tract system.
- Patient is aware and informed about kidney function and diagnostic tests.

Laboratory assessment
- Hematocrit and hemoglobin are within normal limits (no anemia).
- BUN and creatinine are within normal limits.
- Serum electrolytes are within normal ranges.
- Urinalysis shows no bacteria, blood, sediment, or protein.

GET READY FOR THE NCLEX® EXAMINATION!

KEY POINTS

Review these Key Points for each NCLEX Examination Client Needs Category.

Safe and Effective Care Environment
- Use sterile technique when inserting a catheter or any other instrument into the urinary system.
- Use Contact Precautions with any patient who has drainage from the genitourinary tract.
- Evaluate risk for kidney injury from diagnostic testing by asking about allergy to radiopaque contrast dye, shellfish, or iodine or adverse reactions following the use of diagnostic agents such as gadolinium in MRI.
- Identify prescribed and over-the-counter drugs that increase risk for kidney dysfunction.

Health Promotion and Maintenance
- Teach patients to clean the perineal area after voiding, after having a bowel movement, and after sexual intercourse.
- Urge all patients to maintain an adequate fluid intake (sufficient to dilute urine to a light yellow color). A minimum of 2 L/day may be recommended unless another health problem requires fluid restriction.
- Teach patients who come into contact with chemicals in their workplaces or for leisure time activities to avoid direct skin or mucous membrane contact with these chemicals.

Psychosocial Integrity
- Allow the patient the opportunity to express concerns about tests of the kidney and urinary tract or about a potential change in kidney function.
- Assess the patient's level of comfort in discussing issues related to elimination and the urogenital area.
- Explain all diagnostic procedures, restrictions, and follow-up care to the patient scheduled for tests.
- Provide as much privacy as possible for patients undergoing examination or testing of the kidney/urinary tract.
- Use language and terminology that the patient can understand during discussions of kidney/urinary assessment.

Physiological Integrity
- Ask the patient about kidney problems in any other members of the family, because some problems have a genetic component.
- Ask the patient about current and past drug use (prescribed, over-the-counter, and illicit), and evaluate drug use for potential nephrotoxicity.
- Assess urine output closely after any procedure in which contrast dye is used IV.
- Assess the patient for bleeding or manifestations of infection after any invasive test of kidney/urinary function.

Care of Patients with Urinary Problems

Chris Winkelman

LEARNING OUTCOMES

Safe and Effective Care Environment

1. Assess the appropriateness for continuing therapy with indwelling urinary catheters.
2. Use principles of asepsis during catheter insertion.

Health Promotion and Maintenance

3. Encourage everyone to have a daily fluid intake of 1.5 to 2.5 L unless another health problem requires fluid restriction or to have sufficient fluid intake to result in urine output of 2 to 2.5 L daily.
4. Teach women risk-reduction interventions for urinary tract infections.
5. Teach the proper application of pelvic floor exercises to reduce or prevent urinary incontinence.
6. Encourage anyone who comes into contact with chemicals as part of work or hobbies to use appropriate personal protective equipment to reduce the risk for bladder cancer.

Psychosocial Integrity

7. Use language the patient is comfortable with when discussing urinary and sexual issues.
8. Encourage patients and families to express their feelings and concerns about a change in urinary elimination.
9. Explain to the patient and family what to expect during tests and procedures for urinary problems.
10. Refer patients with long-term urinary problems to appropriate community resources and support groups.

Physiological Integrity

11. Coordinate care to prevent urinary tract infections among hospitalized patients.
12. Compare the pathophysiology and manifestations of stress incontinence, urge incontinence, overflow incontinence, mixed incontinence, and functional incontinence.
13. Coordinate nursing care for the patient who has invasive bladder cancer.

The urinary system consists of the ureters, bladder, and urethra. Their functions are to store the urine made by the kidney and eliminate it from the body. These actions do not contribute to the homeostatic purposes of *urinary elimination*. However, when problems in the urinary system interfere with the mechanics of moving urine out of the body, urinary elimination is inadequate and homeostasis of fluids, electrolytes, nitrogenous wastes, and blood pressure is disrupted.

Urinary problems affect the storage or elimination of urine. Both acute and chronic urinary problems are common and costly. More than 20 million people in the United States are treated annually for urinary tract infections, cystitis, kidney and ureter stones, or urinary incontinence (U.S. Renal Data Systems, 2010). Although life-threatening complications are rare with urinary problems, patients may have significant functional, physical, and psychosocial changes that reduce quality of life. Nursing interventions are directed

TABLE 69-1	FACTORS CONTRIBUTING TO URINARY TRACT INFECTIONS
FACTOR	**MECHANISM**
Obstruction	Incomplete bladder emptying creates a continuous pool of urine in which bacteria can grow, prevents flushing out of bacteria, and allows bacteria to ascend more easily to higher structures.
	Bacteria have a greater chance of multiplying the longer they remain in residual urine.
	Overdistention of the bladder damages the mucosa and allows bacteria to invade the bladder wall.
Stones (calculi)	Large stones can obstruct urine flow.
	The rough surface of a stone irritates mucosal surfaces and creates a spot where bacteria can establish and grow.
	Bacteria can live within stones and cause re-infection.
Vesicoureteral reflux	Bacteria-laden urine is forced backward from the bladder up into the ureters and kidneys, where pyelonephritis can develop.
	Reflux of sterile urine can cause kidney scarring, which may promote kidney dysfunction.
Diabetes mellitus	Excess glucose in urine provides a rich medium for bacterial growth.
	Peripheral neuropathy affects bladder innervation and leads to a flaccid bladder and incomplete bladder emptying.
Characteristics of urine	Alkalotic urine promotes bacterial growth.
	Concentrated urine promotes bacterial growth.
Gender	Women are susceptible to periurethral colonization with coliform bacteria.
	Use of diaphragms, frequency of intercourse, and a new partner within the past year are associated with urinary tract infection (UTI) in women.
	Bladder displacement during pregnancy predisposes women to cystitis and the development of pyelonephritis.
	A diaphragm or pessary that is too large can obstruct urine flow or traumatize the urethra.
Age	Urinary stasis may be caused by incomplete bladder emptying as a result of an enlarged prostate in men and cystocele and prolapse in women.
	Neuromuscular conditions that cause incomplete bladder emptying, such as Parkinson disease and strokes, affect older adults more frequently.
	The use of anticholinergic drugs in older adults contributes to delayed bladder emptying.
	Fecal incontinence contributes to poor perineal hygiene.
	Hypoestrogenism in older women adversely affects the cells of the vagina and urethra, making them more susceptible to infections.
Sexual activity	Irritation of the perineum and urethra during intercourse can promote migration of bacteria from the perineal area to the urinary tract in some women.
	Spermicides can alter vaginal pH, increasing potential numbers of pathogens.
	Inadequate vaginal lubrication may exacerbate potential urethral irritation.
	Bacteria may be introduced into the man's urethra during anal intercourse or during vaginal intercourse with a woman who has a bacterial vaginitis.
Recent use of antibiotics	Antibiotics change normal protective flora, providing opportunity for pathogenic bacterial overgrowth and colonization.

toward prevention, detection, and management of urologic disorders.

INFECTIOUS DISORDERS

Infections of the urinary tract and kidneys are common, especially among women. Manifestations of urinary tract infection (UTI) account for more than 7 million health care visits and 1 million hospital admissions annually in the United States (U.S. Renal Data Systems, 2010). UTIs are the most common health care–acquired infection. Total direct and indirect costs for adult urinary tract infections are estimated at $1.6 billion each year (Centers for Disease Control and Prevention [CDC], 2009).

Urinary tract infections are described by their location in the tract. Acute infections in the urinary tract include *urethritis* (urethra), *cystitis* (bladder), and *prostatitis* (prostate gland). Acute *pyelonephritis* is a kidney infection. The site of infection is important to know because site, along with the specific type of bacteria present, determines treatment. Several risk factors are associated with occurrence of UTIs (Table 69-1).

CYSTITIS

Pathophysiology

Cystitis is an inflammation of the bladder. It can be caused by irritation or, more commonly, by infection from bacteria, viruses, fungi, or parasites. Infectious cystitis is the most common of the UTIs. Noninfectious cystitis is caused by irritation from chemicals or radiation. Interstitial cystitis is an inflammatory disease that has no known cause.

Infectious agents, most commonly bacteria, move up the urinary tract from the external urethra to the bladder. Less common, spread of infection through the blood and lymph fluid can occur. Once bacteria enter the urinary tract, several factors influence the outcome (Table 69-2).

The presence of bacteria in the urine is bacteriuria and can occur with any urologic infection. When bacteriuria is without symptoms of infection, it is called *colonization*. Colonization, asymptomatic bacteriuria, is more common in older adults. This problem does not appear to progress to acute infection or kidney impairment unless the patient has other pathologic problems, and then it requires treatment.

TABLE 69-2	IMPORTANT FACTORS INFLUENCING THE OUTCOME OF URINARY TRACT INFECTION
FACILITATING ASPECTS	**PROTECTIVE ASPECTS**
Anatomy	
Females: Short length of the urethra and its proximity to the vagina and rectum facilitate colonization of coliform bacteria.	
Males: With age, the prostate enlarges and may obstruct the normal flow of urine, producing stasis.	Males: Long length of the urethra and its distance from the rectum provide protection from colonization with coliform bacteria.
Physiology	
Females: Pregnancy predisposes a woman to ureteral reflux and subsequent pyelonephritis; with age, the decline in estrogen facilitates colonization of *Escherichia coli*. In addition, vaginal atrophy can alter urethral competency.	Females: Well-estrogenized mucosa in the urethra and trigone may inhibit bacterial colonization and enhance urogenital blood flow.
Males: With age, prostatic secretions lose their antibacterial characteristics and predispose to bacterial proliferation in the urine.	Males: Normal prostatic secretions inhibit bacterial growth.
	Both males and females: Mucin is produced by urothelial cells lining the bladder—this helps maintain mucosal integrity and prevent cellular damage; mucin may also prevent bacteria from adhering to urothelial cells.
Trauma	
Females: Vaginal penetration with sexual intercourse may traumatize the urethra and bladder base, leading to postcoital (or "honeymoon") cystitis; a vaginal diaphragm that is too large can place pressure on the urethra, causing trauma; vaginal childbirth can cause permanent damage to the urethra.	Females: Adequate lubrication, either natural or artificial, with intercourse may prevent any trauma.
Males: Sexually transmitted diseases may cause urethral strictures that obstruct the flow of urine and predispose to urinary stasis.	
Both males and females: Urethral instrumentation (e.g., catheterization) may disturb the urothelial surface and predispose to adherence of bacteria that would ordinarily not be pathogenic.	
Infectious Agent	
Some organisms are better able to adhere to host cells and secrete substances that induce inflammation.	A small inoculum (number of microorganisms introduced into the body) is more easily flushed away by the flow of urine.

Etiology and Genetic Risk

UTIs, like other infections, are the result of interactions between a pathogen and the host. Usually, a high bacterial *virulence* (ability to invade and infect) is needed to overcome normal strong host resistance. However, a compromised host is more likely to become infected even with bacteria that have low virulence. Genetically, invading bacteria with special adhesions are more likely to cause ascending UTIs that start in the urethra or bladder and move up into the ureter and kidney. Patient-specific genetic factors such as blood type and ability to produce bladder surface biofilms that protect bacteria may influence the risk for UTI (Bowen & Hellstrom, 2007).

Infectious cystitis is most commonly caused by organisms from the intestinal tract. About 90% of UTIs are caused by *Escherichia coli*. Less common organisms include *Staphylococcus saprophyticus, Klebsiella pneumoniae,* and organisms from the *Proteus* and *Enterobacter* species (Bowen & Hellstrom, 2007).

In most cases, organisms first grow in the perineal area, then move into the urethra as a result of irritation, trauma, or catheterization of the urinary tract, and finally ascend to the bladder. Catheters are the most common factor placing patients at risk for UTIs in the hospital setting. Within 48 hours of catheter insertion, bacterial colonization begins. About 50% of patients with indwelling catheters become infected within 1 week of catheter insertion.

How a catheter-related infection occurs varies between genders. Bacteria from a woman's perineal area are more likely to ascend to the bladder by moving along the outside of the catheter. In men, bacteria tend to gain access to the bladder from inside the lumen of the catheter. Any break in the closed urinary drainage system allows bacteria to move through the urinary tract. Best practices to reduce the risk for catheter contamination and catheter-related UTIs are listed in Chart 69-1.

Organisms other than bacteria also can cause cystitis. Fungal infections, such as those caused by *Candida,* can occur during long-term antibiotic therapy, because antibiotics reduce normal protective flora. Patients who are severely immunosuppressed, are receiving corticosteroids or other immunosuppressive agents, or have diabetes mellitus or acquired immune deficiency syndrome (AIDS) are at higher risk for fungal UTIs.

Viral and parasitic infections are rare and usually are transferred to the urinary tract from an infection at another body site. For example, *Trichomonas,* a parasite found in the vagina, can also be found in the urine. Treatment of the vaginal infection (see Chapter 74) also resolves the UTI.

Noninfectious cystitis may result from chemical exposure, such as to drugs (e.g., cyclophosphamide [Cytoxan, Procytox ✦]), from radiation therapy, and from immunologic responses, as with systemic lupus erythematosus (SLE).

Interstitial cystitis is a rare, chronic inflammation of the bladder, urethra, and adjacent pelvic muscles that is not a result of infection. The condition affects women ten times more often than men, and the diagnosis is difficult to make. Manifestations are similar to those of infectious cystitis with voiding occurring as often as 60 times daily, more intense urgency preceding urination, and suprapubic or pelvic pain,

CHART 69-1 BEST PRACTICE FOR PATIENT SAFETY & QUALITY CARE

Minimizing Catheter-Related Infection

- Assess patients daily for those who no longer need indwelling catheters.
- Consider appropriate alternatives to an indwelling catheter.
- Use aseptic routine when handling catheter devices; manipulation can promote an environment favorable to pathogens.
- Select a small-size catheter (14 to 18 Fr with a 5-mL balloon).
- Use strict sterile technique to insert the catheter (in the hospital setting); a break in technique can introduce pathogens into the urinary tract.
- Do not inject more than 10 mL into the balloon.
- Maintain a closed-system irrigation by ensuring that catheter tubing connections are sealed securely; disconnections can introduce pathogens into the urinary tract.
- Avoid routine catheter irrigation.
- Keep urine collection bags below the level of the bladder at all times; elevating the collection bag above the bladder causes reflux of pathogens from the bag into the urinary tract.
- Secure the catheter to the patient's thigh (women) or lower abdomen (men); catheter movement can cause urethral friction and irritation.
- Perform daily catheter care by washing the perineum and proximal portion of the catheter with soap and water and drying gently (removes pathogens and reduces pathogenic population).
- Consider the use of coated catheters for patients requiring indwelling catheters for more than 3 to 5 days. This coating reduces bacterial colonization along the catheter.

Application of antiseptic solutions or antibiotic ointments to the perineal area of catheterized patients has not been demonstrated to have any beneficial effect.

Data from Smith, J. (2003). Indwelling catheter management: From habit to evidence-based practice. *Ostomy and Wound Management, 49*(12), 34-45.

---

sometimes radiating to the groin, vulva or rectum, that is relieved by voiding. Results from urinalysis and urine culture are negative for infection (Evans & Sant, 2007; Siegel et al., 2008).

Although cystitis is not life threatening, infectious cystitis can lead to life-threatening complications, including pyelonephritis and sepsis. Severe kidney damage is a rare complication unless the patient also has other predisposing factors, such as anatomic abnormalities, pregnancy, obstruction, reflux, calculi, or diabetes.

The spread of the infection from the urinary tract to the bloodstream is termed urosepsis and is more common among older adults (Kessenich, 2010). Sepsis from any source is a systemic infection that can lead to overwhelming organ failure, shock, and death. The most common cause of sepsis in the hospitalized patient is a UTI (CDC, 2009). Sepsis has a high mortality and prolongs hospital stays (see Chapter 39).

Incidence/Prevalence

The incidence of UTI is second only to that of upper respiratory infections in primary care. Patients who have frequency (an urge to urinate frequently in small amounts), dysuria (pain or burning with urination), and urgency (the feeling that urination will occur immediately) account for more than 5 million health care visits annually. About 50% of these patients will have a confirmed UTI (U.S. Renal Data Systems, 2010).

CONSIDERATIONS FOR OLDER ADULTS

The prevalence of UTIs varies with age and gender. Women of any age are more commonly affected with UTIs than are men. In men, the incidence of UTI greatly increases after 73 years of age. In women, the prevalence of UTIs increases from 20% among all women to 50% in those older than 80 years (U.S. Renal Data Systems, 2010). Skin and mucous membrane changes from a lack of estrogen appear to account for much of the increased risk in older women. Prostate disease increases risk for UTIs in men.

Health Promotion and Maintenance

Although cystitis is common, in many cases it is preventable. In the health care setting, reducing the use of indwelling urinary catheters is a major prevention strategy (Gray, 2010). When catheters must be used, strict attention to sterile technique during insertion can reduce the risk for UTIs as can consistent and adequate perineal and catheter care (see Chart 69-1).

! NURSING SAFETY PRIORITY

Action Alert

Ensuring that urinary catheters are used appropriately and discontinued as early as possible is everyone's responsibility. Do not allow catheters to remain in place for staff convenience.

Changes in fluid intake patterns, urinary elimination patterns, and hygiene patterns can help prevent or reduce cystitis in the general population. Teach all people to have a minimum fluid intake of 1.5 to 2.5 L daily unless fluid restriction is required for other health problems. Another strategy is to have sufficient fluid intake to cause 2 to 2.5 L of urine daily. Encourage people to drink more water rather than sugar-containing drinks. Teach people to avoid urinary stasis by urinating every 3 to 4 hours rather than waiting until the bladder is greatly distended. Encourage everyone either to shower daily or to wash the perineal and urethral areas daily with mild soap and a water rinse. Teach women to avoid the use of vaginal washes. Other hygiene measures that specifically reduce the risk for cystitis and other UTIs are listed in Chart 69-2.

PATIENT-CENTERED COLLABORATIVE CARE

ASSESSMENT

Physical Assessment/Clinical Manifestations

Frequency, urgency, and dysuria are the common manifestations of a urinary tract infection (UTI), but other manifestations may be present (Chart 69-3). Urine may be cloudy, foul smelling, or blood tinged. Ask the patient about risk factors for UTI during the assessment (see Table 69-1). For noninfectious cystitis, the Pelvic Pain and Urgency/Frequency (PUF) Patient Symptom Scale can identify patients with interstitial cystitis.

Before performing the physical assessment, ask the patient to void so that the urine can be examined and the bladder emptied before palpation. Assess vital signs to help rule out sepsis. Inspect the lower abdomen, and palpate the urinary

Preventing a Urinary Tract Infection

- Drink at least 2 to 3 L of sugarless fluid every day.
- Be sure to get enough sleep, rest, and nutrition daily.
- [For women] Clean your perineum (the area between your legs) from front to back.
- [For women] Avoid using or wearing irritating substances, such as bubble bath, nylon underwear, and scented toilet tissue. Wear loose-fitting cotton underwear.
- [For women] Empty your bladder before and after intercourse.
- For both women and men, gently wash the perineal area before intercourse.
- Avoid the use of scented or flavored lubricants.
- If you experience burning when you urinate, if you have to urinate frequently, or if you find it difficult to begin urinating, notify your physician or other health care provider right away, especially if you have a chronic medical condition (e.g., diabetes) or are pregnant.
- Empty your bladder as soon as you feel the urge to urinate.
- Empty your bladder regularly (every 4 hours), even if you do not feel the urge to urinate.
- You may try these home therapies:
  - Cranberry juice (pure), 50 mL daily
  - Apple cider vinegar, 2 tablespoons three times daily in juice
  - Vitamin C, 500 mg daily to acidify the urine
- To prevent recurrent infection:
  - Take your prescribed antibiotic or other drug as directed, even after the symptoms go away.
  - Schedule a follow-up appointment for 10 to 14 days after you finish taking the drug. At your follow-up visit, another urine sample may be taken for analysis or culture.

CHART 69-3 KEY FEATURES

Urinary Tract Infection

Common Clinical Manifestations	Rare Clinical Manifestations
• Frequency	• Fever
• Urgency	• Chills
• Dysuria	• Nausea or vomiting
• Hesitancy or difficulty in initiating urine stream	• Malaise
• Low back pain	• Flank pain
• Nocturia	**Clinical Manifestations that May Occur in the Older Adult**
• Incontinence	
• Hematuria	• The only symptom may be something as vague as increasing mental confusion or frequent, unexplained falls.
• Pyuria	
• Bacteriuria	• A sudden onset of incontinence or a worsening of incontinence may be the only symptom of an early UTI.
• Retention	
• Suprapubic tenderness or fullness	• Fever, tachycardia, tachypnea, and hypotension, even without any urinary symptoms, may be signs of urosepsis.
• Feeling of incomplete bladder emptying	
	• Loss of appetite, nocturia, and dysuria are common symptoms.

UTI, Urinary tract infection.

bladder. Distention after voiding indicates incomplete bladder emptying.

Using Standard Precautions, examine any lesions around the urethral meatus and vaginal opening. To help differentiate between a vaginal and a urinary tract infection, note whether there is any vaginal discharge (vaginal discharge and irritation are more indicative of vaginal infection). Women often report burning with urination when normal acidic urine touches labial tissues that are inflamed or ulcerated by vaginal infections or sexually transmitted diseases (STDs). Maintain privacy with drapes during the examination.

The prostate is palpated by digital rectal examination (DRE) for size, change in shape or consistency, and tenderness. The physician or advanced practice nurse performs the DRE.

Laboratory Assessment

Laboratory assessment for a UTI is a urinalysis with testing for leukocyte esterase and nitrate. The combination of a positive leukocyte esterase and nitrate is 68% to 88% sensitive in the diagnosis of a UTI (Bowen & Hellstrom, 2007). Although a urinalysis can include a microscopic count of bacteria, white blood cells (WBCs), and red blood cells (RBCs), this additional testing is more expensive, is time consuming, and may not improve diagnostic accuracy. The presence of more than 20 epithelial cells/high power field (hpf) suggests contamination. The presence of 100,000 colonies/mL or the presence of three or more WBCs (pyuria) with RBCs (hematuria) indicates infection.

A urinalysis is performed on a clean-catch midstream specimen. If the patient cannot produce a clean-catch specimen, you may need to obtain the specimen with a small-diameter (6 Fr) catheter. For a routine urinalysis, 10 mL of urine is needed; smaller quantities are sufficient for culture.

A urine culture confirms the type of organism and the number of colonies. Urine culture is expensive, and results take at least 48 hours. It is indicated when the UTI is complicated or does not respond to usual therapy or the diagnosis is uncertain. A UTI is confirmed when more than 10^5 colony-forming units are in the urine from any patient. In patients who also have symptoms of UTI, as few as 10^3 colony-forming units may allow the diagnosis to be made. The presence of many different types of organisms in low colony counts usually indicates that the specimen is contaminated. Sensitivity testing follows culture results when complicating factors are present (e.g., stones or recurrent infection), when the patient is older, or to ensure the appropriate antibiotics are prescribed.

Occasionally the serum WBC count may be elevated, with the differential WBC count showing a "left shift" (see Chapter 19). This shift indicates that the number of immature WBCs is increasing in response to the infection. As a result, the number of bands, or immature WBCs, is elevated. Left shift most often occurs with urosepsis and rarely occurs with uncomplicated cystitis, which is a local rather than a systemic infection.

Other Diagnostic Assessment

The diagnosis of cystitis is based on the history, physical examination, and laboratory data. If urinary retention and obstruction of urine outflow are suspected, urography, abdominal sonography, or computed tomography (CT) may be needed to locate the site of obstruction or the presence of calculi. Voiding cystourethrography (see Chapter 68) is needed when ureteral reflux is suspected.

Cystoscopy (see Chapter 68) may be performed when the patient has recurrent UTIs (more than three or four a year).

A urine culture is performed first to ensure that no infection is present. If infection is present, the urine is sterilized with antibiotic therapy before the procedure to reduce the risk for sepsis. Cystoscopy identifies abnormalities that increase the risk for cystitis. Such abnormalities include bladder calculi, bladder diverticula, urethral strictures, foreign bodies (e.g., sutures from previous surgery), and trabeculation (an abnormal thickening of the bladder wall caused by urinary retention and obstruction). Retrograde pyelography, along with the cystoscopic examination, shows outlines and images of the drainage tract. Areas of obstruction or malformation and the presence of reflux are then identified early.

Cystoscopy is needed to accurately diagnose interstitial cystitis. A urinalysis usually shows WBCs and RBCs but no bacteria. Common findings in interstitial cystitis are a small-capacity bladder, the presence of Hunner's ulcers (a type of bladder lesion), and small hemorrhages after bladder distention.

INTERVENTIONS

Nonsurgical Management

The expected outcome is to maintain an optimal urinary elimination pattern. Nursing interventions for the management of cystitis focus on comfort and teaching about drug therapy, nutrition therapy, and prevention measures.

Drug Therapy. Drugs used to treat bacteriuria and promote patient comfort include urinary antiseptics or antibiotics, analgesics, and antispasmodics. Cure of a UTI depends on the antibiotic levels achieved in the urine (Chart 69-4). Oral antifungal agents are usually prescribed for fungal infections. When oral antifungal therapy is not sufficient, amphotericin B is most often given in daily bladder instillations. Antispasmodic drugs decrease bladder spasm and promote complete bladder emptying.

Antibiotic therapy is used for bacterial UTIs (see Chart 69-4). Guidelines indicate that a 3-day, high-dose course of trimethoprim/sulfamethoxazole or a fluoroquinolone is effective in treating uncomplicated, community-acquired UTIs in women (Bowen & Hellstrom, 2007). Fluoroquinolones cannot be used to treat UTIs during pregnancy because

! NURSING SAFETY PRIORITY

Drug Alert

Two of the fluoroquinolone antibiotics, Tequin and Noroxin, are designated as sound-alike, look-alike agents with other drugs and could easily be administered in error. Take care to not confuse Tequin with Tegretol, an oral anticonvulsant, or with Ticlid, a platelet inhibitor. Take care to not confuse Noroxin with Neurontin, an oral anticonvulsant.

? NCLEX EXAMINATION CHALLENGE

Safe and Effective Care Environment

The client prescribed cephalexin (Keflex) for cystitis reports that she has had a severe allergic reaction to penicillin in the past. What is the nurse's best action?
A. Reassure the client that Keflex is not penicillin.
B. Place an allergy alert band on the client's wrist.
C. Notify the prescriber before administering the first Keflex dose.
D. Highlight this important information in the client's medical record.

of the potential for birth defects. The shorter courses increase adherence and reduce cost. Longer antibiotic treatment (7 to 21 days) and/or different agents are required for hospitalized patients; those with complicating factors, such as pregnancy, indwelling catheters, or stones; and those with diabetes or immunosuppression.

Long-term, low-dose antibiotic therapy is used for chronic, recurring infections caused by structural abnormalities or stones. Trimethoprim 100 mg daily may be used for long-term management of the older patient with frequent UTIs. For women who have recurrent UTIs after intercourse, one low-dose tablet of trimethoprim (TMP) (Proloprim, Trimpex) or TMP/sulfamethoxazole (half or single-strength Bactrim, Cotrim, Septra) or nitrofurantoin (Macrodantin, Nephronex ✚, Novofuran ✚) after intercourse is often prescribed. Estrogen used as an intravaginal cream may prevent recurrent UTIs in the postmenopausal woman, although this therapy is controversial.

WOMEN'S HEALTH CONSIDERATIONS

Pregnant women with a bacterial UTI require prompt and aggressive treatment because simple cystitis can lead to acute pyelonephritis during pregnancy. Pyelonephritis in pregnancy can cause preterm labor and adversely affect the fetus.

Nutrition Therapy. The diet should include all food groups and include more calories for the increased metabolism caused by infection. Urge patients to drink enough fluid to maintain a diluted urine throughout the day and night unless fluid restriction is required for other health problems. The drinking of 50 mL of concentrated cranberry juice daily appears to decrease the ability of bacteria to adhere to the epithelial cells lining the urinary tract, decreasing the incidence of symptomatic UTIs in some patients. Cranberry juice must be consumed for 3 to 4 weeks to be effective, and the efficacy of cranberry tablets has not been established (Bowen & Hellstrom, 2007). It is important to note that cranberry juice is an irritant to the bladder with interstitial cystitis and should be avoided by patients with this condition. Avoiding caffeine, carbonated beverages, and tomato products may decrease bladder irritation during cystitis.

Comfort Measures. A warm sitz bath taken two or three times a day for 20 minutes may provide comfort and some relief of local symptoms. If burning with urination is severe or urinary retention occurs, teach the patient to sit in the sitz bath and urinate into the warm water.

Surgical Management

Surgery for cystitis treats the conditions that increase the risk for recurrent UTIs (e.g., removal of obstructions and repair of vesicoureteral reflux). Procedures may include cystoscopy (see Chapter 68) to identify and remove calculi or obstructions.

Community-Based Care

Assess the patient's level of understanding of the problem. His or her knowledge about factors that promote the development of cystitis determines the teaching interventions planned.

Teach the patient how to take prescribed drugs. Stress the need for correct spacing of doses throughout the day and the

CHART 69-4	COMMON EXAMPLES OF DRUG THERAPY

Urinary Tract Infections

DRUG/DOSAGE	PURPOSE/ACTION	NURSING INTERVENTIONS	RATIONALES
Antimicrobials *Sulfonamides* Trimethoprim*/ sulfamethoxazole (Bactrim, Bacter-Aid, Septra, Sulfatrim, Sultrex, Roubac 🍁) 160 mg trimethoprim/800 mg sulfamethoxazole orally every 12 hr	Drug reduces bacteria in the urinary tract by direct killing (trimethoprim) and by inhibiting bacterial reproduction (sulfamethoxazole).	Ask patients about drug allergies, especially to sulfa drugs, before beginning drug therapy. Teach patients to drink a full glass of water with each dose and to have an overall fluid intake of at least 3 L daily. Teach patients to keep out of the sun or to wear protective clothing outdoors and use a sunscreen. Caution patients to complete the drug regimen even if the symptoms improve or disappear sooner.	Allergies to sulfa drugs are common and require changing the drug therapy. Sulfamethoxazole can form crystals that precipitate in the kidney tubules. Fluid intake prevents this complication. This drug increases skin sensitivity to the sun and can lead to severe sunburns, even in darker-skinned patients. Not completing the drug regimen can lead to an infection recurrence and to bacterial drug resistance.
Fluoroquinolones Ciprofloxacin (Cipro, ProQuin) 250 mg orally twice daily Gatifloxacin 🍁 (Tequin, Zymar) 200-400 mg orally or IV once daily Levofloxacin (Levaquin) 400 mg orally daily Lomefloxacin (Maxaquin) 250 mg orally daily Norfloxacin (Noroxin) 400 mg orally twice daily Ofloxacin (Floxin) 200 mg orally twice daily Sparfloxacin (Zagam) 200-400 mg orally daily	Drugs from this class reduce bacteria in the urinary tract by direct killing (bactericidal actions) and by inhibiting bacterial reproduction (bacteriostatic actions).	Teach patients taking the extended- release drugs to swallow them whole, not to crush or chew the tablets. Warn patients to not take the drug within 2 hours of taking an antacid. Teach patients how to take their pulse, to monitor it twice daily while on this drug, and to notify the prescriber if new-onset irregular heartbeats occur. Teach patients to keep out of the sun or to wear protective clothing outdoors and use a sunscreen. Caution patients to complete the drug regimen even if the symptoms improve or disappear sooner.	Crushing or chewing the tablet releases all the drug at once, ruining the extended effect. Many antacids (especially those containing magnesium or aluminum) interfere with drug absorption. This class of drugs can induce serious cardiac dysrhythmias. Most quinolones increase skin sensitivity to the sun and can lead to severe sunburns even in darker-skinned patients. Not completing the drug regimen can lead to an infection recurrence and to bacterial drug resistance.
Penicillins Amoxicillin (Amoxil) 500 mg orally every 12 hr Amoxicillin/clavulanate (Augmentin, Clavulin 🍁) 500 mg/125 mg orally every 12 hr	Drugs from this class reduce bacteria in the urinary tract by direct killing (bactericidal actions) as a result of interrupting bacterial cell wall synthesis.	Ask patients about drug allergies to penicillin before beginning drug therapy. Teach patients to take the drug with food. Instruct patients to call the prescriber if severe or watery diarrhea develops. Suggest that women who take oral contraceptives use an additional method of birth control while taking this drug. Caution patients to complete the drug regimen even if the symptoms improve or disappear sooner.	Allergies to penicillin are common and require changing the drug therapy. Taking it with food reduces the risk for GI upset. A complication of penicillin therapy is pseudomembranous colitis, which may require discontinuing the drug. Penicillin appears to reduce the effectiveness of estrogen-containing oral contraceptives. Not completing the drug regimen can lead to an infection recurrence and to bacterial drug resistance.
Cephalosporins Cefadroxil (Duricef) 1-2 g orally every 12 hr Cefixime (Suprax) 400 mg orally every 12 to 24 hr	Drugs from this class reduce bacteria in the urinary tract by direct killing (bactericidal actions) as a result of interrupting bacterial cell wall synthesis.	Ask about drug allergies to penicillin or cephalosporins before beginning drug therapy. Instruct patients to call the prescriber if severe or watery diarrhea develops. Caution patients to complete the drug regimen even if the symptoms improve or disappear sooner.	Drugs in this class are structurally similar to penicillin. Anyone with allergies to penicillin is likely to be allergic to the cephalosporins. A complication of penicillin therapy is pseudomembranous colitis, which may require discontinuing the drug. Not completing the drug regimen can lead to an infection recurrence and to bacterial drug resistance.

Continued

CHART 69-4 **COMMON EXAMPLES OF DRUG THERAPY**

Urinary Tract Infections—cont'd

DRUG/DOSAGE	PURPOSE/ACTION	NURSING INTERVENTIONS	RATIONALES
Fosfomycin (Monurol) 3 g orally as a one-time dose	This drug reduces bacteria in the urinary tract by direct killing (bactericidal actions) as a result of interrupting bacterial cell wall synthesis.	Instruct patients to mix the contents of a package in about ½ cup of cold water, stir well, and drink all the liquid. Avoid taking this drug when also taking metoclopramide or any other drug that increases GI motility.	This oral drug is available as granules that must be dissolved before taking. Drugs that increase GI motility reduce the absorption of fosfomycin.
Urinary Antiseptics Nitrofurantoin (Furadantin, Macrobid, Macrodantin, Nephronex ✤, Urotoin) 100 mg orally every 12 hr	Drugs from this class usually reduce bacteria in the urinary tract by inhibiting bacterial reproduction (bacteriostatic actions).	Teach patients to shake the bottle well before measuring the drug. Suggest that patients obtain a calibrated spoon for liquid drugs and to not use household spoons. Teach patients to drink a full glass of water with each dose and to have an overall fluid intake of at least 3 L daily. Caution patients to complete the drug regimen even if the symptoms improve or disappear sooner.	Drug is a suspension and requires shaking to ensure homogeneity. Household spoons are not accurate for measuring drugs. Drug precipitates in the kidney tubules and damages the kidney. Fluid intake prevents this complication. Not completing the drug regimen can lead to an infection recurrence and to bacterial drug resistance.
Bladder Analgesics Phenazopyridine (Azo-Dine, Prodium, Pyridiate, Pyridium, Uristat, Phenazo ✤) 200 mg orally 3 times daily, after meals	Drug reduces bladder pain and burning on urination by exerting a topical analgesic or local anesthetic effect on the mucosa of the urinary tract.	Remind patients that this drug will not treat an infection, only the symptoms. Teach patients to take the drug with or immediately after a meal. Warn patients that urine will turn red or orange.	Drug does not have any antibacterial actions. Food reduces the risk for GI disturbances. This expected response to the drug may stain clothing or toilets.
Antispasmodics Hyoscyamine (Anaspaz, Cystospaz, many others) 0.125 mg-0.25 mg orally 3 to 4 times daily	Drug relieves bladder spasms by inhibiting nerve stimulation to the bladder muscle.	Teach patients to notify the prescriber if blurred vision or other eye problems, confusion, dizziness or fainting spells, fast heartbeat, fever, or difficulty passing urine occurs. Teach patients to wear dark glasses in sunlight or other bright-light areas.	These are manifestations of drug toxicity. Drug dilates the pupil and increases eye sensitivity to light.

*Trimethoprim can be given alone to patients with a sulfa allergy.

need to complete all of the prescribed drugs. If the drug will change the color of the urine, as it does with phenazopyridine (Pyridium, Urogesic, Phenazo ✤), inform the patient to expect this change. Offer techniques for remembering the drug schedule, such as the use of a daily calendar or the association of drugs with usual activities (e.g., mealtimes).

Patients may associate symptoms of discomfort with sexual activities and have feelings of guilt and embarrassment. Open and sensitive discussions with a woman who has recurrences of UTI after sexual intercourse can help her find techniques to handle the problem (see Chart 69-2). Explore with her the factors that contribute to her infections, such as sexual penetration when the bladder is full, diaphragm use, and her general resistance to infection. Some positions during intercourse may reduce urethral irritation and subsequent cystitis. Remind the patient that although perineal washing before intercourse is helpful, vigorous cleaning of the perineum with harsh soaps and vaginal douching may irritate the perineal tissues and increase the risk for UTI. At the patient's request, discuss the problem with her and her partner to help them find ways of maintaining their intimate relationship.

? **DECISION-MAKING CHALLENGE**

Patient-Centered Care; Evidence-Based Practice

The 26-year-old female patient with recurrent cystitis tells you that she now "holds" her urine all day and drinks very little to prevent the need to use the public toilet while at work. She is convinced that the toilet is the source of her repeated bladder infections.

1. Is this patient's understanding of the cause of recurrent cystitis correct? Why or why not?
2. What other assessment data should you obtain and why?
3. What will you tell her about the effectiveness of her actions to reduce the need to urinate at a public toilet?
4. What techniques could you suggest for her to use a public toilet for urination?

URETHRITIS

Pathophysiology

Urethritis is an inflammation of the urethra that causes symptoms similar to urinary tract infection (UTI). In men, manifestations include burning or difficulty urinating and a discharge from the urethral meatus. The most common cause of urethritis in men is sexually transmitted diseases (STDs). These include gonorrhea or nonspecific urethritis caused by *Ureaplasma* (a gram-negative bacterium), *Chlamydia* (a sexually transmitted gram-negative bacterium), or *Trichomonas vaginalis* (a protozoan found in both the male and female genital tract).

In women, urethritis causes manifestations similar to those of bacterial cystitis. Urethritis is known by several other terms: *pyuria-dysuria syndrome, frequency-dysuria syndrome, trigonitis syndrome,* and *urethral syndrome.* Urethritis is most common in postmenopausal women and appears to be caused by tissue changes related to low estrogen levels.

PATIENT-CENTERED COLLABORATIVE CARE

Ask the patient about a history of STD, painful or difficult urination, discharge from the penis or vagina, and discomfort in the lower abdomen. Urinalysis may show pyuria (white blood cells [WBCs] in the urine) without a large number of bacteria. However, results of urethral culture may indicate an STD. In women, the diagnosis may be made by excluding cystitis when urinalysis and urethral culture are negative for bacteria but symptoms persist. In such cases, pelvic examination may reveal tissue changes from low estrogen levels in the vagina. Urethroscopy may show low estrogen changes with inflammation of urethral tissues.

STDs and infection are treated with antibiotic therapy. More information on STDs can be found in Chapter 76.

Postmenopausal women often have improvement in their urethral symptoms with the use of estrogen vaginal cream. Estrogen cream applied locally to the vagina increases the amount of estrogen in the urethra as well, and irritating symptoms are reduced.

NONINFECTIOUS DISORDERS

URETHRAL STRICTURES

Urethral strictures are narrowed areas of the urethra. These problems may be caused by complications of an STD (usually gonorrhea) and by trauma during catheterization, urologic procedures, or childbirth. About one third of urethral strictures have no obvious cause. Strictures occur more often in men than in women. They may be a factor in other urologic problems, such as recurrent UTIs, urinary incontinence, and urinary retention.

The most common symptom of urethral stricture is obstruction of urine flow. Strictures rarely cause pain. Because urine stasis can result when flow is obstructed, the patient with a stricture is at risk for developing a UTI and may have overflow incontinence. Overflow incontinence is the involuntary loss of urine when the bladder is overdistended. Assess the patient for these two problems.

A urethral stricture is treated surgically. Dilation of the urethra (using a local anesthetic) is only a temporary measure, not a curative one. Stent placement can be used in some patients. The best chance of long-term cure is with urethroplasty, which is the surgical removal of the affected area with or without grafting to create a larger opening. The recurrence rate after surgery is still high, and most patients need repeated procedures. The urethral stricture location and length are the most important factors affecting choice of interventions and recovery.

URINARY INCONTINENCE
Pathophysiology

Continence is the control over the time and place of urination and is unique to humans and some domestic animals. It is a learned behavior in which a person can suppress the urge to urinate until a socially appropriate location is available (e.g., a toilet). Efficient bladder emptying (i.e., coordination between bladder contraction and urethral relaxation) is needed for continence.

Incontinence is an involuntary loss of urine severe enough to cause social or hygienic problems. It is *not* a normal consequence of aging or childbirth and often is a stigmatizing and an underreported health problem. Many people suffer in silence, are socially isolated, and may be unaware that treatment is available. In addition, the cost of incontinence can be enormous.

Continence occurs when pressure in the urethra is greater than pressure in the bladder. For normal voiding to occur, the urethra must relax and the bladder must contract with enough pressure and duration to empty completely. Voiding should occur in a smooth and coordinated manner under a person's conscious control. Incontinence has several possible causes and can be either temporary or chronic (Table 69-3). Temporary causes usually do not involve a disorder of the urinary tract. The most common forms of adult urinary incontinence are stress incontinence, urge incontinence, overflow incontinence, functional incontinence, and a mixed form.

Stress incontinence is the most common type. Its main feature is the loss of small amounts of urine during coughing, sneezing, jogging, or lifting. In the continent person, the urethra can be relaxed and tightened under conscious control because skeletal muscles of the pelvic floor surround it. When a person feels the urge to urinate, the conscious contraction of the urethra can override a bladder contraction if the urethral contraction is strong enough.

Patients with *stress incontinence* cannot tighten the urethra enough to overcome the increased bladder pressure caused by contraction of the detrusor muscle. This is common after childbirth, when the pelvic muscles are stretched and weakened. The weakened pelvic floor allows the urethra to move during exertion. If the pelvic muscles are not strengthened, this condition continues. Low estrogen levels after menopause also contribute to stress incontinence. Vaginal, urethral, and pelvic floor muscles become thin and weak without estrogen.

Urge incontinence is the perception of an urgent need to urinate as a result of bladder contractions regardless of the volume of urine in the bladder. Normally when the bladder is full, contraction of the smooth muscle fibers of the bladder detrusor muscle signals the brain that it is time to urinate. Continent persons override that signal and relax the detrusor muscle for the time it takes to locate a toilet. Those who suffer from urge incontinence cannot suppress the signal and have a sudden strong urge to void and often leak large amounts of urine at this time. Urge incontinence is also known as an *overactive bladder* (OAB). Overactivity may have no known cause or may be the result of abnormal detrusor contractions

TABLE 69-3 TYPES OF URINARY INCONTINENCE

TYPE	DEFINITION/DESCRIPTION	CAUSE	CLINICAL MANIFESTATIONS
Stress incontinence	The involuntary loss of urine during activities that increase abdominal and detrusor pressure. Patients cannot tighten the urethra sufficiently to overcome the increased detrusor pressure; leakage of urine results.	Weakening of bladder neck supports; associated with childbirth. Intrinsic sphincter deficiency caused by such congenital conditions as epispadias (abnormal location of the urethra on the dorsum of the penis) or myelomeningocele. Acquired anatomic damage to the urethral sphincter (from repeated incontinence surgeries, prostatectomy, radiation therapy, and trauma).	Urine loss with physical exertion, cough, sneeze, or exercise. Usually only small amounts of urine are lost with each exertion. Normal voiding habits (≤8 times per day, ≤2 times per night). Post-void residual usually ≤50 mL. Pelvic examination shows hypermobility of the urethra or bladder neck with Valsalva maneuvers.
Urge incontinence	The involuntary loss of urine associated with a strong desire to urinate. Patients cannot suppress the signal from the bladder muscle to the brain that it is time to urinate.	Unknown.	An abrupt and strong urge to void. May have loss of large amounts of urine with each occurrence.
Detrusor hyperreflexia (reflex incontinence)	The abnormal detrusor contractions result from neurologic abnormalities.	Central nervous system (CNS) lesions from stroke, multiple sclerosis, and parasacral spinal cord lesions. Local irritating factors such as caffeine, medications, or bladder tumor.	Post-void residual ≤50 mL.
Overflow incontinence	The involuntary loss of urine associated with overdistention of the bladder when the bladder's capacity has reached its maximum. The urethra is obstructed, so it fails to relax sufficiently to allow urine to flow, resulting in incomplete bladder emptying or complete urinary retention, causing overflow incontinence.	Diabetic neuropathy; side effects of medication; after radical pelvic surgery or spinal cord damage; outlet obstruction. Causes external to the mechanism of the urethra: an enlarged prostate (male patients) and large genital prolapse (female patients). When the cause is intrinsic to the urethra, abnormal contraction of the skeletal muscle occurs, causing obstruction. This condition, called detrusor dyssynergia, is seen in patients with spinal cord injuries and multiple sclerosis.	Bladder distention, often up to the level of the umbilicus. Constant dribbling of urine.
Mixed incontinence	A combination of stress, urge, and overflow incontinence.	As with each separate disorder.	As with each separate disorder.
Functional incontinence	Leakage of urine caused by factors other than disease of the lower urinary tract.		Quantity and timing of urine leakage vary; patterns are difficult to discern.
Transient causes	Transient causes improve with treatment of the underlying condition.	Loss of cognitive functioning. Loss of awareness that urination is to occur in a socially acceptable place. Abnormal openings in the urinary tract, such as a fistula or diverticulum. Drugs, such as sedatives, hypnotics, diuretics, anticholinergics, decongestants, antihypertensives, and calcium channel blockers. Diabetes insipidus or psychogenic polydipsia. Inability to get to toileting facilities. Direct bladder pressure or urethral obstruction.	Altered mental state, as in delirium, confusion, depression, dementia, sepsis, mental illness, or severe psychological stress. Urinary drainage noted from areas other than the urinary meatus. Some drugs cause altered mental state; others cause increased urine production. Increased urine output. Restraints, restricted mobility. Constipation or fecal impaction.
Permanent causes	Permanent causes are organic but may be improved with treatment.	Cognitive impairment. Traumatic or surgical effects. Those factors contributing to stress incontinence, urge incontinence, and overflow incontinence. Structural or functional defects of the bladder or the sphincters. Injuries or diseases of the spinal cord, brainstem, or cerebral cortex (neurogenic bladder). Congenital defects, including exstrophy of the bladder (bladder turned "inside out") and spina bifida.	Clinical manifestations depend on the cause.

related to other problems. Such problems include stroke and other neurologic problems, other urinary tract problems, and irritation from concentrated urine or artificial sweeteners, caffeine, alcohol, and citric intake. Drugs, such as diuretics, and nicotine can also irritate the bladder.

Mixed incontinence is the presence of more than one type of incontinence. Often urine loss is related to both stress and urge incontinence. The manifestations mimic more than one subtype. This category is more common in older women.

Overflow incontinence occurs when the detrusor muscle fails to contract and the bladder becomes overdistended. This type of incontinence (also known as *reflex incontinence*) occurs when the bladder has reached its maximum capacity and some urine must leak out to prevent bladder rupture. Causes for the underactive (acontractile) bladder may or may not be determined.

The urethra can be obstructed and fail to relax enough to allow urine flow. Incomplete bladder emptying or urinary retention from urethral obstruction results in overflow incontinence.

Functional incontinence is incontinence occurring as a result of factors other than the abnormal function of the bladder and urethra. A common factor is the loss of cognitive function in patients affected by dementia. To maintain continence, a person must be aware that urination needs to occur in a socially acceptable place. Patients with dementia may not have that awareness.

Etiology and Genetic Risk

Incontinence may have temporary or permanent causes. Evaluation of the incontinent patient means considering all possible causes, beginning with those that are temporary and correctable. Surgical and traumatic causes of urinary incontinence are related to procedures or surgery in the lower pelvic structures, areas that contain complex nerve pathways. Radical urologic, prostatic, and gynecologic procedures for treatment of pelvic cancers may result in urinary incontinence. Injury to segments S2 to S4 of the spinal cord may cause incontinence from impairment of normal nerve pathways.

Inappropriate bladder contraction may result from disorders of the brain and nervous system or from bladder irritation due to chronic infection, stones, chemotherapy, or radiation therapy. Failure of bladder contraction occurs with neuropathy of diabetes mellitus and syphilis.

CONSIDERATIONS FOR OLDER ADULTS

Many factors contribute to urinary incontinence in older adults (Chart 69-5). An older person may have decreased mobility from many causes. In inpatient settings, mobility is limited when the older patient is restrained or placed on bedrest. Vision and hearing impairments may also prevent the patient from locating a call light to notify the nurse or assistive personnel of the need to void. Assess for these factors, and minimize them to prevent urinary incontinence. Getting out of bed to urinate is a common cause of falls among older adults.

Incidence/Prevalence

Incontinence is a major health problem that affects more than 13 million people of all ages in the United States (Agency for Health Care Policy and Research [AHCPR], 2001a); about 85% are women. It is most common in older adults, including

---

CHART 69-5 NURSING FOCUS ON THE OLDER ADULT

*Factors Contributing to Urinary Incontinence**

Drugs
- Central nervous system depressants, such as opioid analgesics, decrease the patient's level of consciousness and the urge to void, and they contribute to constipation.
- Diuretics cause frequent voiding, often of large amounts of urine.
- Multiple drugs can contribute to changes in mental status or mobility, and they can irritate the bladder.
- Anticholinergic drugs or drugs with anticholinergic side effects are especially challenging, because they affect both cognition and the ability to void. Monitor patient responses to these drugs early in treatment.

Disease
- Cerebrovascular accidents and other neurologic disorders decrease mobility, sensation, or cognition.
- Arthritis decreases mobility and causes pain.
- Parkinson disease causes muscle rigidity and an inability to initiate movement.

Depression
- Depression decreases the energy necessary to maintain continence.
- Decreased self-esteem and feelings of self-worth decrease the importance to the patient of maintaining continence.

Inadequate Resources
- Patients who need assistive devices (e.g., eyeglasses, cane, walker) may be afraid to ambulate without them or without personal assistance.
- Products that help patients manage incontinence are often costly.
- No one may be available to assist the patient to the bathroom or help with incontinence products.

*These factors are in addition to the physiologic changes of aging given in Chapter 3.

15% to 30% of community-dwelling older people and at least one half of all nursing home residents (AHCPR, 2001a).

In adult patients younger than 65 years, urinary incontinence occurs twice as often in women as in men. Incontinence in women may occur after one or more pregnancies. Men in this age-group rarely experience incontinence unless they have prostate disease or a spinal cord injury.

PATIENT-CENTERED COLLABORATIVE CARE

ASSESSMENT

History

Effective screening includes asking patients to respond "always," "sometimes," or "never" to these questions:
- Do you ever leak urine or water when you don't want to?
- Do you ever leak urine or water when you cough, laugh, or exercise?
- Do you ever leak urine or water on the way to the bathroom?
- Do you ever use pads, tissue, or cloth in your underwear to catch urine?

If any answer is "always" or "sometimes," proceed with a focused assessment (AHCPR, 2001b) (Chart 69-6).

CHART 69-6 FOCUSED ASSESSMENT

The Patient with Urinary Incontinence

Note the presence of risk factors for urinary incontinence:
- Age
- If female, menopausal status
- Neurologic disease:
  Parkinson disease
  Dementia
  Multiple sclerosis
  Stroke
  Spinal injury
- Diabetes mellitus
- Childbirth
- Urologic procedures
- Prescribed and over-the-counter drugs
- Bowel patterns
- Stress/anxiety level

Detail the symptoms of urinary incontinence:
- Leakage
- Frequency
- Urgency
- Nocturia
- Sensation of full bladder before leakage

Obtain a 24-hour intake and output record or a voiding diary:
- Time and amount of oral intake and continent voidings
- Time and estimated amount of incontinent leakages
- Activity around the time of leakage

Assess the patient's:
- Mobility
- Self-care ability
- Cognitive ability
- Communication patterns

Assess the environment for barriers to toileting:
- Privacy
- Restrictive clothing
- Access to toilet

Data from Mather, K. (2002). Nursing assistants' perceptions of their ability to provide continence care. *Geriatric Nursing, 23*(2), 76-81; and Agency for Health Care Policy and Research (AHCPR). (1996; revised 2001). *Urinary incontinence in adults: Acute and chronic management. Clinical practice guideline.* AHCPR Publication No. 96-0682. Rockville, MD: Agency for Health Care Policy and Research, Public Health Service, U.S. Department of Health and Human Services; www.ahcpr.gov/clinic/uhistory.html (*Clinical Practice Guidelines Online: Urinary Incontinence Guideline: Real World Examples of Use*).

Incontinence may be underreported because health care professionals do not ask patients about urine loss. *Do not assume that patients will volunteer the information without specifically being asked.*

Physical Assessment/Clinical Manifestations

Assess the abdomen to estimate bladder fullness, to rule out palpable hard stool, and to evaluate bowel sounds. Determine the amount of *residual urine* (urine remaining in the bladder immediately after voiding) by portable ultrasound. With a health care provider's order, catheterizing the patient immediately after voiding can also be used to determine residual volume. Urinary incontinence is confirmed by evaluating the force and character of the urine stream during voiding. Asking the patient to cough while wearing a perineal pad is useful in evaluating stress incontinence; a wet pad on forceful coughing may indicate stress incontinence. A cystometrogram (see Chapter 68) is used most often for diagnosis.

For women, inspect the external genitalia to determine whether there is apparent urethral or uterine prolapse, cystocele (herniation of the bladder into the vagina), or rectocele. These conditions occur with pelvic floor muscle weakness. An advanced practice nurse puts on an examination glove and inserts two fingers into the vagina to assess the strength of these muscles. Strength is described as *weak, adequate,* or *strong* based on the amount of pressure felt by the nurse as the patient tightens her vaginal muscles. Describe and document the color, consistency, and odor of any secretions from the genitourinary orifices. The urine stream

interruption test (see Chapter 68) is another method of determining pelvic muscle strength. For men, inspect the urethral meatus for any discharge.

A digital rectal examination (DRE) is performed by the physician or advanced practice nurse on both male and female patients. It provides information about the nerve integrity to the bladder. The examiner determines whether there is tactile sensation in the anal area by observing whether the rectal sphincter is relaxed or contracted on digital insertion. Because nerve supply to the bladder is similar to nerve supply to the rectum, the presence of tactile sensation and a rectal sphincter that contracts suggest that the nerve supply to the bladder is intact. The health care provider assesses for prostate enlargement in men as a possible cause of incontinence.

Laboratory Assessment

A urinalysis is useful to rule out infection. This test is the first step in the assessment of incontinent patients of any age. The presence of red blood cells (RBCs), white blood cells (WBCs), leukocyte esterase, or nitrites is an indication for culturing the urine. Any infection is treated before further assessment of incontinence.

Imaging Assessment

Imaging is rarely needed unless surgery is being considered. Urography is most useful for locating the kidneys and ureters. A voiding cystourethrogram (VCUG) may be performed to assess the size, shape, support, and function of the bladder. Problems identified by this test include obstruction (especially prostate obstruction in men) and post-void residual (PVR). Assessment of PVR also can be made with a portable ultrasonographic bladder scanner.

Other Diagnostic Assessment

Patients who have unusual symptoms, medical complications, or a history of failed incontinence surgery may need urodynamic studies to determine the cause of their incontinence. These studies are not standardized procedures and may consist of any combination of these tests:

- Cystourethroscopy to examine the inside of the bladder and urethra directly
- Cystometrogram (CMG) to measure the pressure inside the bladder as it fills
- Urethral pressure profilometry (UPP) to measure the pressure in the urethra in relation to the bladder pressure during various activities
- Uroflowmetry to measure rate and degree of bladder emptying

Testing may take several hours and more than one visit.

Electromyography (EMG) of the pelvic muscles may be a part of the urodynamic studies. A perineometer is a tampon-shaped instrument inserted into the vagina to measure the strength of pelvic muscle contractions. The graph shows the amplitude of muscle contraction to the patient as a method of biofeedback.

❙ ANALYSIS

Priority problems for patients with urinary incontinence include:

1. Stress Urinary Incontinence related to weak pelvic muscles and structural supports

2. Urge Urinary Incontinence related to decreased bladder capacity, bladder spasms, diet, and neurologic impairment
3. Reflex Urinary Incontinence related to neurologic impairment
4. Functional Urinary Incontinence related to impaired cognition or neuromuscular limitations
5. Complete urinary incontinence (mixed) related to many causes

PLANNING AND IMPLEMENTATION

Several interventions are useful for each type of incontinence in addition to drugs, surgical repair, and nutrition therapy.

Reducing Stress Urinary Incontinence

Planning: Expected Outcomes. With appropriate therapy, the patient with urinary incontinence is expected to develop urinary continence. Indicators include that the patient rarely or never demonstrates these actions:

- Urine leakage between voidings
- Urine leakage with increased abdominal pressure (e.g., sneezing, laughing, lifting)

Interventions. Initial interventions for patients with stress incontinence include keeping a diary, behavioral interventions, and drugs. Surgery also may be an option if other interventions are not effective. Explain the purpose of a detailed diary in which the patient records times of urine leakage, activities, and foods eaten. The diary is then used by the health care provider to plan and evaluate interventions. Collection devices, absorbent pads, and undergarments may be used during the sometimes lengthy process of assessment and treatment and by those patients who elect not to pursue further interventions.

Nonsurgical Management. Drug therapy and behavioral interventions (primarily diet and exercise) for stress incontinence require the patient's active participation for success. Nursing interventions focus on teaching patients about the drugs and behavioral strategies and on providing ongoing encouragement, clarification, and support to maximize intervention effects.

Pelvic floor (Kegel) exercise therapy for women with stress incontinence strengthens the muscles of the pelvic floor (circumvaginal muscles). These muscles become strengthened, as any other skeletal muscle does, by frequent, systematic, and repeated contractions.

The most important step in teaching pelvic muscle exercises is to help the patient learn which muscle to exercise. During the pelvic examination in women and the rectal examination in men or women, instruct the patient to tighten the pelvic muscles around your fingers. Then provide feedback about the strength of the contraction. Biofeedback devices, such as electromyography or perineometers (see discussion on p. 1500 in the Other Diagnostic Assessment section), measure the strength of contraction. Retention of a vaginal weight also shows that the patient has identified the proper muscle. Starting and stopping the urine stream or stopping the passage of flatus also indicates that the patient has correctly identified the pelvic muscles.

Instructions for pelvic muscle exercises are given in Chart 69-7. Although improvement may take several months, most patients notice a positive change after 6 weeks. Teach patients to continue the exercises to maintain the improvement.

CHART 69-7 PATIENT AND FAMILY EDUCATION: PREPARING FOR SELF-MANAGEMENT

Pelvic Muscle Exercises

- The pelvic muscles are composed of a sling of muscles that support your bladder, urethra, and vagina. Like any other muscles in your body, you can make your pelvic muscles stronger by alternately contracting (tightening) and relaxing them in regular exercise periods. By strengthening these muscles, you will be able to stop your urine flow more effectively.
- To identify your pelvic muscles, sit on the toilet with your feet flat on the floor about 12 inches apart. Begin to urinate, and then try to stop the urine flow. Do not strain down, lift your bottom off the seat, or squeeze your legs together. When you start and stop your urine stream, you are using your pelvic muscles.
- To perform pelvic muscle exercises, tighten your pelvic muscles for a slow count of 10 and then relax for a slow count of 10. Do this exercise 15 times while you are lying down, sitting up, and standing (a total of 45 exercises). Repeat—and this time rapidly contract and relax the pelvic muscles 10 times. This should take no more than 10 to 12 minutes for all three positions, or 3 to 4 minutes for each set of 15 exercises.
- Begin with 45 exercises a day in three sets of 15 exercises each. You will notice faster improvement if you can do this twice a day, or a total of 20 minutes each day. Remember to exercise in all three positions so your muscles learn to squeeze effectively despite your position. At first, it is helpful to have a designated time and place to do these exercises because you will have to concentrate to do them correctly. After you have been doing them for several weeks, you will notice improvement in your control of urine. However, many people report that improvement may take as long as 3 months.

Nutrition therapy in the form of weight reduction is helpful for obese patients because stress incontinence is made worse by increased abdominal pressure from obesity. Teach the patient to avoid alcohol, nicotine, artificial sweeteners, citrus, and caffeine (bladder irritants). Stress the importance of maintaining an adequate fluid intake, especially water. Refer the patient to the dietitian as needed.

Drug therapy can be useful for some people with stress incontinence. Because bladder pressure is greater than urethral resistance in patients with stress incontinence, drugs may be used to improve urethral resistance (Chart 69-8).

Estrogen is used to treat postmenopausal women with stress incontinence, although it is not known exactly how this drug helps improve continence. Estrogen may increase the blood flow and tone of the muscles around the vagina and urethra, thus improving the patient's ability to contract those muscles during times of increased intra-abdominal stress.

Vaginal cone therapy involves using a set of five small, cone-shaped weights. They are of equal size but of varying weights and are used together with pelvic muscle exercise. The woman inserts the lightest cone, labeled *1*, into her vagina (Fig. 69-1), with the string to the outside, for a 1-minute test period. If she can hold the first cone in place without its slipping out while she walks around, she proceeds to the second cone, labeled *2*, and repeats the procedure. The patient begins her treatment with the heaviest cone she can comfortably hold in her vagina for the 1-minute test period. Treatment periods are 15 minutes twice a day. When the patient can comfortably hold the cone in her vagina for the

15-minute period, she progresses to the next heaviest weight. Treatment is completed with the cone labeled 5.

Weighted vaginal cones can help strengthen the pelvic muscles and decrease stress incontinence but may not help pelvic prolapse. Vaginal cones do not require a prescription.

Other interventions for stress incontinence include behavior modification, psychotherapy, electrical stimulation devices to strengthen urethral contractions, and urethral plugs. Many intravaginal and intrarectal electrical stimulation devices have been used with varying degrees of success. More research is needed to determine the ideal level of stimulation and methods of reducing discomfort before electrical stimulation becomes a standard treatment for incontinence.

One brand of urethral plug is the Reliance insert. It is like a tiny tampon that the patient inserts into the urethra. After insertion, the patient inflates a tiny balloon, which rests at the bladder neck and prevents the flow of urine. To void, the patient pulls a string to deflate the balloon and removes the device. The applicator is reusable, although the tampon part is disposed of after each void.

Surgical Management. Stress incontinence may be corrected by vaginal, abdominal, or retropubic surgeries. Success rates vary between 50% and 90% for most procedures, but these rates are difficult to evaluate because of the varying definitions of cure. Cure also may vary between short-term and long-term (over 5 years) results. Complications can be significant, with rates ranging from less than 2% for collagen or siloxane injection to 50% for bladder neck suspension.

Preoperative Care. Teach the patient about the procedure, and clarify the surgeon's explanation of events surrounding the surgery. Extensive urodynamic testing (see Chapter 68) is often performed before surgery, and you must explain the need for such thorough assessment to the patient and family.

Operative Procedures. The procedures used for women include repositioning the urethra and bladder, changing the structure of the involved tissues, or inserting artificial devices to improve function (Table 69-4).

Postoperative Care. After surgery, assess for and intervene to prevent or detect complications. For prevention of movement or traction on the bladder neck, secure the urethral catheter with tape or a tube holder. If a suprapubic catheter is used instead of a urethral catheter, monitor the dressing for urine leakage and other drainage. Catheters are usually in place until the patient can urinate easily and has residual urine volume after voiding of less than 50 mL. (See Chapters 16 and 18 for a discussion of general care before and after surgery.)

CHART 69-8 **COMMON EXAMPLES OF DRUG THERAPY**

Urinary Incontinence

DRUG/DOSAGE	PURPOSE/ACTION	NURSING INTERVENTIONS	RATIONALES
Estrogen (Cenestin, Cenestin, Enjuvia, Premarin, C.E.S. ♣) 0.3-1.25 mg orally daily **OR** 2-4 g vaginal cream every other day	This drug reduces incontinence, possibly by improving vaginal and urethral blood flow and tone.	Teach patients to report any unusual vaginal bleeding to their health care provider. Teach patients to avoid smoking while on this drug and to report any calf pain or swelling.	Estrogen increases the risk for endometrial cancer. Estrogen increases the risk for thrombophlebitis, especially among women who smoke.
Anticholinergics/Antispasmodics Oxybutynin (Ditropan) 5 mg orally 3-4 times daily; (Ditropan XL) 5-10 mg orally daily Tolterodine (Detrol) 2 mg orally twice daily; (Detrol LA) 4 mg orally daily Propantheline (Pro-Banthine, Propanthel ♣) 7.5-30 mg orally 3-4 times daily Dicyclomine (Barmine, Bentyl) 10-40 mg orally 3-4 times daily Trospium (Sanctura) 20 mg orally every 12 hr	These drugs reduce incontinence by causing bladder muscle relaxation and suppressing the urge to void.	Ask whether the patient has glaucoma before starting the drug. Suggest that patients increase fluid intake and use hard candy to moisten the mouth. Teach patients to increase fluid intake and the amount of dietary fiber. Teach patients to monitor urine output and to report an output significantly lower than intake to the health care provider. Instruct patients taking the extended-release forms of these drugs not to chew or crush the tablet/capsule	Anticholinergics can increase intraocular pressure and make glaucoma worse. Dry mouth is a common side effect of drugs in this category. Constipation is a common side effect of drugs in this category. Drugs in this category can cause urinary retention. Crushing or chewing the tablet/capsule releases all the drug at once, ruining the extended effect and increasing the possibility of side effects
Tricyclic Antidepressants Imipramine (Tofranil, Novo-Pramine ♣) 25-100 mg orally 4 times daily Desipramine (Norpramin) 10-25 mg orally 3 times daily Nortriptyline (Pamelor, Aventyl) 10-25 mg orally 3 times daily	Drugs from this class have some anticholinergic actions and also block acetylcholine receptors. Both actions can relieve urinary incontinence.	Warn patients not to take these drugs with any other tricyclic antidepressants or MAO inhibitors. Teach patients to change positions slowly, especially in the morning. Teach patients the same interventions as for anticholinergic agents.	These drugs prolong the effects of catecholamines (epinephrine and norepinephrine) and lead to hypertensive crisis. These drugs cause dizziness and orthostatic hypotension and can increase the risk for falls. These drugs have anticholinergic activity and produce the same side effects.

MAO, Monoamine oxidase.

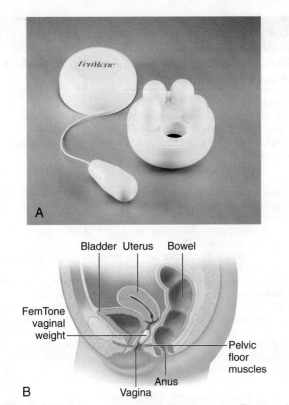

FIG. 69-1 A, FemTone vaginal weights, or cones. The number on the top of each cone represents increasing weight up to the heaviest cone, a 5. **B,** Diagram showing the correct positioning of a vaginal weight, or cone, in place.

Reducing Urge Urinary Incontinence

Planning: Expected Outcomes. The patient with urinary incontinence is expected to use techniques to prevent or manage urge incontinence. Indicators include that the patient often or consistently demonstrates these behaviors:

- Responds to urge in a timely manner
- Gets to toilet between urge and passage of urine
- Avoids substances that stimulate the bladder (e.g., caffeine, alcohol)

Interventions. Interventions for patients with urge incontinence or overactive bladder include behavioral interventions and drugs. Surgery is not the recommended treatment of this condition. Collection devices and absorbent pads and undergarments may be used.

Drug Therapy. Because the hypertonic bladder contracts involuntarily in patients with urge incontinence, drugs that relax the smooth muscle and increase the bladder's capacity are prescribed (see Chart 69-8).

The most effective drugs are anticholinergics, such as propantheline (Pro-Banthine, Propanthel ♣), and anticholinergics with smooth muscle relaxant properties, such as oxybutynin (Ditropan and Ditropan XL), tolterodine (Detrol and Detrol LA), and dicyclomine hydrochloride (Barmine, Bentyl, Spasmoban ♣), all of which inhibit the nerve fibers that stimulate bladder contractions. Anticholinergic drugs have serious side effects and are used along with behavioral interventions. Tricyclic antidepressants with anticholinergic and alpha-adrenergic agonist activity, such as imipramine (Tofranil, Novopramine ♣), have been used successfully. The effectiveness of other drugs, such as flavoxate (Urispas) and

TABLE 69-4	SURGICAL PROCEDURES FOR STRESS INCONTINENCE	
PROCEDURE	**PURPOSE**	**NURSING CONSIDERATIONS**
Anterior vaginal repair (colporrhaphy)	Elevates the urethral position and repairs any cystocele.	Because the operation is performed by vaginal incision, it is often done in conjunction with a vaginal hysterectomy. Recovery is usually rapid, and a urethral catheter is in place for 24-48 hr.
Retropubic suspension (Marshall-Marchetti-Krantz or Burch colposuspension)	Elevates the urethral position and provides longer-lasting results.	The operation requires a low abdominal incision and a urethral or suprapubic catheter for several days postoperatively. Recovery takes longer, and urinary retention and detrusor instability are the most frequent complications.
Needle bladder neck suspension (Pereyra or Stamey procedure)	Elevates the urethral position and provides longer-lasting results without a long operative time.	The combined vaginal approach with a needle and a small suprapubic skin incision does not allow direct vision of the operative site; however, the high complication rates may be due to the selection of patients who, because of their medical condition, are not good candidates for longer retropubic procedures.
Pubovaginal sling procedures	A sling made of synthetic or fascial material is placed under the urethrovesical junction to elevate the bladder neck.	The operation uses an abdominal, vaginal, or combined approach to treat intrinsic sphincter deficiencies. Temporary or permanent urinary retention is common postoperatively.
Midurethral sling procedures	A tensionless vaginal sling is made from polypropylene mesh (or other materials) and placed near the urethrovesical junction to increase the angle, which inhibits movement of urine into the urethra with lower intravesicular pressures.	This outpatient procedure uses a vaginal approach to improve symptoms of stress incontinence. Temporary or permanent urinary retention is common postoperatively.
Artificial sphincters	A mechanical device to open and close the urethra is placed around the anatomic urethra.	The operation is done more frequently in men. The most common complications include mechanical failure of the device, erosion of tissue, and infection.
Periurethral injection of collagen or Siloxane	Implantation of small amounts of an inert substance through several small injections provides support around the bladder neck.	The procedure can be done in an ambulatory care setting and can be repeated as often as necessary. Certain compounds may migrate after injection; an allergy test to bovine collagen must be performed before implantation.

the antihistamines, NSAIDs, beta-adrenergic agonists, and calcium channel blockers, has yet to be determined.

! NURSING SAFETY PRIORITY

Drug Alert

Teach patients taking the extended-release forms of anticholinergic drugs to swallow the tablet or capsule whole without chewing it or crushing it. Chewing or crushing the tablet/capsule ruins the extended-release feature, allowing the entire dose to be absorbed quickly, which increases drug side effects.

? NCLEX EXAMINATION CHALLENGE

Safe and Effective Care Environment

While assessing a client with overactive bladder, the nurse discovers the client also has the following health problems. Which health problem could be made worse by the drug *tolterodine* (Detrol)?
A. Asthma
B. Glaucoma
C. Hypotension
D. Diabetes mellitus

Nutrition Therapy. Teach the patient to avoid foods that have a direct bladder-stimulating or diuretic effect, such as caffeine and alcohol. Spacing fluids at regular intervals throughout the day (e.g., 120 mL every hour or 240 mL every 2 hours) and limiting fluids after the dinner hour (e.g., only 120 mL at bedtime) help avoid fluid overload on the bladder and allow urine to collect at a steady pace.

Behavioral Interventions. Behavioral interventions for urge incontinence include bladder training, habit training, exercise therapy, and electrical stimulation.

Interventions for urinary bladder training and urinary habit training are listed in Chart 69-9. It can be difficult for patients to use these interventions because they involve a great deal of patient participation. Provide ongoing encouragement, clarification, and support to increase the effects of all interventions. Behavioral interventions are often combined with drug therapy for greatest effect.

Bladder training is an education program for the patient that begins with a thorough explanation of the problem of urge incontinence. Instead of the bladder being in control of the patient, the patient learns to control the bladder. For the program to succeed, he or she must be alert, aware, and able to resist the urge to urinate.

Start a schedule for voiding, beginning with the longest interval that is comfortable for the patient, even if the interval is only 30 minutes. Instruct the patient to void every 30 minutes and to ignore any urge to urinate between the set intervals. Once he or she is comfortable with the starting schedule, increase the interval by 15 to 30 minutes. Instruct the patient to follow the new schedule until he or she achieves success again. As the interval increases, the bladder gradually tolerates more volume. Teach him or her relaxation and distraction techniques to maximize success in the retraining. Provide positive reinforcement for maintaining the prescribed schedule.

Habit training (scheduled toileting) is a type of bladder training that is successful in reducing incontinence in cognitively impaired patients. To use habit training, caregivers assist the patient in voiding at specific times (e.g., every 2

CHART 69-9   BEST PRACTICE FOR PATIENT SAFETY AND QUALITY CARE

Bladder Training and Habit Training to Reduce Urinary Incontinence

Bladder Training
- Assess patient's awareness of bladder fullness and ability to cooperate with training regimen.
- Assess the patient's 24-hour voiding pattern for 2 to 3 consecutive days.
- Base the initial interval of toileting on the voiding pattern (e.g., 45 minutes).
- Teach the patient to void every 45 minutes on the first day and to ignore or suppress the urge to urinate between the 45-minute intervals.
- Take the patient to the toilet or remind him or her to urinate at the 45-minute intervals.
- Provide privacy for toileting and run water in the sink to promote the urge to urinate at this time.
- If the patient is not consistently able to resist the urge to urinate between the intervals, reduce the intervals by 15 minutes.
- Continue this regimen for at least 24 hours or for as many days as it takes for the patient to be comfortable with this schedule and not urinate between the intervals.
- When the patient remains continent between the intervals, increase the intervals by 15 minutes daily until a 3- to 4-hour interval is comfortable for the patient.
- Praise successes. If incontinence occurs, work with the patient to re-establish an acceptable toileting interval.

Habit Training
- Assess the patient's 24-hour voiding pattern for 2 to 3 days.
- Base the initial interval of toileting on the voiding pattern (e.g., 2 hours).
- Assist the patient to the toilet or provide a bedpan/urinal every 2 hours (or whatever has been determined to be an appropriate toileting interval for the individual patient).
- During the toileting, remind the patient to void and provide cues such as running water.
- If the patient is incontinent between scheduled toileting, reduce the time interval by 30 minutes until the patient is continent between voidings.
- Assist the patient to toilet and prompt to void at prescribed intervals.
- Do not leave the patient on the toilet or bedpan for longer than 5 minutes.
- Ensure that all nursing staff members comply with the established toileting schedule and do not apply briefs or encourage the patient to "just wet the bed."
- Reduce toileting interval by 30 minutes if there are more than two incontinence episodes in 24 hours.
- If the patient remains continent at the toileting interval, attempt to increase the interval by 30 minutes until a 3- to 4-hour continence interval is reached.
- Praise the patient for successes, and spend extra time socializing with the patient.
- When incontinence occurs, ensure that the patient and bed are cleaned appropriately but do not spend extra time socializing with the patient.
- Discuss daily record of continence with staff to provide reinforcement and encourage compliance with toileting schedule.
- Include unlicensed assistive personnel in all aspects of the habit training.

hours on the even hours). The goal is to get the patient to the toilet before incontinence occurs. The focus is on reducing incontinence. When that has been achieved, the focus may change to increase bladder capacity by gradually lengthening the voiding intervals, but this is only secondary.

! NURSING SAFETY PRIORITY

Action Alert

> Habit training is undermined when unlicensed assistive personnel (UAP) apply absorbent briefs or tell patients to "just wet the bed." This practice also increases the risk for falls because patients may try to get out of bed unassisted to use the toilet. Work with all staff members, including UAP, to implement consistently the toileting schedule for habit training.

Prompted voiding, a supplement to habit training, attempts to increase the patient's awareness of the need to void and to prompt him or her to ask for toileting assistance. Habit training otherwise relies completely on a time schedule.

Exercise therapy with pelvic muscle exercises for urge incontinence has been helpful and is taught in the same way as for stress incontinence (see Chart 69-7). Improved urethral resistance helps the patient overcome abnormal detrusor contractions long enough to get to the toilet.

Electrical stimulation with either an intravaginal or intrarectal electrical stimulation device is available to treat both urge and stress incontinence.

Reducing Reflex Urinary Incontinence

Planning: Expected Outcomes. With appropriate intervention, the patient with reflex incontinence is expected to achieve continence. Indicators include that the patient often or consistently demonstrates these behaviors:

- Recognizes the urge to void
- Maintains a predictable pattern of voiding
- Responds to urge in a timely manner
- Empties bladder completely
- Keeps urine volume in the bladder under 300 mL to prevent overdistention

Interventions. Interventions for the patient with reflex (overflow) incontinence caused by obstruction of the bladder outlet may include surgery to relieve the obstruction. The most common surgical procedures are prostate removal (see Chapter 75) and repair of uterine prolapse (see Chapter 74). For overflow incontinence related to detrusor muscle weakness, the most effective methods of treatment are the behavioral interventions of bladder compression and intermittent self-catheterization.

Drug Therapy. Drugs are prescribed for short-term management of urinary retention, often after surgery. They are not used in long-term management of overflow incontinence caused by a hypotonic bladder. The most commonly used drug is bethanechol chloride (Urecholine), an agent that increases bladder pressure.

Behavioral Interventions. The most common behavioral interventions are bladder compression and intermittent self-catheterization.

Bladder compression uses techniques that promote bladder emptying and include the Credé method, the Valsalva maneuver, double-voiding, and splinting.

For the Credé method, teach the patient how to press over the bladder area, increasing its pressure, or to trigger nerve stimulation by tugging at pubic hair or massaging the genital area. These techniques manually assist the bladder in emptying. In the Valsalva maneuver, breathing techniques increase chest and abdominal pressure. This increased pressure is then directed toward the bladder during exhalation. With the technique of double-voiding, the patient empties the bladder and then, within a few minutes, attempts a second bladder emptying.

For women who have a large *cystocele* (prolapse of the bladder into the vagina), a technique called *splinting* both compresses the bladder and moves it into a better position. The woman inserts her fingers into her vagina, gently lifts the cystocele, and begins to urinate.

Intermittent self-catheterization is often used to help patients with long-term problems of incomplete bladder emptying. It is effective, can be learned fairly easily, and remains the preferred method of bladder emptying in patients who have incontinence as a result of a neurogenic bladder (Newman & Willson, 2011). These points are important in teaching the technique:

- Proper handwashing and cleaning of the catheter reduce the risk for infection.
- A small lumen and good lubrication of the catheter prevent urethral trauma.
- A regular schedule for bladder emptying prevents distention and mucosal trauma.

Patients must be able to understand instructions and have the manual dexterity to manipulate the catheter. Caregivers or family members in the home can also be taught to perform straight catheterization using a clean (rather than sterile) technique with good outcomes (Kannankeril et al., 2011).

Reducing Functional Urinary Incontinence

Planning: Expected Outcomes. The patient with functional urinary incontinence is expected to remain dry. Indicators include that the patient often or consistently demonstrates these behaviors:

- Uses urine containment or collection measures to ensure dryness
- Manages clothing independently

Interventions. Causes of functional (or chronic intractable) incontinence vary greatly. Some are reversible, and others are not. The focus of intervention is treatment of reversible causes. When incontinence is not reversible, urinary habit training (see discussion of habit training, p. 1504) is used to establish a predictable pattern of bladder emptying to prevent incontinence. A final strategy focuses on containment of the urine and protection of the patient's skin. Nonsurgical interventions include applied devices, containment, and catheterization.

Applied devices include intravaginal pessaries for women and penile clamps for men. The intravaginal pessary supports the uterus and vagina and helps maintain the correct position of the bladder. (See Chapter 74 for further discussion of pessaries.) The penile clamp is applied around the outside of the penis to compress the urethra and prevent urine leakage.

The dangers of pessaries and penile clamps include damage to the tissues and infection from constant pressure in sensitive areas. Both devices require either that the patient has manual dexterity or that a caregiver applies and removes the device. Instruct the patient or caregivers in the use of these devices. Male patients may use an external collecting device, such as a condom catheter. Design of an effective external collecting device for women has not been as successful.

Containment is achieved with absorbent pads and briefs designed to collect urine and keep the patient's skin and clothing dry. Many types and sizes of pads are available:

- Shields or liners inserted inside a panty
- Undergarments consisting of full-size pads with waist straps
- Plastic-lined protective underpants with or without elastic legs
- Combination pad and pant systems
- Absorbent bed pads

A major concern with the use of protective pads is the risk that skin breakdown will occur. Materials and costs vary. Some are reusable; others are disposable. The disposal of these products raises ecologic concerns. Avoid use of the word "diaper" when discussing these adult protective pants, however, because of the usual association of diapers with a baby.

Catheterization for control of incontinence may be intermittent or involve an indwelling catheter. Intermittent catheterization is preferred to an indwelling catheter because of the reduced risk for infection. An indwelling urinary catheter is appropriate for patients with skin breakdown who need a dry environment for healing, for those who are terminally ill and need comfort, and for those who are critically ill and require careful measurement of urine output.

Reducing Total or Mixed Urinary Incontinence

Total or mixed urinary incontinence is a combination of two or more types of involuntary urine loss syndromes. For example, stress incontinence and urge incontinence often occur together in women during and after menopause. For the patient with total or mixed incontinence, combinations of assessment techniques (as discussed under each syndrome) are used. Interventions are also combined to promote continence. The problems and interventions for mixed incontinence are the same as for each specific type of incontinence separately. After identifying the specific types of incontinence an individual patient has, apply the appropriate priority patient problems, interventions, and expected outcomes discussed earlier with each incontinence type.

❓ DECISION-MAKING CHALLENGE

Patient-Centered Care; Evidence-Based Practice

The patient is a 32-year-old woman who is 8 weeks postpartum from a vaginal delivery of her first child, a 9-pound boy. She has recently taken up running again and reports a small loss of urine with every running step. She states her mother has had a continuing problem with incontinence for years and seldom leaves her home. The patient is worried that this problem is genetic and will only get worse with time. She is also worried that if surgery is needed to correct the problem, she will have to stop breast-feeding her infant.

1. What other information should you obtain from this patient?
2. What type or types of incontinence is she most likely to have from the information she has provided thus far?
3. Is this problem likely to be genetic? Why or why not?
4. What will you tell her regarding surgery and her concern about being separated from her infant?
5. What measures can you recommend to help reduce her incontinence?

Community-Based Care

Community-based care for the patient with urinary incontinence considers his or her personal, physical, emotional, and social resources. Important personal resources for self-care include mobility, vision, and manual dexterity. When planning care, consider who will be the primary caregiver and what factors may influence the effectiveness of the plan.

Home Care Management

Assess the home environment for barriers that limit access to the bathroom. Eliminate hazards that might slow walking or lead to a fall. Such hazards include throw rugs, furniture with legs that extend into the walking area, slippery waxed or polished floors, and poor lighting.

If the patient must climb stairs to reach a bathroom, handrails should be installed and stairs kept free of obstacles. Toilet seat extenders may help provide the right level of seating so that maximal abdominal pressure may be applied for voiding. Portable commodes may be obtained when ambulatory access to toilets is impractical or impossible. Physical and occupational therapists are valuable resources for assisting with home care management.

Teaching for Self-Management

Teach the patient and family about the cause of the specific type of incontinence, and discuss available treatment options for its management. The teaching plan addresses the prescribed drugs (purpose, dosage, method and route of administration, and expected and potential side effects). Instruct the patient and family about the importance of weight reduction and dietary modification to help control urinary incontinence. Remind the patient who smokes that nicotine can contribute to bladder irritation and that smoker's cough can cause urine leakage.

When external devices or protective pads are needed, describe the possible options, discuss the advantages and disadvantages of each, and help the patient make a selection best for his or her lifestyle and resources. For patients who will use intermittent catheterization or those with artificial urinary sphincters, demonstrate the correct technique to the patient or caregiver. Evaluate return demonstrations for correct technique. Chart 69-10 also addresses teaching.

Psychosocial Preparation

The embarrassment of incontinence can be devastating to a patient's self-esteem, body image, and relationships. Sexual intimacy is often adversely affected by incontinence. The unpredictable nature of incontinence creates anxiety. Patients are often embarrassed to seek help, and even when resources are identified, they may need help to feel comfortable in using the resources. Buying supplies at a local store may threaten privacy.

Accept and acknowledge the personal concerns of the patient and caregiver. Never make their concerns seem trivial. Help the patient learn methods of managing the fear or anxiety. As he or she learns the specifics of the plan that will allow control of urinary incontinence, the confidence to resume social interactions should return.

Health Care Resources

Referral to home care agencies for help with personal care and to continence clinics that specialize in evaluation and treatment may be helpful. In many continence clinics, nurses

Urinary Incontinence

- Maintain a normal body weight to reduce the pressure on your bladder.
- Do not try to control your incontinence by limiting your fluid intake. Adequate fluid intake is necessary for kidney function and health maintenance.
- If you have a catheter in your bladder, follow the instructions given to you about maintaining the sterile drainage system.
- If you are discharged with a suprapubic catheter in your bladder, inspect the entry site for the tube daily, clean the skin around the opening gently with warm soap and water, and place a sterile gauze dressing on the skin around the tube. Report any redness, swelling, drainage, or fever to your physician.
- Do not put anything into your vagina, such as tampons, drugs, hygiene products, or exercise weights, until you check with your physician at your 6-week checkup after surgery.
- Do not have sexual intercourse until after your 6-week postoperative checkup.
- Do not lift or carry anything heavier than 5 pounds or participate in any strenuous exercise until your physician gives you postoperative clearance. In some cases, this could be as long as 3 months.
- Avoid exercises, such as running, jogging, step or dance aerobic classes, rowing, cross-country ski or stair-climber machines, and mountain biking. Brisk walking without any additional hand, leg, or body weights is allowed. Swimming is allowed after all drains and catheters have been removed and your incision is completely healed.
- If Kegel exercises are recommended, ask your nurse for specific instructions.

collaborate with physicians and other health care professionals to evaluate and manage patients. The treatment plan is specific for each patient; supplies and products are custom selected.

Patients may benefit from education and from the support of others who experience similar concerns. The National Association for Continence (NAFC) (www.nafc.org), Access to Continence Care and Treatment (www.wellweb.com/INCONT/acct/contents.htm), and the Wound, Ostomy, and Continence Nurses (www.wocn.org) publish newsletters and educational materials written with simple, easy-to-understand explanations. The American Foundation for Urologic Disease (www.afud.com) provides information on many areas of bladder dysfunction. The Agency for Healthcare Research and Quality (AHRQ) has also published a caregiver guide (AHCPR Publication No. 96-0683) for the public that is available on the Internet or by calling (800) 358-9295. Local hospitals often have local NAFC-approved support groups.

? NCLEX EXAMINATION CHALLENGE

Physiological Integrity

For which client living at home is intermittent self-catheterization an inappropriate method for incontinence management?
A. 36-year-old woman who is blind
B. 46-year-old man who has paraplegia
C. 56-year-old woman who has diabetes
D. 66-year-old man who has severe osteoarthritis

▌EVALUATION: OUTCOMES

Evaluate the care of the patient with urinary incontinence based on the identified priority patient problems. The expected outcomes are that the patient will:

- Describe the type of urinary incontinence experienced
- Demonstrate knowledge of proper use of drugs and correct procedures for self-catheterization, use of the artificial sphincter, or care of an indwelling urinary catheter
- Demonstrate effective use of the selected exercise or bladder-training program
- Select and use incontinence devices and products
- Have a reduction in the number of incontinence episodes

Specific indicators for these outcomes are listed for each priority patient problem under the Planning and Implementation section (see earlier).

UROLITHIASIS

Pathophysiology

Urolithiasis is the presence of *calculi* (stones) in the urinary tract. Stones often do not cause symptoms until they pass into the urinary tract, where they can cause excruciating pain. Nephrolithiasis is the formation of stones in the kidney. Formation of stones in the ureter is ureterolithiasis.

Urologic stones are caused by many disorders. However, the exact mechanism of stone formation is not entirely understood. Everyone excretes crystals in the urine at some time, but fewer than 10% of people form stones. Most stones contain calcium (calcium oxalate or calcium phosphate) as one part of the stone complex. Struvite (15%), uric acid (8%), and cystine (3%) are more rare compositions of stones. Formation of stones involves three conditions:

- Slow urine flow, resulting in supersaturation of the urine with the particular element (e.g., calcium) that first becomes crystallized and later becomes the stone
- Damage to the lining of the urinary tract (e.g., abrasion from crystals)
- Decreased amounts of inhibitor substances in the urine that would otherwise prevent supersaturation and crystal aggregation

High urine acidity (as with uric acid and cystine stones) or alkalinity (as with calcium phosphate and struvite stones) and drugs (as with triamterene, indinavir, and acetazolamide) contribute to stone formation.

One example of a metabolic problem causing stone formation begins when excessive amounts of calcium are absorbed through the intestinal tract (the most common cause of hypercalciuria). As blood circulates through the kidneys, the excess calcium is filtered into the urine, causing supersaturation of calcium in the urine. If fluid intake is poor, such as when a patient is dehydrated, supersaturation is more likely to occur and the risk for calcium combining with another compound to form a larger molecule increases. Calcium complexes often serve as a center for other deposits, and eventually a stone forms.

Stones that form in the kidney and then pass into the ureter often lodge in areas where the ureter bends or slightly changes shape. When the stone occludes the ureter and blocks the flow of urine, the ureter dilates. Enlargement of the ureter is called hydroureter.

The pain associated with ureteral spasm is excruciating and may cause the patient to go into shock from stimulation of nearby nerves. In addition, hematuria (bloody urine) may result from damage to the urothelial lining. If the obstruction is not removed, urinary stasis can cause infection and impair kidney function on the side of the blockage. As the blockage persists, hydronephrosis (enlargement of the kidney caused by blockage of urine lower in the tract and filling of the kidney with urine) and permanent kidney damage may develop.

Etiology and Genetic Risk

The cause of urolithiasis is unknown. At least 90% of patients who form stones have a metabolic risk factor. Table 69-5 lists some metabolic problems that often cause stone formation.

A diet high in calcium is not believed to cause stones unless a metabolic problem or kidney tubule defect already exists. Data suggest that a normal-calcium diet that is relatively low in animal protein, sodium, or both may help prevent stone formation. A low-calcium diet does not prevent stone formation (Brenner, 2008). Urinary stasis, urinary retention, immobility, and dehydration all increase the risk for stones to form. Except for the use of the thiazides for calcium oxalate stones, diuretics can cause volume depletion and thus may promote the formation of stones. Generally, fluid intake sufficient to cause a urine output of 2 to 2.5 L daily is recommended.

TABLE 69-5	METABOLIC DEFECTS THAT COMMONLY CAUSE CALCULI
METABOLIC DEFICIT	**ETIOLOGY**
Hypercalcemia	
Primary	Absorptive: increased intestinal calcium absorption
	Renal: decreased kidney tubular excretion of calcium
Secondary	Resorptive: hyperparathyroidism, vitamin D intoxication, kidney tubular acidosis, prolonged immobilization
Hyperoxaluria	
Primary	Genetic: autosomal recessive trait resulting in high oxalate production
Secondary	Dietary: excess oxalate from foods such as spinach, rhubarb, Swiss chard, cocoa, beets, wheat germ, pecans, peanuts, okra, chocolate, and lime peel
Hyperuricemia	
Primary	Gout is an inherited disorder of purine metabolism (20% of patients with gout have uric acid calculi)
Secondary	Increased production or decreased clearance of purine from myeloproliferative disorders, thiazide diuretics, carcinoma
Struvite	Made of magnesium ammonium phosphate and carbonate apatite; formed by urea splitting by bacteria, most commonly, Proteus mirabilis; needs an alkaline urine to form
Cystinuria	Autosomal recessive defect of amino acid metabolism that precipitates insoluble cystine crystals in the urine

GENETIC/GENOMIC CONSIDERATIONS

More than 30 genetic variations are associated with the formation of kidney stones. Single gene disorders are rare. More commonly, nephrolithiasis is a complex disease, with genetic variation in intestinal calcium absorption, kidney calcium transport, or kidney phosphate transport all associated with stone formation (Brenner, 2008). Always ask a patient with a kidney or ureteral stone whether other family members have also had this problem.

Incidence/Prevalence

The incidence of stone disease is high and varies with geographic location, race, and family history. About 12% of adults will have at least one episode of kidney stone disease. The incidence is higher in men; however, struvite stones are twice as common in women. Recurrence rates vary depending on the type of treatment. The recurrence rate of untreated calcium oxalate stones is 35% to 50% in 5 to 10 years. A higher recurrence of stones occurs in patients with a family history of stone disease and in those who had their first occurrence by age 25 years.

🌐 CULTURAL AWARENESS

The incidence of stone disease is most common in the southeastern United States, Japan, and Western Europe. Calcium stone disease is more common in men than in women and tends to occur in young adults or during early middle adulthood. Kidney stone disease occurs more often in younger adults than older adults and more commonly among white people (Brenner, 2008). For patients in these higher-risk groups, nursing care includes teaching family members, as well as patients, about the manifestations of a stone and interventions to reduce stone formation.

PATIENT-CENTERED COLLABORATIVE CARE

ASSESSMENT

Ask the patient about a personal or family history of urologic stones. Obtain a diet history, including fluid intake patterns. If he or she has a history of stone formation, ask about past treatment, whether chemical analysis of the stone was performed, and what preventive measures are followed.

The major manifestation of stones is severe pain, commonly called renal colic. Flank pain suggests that the stone is in the kidney or upper ureter. Flank pain that extends toward the abdomen or to the scrotum and testes or the vulva suggests that stones are in the ureters or bladder. Pain is most intense when the stone is moving or when the ureter is obstructed.

Renal colic begins suddenly and is often described as "unbearable." Nausea, vomiting, pallor, and diaphoresis often accompany the pain. A large stationary stone in the kidney (staghorn calculus), however, rarely causes much pain because it is not moving. Frequency and dysuria occur when a stone reaches the bladder. Oliguria (scant urine output) or anuria (absence of urine output) suggests obstruction, possibly at the bladder neck or urethra. *Urinary tract obstruction is an emergency and must be treated immediately to preserve kidney function.*

Examine the patient to detect bladder distention. The patient may appear pale, ashen, and diaphoretic and may suffer from excruciating pain. Vital signs may be moderately elevated with pain; body temperature and pulse are elevated with infection. Blood pressure may decrease if the severe pain causes shock.

Urinalysis is performed in patients with suspected stones. Hematuria is common, and blood may make the urine appear smoky or rusty. The presence of RBCs is usually caused by stone-induced trauma on the lining of the ureter, bladder, or urethra. WBCs and bacteria may be present as a result of urinary stasis. Increased *turbidity* (cloudiness) and odor indicate that infection may also be present. Microscopic examination of the urine may identify crystals from which stones could form. Urinary pH is measured to determine acidity or alkalinity.

The serum WBC count is elevated with infection. Increases in the serum calcium, serum phosphate, or serum uric acid levels indicate excess minerals are present and may contribute to stone formation.

Stones are easily seen on x-rays of the kidneys, ureters, and bladder (KUB) (Fig. 69-2); IV urograms; or computed tomography (CT). Noncontrast CT is the most sensitive test to identify urinary tract stones. These procedures confirm the presence and location of the stones.

IV urography is useful for identifying whether the urinary tract is obstructed. However, because of the risk for acute kidney injury (AKI) induced by contrast dye, other diagnostic tests may be chosen for high-risk patients (older adults and patients with diabetes mellitus, multiple myeloma, or elevated serum creatinine levels).

Renal ultrasonography creates images from sound waves hitting structures of different densities. Solid structures, such as stones, are extremely dense, and the images of stones are clear. Small stones are harder to identify and locate. Ultrasound is the main method used to identify hydronephrosis from any cause.

INTERVENTIONS

Nursing interventions focus on pain management and prevention of infection and urinary obstruction. Most patients can expel the stone without invasive procedures. The most important factors regarding whether a stone will pass on its own are its composition, size, and location. The larger the stone and the higher up in the urinary tract it is, the less likely it is to be passed. When the stone is passed, it should be captured and sent to the laboratory for analysis. Other interventions are needed when the patient does not pass the stone spontaneously (Fig. 69-3).

Managing Pain

Nonsurgical and surgical approaches are used to assist the patient with a kidney stone achieve an acceptable degree of pain relief.

Nonsurgical Management. Nonsurgical measures to relieve pain include strategies to enhance stone passing, as well as direct pain management.

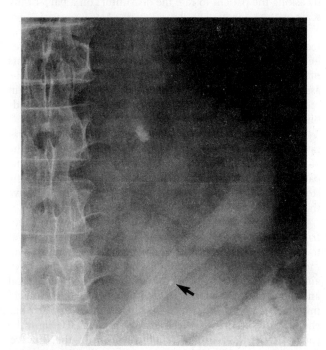

FIG. 69-2 Urinary stones on x-ray of the kidneys, ureters, and bladder (KUB).

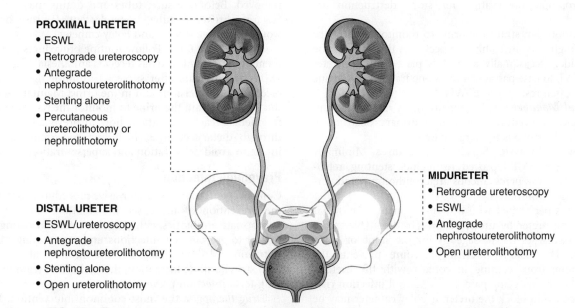

PROXIMAL URETER
- ESWL
- Retrograde ureteroscopy
- Antegrade nephrostoureterolithotomy
- Stenting alone
- Percutaneous ureterolithotomy or nephrolithotomy

DISTAL URETER
- ESWL/ureteroscopy
- Antegrade nephrostoureterolithotomy
- Stenting alone
- Open ureterolithotomy

MIDURETER
- Retrograde ureteroscopy
- ESWL
- Antegrade nephrostoureterolithotomy
- Open ureterolithotomy

FIG. 69-3 Treatment options for ureteral stones. *ESWL,* Extracorporeal shock wave lithotripsy.

Drug therapy is needed most in the first 24 to 36 hours when pain is most severe. Opioid analgesics are often needed to control the severe pain caused by stones in the urinary tract. Opioid agents, such as morphine (Statex ✚), are often given IV for rapid pain relief. NSAIDs such as ketorolac (Toradol) in the acute phase may be quite effective. When NSAIDs are used, the risk for bleeding is increased and the use of extracorporeal shock wave lithotripsy is delayed.

Control of pain is more effective when drugs are given at regularly scheduled intervals or by a constant delivery system (e.g., skin patch) instead of PRN. Spasmolytic drugs, such as oxybutynin chloride (Ditropan) and propantheline bromide (Pro-Banthine, Propanthel ✚), are important for control of pain (see Chart 69-8). Give the drugs, and assess the response by asking the patient to rate the discomfort on a pain-rating scale.

Complementary and alternative therapy with relaxation techniques, such as hypnosis and imagery, therapeutic or healing touch, and acupuncture, can reduce pain. Patients often have difficulty finding a comfortable position. Thus assisting the patient with positioning can often aid in pain reduction. Breathing techniques, such as those used in childbirth, can also help him or her relax.

Other management techniques include avoiding overhydration and underhydration in the acute phase to help make the passage of a stone less painful. Strain the urine and teach the patient to strain it to monitor for stone passage. Send any stone passed to the laboratory for analysis, because preventive therapy is based on stone composition.

Lithotripsy, also known as *extracorporeal shock wave lithotripsy (ESWL)*, is the use of sound, laser, or dry shock waves to break the stone into small fragments. The patient receives moderate sedation and lies on a flat table with the lithotriptor aimed at the stone, which is located by fluoroscopy. A local anesthetic cream is applied to the skin site over the stone 45 minutes before the procedure. During the procedure, cardiac rhythm is monitored by electrocardiography (ECG) and the shock waves are delivered in synchrony with the R wave. About 500 to 1500 shock waves are applied in 30 to 45 minutes. Continuous ECG monitoring for dysrhythmia and fluoroscopic observation for stone destruction are maintained.

After lithotripsy, strain the urine to monitor the passage of stone fragments. Bruising may occur on the flank of the affected side. Occasionally a stent is placed in the ureter before ESWL to ease passage of the stone fragments. Cystine stones are often resistant to ESWL.

Surgical Management. Minimally invasive surgical and open surgical procedures are used if urinary obstruction occurs or if the stone is too large to be passed.

Minimally Invasive Surgical Procedures. Minimally invasive surgical (MIS) procedures include stenting, retrograde ureteroscopy, percutaneous ureterolithotomy, and percutaneous nephrolithotomy.

Stenting is performed with a stent—a small tube that is placed in the ureter by ureteroscopy. The stent dilates the ureter and enlarges the passageway for the stone or stone fragments. This totally internal procedure prevents the passing stone from coming in contact with the ureteral mucosa, thereby reducing pain, bleeding, and infection risk, all of which could block the ureter. A Foley catheter may be placed to facilitate passage of the stone through the urethra.

Retrograde ureteroscopy is an endoscopic procedure. The ureteroscope is passed through the urethra and bladder into the ureter. Once the stone is seen, it is removed using grasping baskets, forceps, or loops. Lithotripsy also can be performed through the ureteroscope. A Foley catheter may be placed to facilitate passage of the stone fragments through the urethra.

Percutaneous ureterolithotomy or nephrolithotomy is the removal of a stone in the kidney or ureter through the skin. The patient lies prone or on the side and receives local or general anesthesia. The physician identifies the ideal entry point with fluoroscopy and then passes a needle into the collecting system of the kidney. Once a tract has been made in the kidney, other equipment, such as an intracorporeal (inside the body) ultrasonic or laser lithotriptor, can be used to break up and remove the stone. An endoscope with a special attachment to grasp and extract the stone can be used. Often a nephrostomy tube is left in place at first to prevent the stone fragments from passing through the urinary tract.

Provide routine nephrostomy tube care and monitor the patient for complications after the procedure. Complications include bleeding at the site or through the tube, pneumothorax, and infection.

Open Surgical Procedures. When other stone removal attempts have failed or when risk for a lasting injury to the ureter or kidney is possible, an *open ureterolithotomy* (into the ureter), *pyelolithotomy* (into the kidney pelvis), or *nephrolithotomy* (into the kidney) procedure may be performed. These procedures are used for a large or impacted stone.

Preoperative Care. Prepare the patient for the selected procedure by explaining how, when, and where the procedure will be performed. Describe what he or she can expect to see, hear, and feel before and after the procedure. The patient is given nothing by mouth and also receives a bowel preparation before the procedure. (See Chapter 16 for routine care before surgery.)

Operative Procedures. The retroperitoneal area is entered through a large flank incision, as for nephrectomy (see Chapter 70), pyelolithotomy, or nephrolithotomy, and through a lower abdominal incision for ureterolithotomy. The urinary tract is entered surgically, and the stone is removed. Before closure, tubes and drains may be placed (e.g., nephrostomy tube, ureteral stent, Penrose or other wound drainage device, and Foley catheter).

Postoperative Care. Follow routine procedures for assessment of the patient who has received anesthesia. (See Chapter 18 for routine care after surgery.) Monitor the amount of bleeding from incisions and in the urine. Maintain adequate fluid intake. Strain the urine to monitor the passage of stone fragments. Teach the patient how to prevent future stones through dietary changes, including consistent daily fluid intake to avoid dehydration and supersaturation.

Preventing Infection

Control of infections before invasive procedures is critical for the prevention of urosepsis. Interventions include giving appropriate antibiotics, either to eliminate an existing infection or to prevent new infections, and maintaining adequate nutrition and fluid intake. Because infection always occurs with struvite stone formation, the health care team plans for long-term infection prevention.

Drug therapy is the most common intervention. Broad-spectrum antibiotics, such as the aminoglycosides (e.g., gentamicin [Garamycin]) and cephalosporins (e.g., cephalexin [Keflex, Novo-Lexin ✦]), are first prescribed for infections occurring with stone disease. The broad coverage is effective against gram-negative organisms. After the results of the culture and sensitivity (C&S) studies are obtained, more specific antibiotics may be prescribed. C&S studies are often done 48 hours after the start of antibiotic therapy and again 48 hours after completion of the prescribed course of therapy.

Blood levels of antibiotics may be measured to ensure that adequate levels have been reached. If the desired blood level of these antibiotics is exceeded, toxic effects and kidney damage may result. If the blood level of the antibiotic is not adequate, organisms may not be completely eliminated. Evidence of a new infection (e.g., chills, fever, altered mental status) warrants the collection of a urine sample for repeat C&S tests.

For the patient with struvite stones, periodic and long-term monitoring of the urine for infection is needed. Urine cultures are checked monthly for 3 months and then quarterly for 1 year. Drugs that prevent bacteria from splitting urea, such as acetohydroxamic acid (Lithostat) and hydroxyurea (Hydrea), are often prescribed long-term for patients with struvite stones. Serum creatinine levels are monitored in patients receiving acetohydroxamic acid. This drug is stopped if creatinine levels are above 2 mg/dL. Review interventions aimed at preventing urinary tract infection (UTI). (See Interventions discussion on p. 1494 in the Cystitis section.)

Nutrition therapy ideally includes adequate calorie intake with a balance of all food groups. Encourage a fluid intake sufficient to dilute urine to a light color throughout the 24-hour day (typically 2 to 3 L/day) unless another health problem requires fluid restriction.

Preventing Obstruction

Measures to prevent urinary obstruction by stones include a high intake of fluids (3 L/day or more) and careful measures of intake and output. Fluid intake sufficient to provide a diluted urine helps prevent dehydration, promotes the flow of urine, and decreases the chance of crystals forming a stone. Interventions also depend on the type of stone the patient has formed. Drugs, diet modification, and fluid intake are the major strategies used to prevent future stones.

Drug therapy to prevent obstruction depends on what is causing stone formation and the type of stone formed. Teach the patient the reason for the drug, and assess for side effects or adverse drug reactions. Some drugs may need to be avoided because they may contribute to stone formation.

Drugs to treat *hypercalciuria* (high levels of calcium in the urine) include thiazide diuretics (e.g., chlorothiazide [Diuril] or hydrochlorothiazide [HydroDIURIL, Urozide ✦]), orthophosphate, and sodium cellulose phosphate. Thiazide diuretics promote calcium resorption from the kidney tubules back into the body, thereby reducing urine calcium loads. Orthophosphates alter calcium-phosphorus metabolism, resulting in decreased urine saturation of calcium oxalate. Sodium cellulose phosphate reduces intestinal absorption of calcium.

For patients with *hyperoxaluria* (high levels of oxalic acid in the urine), allopurinol (Zyloprim) and vitamin B_6 (pyridoxine) are used.

For patients with chronic gout, allopurinol helps prevent the formation of urate (uric acid) stones. To alkalinize the urine, drugs such as potassium citrate, 50% sodium citrate, and sodium bicarbonate are used. The desired urine pH is 6 to 6.5. Because the normal urine pH averages 5 to 6, the desired values are termed *alkaline*.

For patients with *cystinuria* (high levels of cystine in the urine), both alpha-mercaptopropionylglycine (AMPG) and captopril (Capoten) lower urine cystine levels. They are used when hydration and urine alkalinization have not been successful.

Nutrition therapy depends on the type of stone formed (Table 69-6). Collaborate with the dietitian to plan for and teach the appropriate diet to the patient.

Other measures can help the patient pass the stone more quickly. Encourage the patient to walk as often as possible. Walking promotes passage of stones and reduces bone calcium resorption. Check the urine pH daily, and strain all urine with filter paper to collect passed stones and fragments.

TABLE 69-6	DIETARY TREATMENT FOR KIDNEY AND URINARY STONES	
STONE TYPE	**DIETARY INTERVENTIONS**	**RATIONALES**
Calcium oxalate	Avoid oxalate sources, such as spinach, black tea, and rhubarb.	Reduction of urinary oxalate content may help prevent these stones from forming. Urinary pH is not a factor.
	Decrease sodium intake.	High sodium intake reduces kidney tubular calcium reabsorption.
Calcium phosphate	Limit intake of foods high in animal protein to 5-7 servings per week and never more than 2 per day.	Reduction of protein intake reduces acidic urine and prevents calcium precipitation.
	Some patients may benefit from a reduced calcium intake (milk, other dairy products).	Reduction of urine calcium concentration may prevent calcium precipitation and crystallization.
	Decrease sodium intake.	High sodium intake reduces kidney tubular calcium reabsorption.
Struvite (magnesium ammonium phosphate)	Limit high-phosphate foods, such as dairy products, organ meats, and whole grains.	Reduction of urinary phosphate content may help prevent these stones from forming.
Uric acid (urate)	Decrease intake of purine sources, such as organ meats, poultry, fish, gravies, red wines, and sardines.	Reduction of urinary purine content may help prevent these stones from forming.
Cystine	Limit animal protein intake (as above).	Reduces urinary uric acid.
	Encourage oral fluid intake (500 mL every 4 hours while awake and 750 mL at night).	Increased fluid helps dilute the urine and prevents the cystine crystals from forming.

CHART 69-11   PATIENT AND FAMILY EDUCATION: PREPARING FOR SELF-MANAGEMENT

Urinary Calculi

- Finish your entire prescription of antibiotics to ensure that you will not get a urinary tract infection.
- You may resume your usual daily activities.
- Remember to balance regular exercise with sleep and rest.
- You may return to work 2 days to 6 weeks after surgery, depending on the type of intervention, your personal tolerance, and your physician's directives.
- Depending on the type of stone you had, your diet may be restricted to prevent further stone formation.
- Remember to drink at least 3 L of fluid a day to dilute potential stone-forming crystals, prevent dehydration, and promote urine flow.
- Monitor urine pH as directed (possibly up to three times per day).
- Expect bruising after lithotripsy. The bruising may be quite extensive and may take several weeks to resolve.
- Your urine may be bloody for several days after surgery.
- Pain in the region of the kidneys or bladder may signal the beginning of an infection or the formation of another stone. Report any pain, fever, chills, or difficulty with urination immediately to your physician or nurse.
- Keep follow-up appointments to check on infection, and have repeat cultures done.

Teaching for self-management includes the key points listed in Chart 69-11. Follow-up care to evaluate effects of intervention includes a 24-hour urine collection and serum chemical analysis. The patient often has great anxiety and fear that a stone and its pain may recur. In addition to anxiety about the pain, the risk for repeated surgical interventions or permanent and serious kidney damage is of major concern. Psychosocial preparation is enhanced when patients know what to expect and what actions to take if problems develop. Reassure the patient that preventive and health promotion activities help prevent recurrence.

UROTHELIAL CANCER

Pathophysiology

Urothelial cancers are malignant tumors of the *urothelium*—the lining of transitional cells in the kidney, renal pelvis, ureters, urinary bladder, and urethra. Most urothelial cancers occur in the bladder. Thus the term *bladder cancer* is often used to describe this condition.

In the United States, about 73% of urinary tract cancers are transitional cell carcinomas of the bladder (American Cancer Society [ACS], 2011). The second most common site of urinary tract cancer is the kidney and renal pelvis. Urothelial cancers are usually low grade, have multiple points of origin (*multifocal*), and are recurrent. Once the cancer spreads beyond the transitional cell layer, it is highly invasive and can spread beyond the bladder. Because of the nature of this cancer, patients may have recurrence up to 10 years after being cancer-free (ACS, 2011).

Tumors confined to the bladder mucosa are treated by simple excision, whereas those that are deeper but not into the muscle layer are treated with excision plus intravesical (inside the bladder) chemotherapy. Cancer that has spread deeper into the bladder muscle layer is treated with more extensive surgery, often a radical cystectomy (removal of the bladder and surrounding tissue) with urinary diversion. Chemotherapy and radiation therapy are used in addition to surgery. If untreated, the tumor invades surrounding tissues, spreads to distant sites (liver, lung, and bone), and ultimately leads to death.

Exposure to toxins, especially chemicals used in the hairdressing, rubber, paint, electric cable, and textile industries, increases the risk for bladder cancer. The greatest risk factor for bladder cancer is tobacco use. Other risks include *Schistosoma haematobium* (a parasite) infection, excessive use of drugs containing phenacetin, and long-term use of cyclophosphamide (Cytoxan, Procytox ♦).

About 67,000 new cases of bladder cancer are diagnosed each year in the United States, and about 13,000 deaths occur each year from the disease (ACS, 2011). This cancer is rare in adults younger than 40 years and is most common after 60 years of age.

Health Promotion and Maintenance

Many people believe that tobacco use is associated with cancers only of organs that come into direct contact with it, such as the lungs. However, many compounds in tobacco enter the bloodstream and affect distant organs, such as the bladder. Therefore encourage everyone who smokes to quit and nonsmokers to not start. Just as important, encourage anyone who comes into contact with dry, liquid, or gaseous chemicals to take precautions. Some people work with chemicals, and others may come into contact with them while engaging in hobbies, such as refinishing furniture. Many chemicals and fumes can enter the body through contact with skin and with mucous membranes in the respiratory tract. Use of personal protective equipment, such as gloves and masks, can reduce this contact. Also encourage anyone who works with chemicals to shower or bathe and change clothing as soon as contact is completed.

PATIENT-CENTERED COLLABORATIVE CARE

ASSESSMENT

Physical Assessment/Clinical Manifestations

Ask about the patient's perception of his or her general health. Document the gender and age of the patient. Ask about active and passive exposure to cigarette smoke. To detect exposure to harmful environmental agents, ask the patient to describe his or her occupation and hobbies in detail. Also ask the patient to describe any change in the color, frequency, or amount of urine and any abdominal discomfort.

Observe the overall appearance of the patient, especially skin color and general nutritional status. Inspect, percuss, and palpate the abdomen for asymmetry, tenderness, and bladder distention.

Examine the urine for color and clarity. Blood in the urine is often the first major sign of bladder cancer. It may be gross or microscopic and is usually painless and intermittent. Dysuria, frequency, and urgency occur when infection or obstruction is also present.

Psychosocial Assessment

Assess the patient's emotions, including his or her response to a tentative diagnosis of bladder cancer, and note anxiety, fear, sadness, anger, or guilt. Early manifestations are painless, and many patients ignore the blood in the urine because it is intermittent. They also may be reluctant to seek treatment because they suspect a sexually transmitted disease (STD). As a result, they may have guilt or anger about their own delays in seeking medical attention.

Assess the patient's methods of coping and the degree of support from family members. Social support may provide motivation and improve coping during recovery from treatment.

Diagnostic Assessment

The only significant finding on a routine urinalysis is gross or microscopic hematuria. Cytologic testing on voided urine specimens is not usually helpful. Bladder-wash specimens and bladder biopsies are the most specific tests for cancer.

Cystoscopy with retrograde urography is usually performed to evaluate painless hematuria. A biopsy of a visible bladder tumor can be performed during cystoscopy. This is essential for staging and is usually performed in a day-surgery unit before admission to the hospital for treatment. IV urography may be used when there is blood in the urine. Excretory urography is useful in identifying obstructions, especially where the ureter joins the bladder. Computed tomography (CT) scans show tumor invasion of surrounding tissues. Ultrasonography shows masses but is less valuable for tumor staging. Magnetic resonance imaging (MRI) may help assess deep, invasive tumors.

▌INTERVENTIONS

Therapy for the patient with bladder cancer usually begins with surgical removal of the tumor for diagnosis and staging of disease. For tumors extending beyond the mucosa, surgery is followed by intravesical chemotherapy or immunotherapy. High-grade or recurrent tumors are treated with more radical surgery plus intravesical chemotherapy, radiotherapy, or both. Systemic chemotherapy is reserved for patients with distant metastases. (See Chapter 24 for general care of the patient receiving chemotherapy or radiation therapy.)

Nonsurgical Management

Prophylactic immunotherapy with intravesical instillation of bacille Calmette-Guérin (BCG), a live virus compound, is used to prevent tumor recurrence of superficial cancers. This procedure is more effective than single-agent chemotherapy. Usually the agent is instilled in an outpatient clinic and allowed to dwell in the bladder for a specified length of time, usually 2 hours. When the patient urinates, live virus is excreted with the urine.

Teach patients receiving this treatment to prevent contact of the live virus with other members of the household by not sharing a toilet with others for at least 24 hours after instillation. Instruct men to urinate while sitting down to avoid splashing the urine. After 24 hours, the toilet should be completely cleaned using a solution of 10% liquid bleach. If only one toilet is available in the household, teach the patient to flush the toilet after use and follow this by adding one cup of undiluted bleach to the bowl water. The bowl is then flushed after 15 minutes and the seat and flat surfaces of the toilet wiped with a cloth containing a solution of 10% liquid bleach. Teach the patient to wear gloves during the cleaning and to dispose of the cloth after sealing it in a plastic bag.

Underwear or other clothing that has come into contact with the urine during the 24 hours after instillation should be washed separately from other clothing in a solution of 10% liquid bleach. Sexual intercourse is avoided for 24 hours after the instillation.

Multiagent chemotherapy is successful in prolonging life after distant metastasis has occurred but rarely results in a cure. Radiation therapy is also useful in prolonging life.

Surgical Management

The type of surgery for bladder cancer depends on the type and stage of the cancer and the patient's general health. Complete bladder removal (cystectomy) with additional removal of surrounding muscle and tissue offers the best chance of a cure for large, invasive bladder cancers. Four alternatives are used after cystectomy: ileal conduit; continent pouch; bladder reconstruction, also known as *neobladder;* and ureterosigmoidostomy.

Preoperative Care. Specific patient education depends on the type and extent of the planned surgical procedure. Coordinate education before surgery with the patient, surgeon, and enterostomal therapist (ET). Discuss the type of planned urinary diversion and the selection of a site for the stoma. Including the patient in this planning improves the chances for the patient to have a positive attitude about body image and a positive self-image. Use educational counseling to ensure understanding about self-care practices, methods of pouching, control of urine drainage, and management of odor.

The site selected for the stoma should be visible and avoid folds of skin, bones, and scar tissue. When possible, the patient's waistline or belt area is avoided. Prepare the patient for the number and type of drains that will be present after surgery. General care before surgery is discussed in Chapter 16.

Operative Procedures. Transurethral resection of the bladder tumor (TURBT) or partial cystectomy is performed for small, early, superficial tumors. In a partial (segmental) cystectomy, a portion of the bladder is removed. This procedure is used when there is only a single isolated bladder tumor.

When the entire bladder must be removed (complete cystectomy), the ureters are diverted into a collecting reservoir. Techniques for urinary diversion are shown in Fig. 69-4. With an ileal conduit, the ureters are surgically placed in the ileum and urine is collected in a pouch on the skin around the stoma. More often, continent reservoirs or "neobladders" are created from an intestinal graft. With cutaneous ureterostomy or ureteroureterostomy, the ureter opening is brought out onto the skin. The cutaneous ureterostomies may be located on either side of the abdomen or side by side.

Postoperative Care. After cutaneous ureterostomy, an external pouch covers the ostomy to collect urine. Work with the ET to focus care on the wound, the skin, and urinary drainage. (See Chapters 59 and 60 for ostomy care.)

The patient with a Kock's pouch, a continent reservoir, may have a Penrose drain and a plastic Medena catheter in the stoma. The drain removes lymphatic fluid or other secretions; the catheter ensures urine drainage so that suture lines can heal. The patient with a neobladder usually requires 2 to 4 days in the intensive care unit (ICU) and will have a drain at first in the event the neobladder requires irrigation. Later, irrigation can be performed with intermittent catheterization. Irrigation is performed to ensure patency. There is no sensation of bladder fullness with a neobladder because sensory nerves are not attached. As a result, the patient will need to learn new cues to void, such as prescribed times or

Ureterostomies divert urine directly to the skin surface through a ureteral skin opening (stoma). After ureterostomy, the patient must wear a pouch.

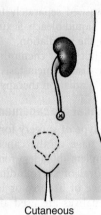

Cutaneous ureterostomy

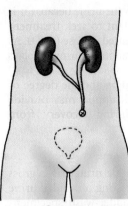

Cutaneous ureteroureterostomy

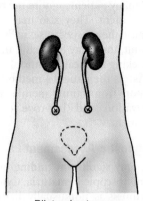

Bilateral cutaneous ureterostomy

Conduits collect urine in a portion of the intestine, which is then opened onto the skin surface as a stoma. After the creation of a conduit, the patient must wear a pouch.

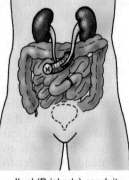

Ileal (Bricker's) conduit

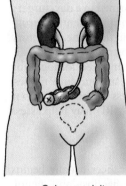

Colon conduit

Ileal reservoirs divert urine into a surgically created pouch, or pocket, that functions as a bladder. The stoma is continent, and the patient removes urine by regular self-catheterization.

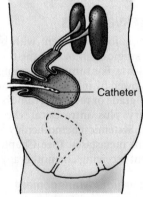

Catheter

Continent internal ileal reservoir (Kock's pouch)

Sigmoidostomies divert urine to the large intestine, so no stoma is required. The patient excretes urine with bowel movements, and bowel incontinence may result.

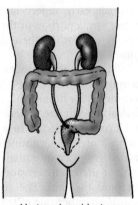

Ureterosigmoidostomy

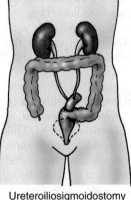

Ureteroiliosigmoidostomy

FIG. 69-4 Urinary diversion procedures used in the treatment of bladder cancer.

noticing a feeling of neobladder pressure. General care after surgery is discussed in Chapter 18.

Different types of drains and nephrostomy catheters are used, sometimes on a temporary basis, to drain urine from the kidney. Some are totally internal, with no drainage to the outside. Others may drain exclusively to the outside and urine is collected in a pouch or bag. For this type of drainage system, urine output remains constant. A decrease in amount or no drainage is cause for concern and must be reported to the surgeon or nephrologist, as is leakage around the catheter.

Some nephrostomy tubes are connected both to the new bladder (internal drainage) and to an external drainage system. With this type of system, urine output from the external portion of the catheter is variable. With any drainage system, intervention is needed if the external catheter is accidentally partially or completely pulled out. Immediately notify the surgeon or nephrologist. If the catheter remains partially in place, secure it from further movement. This action may result in a re-insertion process rather than a total replacement.

Community-Based Care

Teaching for Self-Management

Teach the patient and family about drugs, diet and fluid therapy, the use of external pouching systems, and the technique for catheterizing a continent reservoir.

With some procedures, the patient may need electrolyte replacement to prevent long-term deficits. Teach him or her to avoid foods that are known to produce gas if the urinary diversion uses the intestinal tract. When intestinal production of gas is excessive, flatus can induce incontinence.

Patients who have a neobladder created often have extreme weight loss during the first few weeks after surgery. Collaborate with a dietitian to develop a diet plan specific to the patient to meet his or her caloric needs.

! NURSING SAFETY PRIORITY

Action Alert

Infection is common in patients who have a neobladder. Teach patients and family members the manifestations of infection and the importance of reporting the infection immediately to the surgeon.

Instruct the patient and family about any changes in self-care activities related to the urinary diversion. In collaboration with the enterostomal therapist, demonstrate external pouch application, local skin care, pouch care, methods of adhesion, and drainage mechanisms. If a Kock's pouch has been created, teach the patient how to use a catheter to drain the pouch. For all instruction, observe at least one return demonstration by the patient or the caregiver. Ideally, the patient assumes responsibility for self-care before discharge.

Assist the patient to prepare for the impact of urinary diversion on self-image, body image, sexual functioning, and self-esteem. Counseling provides information and support to reduce feelings of powerlessness.

Through discussions with the patient about usual social situations, help him or her gain control over new toileting practices. Men with a urinary diversion into the sigmoid colon need to learn the habit of sitting to urinate. For patients of either gender, promote confidence in social situations by encouraging frequent emptying of urinary collection devices before traveling or attending social functions. Resumption of sexual activity is a major concern for many, regardless of age, and may remain problematic for many years after surgery (Gemmill et al., 2010) (see the Evidence-Based Practice Box at right). Address this topic openly and with sensitivity. Cystectomy causes impotence in men, but treatment is available (see Chapter 75).

Health Care Resources

The United Ostomy Association and the American Cancer Society have educational materials that may be useful to patients. Refer patients and family members to local chapters or units of these organizations. In some areas, local support groups have meetings to assist others and to send visitors to provide peer counseling and support. Home care personnel may assist with follow-up, easing the transition from hospital to home. The Wound, Ostomy, and Continence Nurses Society has educational programs and a journal for the care of patients with ostomies.

EVIDENCE-BASED PRACTICE

How Does Urinary Diversion for Bladder Cancer Affect Sexual Expression and Quality of Life?

Gemmill, R., Ferrell, B., Krouse, R., & Grant, M. (2010). Going with the flow: Quality-of-life outcomes of cancer survivors with urinary diversion. *Journal of the Wound, Ostomy and Continence Nurses, 37*(1), 65-72.

Urinary diversion (UD) is a common outcome after treatment of bladder cancer and requires continued daily personal attention. In addition, the urinary system is anatomically associated with many of the physical aspects of sexual expression and behavior for both men and women. As survival rates from bladder cancer increase, more individuals are long-term with UD. One purpose of this descriptive study was to describe health-related quality of life (HRQOL) concerns among cancer survivors with different types of UD (continent or incontinent).

The study methods involved distribution of a HRQOL questionnaire that had been developed, tested, revised, and retested over many years at multiple sites for its utility in assessing the four dimensions of physical well-being, psychological well-being, social well-being, and spiritual well-being among cancer patients. This highly valid questionnaire was revised to include issues that were specifically ostomy-related. The revised tool had acceptable levels of reliability and validity as indicated by a subscale Cronbach alpha ranging between 0.77 to 0.90 and an overall Cronbach alpha of $r = 0.95$.

Data obtained from a total of 307 respondents meeting study criteria were analyzed using univariate logistical regression and multivariate logistical regression methods. The median time of having a UD in this sample was 9.5 years (range of 3 to 13 years). Only one third of respondents reported having an overall "excellent" HRQOL. Common areas of dissatisfaction were related to reduced sexual activity, daily time involved with care related to the UD, peristomal irritation, bowel changes, urine leakage, fear of disease recurrence, and embarrassment related to urine leakage or body image. A major finding of this study was that these issues were not limited to the immediate postoperative period but persisted for years.

Level of Evidence: 4

Although very large, the study was descriptive in nature without randomization of subject selection or assignment. The information collected relied on subject self-report. The methods of statistical analysis were appropriate for the research questions posed. A major strength of the study was the collection of data from long-term recipients of UD.

Commentary: Implications for Practice and Research

The results of this study indicate that adjustment of patients to UD requires considerable time and that quality of life is affected for years. The problems associated with sexuality were experienced by both men and women. Many of the issues identified by the respondents could be made easier by nursing interventions that include adequate patient teaching, long-term support, and continued access to wound and ostomy care nurses.

? NCLEX EXAMINATION CHALLENGE

Health Promotion and Maintenance

Which statement made by the client who is receiving intravesicular instillations of BCG for bladder cancer indicates to the nurse that more teaching is needed?

A. "Holding my urine for at least 8 hours after the treatment keeps the drug in contact with my bladder."

B. "Drinking plenty of fluids during the evening after the treatment helps get the drug out of my system."

C. "Sitting to urinate for 24 hours after treatment prevents exposure of other people to the drug."

D. "Avoiding intercourse for 24 hours after treatment reduces my wife's exposure to the drug."

BLADDER TRAUMA

Pathophysiology

Bladder trauma can be caused by penetrating or blunt injury to the lower abdomen. Penetrating injury may occur by stabbing, gunshot wound, or other trauma in which objects pierce the abdominal wall. A fractured pelvis with puncture of the bladder by bone fragments is the most common cause of bladder trauma. Bladder trauma may also be a result of sexual assault.

Blunt trauma compresses the abdominal wall and the bladder. A seat belt may compress the bladder hard enough to cause injury, especially if the bladder is full or distended.

PATIENT-CENTERED COLLABORATIVE CARE

Patients with a penetrating bladder wound often have anuria or hematuria. In the emergency department, initial assessment includes inspection of the urinary meatus for blood.

Diagnostic tests include cystography and voiding cysto-urethrography (VCUG). If kidney or ureteral trauma is suspected, IV urography is scheduled before cystography so that any leakage of bladder contrast medium does not mask the outlines of the kidneys or ureters. The cystogram shows whether there is a defect in bladder filling; the voiding cysto-urethrogram defines bladder emptying.

Bladder trauma, other than a simple contusion, requires surgical intervention. When bone fractures are present, they are stabilized before bladder repair to prevent further bladder damage. Surgical interventions include repairing the bladder wall and peritoneal membrane. Usually, repairs of the bladder are closure procedures.

Patients with an anterior bladder wall injury usually have a Penrose drain and a Foley catheter in place after surgery. Those with a posterior bladder wall injury have a Penrose drain and Foley or suprapubic catheter after surgery. In some instances, vaginal or rectal fistulas may also require repair.

Psychosocial support is critical for patients who have sustained traumatic injuries. Refer them to counseling resources to assist in dealing with psychosocial issues.

NURSING CONCEPT REVIEW

What might you NOTICE if the patient is experiencing urinary elimination problems as a result of cystitis?
- Patient urinates frequently in small amounts.
- Patient reports pain and burning on urination.
- Patient reports suprapubic pain.
- Urine is cloudy and foul-smelling.
- Urine may be darker or smoky or have obvious blood in it.

What should you INTERPRET and how should you RESPOND to a patient experiencing urinary elimination problems as a result of a UTI?

Perform and interpret physical assessment, including:
- Ask how long manifestations have been present.
- Ask about low back pain (midline in men) or flank pain.
- Ask whether he or she has had a UTI in the past; how long ago; how it was treated; and if antibiotics were prescribed, whether the drug course was completed.
- Ask about the presence of pregnancy or any chronic health problem, especially diabetes.
- Determine fluid intake and output volumes.
- Assess for bladder distention by palpation or with a bedside bladder ultrasound scanner (see Chapter 68).

- Assess for pain over the right and left kidneys.
- Examine the meatus for irritation.
- If a Foley catheter is in place, determine why it is in use and how long it has been present.
- Interpret laboratory values:
  - Is the complete blood count within normal limits?
  - Is the urinalysis positive for bacteria, leukocyte esterase, nitrate, red blood cells, or white blood cells?

Respond by:
- Assessing the need for continuing indwelling catheter
- Teaching the patient comfort measures
- Teaching the patient the importance of completing the prescribed drug regimen

On what should you REFLECT?
- Observe patient for evidence of improved urinary output (see Chapter 68).
- Think about what may have caused this infection in a hospitalized patient (or long-term care resident) and what steps could be taken to prevent a similar episode.
- Think about what patient-teaching focus could help reduce the risk for future UTI.

GET READY FOR THE NCLEX® EXAMINATION!

KEY POINTS

Review these Key Points for each NCLEX Examination Client Needs Category.

Safe and Effective Care Environment
- Use sterile technique when inserting a catheter or any other instrument into the urinary system.

- Use Contact Precautions with any drainage from the genitourinary tract.

Health Promotion and Maintenance
- Teach patients to clean the perineal area daily, after voiding, after having a bowel movement, and after sexual intercourse.

- Encourage all patients to maintain an adequate fluid intake (minimum of 1.5 to 2.5 L daily unless another health problem requires fluid restriction).
- Instruct women who have stress incontinence the proper way to perform pelvic floor strengthening exercises.
- Teach patients who come into contact with chemicals in their workplaces or with leisure-time activities to avoid direct skin and mucous membrane contact with these chemicals.

Psychosocial Integrity

- Allow the patient the opportunity to express feelings or concerns regarding a potential cancer diagnosis.
- Use a nonjudgmental approach in caring for patients with urinary incontinence.
- Avoid referring to protective pads or pants as "diapers."
- Recognize the need for the patient undergoing cystectomy and urinary diversion to grieve about the body image change.
- Assess the patient's level of comfort in discussing issues related to elimination and the urogenital area.

- Use language and terminology during kidney and urinary assessment that the patient is comfortable using.
- Refer patients to community resources and support groups.

Physiological Integrity

- Identify hospitalized patients at risk for bacteriuria and urosepsis.
- Report immediately any condition that obstructs urine flow.
- Instruct patients with UTI to complete all prescribed antibiotic therapy even when symptoms of infection are absent.
- Evaluate daily the indications for maintaining indwelling catheters, and discontinue their use as soon as possible.
- Teach patients the expected side effects and any adverse reactions to prescribed drugs.
- Assess the patient's manual dexterity and cognitive awareness before teaching a regimen of intermittent self-catheterization.

CHAPTER 70

Care of Patients with Renal Disorders

Chris Winkelman

LEARNING OUTCOMES

Health Promotion and Maintenance

1. Encourage patients with diabetes to achieve tight glycemic control.
2. Encourage patients with hypertension to follow their treatment regimens to maintain blood pressure within the target range.
3. Teach patients at risk for urinary tract infection (UTI) to maintain a daily fluid intake of 2 L unless another health problem requires fluid restriction.
4. Teach patients on antibiotic therapy for a UTI to complete the drug regimen.
5. Teach all people strategies to prevent kidney trauma.

Psychosocial Integrity

6. Use language the patient is comfortable with during assessment of the kidney and urinary system.

7. Encourage the patient to express feelings or concerns about a change in kidney function.
8. Explain treatment procedures to patients and families.

Physiological Integrity

9. Explain the genetics of autosomal dominant polycystic kidney disease.
10. Use laboratory data and clinical manifestations to determine the effectiveness of therapy for pyelonephritis.
11. Describe the clinical manifestations of hydronephrosis.
12. Explain the relationship between hypertension and kidney disease.
13. Coordinate nursing care for the patient with pyelonephritis.
14. Coordinate nursing care for the patient during the first 24 hours after a nephrectomy.

The kidneys participate in *urinary elimination* by filtering wastes and balancing fluids, electrolytes, acids, and bases. Any problem that disrupts kidney function limits the ability to meet that need and has the potential to impair general homeostasis (Fig. 70-1). The kidneys work together with many other organ systems. Thus kidney disorders affect systemic health and can lead to life-threatening outcomes. Kidney disorders are classified as congenital, obstructive, infectious, glomerular, and degenerative. Kidney tumors and kidney trauma are also described in this chapter. Acute kidney injury and chronic kidney disease are discussed in Chapter 71.

CONGENITAL DISORDERS

POLYCYSTIC KIDNEY DISEASE

Pathophysiology

Polycystic kidney disease (PKD) is an inherited disorder in which fluid-filled cysts develop in the nephrons. In the dominant form, only a few nephrons have cysts until the person reaches his or her 30s. In the recessive form of the disease, nearly 100% of nephrons have cysts from birth. Cysts develop anywhere in the nephron as a result of abnormal kidney cell division.

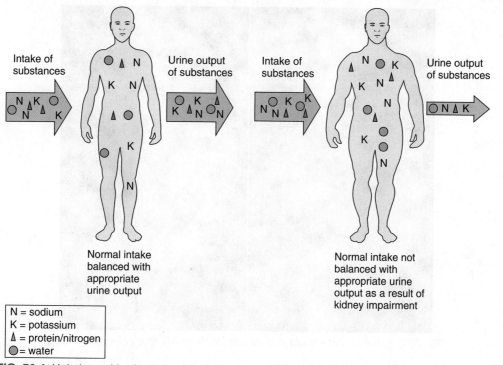

Intake of substances | Urine output of substances | Intake of substances | Urine output of substances

Normal intake balanced with appropriate urine output

Normal intake not balanced with appropriate urine output as a result of kidney impairment

N = sodium
K = potassium
Δ = protein/nitrogen
● = water

FIG. 70-1 Unbalanced body water, electrolytes, and waste products as a result of kidney problems that prevent adjustments in urinary elimination.

Over time, small cysts become much larger (up to a few centimeters in diameter) and more widely distributed. The growing cysts damage the glomerular and tubular membranes. As the cysts fill with fluid and enlarge, the nephron and kidney function become less effective.

The kidney tissue is eventually replaced by nonfunctioning cysts, which look like clusters of grapes (Fig. 70-2). The kidneys become very large. Each cystic kidney may enlarge to two or three times its normal size, becoming as large as a football, and may weigh 10 pounds or more each. Other abdominal organs are displaced, and the patient has pain. The fluid-filled cysts are also at increased risk for infection, rupture, and bleeding, which increase pain.

Most patients with PKD have high blood pressure. The cause of hypertension is related to kidney ischemia from the enlarging cysts. As the vessels are compressed and blood flow to the kidneys decreases, the renin-angiotensin system is activated, raising blood pressure. Control of hypertension is a top priority because proper treatment can disrupt the process that leads to further kidney damage.

Cysts may occur also in other tissues, such as the liver and blood vessels. They may reduce liver function. In addition, the incidence of cerebral *aneurysms* (outpouching and thinning of an artery wall) is higher in patients with PKD. These aneurysms may rupture, causing bleeding and sudden death. For reasons as yet unknown, kidney stones occur in 8% to 36% of the patients with PKD. Heart valve problems (e.g., mitral valve prolapse), left ventricular hypertrophy, and colonic diverticula also are common in patients with PKD.

Etiology and Genetic Risk

PKD has several forms and can be inherited as either an autosomal dominant trait or, less commonly, as an autosomal recessive trait. People who inherit the recessive form of PKD

usually die in early childhood. The 5% to 10% incidence of PKD in patients with no family history occurs as a result of a new gene mutation.

GENETIC/GENOMIC CONSIDERATIONS

The autosomal dominant form of PKD (ADPKD) is the most common form of polycystic disease. Children of parents who have the autosomal dominant form of PKD have a 50% chance of inheriting the gene that causes the disease. Fig. 70-3 shows a typical pedigree for a family with ADPKD. Presentation of ADPKD can vary for age of onset, manifestations, and illness severity, even within one family. However, it is highly penetrant, meaning that nearly 100% of people who inherit a PKD gene will develop kidney cysts by age 30 (Nussbaum et al., 2007). Half of these people develop chronic kidney disease by age 50 years. ADPKD-1 is the most common and most severe form of the autosomal dominant disease. ADPKD-2 has a slower rate of cyst formation, so symptoms occur later in life and progression to end-stage kidney disease and other complications is delayed.

Autosomal recessive PKD is rare, and most people with the disease die in early childhood. It is caused by a gene mutation different from the dominant form. To inherit a recessive gene, both parents must carry a copy of the mutated allele and both mutated alleles must be inherited. Thus each child has a 1-in-4 chance of inheriting autosomal recessive polycystic disease.

There is no way to prevent PKD, although early detection and management of hypertension may slow the progression of kidney damage. Genetic counseling may be useful for adults who have one parent or both parents with PKD. Family history analysis is a simple assessment that can be used to help identify people at risk for PKD (see Fig. 70-3).

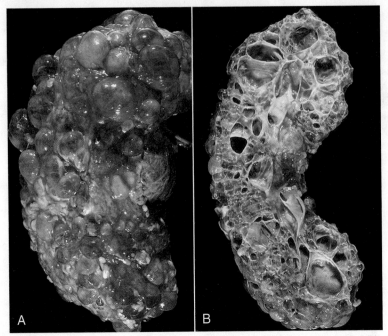

FIG. 70-2 External surface **(A)** and internal surface **(B)** of a polycystic kidney.

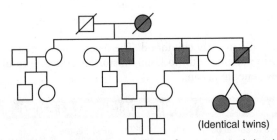

(Identical twins)

FIG. 70-3 Four-generation pedigree for autosomal dominant polycystic kidney disease (ADPKD). Colored-in symbols indicate family members with ADPKD. Slashes indicate the person has died.

Incidence/Prevalence

PKD is a common disorder, affecting 250,000 to 500,000 people in the United States. It is more common in white people than in people of other races. Men and women have an equal chance of inheriting the disease because the gene responsible for PKD is not located on the sex chromosomes (Polycystic Kidney Disease Foundation, 2011).

PATIENT-CENTERED
COLLABORATIVE CARE

ASSESSMENT

History

Explore the family history of a patient with suspected or actual PKD, and ask whether either parent was known to have PKD or whether there is any family history of kidney disease. The age at which the problem was diagnosed in the parent and any related complications are important to obtain. Ask about constipation, abdominal discomfort, a change in urine

CHART 70-1	KEY FEATURES

Polycystic Kidney Disease

- Abdominal or flank pain
- Hypertension
- Nocturia
- Increased abdominal girth
- Constipation
- Bloody or cloudy urine
- Kidney stones

color or frequency, high blood pressure, headaches, and a family history of sudden death from a stroke.

Physical Assessment/Clinical Manifestations

Chart 70-1 lists key features of PKD. Pain is often the first manifestation. Inspect the abdomen. A distended abdomen is common as the cystic kidneys swell and push the abdominal contents forward. Polycystic kidneys are easily palpated because of their increased size. Proceed with *gentle* abdominal palpation because the cystic kidneys and nearby tissues may be tender and palpation is uncomfortable.

The patient also may have flank pain as a dull ache or as sharp and intermittent discomfort. Dull, aching pain is caused by increased kidney size with distention or by infection within the cyst. Sharp, intermittent pain occurs when a cyst ruptures or a stone is present. When a cyst ruptures, the patient may have bright red or cola-colored urine. Infection is suspected if the urine is cloudy or foul smelling or if there is dysuria (pain on urination).

Nocturia (the need to urinate excessively at night) is an early manifestation and occurs because of decreased urine concentrating ability. As kidney function further declines, the patient has increasing hypertension, edema, and uremic manifestations such as anorexia, nausea, vomiting, pruritus, and fatigue (see Chapter 71). Because berry aneurysms often occur in patients with PKD, a severe headache with or without neurologic or vision changes requires attention.

Psychosocial Assessment

As an inherited disorder, PKD may cause psychosocial responses. The patient often has seen the effects and problems of the disease in close family members. He or she may have had a parent who died or close relatives who required dialysis or transplantation. While obtaining the family history, listen carefully for spoken and unspoken feelings of anger, resentment, futility, sadness, or anxiety. Such feelings may need further exploration. The focus of the feelings may be one or both parents or the process of diagnosis and treatment. Feelings of guilt and concern for the patient's children may also complicate the issue.

Diagnostic Assessment

Urinalysis shows proteinuria (protein in the urine) once the glomeruli are involved. Hematuria (blood in the urine) may be gross or microscopic. Bacteria in the urine indicate infection, usually in the cysts. Obtain a urine sample for culture and sensitivity testing when there is evidence of infection. As kidney function declines, serum creatinine and blood urea nitrogen (BUN) levels rise. With decreasing kidney function, creatinine clearance decreases. Changes in kidney handling of sodium may cause either sodium losses or sodium retention.

Diagnostic studies include renal sonography, computed tomography (CT), and magnetic resonance imaging (MRI). Small cysts are detected by sonography, CT, or MRI. Renal sonography shows evidence of PKD, with minimal risk.

❓ DECISION-MAKING CHALLENGE

Patient-Centered Care; Teamwork and Collaboration

The 36-year-old unaffected daughter of a 63-year-old man with PKD is visiting her two 31-year-old sisters (identical twins) who are both hospitalized with acute complications of their PKD (see Fig. 70-3). You find the unaffected sister in the hallway crying. She tells you that she feels sad that her sisters are suffering so much and guilty that she has escaped the disease. She also tells you that, although she wants to donate a kidney to the sister whose disease has already progressed to end-stage kidney disease (ESKD), she is not a blood type match. (Both parents have type A blood, the unaffected sister has type A blood, and the affected twin sisters have type O blood.) In addition, she has a 2-year-old son and a 6-week-old son, and she fears that they may either develop the disease or pass it on to their children. She also tells you that she is grateful that her father's PKD is not as severe as her sisters' disease.

1. What is the pattern of inheritance for the PKD depicted in Fig. 70-3 (and explain why it could not be another pattern of inheritance)?

2. Are the unaffected sister's fears of passing the disease on to her children or grandchildren founded or unfounded? Provide a rationale for your decision.

3. Is the unaffected sister correct in thinking that her blood type difference eliminates the possibility that she could donate a kidney to one of her sisters? Why or why not? (You may need to review blood type issues in Chapter 42 and kidney transplantation issues in Chapter 71.)

4. What comments or suggestions could you make to help the unaffected sister feel less guilty about her own good health?

❚ INTERVENTIONS

Interventions for the patient with PKD include pain management and prevention of infection, constipation, hypertension, and chronic kidney disease. When the disease progresses to the point that the kidneys no longer function to clear wastes, care becomes similar to that needed for the patient with end-stage kidney disease (see Chapter 71).

Managing Pain

Comfort strategies include drug therapy and complementary approaches. A combination may be most effective. NSAIDs are used cautiously because of their tendency to reduce kidney blood flow. Aspirin-containing compounds are avoided to reduce the risk for bleeding.

If cyst infection causes discomfort, antibiotics such as trimethoprim/sulfamethoxazole (Bactrim, Septra, Trimpex) or ciprofloxacin (Cipro) are prescribed. (See Chart 69-4 in Chapter 69.) These drugs enter the cyst wall. Monitor the serum creatinine levels because antibiotic therapy can be nephrotoxic. Apply dry heat to the abdomen or flank to promote comfort when kidney cysts are infected. When pain is severe, cysts can be reduced by needle aspiration and drainage; however, they usually refill.

Teach the patient methods of relaxation and comfort using deep breathing, guided imagery, or other strategies. The expected outcome is patient self-management. (See Chapter 5 for pain management.)

Preventing Constipation

Teach the patient who has adequate urine output how to prevent constipation by maintaining adequate fluid intake, increasing dietary fiber when fluid intake is more than 2500 mL/24 hr, and exercising regularly. Explain that pressure on the large intestine may occur as the polycystic kidneys increase in size. The patient should know that these recommendations for bowel management might change, particularly if end-stage kidney disease also develops. Advise him or her about the use of stool softeners and bulk agents, including the careful use of laxatives, to prevent chronic constipation.

Controlling Hypertension and Preventing End-Stage Kidney Disease

Blood pressure control is necessary to reduce cardiovascular complications and slow the progression of kidney dysfunction. Nursing interventions include education to promote self-management and understanding. When kidney impairment results in decreased urine concentration with nocturia and low urine specific gravity, urge the patient to drink at least 2 L of fluid per day to prevent dehydration, which can further reduce kidney function. Restricting sodium intake may help control blood pressure. See Chapter 38 for a detailed discussion about the causes and management of hypertension.

Drug therapy for blood pressure control includes antihypertensive agents and diuretics. Antihypertensive agents include angiotensin-converting enzyme (ACE) inhibitors, calcium channel blockers, beta blockers, and vasodilators (see Chapter 38). ACE inhibitors may help control the cell growth aspects of PKD and reduce microalbuminuria.

Teach the patient and family how to measure and record blood pressure. Help the patient establish a schedule for self-administering drugs, monitoring daily weights, and keeping blood pressure records (Chart 70-2). Explain the potential side effects of the drugs. Make available written materials, such as drug teaching cards and booklets.

A low-sodium diet is often prescribed to control the hypertension that usually occurs with PKD. However, some patients may have salt wasting and should not follow a sodium-restricted diet. As the disease progresses, the protein intake may be limited to slow the development of end-stage kidney disease. Assist the patient and family in understanding the diet plan and why it was prescribed. Work closely with the dietitian to foster the patient's understanding. Also refer the patient for nutritional counseling.

Health Care Resources

The Polycystic Kidney Disease Foundation (www.pkdcure.org) and the National Kidney & Urologic Diseases Information Clearinghouse (NKUDIC) of the National Institute of Diabetes and Digestive and Kidney Diseases (www2.niddk.nih.gov) conduct research and provide education about PKD. Many pamphlets are available; there is a fee for some materials. Chapters of the National Kidney Foundation (NKF) and the American Association of Kidney Patients (AAKP) also have resources for information and support.

OBSTRUCTIVE DISORDERS

HYDRONEPHROSIS, HYDROURETER, AND URETHRAL STRICTURE

Pathophysiology

Hydronephrosis and hydroureter are problems of urine outflow obstruction. Urethral strictures also obstruct urine outflow. Prompt recognition and treatment are crucial to prevent permanent kidney damage.

In hydronephrosis, the kidney enlarges as urine collects in the renal pelvis and kidney tissue. Because the capacity of the renal pelvis is normally 5 to 8 mL, obstruction in the pelvis or at the point where the ureter joins the renal pelvis quickly distends the renal pelvis. Kidney pressure increases as the volume of urine increases. Over time, sometimes in only a matter of hours, the blood vessels and kidney tubules can be damaged extensively (Fig. 70-4).

In patients with hydroureter (enlargement of the ureter), the effects are similar but the obstruction is in the ureter rather than in the kidney. The ureter is most easily obstructed where the iliac vessels cross or where the ureters enter the bladder. Ureter dilation occurs above the obstruction and enlarges as urine collects (see Fig. 70-4).

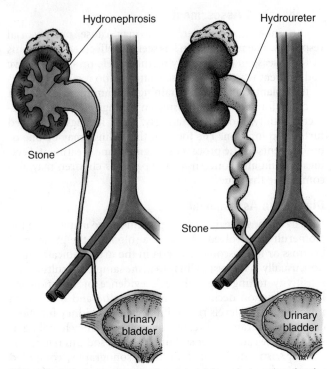

FIG. 70-4 Hydronephrosis is caused by obstruction in the upper part of the ureter. Hydroureter is caused by obstruction in the lower part of the ureter.

In patients with a urethral stricture, the obstruction is very low in the urinary tract, causing bladder distention before hydroureter and hydronephrosis. The problems and kidney damage are similar without prompt treatment.

Urinary obstruction causes damage when pressure builds up directly on kidney tissue. Tubular filtrate pressure also increases in the nephron as drainage through the collecting system is impaired. With this added pressure, glomerular filtration decreases or ceases, and complete necrosis of the affected kidney can occur. Nitrogen waste products (urea, creatinine, and uric acid) and electrolytes (sodium, potassium, chloride, and phosphorus) are retained, and acid-base balance is impaired.

Causes of hydronephrosis or hydroureter include tumors, stones, trauma, structural defects, and fibrosis. In patients with cancer, obstructed ureters may result from the tumors themselves, pelvic radiation, or surgical treatment. Early treatment of the causes can prevent hydronephrosis and hydroureter and thus prevent permanent kidney damage. The specific time needed to prevent permanent damage depends on the patient's kidney health. Permanent damage can occur in less than 48 hours in some patients and after several weeks in other patients.

PATIENT-CENTERED COLLABORATIVE CARE

ASSESSMENT

Obtain a history from the patient, focusing on known kidney or urologic disorders. A history of childhood urinary tract problems may indicate previously undiagnosed structural defects. Ask about his or her usual pattern of urination, especially amount, frequency, color, clarity, and odor. Ask about recent flank or abdominal pain. Chills, fever, and malaise may be present with a urinary tract infection (UTI).

Inspect each flank to identify asymmetry, which may occur with a kidney mass, and *gently* palpate the abdomen to locate areas of tenderness. Palpate and percuss the bladder to detect distention, or use a bedside bladder scanner. Gentle pressure on the abdomen may cause urine leakage, which reflects a full bladder and possible obstruction.

Urinalysis may show bacteria or white blood cells if infection is present. When urinary tract obstruction is prolonged, microscopic examination may show tubular epithelial cells. Blood chemistries are normal unless glomerular filtration decreases. Blood creatinine and blood urea nitrogen (BUN) levels increase with a reduced glomerular filtration rate (GFR). Serum electrolyte levels may be altered with elevated blood levels of potassium, phosphorus, and calcium along with a metabolic acidosis (bicarbonate deficit).

IV urography shows ureteral or renal pelvis dilation. Urinary outflow obstruction can be seen with sonography (renal echography) or computed tomography (CT).

INTERVENTIONS

Urinary retention and potential for infection are the primary problems. Failure to treat the cause of obstruction leads to infection and end-stage kidney disease.

Urologic Interventions

If the stricture is caused by a stone, it can be located and removed using cystoscopic or retrograde urogram procedures. The urologist uses a cystoscope to guide a stone basket over the stone and removes it through the bladder. After stone removal, a plastic stent is usually left in the ureter for a few weeks to improve urine flow in the area irritated by the stone. The stent is later removed by another cystoscopic procedure.

Radiologic Interventions

When a stricture is causing hydronephrosis and cannot be corrected with urologic procedures, a nephrostomy is performed. This procedure diverts urine externally and prevents further damage to the kidney.

Patient Preparation. If possible, the patient is kept NPO for 4 to 6 hours before the procedure. Clotting studies (e.g., international normalized ratio [INR], prothrombin time [PT], and partial thromboplastic time [PTT]) should be normal or corrected. The patient receives moderate sedation for the procedure.

Procedure. The patient is placed in the prone position. The kidney is located under ultrasound or fluoroscopic guidance, and a local anesthetic is given. A needle is placed into the kidney, a soft-tipped guidewire is placed through the needle, and then a catheter is placed over the wire. The catheter tip remains in the renal pelvis, and the external end is connected to a drainage bag. The procedure immediately relieves the pressure and prevents further damage. The nephrostomy tube remains in place until the obstruction is resolved (with or without further intervention).

Follow-up Care. Assess the amount of drainage in the collection bag. The amount of drainage depends on whether a ureteral catheter is also being used (with a separate drainage bag). Patients with ureteral tubes may have all urine pass through to the bladder or may have urine drain into the collection bags. The type of urine drainage expected should be clearly communicated in the chart. If urine is expected to drain into the collection bag, assess the amount of drainage hourly for the first 24 hours. If the amount of drainage decreases and the patient has back pain, the tube may be clogged or dislodged.

Monitor the nephrostomy site for leaking urine or blood. Urine drainage may be red-tinged for the first 12 to 24 hours after the procedure and should gradually clear. Assess the patient for manifestations of infection, including fever or a change in urine character.

> **! NURSING SAFETY PRIORITY**
>
> **Critical Rescue**
>
> After nephrostomy, notify the physician immediately when the drainage decreases or stops, drainage becomes cloudy or foul-smelling, the nephrostomy site leaks blood or urine, or the patient has back pain.

> **? NCLEX EXAMINATION CHALLENGE**
>
> **Safe and Effective Care Environment**
>
> Which laboratory test result for a client who is about to have a nephrostomy for hydronephrosis does the nurse report immediately to the physician?
> A. Serum sodium 137 mEq/L
> B. Serum potassium 4.8 mEq/L
> C. Blood urea nitrogen (BUN) 23 mg/dL
> D. International normalized ratio (INR) 4.6

INFECTIOUS DISORDERS: PYELONEPHRITIS

In the healthy person, urine is normally sterile and remains sterile if there is no obstruction to urine passage in the kidney and urinary tract. When any structural abnormality is present, the risk for damage as a result of infection is greatly increased. Urinary tract infection (UTI) is an infection in this normally sterile system. Pyelonephritis is a bacterial infection in the kidney and renal pelvis.

Pathophysiology

Pyelonephritis is either the presence of active organisms in the kidney or the effects of kidney infections. Acute pyelonephritis is the active bacterial infection, whereas chronic pyelonephritis results from repeated or continued upper urinary tract infections or the effects of such infections. Chronic pyelonephritis often occurs with a urinary tract defect, obstruction, or, most commonly, when urine refluxes from the bladder back into the ureters. The vesicoureteral junction is the point at which the ureter joins the bladder. Reflux is the reverse or upward flow of urine toward the renal pelvis and kidney.

In pyelonephritis, organisms move up from the urinary tract into the kidney tissue. Descending infection transmitted by organisms in the blood may occur, but not often. Bacteria trigger the inflammatory response, and local edema results.

Acute pyelonephritis involves acute tissue inflammation, tubular cell necrosis, and possible abscess formation. Abscesses, which are pockets of infection with pus, can occur anywhere in the kidney. The infection is scattered within the kidney; healthy tissues can lie next to infected areas. Fibrosis and scar tissue develop from the inflammation. The calices thicken, and scars develop in the interstitial tissue.

Reflux of infected urine from the bladder into the ureters and kidney is responsible for most cases of chronic pyelonephritis. Reflux within the kidney can occur when some papillae in the kidney do not close properly. Inflammation and fibrosis lead to deformity of the renal pelvis and calices. Repeated or continuous infections create additional scar tissue, changing blood vessel, glomerular, and tubular structure. As a result, filtration, reabsorption, and secretion are impaired and kidney function is reduced (Fig. 70-5).

Etiology and Genetic Risk

Single episodes of *acute pyelonephritis* may result from the entry of bacteria, especially during pregnancy, obstruction, or reflux. *Chronic pyelonephritis* usually occurs with structural deformities or obstruction with reflux. Reflux or obstruction leading to chronic pyelonephritis is often caused by stones or neurogenic impairment of voiding. Reflux is more common in children who have acquired scarring during acute infection or as a result of anatomic anomalies. Reflux and scarring contribute to chronic pyelonephritis as an adult. Chronic pyelonephritis in adults who did not have reflux as a child usually occurs with spinal cord injury, bladder tumor, prostate enlargement, or urinary tract stones.

Acute or chronic pyelonephritis occurs often in patients who have undergone manipulation of the urinary tract (e.g., placement of a urinary catheter), those with diabetes mellitus or chronic kidney stones, or those who overuse analgesics. In those with diabetes mellitus, the reduced bladder tone increases the risk for pyelonephritis. In patients with chronic stone disease, stones may retain organisms, resulting in ongoing infection and kidney scarring. NSAID use can lead to papillary necrosis and reflux.

The most common pyelonephritis-causing organism is *Escherichia coli*. *Enterococcus faecalis* is common in hospitalized patients. Both organisms are in the intestinal tract. Other organisms that cause pyelonephritis in hospitalized patients include *Proteus mirabilis*, *Klebsiella*, and *Pseudomonas aeruginosa*. When the infection is bloodborne, common infecting organisms include *Staphylococcus aureus* and the *Candida* and *Salmonella* species.

Other causes of kidney scarring leading to kidney function impairment include antibody reactions, cell-mediated immunity against the bacterial antigens, or autoimmune reactions.

Incidence/Prevalence

There are approximately 250,000 cases of acute pyelonephritis each year, resulting in more than 100,000 hospitalizations. Chronic pyelonephritis is commonly associated with vesicoureteral reflux or other anatomic abnormalities and is more common in women, although exact numbers for incidence and prevalence are not available. After 65 years of age, rates of pyelonephritis for men increase greatly because of the increased incidence of prostatitis and enlarged prostate.

PATIENT-CENTERED COLLABORATIVE CARE

ASSESSMENT

History

Ask about a history of urinary tract infections (UTIs), diabetes mellitus, stone disease, and defects of the genitourinary tract. Determine whether the UTIs occurred with pregnancy, and ask the patient about any previous episodes of pyelonephritis or similar symptoms. Ask about disease or treatment that causes immunosuppression, because they can also increase risk for pyelonephritis. Recurrences are common and may lead to a decline of kidney function.

Physical Assessment/Clinical Manifestations

Ask about specific manifestations of acute pyelonephritis (Chart 70-3). Chronic pyelonephritis has a less dramatic presentation, with manifestations related to the infection or kidney function. Ask the patient to describe any vague or nonspecific urinary symptoms or abdominal discomfort. Inquire about any history of repeated low-grade fevers. The patient with chronic pyelonephritis often has bacteriuria that causes no symptoms. Chart 70-4 outlines the kidney effects of chronic pyelonephritis.

CHART 70-3   KEY FEATURES

Acute Pyelonephritis

- Fever
- Chills
- Tachycardia and tachypnea
- Flank, back, or loin pain
- Tender costovertebral angle (CVA)
- Abdominal, often colicky, discomfort
- Nausea and vomiting
- General malaise or fatigue
- Burning, urgency, or frequency of urination
- Nocturia
- Recent cystitis or treatment for urinary tract infection (UTI)

CHART 70-4   KEY FEATURES

Chronic Pyelonephritis

- Hypertension
- Inability to conserve sodium
- Decreased urine concentrating ability, resulting in nocturia
- Tendency to develop hyperkalemia and acidosis

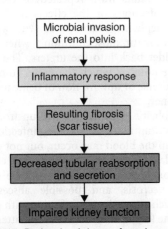

FIG. 70-5 Pathophysiology of pyelonephritis.

Inspect the flanks, and gently palpate the costovertebral angle (CVA). Inspect both CVAs for enlargement, asymmetry, edema, or redness, all of which can indicate inflammation. If there is no tenderness to light palpation in either CVA, an advanced practice nurse firmly percusses each area. Tenderness or discomfort may indicate infection or inflammation.

Psychosocial Assessment

The patient with any problem in the genitourinary area may have feelings of anxiety, embarrassment, or guilt. Listen carefully for signs of anxiety or specific fears, and prevent embarrassment during assessment. Feelings of guilt, often associated with sexual habits or practices, may be masked through delay in seeking treatment or through vague, nonspecific responses to specific or direct questions. Encourage patients to tell their own story in familiar, comfortable language.

Laboratory Assessment

Urinalysis shows a positive leukocyte esterase and nitrite dipstick test and the presence of white blood cells and bacteria. Occasional red blood cells, white blood cell casts, and protein may be present. The urine is cultured to determine whether gram-positive or gram-negative organisms are causing the infection. The urine sample for culture and sensitivity testing, obtained by the clean-catch method, shows the bacterial species and susceptibility or resistance of the specific organism to various antibiotics. In patients with recurrent episodes of pyelonephritis or upper UTIs, more specific testing of bacterial antigens and antibodies may help determine whether the same organism is responsible for the recurrent infections.

Blood cultures are obtained for specific organisms. Other blood tests include the C-reactive protein and erythrocyte sedimentation rate to determine the presence of inflammation.

Imaging Assessment

An x-ray of the kidneys, ureters, and bladder (KUB) and IV urography are performed to diagnose stones or obstructions. A cystourethrogram is indicated for some patients. These procedures define urinary tract structures and identify any defects. Specific defects to be identified include foreign bodies, such as stones; obstruction to the outflow of urine, such as tumors, structural defects, or prostate enlargement; and urine reflux caused by incompetent bladder-ureter valve closure. (See Chapter 68 for more information on imaging assessment.)

Other Diagnostic Assessment

Other diagnostic tests include examining antibody-coated bacteria in urine, certain enzymes (e.g., lactate dehydrogenase isoenzyme 5), and radionuclide scintillation (e.g., gallium scan). Examining urine for antibody-coated bacteria helps identify patients who may need long-term antibiotic therapy. High-molecular-weight enzymes in urine, such as lactate dehydrogenase isoenzyme 5, are present with any kidney tissue deterioration problem and give trend data. The gallium scan can identify active pyelonephritis or abscesses in or around the kidney.

▌ANALYSIS

The priority problems for the patient with pyelonephritis are:
1. Acute Pain (flank and abdominal) related to inflammation and infection

2. Potential for chronic kidney disease and end-stage kidney disease related to infectious tissue destruction

▌PLANNING AND IMPLEMENTATION
Managing Pain

Planning: Expected Outcomes. With proper intervention, the patient with pyelonephritis is expected to achieve an acceptable state of comfort. Indicators include that he or she often or consistently demonstrates these behaviors:
- Uses pharmacologic relief measures
- Uses NSAIDs appropriately
- Reports pain controlled

Interventions. Interventions may be nonsurgical or surgical. The use of several techniques that crush stones, such as lithotripsy and percutaneous ultrasonic pyelolithotomy (see Chapter 69), has decreased the need for surgery.

Nonsurgical Management. Interventions include the use of drug therapy, nutrition and fluid therapy, and teaching to ensure the patient's understanding of the treatment.

Drug therapy with antibiotics is prescribed to treat the infection. At first, the antibiotics are broad spectrum. After urine and blood culture and sensitivity results are known, more specific antibiotics may be prescribed. Urinary antiseptic drugs (e.g., nitrofurantoin [Macrodantin]) may also be prescribed to provide comfort.

Nutrition therapy involves ensuring that the patient's nutritional intake has adequate calories from all food groups for healing to occur. Fluid intake is recommended at 2 L/day unless another health problem requires fluid restriction.

Surgical Management. Surgical interventions can correct structural problems causing urine reflux or obstruction of urine outflow or can remove the source of infection.

Antibiotics are given, usually IV, to achieve adequate blood levels or sterile blood culture results. Teach the patient the nature and purpose of the proposed surgery, the expected outcome, and how he or she can participate.

The surgical procedures may be one of these: pyelolithotomy (stone removal from the kidney), nephrectomy (removal of the kidney), ureteral diversion, or reimplantation of ureter to restore proper bladder drainage.

A pyelolithotomy is needed for removal of a large stone in the renal pelvis that blocks urine flow and causes infection. Nephrectomy is a last resort when all other measures to clear the infection have failed. For patients with poor ureter valve closure or dilated ureters, ureteroplasty (ureter repair or revision) or ureteral reimplantation (through another site in the bladder wall) preserves kidney function and eliminates infections.

See Chapter 69 for nursing care after surgery for the patient undergoing urologic surgery.

Preventing End-Stage Kidney Disease

Planning: Expected Outcomes. The patient is expected to conserve existing kidney function for as long as possible and have a slow progression to end-stage kidney disease once the damage has occurred. Indicators include that he or she consistently demonstrates these behaviors:
- Describes the role of antibiotics and self-administration of drugs
- Explains and offers techniques to ensure adequate nutrition and hydration
- Describes the plan for post-treatment follow-up, including knowledge of recurrent symptoms

- Modifies prescribed regimen as directed by a health care professional

Interventions. Specific antibiotics are prescribed to treat the infection. Stress the importance of completing the drug therapy as directed. Discuss with the patient and family the importance of regular follow-up examinations and completing the recommended diagnostic tests.

Blood pressure control is needed to slow the progression of kidney dysfunction. When kidney impairment decreases concentrating ability, encourage the patient to drink at least 2 L of fluid per day to prevent dehydration (dehydration could further reduce kidney function). When dietary protein is restricted, refer the patient to the dietitian as needed. Other interventions related to the progression of chronic kidney disease are covered in Chapter 71.

Community-Based Care

Pyelonephritis causes fear and anxiety in the patient and family. The severity of the acute process and its potential to develop into a chronic process are frightening. The patient and the family need reassurance that treatment and preventive measures can be successful.

Home Care Management

If no surgery is performed, the patient may need help with self-care, nutrition, and drug management at home. If surgery is performed, he or she may need help with incision care, self-care, and transportation for follow-up appointments.

Teaching for Self-Management

After assessing the patient's and family's understanding of pyelonephritis and its therapy, explain:

- Drug regimen (purpose, timing, frequency, duration, and possible side effects)
- The role of nutrition and adequate fluid intake
- The need for a balance between rest and activity, including any limitations after surgery
- The manifestations of disease recurrence
- The use of previously successful coping mechanisms

Advise the patient to complete all prescribed antibiotic regimens and to report any side effects or unusual symptoms to the physician rather than stopping the drugs. Refer the patient and family for nutritional counseling as needed, because many patients have special nutritional requirements, such as those for diabetes or pregnancy.

Health Care Resources

The patient may also briefly need a home health nurse to help with drug or nutrition therapy at home. Housekeeping services may be helpful while he or she is regaining strength.

EVALUATION: OUTCOMES

Evaluate the care of the patient with pyelonephritis based on the identified priority patient problems. Expected outcomes may include that the patient will:

- Report that pain is controlled
- Be knowledgeable about the disease, its treatment, and interventions to prevent or reduce disease progression

Specific indicators for these outcomes are listed for each priority patient problem in the Planning and Implementation section (see earlier).

❓ NCLEX EXAMINATION CHALLENGE
Health Promotion and Maintenance

Which statement made by a client who has acute pyelonephritis indicates to the nurse correct understanding of the antibiotic therapy?
A. "If my temperature is normal for 3 days in a row, the infection is gone and I can stop taking the drug."
B. "If my temperature goes above 100° for 2 days, I should take double the dose of the drug."
C. "Even if I feel completely well, I should take the drug exactly as prescribed until it is gone."
D. "I should notify my prescriber to change the medication if I develop diarrhea while taking this drug."

IMMUNOLOGIC KIDNEY DISORDERS

Glomerulonephritis (GN) is the third leading cause of end-stage kidney disease (ESKD) (U.S. Renal Data Systems, 2010). Whether the disease starts in the kidney or occurs as the result of other health problems, the glomeruli are usually injured (Table 70-1). For disease that starts in the kidney, a genetic basis and immune problem are common. In addition, systemic diseases and infections can have kidney effects and cause glomerular injury (Table 70-2). Conditions that lead to glomerular disease include systemic lupus erythematosus and diabetic nephropathy.

Each type of disease or syndrome has a specific pathophysiology and clinical manifestations. Their *glomerular* effects are caused by injury to the glomeruli and result in

TABLE 70-1   PRIMARY GLOMERULAR DISEASES AND SYNDROMES
- Acute glomerulonephritis - Rapidly progressive glomerulonephritis (RPGN) - Chronic glomerulonephritis - Nephrotic syndrome - Persistent, vague urinary abnormalities with few or no symptoms

TABLE 70-2   SECONDARY GLOMERULAR DISEASES AND SYNDROMES
- Systemic lupus erythematosus (SLE) - Schönlein-Henoch purpura - Goodpasture's syndrome - Systemic necrotizing vasculitis - Wegener's granulomatosis - Periarteritis nodosa (also called *polyarteritis nodosa*) - Amyloidosis - Diabetic glomerulopathy - HIV-associated nephropathy - Alport's syndrome - Multiple myeloma - Viral hepatitis B - Viral hepatitis C - Cirrhosis - Sickle-cell disease - Nonstreptococcal postinfectious acute glomerulonephritis - Infective endocarditis - Hemolytic-uremic syndrome - Thrombotic thrombocytopenic purpura

proteinuria, hematuria, decreased glomerular filtration rate (GFR), edema, and hypertension. The extent and duration of kidney injury, prognosis, and specific cause vary among these syndromes.

Immunologic changes injure the glomeruli, interstitium, or tubules, and the effects may be acute or chronic. Both antibody and cellular immune responses are involved. The resultant kidney disorder can be systemic or confined to the kidneys.

Most forms of glomerulonephritis (GN) occur with a collection of immune complexes in the glomeruli (Fig. 70-6). An immune complex is made up of antigens (foreign substances within the body) and antibodies. The antigen can be part of any normal kidney tissue, or it can be dissolved in a body fluid (e.g., blood). Bacteria and viruses are also antigens. Exposure to bacteria, viruses, drugs, or other toxins is believed to be the trigger for glomerular injury.

Antibody reaction with antigens can cause immune complexes to form and become deposited in glomerular tissue. These complexes trigger many inflammatory mediators, such as complement, white blood cells, and blood clotting proteins, which also damage the kidney tissue. Actions that cause tissue injury include damage to cell membranes, local edema, movement of white blood cells to the site of inflammation, and platelet activation.

ACUTE GLOMERULONEPHRITIS

Pathophysiology

An infection often occurs before the kidney manifestations of acute glomerulonephritis (GN). The onset of symptoms is about 10 days from the time of infection. Usually, patients recover quickly and completely from acute GN. The term *acute nephritic syndrome* also describes this disorder.

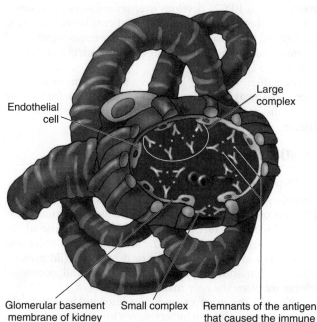

FIG. 70-6 An immune complex precipitating in the glomerulus of a patient with glomerulonephritis.

Labels on figure:
Endothelial cell
Large complex
Glomerular basement membrane of kidney
Small complex
Remnants of the antigen that caused the immune complexes to form

Most causes of acute GN are infectious (Table 70-3) or are related to other systemic diseases (see Table 70-2). The incidence of acute GN is unknown. GN after a systemic streptococcal infection is more common in men.

PATIENT-CENTERED COLLABORATIVE CARE

ASSESSMENT

History

Ask about recent infections, particularly of the skin or upper respiratory tract, and about recent travel or other possible exposures to viruses, bacteria, fungi, or parasites. Recent illnesses, surgery, or other invasive procedures may suggest infections. Ask about any known systemic diseases, such as systemic lupus erythematosus (SLE), which could cause acute GN.

Physical Assessment/Clinical Manifestations

Inspect the patient's skin for lesions or recent incisions (including body piercings). Assess the face, eyelids, hands, and other areas for edema (present in about 75% of the patients with acute GN). Assess for fluid overload and circulatory congestion (which may accompany the sodium and fluid retention occurring with acute GN). Ask about any difficulty in breathing or shortness of breath. Assess for crackles in the lung fields, an S_3 heart sound (gallop rhythm), and neck vein distention.

Ask about changes in urination pattern and any change in urine color. Microscopic blood in the urine occurs most of the time, and patients often describe their urine as smoky, reddish brown, rusty, or cola colored. Ask about dysuria or oliguria. Weigh him or her to assess for fluid retention.

Take the patient's blood pressure and compare it with the baseline blood pressure. Mild to moderate hypertension often occurs with acute GN as a result of sodium and fluid retention. The patient may have fatigue, a lack of energy, anorexia, nausea, and/or vomiting if uremia from severe kidney impairment is present.

TABLE 70-3	INFECTIOUS CAUSES OF ACUTE GLOMERULONEPHRITIS

- Group A beta-hemolytic *Streptococcus*
- Staphylococcal or gram-negative bacteremia or sepsis
- Pneumococcal, *Mycoplasma*, or *Klebsiella* pneumonia
- Syphilis
- Visceral abscesses
- Infective endocarditis
- Hepatitis B
- Infectious mononucleosis
- Measles
- Mumps
- Rocky Mountain spotted fever
- Cytomegalovirus infection
- Histoplasmosis
- Toxoplasmosis
- Varicella
- *Chlamydia psittaci* infection
- Coxsackievirus infection
- Any bacterial, parasitic, fungal, or viral infection (potentially)

CONSIDERATIONS FOR OLDER ADULTS

The less common manifestations of acute GN are more likely to occur in older adults. Circulatory congestion often is present, causing acute GN to be easily confused with congestive heart failure.

Laboratory Assessment

Urinalysis shows red blood cells (*hematuria*) and protein (*proteinuria*). An early morning specimen of urine is preferred for urinalysis because the urine is most acidic and formed elements are more intact at that time. Microscopic examination often shows red blood cell casts, as well as casts from other substances. The urine sediment assay is usually positive.

The glomerular filtration rate (GFR), either estimated from a single serum and urine creatinine value or measured by the 24-hour urine test for creatinine clearance, may be decreased to 50 mL/min. Blood urea nitrogen (BUN) levels are usually increased. The older patient may have a greater decline in GFR.

A 24-hour urine collection for total protein assay is obtained. The protein excretion rate for patients with acute GN may be increased from 500 mg to 3 g/24 hr in most patients. Serum albumin levels are decreased because of the protein lost in the urine and because of fluid retention causing dilution.

Specimens from the blood, skin, or throat are obtained for culture, if indicated. Other serologic tests include antistreptolysin-O titers, C3 complement levels, cryoglobulins (immunoglobulin G [IgG]), antinuclear antibodies (ANAs), and circulating immune complexes.

Antistreptolysin-O titers are increased after group A beta-hemolytic *Streptococcus* infections. Complement levels are decreased when the complement system is activated. Type III cryoglobulins may be found during acute illness. ANAs suggest an autoimmune response, and SLE is just one possibility. Immune complexes containing IgG and C3 are often detected.

Other Diagnostic Assessment

A kidney biopsy provides a precise diagnosis of the condition, assists in determining the prognosis, and helps outline treatment (see Chapter 68). The specific tissue features are determined by light microscopy, immunofluorescent stains, and electron microscopy to identify cell type, the presence of immunoglobulins, or the type of tissue deposits.

INTERVENTIONS

Interventions focus on managing infection, preventing complications, and providing appropriate patient education.

Managing infection as a cause of acute GN begins with appropriate antibiotic therapy. Penicillin, erythromycin, or azithromycin is prescribed for GN caused by streptococcal infection. Check the patient's known allergies before giving any drug. To prevent infection spread, antibiotics for people in immediate close contact with the patient also may be prescribed. Stress personal hygiene and basic infection control principles (e.g., handwashing) to prevent spread of the organism. Teach patients the importance of completing the entire course of the prescribed antibiotic.

Preventing complications is an important nursing intervention. For patients with fluid overload, hypertension, and edema, diuretics and a sodium and water restriction are prescribed. Antihypertensive drugs may be needed to control hypertension (see Chapter 38). The usual fluid allowance is equal to the 24-hour urine output plus 500 to 600 mL. Patients with oliguria usually have increased serum levels of potassium and blood urea nitrogen (BUN). Potassium and protein intake may be restricted to prevent hyperkalemia and uremia as a result of the elevated BUN.

Nausea, vomiting, or anorexia indicates that uremia is present. Dialysis is necessary if uremic symptoms or fluid volume excess cannot be controlled (see Chapter 71). Plasmapheresis (removal and filtering of the plasma to eliminate antibodies) also may be used (see Chapter 42).

To conserve the patient's energy, assist him or her in maintaining a restful environment, balancing activity and rest, and coordinating needed activities. Urge the patient to practice relaxation techniques and to participate in diversional activities to reduce emotional stress.

Preparing for self-management includes teaching the patient and family members about the purpose of prescribed drugs, the dosage and schedule, and potential adverse side effects. Ensure that they understand dietary or fluid restrictions, including methods of detecting fluid retention. Advise the patient to measure weight and blood pressure daily at the same time each day. Instruct him or her to notify the health care provider of any sudden increase in weight or blood pressure.

If short-term dialysis is required to control fluid volume or uremic symptoms, explain peritoneal or vascular access care and dialysis schedules and routines (also see Chapter 71).

RAPIDLY PROGRESSIVE GLOMERULONEPHRITIS

Rapidly progressive glomerulonephritis (RPGN), a type of acute nephritis, is also called *crescentic glomerulonephritis* because of the presence of crescent-shaped cells in the Bowman's capsule. RPGN develops over several weeks or months and causes loss of kidney function. Patients become quite ill quickly and have manifestations of kidney impairment (fluid volume excess, hypertension, oliguria, electrolyte imbalances, and uremic symptoms).

The patient may have had previous infection or systemic disease, such as systemic lupus erythematosus (SLE). The kidney function decline often progresses to end-stage kidney disease.

CHRONIC GLOMERULONEPHRITIS

Pathophysiology

Chronic glomerulonephritis, or *chronic nephritic syndrome*, develops over 20 to 30 years or even longer. The exact onset of the disorder is rarely identified. Often the cause of the disease is not known because the kidneys are atrophied and tissue is not available for biopsy or diagnosis. Mild proteinuria and hematuria, hypertension, fatigue, and occasional edema are often the only manifestations.

Although the exact cause is not known, changes in the kidney tissue result from hypertension, infections and inflammation, or poor blood flow to the kidneys. Kidney tissue atrophies, and the number of functional nephrons is greatly reduced. Biopsy in the late stages of atrophy may show glomerular changes, cell loss, protein and collagen deposits, and fibrosis of the kidney tissue. Microscopic examination shows deposits of immune complexes.

The loss of nephrons reduces glomerular filtration. Hypertension and renal arteriole sclerosis are often present. The glomerular damage allows proteins to enter the urine. Chronic glomerulonephritis always leads to end-stage kidney disease (see Chapter 71).

PATIENT-CENTERED COLLABORATIVE CARE

ASSESSMENT

History

Ask about other health problems, including systemic diseases, kidney or urologic disorders, infectious diseases (e.g., streptococcal infections), and recent exposures to infections. Ask about overall health status and whether increasing fatigue and lethargy have occurred.

Identify the patient's voiding pattern. Ask whether the frequency of voiding has increased or the quantity of urine has decreased. Ask about changes in urine color, odor, or clarity and whether dysuria or incontinence has occurred. Nocturia also is a common symptom.

Assess the patient's general comfort, and ask whether any dyspnea at rest or with exertion has occurred, because fluid overload can occur with decreased urine output. Ask about and observe for changes in mental functioning, such as irritability or an inability to read or to perform job-related functions or other processes requiring concentration. Changes in memory and the ability to concentrate occur as waste products collect in the blood.

Physical Assessment/Clinical Manifestations

Assess for systemic circulatory overload. Auscultate lung fields for crackles, observe the respiratory rate and depth, and measure blood pressure and weight. Auscultate the heart for rate, rhythm, and the presence of an S_3 heart sound. Inspect the neck veins for venous engorgement, and check for edema of the foot and ankle, on the shin, and over the sacrum.

Assess for uremic symptoms, such as slurred speech, ataxia, tremors, or asterixis (flapping tremor of the fingers or the inability to maintain a fixed posture with the arms extended and wrists hyperextended). Inspect skin for a yellowish color, texture, bruises, rashes, or eruptions. Ask about itching, and document areas of dryness or any excoriation from scratching.

Diagnostic Assessment

Urine output decreases, but the urine appears normal unless a urinary tract infection (UTI) also is present. Urinalysis shows protein, usually less than 2 g in a 24-hour collection. The specific gravity is fixed at a constant level of dilution (around 1.010). Red blood cells and casts may be in the urine.

The glomerular filtration rate (GFR), measured by creatinine clearance, is low. The serum creatinine level is elevated, usually greater than 6 mg/dL but may be as high as 30 mg/dL or more. The BUN is increased, often as high as 100 to 200 mg/dL.

Decreased kidney function causes abnormal serum electrolyte levels. Sodium retention is common, but dilution of the plasma from excess fluid can result in a falsely normal serum sodium level (135 to 145 mEq/L) or a low sodium level (less than 135 mEq/L). When oliguria develops, potassium is not excreted and hyperkalemia occurs when levels exceed 5.4 mEq/L.

Hyperphosphatemia develops with serum levels greater than 4.7 mg/dL. Serum calcium levels are usually at the lower end of the normal range or are slightly below normal.

Acidosis develops from hydrogen ion retention and loss of bicarbonate. However, there may be a decrease in serum carbon dioxide (CO_2) levels as patients breathe more rapidly to compensate for the acidosis. If respiratory compensation is present, the pH of arterial blood is between 7.35 and 7.45. A pH of less than 7.35 means that the patient's respiratory system is not completely compensating for the acidosis (see Chapter 14).

The kidneys are abnormally small on x-ray and on IV urography and when measured by sonography or computed tomography (CT).

A kidney biopsy is important in the early stages of glomerulonephritis, when protein or blood is first present in the urine. Tissue changes include a variety of cells infiltrating the glomerular tissue, deposits of immune complexes, and blood vessel sclerosis. In advanced disease, when the kidneys are small, biopsy is not usually performed.

INTERVENTIONS

Interventions focus on slowing the progression of the disease and preventing complications. Management consists of diet changes, fluid intake sufficient to prevent reduced blood flow volume to the kidneys, and drug therapy to control the problems from uremia. Eventually, the patient requires dialysis or transplantation to prevent death from uremia. (Care for the patient with ESKD requiring dialysis or transplantation is discussed in Chapter 71.)

NEPHROTIC SYNDROME

Pathophysiology

Nephrotic syndrome (NS) is a condition of increased glomerular permeability that allows larger molecules to pass through the membrane into the urine and then be excreted. This process causes massive loss of protein into the urine, edema formation, and decreased plasma albumin levels. Many agents and disorders are possible causes of NS.

The most common cause of glomerular membrane changes is an immune or inflammatory process. Defects in glomerular filtration can also occur as a result of genetic defects of the glomerular filtering system, such as Fabry disease. Altered liver activity may occur with nephrotic syndrome, resulting in increased lipid production and hyperlipidemia.

PATIENT-CENTERED COLLABORATIVE CARE

The main feature of nephrotic syndrome (NS) is severe proteinuria (more than 3.5 g of protein in 24 hours). Patients also have low serum albumin levels (serum albumin is less than 3 g/dL), high serum lipid levels, fats in the urine, edema, and hypertension (Chart 70-5). Renal vein thrombosis often occurs at the same time as NS, either as a cause of the problem

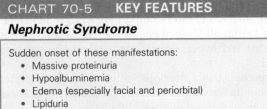

Nephrotic Syndrome

Sudden onset of these manifestations:
- Massive proteinuria
- Hypoalbuminemia
- Edema (especially facial and periorbital)
- Lipiduria
- Hyperlipidemia
- Increased coagulation
- Reduced kidney function

or as an effect. NS may progress to ESKD, but this can be prevented with treatment.

Management varies depending on what process is causing the disorder (identified by kidney biopsy). Immunologic processes may improve with suppressive therapy using steroids and cytotoxic or immunosuppressive agents. Angiotensin-converting enzyme (ACE) inhibitors can decrease protein loss in the urine, and cholesterol-lowering drugs can improve blood lipid levels. Heparin may reduce urine protein loss and improve kidney function. Diet changes are often prescribed. If the glomerular filtration rate (GFR) is normal, dietary intake of complete proteins is needed. If the GFR is decreased, dietary protein intake must be decreased. Mild diuretics and sodium restriction may be needed to control edema and hypertension. Assess the patient's hydration status, because vascular dehydration is common. If the plasma volume is depleted, kidney problems worsen. Acute kidney injury (AKI) may be avoided if good blood flow to the kidney is maintained.

IMMUNOLOGIC INTERSTITIAL AND TUBULOINTERSTITIAL DISORDERS

Problems can arise in the kidney tissues around the nephrons, as well as in the nephron tissues. These interstitial and tubulointerstitial disorders in the kidney are usually caused by immune problems. The kidney changes may be acute or chronic. The acute effects often occur with drugs such as penicillins, cephalosporins, sulfonamides, or NSAIDs. Chronic interstitial nephritis has many causes, including analgesic use, complement activation, cyclosporin use, polycystic kidney disease, autoimmune disorders, multiple myeloma, sickle cell disease, obstructive disorders, and radiation nephritis. Drug-induced problems often occur with a rash or an elevated eosinophil count. Fever is common in interstitial nephritis of unknown cause. Progression to ESKD occurs unless the cause is identified and removed.

DEGENERATIVE DISORDERS

Degenerative disorders that change kidney function often occur with a multisystem disorder. Many of these degenerative disorders result from changes in kidney blood vessels.

NEPHROSCLEROSIS

Pathophysiology

Nephrosclerosis is a problem of thickening in the nephron blood vessels, resulting in narrowing of the vessel lumens. This change decreases kidney blood flow, and the tissue is chronically hypoxic. Ischemia and fibrosis develop over time.

Nephrosclerosis occurs with all types of hypertension, atherosclerosis, and diabetes mellitus. The more severe the hypertension, the greater the risk for severe kidney damage. Nephrosclerosis is rarely seen when blood pressure is consistently below 160/110 mm Hg. The changes caused by hypertension may be reversible or may progress to end-stage kidney disease (ESKD) within months or years.

Hypertension is the second leading cause of ESKD, with about 30% of patients requiring kidney replacement therapy (e.g., dialysis or transplantation).

⊕ CULTURAL CONSIDERATIONS

Hypertension is more common in African Americans and American Indians, and the risks for ESKD from hypertension are also greater for these ethnic groups (U.S. Renal Data Systems, 2010). Between 25 and 45 years of age, the ratio of African Americans to Caucasians at risk for ESKD from hypertension is nearly 20 : 1. At any health care encounter with an African-American patient or an American Indian patient, blood pressure should always be assessed. If hypertension is present, treatment and patient education can help reduce the risk for development of ESKD.

PATIENT-CENTERED COLLABORATIVE CARE

Management focuses on controlling high blood pressure and reducing albuminuria to preserve kidney function. Although many antihypertensive drugs may lower blood pressure, the patient's response is important in ensuring long-term adherence to the prescribed therapy. Factors that promote adherence include once-a-day dosing, low cost, and minimal side effects.

Lack of knowledge or misinformation about hypertension poses many challenges to health care providers working with patients who have hypertension. When kidney disease occurs, adherence to therapy is even more important for preserving health.

Many drugs can control high blood pressure (see Chapter 38), and more than one agent may be needed for best control. Angiotensin-converting enzyme (ACE) inhibitors are very useful in reducing hypertension and preserving kidney function. Diuretics can maintain fluid and electrolyte balance in the presence of kidney function insufficiency. Hyperkalemia needs to be prevented when potassium-sparing diuretics, alone or in combination, are used to treat hypertensive patients with known kidney disease.

RENOVASCULAR DISEASE

Pathophysiology

Processes affecting the renal arteries may severely narrow the lumen and greatly reduce blood flow to the kidney tissues. Uncorrected renovascular disease, such as renal artery stenosis, atherosclerosis, or thrombosis, causes ischemia and atrophy of kidney tissue (Russell, 2008).

Patients with renovascular disease often have a sudden onset of hypertension, particularly in patients older than 50 years. Patients with high blood pressure but with no family history of hypertension also may potentially have renal artery stenosis (RAS). RAS from atherosclerosis or blood vessel hyperplasia is the main cause of renovascular disease. Other causes include thrombosis and renal vessel aneurysms.

Atherosclerotic changes in the renal artery often occur along with sclerosis in the aorta and other major vessels. Changes in the renal artery are often located where the renal artery and aorta meet. Fibrotic changes of the blood vessel wall occur throughout the length of the renal artery.

PATIENT-CENTERED COLLABORATIVE CARE

ASSESSMENT

Key features of renovascular disease are listed in Chart 70-6. Hypertension usually first occurs after 40 to 50 years of age, and often the patient does not have a family history of hypertension. Diagnosis is made by magnetic resonance angiography (MRA), renal duplex ultrasonography, radionuclide imaging, renal arteriography, and renal vein renin levels. MRA provides an excellent image of the renal vasculature and kidney anatomy. Radionuclide imaging is a noninvasive way of evaluating kidney blood flow and excretory function. Combining radionuclide imaging with ingestion of an angiotensin-converting enzyme (ACE) inhibitor such as captopril improves the accuracy of the test. A renal arteriogram makes the features of the renal blood vessels visible. The comparison of renal vein renin levels *may* reveal which kidney is producing more renin.

INTERVENTIONS

Identifying the type of defect, extent of narrowing, and condition of the surrounding blood vessels is critical for treatment choice. The patient's overall health and the size of the atrophied kidney also affect management decisions. Many patients with renovascular disease also have cardiovascular disease, and both conditions require treatment.

RAS may be managed by drugs to control high blood pressure and by procedures to restore the blood supply to the kidney. Drugs may control high blood pressure but may not lead to long-term preservation of kidney function. In young and middle-aged adults, a lifetime of treatment with many drugs for high blood pressure makes treatment difficult and the outcomes uncertain.

Balloon angioplasty with or without stent placement to open renal vessels is less risky and requires less time for recovery than does renal artery bypass surgery (see Chapter 38). Renal artery bypass surgery is a major procedure and requires 2 or more months for recovery. A bypass may be performed for either one or both renal arteries.

Renal angioplasty with metal stent placement is one safe and effective method to repair RAS. After the procedure, the patient usually remains in ICU for 24 hours to monitor for sudden blood pressure fluctuations as the kidneys adjust to increased blood flow.

A synthetic blood vessel graft is inserted to redirect blood flow from the abdominal aorta into the renal artery, beyond the area of narrowing. A splenorenal bypass can also restore blood flow to the kidney. The process is similar to other arterial bypass procedures (see Chapter 37).

DIABETIC NEPHROPATHY

Pathophysiology

Diabetes mellitus is the leading cause of end-stage kidney disease (ESKD) among white people in North America. About 36% of patients requiring dialysis or kidney transplantation have diabetes mellitus (U.S. Renal Data Systems, 2010). Diabetic nephropathy occurs with either type 1 or type 2 diabetes mellitus. Severity of diabetic kidney disease is related to the degree of hyperglycemia the patient generally experiences. With poor control of hyperglycemia, the complicating problems of atherosclerosis, hypertension, and neuropathy (which promotes loss of bladder tone, urinary stasis, and urinary tract infection) are more severe and more likely to cause kidney damage.

PATIENT-CENTERED COLLABORATIVE CARE

Diabetic nephropathy is a vascular complication of diabetes. Its first manifestation is persistent albuminuria (as shown by dipstick or a urinary albumin excretion rate above 0.3 g/dL), without evidence of other kidney disease. Diabetic kidney disease is progressive (Table 70-4).

Structural and functional changes occur in the kidneys of diabetic patients. Initially, kidney size is slightly increased and glomerular filtration rates (GFRs) are higher than normal. Microlevels of albumin are first detected in the urine. Progressive kidney damage occurs before dipstick procedures can detect protein in the urine. For most patients, proteinuria (albuminuria) indicates the need for follow-up and possibly a kidney biopsy for further diagnosis. See Chapter 67 for a detailed discussion of kidney issues in patients with diabetes.

Proteinuria may be mild, moderate, or severe. Patients with diabetes are always considered to be at risk for end-stage

---

CHART 70-6   KEY FEATURES

Renovascular Disease

- Significant, difficult-to-control high blood pressure
- Poorly controlled diabetes or sustained hyperglycemia
- Elevated serum creatinine
- Decreased creatinine clearance

TABLE 70-4   THE STAGES OF PROGRESSION OF TYPE 1 DIABETIC KIDNEY DISEASE

Stage I, at the time diabetes is diagnosed. Kidney size and glomerular filtration rate are increased. Blood sugar control can reverse the changes.

Stage II, 2 to 3 years after diagnosis. Glomerular and tubular capillary basement membrane changes result in microscopic changes, with loss of filtration surface area and scar formation. Glomerular changes are referred to as *glomerulosclerosis*.

Stage III, 7 to 15 years after diagnosis. Microalbuminuria is present. The glomerular filtration rate (GFR) may still be normal or may be increased.

Stage IV. Albuminuria is detectable by dipstick. GFR is decreased. Blood pressure is increased, and retinopathy is present.

Stage V. GFR decreases at an average rate of 10 mL/min/yr.

NOTE: Progression of chronic kidney disease related to type 1 diabetes mellitus can be delayed by maintaining glycemic control with HbA$_{1c}$ levels below 8%.

kidney disease (ESKD). If possible, nephrotoxic agents (e.g., radiopaque contrast media or aminoglycosides) and dehydration are avoided. Patients with worsening kidney function may begin to have frequent hypoglycemic episodes and a reduced need for insulin or antidiabetic agents. Explain that the kidneys metabolize and excrete insulin. When kidney function is reduced, the insulin is available for a longer time and thus less of it is needed. Unfortunately, many patients believe this means their diabetes is improving. The result is a more rapid progression to ESKD. (See Chapter 67 for specific information on diabetic nephropathy.)

? NCLEX EXAMINATION CHALLENGE

Health Promotion and Maintenance

The client with diabetes who also has persistent proteinuria asks what he could do to prevent eventual kidney failure. What is the nurse's best response?
A. "Wear pads and other protective gear around your lower back when engaging in contact sports."
B. "Drink at least 3 L of water daily and avoid carbonated beverages."
C. "Limit your intake of proteins to less than 100 g daily."
D. "Keep your blood glucose levels in the target range."

RENAL CELL CARCINOMA

Pathophysiology

Renal cell carcinoma (RCC) is the most common type of kidney cancer and is also known as *adenocarcinoma of the kidney.* As with other cancers, the healthy tissue of the kidney is damaged and replaced by cancer cells.

Systemic effects occurring with this cancer type are called *paraneoplastic syndromes* and include anemia, erythrocytosis, hypercalcemia, liver dysfunction with elevated liver enzymes, hormonal effects, increased sedimentation rate, and hypertension.

Anemia and erythrocytosis may seem confusing; however, most patients with this cancer have *either* anemia or erythrocytosis, not both at the same time. There is some blood loss from hematuria, but the small amount lost does not cause anemia. The cause of the anemia and the erythrocytosis is related to kidney cell production of erythropoietin. At times, the tumor cells produce large amounts of erythropoietin, causing erythrocytosis. Other times, the tumor cells destroy the erythropoietin-producing kidney cells and anemia results. Hypertension may result from increased blood levels of renin.

Parathyroid hormone produced by tumor cells can cause hypercalcemia. Other hormone changes include increased renin levels (causing hypertension) and increased human chorionic gonadotropin (hCG) levels, which decrease libido and change secondary sex features.

RCC has four distinct cell types. Genetic differences cause a predisposition to develop tumors of each of these types. The most well known genetic familial syndrome that includes kidney cancer is von Hippel-Lindau syndrome. These cancers are highly vascular and may occur with cancers of the pancreas, central nervous system, and adrenal glands.

Kidney tumors are classified into four stages (Table 70-5). Complications include metastasis and urinary tract obstruction. The cancer usually spreads to the adrenal gland, liver, lungs, long bones, or the other kidney (Moldawer & Figlin,

TABLE 70-5 STAGING KIDNEY TUMORS

Stage I. Tumors up to 2.5 cm are situated within the capsule of the kidney. The renal vein, perinephric fat, and adjacent lymph nodes have no tumor.

Stage II. Tumors are larger than 2.5 cm and extend beyond the capsule but are within Gerota's fascia. The renal vein and lymph nodes are not involved.

Stage III. Tumors extend into the renal vein, lymph nodes, or both.

Stage IV. Tumors include invasion of adjacent organs beyond Gerota's fascia or metastasize to distant tissues.

Data from American Cancer Society. (2011). *Cancer facts and figures 2011.* Report No. 00-300M–No. 5008.11. Atlanta: Author.

2008). When the cancer surrounds a ureter, hydroureter and obstruction may result.

The exact cause of RCC is unknown, but the risk is slightly higher for people who use tobacco or are exposed to lead, phosphate, and cadmium.

Kidney cancers account for about 51,190 new cases and 12,890 deaths annually in the United States. The 5-year survival rate is 60% in the United States. Renal cell carcinoma occurs most often in patients between 55 and 60 years of age (Jemal et al., 2007).

PATIENT-CENTERED COLLABORATIVE CARE

ASSESSMENT

History

Ask the patient about age, known risk factors (e.g., smoking or chemical exposures), weight loss, changes in urine color, abdominal or flank discomfort, and fever. Also ask whether any other family member has ever been diagnosed with cancer of the kidney, bladder, ureter, prostate gland, uterus, or ovary.

Physical Assessment/Clinical Manifestations

Only about 5% to 10% of patients with renal cell cancer have flank pain, obvious blood in the urine, and a kidney mass that can be palpated. Ask about the nature of the flank or abdominal discomfort. Patients often describe the pain as dull and aching. The pain may be more intense if bleeding into the tumor or kidney occurs. Inspect the flank area, checking for asymmetry or an obvious bulge. An abdominal mass may be felt through *gentle* palpation. A renal bruit may be heard on auscultation.

Bloody urine is a *late* common sign. Blood may be visible as bright red flecks or clots, or the urine may appear smoky or cola colored. Without gross hematuria, microscopic examination may or may not reveal red cells.

Inspect the skin for pallor, darkening of the nipples, and, in men, breast enlargement (*gynecomastia*) caused by changing hormone levels. Other findings may include muscle wasting, weakness, poor nutritional status, and weight loss. All tend to occur late in the disease.

Diagnostic Assessment

Urinalysis may show red blood cells. Hematologic studies show decreased hemoglobin and hematocrit values, hypercalcemia, increased erythrocyte sedimentation rate, and increased levels of adrenocorticotropic hormone, human chorionic gonadotropin (hCG), cortisol, renin, and parathyroid hormone.

Kidney masses may be detected by surgical exploration, IV urogram with nephrograms, or sonography. The mass and surrounding tissues may be outlined by CT with contrast or by magnetic resonance imaging (MRI). Complete diagnosis requires a biopsy of the tumor.

INTERVENTIONS

Interventions focus on controlling the cancer and preventing metastasis.

Nonsurgical Management

Radiofrequency ablation can slow tumor growth. It is a minimally invasive procedure carried out after MRI has precisely located the tumor. The procedure is used most commonly for patients who have only one kidney or who are poor surgical candidates.

Chemotherapy has limited effectiveness against this cancer type. Use of biological response modifiers (BRMs) such as interleukin-2 (IL-2), interferon (INF), and tumor necrosis factor (TNF) has lengthened survival time (see Chapters 19 and 24). Newer targeted therapy agents, sorafenib (Nexavar) and temsirolimus (Torisel), were approved as treatment for patients with advanced renal cell carcinoma. Sorafenib, an oral drug taken daily, is a multikinase inhibitor that slows cancer cell division and inhibits blood vessel growth in the tumor. Temsirolimus is a weekly IV infusion and works by inhibiting cell division. These drugs have increased survival time of patients with advanced cancer.

Surgical Management

Renal cell carcinoma is usually treated surgically by *nephrectomy* (kidney removal). Renal cell tumors are highly vascular, and blood loss during surgery is a major concern. Before surgery, the arteries supplying the kidney may be occluded (embolized) by radiation to reduce bleeding during nephrectomy.

Preoperative Care. Instruct the patient about surgical routines (see Chapters 16, 17, and 18). Explain the probable site of incision and the presence of dressings, drains, or other equipment after surgery. Reassure the patient about pain relief. Care before surgery may include giving blood and fluids IV to prevent shock.

Operative Procedures. The patient is placed on his or her side with the kidney to be removed uppermost. The trunk area is flexed to increase exposure of the kidney area. Removal of the eleventh or twelfth rib may be needed to provide better access to the kidney. The surgeon removes the entire kidney and all visible tumor, renal artery and vein, and fascia after tying off the ureter. The adrenal gland is left intact. A drain may be placed in the wound before closure.

When a *radical* nephrectomy is performed, local and regional lymph nodes are also removed. The surgical approach may be transthoracic (as discussed in the previous paragraph), lumbar, or through the abdomen, depending on the size and location of the tumor. Radiation therapy may follow a radical nephrectomy.

Postoperative Care. Refer to Chapter 18 for care of the patient after surgery. Nursing priorities are focused on assessing kidney function to determine effectiveness of the remaining kidney, pain management, and preventing complications.

Monitoring includes assessing for hemorrhage and adrenal insufficiency. Inspect the patient's abdomen for distention from bleeding. Check the bed linens under the patient, because blood may pool there. Hemorrhage or adrenal insufficiency causes hypotension, decreased urine output, and an altered level of consciousness.

A decrease in blood pressure is an early sign of both hemorrhage and adrenal insufficiency. With hypotension, urine output also decreases immediately. Large water and sodium losses in the urine occur in patients with adrenal insufficiency. As a result, a large urine output is followed by hypotension and oliguria (less than 400 mL/24 hr or less than 25 mL/hr). IV replacement of fluids and packed red blood cells may be needed.

The second kidney is expected to provide adequate function, but this may take days or weeks. Assess urine output hourly for the first 24 hours after surgery (urine output of 0.5 mL/kg/hr or about 30 to 50 mL/hr is acceptable). Output of less than 25 to 30 mL/hr suggests decreased blood flow to the kidney and the onset or worsening of acute kidney injury. The hemoglobin level, hematocrit values, and white blood cell count may be measured every 6 to 12 hours for the first day or two after surgery.

Monitor the patient's temperature, pulse rate, and respiratory rate at least every 4 hours. Accurately measure and record fluid intake and output. Weigh the patient daily.

The patient may be in a special care unit for 24 to 48 hours after surgery for monitoring of bleeding and adrenal insufficiency. A drain placed near the site of incision removes residual fluid. Because of the discomfort of deep breathing, the patient is at risk for atelectasis. Fever, chills, thick sputum, or decreased breath sounds suggest pneumonia.

Managing pain after surgery usually requires opioid analgesics (e.g., hydromorphone [Dilaudid] and morphine [Statex ✦]) given intravenously. The incision was made through major muscle groups used with breathing and movement. Liberal use of analgesics is needed for 3 to 5 days after surgery to manage pain. Oral agents may be tried when the patient can eat and drink.

Preventing complications focuses on infection and management of adrenal insufficiency. Antibiotics may be prescribed during and after surgery to prevent infection. The need for additional antibiotics is based on evidence of infection. Assess the patient at least every 8 hours for manifestations of systemic infection or local wound infection.

Adrenal insufficiency is possible as a complication of kidney and adrenal gland removal. Although only one adrenal gland may be affected, the remaining gland may not be able to secrete sufficient glucocorticoids immediately after surgery. Steroid replacements may be needed in some patients. Chapter 65 discusses the manifestations of acute adrenal insufficiency in detail along with specific nursing interventions.

KIDNEY TRAUMA

Pathophysiology

Trauma to one or both kidneys is always a concern in penetrating wounds or blunt injuries to the back, flank, or abdomen. Blunt trauma to the back, flank, or abdomen

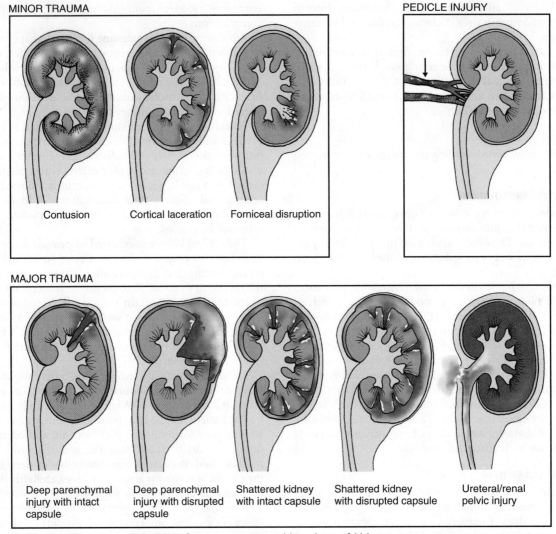

MINOR TRAUMA

Contusion   Cortical laceration   Forniceal disruption

PEDICLE INJURY

MAJOR TRAUMA

Deep parenchymal injury with intact capsule   Deep parenchymal injury with disrupted capsule   Shattered kidney with intact capsule   Shattered kidney with disrupted capsule   Ureteral/renal pelvic injury

FIG. 70-7 Common types and locations of kidney trauma.

CHART 70-7 PATIENT AND FAMILY EDUCATION: PREPARING FOR SELF-MANAGEMENT

Preventing Kidney and Genitourinary Trauma

- Wear a seat belt.
- Practice safe walking habits.
- Use caution when riding bicycles and motorcycles.
- Wear appropriate protective clothing when participating in contact sports.
- Avoid all contact sports and high-risk activities if you have only one kidney.

---

accounts for most kidney injuries. Injury can be minor, major, or pedicle (Fig. 70-7). Anyone can suffer kidney trauma. Strategies to prevent trauma are reviewed in Chart 70-7.

Minor injuries include contusions, small lacerations, and tearing of the parenchyma and the calyx (forniceal disruption) caused by falls, contact sports, and blows to the back and torso. With a contusion, one or both kidneys are bruised because of impact. Small blood vessels may be damaged, causing some hematuria. Small lacerations may result in small, local hematomas. A small hematoma also may occur at the site of forniceal disruption.

Major injuries include lacerations to the cortex, medulla, or branches of the renal artery or vein. Deep tissue injuries may extend throughout the kidney and cause hematomas within or through the capsule. Injuries involving the cortex can cause tissue shattering. The capsule may remain intact or be ruptured.

A major injury often follows penetrating abdominal, flank, or back wounds (e.g., as is seen with gunshot wounds, knife wounds, or motor vehicle crashes). Bleeding is extensive, and surgical exploration is often needed. Because of the hemorrhage, decreased blood flow to the kidney can produce short-term or long-term renin-induced hypertension.

Pedicle injuries are lacerations or breaks in the renal artery or renal vein. Hemorrhage is extensive and rapid, and death may occur unless diagnosis and intervention are prompt.

PATIENT-CENTERED COLLABORATIVE CARE

ASSESSMENT

Obtain a history of the patient's usual health and the events involved in the trauma from the patient, a witness, or emergency personnel. Critical information to know is a history of kidney or urologic disease, surgical intervention, or health problems such as diabetes mellitus or hypertension.

Ureteral or renal pelvic injury often causes diffuse abdominal pain, local collections of urine, and infection. Ask the patient about pain in the flank or abdominal pain. Is the pain dull? Sharp? Constant? Intermittent? Made worse by coughing?

Take the patient's blood pressure, apical and peripheral pulses, respiratory rate, and temperature. Inspect both flanks for asymmetry or penetrating injuries of the lower chest or back. Also inspect the abdomen for bruising or penetrating wounds. Percuss the abdomen for distention. Inspect the urethra for gross bleeding.

Urinalysis usually shows hemoglobin or red blood cells from renal blood vessel rupture. Microscopic examination may also show red blood cell casts, which suggest tubular damage. Hemoglobin and hematocrit values decrease with blood loss. If inflammation or infection is present, the white blood cell count is elevated.

Diagnostic procedures include IV urography and computed tomography (CT). CT scan shows the location of the injury and blood vessel and tissue integrity. Hematomas within or through the kidney capsule are seen with CT scan. A urogram reveals the integrity and patency of the collecting system. Sonography can be used instead if there is a need to avoid contrast dye, especially in patients with elevated serum creatinine levels.

INTERVENTIONS

Nonsurgical Management

Drug therapy is used for bleeding prevention or control. The need for clotting factors such as vitamin K and platelets is assessed, and they are given as needed.

Fluid therapy is given to restore circulating blood volume and ensure adequate blood flow to the kidneys. *Crystalloid solutions* replace water and some electrolytes and include 0.9% sodium chloride (normal saline solution [NSS]), 5% dextrose in 0.45% sodium chloride, and lactated Ringer's solution. When bleeding is extensive, whole blood or packed red cell replacement restores hemoglobin and promotes oxygenation. *Plasma volume expanders,* such as dextran or albumin, help restore plasma oncotic pressure and reduce fluid shift to the interstitial fluid space.

During fluid restoration, give fluids at the prescribed rate and monitor the patient for shock. Take vital signs as often as every 5 to 15 minutes. Measure and record urine output hourly. Output should be greater than 0.5 mL/kg/hr.

> ## ! NURSING SAFETY PRIORITY
> ### Action Alert
> If the urethral opening is bleeding, consult with the physician before attempting urinary catheterization.

Surgical Management

Nephrectomy or partial nephrectomy may be needed. When major blood vessels are torn, the kidney may be removed, repaired outside of the patient, and then reimplanted, a process known as "bench surgery."

Community-Based Care

Teach the patient and family about the effects of the injury and how to assess for infection or other complications, such as the onset of bleeding or urinary retention. Instruct the patient to check the pattern and frequency of urination and to note whether the color, clarity, and amount appear normal. Also instruct the patient to seek medical attention if anything appears abnormal or if bladder distention or inadequate bladder emptying occurs, which suggests an obstruction. Chills, fever, lethargy, or cloudy, foul-smelling urine indicates a urinary tract infection. Warn the patient to not ignore these manifestations and to seek medical care promptly if they occur.

NURSING CONCEPT REVIEW

What might you NOTICE if the patient is experiencing problems with urinary elimination as a result of acute pyelonephritis?

- Patient urinates frequently in small amounts.
- Patient reports pain and burning on urination.
- Patient reports back or flank pain.
- Urine is cloudy and foul smelling.
- Urine may be darker or smoky or have obvious blood in it.

What should you INTERPRET and how should you RESPOND to a patient experiencing problems with urinary elimination as a result of acute pyelonephritis?

Perform and interpret physical assessment, including:
- Ask how long manifestations have been present.
- Ask about low back pain (midline in men) or flank pain.

- Ask whether he or she has had a UTI in the past; how long ago; how it was treated; and if antibiotics were prescribed, whether the drug course was completed.
- Ask about the presence of pregnancy or any chronic health problem, especially diabetes.
- Ask about any nausea or vomiting and its duration.
- Determine fluid intake and output volumes.
- Assess for pain over the right and left kidneys.
- Weigh the patient, and ask whether this weight is more or less than his or her usual weight.
- Assess for fever and chills.
- Assess for tachycardia.
- Interpret laboratory values:
  - Is the complete blood count with differential elevated?

NURSING CONCEPT REVIEW—cont'd

- Are the BUN and serum creatinine levels elevated?
- Is the urinalysis positive for bacteria, leukocyte esterase, nitrate, red blood cells, white blood cells, or casts?

Respond by:
- Providing for pain control
- Teaching the patient the importance of completing the prescribed antibiotic drug regimen

On what should you REFLECT?
- Observe patient for evidence of improved urinary output (see Chapter 68).
- Think about what may have caused this infection and what steps could be taken to prevent a similar episode.
- Think about what patient teaching focus could help reduce the risk for future pyelonephritis and its complications.

GET READY FOR THE NCLEX® EXAMINATION!

KEY POINTS

Review these Key Points for each NCLEX Examination Client Needs Category.

Health Promotion and Maintenance
- Encourage all patients to maintain an adequate fluid intake (2-3 L/day unless another condition requires fluid restriction).
- Encourage patients with diabetes to adhere to regimens for glucose control and blood pressure control to prevent kidney disease.

Psychosocial Integrity
- Allow the patient the opportunity to express fear or anxiety regarding the potential for chronic kidney disease and end-stage kidney disease.
- Assess the patient's level of comfort in discussing issues related to elimination and the genitourinary area.
- Refer patients with polycystic kidney disease to a geneticist or a genetic counselor.
- During kidney/urinary assessment, use language and terminology that is comfortable for the patient.
- Refer patients to community resources, support groups, and information organizations such as the National Kidney Foundation, the Polycystic Kidney Disease Foundation, and the American Association of Kidney Patients.

Physiological Integrity
- Report immediately any condition that obstructs urine flow.
- Instruct patients with UTI to complete all prescribed antibiotic therapy even when symptoms of infection are absent.
- Check the blood pressure and urine output frequently in patients who have any type of kidney problem.
- Report immediately to the health care provider any sudden decrease of urine output in a patient with kidney disease or kidney trauma. In general, adult urine output expectations are 0.5-1 mL/kg/hr.
- Instruct patients with any type of kidney problem to weigh daily and to notify their health care provider if there is a sudden weight gain.
- Teach patients the expected side effects and any adverse reactions to prescribed drugs.
- Teach patients the manifestations of disease recurrence and when to seek medical help.

Care of Patients with Acute Kidney Injury and Chronic Kidney Disease

Linda LaCharity

ⓔvolve WEBSITE

http://evolve.elsevier.com/Iggy/

Animation: Renal and Urinary Disorders
Answer Key for NCLEX Examination Challenges and
    Decision-Making Challenges
Audio Glossary

Concept Map Creator
Concept Map: End-Stage Kidney Disease
Key Points
Review Questions for the NCLEX® Examination

LEARNING OUTCOMES

Safe and Effective Care Environment

1. Evaluate patient risk for dehydration, shock, and acute kidney injury.
2. Collaborate with members of the health care team to reduce patient exposure to nephrotoxins in the acute care setting.
3. Prevent injury in the patient who has bone density loss or skin changes from kidney disease.
4. Apply principles of infection control to prevent infection in patients receiving immunosuppressive therapy.

Health Promotion and Maintenance

5. Teach everyone to drink fluids to prevent dehydration during hot weather and when engaging in heavy work or exercise.
6. Assess intake and output for anyone at risk for or with hypovolemia.
7. Teach transplant recipients and their families about the importance of adhering to anti-rejection therapy.

Psychosocial Integrity

8. Encourage patients and families to express any concerns about the risk for death and the disruption of lifestyle as a result of treatment for kidney dysfunction.

9. Assess the patient for depression and nonacceptance of the diagnosis or treatment plan.
10. Refer patients to community resources and support groups.

Physiological Integrity

11. Compare the pathophysiology and causes of acute kidney injury (AKI) with those of chronic kidney disease (CKD).
12. Use laboratory data and clinical assessment to determine the effectiveness of therapy for kidney dysfunction.
13. Discuss interventions to prevent AKI.
14. Discuss the mechanisms of peritoneal dialysis (PD) and hemodialysis (HD) as renal replacement therapies.
15. Coordinate nursing care for the patient with severe CKD or end-stage kidney disease (ESKD).
16. Plan prevention strategies for the complications of PD.
17. Coordinate nursing care for the patient during the first 24 hours after kidney transplantation.

Severe kidney disease leading to renal failure is common in North America. Acute kidney injury (AKI) is most common in the acute care setting, and chronic kidney disease (CKD), which may take years to develop, is more common in the community. Both types of kidney dysfunction cause problems by interfering with urinary elimination and disrupting homeostasis of fluid volume, blood pressure, electrolytes, wastes, and acid-base balance (see Fig. 70-1 in Chapter 70). These problems can reduce general function, shorten life, and decrease quality of life. Diabetes, hypertension, and

TABLE 71-1	CHARACTERISTICS OF ACUTE KIDNEY INJURY AND CHRONIC KIDNEY DISEASE	
CHARACTERISTIC	ACUTE KIDNEY INJURY	CHRONIC KIDNEY DISEASE
Onset	Sudden (hours to days)	Gradual (months to years)
% of nephron involvement	≈50%	90%-95%
Duration	2-4 wks; less than 3 months	Permanent
Prognosis	Good for return of kidney function with supportive care; high mortality in some situations	Fatal without a renal replacement therapy such as dialysis or transplantation

cardiovascular disease are much more common in people with CKD, and their incidence increases as the stage of CKD worsens (U.S. Renal Data Systems [USRDS], 2010). Between 2003 and 2006, the number of patients with stage 3 CKD rose by 1.8% (USRDS, 2010). Thus overall, the incidence has increased only slightly and is most likely related to the use of kidney protective therapy with antihypertensive drugs such as angiotensin-converting enzyme (ACE) inhibitors and angiotensin II receptor blocker (ARB) drugs, as well as the benefits associated with use of beta-blocker drugs in the treatment of heart failure. The incidence is expected to continue to rise as a result of the aging population and the huge increase in the incidence of type 2 diabetes. In the United States, about half a million people with end-stage-kidney disease (ESKD) are treated yearly with dialysis or kidney transplantation (Okusa et al., 2009). Kidney dysfunction has many causes. CKD is most commonly caused by hypertension (HTN) and diabetes.

As described in Chapter 68, kidney functions include excretion of waste, water and salt balance, acid-base balance, and hormone secretion. When kidney function declines gradually, as occurs most often with CKD (also known as *chronic renal failure [CRF]*), 90% to 95% of the nephrons must be destroyed before kidney dysfunction is obvious. The patient may have many years of reduced kidney function (*renal insufficiency*) before the uremia of ESKD develops. During this time of decreased kidney function, the patient is at increased risk for acute kidney injury because of the stress on remaining nephrons.

When kidney decline is sudden, the functioning nephrons are overworked and kidney dysfunction may develop with the loss of only 50% of functioning nephrons. Acute kidney injury and chronic kidney disease are compared in Table 71-1. Acute kidney injury affects *many* body systems. Chronic kidney disease affects *every* body system. The problems that occur with loss of kidney function are related to fluid overload, electrolyte and acid-base abnormalities, buildup of nitrogen-based wastes, and loss of kidney hormone function.

When kidney function declines to the point that the kidneys can no longer maintain homeostasis by urine elimination, renal replacement therapy is needed to prevent death.

ACUTE KIDNEY INJURY

Pathophysiology

Acute kidney injury (AKI), which used to be known as acute renal failure (ARF) is a rapid decrease in kidney function, leading to the collection of metabolic wastes in the body. AKI can result from conditions that reduce blood flow to the kidneys (prerenal acute kidney injury); damage to the glomeruli, interstitial tissue, or tubules (intrarenal/intrinsic acute kidney injury); or obstruction of urine flow (postrenal acute kidney injury). When AKI occurs in patients who already have reduced kidney function, it may lead to end-stage kidney disease (ESKD) or it may resolve to nearly the pre-AKI level of kidney function. Many factors contribute to kidney insults in AKI, but the acute syndrome may be reversible, especially with prompt intervention.

The pathologic process of AKI is related to the cause of the sudden decrease in kidney function and to the affected kidney site(s). Reduced blood flow (poor perfusion), toxins, tubular ischemia, infections, and obstruction have different effects on the kidney and its function. Any of these processes can reduce glomerular filtration rate (GFR), damage nephron cells, and obstruct urine flow in the kidney tubules.

With shock or other problems causing an acute reduction in blood flow to the kidney *(hypoperfusion)*, the kidney compensates by constricting renal blood vessels, activating the renin-angiotensin-aldosterone pathway, and releasing antidiuretic hormone (ADH). These responses increase blood volume and improve kidney perfusion. However, these same responses reduce urine volume, resulting in oliguria (urine output less than 400 mL/day) and azotemia (the retention and buildup of nitrogenous wastes in the blood). Nephron cell injury is more likely to occur from the lack of oxygen *(ischemia)* related to reduced blood flow (McCance et al., 2010). Toxins can cause blood vessel constriction in the kidney, leading to reduced kidney blood flow and kidney ischemia.

Kidney tissue inflammation caused by infection, drugs, or cancer results in immune-mediated changes in kidney tissue. With extensive tubular damage, tubular cells slough and combine with other formed elements (e.g., red blood cell [RBC] casts), which then obstruct tubular lumens and prevent urine outflow. *Obstruction anywhere within the urinary tract may result in reduced urine formation and full or partial obstruction to urine outflow.*

When pressure in the kidney tubules *(intrarenal pressure)* exceeds glomerular pressure, glomerular filtration stops. This problem allows nitrogen-based wastes to collect in the blood, increasing the blood urea nitrogen (BUN) and serum creatinine levels. When the BUN rises faster than the serum creatinine level, the cause is usually related to protein breakdown or dehydration. When both the BUN and the creatinine levels rise and the ratio between the two remains constant, this indicates kidney dysfunction.

Classification of Acute Kidney Injury Risk

The recent change in terminology from *acute renal failure* to *acute kidney injury* resulted in the development of standardized criteria to recognize the changes associated with the problem earlier, when interventions are more likely to reverse the process and prevent permanent kidney damage (Dirkes, 2011; Martin, 2010). This change was aimed at preventing

TABLE 71-2   THE RIFLE CLASSIFICATION SYSTEM FOR DIAGNOSIS AND SEVERITY OF ACUTE KIDNEY INJURY

RIFLE CLASSIFICATION	SERUM CREATININE LEVEL	GLOMERULAR FILTRATION RATE (GFR)	URINE OUTPUT
Severity Level			
Risk	Increased 1.5 times above normal (or the patient's normal when chronic kidney disease is known to exist) OR	Decreased by at least 25% of the standard normal or the patient's normal	<0.5 mL/kg hourly for 6 hours
Injury	Increased 2.5 times standard normal or the patient's normal OR	Decreased by at least 50% of the standard normal or the patient's normal	<0.5 mL/kg hourly for 12 hours
Failure	Increased 3 times standard normal or the patient's normal OR	Decreased by more than 50% of the standard normal or the patient's normal	<0.5 mL/kg hourly for 24 hours or no urine output (anuria) for 12 hours
Outcome Level			
Loss	Complete loss of kidney function that persists for more than 4 weeks		None without renal replacement therapy
End-stage kidney disease	Complete loss of kidney function that persists for more than 3 months		None without renal replacement therapy

kidney damage both in people who had healthy kidneys before a specific precipitating event and in those who already had some degree of chronic kidney disease (CKD). (An acute kidney injury occurring in a person with CKD can greatly increase the rate of progression to end-stage kidney disease.)

Table 71-2 lists the criteria for classification of acute kidney injury based on the five RIFLE categories of changes in glomerular filtration, serum creatinine levels, and reduction of hourly urine output. (RIFLE stands for **R**isk, **I**njury, **F**ailure, **L**oss, and **E**nd-stage kidney disease.) These criteria apply to patients with no known kidney problems and to patients with CKD. The first three criteria (R,I,F), are injury severity levels. Identification of AKI at these levels and proper management can prevent progression to more serious injury that may not be reversible. The last two criteria (L,E) indicate serious injury that requires renal replacement therapy at least on a temporary basis. Even at level L, some people have return of kidney function. It is the responsibility of all health care professionals to be alert to the possibility of AKI, implement prevention strategies, and identify the need to implement appropriate interventions to prevent permanent impairment of kidney function.

Types of Acute Kidney Injury

The types of AKI are described by their causes. These include prerenal azotemia, intrarenal *(intrinsic)* AKI, and postrenal azotemia. Table 71-3 lists causes of AKI.

Prerenal azotemia is kidney injury caused by poor blood flow to the kidneys. The most common problems leading to AKI are hypovolemic shock and heart failure (Ali & Gray-Vickrey, 2011). Early AKI (levels R and I) often can be reversed by correcting blood volume, increasing blood pressure, and improving cardiac output. When the reduced blood flow is prolonged, the kidneys are severely damaged and intrarenal kidney injury results.

The term *intrarenal AKI* is often referred to as *oliguric AKI* in the clinical setting. Other terms include *acute tubular necrosis (ATN)* and *lower nephron nephrosis*. Infections (bacteria, viral, fungal), drugs (especially aminoglycoside antibiotics and NSAIDs), and invading tumors (e.g., lymphomas or leukemias) can cause acute interstitial nephritis. Other

TABLE 71-3   CAUSES OF THE THREE TYPES OF ACUTE KIDNEY INJURY

Prerenal Acute Kidney Injury
Any condition decreasing blood flow to the kidneys and leading to ischemia in the nephrons, such as:
- Shock (hypovolemia, hemorrhage, distributive, obstructive)
- Heart failure
- Pulmonary embolism
- Anaphylaxis
- Sepsis
- Pericardial tamponade

Intrarenal (Intrinsic) Acute Kidney Injury
Actual physical, chemical, hypoxic, or immunologic damage directly to the kidney tissue, such as:
- Acute interstitial nephritis
- Exposure to nephrotoxins
- Acute glomerular nephritis
- Vasculitis
- Acute tubular necrosis
- Renal artery or vein stenosis
- Renal artery or vein thrombosis
- Formation of crystals or precipitates in the nephron tubules

Postrenal Acute Kidney Injury
Obstruction of the urine collecting system anywhere from the calyces to the urethral meatus (obstruction of the ureter must be bilateral to cause postrenal failure unless only one kidney is functional), such as:
- Ureter, bladder, or urethral cancer
- Kidney, ureter, or bladder stones
- Bladder atony
- Prostatic hyperplasia or cancer
- Urethral stricture
- Cervical cancer

causes of intrarenal AKI include inflammation of the glomeruli *(glomerulonephritis)* or of the small vessels of the kidneys *(vasculitis)* or an obstruction of blood flow to the kidneys.

Postrenal azotemia develops from obstruction to the outflow of formed urine anywhere within the kidney or urinary tract.

TABLE 71-4	THE PHASES OF OLIGURIC ACUTE KIDNEY INJURY	
PHASE	**DESCRIPTION**	**CHARACTERISTICS**
Onset phase	Begins with the precipitating event and continues until oliguria develops. Lasts hours to days.	The gradual accumulation of nitrogenous wastes, such as increasing serum creatinine and BUN, may be noted.
Oliguric phase	Characterized by a urine output of 100-400 mL/24 hr that does not respond to fluid challenges or diuretics. Lasts 1-3 weeks.	Laboratory data include increasing serum creatinine and BUN levels, hyperkalemia, bicarbonate deficit (metabolic acidosis), hyperphosphatemia, hypocalcemia, and hypermagnesemia. Sodium retention occurs, but this is masked by the dilutional effects of water retention. Urinary indices are typically low and fixed; regulation of water balance by the kidneys is impaired, so urine specific gravity and urine osmolarity do not vary as plasma osmolarity changes.
Diuretic phase (high-output phase)	Often has a sudden onset within 2-6 wk after oliguric stage. Urine flow increases rapidly over a period of several days. The diuresis can result in an output of up to 10 L/day of dilute urine.	Electrolyte losses typically precede clearance of nitrogenous wastes. Later in the diuretic phase, the BUN level starts to fall and continues to fall until the level reaches normal limits or reaches a plateau. Normal kidney tubular function is re-established during this phase.
Recovery phase (convalescent phase)	In this phase, the patient begins to return to normal levels of activity. Complete recovery may take up to 12 months.	The patient functions at a lower energy level and has less stamina than before the illness. Residual kidney dysfunction may be noted through regular monitoring of kidney function. Kidney function may never return to pre-illness levels, but function sufficient for a long and healthy life is likely.

BUN, Blood urea nitrogen.

When kidney function declines, the oliguric phases of AKI begin (Table 71-4). Some patients have a *nonoliguric* form of AKI in which urine output remains near normal but serum creatinine levels rise. Ideally, interventions to restore circulating volume, improve cardiac output, and increase blood pressure prevent progression to a more severe level of kidney injury.

Etiology

Many types of problems can reduce kidney function. Severe hypotension from shock or dehydration reduces kidney blood flow and can lead to prerenal AKI. Cardiac disease or heart failure also can reduce kidney blood flow. The patient may be oliguric or even anuric (less than 100 mL/24 hr) if kidney blood flow reduction is severe. Conditions causing AKI are listed in Table 71-3.

Incidence/Prevalence

Health care–acquired AKI occurs in as many as 4% of hospital admissions and 20% of critical care admissions (Peacock & Sinert, 2010). Most AKI episodes are due to events that lead to hypotension with poor kidney perfusion and worsening of chronic kidney problems. For patients who survive the precipitating event, the chance for return of kidney function is good. However, complications during the course of AKI can greatly increase the risk for death. Bloodstream infections from IV line contamination are frequent complications that lead to death. However, the highest death rate occurs with trauma (70%) and surgery. AKI caused by nephrotoxic (kidney damaging) substances (Table 71-5) has the lowest rates of recovery. The prognosis for AKI caused by obstruction or glomerulonephritis is much better.

Health Promotion and Maintenance

Keep in mind that severe blood volume depletion can lead to kidney injury even in people who have no known kidney problems. Urge all people to avoid dehydration by drinking at least

TABLE 71-5	SOME POTENTIALLY NEPHROTOXIC SUBSTANCES

Drugs
Antibiotics/Anti-infectives
- Amphotericin B
- Colistimethate
- Methicillin
- Polymyxin B
- Rifampin
- Sulfonamides
- Tetracycline hydrochloride
- Vancomycin

Aminoglycoside Antibiotics
- Gentamicin
- Kanamycin
- Neomycin
- Netilmicin sulfate
- Tobramycin

Chemotherapy agents
- Cisplatin
- Cyclophosphamide
- Methotrexate

Nonsteroidal Anti-inflammatory Drugs (NSAIDs)
- Celecoxib
- Flurbiprofen
- Ibuprofen
- Indomethacin
- Ketorolac
- Meclofenamate
- Meloxicam
- Nabumetone
- Naproxen
- Oxaprozin
- Rofecoxib
- Tolmetin

Other Drugs
- Acetaminophen
- Captopril
- Cyclosporine
- Fluorinate anesthetics
- Metformin
- *D*-Penicillamine
- Phenazopyridine hydrochloride
- Quinine

Other Substances
Organic Solvents
- Carbon tetrachloride
- Ethylene glycol

Non-drug Chemical Agents
- Radiographic contrast dye
- Pesticides
- Fungicides
- Myoglobin (from breakdown of skeletal muscle)

Heavy Metals and Ions
- Arsenic
- Bismuth
- Copper sulfate
- Gold salts
- Lead
- Mercuric chloride

2 to 3 L of fluids daily. This is especially important for athletes or any person who performs strenuous exercise or work and sweats heavily.

Nurses have an essential role in the prevention of acute kidney injury in hospitalized patients. Always be on the lookout for signs of reduced kidney function through careful physical assessment (especially of urine output and weight), close monitoring of laboratory values, and evaluation of fluid status. Early recognition and correction of problems causing reduced kidney blood flow usually restore function before tissue damage can occur. Evaluate the patient's fluid status. Accurately measure intake and output and check body weight to identify changes in fluid balance.

! NURSING SAFETY PRIORITY

Critical Rescue

In any acute care setting, preventing volume depletion is a nursing priority because this is the most common cause of AKI. Recognizing the manifestations of volume depletion (low urine output, decreased systolic blood pressure, decreased pulse pressure, orthostatic hypotension, thirst, rising blood osmolarity) and intervening early to restore volume can reverse AKI and prevent permanent kidney damage.

Also monitor laboratory values for any changes that reflect poor kidney function. Decreased urine specific gravity indicates a loss of urine-concentrating ability and is the earliest sign of kidney tubular damage. Other laboratory values that are helpful in monitoring kidney function include serum creatinine, urine and serum electrolytes, and blood urea nitrogen (BUN).

Be aware of nephrotoxic substances that the patient may ingest or be exposed to (see Table 71-5). Question any prescription for potentially nephrotoxic drugs, and validate the dose before the patient receives the drug. Antibiotics are common drugs that have nephrotoxic side effects. NSAIDs can cause or increase the risk for AKI. Combining two or more nephrotoxic drugs dramatically increases the risk for AKI. If a patient must receive a known nephrotoxic drug, closely monitor laboratory values, including BUN, creatinine, and drug peak and trough levels, for indications of reduced kidney function.

PATIENT-CENTERED COLLABORATIVE CARE

ASSESSMENT

History

The accurate diagnosis of AKI, including its type and its cause, depends on a detailed history of potential causes of AKI. Ask the patient about exposure to nephrotoxins, recent surgery or trauma, transfusions, or other factors that might lead to reduced kidney blood flow. Obtain a drug history, especially treatment with antibiotics, ACE inhibitors, and NSAIDs. Ask about recent imaging procedures requiring injection of a contrast dye. These dyes can cause AKI, especially in older patients with reduced kidney function. AKI must be differentiated from chronic kidney disease (CKD). Ask the patient about diseases that impair kidney function, such as diabetes mellitus, long-term hypertension, systemic lupus erythematosus, and other connective tissue diseases.

To identify possible acute glomerulonephritis, ask about acute illnesses such as influenza, colds, gastroenteritis, and sore throats. Ask whether urine color is darker or appears smoky.

Reversible prerenal azotemia may occur after any episode of acute hypotension, hemorrhage or shock, burns, heart failure, or any problem in which the blood volume is depleted. Extensive bowel preparations, being NPO before surgery without fluid replacement, and fluid loss during surgery can cause prerenal AKI in some patients.

Postrenal kidney injury is identified by focusing on urinary obstructive problems. Ask the patient about any difficulty in starting the urine stream, changes in the amount or appearance of the urine, narrowing of the urine stream, nocturia, urgency, or symptoms of kidney stones. Also ask about any cancer history that may cause urinary obstruction.

Physical Assessment/Clinical Manifestations

The manifestations of AKI are related to the buildup of nitrogenous wastes (azotemia), as well as to as the underlying cause (Chart 71-1). Manifestations of *prerenal* azotemia are hypotension, tachycardia, decreased urine output, decreased cardiac output, decreased central venous pressure (CVP), and

---

CHART 71-1 KEY FEATURES

Acute Kidney Injury

Prerenal Azotemia
- Hypotension
- Tachycardia
- Decreased cardiac output
- Decreased central venous pressure
- Decreased urine output
- Lethargy

Intrarenal (Intrinsic) AKI and Postrenal Azotemia
- Renal manifestations:
  - Oliguria or anuria
  - Increased urine specific gravity
- Cardiac manifestations:
  - Hypertension
  - Tachycardia
  - Jugular venous distention
  - Increased central venous pressure
  - ECG changes: tall T waves
- Respiratory manifestations:
  - Shortness of breath
  - Orthopnea
  - Crackles
  - Pulmonary edema
  - Friction rub
- Gastrointestinal manifestations:
  - Anorexia
  - Nausea
  - Vomiting
  - Flank pain
- Neurologic manifestations:
  - Lethargy
  - Headache
  - Tremors
  - Confusion
- General manifestations:
  - Generalized edema
  - Weight gain

AKI, Acute kidney injury; *ECG,* electrocardiogram.

lethargy. The appearance of a patient with prerenal azotemia is similar to that of a patient with heart failure or dehydration, depending on the cause of the poor kidney blood flow.

Intrarenal (intrinsic) AKI usually occurs with damage to the glomeruli, interstitial tissue, or tubules. Manifestations are related to the retention of fluid and nitrogenous wastes. These include oliguria (decreased urine output) or anuria (absence of urine), edema, hypertension, tachycardia, shortness of breath, distended neck veins, elevated CVP, weight gain, respiratory crackles, anorexia, nausea, vomiting, and lethargy or changes in levels of consciousness. Manifestations of electrolyte imbalances (particularly elevated potassium levels and low calcium levels), such as electrocardiographic (ECG) changes, may also be present.

In patients with *postrenal* AKI, monitor for oliguria or intermittent anuria, symptoms of uremia, and lethargy. Report changes in the urine stream, difficulty starting urination, and the presence of blood or particles in the urine.

Laboratory Assessment

The many changes in laboratory values in the patient with AKI are similar to those occurring in chronic kidney disease (CKD) (Chart 71-2; see also p. 1552 in the discussion of Laboratory Assessment in the Chronic Kidney Disease section). Expect to see rising BUN and serum creatinine levels and abnormal blood electrolyte values. Patients with AKI, however, usually do *not* have the anemia associated with CKD unless there is hemorrhagic blood loss or unless blood urea levels are high enough to break (lyse) red blood cells.

In early AKI, urine tests provide important information. Urine sodium levels are often less than 10 to 20 mEq/L in patients with prerenal azotemia. The urine is concentrated, with a specific gravity greater than 1.030. The presence of urine sediment (e.g., red blood cells [RBCs], RBC casts, and tubular cells), myoglobin, or hemoglobin; a urine sodium level lower than 40 mEq/L; and a specific gravity of less than 1.010 indicate intrarenal kidney injury. In postrenal AKI,

---

CHART 71-2	**LABORATORY PROFILE**

Kidney Disease

TEST	NORMAL RANGE FOR ADULTS	VALUES IN KIDNEY DISEASE
Serum creatinine	*Male:* 0.6-1.2 mg/dL *Female:* 0.5-1.1 mg/dL *Older adults:* Decreased	**In Chronic Kidney Disease** May increase by 0.5-1.0 mg/dL every 1-2 yr May be as high as 15-30 mg/dL *before* symptoms of severe CKD are present **In Acute Kidney Injury** Gradual increase of 1-2 mg/dL every 24-48 hr May increase 1-6 mg/dL in 1 wk or less
Blood urea nitrogen	10-20 mg/dL *Older adults:* May be slightly increased	**In Chronic Kidney Disease** May reach 180-200 mg/dL *before* symptoms develop **In Acute Kidney Injury** Often increases by 10-20 mg/dL at same pace as serum creatinine level May reach 80-100 mg/dL within 1 wk
Serum sodium	136-145 mEq/L; 136-145 mmol/L (SI units)	Normal, increased, or decreased
Serum potassium	3.5-5.0 mEq/L; 3.5-5.0 mmol/L (SI units)	Increased
Serum phosphorus (phosphate)	3.0-4.5 mg/dL; 0.97-1.45 mmol/L (SI units) *Older adults:* May be slightly decreased	Increased
Serum calcium	Total calcium: 9.0-10.5 mg/dL; 2.25-2.75 mmol/L (SI units) Ionized calcium: 4.5-5.6 mg/dL; 1.05-1.3 mmol/L (SI units) *Older adults:* Slightly decreased	Decreased
Serum magnesium	1.3-2.1 mEq/L; 0.65-1.05 mmol/L	Increased
Serum carbon dioxide combining power (bicarbonate)	23-30 mEq/L (venous); 23-30 mmol/L (SI units)	Decreased
Arterial blood pH	7.35-7.45	Decreased (in metabolic acidosis) or normal
Arterial blood bicarbonate (HCO_3)	21-28 mEq/L	Decreased
Arterial blood $Paco_2$	35-45 mm Hg	Decreased
Hemoglobin	*Female:* 12-16 g/dL; 7.4-9.9 mmol/L (SI units) *Male:* 14-18 g/dL; 8.7-11.2 mmol/L (SI units) *Older adults:* Slightly decreased	Decreased
Hematocrit	*Female:* 37%-47% *Male:* 42%-52% *Older adults:* May be slightly decreased	Decreased to 20%
Blood osmolarity	285-295 mOsm/kg or mmol/kg (SI)	Elevated in volume-depleted states, increasing the risk for acute tubular necrosis.

CKD, Chronic kidney disease; *SI,* International System of Units.

urine sodium levels may be normal (about 40 mEq/L), with a specific gravity of 1.000 to 1.010.

Imaging Assessment

X-rays help determine the cause of AKI. An abdominal x-ray is used to check the size of the kidneys. Enlarged kidneys, possibly due to obstruction, may result from hydronephrosis. X-rays may show stones obstructing the renal pelvis, ureters, or bladder.

Renal ultrasonography is a noninvasive procedure using high-energy sound waves. It is useful in the diagnosis of urinary tract obstruction. Dilation of the renal calyces and collecting ducts, as well as stones, can be detected. Ultrasonography can show kidney size and patency of the ureters.

CT scans without contrast dye can identify obstruction or tumors. Contrast dyes are usually avoided to prevent further kidney damage. A nuclear medicine study called *MAG3* may be used to determine the nature of the renal failure, GFR, or tubular function and its severity. A renal scan can determine whether blood flow to the kidneys is sufficient. Cystoscopy or retrograde pyelography may be needed to identify obstructions of the lower urinary tract.

Other Diagnostic Assessment

Kidney biopsy is performed if the cause of AKI is uncertain, an immunologic disease is suspected, or the reversibility of the kidney dysfunction needs to be determined after AKI has persisted for an extended period. Prepare the patient before the test, and provide follow-up care. Be aware of all test results and understand how they might affect the treatment regimen. (See Chapter 68 for a detailed discussion of renal diagnostic tests.)

? NCLEX EXAMINATION CHALLENGE

Safe and Effective Care Environment

The client admitted to the emergency department 1 hour after a motorcycle crash has all of the following laboratory test results. Which result does the nurse report to the health care provider immediately?
A. Blood glucose level of 138 mg/dL
B. Blood urea nitrogen of 22 mg/dL
C. Blood osmolarity of 330 mOsm
D. Serum potassium of 4.9 mEq/L

INTERVENTIONS

The patient with AKI may move from the oliguric phase (in which fluid and electrolytes are retained) to the diuretic phase. In the oliguric phase, the plan of care focuses on close monitoring for life-threatening electrolyte changes and nitrogen retention that may require intervention. During the diuretic phase, hypovolemia and electrolyte *loss* are the main problems. The patient in the diuretic phase of AKI needs a plan of care that focuses on fluid and electrolyte *replacement* and monitoring.

These examples of output variation reflect the continually changing nature of AKI and the need for the plan of care to be constantly updated to reflect the stages of the disease process. Drug therapy, nutrition therapy, and renal replacement therapy (peritoneal dialysis [PD], hemodialysis [HD], or hemofiltration) are commonly used to manage AKI.

Drug Therapy

Patients with AKI receive many drugs. As kidney function changes, drug dosages are changed. It is important to be knowledgeable about the site of drug metabolism and especially careful when giving drugs. Constantly monitor for possible side effects and interactions of the drugs that the patient with AKI is receiving (Chart 71-3; see also the discussion of drug therapy on pp. 1553, 1556, and 1557 in the Chronic Kidney Disease section). Diuretics may be used to increase urine output.

In patients with prerenal azotemia, fluid challenges and diuretics are often used to promote kidney blood flow. In the patient without fluid overload, 500 to 1000 mL of normal saline may be infused over 1 hour. In prerenal azotemia, the patient responds to the fluid challenge by producing urine soon after the initial bolus. Diuretics such as furosemide (Lasix) also may be prescribed along with a fluid bolus. If oliguric kidney injury is diagnosed, the fluid challenges and diuretics are discontinued. Patients often require central venous pressure (CVP) monitoring or measurement of pulmonary arterial pressure by means of a pulmonary artery catheter for accurate evaluation of their hemodynamic status. They also require constant nursing supervision for assessment of the response to fluid and drug therapy. Carefully monitor for signs of possible fluid overload.

Calcium channel blockers may be used to treat AKI resulting from nephrotoxic acute tubular necrosis (ATN). These drugs prevent the movement of calcium into the kidney cells, maintain kidney cell integrity, and improve the glomerular filtration rate (GFR) by improving kidney blood flow.

? DECISION-MAKING CHALLENGE

Patient-Centered Care; Evidence-Based Practice; Quality Improvement

The patient is a 67-year-old woman who has type 2 diabetes (for which she takes metformin) and had a CT scan with contrast material 3 days ago for a pulmonary problem. Today she is sent to the emergency department by her primary care physician because she has gained 8 pounds since the scan and has symptoms of heart failure. She describes her urine output for the past 24 hours as being "about a teacup full." Her admitting diagnosis is possible acute kidney injury. Her vital signs are as follows: temperature 100° F; pulse 108 and irregular; respirations 32; blood pressure 166/110.
1. What additional assessment data should you obtain? Provide a rationale for your choices.
2. What risk factors does she have for acute kidney injury?
3. Is her risk greatest for prerenal acute kidney injury, intrarenal azotemia, or postrenal acute kidney injury? Explain your answer.
4. What questions will you ask her about her urine output?
5. What resources or changes in policy could have helped prevent this problem and future problems?

Nutrition Therapy

Patients who have AKI often have a high rate of protein breakdown. The exact cause for this state is not known. Increases in metabolism and protein breakdown may be related to the stress of a critical illness, causing an increase in blood levels of catecholamines, cortisol, and glucagon. The rate of protein breakdown correlates with the severity of uremia and azotemia. This state causes the breakdown of muscle for protein, which leads to an increase in azotemia and an even more elevated blood urea nitrogen (BUN) level.

CHART 71-3 **COMMON EXAMPLES OF DRUG THERAPY**

Kidney Disease

DRUG/DOSAGE	ACTION/PURPOSE	NURSING INTERVENTIONS	RATIONALES
Cardiac Glycosides			
Digoxin (Digitek, Lanoxicaps, Lanoxin, Novodigoxin ♦) 0.125-0.25 mg orally or IV daily or every other day *Older adults:* 0.0625-0.125 mg orally or IV daily or every other day	Used when heart failure induces kidney injury/disease or makes it worse. Improves ventricular contraction, increasing stroke volume and cardiac output.	Teach patients to take pulse daily before taking the drug and to notify the prescriber if it is below 60.	Drug slows the heart rate and can cause severe bradycardia.
		Instruct patients to notify prescriber if any of these manifestations occur: changes in color vision (more yellow color), blurred vision, eyes sensitive to light, light flashes, or halos around bright lights; changes in behavior, mood, or mental ability; chest pain or palpitations.	These are manifestations of drug toxicity and require the drug be stopped or the dose decreased temporarily.
		Teach patients to not take antacids within 2 hours of taking this drug.	Antacids prevent drug absorption and may delay or inhibit drug effectiveness.
Vitamins and Minerals			
Folic acid (vitamin B₉, Folvite, Novofolacid ♦) 1 mg orally daily Ferrous sulfate (Feosol, Novoferrosulfa ♦) 325 mg orally three or four times daily	When the patient is receiving dialysis, many essential vitamins and minerals are removed from the blood. Replacement is needed to prevent severe deficiencies.	Teach patients to take the drugs after dialysis.	Dialysis removes the drug from the blood.
		Teach patients to take iron supplements (ferrous sulfate) with meals.	Food reduces nausea and abdominal discomfort.
		Teach patients to take stool softeners daily while taking iron supplements.	Oral iron preparations cause constipation, and most patients with kidney disease failure must reduce their fluid intake, further increasing the risk for constipation.
		Remind patients that iron supplements change the color of the stool.	Knowing the expected side effects decreases anxiety when they appear.
Synthetic Erythropoietin			
Epoetin alfa (Epogen, Procrit) 50-100 units/kg subcutaneously or IV three times a week for patients on dialysis Darbepoetin alfa (Aranesp) 0.45 mcg/kg subcutaneously or IV once weekly for patients on dialysis	Drug prevents anemia by stimulating red blood cell growth and maturation in the bone marrow.	Teach patients to report any of these side effects to the prescriber as soon as possible: chest pain, difficulty breathing, high blood pressure, rapid weight gain, seizures, skin rash or hives, swelling of feet or ankles.	Drug can induce serious cardiovascular problems, such as myocardial infarction (MI).
		Reinforce to patients that they must have hemoglobin levels monitored weekly.	Drug can raise hemoglobin and hematocrit levels to the point that blood viscosity increases, raising blood pressure and increasing the risk for MI. Drug dosage is reduced to prevent hemoglobin levels higher than 10 to 12 mg/dL.
Phosphate Binders			
Aluminum hydroxide gel (Amphojel, AlternaGEL, Alu-Cap, Nephrox) 300-600 mg orally two to four times daily Aluminum carbonate gel (Basaljel) 500 mg-2 g orally two to four times daily	High blood phosphate levels cause hypocalcemia and osteodystrophy. Drugs lower serum phosphate levels by binding phosphorus present in food.	Teach patients to take drugs with meals.	Drug action is to bind phosphate in food, preventing its absorption.
		Remind patients taking digoxin to separate the drugs by at least 2 hours.	These drugs reduce digoxin absorption and effects.
		Teach patients to take stool softeners daily while taking these drugs.	These drugs cause constipation, and most patients with severe kidney disease must reduce their fluid intake, further increasing the risk for constipation.
		Teach patients to report muscle weakness, slow or irregular pulse, or confusion to the prescriber.	These are manifestations of hypophosphatemia, which require dosage adjustment.

If the patient with AKI has a good dietary intake (see discussion of Enhancing Nutrition on pp. 1555-1556 in the Chronic Kidney Disease section), nutritional support may not be needed. A dietary consult with a dietitian, who will calculate the patient's caloric needs, may be prescribed. Work with the dietitian to provide a diet with specified amounts of protein, sodium, and fluids. For the patient who does not require dialysis, 0.6 g/kg of body weight or 40 g/day of protein is usually prescribed. For patients who do require dialysis, the protein level needed will range from 1 to 1.5 g/kg. The amount of dietary sodium ranges from 60 to 90 mEq. If high blood potassium levels are present, dietary potassium is restricted to 60 to 70 mEq. The amount of fluid permitted is generally calculated to be equal to the urine volume plus 500 mL. Assess food intake every shift to ensure that caloric intake is adequate.

Many patients with AKI are too ill or their appetite is too poor to eat enough food. For these patients, some form of nutritional support (e.g., total parenteral nutrition [TPN] or hyperalimentation) is needed. The purposes of nutritional support in AKI are to provide sufficient nutrients to maintain or improve nutritional status, to preserve lean body mass, to restore or maintain fluid balance, and to preserve kidney function.

If TPN is used, the solutions are mixed to meet the patient's specific needs. Because kidney function is unstable in AKI, constantly monitor the serum electrolyte levels to indicate when the TPN solution needs to be changed. IV fat emulsion (Intralipid) infusions can provide a nonprotein source of calories. In uremic patients, fat emulsions are used in place of glucose to avoid the problems of excessive sugars.

Dialysis Therapies

Hemodialysis (HD) and peritoneal dialysis (PD) are used for patients with L and E levels of AKI. Indications for dialysis use include the presence of uremia, persistent high potassium levels, metabolic acidosis, continued fluid overload, uremic pericarditis, and encephalopathy.

Immediate vascular access for HD in patients with AKI is made by placement of a dual- or triple-lumen catheter specific for HD. When HD is expected to be used for several weeks, the catheter is usually placed in the subclavian or internal jugular vein. If only one or two HD treatments are needed, as for removal of drugs or toxins, a femoral site may be selected. Longer use of the femoral site is avoided because the patient's mobility is restricted and complications, such as hematomas and infection, are common. Repeatedly accessing the femoral site increases the risk for hematoma formation and makes repeated use of the vein impossible.

The subclavian vein is used, when possible, instead of the femoral site because the catheter can be left in place between dialysis treatments. However, the longer the catheter is left in this place, the greater the chance for infection. The subclavian dialysis catheter (Fig. 71-1) is inserted at the bedside. A physician or nurse practitioner performs the sterile procedure, and then the catheter is covered with a sterile dressing. Monitor for manifestations of procedure complications such as pneumothorax (reduced breath sounds, tracheal deviation away from midline, prominence and poor movement of one side of the chest) or subcutaneous emphysema (crackling and swelling of tissue around the site). Catheter placement is checked by chest x-ray before its use.

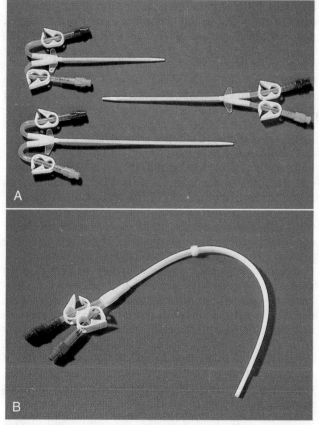

FIG. 71-1 Subclavian dialysis catheters. These catheters are radiopaque tubes that can be used for hemodialysis access. The Y-shaped tubing allows arterial outflow and venous return through a single catheter. **A,** Mahurkar catheters, made of polyurethane and used for short-term access. **B,** A PermCath catheter, made of silicone and used for long-term access.

If hemodialysis is needed for more than a few days, a long-term dialysis catheter may be used. Most of these catheters are placed in the radiology department using a tunneling technique. The patient receives moderate sedation. Under sonographic or fluoroscopic guidance, the physician makes a small incision where the internal jugular vein passes behind the clavicle. A 6- to 8-cm tunnel is created out from the side of the incision. A long-term hemodialysis catheter is inserted through the tunnel and into the jugular vein. Keeping a segment of the catheter within the subcutaneous tissues before entering the jugular vein reduces the risk for infection.

Hemodialysis catheters have two lumens, one for outflow and one for inflow. This allows the outflow of blood for dialysis to be separated from the dialyzed blood returned through the inflow lumen. A triple-lumen catheter for HD is available. The third lumen is an access for drawing venous blood or giving drugs and fluid without interrupting dialysis.

Peritoneal dialysis (PD) may also be used in the treatment of AKI, although some patients, such as those being mechanically ventilated, may not be able to tolerate the abdominal distention that occurs with PD. PD uses the peritoneum as the dialyzing membrane. The dialysate is infused through a catheter implanted in the peritoneum. A complete discussion of PD is provided in the Chronic Kidney Disease section, pp. 1564-1567.

Continuous Renal Replacement Therapy

Continuous renal replacement therapies (CRRTs) are the standard treatment for AKI levels L and E. Renal replacement therapies in the form of hemofiltration are often better tolerated than HD for critically ill patients because this method avoids rapid shifts of fluids and electrolytes.

Continuous venovenous hemofiltration (CVVH), continuous venovenous hemodiafiltration (CVVHD), continuous arteriovenous hemofiltration (CAVH), and continuous arteriovenous hemofiltration with dialysis (CAVHD) are the renal replacement therapies most commonly used for patients with AKI. The venovenous methods are being used more often than the arteriovenous methods. These procedures are similar to HD but their use is temporary.

Continuous venovenous hemofiltration (CVVH) is often used with critically ill patients. CVVH uses only a double-lumen venous catheter for access and is powered by a pump, making the rate of filtration more reliable than methods using mean arterial pressure. The pump increases the risk for an air embolus, but most pumps have alarms that detect air. These systems also require the use of anticoagulants but at lower doses than needed for AV systems. These procedures are used in critical care units, and patients require continuous nursing care.

The technique of CVVHD is a very common method of renal replacement therapy. It uses an infusion pump, hemodialysis membrane, and dialysate solution, as well as the same type of blood access as the CVVH technique. Similar to the CAVHD system, CVVHD adds the dialysis membrane and the dialysate solution instead of just filtering the blood and, as a result, increases the efficiency of removing waste products from the blood. CVVHD is somewhat less effective than CAVHD because the lower pressure in the venous system compared with the arterial system does not filter as much blood in the same amount of time. Thus CVVHD needs to be performed for longer periods to achieve the same effects as CAVHD. However, because the removal is slower, fewer adverse changes in blood volume and blood pressure are likely to occur.

CAVH is used for patients who have fluid volume overload, are resistant to diuretics, and have unstable blood pressures and cardiac output. The use of CAVH requires placement of both arterial and venous catheters and that the patient have a mean arterial pressure (MAP) of at least 60 mm Hg. (**Mean arterial pressure** is a person's average arterial pressure and is based on cardiac output and systemic vascular resistance. The normal adult MAP is 100 mm Hg.) CAVH continuously removes large amounts of plasma water, wastes, and electrolytes. Electrolytes are replaced through prescribed amounts of IV electrolyte solutions. A major disadvantage of arteriovenous (AV) filtration is the risk for bleeding caused by anticoagulants used to prevent membrane clotting.

A double-lumen dialysis catheter is inserted into a large vein (subclavian, jugular) for CAVHD. A **dialysate** (a solution composed of water, glucose, sodium chloride, potassium, magnesium, calcium, and bicarbonate) delivery system is used to remove waste products in addition to plasma water in patients with limited cardiac output, those with severe

hypotension, or those who do not respond to diuretic therapy. These patients cannot tolerate HD, and PD could not remove the large amount of excess fluid.

? NCLEX EXAMINATION CHALLENGE

Safe and Effective Care Environment

> When performing an hourly assessment of a client who had a subclavian catheter placed 6 hours ago for continuous arteriovenous hemofiltration with dialysis (CAVHD), the nurse observes these findings. For which finding does the nurse stop the CAVHD?
> A. The right foot and ankle appear slightly more edematous than the left foot and ankle.
> B. Blood pressure has decreased from 148/90 to 90/60.
> C. Pulse oximetry is increased from 89% to 91%.
> D. The trachea is in a midline position.

Posthospital Care

The care for a patient with AKI after discharge from the hospital varies, depending on the status of the disorder when the patient is discharged. The course of AKI varies, with recovery lasting up to several months. If the kidney injury is resolving, follow-up care may be provided by a nephrologist or by the family physician in consultation with the nephrologist. However, AKI may result in permanent kidney damage and CKD with the need for chronic dialysis or even transplantation. In these cases, follow-up care is similar to that needed for patients with chronic kidney disease (see Community-Based Care, pp. 1571-1572).

If the AKI is beginning to resolve, the follow-up care may involve many services. Frequent medical visits are necessary, as are scheduled laboratory blood and urine tests to monitor kidney function. A dietitian is needed to modify the patient's diet according to the degree of kidney function and ongoing nutritional needs. Teach patients continuing dialysis after discharge to limit foods high in potassium, sodium, and phosphorus and to observe protein restrictions. Also teach about any needed fluid intake limitation. Instruct patients to weigh themselves daily, keep a daily log, and report any daily weight gain of 2 pounds or more immediately to the health care provider.

Some patients may need temporary dialysis until their kidneys can eliminate fluid and waste products. The dialysis started while the patient was an inpatient can be continued at an outpatient dialysis center. Teaching about the type of dialysis, how to care for vascular access sites, dietary restrictions, fluid restrictions, and prevention of complications is ongoing throughout the recovery phase. Depending on their level of independence and family support, some patients may also need home care nursing or social work assistance.

? NCLEX EXAMINATION CHALLENGE

Health Promotion and Maintenance

> What is the most important precaution for the nurse to teach the client with continuing kidney impairment on discharge after treatment for acute kidney injury?
> A. Avoid fluids that contain either alcohol or caffeine.
> B. Weigh yourself daily and report any rapid weight gain.
> C. Drink at least 3 liters of fluid daily to prevent dehydration.
> D. Use a dipstick to check for glucose in your urine at least once daily.

CHART 71-4 KEY FEATURES

Uremia

- Metallic taste in the mouth
- Anorexia
- Nausea
- Vomiting
- Muscle cramps
- Uremic "frost" on skin
- Itching
- Fatigue and lethargy
- Hiccups
- Edema
- Dyspnea
- Muscle cramps
- Paresthesias

TABLE 71-6 PROGRESSION OF CHRONIC KIDNEY DISEASE

STAGE OF CHRONIC KIDNEY DISEASE (CKD)	ESTIMATED GLOMERULAR FILTRATION RATE	INTERVENTION
Stage 1 At risk; normal kidney function (early kidney disease may or may not be present)	>90 mL/min	Screening for risk factors Uncontrolled hypertension Diabetes mellitus Chronic kidney or urinary tract infection Presence of genetic kidney diseases Exposure to nephrotoxic substances
Stage 2 Mild CKD	60-89 mL/min	Focus on reduction of risk factors
Stage 3 Moderate CKD	30-59 mL/min	Implement strategies to slow disease progression
Stage 4 Severe CKD	15-29 mL/min	Manage complications, and prepare for eventual renal replacement therapy
Stage 5 End-stage kidney disease (ESKD)	<15 mL/min	Implement renal replacement therapy/ kidney transplantation

CHRONIC KIDNEY DISEASE

Pathophysiology

Unlike acute kidney injury (AKI), chronic kidney disease (CKD) is a progressive, irreversible disorder and kidney function does *not* recover. When kidney function is too poor to sustain life, CKD becomes end-stage kidney disease (ESKD). Terms used with kidney dysfunction include azotemia (buildup of nitrogen-based wastes in the blood), uremia (azotemia with clinical symptoms [Chart 71-4]), and uremic syndrome. Table 71-1 compares AKI and CKD.

Stages of Chronic Kidney Disease

The kidneys lose function (fail) in an organized fashion involving five stages based on estimated glomerular filtration rate (GFR). Progression toward ESKD usually starts with a gradual decrease in GFR (Table 71-6). In this first stage, the person may have a normal GFR (greater than 90 mL/min) with normal kidney function and no obvious kidney disease. However, there may be a *reduced renal reserve* in which

reduced kidney function occurs *without* buildup of wastes in the blood because the unaffected nephrons overwork to compensate for the diseased nephrons. Although no manifestations of kidney dysfunction are usually present at this stage, if the patient is stressed with infection, fluid overload, pregnancy, or dehydration, kidney function at this stage can appear reduced.

In the next stage, *mild CKD*, GFR is reduced, ranging between 60 and 89 mL/min. Kidney nephron damage has occurred, and there may be slight elevations of metabolic wastes in the blood because not enough healthy nephrons remain to compensate completely for the damaged nephrons. Levels of blood urea nitrogen (BUN), serum creatinine, uric acid, and phosphorus are not sensitive enough to define this stage, however, and reduced GFR is the best measure of CKD. Increased output of dilute urine may occur at this stage of CKD and, if the problem is untreated at this stage, can cause severe dehydration.

! NURSING SAFETY PRIORITY

Action Alert

Teach patients with mild CKD that carefully managing fluid volume, blood pressure, electrolytes, and other kidney-damaging diseases (e.g., hypertension, diabetes mellitus) by following prescribed drug and nutrition therapies can prevent damage and slow the progression to ESKD.

In *moderate CKD*, GFR reduction continues and ranges between 30 and 59 mL/min. Nephron damage has continued, and the remaining nephrons cannot manage metabolic wastes, fluid balance, and electrolyte balance. Restriction of fluids, proteins, and electrolytes is needed.

Over time, patients progress to *severe CKD* (the fourth stage) and *end-stage kidney disease* (ESKD) (the fifth stage). Excessive amounts of urea and creatinine build up in the blood, and the kidneys cannot maintain homeostasis. Severe fluid, electrolyte, and acid-base imbalances occur (Pradeep & Verrelli, 2010). Without renal replacement therapy, fatal complications occur.

Kidney Changes

Kidney dysfunction with greatly reduced GFR causes many problems, including abnormal urine production, poor water excretion, electrolyte imbalances, and metabolic abnormalities. Because the healthy nephrons become larger and work harder, the GFR is effective until about three fourths of kidney function is lost. Homeostasis of electrolytes, acid-base, and nitrogenous wastes is maintained until late in the course of kidney disease.

As the disease progresses, the ability to produce dilute urine is reduced, resulting in urine with a fixed osmolarity (isosthenuria). As kidney function continues to decline, the BUN increases and urine output decreases. At this point, the patient is at risk for fluid overload.

Metabolic Changes

Urea and creatinine excretion are disrupted by kidney dysfunction. Creatinine comes from proteins present in skeletal muscle. The rate of creatinine excretion depends on muscle mass, physical activity, and diet. Without major changes in diet or physical activity, the serum creatinine level is constant.

Creatinine is partially excreted by the kidney tubules, and a decrease in kidney function leads to a buildup of serum creatinine. Urea is made from protein metabolism and is excreted by the kidneys. The BUN level normally varies directly with protein intake and hydration status.

The method for assessing the GFR is the use of a formula that considers the serum creatinine level, age, gender, race, and body size. The most common formula is the Cockcroft-Gault equation.

Sodium excretion changes are common. Early in CKD, the patient is at risk for *hyponatremia* (sodium depletion) because there are fewer healthy nephrons to reabsorb sodium. Thus sodium is lost in the urine. The polyuria of early kidney dysfunction also causes sodium loss.

In the later stages of CKD, kidney excretion of sodium is reduced as urine production decreases. Then sodium retention and high serum sodium levels *(hypernatremia)* can occur with only modest increases in dietary sodium intake. This problem leads to severe fluid and electrolyte imbalances (see Chapter 13). Sodium retention causes hypertension and edema.

Even with sodium retention, the serum sodium level may appear normal because plasma water is retained at the same time. If fluid retention occurs at a greater rate than sodium retention, the serum sodium level is falsely low because of dilution (see Chart 71-2).

Potassium excretion occurs mainly through the kidney. Any increase in potassium load during the later stages of CKD can lead to hyperkalemia (high serum potassium levels). Normal serum potassium levels of 3.5 to 5 mEq/L are maintained until the 24-hour urine output falls below 500 mL. High potassium levels then develop quickly, reaching 7 to 8 mEq/L or greater. Severe ECG changes result from this elevation, and fatal dysrhythmias can occur. Other factors contribute to high potassium levels in CKD, including the ingestion of potassium in drugs, failure to restrict dietary potassium, tissue breakdown, blood transfusions, and bleeding or hemorrhage. (See Chapter 13 for discussion of potassium problems.)

Acid-base balance is affected by CKD. In the early stages, blood pH changes little because the remaining healthy nephrons increase their rate of acid excretion. As more nephrons are lost, acid excretion is reduced and metabolic acidosis results (see Chapter 14).

Many factors lead to acidosis in CKD. First, the kidneys cannot excrete excessive hydrogen ions (acids). Normally, tubular cells move hydrogen ions into the urine for excretion, but ammonium and bicarbonate are needed for this movement to occur. In patients with CKD, ammonium production is decreased and reabsorption of bicarbonate does not occur. This process leads to a buildup of hydrogen ions and reduced levels of bicarbonate *(base deficit)*. High potassium levels further reduce kidney ammonium production and excretion.

As CKD worsens and acid retention increases, increased respiratory action is needed to keep blood pH normal. The respiratory system adjusts or compensates for the increased blood hydrogen ion levels (decreased pH) by increasing the rate and depth of breathing to excrete carbon dioxide through the lungs. This breathing pattern, called Kussmaul respiration, increases with worsening kidney disease. Although hydrogen ions (acids) can leave the body this way, when too much carbon dioxide is "blown off," respiratory alkalosis results. Serum bicarbonate measures the extent of metabolic acidosis (bicarbonate deficit). Patients with CKD usually need alkali replacement to counteract acidosis.

Calcium and phosphorus balance is disrupted by CKD. A complex, balanced normal relationship exists between calcium and phosphate and is influenced by vitamin D (see Chapter 13). The kidney produces calcitriol, the active form of vitamin D, which then enhances intestinal absorption of calcium.

In CKD, phosphate retention and a deficiency of active vitamin D disrupt the calcium and phosphate balance. Normally, excessive dietary phosphate is excreted by the kidneys in the urine. Parathyroid hormone (PTH) controls the amount of phosphate in the blood by causing tubular excretion of phosphate when there is an excess. An early effect of CKD is reduced phosphate excretion (Fig. 71-2). As plasma

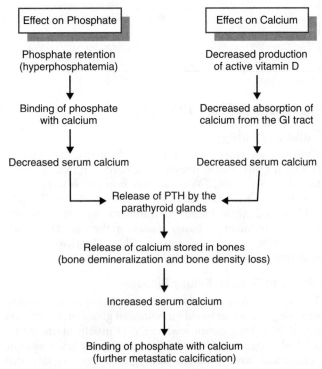

FIG. 71-2 The effects of kidney dysfunction on phosphate and calcium balance. *PTH*, Parathyroid hormone.

phosphate levels increase *(hyperphosphatemia),* calcium levels decrease *(hypocalcemia).* Chronic low blood calcium levels stimulate the parathyroid glands to release more PTH. Under the influence of additional PTH, calcium is released from storage areas in bones (bone resorption), which results in bone density loss. The extra calcium from the bone is needed to balance the excess plasma phosphate level. The problem of low blood calcium levels is made worse with severe CKD because kidney cell damage also reduces production of active vitamin D. Thus less calcium is absorbed through the intestinal tract in the absence of sufficient vitamin D.

The problems in bone metabolism and structure caused by CKD-induced low calcium levels and high phosphorus levels are called renal osteodystrophy. Bone mineral loss causes bone pain, spinal sclerosis, fractures, bone density loss, osteomalacia, and tooth calcium loss.

Crystals formed from excessive calcium phosphate are called *metastatic calcifications* and may precipitate in many body areas. When the plasma level of the calcium-phosphate product (serum calcium level multiplied by the serum phosphate level) exceeds 70 mg/dL, the crystals may lodge in the kidneys, heart, lungs, major blood vessels, joints, eyes (causing conjunctivitis), and brain. Skin itching increases with calcium-phosphate imbalances.

Cardiac Changes

Hypertension is common in most patients with CKD. This problem may be either the cause or the result of CKD. In patients who have other causes of hypertension such as atherosclerosis, the increased blood pressure damages the delicate capillaries in the glomerulus, and eventually ESKD results.

CKD itself elevates blood pressure by causing fluid and sodium overload and dysfunction of the renin-angiotensin-aldosterone system. The retention of sodium and water causes circulatory overload, which elevates blood pressure. The kidneys respond to a decrease in kidney blood flow or to low serum sodium levels by trying to improve blood flow to the kidney. The release of renin triggers the production of more angiotensin and aldosterone. Angiotensin causes blood vessel constriction and increases blood pressure. Aldosterone, a hormone released by the adrenal glands, stimulates kidney tubules to reabsorb sodium and water. These actions increase plasma volume and raise blood pressure. The damaged kidneys do not recognize the increase in blood pressure and continue to produce renin. The result is severe hypertension that is difficult to treat and worsens kidney function. Many patients with CKD also have heart damage and heart enlargement from the long-term hypertension.

Hyperlipidemia occurs in CKD from changes in fat metabolism that increase triglyceride, total cholesterol, and low-density lipoprotein (LDL) levels. These changes increase the patient's risk for coronary artery disease and acute cardiac events. Problems with lipids and atherosclerosis are increased for the patient CKD and diabetes (Brites et al., 2007).

Heart failure may occur in CKD because it increases the workload on the heart as a result of anemia, hypertension, and fluid overload. Left ventricular enlargement and heart failure are common in ESKD. Uremia may cause *uremic cardiomyopathy,* the uremic toxin effect on the myocardium. Heart failure also may occur in these patients because of hypertension and coronary artery disease. Cardiac disease continues to be the leading cause of death in patients with ESKD (USRDS, 2010).

Pericarditis also occurs in patients with CKD. The pericardial sac becomes inflamed by uremic toxins or infection. If it is not treated, this problem leads to pericardial effusion, cardiac tamponade, and death. Manifestations include severe chest pain, increased pulse rate, low-grade fever, and a pericardial friction rub that can be heard with a stethoscope placed over the left sternal border.

As the pericarditis continues and the pericardial effusion worsens, dysrhythmias may develop. The fluid around the heart makes heart tones softer and harder to hear. Blood pressure decreases, and the patient may have shortness of breath. If left untreated, pericardial effusion causes cardiac tamponade, an emergency in which pulse pressure decreases and bradycardia results. Treatment of tamponade requires removal of pericardial fluid by placement of a needle, catheter, or drainage tube into the pericardium.

Hematologic Changes

Anemia is a common problem in patients in the later stages of CKD, and it worsens the CKD manifestations. The causes of anemia include a decreased erythropoietin level that decreases red blood cell (RBC) production, decreased RBC survival time resulting from uremia, iron and folic acid deficiencies, and increased bleeding as a result of impaired platelet function.

Gastrointestinal Changes

Uremia affects the entire GI system. The normal flora of the mouth changes with uremia. The mouth contains the enzyme *urease,* which breaks down urea into ammonia. The ammonia generated from this reaction causes halitosis (bad breath) and may also cause stomatitis (mouth inflammation).

Anorexia, nausea, vomiting, and hiccups are common in patients with uremia. The specific cause of these problems is unknown but may be related to high BUN and creatinine levels as well as acidosis.

Peptic ulcer disease is common in patients with uremia, but the exact cause is unclear. Uremic colitis with watery diarrhea or constipation may also be present with uremia. Ulcers may occur in the stomach or small or large intestine, causing erosion of blood vessels. The blood loss caused by these erosions may lead to hemorrhagic shock from severe GI bleeding.

Etiology and Genetic Risk

The causes of CKD are complex (Table 71-7). More than 100 different disease processes can result in progressive loss of kidney function (see also Chapter 70). Two main causes of ESKD are hypertension and diabetes mellitus (USRDS, 2010). Infection and genetic kidney diseases also can lead to ESKD (Nussbaum et al., 2007). African-American patients are four times more likely to develop ESKD and seven times more likely to have hypertensive ESKD.

Incidence/Prevalence

The number of patients being treated for CKD is increasing. The 2010 U.S. Renal Data Systems' annual report stated that 527,283 people in the United States were under treatment for ESKD. In 2007, the reported incidence of kidney disease (new patients per year requiring renal replacement therapy)

TABLE 71-7   SELECTED CAUSES OF CHRONIC KIDNEY DISEASE

Glomerular Disease
- Glomerulonephritis
- Basement membrane disease
- Goodpasture's syndrome
- Intercapillary glomerulosclerosis

Tubular Disease
- Chronic hypercalcemia
- Chronic potassium depletion
- Fanconi's syndrome
- Heavy metal (lead) poisoning

Vascular Disease of the Kidney
- Ischemic disease of the kidney
- Bilateral renal artery stenosis
- Nephrosclerosis
- Hyperparathyroidism

Urinary Tract Disease
- Obstructive uropathy

Inherited or Genetic Conditions
- Hypoplastic kidneys
- Medullary cystic disease
- Polycystic kidney disease

Infection
- Pyelonephritis
- Tuberculosis

Systemic Vascular Disease
- Intrarenal renovascular hypertension
- Extrarenal renovascular hypertension

Metabolic Kidney Disease
- Amyloidosis
- Gout (hyperuricemic nephropathy)
- Diabetic nephropathy
- Milk-alkali syndrome
- Sarcoidosis

Connective Tissue Disease
- Progressive systemic sclerosis
- Systemic lupus erythematosus
- Polyarteritis

NOTE: List is not all-inclusive.

CHART 71-5   PATIENT AND FAMILY EDUCATION: PREPARING FOR SELF-MANAGEMENT

Prevention of Kidney and Urinary Problems

- Be alert to the general appearance of your urine. Note any changes in its color, clarity, or odor.
- Changes in the frequency or volume of urine passage occur with changes in fluid intake. More frequent or infrequent voiding not associated with changes in fluid intake may signal potential problems.
- Any discomfort or distress with the passage of urine is not normal. Pain, burning, urgency, aching, or difficulty with initiating urine flow or complete bladder emptying is of some concern.
- The kidneys need 1 to 2 quarts of fluid a day to flush out your body wastes. Water is the ideal flushing agent.
- Reduce your intake of carbonated soft drinks.
- Changes in kidney function are often silent for many years. Periodically ask your health care provider to measure your kidney function with a blood test (serum creatinine) and a urinalysis.
- If you have a history of kidney disease, diabetes mellitus, hypertension (high blood pressure), or a family history of kidney disease, you should know your serum creatinine level and your 24-hour creatinine clearance. At least one checkup per year that includes laboratory blood and urine testing of kidney function is recommended.
- If you are identified as having decreased kidney function, ask about whether any prescribed drug, diet, diagnostic test, or therapeutic procedure will present a risk to your current kidney function. Check out all nonprescription drugs with your physician or pharmacist before using them.

---

was close to 110,000. More than 24% of patients with ESKD die during the first year of treatment. ESKD occurs more often in men than in women (USRDS, 2010). The greatest increase in ESKD is in patients 65 years of age and older. Chart 71-5 addresses prevention of kidney and urinary problems.

Health Promotion and Maintenance

The health-promotion activities to prevent or delay the onset of CKD focus on controlling the diseases that lead to its development, such as diabetes and hypertension. Identifying patients who have these disorders at an early stage is critical to CKD prevention. Teach patients to adhere to drug and diet regimens and engage in regular physical activity to prevent the blood vessel changes that lead to kidney damage. Instruct patients with diabetes to keep their blood glucose levels within the prescribed range. Teach patients with hypertension that drug therapy is not a cure and must be continued along with lifestyle changes. Urge patients with diabetes or hypertension to have yearly testing for microalbuminuria.

Teach everyone treated for an infection anywhere in the kidney/urinary system to take all antibiotics as prescribed. Urge everyone to drink at least 3 L of water daily unless a health problem requires fluid restriction. Caution people who use over-the-counter NSAIDs to avoid abusing these drugs because they reduce blood flow to the kidney and their long-term use reduces kidney function (Solomon, 2010). Chart 71-5 is a patient education guide for prevention of kidney and urinary problems.

PATIENT-CENTERED COLLABORATIVE CARE

ASSESSMENT

History

When taking a history from a patient with suspected chronic kidney disease (CKD), document the patient's age and gender. Accurately measure weight and height, and ask about usual weight and recent weight gain or loss. Weight gain may indicate fluid retention from poor kidney function. Weight loss may be the result of anorexia from high blood urea levels.

Obtain a complete history of known kidney or urologic disorders, long-term health problems, drug use, and current health problems. Ask the patient about any existing kidney disease or family history of kidney disease that might indicate a genetic problem. A history of kidney infection or stones may imply past kidney damage. Explore the possibility of long-term health problems, because illnesses such as hypertension, diabetes, systemic lupus erythematosus, arthritis, cancer, and tuberculosis can cause decreased kidney function.

Document the use of current and past prescription and over-the-counter drugs, because many drugs are nephrotoxic and can cause kidney damage (see Table 71-5).

Examine the patient's dietary habits, and discuss any present GI problems. A change in the taste of foods often occurs with CKD. Patients may report that sweet foods are not as appealing or that meats have a metallic taste. Ask about the presence of nausea, vomiting, anorexia, hiccups, diarrhea, or constipation. These manifestations may be the result of excess wastes that the body cannot excrete because of kidney disease.

Ask about the patient's energy level and any recent injuries or bleeding. Explore changes in his or her daily routine as a possible *result* of fatigue. Weakness, drowsiness, and shortness of breath suggest impending pulmonary edema or neurologic degeneration. Ask about bruising or bleeding, which can be caused by hematologic changes from uremia.

Discuss urine elimination in detail, including frequency of urination, appearance of the urine, and any difficulty starting or controlling urination. These data can help identify urologic problems that may influence existing kidney function.

? NCLEX EXAMINATION CHALLENGE

Health Promotion and Maintenance

A 40-year-old African-American woman is newly diagnosed with mild chronic kidney disease (CKD). She is otherwise very fit and healthy, and no one in her family has CKD. She asks the nurse whether any of the following factors could have caused this problem. Which factor should the nurse indicate may have influenced the development of CKD?

A. She has followed a vegetarian diet that includes eggs but no dairy products for the past 3 years.

B. She has taken 220 mg of naproxen twice daily for 3 years.

C. Her mother and older sister have type 2 diabetes.

D. She drinks 3 liters of water daily.

Physical Assessment/Clinical Manifestations

CKD causes changes in all body systems (Chart 71-6). Most manifestations are related to changes in fluid volume, electrolyte and acid-base imbalances, and buildup of nitrogenous wastes.

Neurologic manifestations of CKD and uremic syndrome vary (see Chart 71-6). Observe for problems ranging from lethargy to seizures or coma, which indicate uremic encephalopathy. Assess for sensory changes that appear in a glove and stocking pattern over the hands and feet. Check for weakness in the upper or lower extremities (e.g., uremic neuropathy).

If untreated, encephalopathy can lead to seizures and coma. Dialysis is used for CKD when neurologic problems result. The manifestations of encephalopathy resolve with dialysis. However, improvement in neuropathy is limited if it is severe and motor function is impaired.

Cardiovascular manifestations of CKD and uremia result from fluid overload, hypertension, heart failure (HF), pericarditis, and potassium-induced dysrhythmias. Assess for signs of reduced sodium and water excretion. Circulatory overload, if untreated, leads to HF, pulmonary edema, peripheral edema, and hypertension.

Assess heart rate and rhythm, listening for extra sounds (particularly an S_3), irregular patterns, or a pericardial friction rub. Unless a hemodialysis (HD) vascular access has been created, measure blood pressure in each arm. Assess the jugular veins for distention, and assess for edema of the feet, shins, and sacrum and around the eyes. Shortness of breath with exertion and at night suggests fluid overload.

Respiratory manifestations of CKD also vary (e.g., breath that smells like urine [*uremic fetor* or uremic halitosis], deep sighing, yawning, shortness of breath). Observe the rhythm, rate, and depth of breathing. Tachypnea (increased rate of

---

CHART 71-6 KEY FEATURES

Severe Chronic Kidney Disease

Neurologic Manifestations
- Lethargy and daytime drowsiness
- Inability to concentrate or decreased attention span
- Seizures
- Coma
- Slurred speech
- Asterixis (jerky movements or "flapping" of the hands)
- Tremors, twitching, or jerky movements
- Myoclonus
- Ataxia (alteration in gait)
- Paresthesias

Cardiovascular Manifestations
- Cardiomyopathy
- Hypertension
- Peripheral edema
- Heart failure
- Uremic pericarditis
- Pericardial effusion
- Pericardial friction rub
- Cardiac tamponade

Respiratory Manifestations
- Uremic halitosis
- Tachypnea
- Deep sighing, yawning
- Kussmaul respirations
- Uremic pneumonitis
- Shortness of breath
- Pulmonary edema
- Pleural effusion
- Depressed cough reflex
- Crackles

Hematologic Manifestations
- Anemia
- Abnormal bleeding and bruising

Gastrointestinal Manifestations
- Anorexia
- Nausea
- Vomiting
- Metallic taste in the mouth
- Changes in taste acuity and sensation
- Uremic colitis (diarrhea)
- Constipation
- Uremic gastritis (possible GI bleeding)
- Uremic fetor (breath odor)
- Stomatitis

Urinary Manifestations
- Polyuria, nocturia (early)
- Oliguria, anuria (later)
- Proteinuria
- Hematuria
- Diluted, straw-colored appearance (early)
- Concentrated and cloudy appearance (later)

Integumentary Manifestations
- Decreased skin turgor
- Yellow-gray pallor
- Dry skin
- Pruritus
- Ecchymosis
- Purpura
- Soft-tissue calcifications
- Uremic frost (late, premorbid)

Musculoskeletal Manifestations
- Muscle weakness and cramping
- Bone pain
- Pathologic fractures
- Renal osteodystrophy

Reproductive Manifestations
- Decreased fertility
- Infrequent or absent menses
- Decreased libido
- Impotence

---

breathing) and hyperpnea (increased depth of breathing) occur with metabolic acidosis.

With severe metabolic acidosis, extreme increases in rate and depth of ventilation (Kussmaul respirations) occur. A few patients have pneumonitis, or *uremic lung*. In these patients, assess for thick sputum, reduced coughing, tachypnea, and fever. A pleural friction rub may be heard with a stethoscope. Patients often have pleuritic pain with breathing. Auscultate the lungs for crackles, which indicate fluid overload (Martchev, 2008).

Hematologic manifestations of CKD include anemia and abnormal bleeding. Check for indicators of anemia (e.g., fatigue, pallor, lethargy, weakness, shortness of breath, dizziness). Check for abnormal bleeding by observing for bruising, petechiae, purpura, mucous membrane bleeding in the nose or gums, or intestinal bleeding (black, tarry stools [melena]).

GI manifestations of CKD include foul breath and mouth ulceration or inflammation. Document any abdominal pain, cramping, or vomiting. Test all stools for occult blood.

Skeletal manifestations of CKD are related to osteodystrophy from poor absorption of calcium and continuous bone calcium resorption. Adults with osteodystrophy have thin, fragile bones that are at risk for pathologic fractures. These bones break easily with even slight trauma. Vertebrae become more compact and may bend forward, leading to an overall loss of height. Ask about changes in height and any unexplained bone pain. Observe for spinal curvatures and any unusual bumps or protrusions in bone areas that may indicate old fractures. Handle the patient carefully during examination and care.

Urine manifestations in CKD failure reflect the kidneys' decreasing function. At first, the amount, frequency, and appearance of the urine change. Protein or blood may be in the urine.

The amount and composition of the urine change as kidney function decreases. With the onset of mild to moderate CKD, the urine may be more dilute and clearer because tubular reabsorption of water is reduced. The actual urine output in a patient with CKD varies with the amount of remaining kidney function. The patient with severe CKD or ESKD usually has oliguria, but some patients continue to produce 1 L or more per 24 hours. Daily urine volume usually changes again after dialysis is started.

Skin manifestations of CKD occur as a result of uremia. Pigment is deposited in the skin, causing a yellowish coloration. Some African Americans report a darkening of the skin. The anemia of CKD causes a sallowness, appearing as a faded suntan on lighter-skinned patients.

Skin oils and turgor are decreased in patients with uremia. A distressing problem of uremia is severe *pruritus* (itching). Uremic frost, a layer of urea crystals from evaporated sweat, may appear on the face, eyebrows, axilla, and groin in patients with advanced uremic syndrome. Assess for bruises (*ecchymoses*), purple patches (*purpura*), and rashes.

Psychosocial Assessment

Chronic kidney disease (CKD) and its treatment disrupt many aspects of a patient's life. You are in a unique position to evaluate the patient with newly diagnosed kidney failure and to assist with adjustments.

Psychosocial assessment and support are part of the nurse's role from the time that CKD is first diagnosed. Ask about the patient's understanding of the diagnosis and what the treatment regimen means to him or her (e.g., diet, drugs, dialysis). Assess for anxiety and for the coping styles used by the patient or family members. Psychosocial issues affected by CKD include family relations, social activity, work patterns, body image, and sexual activity. The long-term nature of severe CKD and ESKD, the many treatment options, and the uncertainties about the course of the disease and its treatment require ongoing psychosocial assessment.

Laboratory Assessment

CKD causes extreme changes in many laboratory values (see Chart 71-2). Monitor the following blood values: creatinine, blood urea nitrogen (BUN), sodium, potassium, calcium,

phosphate, bicarbonate, hemoglobin, and hematocrit. Also monitor GFR for trends.

A urinalysis is performed. In the early stages of CKD, urinalysis may show excessive protein, glucose, red blood cells (RBCs), white blood cells (WBCs), and decreased or fixed specific gravity. Urine osmolarity is usually decreased. Glomerular filtration rate (GFR) is calculated based on serum creatinine levels, age, gender, race, and body size. A 24-hour creatinine clearance also may be calculated after blood and urine creatinine levels are collected and quantified. As CKD progresses, the urine output decreases dramatically.

In severe CKD, measurements of the serum creatinine and BUN levels may be used to determine the presence and degree of uremia. Serum creatinine levels may increase gradually over a period of years, reaching levels of 15 to 30 mg/dL or more, depending on the patient's muscle mass. BUN levels are directly related to dietary protein intake. Without protein restriction, BUN levels may rise 10 to 20 times the value of the serum creatinine level. With dietary protein restriction, BUN levels are elevated but less than those of non–protein-restricted patients. Fluid balance also affects BUN. Chapter 68 describes the significance of BUN and creatinine levels, as well as creatinine clearance.

Imaging Assessment

Few x-ray findings are abnormal with CKD. Bone x-rays of the hand can show renal osteodystrophy. With long-term end-stage kidney disease (ESKD), the kidneys have shrunk (except for ESKD caused by polycystic kidney disease) and may be 8 to 9 cm or smaller. This small size results from atrophy and fibrosis. If CKD progresses suddenly, a kidney ultrasound or CT scan without contrast medium may be used to rule out an obstruction. (See Chapter 68 for a complete description of diagnostic tests for kidney function.)

ANALYSIS

The patient with CKD has usually had a progressive reduction of kidney function and is often hospitalized for adjustment of the treatment plan. The focus of care is to manage symptoms and prevent complications. Priority problems for patients with CKD are:

1. Fluid overload related to the inability of diseased kidneys to maintain body fluid balance
2. Potential for pulmonary edema related to fluid overload
3. Decreased Cardiac Output related to reduced stroke volume, dysrhythmias, fluid overload, and increased peripheral vascular resistance
4. Inadequate nutrition related to inability to ingest, digest food, or absorb nutrients as a result of physiologic factors
5. Potential for infection related to skin breakdown, chronic disease, or malnutrition
6. Potential for injury related to effects of kidney disease on bone density, blood clotting, and drug elimination
7. Fatigue related to kidney disease, anemia, and reduced energy production
8. Anxiety related to threat to or change in health status, economic status, relationships, role function, systems, or self-concept; situational crisis; threat of death; lack of knowledge about diagnostic tests, disease process, treatment; loss of control; or disrupted family life

PLANNING AND IMPLEMENTATION

The Concept Map on p. 1554 discusses nursing care issues related to patients who have end-stage kidney disease (ESKD).

Managing Fluid Volume

Planning: Expected Outcomes. The patient with CKD is expected to achieve and maintain an acceptable fluid balance. Indicators include that the blood pressure, body weight, central venous pressure, and serum electrolytes are normal or nearly normal.

Interventions. Management of the patient with CKD includes drug therapy, nutrition therapy, fluid restriction, and dialysis. Nutrition therapy is discussed in the Enhancing Nutrition section, pp. 1555-1556, and dialysis is discussed in the Renal Replacement Therapies section, pp. 1558-1567).

The purpose of fluid management is to attain fluid balance and prevent complications of fluid overload (Chart 71-7). Monitor the patient's intake and output and hydration status. Assess for manifestations of fluid overload (e.g., crackles in the bases of the lungs, edema, and distended neck veins).

Drug therapy with diuretics is prescribed for patients with some kidney impairment to manage fluid retention or help control blood pressure. The increased urine output produced from these drugs helps reduce fluid overload in patients who still have some urine output. Diuretics are seldom used in ESKD after dialysis is started because, as kidney function is reduced, these drugs can have harmful side effects on the remaining kidney cells and on a patient's hearing.

Assess fluid status by obtaining daily weights and reviewing intake and output. Daily weight gain in these patients indicates fluid retention rather than true body weight gain. Estimate the amount of fluid retained: 1 kg of weight equals about 1 L of fluid retained. Weigh the patient daily at the same time each day, on the same scale, wearing the same amount of clothing, and after voiding (if the patient is not anuric). Monitor weight for changes before and after dialysis.

Fluid restriction is often needed. The amount of fluid restricted is reviewed in the discussion of sodium restriction on p. 1556. Consider all forms of fluid intake, including oral, IV, and fluid or drugs given through gastric tubes, when calculating fluid intake. Assist the patient in spreading oral fluid intake over a 24-hour period. Monitor his or her response to fluid restriction, and notify the health care provider if manifestations of fluid overload persist or worsen.

Preventing Pulmonary Edema

Planning: Expected Outcomes. The patient with CKD is expected to remain free of pulmonary edema by maintaining optimal fluid balance. Indicators include that the patient will have no breathing difficulty, no adventitious lung sounds (e.g., crackles, wheezes) are present on auscultation, and oxygen saturation remains within the patient's usual range.

Interventions. In the patient with CKD, pulmonary edema can result from left-sided heart failure related to fluid overload or from blood vessel injury. In left-sided heart failure, the heart is unable to eject blood adequately from the left ventricle, leading to an increased pressure in the left atrium and in the pulmonary blood vessels. The increased pressure causes fluid to cross the capillaries into the pulmonary tissue, forming edema. Pulmonary edema can also occur from injury to the lung blood vessels as a result of uremia. This condition causes inflammation and capillary leak. Fluid then leaks from pulmonary circulation into the lung tissue and the alveoli.

Assess the patient for early signs of pulmonary edema, such as restlessness, anxiety, rapid heart rate, shortness of breath, and crackles that begin at the base of the lungs. As pulmonary edema worsens, the level of fluid in the lungs rises. Auscultation reveals increased crackles and decreased gas exchange. The patient may have frothy, blood-tinged sputum. As cardiac and pulmonary function decrease further, the patient becomes diaphoretic and cyanotic.

The patient with pulmonary edema usually is admitted to the ICU for aggressive treatment and continuous cardiac monitoring. Place the patient in a high-Fowler's position, and give oxygen to improve gas exchange. Drug therapy with kidney failure and pulmonary edema is difficult because of potential adverse drug effects on the kidneys. Treatment of pulmonary edema involves giving loop diuretics, such as furosemide (Lasix), IV. Kidney impairment increases the risk for *ototoxicity* (ear damage with hearing loss) with the use of furosemide; thus IV doses are given cautiously. Diuresis usually begins within 5 minutes of giving IV furosemide. Measure urine output every 15 to 30 minutes during the acute episode and every hour thereafter until the patient is stabilized. Monitor vital signs and assess breath sounds at least every 2 hours to evaluate the patient's response to this treatment.

IV morphine sulfate (1 to 2 mg) is often prescribed to reduce myocardial oxygen demand by triggering blood vessel dilation and to provide sedation. Dosage adjustments are needed to achieve the desired response and avoid respiratory depression. Monitor the patient's respiratory rate, oxygen saturation, and blood pressure hourly during this therapy. Other drugs that dilate blood vessels, such as nitroglycerin, also may be given as a continuous infusion to reduce

Concept Map: End–Stage Kidney Disease

Concept Map by Deanne A. Blach, MSN, RN

INTERVENTIONS

1 Assessment

Assess for presence of S_3 or pericardial friction rub, chest pain, JVD, edema fatigue, dyspnea, crackles, weight change, skin integrity, pruritus, skin discoloration, mental status, seizure activity, sensory changes, LE weakness, anorexia, nausea, vomiting, stomatitis, melena, urine amount/frequency/appearance, bone pain, presence of hyperglycemia secondary to diabetes, signs of bleeding disorders (petechiae, purpura, ecchymosis). *Guides patient care; assesses for signs of kidney failure.*

2 Vital Signs

Monitor VS; treat hypertension with ACE inhibitor or ARBs. Treat CHF with digoxin and beta blockers.

3 Nursing Safety Priority: Drug Alert!

Monitor for drug-related complications; ensure dosages are adjusted as needed. *Assesses for SE, drug toxicity. Dosages of drugs adjusted according to degree of remaining kidney function.*

4 Lab Findings

Monitor lab values — BUN, serum creatinine, creatinine clearance, CBC, electrolytes. *Determines the effectiveness of therapy for kidney failure.*

5 Fluid Status

Evaluate fluid status. Accurately measure I/O and check body weight to identify changes in fluid balance. *Fluid overload common in patients with ESKD; sodium retention causes hypertension and edema.*

6 Dialysis

Ensure participation in renal replacement therapies, either peritoneal dialysis (PD) or hemodialysis (HD). *Improves fluid, electrolyte, and acid-base balance; removes nitrogen-based wastes.*

7 Nursing Safety Priority: Action Alert!

Monitor for complications with PD or HD. *Early recognition and treatment may prevent a life-threatening situation.*

8 Health Promotion and Maintenance

Teach patient and family the importance of adhering to prescribed fluid and dietary restrictions, medications, and dialysis as scheduled. *Promotes health and reduces complications.*

9 Psychosocial Integrity

Encourage expression of concerns about risks for death and lifestyle disruption; determine presence of anxiety or maladaptive behavior. Refer to community health or support groups. *Minimizes the impact that depression, anxiety, and nonacceptance have on mental well-being.*

EXPECTED OUTCOMES

- Decreased apprehension (seeks information to reduce anxiety, uses effective coping strategies, reports no signs of anxiety)
- Decreased fatigue (participates in self-care, interested in life, demonstrates mental concentration)
- Remains free of injury (no pathologic fractures, toxic SE from drugs, or bleeding)
- Remains free of infection (mild to no fever, no lymph node enlargement, negative urine culture, negative dialysis access site, WBC within normal limits or slightly elevated)

Planning

History

- Age 56, male, height 5'9", 225 lbs; recent weight gain of 8 lbs.
- History of kidney stones, uncontrolled DM type 2, drug use, HTN, and hyperlipidemia. Family history of polycystic kidney disease.
- Chronic use of NSAIDs for arthritis pain.
- He reports that desserts "don't taste sweet like before" and meat leaves a metallic taste. Some nausea and anorexia.
- He reports feeling weak and tired and is often short of breath. He has several bruises on his arms and legs at different stages.
- He states he urinates dark-colored urine in small amounts a few times a day.

Carl Brown is a 56-year-old African-American man who has a lengthy history of type 2 diabetes, coronary artery disease, and hyperlipidemia. He has had complete loss of kidney function for 4 months. His VS are T – 100°F; P – 104 and irregular, R – 32; BP – 160/100 mm Hg.

pulmonary pressure. Monitor vital signs at least hourly because this drug combination may cause severe hypotension.

Monitor serum electrolyte levels daily, and report abnormalities to the health care provider so that imbalances can be corrected quickly. Monitor ECG tracings at least every 2 hours to identify any dysrhythmias. Monitor oxygen saturation levels by pulse oximetry and arterial blood gas values. Adjust oxygen delivery to maintain adequate oxygen saturation levels. Monitor the patient for worsening of the condition, manifested as increasing hypoxemia. He or she may require temporary intubation and mechanical ventilation to prevent death.

Patients with CKD who have existing cardiac problems, high blood pressure, or chronic fluid retention are at increased risk for developing pulmonary edema. They are less likely to respond quickly to treatment and are more likely to develop problems related to drug therapy. Ultrafiltration may be used with these patients to reduce fluid volume.

? NCLEX EXAMINATION CHALLENGE

Safe and Effective Care Environment

The client with end-stage kidney disease (ESKD) appears to have pulmonary edema. Which intervention does the nurse perform first?
A. Raise the head of the bed
B. Apply oxygen by nasal cannula
C. Notify the Rapid Response Team
D. Measure oxygen saturation by pulse oximetry

Increasing Cardiac Output

Planning: Expected Outcomes. The patient with CKD is expected to attain and maintain adequate cardiac output. Indicators include that systolic and diastolic blood pressures, ejection fraction, peripheral pulses, and cognitive status are either normal or nearly normal.

Interventions. Many patients with long-standing hypertension are at risk for kidney disease and have mild CKD. Some progress to severe CKD and ESKD. *Therefore blood pressure control is essential in preserving kidney function.* To control blood pressure, calcium channel blockers, angiotensin-converting enzyme (ACE) inhibitors, alpha-adrenergic and beta-adrenergic blockers, and vasodilators may be prescribed. ACE inhibitors appear to be the most effective drugs to slow the progression of kidney failure. Calcium channel blockers seem to improve the GFR and blood flow within the kidney.

More information on the specific drugs for blood pressure control can be found in Chapter 38. Indications vary depending on the patient, and these drugs are used carefully to avoid complications. Different combinations and doses may be tried until blood pressure control is adequate and side effects are minimized.

Teach the patient and family to measure blood pressure daily. Evaluate their ability to measure and record blood pressure accurately using their own equipment. Re-check measurement accuracy on a regular basis. The patient and family must understand the relationship of blood pressure control to diet and drug therapy. Also instruct the patient to weigh daily and to bring records of blood pressure measurements, drug administration times, and weights for discussion with the physician, nurse, or dietitian.

Assess the patient on an ongoing basis for manifestations of reduced cardiac output, heart failure, and dysrhythmias. These topics are discussed in Chapters 36 through 38.

Enhancing Nutrition

Planning: Expected Outcomes. The patient with CKD is expected to maintain adequate nutrition. The patient should have a caloric intake appropriate for his or her weight-to-height ratio, muscle tone, and laboratory values (serum albumin, hematocrit, hemoglobin).

Interventions. The nutritional needs and diet restrictions for the patient with CKD vary according to the degree of remaining kidney function and the type of renal replacement therapy used (Table 71-8).

The purpose of nutrition therapy is to provide the food and fluids needed to prevent malnutrition. Patients starting hemodialysis (HD) have an increase in protein breakdown and a decrease in intake that results in a loss of lean body mass.

The patient is referred to a dietitian for dietary teaching and planning. Work with the dietitian to teach the patient about diet changes that are needed as a result of CKD. Common changes include control of protein intake; fluid intake limitation; restriction of potassium, sodium, and phosphorus intake; taking vitamin and mineral supplements; and eating enough calories to meet metabolic need.

If adequate calories are not supplied, the body will use muscle protein for energy, which leads to a negative nitrogen balance and malnutrition. The dietitian determines the number of calories and types of nutrients required to meet body needs.

Protein restriction early in the course of the disease prevents some of the symptoms of CKD and may preserve

TABLE 71-8 DIETARY RESTRICTIONS FOR THE PATIENT WITH SEVERE KIDNEY DISEASE AND END-STAGE KIDNEY DISEASE

DIETARY COMPONENT	WITH CHRONIC UREMIA	WITH HEMODIALYSIS	WITH PERITONEAL DIALYSIS
Protein	0.55-0.60 g/kg/day	1.0-1.5 g/kg/day	1.2-1.5 g/kg/day
Fluid	Depends on urine output but may be as high as 1500-3000 mL/day	500-700 mL/day plus amount of urine output	Restriction based on fluid weight gain and blood pressure
Potassium	60-70 mEq/day	70 mEq/day	Usually no restriction
Sodium	1-3 g/day	2-4 g/day	Restriction based on fluid weight gain and blood pressure
Phosphorus	700 mg/day	700 mg/day	800 mg/day

kidney function. Protein is restricted on the basis of the degree of kidney impairment (reduced GFR) and the severity of the symptoms. Buildup of waste products from protein breakdown is the main cause of uremia. Although lower protein levels are recommended, protein-calorie malnutrition must be avoided in patients receiving hemodialysis (HD). At least 1.5 g of protein per kilogram of body weight per day may be needed for weight gain and improved nutritional status in patients receiving maintenance HD.

The glomerular filtration rate (GFR) is used as an indicator of kidney function and as a guide to safe levels of protein intake. A patient with a severely reduced GFR who is *not* undergoing dialysis is usually permitted 0.55 to 0.60 g of protein per kilogram of body weight (e.g., 40 g of protein daily for a 150-pound [about 70-kg] adult). If protein is lost in the urine, protein is added to the diet in amounts equal to that lost in the urine. Protein requirements are calculated based on actual body weight (corrected for edema), not ideal body weight.

The patient receiving dialysis needs more protein because some protein is lost through dialysis. While receiving HD, protein requirements are tailored according to the patient's post-dialysis, or "dry," weight. Generally, HD patients are allowed about 1 to 1.5 g of protein/kg/day. Peritoneal dialysis (PD) patients are allowed 1.2 to 1.5 g of protein/kg/day because protein is lost with each exchange. Suggested protein-containing foods are milk, meat, or eggs. If protein intake is not adequate, a negative nitrogen balance develops and causes muscle wasting. BUN and serum prealbumin levels and albumin levels are used to monitor the adequacy of protein intake. Decreased serum prealbumin or albumin levels indicate poor protein intake. Excessive protein intake increases BUN levels in patients with CKD.

Sodium restriction is needed in patients with little or no urine output. Both fluid and sodium retention cause edema, hypertension, and heart failure (HF). Most patients with CKD retain sodium; a few cannot conserve sodium.

Estimate fluid and sodium retention status by monitoring the patient's body weight and blood pressure. In uremic patients not receiving dialysis, sodium is limited to 1 to 3 g daily and fluid intake depends on urine output. In patients receiving dialysis, the sodium restriction is 2 to 4 g daily and fluid intake is limited to 500 to 700 mL plus the amount of any urine output. Instruct the patient not to add salt at the table or during cooking. Foods high in sodium (e.g., processed foods, fast foods, potato chips, pretzels, pickles, ham, bacon, sausage) are permitted in moderation. Herbs and spices can be used in place of salt to enhance food flavor.

Potassium restriction may be needed because high blood potassium levels can cause dangerous cardiac dysrhythmias. Monitor the ECG for tall, peaked T waves caused by hyperkalemia. Document serum potassium levels. Instruct the patient with ESKD to limit potassium intake to 60 to 70 mEq/day. Teach him or her to read labels of seasoning agents carefully for sodium and potassium content. Chart 13-8 in Chapter 13 lists common foods that are low in potassium along with foods that are high in potassium and should be avoided. Instruct patients to avoid salt substitutes composed of potassium chloride. Those receiving PD or who are producing urine may not need potassium restriction.

Phosphorus restriction for control of phosphate levels is started early in CKD to avoid osteodystrophy (bone defects).

Monitor serum phosphate levels. Dietary phosphorus restrictions and drugs to assist with phosphate control may be prescribed. Phosphate binders must be taken at mealtimes. Most patients with CKD already restrict their protein intake, and because high-protein foods are also high in phosphorus, this reduces phosphorus intake. Chapter 13 lists foods high in potassium, sodium, and phosphorus.

Vitamin supplementation is needed daily for most patients with CKD. Low-protein diets are also low in vitamins, and water-soluble vitamins are removed from the blood during dialysis. Anemia also is a problem in patients with CKD because of the limited iron content of low-protein diets and decreased kidney production of erythropoietin. Thus supplemental iron is needed. Calcium and vitamin D supplements may be needed, depending on the patient's serum calcium levels and bone status.

Nutritional needs for patients undergoing PD are slightly different from those undergoing HD. Because protein is lost with the dialysate in PD, replacing lost protein is needed. Often 1.2 to 1.5 g of protein per kilogram of body weight per day is recommended. Patients may have anorexia and have difficulty eating enough protein. High-calorie enteral supplements may also be needed (e.g., Magnacal Renal, Ensure Plus). Sodium restriction varies with fluid weight gain and blood pressure. Usually dietary potassium does not need to be restricted because the dialysate is potassium-free. Any potassium restriction is determined by serum potassium levels.

Collaborate with the dietitian to assess each patient's nutritional needs. Teach the patient and evaluate his or her understanding of and adherence with dietary regimens. Give the patient and family written examples of the diet to promote adherence. Help patients adapt the diet to their budget, ethnic background, and food preferences to meet the diet's restrictions.

Preventing Infection

Planning: Expected Outcomes. The patient with CKD is expected to remain free of infection. Indicators include that the patient will have only mild or no fever, no lymph node enlargement, negative urine culture, negative dialysis access site culture, and white blood cell count either within the normal range or only slightly elevated.

Interventions. Provide meticulous care to any areas where skin is not intact (e.g., AV grafts and fistulas, incisions, site of drains, puncture sites, cracked or excoriated skin, pressure sores), and provide preventive skin care to intact areas. For patients undergoing dialysis, inspect the vascular access site or peritoneal dialysis (PD) catheter insertion site every shift for redness, swelling, pain, and drainage. Monitor vital signs for any manifestation of infection (e.g., fever, tachycardia).

Preventing Injury

Planning: Expected Outcomes. The patient with CKD is expected to remain free of injury. Indicators include that the patient should not have any of the following problems:

- Pathologic fractures
- Toxic side effects from drug therapy
- Bleeding

Interventions. Injury prevention strategies are needed because the patient with long-standing CKD may have brittle, fragile bones that fracture easily and cause little pain. When lifting or moving a patient with fragile bones, use a lift sheet rather than pulling the patient. Teach unlicensed assistive personnel (UAP) the correct use of lift sheets. Observe for normal range of joint motion and for unusual surface bumps or depressions over bones, which may indicate fractures.

Managing drug therapy in patients with CKD is a complex clinical problem. Many over-the-counter drugs contain agents that alter kidney function. Therefore it is important to obtain a detailed drug history. Know the use of each drug, its side effects, and its site of metabolism.

Certain drugs must be avoided, and the dosages of others must be adjusted according to the degree of remaining kidney function. As the patient's kidney function decreases, repeated dosage adjustments are necessary. Assess for side effects and signs of drug toxicity, and notify the prescriber as appropriate.

> **❗ NURSING SAFETY ALERT**
>
> **Drug Alert**
>
> Monitor the patient with severe CKD or ESKD closely for drug-related complications, and ensure that dosages are adjusted as needed.

Many drugs are routinely given to patients with CKD (see Chart 71-3). Know the rationale for these drugs and the indicated nursing interventions. Many patients also have cardiac disease and may require cardiac drugs such as digoxin. Patients with severe CKD and ESKD are particularly at risk for digoxin toxicity because the drug is excreted by the kidneys. When caring for patients with CKD who are receiving digoxin, monitor for signs of toxicity, such as nausea, vomiting, anorexia, visual changes, restlessness, headache, fatigue, confusion, *bradycardia* (pulse rate less than 50 to 60 beats/min), and *tachycardia* (pulse rate greater than 100 beats/min). Monitor the serum drug levels to be certain they are in the therapeutic range (0.8-2 ng/mL). Also closely monitor the serum potassium levels of any patient receiving digoxin.

> **❗ NURSING SAFETY PRIORITY**
>
> **Drug Alert**
>
> Doses of digoxin are generally much lower than for most drugs. When digoxin is administered to older adults with kidney disease, the prescribed dose may be even lower (0.0625-0.125 mg). Check and re-check the dosage before administering digoxin to a patient with kidney disease.

Drugs to control an excessively high phosphate level include phosphate-binding agents. Calcium acetate, calcium carbonate, and aluminum hydroxide are used as phosphate-binding agents in patients with impaired kidney function or CKD. These drugs help prevent renal osteodystrophy and related injuries. Stress the importance of taking these agents and all prescribed drugs.

Hypophosphatemia (low serum phosphorus levels) is a complication of phosphate binding, especially in patients who are not eating adequately but who are continuing to take phosphate-binding drugs. *Hypercalcemia* (high serum calcium levels) also is a possible complication for patients taking calcium-containing compounds to control phosphate excess. In patients taking aluminum-based phosphate binders

for prolonged periods, aluminum deposits may cause bone disease or permanent neurologic problems. Monitor the patient for muscle weakness, anorexia, malaise, tremors, or bone pain.

Teach patients with kidney disease to avoid antacids containing magnesium. These patients cannot excrete magnesium and thus should avoid additional intake.

Some drugs, in addition to those used to manage CKD, require special attention. These drugs include antibiotics, opioids, antihypertensives, diuretics, insulin, and heparin.

Many antibiotics are safe for patients with CKD, but those excreted by the kidney require dose adjustment. To prevent complications of bloodstream infections from mouth bacteria, prophylactic antibiotic treatment is given to patients with CKD before any dental procedures. The antibiotic used varies with the patient's needs and the physician's preference.

Give opioid analgesics cautiously in patients with severe CKD or ESKD because the effects often last longer than in those with healthy kidneys. Patients with uremia are sensitive to the respiratory depressant effects of these drugs. Because opioids are broken down by the liver and not the kidneys, the dosages are often the same regardless of the level of kidney function. Monitor the patient's reactions closely after opioids are given to determine whether adjustments are needed.

As CKD progresses, the patient with diabetes often requires reduced doses of insulin or antidiabetic drugs because the failing kidneys do not excrete or metabolize these drugs well. Thus the drugs are effective longer, increasing the risk for hypoglycemia. Monitor blood glucose levels at least four times per day to determine whether a dosage change is needed.

Poor platelet function and capillary fragility in CKD make anticoagulant therapy risky. Monitor patients receiving heparin, warfarin, or any anticoagulant every shift for bleeding. See Chapter 42 for more information on caring for patients at increased risk for bleeding.

Minimizing Fatigue

Planning: Expected Outcomes. The patient with chronic kidney disease (CKD) is expected to conserve energy by balancing activity and rest. Indicators include that the patient will be able to participate in self-care activities, have interest in surroundings, and demonstrate mental concentration.

Interventions. Some causes of fatigue in the patient with CKD are vitamin deficiency, poor nutrition, anemia, and buildup of urea. All patients are given some type of vitamin and mineral supplement because of diet restrictions and vitamin losses from dialysis. Avoid giving these supplements before hemodialysis (HD) treatment because they will be dialyzed out of the body and the patient will receive no benefit.

The anemic patient with CKD is treated with erythropoietin (Epogen, Procrit). The outcome of this therapy is to maintain a hematocrit of 30% to 35%. This therapy is effective in triggering bone marrow production of red blood cells if the patient has adequate iron stores. Iron supplements may be needed if patients are iron deficient. Many who receive erythropoietin report improved appetite and sexual function along with decreased fatigue. The increased production of all blood cells from this therapy may increase blood pressure. The improved appetite challenges patients in their attempts to maintain protein, potassium, and fluid restrictions and requires additional education.

Reducing Anxiety

Planning: Expected Outcomes. The patient with CKD is expected to have reduced tension and apprehension. Indicators include that the patient consistently demonstrates these behaviors:

- Seeks information to reduce anxiety
- Uses effective coping strategies
- Reports an absence of physical manifestations of anxiety

Interventions. The nurse coordinates a team of health care professionals to support and counsel the patient and family, often over many years of treatment. The nurse has the most contact with the patient with severe CKD and ESKD when the patient is hospitalized or undergoing in-center dialysis treatments. Perform an ongoing assessment of the patient's anxiety level to determine the level of nursing intervention required. Observe his or her behavior for cues indicating anxiety (e.g., anxious facial expressions, clenching of hands, tapping of feet, withdrawn posture, absence of eye contact, an increased pulse rate). Evaluate the support systems, such as the involvement of family and friends with the patient's care.

Unfamiliar settings and lack of knowledge about treatments and tests can increase the patient's anxiety level. Explain all procedures, tests, and treatments. Identify the patient's knowledge needs about kidney function and kidney disease. Provide instruction at a level he or she can understand using a variety of written and visual materials.

Provide continuity of care, whenever possible, by using a consistent nurse-patient relationship to decrease anxiety and promote discussions of concerns. As you develop the nurse-patient relationship, encourage the patient to discuss current problems or concerns.

Encourage the patient to ask questions and discuss fears about the diagnosis of severe kidney disease or ESKD. An open atmosphere that allows for discussion can decrease anxiety. Facilitate discussions with family members about the prognosis and the impact on lifestyle. Assist the patient to identify strategies for maintaining quality of life.

Renal Replacement Therapies

Renal replacement therapy is needed when the pathologic changes of stage 4 and stage 5 chronic kidney disease (CKD) are life threatening or pose continuing discomfort to the patient. When he or she can no longer be managed with conservative therapies, such as diet, drugs, and fluid restriction, dialysis is indicated. Transplantation may be discussed at any time.

Hemodialysis

Hemodialysis (HD) is the most common renal replacement therapy used with ESKD and kidney failure (Table 71-9). Dialysis removes excess fluids and waste products and restores chemical and electrolyte balance. HD involves passing the patient's blood through an artificial semipermeable membrane to perform the filtering and excretion functions of the kidney.

Patient Selection. Any patient may be considered for HD therapy. Starting this therapy depends on symptoms, not on the glomerular filtration rate (GFR). Dialysis is started immediately for patients who have the following: fluid overload that does not respond to diuretics, pericarditis, uncontrolled

TABLE 71-9 A COMPARISON OF HEMODIALYSIS AND PERITONEAL DIALYSIS AS RENAL REPLACEMENT THERAPY OPTIONS

HEMODIALYSIS	PERITONEAL DIALYSIS
Advantages	
More efficient clearance	Easy access
Short time needed for treatment	Few hemodynamic complications
Complications	
Disequilibrium syndrome	Protein loss
Muscle cramps	Peritonitis
Hemorrhage	Hyperglycemia
Air embolus	Respiratory distress
Hemodynamic changes (hypotension, anemia)	Bowel perforation
Cardiac dysrhythmias	Infection
Infection	
Contraindications	
Hemodynamic instability	Extensive peritoneal adhesions
	Peritoneal fibrosis
	Recent abdominal surgery
Access	
Vascular access route	Intra-abdominal catheter
Procedure	
Complex	Simple
Specially trained registered nurses required	Training less complex than for hemodialysis
Nursing Implications	
Vascular access care	Abdominal catheter care
Restrict diet	More flexible diet

hypertension, neurologic problems, and development of bleeding. Most commonly, dialysis is started when uremic manifestations, such as nausea and vomiting, decreased attention span, decreased cognition, worsening anemia, and pruritus, are present.

Many patients survive for years with HD therapy, and others may live only a few months. How long the patient survives using HD therapy depends on his or her age, the cause of kidney failure, and the presence of other diseases, such as coronary artery disease, hypertension, or diabetes. General patient selection criteria are:

- Irreversible kidney failure when other therapies are unacceptable or ineffective
- Absence of illnesses that would seriously complicate HD
- Expectation of rehabilitation
- The patient's acceptance of the regimen

Dialysis Settings. Patients with CKD may receive HD treatments in many settings, depending on specific needs. Regardless of the setting for therapy, they need ongoing nursing support to maintain this complex and lifesaving treatment.

Patients may be dialyzed in a hospital-based center if they have recently started treatment or have complicated conditions that require close supervision. Stable patients not requiring intense supervision may be dialyzed in a community or freestanding HD center. Selected patients may participate in complete or partial self-care in an outpatient center or in in-home HD.

In-home HD is the least disruptive and allows the patient to adapt the regimen to his or her lifestyle. Unfortunately, many cannot participate in in-home dialysis because they lack a skilled partner to assist with the therapy and manage the dialysis machine. Some patients and partners find the use of in-home dialysis to be too stressful. In addition, a water treatment system must be installed in the home to provide a safe, clean water supply for the dialysis process.

Procedure. Dialysis works using the passive transfer of toxins by diffusion. Diffusion is the movement of molecules from an area of higher concentration to an area of lower concentration. The rate of diffusion during dialysis occurs more rapidly when the membrane pores are large, there is a large surface area of membrane, the temperature of the solutions is higher, and there is a greater difference in the solute concentrations between the patient's blood and the dialysate. Large molecules, such as RBCs and most plasma proteins, cannot pass through the membrane.

When HD is started, blood and dialysate (dialyzing solution) flow in opposite directions across an enclosed semipermeable membrane. The dialysate contains a balanced mix of electrolytes and water that closely resembles human plasma. On the other side of the membrane is the patient's blood, which contains nitrogen waste products, excess water, and excess electrolytes. During HD, the waste products move from the blood into the dialysate because of the difference in their concentrations (diffusion). Excess water is also removed from the blood into the dialysate by *osmosis* (movement of water across a semipermeable membrane from a solution that has a lower osmolarity or concentration to a solution with a higher osmolarity or concentration). Electrolytes can move in either direction, as needed, and take some fluid with them. Potassium and sodium typically move out of the plasma into the dialysate. Bicarbonate and calcium generally move from the dialysate into the plasma. This circulating process continues for a preset length of time, restoring water, electrolyte, and acid-base balance and removing nitrogenous wastes. Water volume may be removed from the plasma by applying positive or negative pressure to the system.

The HD system includes a dialyzer, dialysate, vascular access routes, and an HD machine. The artificial kidney, or dialyzer (Fig. 71-3), has four parts: a blood compartment, a dialysate compartment, a semipermeable membrane, and an enclosed support structure.

Dialysate is made from clear water and chemicals and is free of any waste products or drugs. Because bacteria and other organisms are too large to pass through the membrane, dialysate is not sterile. The water used in dialysate must meet specific standards and usually requires special treatment before mixing the dialysate. The dialysate composition may be altered according to the patient's needs for management of electrolyte imbalances. During HD, the dialysate is warmed to 100° F (37.8° C) to increase the diffusion rate and to prevent hypothermia.

The HD machine has alarm systems to monitor for potential problems, including changes in dialysate temperature, air in the blood tubing, a blood leak in the dialysate compartment, changes in the pressure in either compartment, and changes in composition of the blood or dialysate. If any of these problems are detected, an alarm sounds to protect the patient from life-threatening complications.

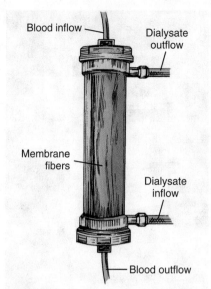

FIG. 71-3 Artificial kidney (dialyzer) used in hemodialysis.

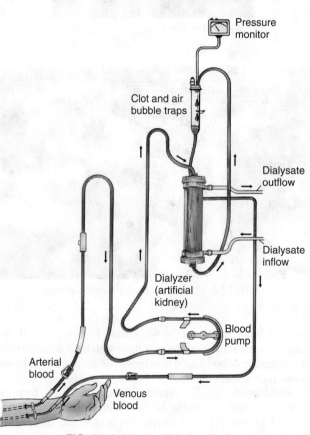

FIG. 71-4 A hemodialysis circuit.

All models of HD machines function in a manner similar to that shown in Fig. 71-4. Fig. 71-5 shows one type of HD machine. Fig. 71-6 shows a patient receiving HD. The number and length of treatments depend on the amount of wastes and fluid to be removed, the clearance capacity of the dialyzer, and the blood flow rate to and from the machine. Most patients require about 12 hours per week of total dialysis time. This time is usually divided into three 4-hour treatments. For those with some ongoing urine production, two

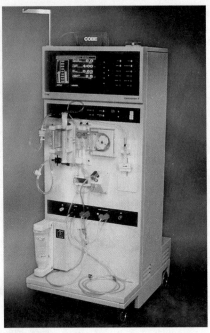

FIG. 71-5 Hemodialysis machine.

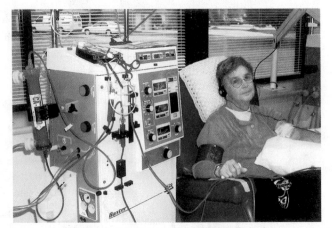

FIG. 71-6 Patient receiving hemodialysis.

TABLE 71-10	**TYPES OF VASCULAR ACCESS FOR HEMODIALYSIS**		
ACCESS TYPE	**DESCRIPTION**	**LOCATION**	**INITIAL USE**
Permanent			
AV fistula	An internal anastomosis of an artery to a vein	Forearm	2-4 mo or longer
AV graft	Synthetic vessel tubing tunneled beneath the skin, connecting an artery and a vein	Forearm Upper arm Inner thigh	1-2 wk
Temporary			
Hemodialysis catheter (dual- or triple-lumen)	A specially designed catheter with two or three lumens Two lumens are for blood outflow and inflow for hemodialysis; a third allows venous access without accessing dialysis lumens	Subclavian, internal jugular, or femoral vein	Immediately after insertion and x-ray confirmation of placement
Subcutaneous device	An internal device with two metallic access ports and two catheters inserted into large central veins	Subclavian	Immediately after insertion

AV, Arteriovenous.

5- to 6-hour treatments a week may be adequate. If the patient gains large amounts of fluid weight, a longer treatment time may be needed to remove the fluid without hypotension or severe side effects.

Anticoagulation. To prevent blood clots from forming within the dialyzer or the blood tubing, anticoagulation is needed during HD treatments. Heparin is the most commonly used drug to prevent clots from forming when blood comes in contact with foreign surfaces. Patient response to heparin varies, and the dose is adjusted based on each patient's need. Those receiving erythropoietin may require additional heparin.

Heparin remains active in the body for 4 to 6 hours after dialysis, making the patient at risk for hemorrhage during and immediately after HD treatments. Invasive procedures must be avoided during that time. Monitor him or her closely for any signs of bleeding or hemorrhage. Clotting tendencies can be monitored during HD with a bedside machine (e.g., the Hemochron), by whole-blood clotting times, or by

activated partial thromboplastin times (aPTTs) during and after HD. Protamine sulfate is an antidote to heparin and always should be available in the dialysis setting.

Vascular Access. Vascular access is required for hemodialysis (Table 71-10). The procedure requires the easy availability of a large amount of blood flow: at least 250 to 300 mL/min, usually for a period of 3 to 4 hours. Normal venous cannulation does not provide this high rate of blood flow.

Long-term vascular access is internal for most patients having long-term HD (see Table 71-10). The two common choices are an internal arteriovenous (AV) fistula or an AV graft (Fig. 71-7). *AV fistulas* are formed by surgically connecting an artery to a vein. The vessels used most often are the radial or brachial artery and the cephalic vein of the nondominant arm. Fistulas increase venous blood flow to 250 to 400 mL/min, the amount needed for effective dialysis.

Time is needed after anastomosis for the AV fistula to develop. As the AV fistula "matures," the increased pressure of the arterial blood flow into the vein causes the vessel walls to thicken. This thickening increases their strength and durability for repeated cannulation. Patients differ in the amount of time needed for the fistula to mature. Some fistulas may not be ready for use for as long as 4 months after the surgery, and a temporary vascular access (AV shunt or HD catheter) is used during this time. Fig. 71-8 shows a mature fistula.

To access a fistula, cannulate it by inserting two needles, one toward the venous blood flow and one toward the arterial blood flow. This procedure allows the HD machine to draw

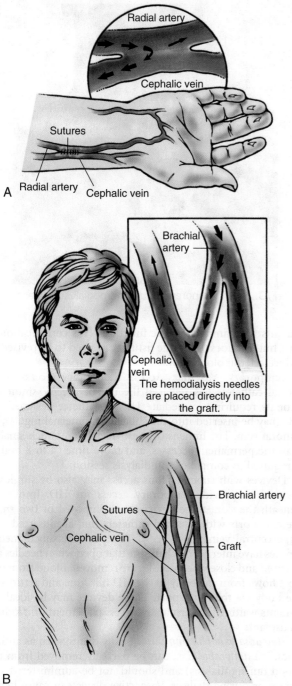

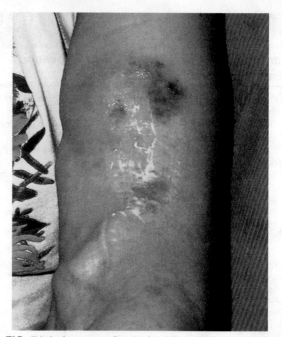

FIG. 71-8 A mature fistula for hemodialysis access.

FIG. 71-7 Options for long-term vascular access for hemodialysis. **A,** A surgically created venous fistula. The increased pressure from the artery forces blood into the vein. This process causes the vein to dilate enough for fistula needles to be placed for hemodialysis. When the vein dilates in this manner, the fistula is said to be "developed" or "mature." **B,** A surgically placed straight vascular graft in the upper arm. The graft creates a shunt between arterial and venous blood.

the blood out through the arterial needle and return it through the venous needle.

Arteriovenous grafts are used when the AV fistula does not develop or when complications limit its use. The poly-tetrafluoroethylene (PTFE) graft is a synthetic material

(GORE-TEX). This type of graft is commonly used for older patients using HD. Fig. 71-7, *B*, shows a patient's AV graft.

Precautions. Some precautions are needed to ensure the functioning of an internal AV fistula or AV graft. First assess for adequate circulation in the fistula or graft as well as in the lower portion of the arm. Check distal pulses and capillary refill in the arm with the fistula or graft. Then check for a *bruit* (swishing sound) by auscultating over the access site or a *thrill* (vibration) by palpating over it. The fistula changes in appearance over time as it dilates, and skin stretching increases the risk for injury in the area. Chart 71-8 lists best practices for care of the patient with an HD access.

> ### ❗ NURSING SAFETY PRIORITY
> #### *Action Alert*
>
> Because repeated compression can result in the loss of the vascular access, avoid taking the blood pressure or performing venipunctures in the arm with the vascular access. Do not use AV fistula or graft for delivery of IV fluids.

Complications. Complications can occur with any type of access. The most common problems are thrombosis or stenosis, infection, aneurysm formation, ischemia, and heart failure.

Thrombosis, or clotting of the AV access, is the most frequent complication. Most grafts fail because of high-pressure arterial flow entering the venous system. The muscle layers of the veins react to this increased pressure by thickening. The venous thickening reduces or occludes blood flow. An interventional radiologist can re-open failing grafts with the injection of a thrombolytic drug (e.g., tPA) to dissolve the clot. The clot usually dissolves within minutes, and often a stricture is revealed at the point where the graft and the vein connect. The stricture can be corrected by balloon angioplasty.

CHART 71-8   BEST PRACTICE FOR PATIENT SAFETY & QUALITY CARE

Caring for the Patient with an Arteriovenous Fistula or Arteriovenous Graft

- Do not take blood pressure readings using the extremity in which the vascular access is placed.
- Do not perform venipunctures or start an IV line in the extremity in which the vascular access is placed.
- Palpate for thrills and auscultate for bruits every 4 hours while the patient is awake.
- Assess the patient's distal pulses and circulation in the arm with the access.
- Elevate the affected extremity postoperatively.
- Encourage routine range-of-motion exercises.
- Check for bleeding at needle insertion sites.
- Assess for manifestations of infection at needle sites.
- Instruct the patient not to carry heavy objects or anything that compresses the extremity in which the vascular access is placed.
- Instruct the patient not to sleep with his or her body weight on top of the extremity in which the vascular access is placed.

AV, Arteriovenous.

TABLE 71-11   NURSING INTERVENTIONS FOR PREVENTION OF COMPLICATIONS IN HEMODIALYSIS VASCULAR ACCESS

ACCESS TYPE	BLEEDING	INFECTION	CLOTTING
AV fistula or AV graft	Apply pressure to the needle puncture sites.	Ensure adequate site cleaning before cannulation.	Avoid constrictive devices. Rotate needle insertion sites with each hemodialysis treatment. Assess for thrill and bruit.
Hemodialysis catheters (temporary and permanent)	Monitor the access site.	Use aseptic technique.	Place a heparin or heparin/saline dwell solution after hemodialysis treatment. Not used between treatments.

AV, Arteriovenous.

Most infections of the vascular access are caused by *Staphylococcus aureus* introduced during cannulation. Use sterile technique during cannulation to prevent infection (Table 71-11).

Aneurysms can form in the fistula and are caused by repeated needle punctures at the same site. Large aneurysms may cause loss of the fistula's function and require surgical repair.

Ischemia occurs in a few patients with vascular access when the fistula decreases arterial blood flow to areas below the fistula. Ischemic symptoms (*"steal syndrome"*) vary from cold or numb fingers to gangrene. If the collateral circulation is inadequate, the fistula may need to be surgically tied off and a new one created in another area to preserve extremity circulation.

Shunting of blood directly from the arterial system to the venous system, through the fistula, can cause heart failure in

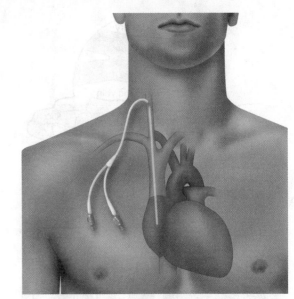

FIG. 71-9 Temporary jugular hemodialysis access.

patients with limited cardiac function. This complication is rare, but if it does occur, the fistula may need to be revised to reduce arterial blood flow.

Temporary Vascular Access. Temporary access with special catheters has replaced the use of the AV shunt for patients requiring immediate HD. A catheter designed for HD may be inserted into the subclavian, internal jugular, or femoral vein. The lumens of these devices are much smaller than the permanent accesses, and more time (4 to 8 hours) is required to complete each dialysis session.

Devices with subcutaneous access may also be surgically inserted to provide temporary access for HD. Implanted beneath the skin, these devices are composed of two small metallic ports with attached catheters that are inserted into large central veins (Fig. 71-9). The ports of subcutaneous devices have internal mechanisms that open when needles are inserted and close when needles are removed. Blood from one port flows from the body to the HD machine and returns to the body via the other port. These devices may be ideal for patients waiting for permanent access placement or a kidney transplant.

Hemodialysis Nursing Care. Many drugs, such as antibiotics, are *dialyzable* (i.e., can be partially removed from the blood during dialysis) and should not be administered just before or during dialysis. Vasoactive drugs can cause hypotension during HD and may also be held until after treatment. Coordinate with the physician to assess the patient's drug regimen and determine which drugs should be held until after HD treatment. Table 71-12 lists common dialyzable and vasoactive drugs that should be given after rather than before HD.

Post-Dialysis Care. Closely monitor the patient immediately and for several hours after dialysis for any side effects from the treatment. Common problems include hypotension, headache, nausea, malaise, vomiting, dizziness, and muscle cramps.

Obtain vital signs and weight for comparison with predialysis measurements. Blood pressure and weight are expected to be reduced as a result of fluid removal. Hypotension may require rehydration with IV fluids, such as normal

TABLE 71-12   DIALYZABLE AND VASOACTIVE DRUGS

Dialyzable Drugs	Vasoactive Drugs
Aminoglycosides	**Antidysrhythmics**
• Amikacin	• Flecainide
• Gentamicin	• Lidocaine
• Tobramycin	• Procainamide
	• Quinidine
Antiviral Agents	
• Acyclovir	**Antihypertensives**
• Ganciclovir	• Atenolol
	• Captopril
Penicillins	• Diltiazem
• Amoxicillin	• Enalapril
• Ampicillin	• Lisinopril
• Cloxacillin	• Methyldopa
• Dicloxacillin	• Nifedipine
• Mezlocillin	• Propranolol
• Penicillin G	• Verapamil
• Ticarcillin	
	Narcotics
Anticonvulsants	• Codeine
• Ethosuximide	• Morphine
• Gabapentin	
• Phenobarbital	**Sedatives**
	• Midazolam
Cephalosporins	• Phenobarbital
• Cefaclor	• Propofol
• Cefazolin	
• Cefoxitin	**Vasodilators**
• Ceftizoxime	• Hydralazine
• Ceftriaxone	• Nitroglycerin
• Cefuroxime	• Nitroprusside
Antituberculosis Agents	
• Ethambutol	
• Isoniazid	
Miscellaneous	
• Aztreonam	
• Cimetidine	
• Vitamins	

CHART 71-9   BEST PRACTICE FOR PATIENT SAFETY & QUALITY CARE

Caring for the Patient Undergoing Hemodialysis

- Weigh the patient before and after dialysis.
- Know the patient's dry weight.
- Discuss with the health care provider whether any of the patient's drugs should be withheld until after dialysis.
- Be aware of events that occurred during previous dialysis treatments.
- Measure blood pressure, pulse, respirations, and temperature.
- Assess for symptoms of orthostatic hypotension.
- Assess the vascular access site.
- Observe for bleeding.
- Assess the patient's level of consciousness.
- Assess for headache, nausea, and vomiting.

short periods with low blood flows so that rapid changes in plasma composition are avoided.

❗ NURSING SAFETY PRIORITY

Critical Rescue

Assess for and document symptoms of disequilibrium syndrome (headache, nausea, vomiting, restlessness, decreased level of consciousness, seizures, coma) during and after HD, because early recognition and treatment with anticonvulsants and barbiturates may prevent a life-threatening situation.

Infectious diseases transmitted by blood transfusion are a serious complication of long-term HD. Two of the most serious blood-transmitted infections are hepatitis and human immune deficiency virus (HIV).

Hepatitis infection (B and C) in patients with chronic kidney disease (CKD) has decreased because the use of erythropoietin has reduced the need for blood transfusions to maintain red blood cell counts. Hepatitis is a problem because of the blood access and the risk for contamination during HD. The viruses can be transmitted through the use of contaminated needles or instruments, by entry of contaminated blood through open wounds in the skin or mucous membranes, or through transfusions with contaminated blood. Monitor all patients receiving HD for manifestations of hepatitis (see Chapter 61).

HIV is a bloodborne virus that poses some risk for patients undergoing HD. Fortunately, the risks for HIV transmission are reduced by the consistent practice of Standard Precautions, routine screening of donated blood for HIV, and decreased need for blood transfusions for patients with CKD and ESKD. Patients who have been undergoing HD or received frequent transfusions during the early to mid-1980s are at risk for acquired immune deficiency syndrome (AIDS) (see also Chapter 21).

CONSIDERATIONS FOR OLDER ADULTS

In 2007, the occurrence of ESKD in patients ages 75 years or older increased to more than 25% of patients beginning ESKD therapy (USRDS, 2010). The overall mean age for new patients is 64.6 years. ESKD incidence caused by diabetes and hypertension continues to grow in older adults. Patients older than 65 years who are receiving HD are more at risk for dialysis-induced hypotension. These patients require more frequent monitoring during and after dialysis.

saline. The patient's temperature may also be elevated because the dialysis machine warms the blood slightly. If he or she has a fever, sepsis may be present and a blood sample is needed for culture and sensitivity.

The heparin required during HD increases the clotting time, which increases the risk for excessive bleeding. All invasive procedures must be avoided for 4 to 6 hours after dialysis. Continually monitor the patient for hemorrhage during and for 1 hour after dialysis (Chart 71-9).

Complications of Hemodialysis. Many fluid-related and infectious complications can occur from HD. The most common complications include disequilibrium syndrome and viral infections.

Dialysis disequilibrium syndrome may develop during HD or after HD has been completed. The cause appears to be the rapid decrease in fluid volume and blood urea nitrogen (BUN) levels during HD. The change in urea levels can cause cerebral edema and increased intracranial pressure. *Neurologic symptoms can result (e.g., headache, nausea, vomiting, restlessness, decreased level of consciousness, seizures, coma, or death).* The problem may be prevented by starting HD for

TABLE 71-13 PERITONEAL DIALYSIS	
ADVANTAGES	**DISADVANTAGES**
Easy to learn	Time-consuming exchanges
Can be done at home	Protein wasting
Ambulatory—no machine needed	Excessive glucose load, causing
When machines are used, they	hyperlipidemia
are small	Sterile technique required
Less stressful on the body	Presence of permanent catheter
Hemodynamic tolerance	Weight gain
Continuous process	Peritonitis risk
Better blood pressure control	Peritoneum injury risk
Less dietary and fluid restrictions	Cannot be done if patient has
Greater freedom in scheduling	had many abdominal surgeries
and traveling	Chronic back pain or
	development of hernia

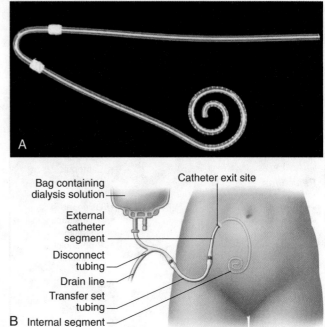

FIG. 71-10 Peritoneal dialysis catheter. **A,** The actual Silastic peritoneal dialysis catheter. **B,** Positioning of the Silastic catheter within the abdominal cavity.

Peritoneal Dialysis

Peritoneal dialysis (PD) allows exchanges of wastes, fluids, and electrolytes to occur in the peritoneal cavity. PD is slower than hemodialysis (HD), however, and more time is needed to achieve the same effect. Advantages and disadvantages are listed in Table 71-13. The use of PD has decreased and currently accounts for only 5% to 6% of dialysis (USRDS, 2010).

Patient Selection. Most patients with chronic kidney disease (CKD) can select either HD or PD. For those who are unstable, those who cannot tolerate anticoagulation, and those with chronic infection, PD is less hazardous than HD. For some patients, vascular access problems may eliminate HD as an option. At times a patient may use PD until a new arteriovenous (AV) fistula matures. PD is also often the treatment of choice for older adults because it offers more flexibility if his or her status changes frequently.

Peritoneal dialysis *cannot* be performed if peritoneal adhesions are present or if extensive intra-abdominal surgery has been performed. In these cases, the surface area of the peritoneal membrane is not sufficient for adequate dialysis exchange. Peritoneal membrane fibrosis may occur after repeated infections, which decreases membrane permeability.

Procedure. Each PD exchange process consists of three phases: fill, dwell, and drain. A siliconized rubber (Silastic) catheter is surgically placed into the abdominal cavity for infusion of dialysate (Fig. 71-10). Usually 1 to 2 L of dialysate is infused by gravity *(fill)* into the peritoneal space over a 10- to 20-minute period, according to the patient's tolerance. The fluid stays *(dwells)* in the cavity for a specified time prescribed by the physician. The fluid then flows out of the body *(drains)* by gravity into a drainage bag. The peritoneal outflow contains the dialysate and the excess water, electrolytes, and nitrogen-based waste products. The dialyzing fluid is called *peritoneal effluent* on outflow. The three phases of the process (infusion, or "fill"; dwell; and outflow, or drain) make up one PD exchange. The number and frequency of PD exchanges are prescribed by the physician, depending on manifestations and laboratory data.

Process. Peritoneal dialysis occurs through diffusion and osmosis across the semipermeable peritoneal membrane and capillaries. The peritoneal membrane is large and porous. It allows solutes and water to move from an area of higher concentration in the blood to an area of lower concentration in the dialyzing fluid (diffusion).

The peritoneal cavity is rich in capillaries and is a ready access to the blood supply. The fluid and waste products dialyzed from the patient move through the blood vessel walls, the interstitial tissues, and the peritoneal membrane and are removed when the dialyzing fluid is drained from the body.

PD efficiency is affected by many factors, such as decreased peritoneal membrane permeability caused by infection or scarring and reduced capillary blood flow resulting from blood vessel constriction, vascular disease, or decreased perfusion of the peritoneum. For PD, water removal depends on the concentration of the dialysate. Increasing the dialysate glucose concentration makes the solution more hypertonic. The more hypertonic the solution, the greater the osmotic pressure (pulling pressure) for water filtration and fluid removal from the patient during an exchange. The dialysate concentration is prescribed based on the patient's fluid status.

Dialysate Additives. Heparin may be added to the dialysate to prevent clotting of the catheter or tubing. Usually intraperitoneal (IP) heparin is needed only after new catheter placement or if peritonitis occurs. IP heparin is not absorbed systemically and does not affect blood clotting.

Other agents that may be given in the dialysate include potassium and antibiotics. Commercially prepared dialysate does not contain potassium. Some patients need potassium added to the dialysate to prevent hypokalemia. Antibiotics may be given by the IP route when peritonitis is present or suspected. Potassium and antibiotics are not mixed in the same dialysate bag because interactions may reduce the antibiotic effect.

Types of Peritoneal Dialysis. Many types of PD are available, including continuous ambulatory PD, multiple-bag continuous ambulatory PD, automated PD, intermittent PD,

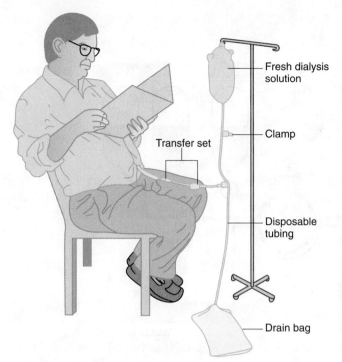

FIG. 71-11 Peritoneal dialysis exchange for control of fluids, electrolytes, nitrogenous wastes, blood pressure, and acid-base balance.

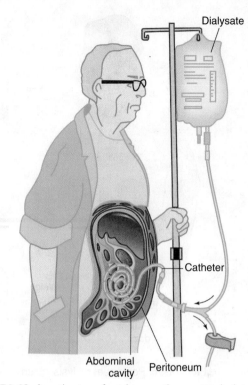

FIG. 71-13 A patient performing continuous ambulatory peritoneal dialysis (CAPD).

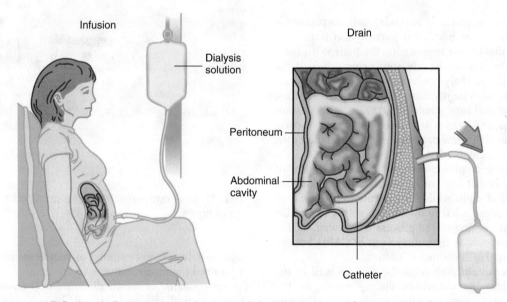

FIG. 71-12 Peritoneal membrane as dialyzing membrane for peritoneal dialysis.

and continuous-cycle PD. The type selected depends on the patient's ability and lifestyle. The two most commonly used types of PD are continuous ambulatory peritoneal dialysis and continuous cycling peritoneal dialysis.

Continuous ambulatory peritoneal dialysis (CAPD) is performed by the patient with the infusion of four 2-L exchanges of dialysate into the peritoneal cavity. Each time, the dialysate remains for 4 to 8 hours, and these exchanges occur 7 days a week (Fig. 71-11 through 71-13). During the dwell period, the patient can use a continuous connect system or a disconnect system.

With the continuous *connect* system (straight transfer set), the dialysate bag is attached to the catheter by 48-inch tubing. The empty bag and tubing are folded and worn beneath the clothing until they are used for outflow. After draining, the patient removes the bag and connects a new bag to repeat the process.

With the *disconnect system* (Y–transfer set), the patient removes the connecting tubing and empty dialysate bag after inflow and attaches a cap to the PD catheter. The disconnect system eliminates the need to wear the tubing and bag but requires opening the system two extra times with each

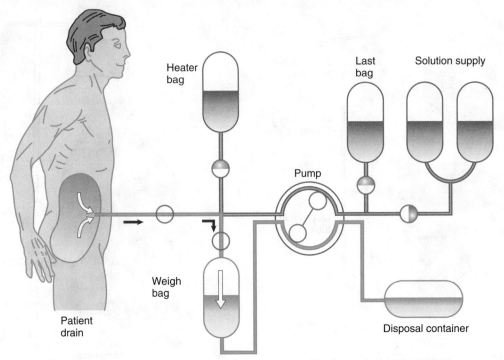

FIG. 71-14 Peritoneal dialysis machine circuit in automated peritoneal dialysis (APD).

exchange. The extra opening of the system increases the risk for infection.

With CAPD, no machine is necessary and no partner is required. However, it is best for a partner also trained in CAPD to be available as a support for the patient if illness occurs. Devices to assist in the safe, sterile connection of the tubing spike with the dialysate bag are available. These are useful for patients with poor vision, limited manual dexterity, or reduced hand and arm strength. CAPD allows constant removal of fluid and wastes and resembles kidney action more closely than HD. Some patients even perform their own exchanges while hospitalized.

Continuous-cycle peritoneal dialysis (CCPD) is a form of automated dialysis that uses an automated cycling machine. Exchanges occur at night while the patient sleeps. The final exchange of the night is left to dwell through the day and is drained the next evening as the process is repeated. CCPD offers the advantage of 24-hour dialysis, as in CAPD, but the sterile catheter system is opened less often.

Automated peritoneal dialysis (APD) may be used in the acute care setting, the outpatient dialysis center, or the patient's home. APD uses a cycling machine for dialysate inflow, dwell, and outflow according to preset times and volumes. A warming chamber for dialysate is part of the machine (Fig. 71-14). The functions are programmed for the patient's specific needs. A typical prescription calls for 30-minute exchanges (10/10/10 for inflow, dwell, and outflow) for a period of 8 to 10 hours. The machines have many safety monitors and alarms and are relatively simple to learn to use (Fig. 71-15).

Automated peritoneal dialysis has several advantages. It permits in-home dialysis while the patient sleeps, allowing him or her to be dialysis-free during waking hours. The incidence of peritonitis is reduced with APD because fewer connections and disconnections are needed. Also, APD can be

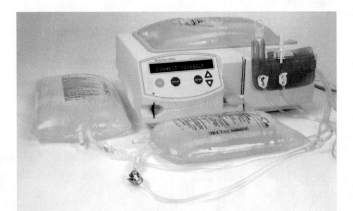

FIG. 71-15 A cycler machine for automated peritoneal dialysis at home.

used to deliver larger volumes of dialysis solution for patients who need higher clearances.

Intermittent peritoneal dialysis (IPD) combines osmotic pressure gradients with true dialysis. The patient usually requires exchanges of 2 L of dialysate at 30- to 60-minute intervals, allowing 15 to 20 minutes of drain time. For most patients, 30 to 40 exchanges of 2 L three times weekly are needed. IPD treatments can be automated or manual.

Complications. Complications are possible with PD, but many can be prevented with meticulous care.

Peritonitis is the major complication of PD. The most common cause of peritonitis is connection site contamination. To prevent peritonitis, use meticulous sterile technique when caring for the PD catheter and when hooking up or clamping off dialysate bags (Chart 71-10).

Manifestations of peritonitis include cloudy dialysate outflow (effluent), fever, abdominal tenderness, abdominal

CHART 71-10 BEST PRACTICE FOR PATIENT SAFETY & QUALITY CARE

Caring for the Patient with a Peritoneal Dialysis Catheter

- Mask yourself and your patient. Wash your hands.
- Put on sterile gloves. Remove the old dressing. Remove the contaminated gloves.
- Assess the area for signs of infection, such as swelling, redness, or discharge around the catheter site.
- Use aseptic technique:
  - Open the sterile field on a flat surface, and place two precut 4 × 4–inch gauze pads on the field.
  - Place three cotton swabs soaked in povidone-iodine on the field. Put on sterile gloves.
- Use cotton swabs to clean around the catheter site. Use a circular motion starting from the insertion site and moving away toward the abdomen. Repeat with all three swabs.
- Apply precut gauze pads over the catheter site. Tape only the edges of the gauze pads.

pain, general malaise, nausea, and vomiting. *Cloudy or opaque effluent is the earliest sign of peritonitis.* Examine all effluent for color and clarity to detect peritonitis early. When peritonitis is suspected, send a specimen of the dialysate outflow for culture and sensitivity study, Gram stain, and cell count to identify the infecting organism.

Pain during the inflow of dialysate is common when patients are first started on PD therapy. Usually this pain no longer occurs after a week or two of PD. Cold dialysate increases discomfort. Warm the dialysate bags before instillation by using a heating pad to wrap the bag or by using the warming chamber of the automated cycling machine. *Microwave ovens are **not** recommended for the warming of dialysate.*

Exit site and tunnel infections are serious complications. The exit site from a PD catheter should be clean, dry, and without pain or inflammation. Exit site infections (ESIs) can occur with any type of PD catheter. These infections are difficult to treat and can become chronic. They can lead to peritonitis, catheter failure, and hospitalization. Dialysate leakage and pulling or twisting of the catheter increase the risk for ESIs. A Gram stain and culture should be performed when exit sites have purulent drainage.

Tunnel infections occur in the path of the catheter from the skin to the cuff. Manifestations include redness, tenderness, and pain. ESIs are treated with antimicrobials. Deep cuff infections may require catheter removal.

Poor dialysate flow is usually related to constipation. To prevent constipation, a bowel preparation is prescribed before placement of the PD. An enema before starting PD may also prevent flow problems. Teach patients to eat a high-fiber diet and use stool softeners to prevent constipation. Other causes of flow difficulty include kinked or clamped connection tubing, the patient's position, fibrin clot formation, and catheter displacement.

Ensure that the drainage bag is lower than the patient's abdomen to enhance gravity drainage. Inspect the connection tubing and PD system for kinking or twisting. Ensure that clamps are open. If inflow or outflow drainage is still inadequate, reposition the patient to stimulate inflow or outflow. Turning the patient to the other side or ensuring that he or she is in good body alignment may help. Having the patient in a supine low-Fowler's position reduces abdominal pressure. Increased abdominal pressure from sitting or standing or from coughing contributes to leakage at the PD catheter site.

Fibrin clot formation may occur after PD catheter placement or with peritonitis. Milking the tubing may dislodge the fibrin clot and improve flow. An x-ray is needed to identify PD catheter placement. If displacement has occurred, the physician repositions the PD catheter.

Dialysate leakage is seen as clear fluid coming from the catheter exit site. When dialysis is first started, small volumes of dialysate are used. It may take patients 1 to 2 weeks to tolerate a full 2-L exchange without leakage around the catheter site. Leakage occurs more often in obese patients, those with diabetes, older adults, and those on long-term steroid therapy. During periods of catheter leak, patients may require hemodialysis (HD) support.

Other complications of PD include bleeding, which is expected when the catheter is first placed, and bowel perforation, which is serious. When PD is first started, the outflow may be bloody or blood tinged. This condition normally clears within a week or two. After PD is well-established, the effluent should be clear and light yellow. Observe for and document any change in the color of the outflow. Brown-colored effluent occurs with a bowel perforation. If the outflow is the same color as urine and has the same glucose level, a bladder perforation is probable. Cloudy or opaque effluent indicates infection.

Nursing Care During Peritoneal Dialysis. In the hospital setting, PD is routinely started and monitored by the nurse. Before the treatment, assess baseline vital signs, including blood pressure, apical and radial pulse rates, temperature, quality of respirations, and breath sounds. Weigh the patient, always on the same scale, before the procedure and at least every 24 hours while receiving treatment. Weight should be checked after a drain and before the next fill to monitor the patient's "dry weight." Baseline laboratory tests, such as electrolyte and glucose levels, are obtained before starting PD and are repeated at least daily during the PD treatment.

Continually monitor the patient during PD. Take and record vital signs every 15 to 30 minutes. Assess for signs of respiratory distress, pain, or discomfort. Check the dressing around the catheter exit site every 30 minutes for wetness during the procedure. Monitor the prescribed dwell time, and initiate outflow. Assess blood glucose levels in patients who absorb glucose.

Observe the outflow pattern (outflow should be a continuous stream after the clamp is completely open). Measure and record the total amount of outflow after each exchange. Maintain accurate inflow and outflow records when hourly PD exchanges are performed. When outflow is less than inflow, the difference is retained by the patient during dialysis and is counted as fluid intake. Weigh the patient daily to monitor fluid status.

Kidney Transplantation

Dialysis and kidney transplant are life-sustaining *treatments* for end-stage kidney disease (ESKD). Kidney transplant is not considered a "cure." Each patient, in consultation with a nephrologist, determines which type of therapy is best suited to his or her physical condition and lifestyle. During 2009,

17,513 kidney transplants had been performed in the United States. In 2010 about 159,000 people were awaiting kidney transplant in North America. The median time on the waiting list was 678 days (USRDS, 2010).

Candidate Selection Criteria. Candidates for transplantation must be free of medical problems that might increase the risks from the procedure. Candidates are accepted for kidney transplant up to 70 years of age. Patients older than 70 years are considered for transplant on an individual basis because complications are more common in the older adult.

The patient is thoroughly assessed before he or she is considered for a kidney transplant. Patients who have advanced, uncorrectable cardiac disease are excluded from the procedure because these problems are made worse by transplantation. Other conditions that preclude kidney transplant include metastatic cancer, chronic infection, and severe psychosocial problems such as alcoholism or chemical dependency. Long-standing pulmonary disease increases the risk for complications and death from respiratory infections. Patients with diseases of the GI system may require treatment before consideration for transplantation. Problems such as peptic ulcer and diverticulosis are made worse by the large doses of steroids used after the surgery.

The urinary system is completely evaluated to ensure normal urine flow. Many patients with ESKD have not used their lower urinary tract for years, and ureteral or bladder problems may require surgical correction before a kidney is transplanted.

Patients with a recent history of cancer are treated with dialysis because of the shortage of donor organs and the uncertain life expectancy of these patients. In addition, the drugs used after the procedure increase the risk for cancer recurrence. If more than 2 to 5 years have passed since eradication of the cancer, the patient can be considered for a transplant.

Diabetes mellitus and other endocrine problems cause even greater risks. Patients with these problems can have a kidney transplant, but they require intense observation and management to limit complications. Other complicating conditions are considered on an individual basis, depending on the patient's current health status. Kidney transplantation can be considered for most patients with ESKD and is the optimal therapy for many people. Most people who have undergone this procedure are satisfied with their quality of life for years after the transplant.

Donors. Kidney donors may be living donors (either related or unrelated to the patient), non–heart-beating donors (NHBDs), and cadaveric donors. The available kidneys are matched on the basis of tissue type similarity between the donor and the recipient. Living donors are most often blood relatives, but unrelated donors have been used. NHBDs are persons declared dead by cardiopulmonary criteria. Kidneys from NHBDs are removed (harvested) immediately after death in cases in which patients have previously given consent for organ donation. If immediate removal must be delayed, the organ is preserved by infusing a cool preservation solution into the abdominal aorta after death is declared and until surgery can be performed. Cadaveric donors are usually individuals who suffered irreversible brain injury and brain death, most often as a result of trauma. These donors are maintained with mechanical ventilation and must have sufficient renal perfusion for the kidneys to remain viable.

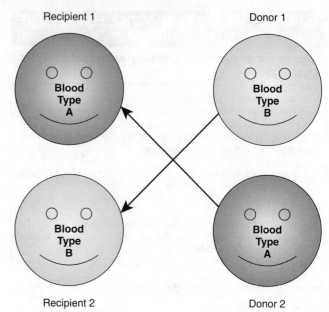

FIG. 71-16 An example of a paired exchange kidney donation. Donor 1 is related to or acquainted with recipient 1 and has agreed to donate a kidney but is not a blood type or tissue type match with recipient. Donor 1 is compatible with recipient 2 and agrees to donate a kidney to recipient 2 if donor 2 agrees to donate a kidney to recipient 1.

The size of the kidney is seldom a problem in adults. Kidneys transplanted from children become larger to meet adult needs within a few months.

Organs from living *related* donors (LRDs) have the highest rates of kidney graft survival (90%). Donors are usually at least 18 years old and are seldom older than 65 years. Physical criteria for donors include:

- Absence of systemic disease and infection
- No history of cancer
- No hypertension or kidney disease
- Adequate kidney function as determined by diagnostic studies

LRDs must express a clear understanding of the surgery and a willingness to give up a kidney. Some transplant centers require a psychiatric evaluation to assess the donor's motivation.

A list-paired exchange donation can be done when two kidney donor/recipient pairs have blood types that are not compatible within one pair. The two recipients trade donors so that each recipient can receive a kidney with a compatible blood type and tissue type (Fig. 71-16). Once the evaluations of all donors and recipients are completed, the two kidney transplant operations are scheduled to occur simultaneously (United Network for Organ Sharing [UNOS], 2011).

Because of advances in immunosuppressant therapy and medical management, the United Network of Organ Sharing (UNOS) reported 1-year kidney transplant graft survival to be almost 95% for all centers in the United States during 2010 (UNOS, 2011).

Preoperative Care. Many issues related to patient health and the actual transplant procedure must be addressed before surgery.

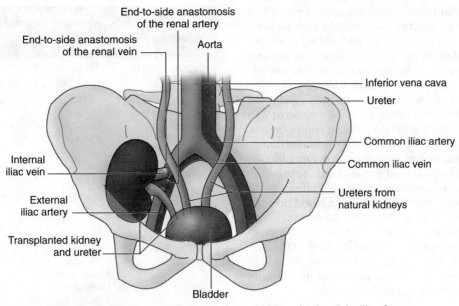

Immunologic studies are needed because the major barrier to transplant success after a suitable donor kidney is available is the body's ability to reject "foreign" tissue. This immunologic process can attack the transplanted kidney and destroy it. For immunologic problems to be overcome, tissue typing is performed on all candidates. These studies include simple blood typing and human leukocyte antigen (HLA) studies, as well as other tests. A donated kidney *must* come from a donor who is the same blood type as the recipient. The HLAs are the main immunologic feature used to match transplant recipients with compatible donors. The more similar the antigens of the donor are to those of the recipient, the more likely the transplant will be successful and rejection will be avoided (see Chapter 19).

Surgical team members for transplantation include circulating and scrub nurses, clinical nurse specialists, transplant surgeons, anesthesiologists, and nephrologists. Nursing actions before surgery include teaching about the procedure and care after surgery, in-depth patient assessment of patient readiness and ability to adhere to the plan of care, coordination of diagnostic tests, and development of treatment plans. See Chapter 16 for more discussion of standard preoperative nursing care.

The patient usually requires dialysis within 24 hours of the surgery. In addition, the recipient often receives a blood transfusion before surgery. Usually blood from the kidney donor is transfused into the recipient. This procedure increases graft survival of organs from living related donors (LRDs).

Operative Procedures. The donor nephrectomy procedure varies depending on whether the donor is a non–heart-beating donor (NHBD), cadaveric donor, or living donor. The NHBD or cadaveric donor nephrectomy is a sterile autopsy procedure performed in the operating room. All arterial and venous vessels and a long piece of ureter are preserved. After removal, the kidneys are preserved until time for implantation into the recipient. The technique for kidney removal from living donors is a delicate procedure that lasts

3 to 4 hours. A flank incision is used, and care is taken to avoid scarring. Donors often have more pain after surgery than do recipients. They also need nursing care and support for the psychological adjustment to loss of a body part.

Transplantation surgery usually takes 4 to 5 hours. The new kidney is usually placed in the right or left anterior iliac fossa (Fig. 71-17) instead of the usual kidney position. This placement allows easier connection of the ureter and the renal artery and vein. It also allows for easier kidney palpation. The recipient's own failed kidneys are not removed unless chronic kidney infection is present or, as in the case of polycystic kidney disease, the nonfunctioning, enlarged kidneys cause pain. After surgery, the patient is taken to the postanesthesia care unit and then, when stable, to a designated unit in the transplant center, to a critical care unit, or to a telemetry unit.

Postoperative Care. Care of the recipient after surgery requires that nurses be knowledgeable about the expected clinical findings and potential complications. Nursing care includes ongoing physical assessment, especially evaluation of kidney function. The transplant recipient requires close attention because the immunosuppressive drug therapy used to prevent tissue rejection impairs healing and increases the risk for infection.

Urologic management is essential to graft success. A large-bore indwelling (Foley) catheter is placed for accurate measurements of urine output and decompression of the bladder. Decompression prevents stretch on sutures and ureter attachment sites on the bladder.

Assess urine output at least hourly during the first 48 hours. An abrupt decrease in urine output may indicate complications such as rejection, acute kidney injury (AKI), thrombosis, or obstruction. Examine the urine color. The urine is pink and bloody right after surgery and gradually returns to normal over several days to several weeks, depending on kidney function. Obtain daily urine specimens for urinalysis, glucose measurement, the presence of acetone, specific gravity measurement, and culture (if needed).

FIG. 71-17 Placement of a transplanted kidney in the right iliac fossa.

Occasionally, a continuous bladder irrigation is prescribed to decrease blood clot formation, which could increase pressure in the bladder and endanger the graft. Perform routine catheter care, according to agency policy, to reduce catheter contamination. The catheter is removed as soon as possible to avoid infection, usually 3 to 7 days after surgery. After surgery, the function of the transplanted kidney (graft) can result in either oliguria or diuresis. Oliguria may occur as a result of ischemia and AKI, rejection, or other complications. To increase urine output, the physician may prescribe diuretics and osmotic agents, such as mannitol. Closely monitor the patient's fluid status because fluid overload can cause hypertension, heart failure, and pulmonary edema. Evaluate his or her fluid status by weighing daily, measuring blood pressure every 2 to 4 hours, and measuring intake and output.

Instead of oliguria, the patient may have diuresis, especially with a kidney from a living related donor (LRD). Carefully monitor intake and output, and observe for serum electrolyte imbalances, such as low potassium and sodium levels. Excessive diuresis may cause hypotension.

⚠ NURSING SAFETY PRIORITY

Critical Rescue

Notify the physician immediately about hypotension or excessive diuresis in the patient who has had a kidney transplant, because hypotension reduces blood flow and oxygen to the new kidney, threatening graft survival.

Complications. Many complications are possible after kidney transplantation. Early detection and intervention improve the chances of graft survival.

Rejection is the most serious complication of transplantation and is the leading cause of graft loss. A reaction occurs between the tissues of the transplanted kidney and the antibodies and cytotoxic T-cells in the recipient's blood. These substances treat the new kidney as a foreign invader and cause tissue destruction, thrombosis, and eventual kidney necrosis.

The three types of rejection are hyperacute, acute, and chronic. Acute rejection is the most common type with kidney transplants. It is treated with increased immunosuppressive therapy and often can be reversible. Rejection is diagnosed by manifestations, a renal scan, and kidney biopsy. Table 71-14 lists the features of the three types of rejection. Chapter 19 discusses their causes and treatment.

Acute tubular necrosis (ATN) after surgery can occur as a result of hypoxic damage when transplantation is delayed after kidneys have been harvested. These patients may need dialysis until adequate urine output returns and the blood urea nitrogen (BUN) and creatinine levels normalize. ATN is often difficult to distinguish from acute rejection, and patients need to undergo weekly biopsies to assess the need for further drug therapy if rejection is occurring.

Thrombosis of the major renal blood vessels may occur during the first 2 to 3 days after the transplant. A sudden decrease in urine output may signal impaired perfusion resulting from thrombosis. Ultrasound examination of the kidney may show decreased or absent blood supply. Emergency surgery is required to prevent ischemic damage or graft loss.

TABLE 71-14	**A COMPARISON OF HYPERACUTE, ACUTE, AND CHRONIC POST-TRANSPLANT REJECTION**	
HYPERACUTE REJECTION	**ACUTE REJECTION**	**CHRONIC REJECTION**
Onset		
Within 48 hr after surgery	1 wk to 2 yr postoperatively (most common in first 2 wk)	Occurs gradually during a period of months to years
Clinical Manifestations		
Increased temperature	Oliguria or anuria	Gradual increase in BUN and serum creatinine levels
Increased blood pressure	Temperature over 100° F (37.8° C)	
Pain at transplant site	Increased blood pressure	Fluid retention
	Enlarged, tender kidney	Changes in serum electrolyte levels
	Lethargy	Fatigue
	Elevated serum creatinine, BUN, potassium levels	
	Fluid retention	
Treatment		
Immediate removal of the transplanted kidney	Increased doses of immunosuppressive drugs	Conservative management until dialysis is required

BUN, Blood urea nitrogen.

Renal artery stenosis may result in hypertension. Other manifestations include a bruit over the artery anastomosis site and decreased kidney function. A renal scan can quantify the blood flow to the kidney. The involved artery may be repaired surgically or by balloon angioplasty in the radiology department. The decision to perform a balloon repair is determined by the amount of healing time after the surgery.

Other vascular problems include vascular leakage or thrombosis, both of which require an emergency transplant nephrectomy.

Other complications may involve the surgical wound or urinary tract. Wound problems, such as hematomas, abscesses, and lymphoceles (lymphocyte cysts containing lymph fluid), increase the risk for infection and exert pressure on the new kidney. Infection is a major cause of death in the transplant recipient. Prevention of infection is essential. Strict aseptic technique and handwashing must be rigorously enforced. Transplant recipients may not have the usual manifestations of infection because of the immunosuppressive therapy. Low-grade fevers, mental status changes, and vague reports of discomfort may be the only manifestations before sepsis. Always consider the possibility of infection with any patient after a kidney transplant. Urinary tract complications include ureteral leakage, fistula, or obstruction; stone formation; bladder neck contracture; and graft rupture. Surgical intervention may be required.

Immunosuppressive Drug Therapy. The success of kidney transplantation depends on changing the patient's immunologic response so that the new kidney is not rejected as a foreign organ. Immunosuppressive drugs protect the transplanted organ and are taken by the transplant recipient for the rest of his or her life. These drugs include corticosteroids, anti-lymphocyte preparations, monoclonal antibodies, and cyclosporine (Cyclosporin A). Chapter 19 discusses the mechanisms of action for these agents and the associated patient responses. Patients taking these drugs are at an increased risk for death by viral, fungal, bacterial, or protozoal infection.

Many patients do not follow the regimen correctly and are at high risk for losing the transplanted kidney. Work with the patient to ensure adherence to the drug regimen.

! NURSING SAFETY PRIORITY

Action Alert

Teach patients and families about the importance of adhering to the anti-rejection drug regimen to prevent transplant rejection.

? DECISION-MAKING CHALLENGE

Safety; Teamwork and Collaboration

The patient is a 62-year-old man with ESKD who has been on hemodialysis for 3 years while waiting for a kidney transplant. He expresses frustration with the wait from time to time and has told you that he fears that he will be considered too old to receive a kidney if much more time goes by. Today, he tells you that he won't be coming to the hemodialysis clinic anymore because he is taking a trip. When you ask him if he would like you to arrange dialysis for him on his trip, he tells you that won't be necessary. He doesn't make eye contact with you when you ask him why it won't be necessary. After a few minutes, he tells you that he is flying to India tonight and has paid to have a kidney transplant this week.

1. How should you respond to this statement?
2. Does the patient have the right to do this?
3. Is he right in thinking that he may be considered too old to receive a kidney?
4. Should you call UNOS and have his name taken off the kidney transplant waiting list?

Community-Based Care

Home Care Management

Because of the complex nature of CKD, its progressive course, and many treatment options, a case manager is helpful in planning, coordinating, and evaluating care. As kidney disease progresses, the patient is seen by a physician or nurse practitioner regularly and may be hospitalized often. Together with the dietitian and social worker, evaluate the home environment and determine equipment needs before discharge. Once the patient is discharged, home care nurses direct care and monitor progress. Chart 71-11 provides a focused assessment guide for the patient after transplantation.

Provide health teaching about the diet in kidney disease and the progression of disease. As CKD approaches end-stage kidney disease (ESKD), one of these courses of treatment is chosen: hemodialysis (HD), peritoneal dialysis (PD), or transplantation. For each form of treatment, the patient and partner must learn about the procedures and consider his or her personal lifestyle, support systems, and methods of coping. Decision making about treatment type or even whether to pursue treatment is difficult for patients and

---

CHART 71-11 FOCUSED ASSESSMENT

The Patient with Chronic Kidney Disease

Assess cardiovascular and respiratory status, including:
- Vital signs, with special attention to blood pressure
- Presence of S_3 or pericardial friction rub
- Presence of chest pain
- Presence of edema (periorbital, pretibial, sacral)
- Jugular vein distention
- Presence of dyspnea
- Presence of crackles, beginning at the bases and extending upward

Assess nutritional status, including:
- Weight gain or loss
- Presence of anorexia, nausea, or vomiting

Assess kidney status, including:
- Amount, frequency, and appearance of urine (in non-anuric patients)
- Presence of bone pain
- Presence of hyperglycemia secondary to diabetes

Assess hematologic status, including:
- Presence of petechiae, purpura, ecchymoses
- Presence of fatigue or shortness of breath

Assess gastrointestinal status, including:
- Presence of stomatitis
- Presence of melena

Assess integumentary status, including:
- Skin integrity
- Presence of pruritus
- Presence of skin discoloration

Assess neurologic status, including:
- Changes in mental status
- Presence of seizure activity
- Presence of sensory changes
- Presence of lower extremity weakness

Assess laboratory data, including:
- BUN
- Serum creatinine
- Creatinine clearance
- CBC
- Electrolytes

Assess psychosocial status, including:
- Presence of anxiety
- Presence of maladaptive behavior

BUN, Blood urea nitrogen; CBC, complete blood count.

---

families. Provide information and emotional support to assist patients with these decisions.

Teach patients who select hemodialysis (HD) about the machine and vascular access care. If in-home HD is selected, preparations are needed for the appropriate equipment, including a water treatment system. Regardless of whether the treatment occurs at home or in a center, provide ongoing assessment and health teaching to promote independence at home.

The patient receiving PD needs extensive training in the procedure. He or she also needs help in obtaining equipment and the many supplies needed. Home care nurses assess patients, monitor vital signs, assess adherence with drug and diet regimens, and monitor for manifestations of peritonitis.

The nurse plays a vital role in the long-term care of the patient with a kidney transplant. This patient is usually discharged 1 to 2 weeks after surgery. Facilitate acceptance and understanding of the anti-rejection drug regimen as a part of daily life. Carefully monitor for signs of graft rejection and for complications, such as infection.

Teaching for Self-Management

Instruct patients and family members in all aspects of nutrition therapy, drug therapy, and complications. Teach them to report complications, such as fluid overload and infection. When a patient requires a more advanced form of therapy, such as dialysis or transplantation, focus teaching on the chosen type of intervention.

Hemodialysis (HD) is the most complex form of therapy for the patient and family to understand. Even if patients receive HD in a dialysis center instead of at home, they are expected to have some knowledge of the HD machine. The patient or a family member must be taught to care for the vascular access and to report signs of infection and stenosis. Those who plan to have in-home HD will need a partner. Both the patient and the partner must be taught the entire process of HD and must be able to perform it independently before the patient is discharged.

Peritoneal dialysis (PD) involves extensive health teaching. This instruction can be given to the patient alone or to the patient and a family member if the patient cannot perform the procedure. Emphasize sterile technique because peritonitis is the most common complication of PD. Instruct patients to report any manifestation of peritonitis, especially cloudy effluent and abdominal pain. If peritonitis develops, teach patients how to give themselves antibiotics by the intraperitoneal (IP) route. Stress the importance of completing the antibiotic regimen. Remind patients that repeated episodes of peritonitis can reduce the effectiveness of PD, which may require the transfer to HD.

The patient receiving a kidney transplant also needs extensive health teaching. Provide instruction about drug regimens, home monitoring, immunosuppression, manifestations of rejection, infection, and prescribed changes in the diet and activity level.

Psychosocial Preparation

Provide psychological support for the patient and family. Help the patient adjust to the diagnosis of kidney failure and eventually accept the treatment regimens.

Many patients view dialysis as a cure instead of lifelong management. For many patients, the reduction of uremic symptoms in the first weeks after starting dialysis treatment creates a sense of well-being (the "honeymoon" period). They feel better physically, and their mood may be happy and hopeful. At this time they tend to overlook the discomfort and inconvenience of dialysis. Use this time to begin health care teaching. Stress that, although the uremic symptoms are reduced, they should not expect a complete return to the previous state of well-being.

Many patients become discouraged during the first year of treatment. This mood state may last a few months to a year or longer. The difficulties of incorporating dialysis into daily life are staggering, and patients may become depressed as problems occur. They may struggle with the idea of having to be permanently dependent on a disruptive therapy. Patients may feel helpless and dependent. Some people retreat into complete or partial denial of the disease and the need for treatment. They may deny the need for dialysis or may not adhere to drug therapy and diet restrictions. Monitor any behaviors that may contribute to nonadherence, and suggest psychiatric referrals. Help the patient and family focus on the positive aspects of the treatments. Continue health care education with patients as active participants and decision makers.

Most patients with CKD eventually enter a phase of acceptance or resignation. The idea of a chronic illness may be devastating for some people, and each person reacts differently. To make this long-term adaptation, the patient must adjust to continuous change. Specific concerns depend on the patient's health and particular treatment method.

After patients have accepted or become resigned to the chronic aspect of their disease, they usually attempt to return to their previous activities. Resuming the previous level of activity, however, may not be possible. Help patients set realistic goals that allow them to lead active, productive lives.

Health Care Resources

Professionals from many disciplines are resources for the patient with kidney failure. Home care nurses monitor the patient's status and evaluate maintenance of the prescribed treatment regimen (HD or PD). Those with advanced disease may need a home care aide to help perform ADLs. Social services are often involved because of the complex process of applying for financial aid to pay for the required medical care. A physical therapist may be beneficial in helping improve the patient's functional health. A dietitian can assist the patient and family members in understanding the special dietary needs. A psychiatric evaluation may be needed if depressive symptoms are present. Clergy and pastoral care specialists offer spiritual support.

Patients with CKD are routinely followed by a physician, usually a nephrologist. Organizations such as the National Kidney Foundation (NKF), the American Kidney Fund, and the National Association of Patients on Hemodialysis and Transplantation (NAPHT) may be helpful to patients and families.

EVALUATION: OUTCOMES

Evaluate the care of the patient with CKD based on the identified priority patient problems. The expected outcomes are that with appropriate management the patient should:
- Achieve and maintain appropriate fluid volume
- Maintain an adequate nutritional status
- Use effective coping strategies
- Report an absence of physical manifestations of anxiety

Specific indicators for these outcomes are listed for each priority problem under the Planning and Implementation section (see earlier).

NURSING CONCEPT REVIEW

What might you NOTICE if the patient is experiencing altered urinary elimination as a result of acute kidney injury?
- Patient urinates infrequently.
- Patient reports back or flank pain.
- Urine may be darker, smoky, or have obvious blood in it.

What should you INTERPRET and how should you RESPOND to a patient experiencing altered urinary elimination as a result of acute kidney injury?

Perform and interpret physical assessment, including:
- Ask how long manifestations have been present.
- Determine fluid intake and output volumes.
- Weigh the patient, and ask whether this weight is more or less than the usual weight.
- Assess for tachycardia.
- Assess for pulmonary congestion.
- Check for presence of generalized and dependent edema.

- Interpret laboratory values:
  - Complete blood count with hemoconcentration
  - BUN and serum creatinine levels elevated
  - Serum potassium level elevated
  - Serum osmolarity abnormal

Respond by:
- Ensuring hemodynamic stability
- Monitoring urine output
- Monitoring for fluid overload

On what should you REFLECT?
- Observe patient for evidence of improved urine output (see Chapter 68).
- Think about what may have caused this problem and what steps could be taken to prevent a similar episode.
- Think about what patient teaching focus could help reduce the risk for future acute kidney injury.

GET READY FOR THE NCLEX® EXAMINATION!

KEY POINTS

Review these Key Points for each NCLEX Examination Client Needs Category.

Safe and Effective Care Environment
- Use sterile technique when cannulating a vascular access or connecting peritoneal dialysis tubing.
- Handle patients with chronic kidney disease gently to prevent fractures.
- Assess all patients at risk for dehydration or hypovolemia for adequacy of kidney perfusion.
- Avoid taking blood pressure measurements or drawing blood from an arm with a vascular access (AV fistula or graft).
- Do not use an AV fistula or graft site to give IV fluids.

Health Promotion and Maintenance
- Encourage patients with chronic kidney disease or kidney failure to follow fluid and dietary restrictions regarding sodium, potassium, and protein.
- Teach patients the expected side effects, any adverse reactions to prescribed drugs, and when to contact the prescriber.
- Teach patients using peritoneal dialysis the manifestations of peritonitis.
- Teach patients on immunosuppressive therapy to assess themselves daily for fever, general malaise, and nausea or vomiting.

Psychosocial Integrity
- Allow patients the opportunity to express concerns about the risk for death and the disruption of lifestyle as a result of treatment for kidney failure.
- Use language and terminology that are comfortable for the patient.
- Assess the patient for depression and nonacceptance of the diagnosis or treatment plan.
- Refer patients to community resources and support groups.

Physiological Integrity
- Report immediately any condition that obstructs urine flow.
- Collaborate with the dietitian to teach patients about needed fluid, sodium, potassium, or dietary protein restriction.
- Teach patients in the early stages of chronic kidney disease the manifestations of dehydration.
- Teach patients in the later stages of chronic kidney disease the manifestations of fluid overload and hyperkalemia.
- Avoid all invasive procedures within 4 to 6 hours after the patient has undergone hemodialysis.
- Use meticulous sterile technique when caring for the peritoneal dialysis catheter and when hooking up or clamping off dialysate bags.

CONCEPT OVERVIEW

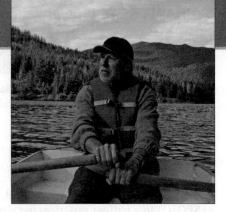

Sexuality

Unlike the physiologic human needs introduced in other section openers of this text, *sexuality* is a complex integration of many physiologic, emotional, social, and cultural aspects of well-being. It is closely associated with self-concept, self-esteem, role relationships, sexual response, and reproduction. Sexuality comprises other related human needs, such as belonging, intimacy (e.g., touching, kissing), sharing, and caring. When these needs are met, a person is sexually healthy (Fig. 1).

External Influences

- **Family** (beliefs, customs, values, educational level)
- **Friends** (e.g., peer group, habits and values)
- **Society** (e.g., media, acceptable practices, legal aspects)

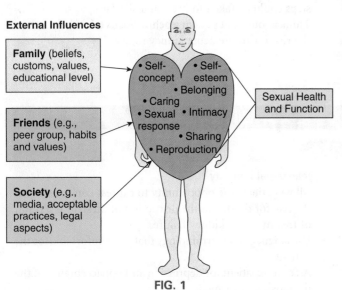

- Self-concept
- Self-esteem
- Belonging
- Caring
- Intimacy
- Sexual response
- Sharing
- Reproduction

→ Sexual Health and Function

FIG. 1

Sexuality, therefore, is a vital part of one's holistic being from birth to death. During the stages of human development, a person's attitudes, beliefs, and values related to sexuality are influenced and shaped by the environment, including family, friends, and society. For example, cultural beliefs affect the nature of physical sexual pleasure. The media also play a large role in developing views on sexuality. Some societies, such as the United States, tend to value youth and beauty more than aging and wisdom. As a result, people in these societies may feel less physically attractive and desirable for intimacy and belonging as they age.

Various external and internal risk factors can alter or impair sexual health. In many cases, they cause physical sexual dysfunction, which then affects emotional needs such as self-esteem (Fig. 2). These factors include:

- Stages of human development
- Physical health problems
- Drugs
- Mental/behavioral health problems

External/Internal Risk Factors

- **Stages of human development** (e.g., menopause)
- **Physical problems** (e.g., pain, trauma, surgeries, illnesses)
- **Drugs** (e.g., antihypertensives, antidepressants, alcohol, illicit drugs)
- **Mental/behavioral problems** (e.g., depression, anxiety)

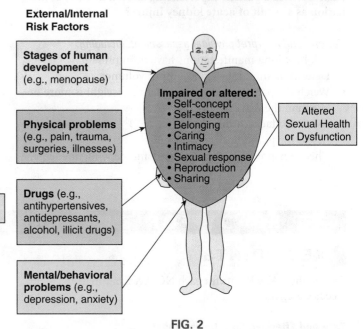

Impaired or altered:
- Self-concept
- Self-esteem
- Belonging
- Caring
- Intimacy
- Sexual response
- Reproduction
- Sharing

→ Altered Sexual Health or Dysfunction

FIG. 2

The *stages of human development* typically influence human sexuality, especially when menopause occurs in middle adulthood. Although each woman's response is different, menopause may result in a decreased libido (desire for sexual contact or intercourse). Relationships with her sexual partner(s) are altered, and interpersonal conflict can occur.

Physical health problems also can negatively affect sexual health. For example, chronic pain may cause decreased physical contact and a lowered self-concept along with chronic fatigue and decreased energy. Sexual dysfunction commonly occurs in people with chronic diseases such as diabetes and hypertension. Reproductive diseases (e.g., sexually transmitted diseases, testicular cancer) and their treatments (e.g., radiation therapy, surgery) can also affect sexuality, both physically and emotionally. Physical trauma such as spinal cord injury may prevent a person from having sexual intercourse.

Certain prescription or recreational *drugs* can cause impotence (inability to have an erection) or infertility. Alcohol and many antihypertensive agents, antidepressants, and illicit drugs interfere with sexual function in men.

Mental/behavioral health problems can also result in altered sexual health. Common examples include depression and severe anxiety states. In some cases, concern about physical performance can lead to sexual dysfunction.

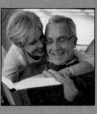

CHAPTER

72

Assessment of the Reproductive System

Donna D. Ignatavicius

evolve WEBSITE

http://evolve.elsevier.com/Iggy/

Animation: Lymphatic Drainage of the Breast
Animation: The Menstrual Cycle
Answer Key for NCLEX Examination Challenges and
    Decision-Making Challenges
Audio Glossary
Key Points

Review Questions for the NCLEX® Examination
Video Clip: Bimanual Examination
Video Clip: External Genitalia
Video Clip: Inguinal Hernia Evaluation
Video Clip: Inspection (Standing)
Video Clip: Speculum Examination

LEARNING OUTCOMES

Health Promotion and Maintenance

1. Teach patients about recommended guidelines for selected reproductive screening tests.
2. Teach pre- and post-test care for diagnostic testing for the reproductive system.

Psychosocial Integrity

3. Identify general psychological responses to reproductive health problems.

Physiological Integrity

4. Briefly review the anatomy and physiology of the male and the female reproductive systems.

5. Identify reproductive changes associated with aging and their implications for nursing care.
6. Perform a focused physical assessment of the patient with male or female reproductive system problems.
7. Explain the use of laboratory testing for patients with suspected or actual reproductive health problems.
8. Develop a teaching plan for a patient undergoing endoscopic studies for reproductive health problems.

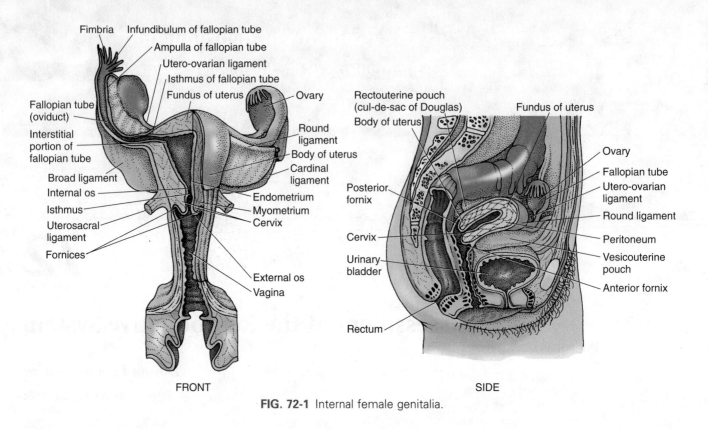

FIG. 72-1 Internal female genitalia.

The nurse is typically the first health care professional to assess the patient with a reproductive system health problem or hear a patient's concern about a reproductive problem. These problems often affect the need for *sexuality,* both its physical and psychosocial aspects, and are difficult for many people to discuss. Assessment of the male and the female reproductive systems should be part of every complete physical assessment. *Be aware of and sensitive to differences in sexual orientation and practices.*

This chapter reviews the focused reproductive system assessment that a nurse generalist performs. An advanced practice nurse or other health care provider performs the comprehensive reproductive examination. A more detailed discussion of human sexuality is found in a fundamentals or basic nursing text.

ANATOMY AND PHYSIOLOGY REVIEW

Structure and Function of the Female Reproductive System

The female reproductive system is located both outside (external) and inside (internal) the body.

External Genitalia

The external female genitalia, or vulva, extend from the mons pubis to the anal opening. The mons pubis is a fat pad that covers the symphysis pubis and protects it during coitus (sexual intercourse).

The labia majora are two vertical folds of adipose tissue that extend posteriorly from the mons pubis to the perineum. The size of the labia majora varies depending on the amount of fatty tissue present. The skin over the labia majora is usually darker than the surrounding skin and is highly vascular. It protects inner vulval structures and enhances sexual arousal.

The labia majora surround two thinner, vertical folds of reddish epithelium called the labia minora. The labia minora are highly vascular and have a rich nerve supply. Emotional or physical stimulation produces marked swelling and sensitivity. Numerous sebaceous glands in the labia minora lubricate the entrance to the vagina. The clitoris is a small, cylindric organ that is composed of erectile tissue with a high concentration of sensory nerve endings. During sexual arousal, the clitoris becomes larger and increases sexual sensation.

The vestibule is a longitudinal area between the labia minora, the clitoris, and the vagina that contains Bartholin glands and the openings of the urethra, Skene's glands (paraurethral glands), and vagina. The two Bartholin glands, located deeply toward the back on both sides of the vaginal opening, secrete lubrication fluid during sexual excitement. Their ductal openings are usually not visible.

The area between the vaginal opening and the anus is the perineum. The skin of the perineum covers the muscles, fascia, and ligaments that support the pelvic structures.

Internal Genitalia

The internal female genitalia are shown in Fig. 72-1. The vagina is a hollow tube that extends from the vestibule to the uterus. In addition to being the channel for the passage of the menstrual flow, the vagina allows for insertion of the penis during intercourse and passage of the fetus during a vaginal birth. Reduced estrogen levels occurring during menopause cause the vaginal wall to become dry, thinner, and smoother. The vagina then atrophies and is prone to pathogenic growth, resulting in a variety of types of infections.

The amounts of glycogen and lubricating fluid secreted by the vaginal cells are influenced by ovarian hormones. The normal vaginal bacteria (flora) interact with the secretions to produce lactic acid and maintain an acidic pH (3.5 to 5) in the vagina. This acidity helps prevent infection in the vagina.

At the upper end of the vagina, the uterine cervix projects into a cup-shaped vault of thin vaginal tissue. The recessed pockets around the cervix permit palpation of the internal pelvic organs. The posterior area provides access into the peritoneal cavity for diagnostic or surgical purposes.

The uterus (or "womb") is a thick-walled, muscular organ attached to the upper end of the vagina. This inverted pear–shaped organ is located within the true pelvis, between the bladder and the rectum. The uterus is made up of the body and the cervix.

The upper segment of the uterine body, between the insertion sites of the fallopian tubes, is referred to as the *fundus*. Although the uterus is a hollow organ, its walls are in such close proximity in the nonpregnant state that its cavity is merely a slit.

The cervix is a short (1 inch [2.5 cm]), narrowed portion of the uterus and extends into the vagina. The surface of the cervix and the canal are the sites for Papanicolaou (Pap) testing. (See discussion on p. 1581.)

The fallopian tubes (uterine tubes) insert into the fundus of the uterus and extend laterally close to the ovaries. They provide a duct between the ovaries and the uterus for the passage of ova and sperm. In most cases, the ovum is fertilized in these tubes.

The ovaries are a pair of almond-shaped organs located near the lateral walls of the upper pelvic cavity. After menopause, they become smaller. These small organs develop and release ova and produce the sex steroid hormones (estrogen, progesterone, androgen, and relaxin). Adequate amounts of these hormones are needed for normal female growth and development and to maintain a pregnancy.

Breasts

The female breasts are a pair of mammary glands that develop in response to secretions from the hypothalamus, pituitary gland, and ovaries. The breasts are an accessory of the reproductive system that nourish the infant after birth.

Breast tissue is composed of a network of glandular and ductal tissue, fibrous tissue, and fat. The proportion of each component of breast tissue depends on genetic factors, nutrition, age, and obstetric history. The breasts are supported by ligaments that are attached to underlying muscles. They have abundant blood supply and lymph flow that drains from an extensive network toward the axilla (Fig. 72-2).

Structure and Function of the Male Reproductive System

The male reproductive system also consists of external and internal genitalia. The primary male hormone for sexual development and function is testosterone. Testosterone production is fairly constant in the adult male. Only a slight and gradual reduction of testosterone production occurs in the older adult male until he is in his 80s. Low testosterone levels decrease muscle mass, reduce skin elasticity, and lead to postural changes and changes in sexual performance.

The penis is an organ for urination and intercourse consisting of the body or shaft and the glans penis (the distal end

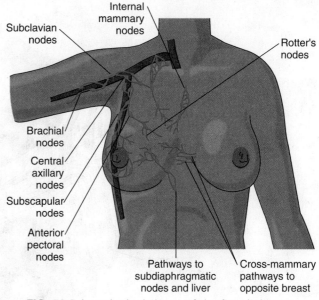

FIG. 72-2 Lymphatic drainage of the female breast.

of the penis). The glans is the smooth end of the penis and contains the slitlike opening of the urethral meatus. The urethra is the pathway for the exit of both urine and semen. A continuation of skin covers the glans and folds to form the prepuce (foreskin). Surgical removal of the foreskin (circumcision) for religious or cultural reasons is a common procedure in the United States and other Western countries.

The scrotum is a thin-walled, fibromuscular pouch that is behind the penis and suspended below the pubic bone. This pouch protects the testes, epididymis, and vas deferens in a space that is slightly cooler than inside the abdominal cavity.

The scrotal skin is darkly pigmented and contains sweat glands, sebaceous glands, and few hair follicles. It contracts with cold, exercise, tactile stimulation, and sexual excitement.

The internal male genitalia are shown in Fig. 72-3. The major organs are the testes and prostate gland. The testes are a pair of oval organs in the scrotum that produce sperm and testosterone. Each testis is suspended in the scrotum by the spermatic cord, which provides blood, lymphatic, and nerve supply to the testis. Sympathetic nerve fibers are located on the arteries in the cord, and sympathetic and parasympathetic fibers are on the vas deferens. When the testes are damaged, these autonomic nerve fibers transmit excruciating pain and a sensation of nausea.

The epididymis is the first portion of a ductal system that transports sperm from the testes to the urethra and is a site of sperm maturation. The vas deferens, or ductus deferens, is a firm, muscular tube that continues from the tail of each epididymis. The end of each vas deferens is a reservoir for sperm and tubular fluids. They merge with ducts from the seminal vesicle to form the ejaculatory ducts at the base of the prostate gland. Sperm from the vas deferens and secretions from the seminal vesicles move through the ejaculatory duct to mix with prostatic fluids in the prostatic urethra.

The prostate gland is a large accessory gland of the male reproductive system. It secretes a milky alkaline fluid that adds bulk to the semen, enhances sperm movement, and neutralizes acidic vaginal secretions. The prostate gland can

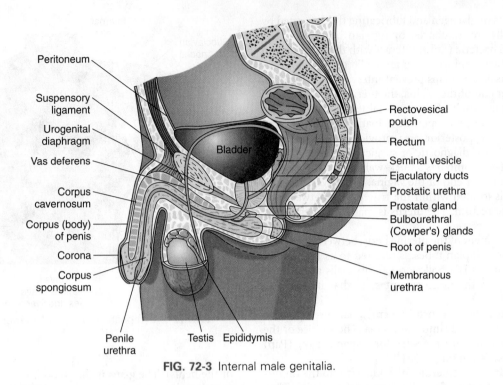

Peritoneum

Suspensory ligament

Urogenital diaphragm

Vas deferens

Corpus cavernosum

Corpus (body) of penis

Corona

Corpus spongiosum

Penile urethra

Testis Epididymis

Rectovesical pouch

Rectum

Seminal vesicle

Ejaculatory ducts

Prostatic urethra

Prostate gland

Bulbourethral (Cowper's) glands

Root of penis

Membranous urethra

Bladder

FIG. 72-3 Internal male genitalia.

be palpated through the rectum and should not project more than ⅜ inch (1 cm) into the rectal lumen.

As men age, the prostate gland becomes clinically significant. Men older than 50 years commonly have an enlarged prostate (benign prostatic hyperplasia [BPH]), which can cause problems such as overflow incontinence and nocturia (nighttime urination). Prostate function depends on adequate levels of testosterone.

The inguinal area (groin) is located between the superior iliac spine and the symphysis pubis and is the junction of the lower abdominal wall and thigh. The area is a common site for a hernia, which is a loop of bowel that protrudes through a weak spot in the muscles.

REPRODUCTIVE CHANGES ASSOCIATED WITH AGING

Age affects the function of both the male and the female reproductive systems. Many changes in the reproductive system occur as people age (Chart 72-1).

ASSESSMENT METHODS

Patient History

Establish a trusting relationship with the patient. Many patients are hesitant to share their reproductive history or concerns about sexuality. Respect their choice to refuse to answer questions and talk about their reproductive problems or sexual practices. Chart 72-2 describes questions to consider when assessing the patient's sexuality and reproductive health using Gordon's Functional Health Patterns.

Assess the patient's health habits, such as diet, sleep, and exercise patterns. Low levels of body fat may be related to ovarian dysfunction. Assess for alcohol, tobacco, and drug use (prescribed, over-the-counter [OTC], and illicit drugs),

because libido (sex drive), sperm production, and the ability to have or sustain an erection can be affected by these substances.

Ask female patients about the date and result of their most recent Pap test, breast self-examination, and vulvar self-examination. Determine when male patients older than 50 years had their last prostate examination and prostate-specific antigen test.

Ask about childhood illnesses that could have an effect on the reproductive system. For example, mumps in men may cause orchitis (painful inflammation and swelling of the testes) and can lead to testicular atrophy and sterility.

Assess for any chronic illnesses or surgeries that could affect reproductive function. For instance, endocrine disorders may affect the hypothalamic-pituitary-gonadal function of men or women. Almost any disease that disturbs a woman's metabolism or nutrition can depress ovarian function and cause amenorrhea (absence of menses). Failure of ovulation is associated with a greater risk for endometrial cancer. Patients with diabetes mellitus may experience physiologic changes such as vaginal dryness or impotence. Chronic disorders of the nervous system, respiratory system, or cardiovascular system can alter the sexual response.

Reproductive system dysfunction can also result from irradiation; prolonged use of corticosteroids, internal or external estrogen, or testosterone; and chemotherapy drugs. In addition, past severe infections can alter a person's reproductive ability. For example, pelvic inflammatory disease or a ruptured appendix followed by peritonitis can cause strictures or adhesions in the fallopian tubes and pelvic scarring. Salpingitis (uterine tube infection) is usually caused by chlamydial infection and can result in female infertility. If a young woman began having intercourse at a very early age and/or has multiple sex partners, she is at high risk for cervical cancer. Breast cancer is more common in women who have

CHART 72-1   NURSING FOCUS ON THE OLDER ADULT

Changes in the Reproductive System Related to Aging

PHYSIOLOGIC CHANGE	NURSING INTERVENTIONS	RATIONALES
Women		
Graying and thinning of the pubic hair Decreased size of the labia majora and clitoris	Discuss changes with the patient (applies to all structures for both women and men).	Education helps prevent problems with body image (applies to all structures for both women and men).
Drying, smoothing, and thinning of the vaginal walls	Provide information about vaginal estrogen therapy and water-soluble lubricants.	Education enables the patient to make informed decisions about the treatment of vaginal dryness, which can cause painful intercourse.
Decreased size of the uterus Atrophy of the endometrium Decreased size and marked convolution of the ovaries Loss of tone and elasticity of the pelvic ligaments and connective tissue	Provide information about Kegel exercises to strengthen pelvic muscles. Urinary incontinence can be a major problem.	Strengthening exercises may prevent or reduce pelvic relaxation and urinary incontinence.
Increased flabbiness and fibrosis of the breasts, which hang lower on the chest wall; decreased erection of the nipples	Teach or reinforce the importance of breast self-awareness, clinical breast examinations, and mammography.	These methods can detect masses or other changes that may indicate the presence of cancer.
Men		
Graying and thinning of the pubic hair Increased drooping of the scrotum and loss of rugae	Teach or reinforce the importance of testicular self-examination (TSE).	TSE may detect changes that may indicate cancer.
Prostate enlargement, with an increased likelihood of urethral obstruction	Teach the patient the signs of urethral obstruction and the importance of prostate cancer screening.	Education helps the patient detect enlargement or obstruction, which may indicate the presence of cancer.

not experienced childbearing. Ask about a history of infections or prolonged fever in males that may have damaged sperm production or caused obstruction of the seminal tract, because these changes cause infertility.

Data about sexual activity are important to obtain as part of the history. Heterosexual activity should not be assumed. Lesbian, gay, bisexual, and transgender (LGBT) issues are often not assessed by health care professionals or shared by the patient. Table 4-3 in Chapter 4 suggests sensitive ways to ask questions about sexual activity.

🌐 CULTURAL AWARENESS

Other cultural beliefs and practices influence lifestyle and sexual activity. For example, a person's religious beliefs often influence specific sexual practices, the acceptable number of sexual partners, and contraceptive use. Be sensitive to these differences by being nonjudgmental and showing acceptance.

Nutrition History

A nutrition history is often critical for an accurate assessment of reproductive system problems. For example, fatigue and low libido may occur with poor diet and anemia. Obesity raises the risk for uterine cancer. High-fat diets may increase the risk for cancer of the breast, ovary, and prostate gland (American Cancer Society [ACS], 2010). Ask the patient to recall his or her dietary intake for a recent 24-hour period to assess quality.

Assess the patient's height, weight, and body mass index. The patient may be hesitant to discuss practices such as bingeing, purging, anorexic behaviors, or excessive exercise. However, these practices may affect the reproductive system. A certain level of body fat and weight is necessary for the

onset of menses and the maintenance of regular menstrual cycles. Decreased body fat results in insufficient estrogen levels.

Women have special nutrition needs. Those who use oral contraceptives need increased sources of folic acid and vitamins B_6, B_{12}, and C. Heavy menstrual bleeding, particularly in women who have intrauterine devices, may require oral iron supplements. Teach all women of any age about their body's need for calcium. Although adequate calcium intake throughout life is needed, it is especially important during and after menopause to help prevent osteoporosis due to decreased estrogen production (see Chapter 53).

Family History and Genetic Risk

The family history helps determine the patient's risk for conditions that affect reproductive functioning. A delayed or early development of secondary sex characteristics may be a familial pattern.

The current age and health status of family members are important. Evidence of medical diseases or reproductive problems in family members (e.g., diabetes, endometriosis, reproductive cancer) allows better interpretation of the patient's current symptoms. For example, daughters of women who were given diethylstilbestrol (DES) to control bleeding during pregnancy are at increased risk for infertility and reproductive tract cancer.

Specific *BRCA1* and *BRCA2* gene mutations increase the overall risk for breast or ovarian cancer (ACS, 2010). Men with first-degree relatives (e.g., father, brother) with prostate cancer are at greater risk for the disease than men in the general population. Testicular cancer can also be familial (ACS, 2010). More information about genetic risks is discussed with specific health problems in later chapters of this unit.

Using Gordon's Functional Health Patterns

Health Perception/Health Management Pattern

- Has anyone in your family had cancer of the breast or reproductive organs? Who and what type of cancer?
- If you engage in sexual activities, do you practice "safer" sex?
- What do you do to keep healthy—regular health checkups, self-examination (breast, genital [vulvar, testicular]), healthy diet, exercise, use of medications or alternative therapies?

Sexuality-Reproductive Pattern
Male and Female

- Are you sexually active? Do you find your sexual relationship satisfying? Have there been any changes in your relationship? Are you having any problems in your sexual relationship?
- Do you use contraceptives? If so, do you have any problems with the method of contraception?
- Have you had any sexually transmitted diseases? If yes, when and what type did you have?

Female

- When did you first start menstruating? When was your last menstrual period? Do you have any menstrual problems?
- Have you ever been pregnant? If so, how many times and what were the outcomes?
- Have you had any symptoms of menopause?

Male

- Do you have any problems with getting and maintaining an erection, or do you have difficulty with ejaculation?
- Have you ever had a hernia or pain in the groin?

Self-Perception/Self-Concept Pattern

- How would you describe yourself? Do you feel good or not so good about yourself?
- Have you experienced changes in your body appearance or function? If so, are these problematic for you? Have you felt anxious, fearful, or depressed about these changes?

Based on Gordon, M. (2011). *Manual of nursing diagnosis* (12th ed.). New York: Jones & Bartlett.

Current Health Problems

Most patients seek medical attention as a result of pain, bleeding, discharge, and masses (Chart 72-3). *Pain* related to reproductive system disorders may be confused with or cause signs and symptoms that are usually associated with GI or urinary health problems (e.g., urinary frequency). Ask the patient to describe the nature of the pain, including its type, intensity, timing and location, duration, and relationship to menstrual, sexual, urinary, or GI function. Assess the factors that exacerbate (worsen) or relieve the pain. Ask about sleeping patterns and if pain or other manifestation is affecting the ability to get adequate rest (Ruhl, 2010).

Heavy *bleeding* or a lack of bleeding may concern the patient. Consider the possibility of pregnancy in any sexually active woman with amenorrhea. Any postmenopausal bleeding needs to be evaluated. Ask the patient to describe the amount and character of abnormal vaginal or penile bleeding. Assess whether the bleeding occurs in relation to the menstrual cycle or menopause, intercourse, trauma, or strenuous exercise. Ask about any associated symptoms, such as pain, cramping or abdominal fullness, a change in bowel habits, urinary difficulties, and weight changes. Many factors

Assessing the Patient with Reproductive Health Problems

PATIENT CONCERN	NURSING ASSESSMENT
Pain	Type and intensity of pain Location and duration of pain Factors that relieve or worsen pain Relationship to menstrual, sexual, urinary, or GI function Medications
Bleeding	Presence or absence of bleeding Character and amount of bleeding Relationship of bleeding to events or other factors (e.g., menstrual cycle) Onset and duration of bleeding Presence of associated symptoms, such as pain
Discharge	Amount and character of discharge Presence of genital lesions, bleeding, itching, or pain Presence of symptoms or discharge in sexual partner
Masses	Location and characteristics of mass Presence of associated symptoms, such as pain Relationship to menstrual cycle

can cause bleeding, and sites other than the genital tract need to be considered.

Discharge from either the male or female reproductive tract can cause severe irritation of the surrounding tissues, itching, pain, embarrassment, and anxiety. Ask about the amount, color, consistency, odor, and chronicity of the discharge. Drugs (e.g., antibiotics) and clothing (e.g., tight jeans, synthetic underwear fabric) may cause or worsen genital discharge. Many types of discharge are caused by sexually transmitted diseases (STDs) (see Chapter 76). The body location of these infections may depend on the patient's sexual practices. Ask the patient about lesions, bleeding, itching, and pain related to the genitals and orifices used during sexual activity. Also inquire about the presence of symptoms in the sexual partner(s).

Any reported *masses* in the breasts, testes, or inguinal area are evaluated. Some masses change in character or size. The patient can often relate these changes to menstrual cycles, heavy lifting, straining, or trauma. Ask about associated symptoms such as tenderness, heaviness, pain, dimpling, and tender lymph nodes.

Physical Assessment

Assessment of the Female Reproductive System

The medical-surgical nurse does not perform a comprehensive female or male reproductive examination. However, perform a focused assessment for specific concerns of the patient. The physician or advanced practice nurse does a more thorough gynecologic assessment as described below. The medical-surgical nurse often assists with the examination.

The physical examination of the reproductive system usually includes the breasts (see Chapter 73). After the breast examination, the examiner generally completes the thoracic and cardiovascular examinations and then inspects, auscultates, and palpates the abdomen. The patient's arms should be at her sides or over her chest to allow better relaxation of the abdominal muscles. During the gynecologic examination, the examiner palpates for symptomatic and asymptomatic abdominopelvic masses. A mass can be of reproductive, intestinal, or urinary tract origin. Careful history-taking combined with the physical examination can usually determine the origin of a mass. Gynecologic masses, such as ovarian masses, may be further differentiated from lesions on the body of the uterus during the bimanual portion of the pelvic examination.

Inspection of the female genitalia and the pelvic examination are usually performed at the end of a head-to-toe physical assessment. The patient is often more apprehensive about these portions of the examination than about any other part. Pain or lack of privacy during previous pelvic or breast examinations may prevent the patient from relaxing.

Other than determining pregnancy or infertility, a pelvic examination is indicated to assess for:
- Menstrual irregularities
- Unexplained abdominal or vaginal pain
- Vaginal discharge, itching, sores, or infection
- Rape trauma or other pelvic injury
- Physical changes in the vagina, cervix, and uterus

Immediately before the pelvic and breast examinations, ask the patient to empty her bladder and undress completely. Drape the woman adequately to protect modesty throughout the examination. If she is not wearing a gown, a small towel can be placed over the breasts under the larger drape. Remove drapes only over the region being examined, and replace them after that area has been assessed. Drapes that prevent eye contact between the examiner and the patient are dehumanizing and prevent comfort during the examination. Mirrors can be used to facilitate teaching if the patient so desires. The examination is performed in a room that has adequate lighting for body inspection, that is a comfortable temperature, and that ensures privacy.

Assessment of the Male Reproductive System

Unless a male patient seeks health care for specific problem, the examiner may not inspect and palpate the male genitalia and rectum during physical examinations, depending on the health care setting and the age of the patient. Men are often embarrassed and anxious when the reproductive system is assessed. This concern may be worse when the examiner is a woman. The patient may be concerned about discomfort, the developmental stage of his genitalia, or the likelihood of an erection during the examination. If he does have an erection, the examiner should assure him that this is a normal response to a tactile stimulus (touch) and should continue the examination.

As with examinations of other body systems, explain each step of the assessment procedure before it is performed. The patient needs to be reassured that the examiner will stop and change the assessment plan or technique if the patient has pain during the examination. Teach relaxation techniques and provide support during the examination to increase comfort.

Psychosocial Assessment

The psychosocial assessment may suggest factors that lead to the patient's health problem. During the social history, ask about sources of support, strengths, and likely reactions to illness or dysfunction.

A patient's personal history or beliefs may negatively influence his or her ability to enjoy a satisfactory sexual life. These factors may include:
- Sexual trauma or abuse inflicted during childhood or adulthood
- Punishment for masturbation
- Psychological trauma
- Cultural influences, such as the idea of female passivity during intercourse
- Concerns about sexual partners or sexual lifestyle
- Use of alcohol or street drugs

Fears may affect the patient's satisfaction with sexuality or body image. He or she may also be concerned about the potential or actual reaction of family members to reproductive health problems (see Chart 72-2).

Diagnostic Assessment

Laboratory Assessment

The Papanicolaou test, or Pap smear, is a cytologic study that is effective in detecting precancerous and cancerous cells from the cervix. It is done immediately before the pelvic examination. A speculum is inserted into the vagina, and several samples of cells from the cervix are obtained with a small brush or spatula. The specimens are placed on a glass slide and sent to the laboratory for examination.

The Pap test should be scheduled between the woman's menstrual periods so that the menstrual flow does not interfere with the test interpretation. Teach women not to douche, use vaginal medications or deodorants, or have sexual intercourse for at least 24 hours before the test.

Based on current evidence, the American Cancer Society (ACS) advises all women to begin having an annual Pap test within 3 years of becoming sexually active or by no later than 21 years of age. Annual screening is recommended until 30 years of age with the conventional Pap test or every 2 years if a liquid-based test is used. After age 30 and three or more consecutive normal test results, Pap tests may be performed every 3 years until 70 years of age. Women 70 years and older who have had normal results for 10 consecutive years may discontinue testing. Those who have had a total hysterectomy, including the cervix, do not need Pap smear testing. Women who have the surgery but still have their cervix should follow the guidelines for other women (ACS, 2011).

Cytologic vaginal *cultures* can detect bacterial, viral, fungal, and parasitic disorders. Examination of cells from the vaginal walls can evaluate estrogen balance.

The human papilloma virus (HPV) test can identify many high-risk types of HPV associated with the development of cervical cancer. This test can be done at the same time as the Pap test for women older than 30 years and for women of any age who have had an abnormal Pap test result. It does not take the place of the Pap test because it tests for the viruses that can cause cell changes in the cervix that, if not treated, could lead to cancer. Cells are collected from the cervix and sent to a laboratory for analysis. Women who have normal Pap test results and no HPV infection are at very low risk for developing cervical cancer. Conversely, women with an abnormal Pap result and a positive HPV test are at higher risk if not treated.

Serum levels of follicle-stimulating hormone (FSH), luteinizing hormone (LH), and prolactin are helpful in the

CHART 72-4   LABORATORY PROFILE

Reproductive Assessment

TEST	NORMAL RANGE FOR ADULTS	SIGNIFICANCE OF ABNORMAL FINDINGS
Serum Studies		
Follicle-stimulating hormone (FSH) (Follitropin)	*Men:* 1.42-15.4 IU/L *Women:* follicular phase, 1.37-9.9 IU/L; midcycle, 6.17-17.2 IU/L; luteal phase, 1.09-9.2 IU/L; postmenopause, 19.3-100.6 IU/L	Decreased levels indicate possible infertility, anorexia nervosa, neoplasm. Elevations indicate possible Turner's syndrome.
Luteinizing hormone (LH) (Lutropin)	*Men:* 1.24-7.8 IU/L *Women:* follicular phase, 1.68-15 IU/L; midcycle, 21.9-56.6 IU/L; luteal phase, 0.61-16.3 IU/L; postmenopause, 14.2-52.3 IU/L	Decreased levels indicate possible infertility, anovulation. Elevations indicate possible ovarian failure, Turner's syndrome.
Prolactin	*Men:* 0-20 ng/mL *Women:* 0-20 ng/mL Pregnant women: 20-400 ng/mL	Elevations indicate possible galactorrhea (breast discharge), pituitary tumor, disease of hypothalamus or pituitary gland, hypothyroidism.
Estradiol	*Men:* 10-50 pg/mL *Women:* follicular phase, 20-350 pg/mL; midcycle, 150-750 pg/mL; luteal phase, 30-450 pg/mL; postmenopause, ≤20 pg/mL	Elevations of estradiol, total estrogens, and estriol in men indicate possible gynecomastia, decreased body hair, increased fat deposits, feminization, testicular tumor; in women, ovarian tumor.
Estriol	Men and nonpregnant women: <2.0 ng/dL	Decreased levels or estradiol, total estrogens, and estriol in women indicate possible amenorrhea, climacteric, impending miscarriage, hypothalamic disorders.
Progesterone	*Men:* 10-50 ng/dL *Women:* follicular phase, <50 ng/dL; luteal phase, 300-2500 ng/dL; postmenopausal, <40 ng/dL	Decreased levels in women indicate possible inadequate luteal phase, amenorrhea. Elevations in women indicate possible ovarian luteal cysts. Decreased levels may indicate ovarian neoplasm, ovarian dysfunction.
Testosterone	*Men:* 280-1080 ng/dL *Women:* <70 ng/dL	Increased levels in men indicate possible testicular tumor, hyperthyroidism. Decreased levels in men indicate possible hypogonadism. Elevations in women indicate possible adrenal neoplasm, ovarian neoplasm, polycystic ovary syndrome.
Prostate-specific antigen	*Men:* <4 ng/mL	Increased levels may indicate prostatitis, benign prostatic hyperplasia, prostate cancer.
Urine Studies		
Total estrogens	*Men:* 4-25 mcg/24 hr *Women:* 4-60 mcg/24 hr	Elevations indicate possible testicular tumors. Decreased levels indicate possible ovarian dysfunction.
Pregnanediol	*Men:* 0-1.9 mg/24 hr *Women:* follicular phase, <2.6 mg/24 hr; luteal phase, 2.6-10.6 mg/24 hr	Elevations indicate possible luteal ovarian cysts, ovarian neoplasms, adrenal disorders. Decreased levels indicate possible amenorrhea.
17-Ketosteroids	Men (20-50 yr): 6-20 mg/24 hr Women (20-50 yr): 6-17 mg/24 hr Values decrease with age	Elevations indicate possible Cushing's syndrome, increased androgen or cortisol production, severe stress. Decreased levels indicate possible Addison's disease, hypopituitarism.

Data from Pagana, K.D., & Pagana, T.J. (2010). *Mosby's manual of diagnostic and laboratory tests* (4th ed.). St. Louis: Mosby.
1 mcg, 1 microgram or 1 millionth of a gram; *1 ng,* 1 nanogram or 1 billionth of a gram; *1 pg,* 1 picogram or 1 trillionth of a gram.

diagnosis of male and female reproductive tract disorders. No nutrition restrictions are necessary before the test. Serum testing can also detect estrogen, progesterone, and testosterone levels in men and women. Chart 72-4 gives the normal values and the significance of abnormal findings.

Serologic studies detect antigen-antibody reactions that occur in response to foreign organisms. This form of diagnostic testing is helpful only after an infection has become well established. Serologic testing can be used in the evaluation of exposure to organisms causing syphilis, rubella, and herpes simplex virus type 2 (HSV2). Results may be read as nonreactive, weakly reactive, or reactive. A single titer is not as revealing as serial titers, which can detect the rise in antibody reactions as the body continues to fight the infection.

Human immune deficiency virus (HIV) testing should be offered to all patients ages 19 to 64 years, especially those with personal risk factors (see Chapter 21 for a detailed discussion of HIV testing). Testing for sexually transmitted diseases should be performed if patients have signs and symptoms associated with these problems. These tests are discussed in other chapters of this unit.

The *prostate-specific antigen (PSA)* test is used to screen for prostate cancer and to monitor the disease after treatment. PSA levels less than 4 ng/mL are normal. Elevated PSA levels, especially above 10 ng/mL, are associated with prostate cancer. Older men, particularly African-American men, often have a higher normal PSA, especially as they age.

The patient should not ejaculate for at least 24 hours before the test to avoid a false-positive result. For the same reason, the blood for the PSA test should be drawn before the digital rectal examination (Pagana & Pagana, 2010).

Imaging Assessment

General X-rays. A kidney, ureter, and bladder (KUB) x-ray of the abdomen shows these structures and is used in the assessment of disorders of either the male or the female reproductive system. Pelvic masses, calcified tumors or fibroids, dermoid cysts, and metastatic bone changes may be seen. No specific preparation is needed.

Bone scans and chest x-rays may also be included in the workup of the patient with suspected metastatic cancer. They help determine the extent of the cancer spread and obstruction or displacement of the organs. These tests are discussed elsewhere in this text.

Computed Tomography. Computed tomography (CT) scans for reproductive system disorders involve the abdomen and the pelvis. They can detect and evaluate masses and lymphatic enlargement from metastasis. This scan can differentiate solid tissue masses from cystic or hemorrhagic structures.

Hysterosalpingography. A hysterosalpingogram is an x-ray of the cervix, uterus, and fallopian tubes and is performed after the injection of a contrast medium. This test is used to evaluate tubal anatomy and patency and uterine problems such as fibroids, tumors, and fistulas. The study should not be attempted for at least 6 weeks after abortion, delivery, or dilation and curettage. Other contraindications include reproductive tract infection and uterine bleeding.

The examination is scheduled in a radiology department 2 to 5 days after the end of the patient's normal menses. The scheduling is important to prevent the accidental flushing of a fertilized ovum from the fallopian tube or the exposure of a fetus to radiation.

The patient is usually instructed to take a laxative the evening before the test, followed by an enema or rectal suppository on the morning of the examination. These procedures reduce the distortion of the x-rays by gas shadows.

On the day of the examination, confirm the date of the patient's last menstrual period and record it in the medical record. Ask about allergies to iodine dye or shellfish. The patient signs a consent form for the procedure. Because discomfort is expected during the examination, premedication with analgesics or NSAIDs may be prescribed. Inform the patient that she may experience some nausea and vomiting, abdominal cramping, or faintness. Provide support and assistance with relaxation techniques.

The patient is placed in the lithotomy position. A speculum is inserted, and the cervix is viewed. Dye is injected through the cervix to fill and highlight the interior of the cervix, uterus, and fallopian tubes. If the fallopian tubes are patent, the contrast material spills into the peritoneal cavity. Usually, only two or three views are obtained to show the path and distribution of the contrast medium.

The patient may experience pelvic pain after the study and should receive analgesic drugs accordingly. She may also have referred pain to the shoulder because of irritation of the phrenic nerve. Provide a perineal pad after the test to prevent the soiling of clothes as the dye drains from the cervix. Instruct the woman to contact her health care provider if bloody discharge continues for 4 days or longer and to report any signs of infection, such as lower quadrant pain, fever, malodorous discharge, or tachycardia.

Mammography. Mammography is an x-ray of the soft tissue of the breast. Mammograms assess differences in the density of breast tissue. They are especially helpful in evaluating poorly defined masses, multiple masses or nodules, nipple changes or discharge, skin changes, and pain. Mammography can detect about 80% to 90% of cancers that are not palpable by physical examination. However, some actual cancers may not appear on mammography or may appear as benign (ACS, 2011).

In young women's breasts, there is little difference in the density between normal glandular tissue and malignant tumors, which makes the mammogram less useful for evaluation of breast masses in these women. For this reason, annual screening mammograms are not recommended for women younger than 40 years (ACS, 2011). In older women, the amount of fatty tissue is higher and the fatty tissue appears lighter than cancers. Cancer and cysts may have the same density. Cysts usually have smooth borders, and cancers often have starburst-shaped margins.

No dietary restrictions are necessary before the mammogram. Remind the patient not to use creams, powders, or deodorant on the breasts or underarm areas before the study because these products can show on the x-ray. If there is any possibility that the patient is pregnant, the test should be rescheduled. Explain the purpose of the examination and its anticipated discomforts. Provide a cover gown and adequate privacy to undress above the waist. The patient also needs support and may need time to express her concerns about the mammogram and the presence of any lumps.

The technician positions the woman next to the x-ray machine with one breast exposed. A film plate and the platform of the machine are placed on opposite sides of the breast to be examined. The technician includes as much breast tissue as possible between the plates. The woman may experience some temporary discomfort when the breast is compressed during the positioning and the test. The test takes about 15 minutes, but the patient is usually asked to wait until the films are developed in case a view needs to be repeated. Some facilities are now using digital imaging rather than films.

The woman should know when to expect the report of the results. Because this is a time when the woman is anxious about the health of her breasts, it is a good opportunity to teach or reinforce the importance of breast self-examination (BSE) and give instructions as needed.

Other Diagnostic Assessment

Ultrasonography. Ultrasonography (US) is a technique that is routinely used to assess problems such as uterine fibroids, ovarian cysts, and pelvic masses. It can be used to monitor the progress of tumor regression after medical treatment. US is also helpful in differentiating solid tumors from cysts in breast examinations. In men, ultrasound can test for varicoceles, scrotal abnormalities, and problems of the ejaculatory ducts and seminal vesicles and the vas deferens (Pagana & Pagana, 2010).

No specific preparations are needed for this study. Women should have a full bladder to help view the uterus and to make the location of other structures more distinct with abdominal ultrasonography. A full bladder is not needed for breast, scrotal, transvaginal, or transrectal scans.

For an abdominal, breast, or scrotal scan, the technician exposes the area and applies oil or gel to the area to be scanned. These substances provide better transmission of sound waves from the transducer through the patient's skin. The transducer is moved in a linear pattern across the area being tested to outline and define soft-tissue masses and to differentiate tumor type, ascites, and encapsulated fluid.

For a *transvaginal* or *transrectal* scan, the transducer is covered with a condom or vinyl glove onto which transmission gel has been placed. The transducer is then inserted into the vagina or rectum as indicated.

The patient may want to watch the viewing screen with a brief explanation of the landmarks and structures seen. There is no special follow-up care for the patient after this procedure except to provide wipes to remove the gel.

Magnetic Resonance Imaging. Magnetic resonance imaging (MRI) uses a magnetic field and radiofrequency energy to scan for pelvic tumors. This scan distinguishes between normal and malignant tissues. MRIs are now being used in the diagnosis of breast cancer in women who have a genetic risk (ACS, 2011). The use of MRI in evaluating patients with dense breast tissue may reduce the need for biopsy.

Endoscopic Studies

Colposcopy. The colposcope allows three-dimensional magnification and intense illumination of epithelium with suspected disease. Colposcopy is suited for inspection of the cervical epithelium, vagina, and vulvar epithelium. This procedure can locate the exact site of precancerous and malignant lesions for biopsy.

The woman is placed in the lithotomy position and provided the same support as for a pelvic examination. The patient should not douche or use vaginal preparations for 24 to 48 hours before the test. This nearly painless procedure is better tolerated if it is explained in advance and if the instrument is shown to the patient.

Colposcopy provides accurate site selection for tissue biopsy. Therefore the patient should also be prepared for a biopsy. Materials for cytologic studies and biopsy should be readily available.

The physician locates the cervix or vaginal site through a speculum examination. Lubricants other than water should not be used. Cells in the area may be stained or left unstained to enhance visibility. The physician cleans and moistens the cervix with normal saline. This increases the visibility of vascular patterns and the junction between the columnar epithelium and the squamous epithelium. Acetic acid, 3%, is applied to the cervix to draw moisture from the tissue and to accentuate important features. The physician then uses a colposcope or colpomicroscope to inspect the area in question.

A biopsy specimen may also be taken if abnormal cells are seen. (See Cervical Biopsy section on p. 1585.)

After the procedure, assist the woman as you would for a pelvic examination and provide supplies to clean the perineum. Also give her a perineal pad to absorb any dye or discharge. If a biopsy specimen is taken, additional follow-up care is needed.

Laparoscopy. Laparoscopy is a direct examination of the pelvic cavity through an endoscope. This procedure can rule out an ectopic pregnancy, evaluate ovarian disorders and pelvic masses, and aid in the diagnosis of infertility and unexplained pelvic pain. Laparoscopy is also used during surgical procedures such as:

- Tubal sterilization
- Ovarian biopsy
- Cyst aspiration
- Removal of endometriosis tissue
- Lysis of adhesions around the fallopian tubes
- Retrieval of "lost" intrauterine devices

A laparoscopy is used instead of a laparotomy for minor surgical procedures because it uses small incisions, involves less discomfort, and does not require overnight hospitalization.

Patient Preparation. The physician explains the procedure, risks (complications associated with the use of general anesthesia, postoperative shoulder pain, and the rare occurrence of infection or electrical burns), and anticipated discomforts and obtains the patient's consent. The procedure can be performed with either a regional or general anesthetic. Patients should expect mild discomfort from the incision site and may experience referred shoulder pain from phrenic nerve irritation.

Procedure. The patient is anesthetized and placed in the lithotomy position. A urinary catheter is inserted to drain the bladder. The operating table is placed in a slight Trendelenburg position to cause the intestines to fall away from the pelvis. The cervix is held with a cannula to allow movement of the uterus during laparoscopy (Fig. 72-4). The surgeon

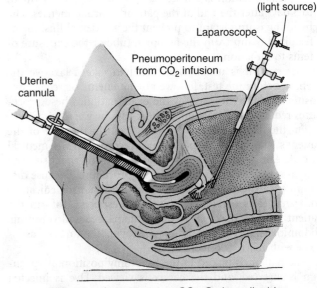

FIG. 72-4 Laparoscopy. CO_2, Carbon dioxide.

inserts a needle below the umbilicus to infuse carbon dioxide (CO_2) into the pelvic cavity, which distends the abdomen and permits better visualization of the organs. After the trocar and cannula are in place in the abdominal cavity, the surgeon removes the trocar and inserts the laparoscope. The surgeon can then visualize the pelvic cavity and reproductive organs. Further instrumentation is possible through one or more small incisions. The laparoscope is removed at the end of the procedure, and the abdomen is deflated. The small incision is closed with absorbable sutures and dressed with an adhesive bandage.

Follow-up Care. Care after surgery is similar to that for other patients after general anesthesia. The patient is usually discharged on the day of the procedure. Discomfort from the incision is managed by oral analgesics. The greatest discomfort is due to referred shoulder pain caused by residual CO_2 in the peritoneal cavity. Most of these sensations disappear within 48 hours. Instruct the patient to change the small adhesive bandage as needed and to observe the incision for signs of infection or hematoma. Remind her to avoid strenuous activity for the first week after the procedure.

Hysteroscopy. Hysteroscopy is an endoscopic examination to view the interior of the uterus and the cervical canal. The hysteroscope includes a fiberoptic camera. Aqueous carbon dioxide is the medium used to distend the uterus. Hysteroscopy can be used for the removal of intrauterine devices and as a complement to other diagnostic tests for infertility and unexplained bleeding.

The surgeon informs the patient of all aspects of the procedure and obtains consent. The preparation is the same as for a pelvic examination. The procedure is best performed 5 days after menses has ceased to reduce the possibility of pregnancy. The woman is placed in the lithotomy position and is usually anesthetized with a paracervical or other regional block.

After she is anesthetized, the cervix is dilated. The physician inserts the hysteroscope through the cervix. Because a medium distends the uterus, cells can be pushed through the fallopian tubes and into the pelvic cavity. Therefore hysteroscopy is contraindicated in patients with suspected cervical or endometrial cancer, in those with infection of the reproductive tract, and in pregnant patients.

Care is the same as that after a pelvic examination. Analgesics may be prescribed if the patient has cramping or shoulder pain.

Biopsy Studies

Cervical Biopsy. In a cervical biopsy, cervical tissue is removed for cytologic study. A biopsy is indicated for an identifiable cervical lesion, regardless of the cytologic findings. The health care provider usually performs a biopsy in conjunction with colposcopy as a follow-up to a suspicious Pap test finding. The procedure may be performed in a clinic or office setting.

Several techniques can be used for a cervical biopsy. If a lesion is clearly visible, an endocervical curettage can be performed as an ambulatory care procedure and with little or no anesthetic. Conization (removal of a cone-shaped sample of tissue) and loop electrosurgical excision procedures (LEEPs) are usually not done unless the cervical biopsy findings are positive or the results of the colposcopy are unsatisfactory (Lowdermilk & Perry, 2011). Conization can be done as a

---

CHART 72-5   PATIENT AND FAMILY EDUCATION: PREPARING FOR SELF-MANAGEMENT

The Patient Recovering from Cervical Biopsy

- Do not lift any heavy objects until the site is healed (about 2 weeks).
- Rest for 24 hours after the procedure.
- Report any excessive bleeding (more than that of a normal menstrual period) to your health care provider.
- Report signs of infection (fever, increased pain, foul-smelling drainage) to your health care provider.
- Do not douche, use tampons, or have vaginal intercourse until the site is healed (about 2 weeks).
- Keep the perineum clean and dry by using antiseptic solution rinses (as directed by your health care provider) and changing pads frequently.

---

cold-knife procedure, a laser excision, or an electrosurgical incision.

The biopsy is usually scheduled when the woman is in the early proliferative phase of the menstrual cycle, when the cervix is least vascular. Because a biopsy evaluates potentially cancerous cells, most women are anxious and need time to discuss their feelings and fears. The use of relaxation techniques may assist comfort. Assist the patient into the lithotomy position and prepare her in the same way as for a pelvic examination. Further preparation depends on the type of procedure to be performed.

The physician may anesthetize the patient according to the needs of the chosen procedure. He or she visualizes the cervix and obtains the tissue sample. All specimens are immediately placed into a formalin solution.

The type of anesthetic used for the procedure determines the type of immediate care needed after the procedure. Discharge instructions are listed in Chart 72-5.

Endometrial Biopsy. Both endometrial biopsy and aspiration are used to obtain cells directly from the lining of the uterus to assess for cancer of the endometrium. Biopsy also helps assess menstrual disturbances (especially heavy bleeding) and infertility (corpus luteum dysfunction).

When menstrual disturbances are being evaluated, the biopsy is generally done in the immediate premenstrual period to provide an index of progesterone influence and ovulation. A biopsy performed in the second half of the menstrual cycle (about days 21 and 22) evaluates corpus luteum function and the presence or absence of a persistent secretory endometrium. Postmenopausal women may undergo biopsies at any time.

Menstrual data are obtained from the patient and are included on the specimen request for the pathologist. The woman has the same preparation as for a pelvic examination. Advise her that she may experience some cramping when the cervix is dilated. Analgesia before the procedure and relaxation and breathing techniques during the procedure may be helpful.

An endometrial biopsy is usually done as an office procedure with or without anesthesia. After the uterus is measured and the cervix dilated, the physician inserts the curette or intrauterine cannula into the uterus. A portion of the endometrium is withdrawn using either the cuplike end of the curette or with suction equipment. The patient usually has moderate cramping. The specimens are placed into a formalin solution and sent for histologic examination.

Allow the woman to rest on the examining table until the cramping has subsided. Provide a perineal pad and a wipe to clean the perineum. Tell her that spotting may be present for 1 to 2 days but any signs of infection or excessive bleeding should be reported to the physician. Instruct the patient to avoid intercourse or douching until all discharge has ceased. Results of the biopsy are usually available within 72 hours.

Breast Biopsy. All breast masses should be evaluated for the possibility of cancer in women or, far less often, in men. Fibrocystic lesions, fibroadenomas, and intraductal papillomas can be differentiated by biopsy. Any discharge from the breasts is examined histologically.

The instructions to the patient depend on the type of biopsy and the type of anesthesia. Explain the procedure. Most biopsies are performed in an ambulatory care setting. Several methods are used to biopsy breast tissue. The patient usually receives a local anesthetic, and the tissue either is aspirated through a large-bore needle (core-needle biopsy) or is removed using a small incision to extract multiple samples of tissue.

Aspirated fluid from benign cysts may appear clear to dark green–brown. Bloody fluid suggests cancer. The specimens also undergo histologic evaluation. If cancer is found, the tissue is evaluated for estrogen receptor analysis. Chapter 73 discusses types of breast cancer and their relationship to estrogen receptors.

❓ NCLEX EXAMINATION CHALLENGE

Physiological Integrity

A client has a left needle breast biopsy with local anesthesia. What post-test teaching will the nurse provide?

A. "Do not use your left arm for at least a week."
B. "You'll likely have some discomfort for about a week."
C. "Do not lift anything over 10 pounds for a week."
D. "Remember to take all of your antibiotics as prescribed."

Discomfort after surgery is usually mild and is controlled with analgesics or the use of ice or heat, depending on the type and extent of the biopsy. Teach the patient how to assess the area or incision for bleeding and edema. Tell women to wear a properly supportive bra continuously for 1 week after surgery. Numbness around the biopsy site may last several weeks. If cancer is identified, provide emotional support as well as information about follow-up treatment alternatives.

Prostate Biopsy. When prostate cancer is suspected, the physician performs a needle aspiration biopsy of the prostate gland for histologic study. This procedure is often performed at the same time as cystoscopy, when the patient is under moderate sedation. The physician can perform needle biopsies without anesthesia or with the patient under local anesthesia.

Preparation for the procedure depends on the technique used to puncture the gland. Explain about the expected discomforts. Teach the patient about breathing and relaxation techniques for use during the examination. Because the purpose of this procedure is to evaluate prostate cells for cancer, the man needs support and time to discuss his fears. Preparation for a transrectal biopsy involves the use of cleansing enemas. Prophylactic antibiotics are given to reduce the risk for bacterial contamination of the blood or prostate tissue. Local anesthesia is used for transperineal biopsy.

The patient is placed in the same position as for a rectal examination. After injecting a local anesthetic for the transperineal biopsy, the physician places a finger in the rectum to help guide the needle to the prostate. For the transrectal biopsy, the physician places the needle against the examining finger and then inserts it into the rectum to the prostate. From this site, the needle is advanced through the rectal mucosa and into the prostate gland. The aspiration may be repeated several times to obtain a satisfactory specimen.

Although not common, sepsis is a life-threatening complication of transrectal biopsy. Teach the patient to report any manifestations of infection (e.g., fever, low back pain). Prophylactic antibiotics may be prescribed.

NURSING CONCEPT REVIEW

What should you expect to see in a patient without reproductive health problems that affect sexuality?

Physical assessment
- No vaginal bleeding other than usual menstruation
- No unusual vaginal discharge
- No penile bleeding or discharge
- No masses or lesions on internal or external genitalia for men or women
- Reports ability to have intercourse without pain

Psychosocial assessment
- Reports satisfaction with sexual activity
- Reports satisfaction with body image

Laboratory assessment
- Sex hormones within normal limits for age
- Prostate-specific antigen within normal limits for age

GET READY FOR THE NCLEX® EXAMINATION!

KEY POINTS

Review these Key Points for each NCLEX Examination Client Needs Category.

Health Promotion and Maintenance

- Encourage all women to follow recommended Pap screening guidelines for early detection of precancerous and cancerous cells from the cervix.
- Assess cultural issues when identifying risks for certain reproductive problems and when evaluating health promotion practices.
- Explain all diagnostic procedures, restrictions, and follow-up care to the patient scheduled for tests.

Psychosocial Integrity

- Allow the patient the opportunity to express fear or anxiety regarding tests of the reproductive system or regarding a potential change in sexual or reproductive function.
- Assess the patient's level of comfort in discussing issues related to reproduction and sexuality.

- Encourage patients to express feelings of anxiety or discomfort related to genital examinations.

Physiological Integrity

- Urge patients with pain, bleeding, discharge, masses, or changes in reproductive function to seek health care advice.
- Provide as much privacy as possible for patients undergoing examination or testing of the reproductive system.
- Recall that reproductive changes occur with aging, as described in Chart 72-1.
- Selected laboratory tests used for diagnosing reproductive health problems are found in Chart 72-4.
- Teach women to report manifestations of infection to their health care provider after endoscopic procedures and biopsies of the breast, cervix, and endometrium.
- Instruct men to report manifestations of infection to their health care provider after a transrectal biopsy of the prostate.

Care of Patients with Breast Disorders

Mary Justice

LEARNING OUTCOMES

Safe and Effective Care Environment

1. Identify community resources for patients with breast cancer.

Health Promotion and Maintenance

2. Describe the three-pronged approach to early detection of breast masses: mammography, clinical breast examination (CBE), and breast self-awareness.
3. Teach a woman who chooses breast self-examination (BSE) as an option to use correct technique.
4. Explain the options available to a person at high genetic risk for breast cancer.
5. Evaluate patient risk factors for breast cancer.

Psychosocial Integrity

6. Explain the psychosocial aspects related to having breast cancer and undergoing treatments for breast cancer.
7. Discuss sexuality issues with the patient having breast surgery.

8. Describe body image changes that can result from breast cancer surgery.

Physiological Integrity

9. Compare assessment findings associated with benign breast lesions with those of malignant breast lesions.
10. Explain the difference between breast reduction and breast augmentation.
11. Discuss treatment options for breast cancer.
12. Develop a postoperative collaborative plan of care for a patient with breast cancer.
13. Describe the role of radiation and drug therapy in the care of patients with breast cancer.
14. Identify the role of complementary and alternative therapies in breast cancer management.
15. Explain what options are available to a woman considering breast reconstruction.

Breast disorders may be benign or cancerous. Western society places a great emphasis on the breast as part of feminine beauty. Any threat to the breast has a significant effect on a woman's self-image and *sexuality*. She may feel unattractive to her partner and worry that their relationship will be negatively affected. She may be embarrassed at how she looks after treatment and refuse to look at herself. Members of the health care team need to be very supportive and acknowledge these feelings and concerns about the woman's perceived

inability to meet her need for *sexuality*. When caring for patients with breast problems, provide privacy and protect their dignity.

BENIGN BREAST DISORDERS

Most breast lumps are benign. Because the incidence of breast disease is related to age, breast disorders are described below in an age-related order (Table 73-1).

TABLE 73-1	**TYPICAL PRESENTATION OF BENIGN BREAST DISORDERS**	
BREAST DISORDER	**DESCRIPTION**	**INCIDENCE**
Fibroadenoma	Most common benign lesion; solid mass of connective tissue that is unattached to the surrounding tissue	During teenage years into the 30s (most commonly)
Fibrocystic breast condition	*First stage:* Characterized by premenstrual bilateral fullness and tenderness *Second stage:* Presence of bilateral multi-centric nodules *Third stage:* Presence of microscopic and macroscopic cysts	Late teens and 20s
Ductal ectasia	Hard, irregular mass or masses with nipple discharge, enlarged axillary nodes, redness, and edema; difficult to distinguish from cancer	Women approaching menopause
Intraductal papilloma	Mass in duct that results in nipple discharge; mass is usually not palpable	Women 40 to 55 yr of age

FIBROADENOMA

Fibroadenomas are the most common benign tumor in women during the reproductive years. However, they also may occur in a few postmenopausal women. A fibroadenoma is a mass of connective tissue that is unattached to the surrounding breast tissue and is usually discovered by the woman herself or during mammography. Although the immediate fear is that of breast cancer, the risk for it occurring within a fibroadenoma is very small. On clinical examination, the tumors are oval, freely mobile, and rubbery. Their size varies from smaller than 1 cm (0.4 inch) in diameter to as large as 15 cm (6 inches) in diameter.

Fibroadenomas may occur anywhere in the breast. The health care provider may request a breast ultrasound examination or may perform a needle aspiration to establish whether the lump is cystic (fluid-filled) or solid. If the lesion is solid, ambulatory care excision using local anesthesia is sometimes the treatment of choice.

FIBROCYSTIC BREAST CONDITION

Pathophysiology

Fibrocystic changes of the breast include a range of changes involving the lobules, ducts, and stromal tissues of the breast. Because these changes affect at least half of women over the life span, they are referred to as fibrocystic breast condition (FBC) rather than fibrocystic disease. This condition most often occurs in premenopausal women between 20 and 50 years of age and is thought to be caused by an imbalance in the normal estrogen-to-progesterone ratio. Typical symptoms include breast pain and tender lumps or areas of thickening in the breasts. The lumps are rubbery, ill defined, and commonly found in the upper outer quadrant of the breast (Lee, 2009).

The two main features of FBC are fibrosis and cysts. Areas of fibrosis are made up of fibrous connective tissue and are firm or hard. Cysts are spaces filled with fluid lined by breast glandular cells. Microcysts are small, nonpalpable cysts inside the breast glands. Macrocysts occur when fluid continues to build up. They often enlarge in response to monthly hormonal changes, stretching the surrounding breast tissue, and become painful. Symptoms usually resolve after menstruation and then recur before the next menstrual period in a cyclic fashion. Breast ultrasound is used to confirm the presence of a cyst. Fine needle aspiration is used to drain the cyst fluid and reduce pressure and pain. Fluid may return, and more aspirations may be necessary.

Postmenopausal women taking hormone replacement therapy (HRT) may develop FBC or experience worsening of symptoms. Having cysts or fibrosis does not increase a woman's chance of developing breast cancer. However, if a lump is very firm or has other features raising the concern about cancer, mammography is indicated. A needle biopsy or a surgical biopsy may be needed to make sure cancer is not present. Biopsy may be indicated in these situations:

- No fluid is aspirated.
- The mammogram shows suspicious findings.
- A mass remains palpable after aspiration.
- The aspirated fluid reveals cancer cells.

Symptoms often resolve after menopause when estrogen decreases.

PATIENT-CENTERED COLLABORATIVE CARE

Management of FBC focuses on the symptoms of the condition. Suggest supportive measures such as the use of mild analgesics or limiting salt intake before menses to help decrease swelling. Wearing a supportive bra can reduce pain by decreasing tension on the ligaments, although some women find that not wearing a bra is more comfortable. Local application of ice or heat may provide temporary relief of pain.

If drug therapy is indicated, oral contraceptives may be prescribed to suppress oversecretion of estrogen, and progestins may be used to correct luteal insufficiency. Danazol (Danocrine, Cyclomen ♣) suppresses ovarian function and estrogen stimulation of breast tissue. However, because danazol does not cure FBC and because its side effects are undesirable, it is generally used only in patients with recurrent and severe FBC.

! NURSING SAFETY PRIORITY
Drug Alert

Explain to women the benefits and risks associated with drug therapy for FBC, such as stroke, liver disease, and increased intracranial pressure. Teach them to seek medical attention immediately if any signs or symptoms of these complications occur.

Treatment for FBC may also include the use of vitamins C, E, and B complex. Diuretics may be prescribed to decrease premenstrual breast engorgement. Reduction of dietary fat and caffeine has been suggested, although the role of caffeine and fat in FBC is unclear.

Encourage the patient to continue prescribed drug therapy, and monitor the effectiveness of these interventions. Teach the patient to become familiar with the normal feel and texture of her breasts so she is aware of any changes.

DUCTAL ECTASIA

Ductal ectasia is a benign breast problem that is usually seen in women approaching menopause. It occurs when a breast duct dilates and its walls thicken, causing the duct to become blocked. The ducts in the subareolar area are most often affected. These ducts become distended and filled with cellular debris, which activates an inflammatory response. Two manifestations result from these changes:

- A mass develops that feels hard, has irregular borders, and may be tender.
- A greenish brown nipple discharge, enlarged axillary nodes, and redness and edema over the site of the mass are noted.

Ductal ectasia does not affect a woman's breast cancer risk. However, if a mass is present, it may be difficult to distinguish it from breast cancer. Because the risk for breast cancer is increased among women in the menopause age-group, accurate diagnosis is vital. A microscopic examination of the nipple discharge is performed to detect any atypical or malignant cells, and the affected area is excised. Nursing care is directed at reducing the anxiety associated with the threat of breast cancer and at supporting the woman through the diagnostic and treatment procedures. Ductal ectasia may improve without treatment. Warm compresses and antibiotics may be helpful. If symptoms do not improve, the abnormal duct may be surgically removed.

INTRADUCTAL PAPILLOMA

Intraductal papilloma occurs most often in women 40 to 55 years of age. A benign process in the epithelial lining of the duct forms a papilloma (pedunculated outgrowth of tissue). As it grows, trauma and erosion within the duct result in a bloody or serous nipple discharge. A mass is rarely palpable.

Diagnosis is aimed first at ruling out breast cancer. Microscopic examination of the nipple discharge and surgical excision of the mass and ductal area are usually indicated.

ISSUES OF LARGE-BREASTED WOMEN

Although Western society emphasizes large breasts as a positive attribute, women with excessive breast tissue often have health problems and discomfort. For instance, a woman with large breasts may have difficulty finding clothes that fit well and in which she feels attractive. The breast size may be out of proportion to the rest of the body, which adds to the problem of finding clothes that fit. Larger bras are expensive and may need to be specially ordered. The woman may have large dents in the shoulders from bra straps. In addition, many large-breasted women develop fungal infections under the breasts, especially in hot weather, because it is difficult to keep this area dry and exposed to air.

Backaches from the added weight are also common. If well-fitting bras do not help and obesity is not part of the problem, the only alternative for this condition may be breast reduction surgery. The surgeon removes excess breast tissue and then repositions the nipple and remaining skin flaps to produce the best cosmetic effect. This operation is a major surgical procedure and is called a reduction mammoplasty.

The decision to have the procedure is usually made after years of living with the discomfort of excessive breast size. Listen to the woman verbalize her feelings, and reinforce information as appropriate. The nursing care after surgery is similar to that for the woman having reconstructive surgery. (See discussion of Breast Reconstruction, p. 1603, in the Surgical Management section.)

ISSUES OF SMALL-BREASTED WOMEN

Some women choose to have breast augmentation surgery to increase or improve the size, shape, or symmetry of their breasts. Most health insurers do not pay for this procedure. Most surgeries involve the implantation of saline-filled or silicon prostheses. Some are constructed from the women's own tissue in much the same way as for reconstruction after mastectomy. *Saline* implants are filled with sterile saline and can be filled with the amount needed to get the shape and firmness the woman wants. If the implant shell leaks, the saline will be safely absorbed by the body. *Silicone* implants are filled with an elastic gel, which can leak into the breast and will not be absorbed. The plastic surgeon reviews the advantages and disadvantages of each implant or natural procedure.

> **! NURSING SAFETY PRIORITY**
>
> ### *Action Alert*
>
> Before breast augmentation surgery, teach the patient to stop smoking (to promote healing), avoid aspirin and other NSAIDs, and avoid herbs that can cause bleeding during the procedure, such as garlic, *Ginkgo biloba*, and ginseng. Tell her that the incisions will be hidden as much as possible, either under the pectoral muscle or directly behind the breast tissue as a submammary placement. One or more wound drains will be inserted during surgery, and she will need to know how to care for those drains at home. Review possible postoperative complications, including infection and prosthesis leakage, which can cause severe pain and possible fever.

After surgery, the patient can be discharged to home the same day or the day after. Remind the family or significant other that someone should stay with her for at least 24 hours after surgery. The incisions may or may not have dressings depending on the surgeon and type of surgery.

> **! NURSING SAFETY PRIORITY**
>
> ### *Action Alert*
>
> Remind the patient after breast augmentation that for the first few days she should expect soreness in her chest and arms. Her breasts will feel tight and sensitive, and the skin over her breasts may feel warm or may itch. Teach the patient that she will have difficulty raising her arms over her head and should not lift, push, or pull anything until the surgeon permits. Teach her to also avoid strenuous activity or twisting above her waist. Remind the patient to walk every few hours to prevent deep vein thrombi. Tell her to expect some swelling of the breasts for 3 to 4 weeks after surgery.

An important issue for patients who have breast augmentation surgery is breast cancer surveillance. Breast

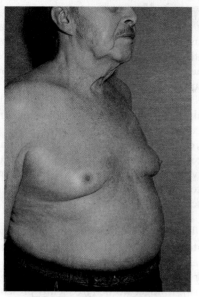

FIG. 73-1 Gynecomastia.

self-examination (BSE) and clinical breast examination (CBE) are easily performed after prostheses are placed. The prosthesis is placed behind the woman's normal breast tissue, actually pushing it forward. However, screening mammography may not be as sensitive because the amount of visualized breast tissue is decreased. Even though breast cancer detection may be impaired, survival rates for augmented women with breast cancer are not affected (Xie et al., 2010). Likewise, there is no association between breast implants and increased risk for breast cancer (American Cancer Society [ACS], 2010a). Teach women desiring cosmetic breast augmentation about the differences in breast cancer screening.

GYNECOMASTIA

Gynecomastia literally means "female breasts" and is a symptom rather than a disease. It is usually a benign condition of breast enlargement in *men* (Fig. 73-1). However, gynecomastia can be a result of a primary cancer such as lung or testicular cancer. The enlargement is usually bilateral but may be asymmetric in a few cases. The condition is caused by abnormal growth of the glandular tissue, including the mammary ducts and ductal tissue. In many instances, it is difficult to determine gynecomastia from breast enlargement related to excess adipose tissue. Other causes of gynecomastia include:

- Drugs, such as anti-androgen agents and corticosteroids
- Aging
- Obesity
- Underlying disease causing estrogen excess, such as malnutrition, liver disease, or hyperthyroidism
- Androgen-deficiency states, such as age, chronic kidney disease, or alcoholism

Although gynecomastia is not common, men with abnormal breast findings, especially a breast mass, should be carefully evaluated for breast cancer.

BREAST CANCER

Pathophysiology

Excluding skin cancers, breast cancer is the most commonly diagnosed cancer in women and is second only to lung cancer as a cause of female cancer deaths (ACS, 2010a). Therefore most references in this section are to women with breast cancer. Because of the high incidence of the disease, almost every woman knows of someone with the disease. Thus most women have strong reactions to the threat of breast cancer. These reactions greatly influence health habits, including breast self-examination (BSE) and the patient's readiness to seek care when a suspicious area is discovered. Nurses play a key role in early detection by educating women about screening guidelines, risk factors for breast cancer, and BSE. Men should also be taught about this disease.

Early detection is the key to effective treatment and survival. The 5-year relative survival rate is lower for women who are diagnosed with an advanced stage of breast cancer. The 5-year survival rate for localized breast cancer is 98%, whereas the rate drops to 84% when the cancer has spread to the regional lymph nodes (ACS, 2010a). Survival drops dramatically when it is metastatic (spread to distant sites).

Cancer of the breast begins as a single transformed cell that grows and multiplies in the epithelial cells lining one or more of the mammary ducts or lobules. It is a heterogeneous disease, having many forms with different clinical presentations and responses to therapy (Weigelt et al., 2010). Some breast cancers will present as a palpable lump in the breast, whereas others will show up only on a mammogram.

There are two broad categories of breast cancer: noninvasive and invasive. About 20% are *noninvasive*; the remaining 80% are invasive. As long as the cancer remains within the duct, it is noninvasive. The cancer is classified as *invasive* when it penetrates the tissue surrounding the duct. Most of these cancers arise from the intermediate ducts. Metastasis occurs when cancer cells leave the breast via the blood and lymph systems, which permits spread of these cells to distant sites. The most common sites of metastatic disease from breast cancer are bone, lungs, brain, and liver. The course of metastatic breast cancer is related to the site affected and to the function impaired. The processes involved in cancer development are described in Chapter 24.

Noninvasive Breast Cancers

Ductal carcinoma in situ (DCIS) is an early *noninvasive* form of breast cancer. In DCIS, cancer cells are located within the duct and have not invaded the surrounding fatty breast tissue. Because of mammography screening and earlier detection, the number of women diagnosed with DCIS has increased. If left untreated, it may spread into the breast tissue surrounding the ducts over a period of years (*invasive breast cancer*). Currently there is no way to determine which DCIS lesions will progress to invasive cancer and which ones will remain unchanged, but research is continuing in this area (Muggerud et al., 2010). *It is important to remember that although DCIS should be treated to prevent it from developing into an invasive breast cancer, it does not metastasize at this stage.*

Another type of noninvasive cancer is lobular carcinoma in situ (LCIS). This cancer type is rare and usually identified incidentally during biopsy for another problem. Having LCIS

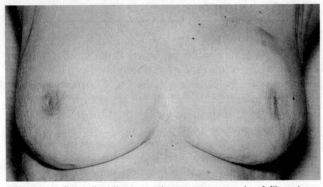

FIG. 73-2 Skin dimpling on a breast as a result of fibrosis or breast cancer.

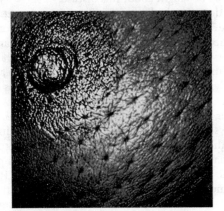

FIG. 73-3 Breast edema giving the skin an "orange peel" (peau d'orange) appearance.

increases one's risk for developing a separate breast cancer later. Traditionally, LCIS has been treated with close observation only. However, emerging evidence suggests that many LCIS lesions will progress to invasive cancer and should be treated with surgical excision (Cangiarella et al., 2008).

Invasive Breast Cancers

The most common type of invasive breast cancer is infiltrating ductal carcinoma. As the name implies, the disease originates in the mammary ducts and grows in the epithelial cells lining these ducts. Once invasive, the cancer grows into the tissue around it in an irregular pattern. If a lump is present, it is felt as an irregular, poorly defined mass. As the tumor continues to grow, fibrosis (replacement of normal cells with connective tissue and collagen) develops around the cancer. This fibrosis may cause shortening of Cooper's ligaments and the resulting typical skin dimpling that is seen with more advanced disease (Fig. 73-2). Another sign, sometimes indicating late-stage breast cancer, is an edematous thickening and pitting of breast skin called *peau d'orange* (orange peel skin) (Fig. 73-3).

A rare but highly aggressive form of invasive breast cancer is inflammatory breast cancer (IBC). Symptoms include swelling, skin redness, and pain in the breasts. IBC seldom presents as a palpable lump and may not show up on a mammogram. Because it is usually diagnosed at a later stage than other types of breast cancer, it is often harder to treat successfully (ACS, 2010b).

Breast Cancer in Men

Male breast cancer is rare, occurring in fewer than 1% of all cases. The average age of onset is 60 years. Most cases occur in those with a genetic mutation in either the *BRCA1* or the *BRCA2* gene. (See discussion of genetic risk below.)

Men usually present with a hard, painless, subareolar mass; gynecomastia may be present. Occasionally the man may have nipple discharge, retraction, erosion, or ulceration. Because *men* usually do not suspect breast cancer when they feel a lump, diagnosis frequently is delayed (Mattarella, 2010). The disease is often advanced when diagnosed; thus men have poorer survival than women (ACS, 2010a). Treatment of breast cancer in men is the same as in women at a similar stage of disease.

Breast Cancer in Young Women

Approximately 5% of breast cancer cases occur in women younger than 40 years (ACS, 2010a). Genetic predisposition is a stronger risk factor for younger women than older women (Pollán, 2010). Younger women frequently present with more aggressive forms of the disease. Screening tools are often less effective for this group because the breasts are denser. Women of childbearing age with breast cancer may be concerned about infertility after treatment. Distress about interrupted childbearing can have a major impact on their quality of life (Camp-Sorrell, 2009). Nurses should discuss issues of fertility with patients before chemotherapy. Younger women who experience abrupt menopause as a result of chemotherapy or ovarian suppression also report a greater effect on their sexuality than do older counterparts (McLachlan, 2009).

Etiology and Genetic Risk

There is no single known cause for breast cancer. *Being an older woman or man is the primary risk factor, although some people are at higher risk than others.* Several breast cancer risk factors have been identified; some are modifiable, whereas others are not (ACS, 2010a). Table 73-2 lists major risk factors for breast cancer development.

Although most breast cancers occur in women with no family history of the disease, having a first-degree relative (mother, sister, or daughter) with breast cancer increases the risk for the disease. Having more than one first-degree relative or a relative diagnosed at a younger age further increases one's risk (ACS, 2010a). Certain genetic factors can increase a woman's risk for both ovarian and breast cancer. Encourage women with a family history of breast or ovarian cancer to discuss this history with their physician.

Breast cancer is usually a *sporadic* (not having a definite genetic pattern) rather than an inherited or a familial disorder. Many personal and environmental interactions are

---

GENETIC/GENOMIC CONSIDERATIONS

Mutations in several genes, such as *BRCA1* and *BCRA2*, are related to hereditary breast cancer. People who have specific mutations in either one of these genes are at a high risk for developing breast cancer as well as ovarian cancer. However, only 5% to 10% of all breast cancers are hereditary. Only women with a strong family history and a reasonable suspicion that a mutation is present have genetic testing for *BRCA* mutations (ACS, 2010a). Encourage women to talk with a genetics counselor to carefully consider the benefits and potential harmful consequences of genetic testing before these tests are done.

TABLE 73-2	RISK FACTORS FOR BREAST CANCER
FACTORS	**COMMENTS**
High Increased Risk (Relative Risk >4.0)	
Female gender	Ninety-nine percent of all breast cancers occur in women.
Age >50 yr	Greatest risk for women is ages 50 to 69 years.
Genetic factors	Inherited mutations of *BRCA1* and/or *BRCA2* increase risk.
Family history	Two or more first-degree relatives with breast cancer at an early age increases risk.
History of a previous breast cancer	The risk for developing a cancer in the opposite breast is 5 times greater than for the average population at risk.
Breast density	Dense breasts contain more glandular and connective tissue, which increases the risk for developing breast cancer.
Moderate Increased Risk (Relative Risk 2.1-4.0)	
Family history	One first-degree relative with breast cancer moderately increases risk.
Biopsy-confirmed atypical hyperplasia	The overactive growth of cells increases risk.
Ionizing radiation	Women who received frequent low-level radiation exposure to the thorax had an increased risk, especially if the exposure occurred during periods of rapid breast formation.
High postmenopausal bone density	High estrogen levels over time both strengthen bone and increase breast cancer risk.
Low Increased Risk (Relative Risk 1.1-2.0)	

Reproductive history
  Nulliparity OR
  First child born after age 30
	Childless women have an increased risk, as do women who bear their first child near or after age 30.

Menstrual history (Early menstruation or late menopause, or both)	The risk for breast cancer rises as the interval between menarche and menopause increases. Women who undergo bilateral oophorectomy before age 35 have less risk for breast cancer than women who undergo natural menopause.
Oral contraceptives	There is a slight increase in breast cancer risk in women taking oral contraceptives.
Hormone replacement therapy (HRT)	Use of estrogen and progestin increases risk; routine use of hormone therapy for osteoporosis and heart disease is no longer recommended.
Obesity	Postmenopausal obesity (especially increased abdominal fat), increased body mass, insulin resistance, and hyperglycemia have been reported to be associated with an increased risk for breast cancer.
Other Risk Factors	
Alcohol	Risk is dose-dependent; consumption of 3 to 14 drinks per week is associated with a slight increase in risk; risk increases with increased consumption.
High socioeconomic status	Breast cancer incidence is greater in women of higher education and socioeconomic background. This relationship is possibly related to lifestyle differences, such as age at first birth.
Jewish heritage	Women of Ashkenazi Jewish heritage have higher incidences of *BRCA1* and *BRCA2* genetic mutations.

Modified from American Cancer Society. (2010). *Breast cancer facts & figures 2009-2010*. Atlanta: Author.

related to its development. Known factors that increase risk include exposure to high-dose ionizing radiation to the thorax (especially before 20 years of age), early menarche (before 12 years of age), and late menopause (after 50 years of age). A history of previous breast cancer, nulliparity (no pregnancies), and first birth after 30 years of age also appear to increase risk.

Other causative risk factors not as well explained are nutrition and hormone replacement therapy (HRT). Alcohol is clearly linked to an increased risk for invasive breast cancer. Having an average of one or more alcoholic drinks a day increases the risk up to one and a half times (ACS, 2010a). Obesity also increases breast cancer risk, especially for women after menopause. Fat tissue becomes the major source of estrogen after the ovaries stop functioning. Having a greater amount of fat tissue increases hormonal influence on breast cancer development (ACS, 2010b). An increase in the risk for breast cancer has been shown in postmenopausal women receiving HRT after 5 or more years of use, with the combination of estrogen and progestin carrying the highest increased risk. However, the use HRT is not considered a major risk factor for breast cancer compared with other breast cancer risks (Bluming & Tavris, 2009). Encourage women seeking help for menopausal symptoms to discuss the benefits and risks of hormonal therapy with their health care provider.

Incidence/Prevalence

In 2010, the projected breast cancer incidence was more than 207,000 women in the United States. Of these, almost 40,000 women are likely to die of the disease (Jemal et al., 2010).

Health Promotion and Maintenance

The American Cancer Society (ACS) establishes evidence-based guidelines for breast cancer screening in women. Guidelines have not been recommended for screening men in the general population because breast cancer in men is so uncommon (ACS, 2010b). Encourage men with a strong family history or known genetic mutations to discuss screening with their health care provider.

🌐 CULTURAL AWARENESS

One of every 8 U.S. women will develop breast cancer by age 70. Euro-American women older than 40 years are at a greater risk than other racial/ethnic groups, but African-American women *younger than 40 years* have breast cancer more often than others in that age-group. African-American women have a higher death rate at any age when compared with other women with the disease (ACS, 2010a). This difference has been attributed to limited access to and lower utilization of services for early detection and treatment (ACS, 2010c). Research has also found differences in tumor characteristics in some African-American women (Cunningham et al., 2010). For example, *triple negative breast cancer* occurs more often in African-American and younger women. In this type of breast cancer, cells lack receptors for estrogen, progesterone, and the protein *HER2*. Triple negative breast cancer tends to be more aggressive than other types of breast cancer, and fewer effective treatments exist for it. Much research is ongoing to better understand this type of breast cancer.

For American Indian and Alaska Native women, 5-year survival rates for breast cancer are very poor (English et al., 2008). These women are less likely than non-Hispanic white women to have mammography screening (Wingo et al., 2008). Health promotion interventions to improve mammography rates should consider cultural customs, transportation, and social support.

Latino and Hispanic women have a lower incidence of breast cancer than Euro-American women but a higher death rate (ACS, 2010d).

Risk factors for Hispanic women are not as well understood as those for non-Hispanic whites, and more research is needed in this area (Hines et al., 2010). Whereas Asian women have better 5-year survival rates than Euro-American women, the rates for Native Hawaiian women are slightly poorer than Euro-American women (ACS, 2010a). Strategies that have increased breast cancer screening in the Native Hawaiian population include the use of lay educators and community cancer outreach programs (Aitaoto et al., 2009).

❓ NCLEX EXAMINATION CHALLENGE

Health Promotion and Maintenance

When teaching women about the risk for breast cancer, which risk factor does the nurse know is the most common for the development of the disease?
A. Having an aunt with breast cancer
B. Being an older adult
C. Being a Euro-American
D. Consuming a low-fat diet

The ACS recommendation for early detection by screening for breast masses is a screening mammogram for women ages 40 years and older and a clinical breast examination (CBE) by a health professional at least every 3 years for women 20 to 40 years old. Monthly breast self-examination (BSE) is less emphasized today than in the past several decades.

❗ NURSING SAFETY PRIORITY

Action Alert

Teach women that no single method for early detection of breast cancer is effective when used alone. The best approach for average-risk women is screening mammogram, clinical breast examination, and breast self-awareness.

Mammography

The use of mammography (x-ray of the breasts) screening for healthy, average-risk women has been a subject of recent controversy among various scientific and advocacy groups. In 2009, the U.S. Preventive Services Task Force (USPSTF)

recommended against routine screening mammography in average-risk women ages 40 to 49 years and older than 75 years, concluding there is only a small net benefit for women in these age-groups (USPSTF, 2009). Scientific evidence shows there are benefits as well as risks associated with mammography, and disagreement exists about the emphasis that should be placed on each one. However, the ACS and The American College of Obstetricians and Gynecologists (ACOG) continue to recommend that all women age 40 and older have a screening mammogram annually (ACOG, 2011). Nurses working with women must be able to educate women on the risks and benefits of breast screening techniques so that they can make informed decisions about the screening methods best suited to their individual situations (Association of Women's Health, Obstetric, and Neonatal Nursing [AWHONN], 2010).

Women with known genetic mutations or other high risk factors for breast cancer should have screening with magnetic resonance imaging (MRI) in addition to annual mammography (ACS, 2010b). Encourage women with moderate risk factors to discuss with their health care provider the benefits and limitations of adding MRI screening to their annual mammograms. MRI screening is not recommended for women with low breast cancer risk factors.

Breast Self-Awareness/Self-Examination

Nurses working with women should teach them the importance of becoming familiar with the appearance and feel of their breasts. Any changes detected by the woman should be reported to her health care provider. Teach a woman that lumps are not necessarily abnormal. For premenopausal women, lumps can come and go with the menstrual cycle. Most lumps that are detected and tested are not cancerous.

Some women may want to practice regular breast self-examination (BSE) as a method for breast self-awareness. Evidence shows that monthly BSE is no more beneficial than women simply being aware of what is normal for their own breasts and women are just as likely to find a lump by chance (ACS, 2010b). However, BSE should be presented as an option to women beginning in their early 20s. In addition to breast self-awareness, emphasis should be placed on mammography and clinical breast examination for early detection of breast cancer. The combined approach is better than any single test (ACS, 2010a). A woman who chooses to perform BSE should be taught the correct technique and have it reviewed by a health care professional during her clinical breast examination.

Teach patients how to perform BSE if they choose. The examination technique is similar for women and men. Use teaching models of normal and abnormal breasts when teaching BSE. Discuss the proper timing for BSE. Instruct premenopausal women to examine their breasts 1 week after the menstrual period. At this time, hormonal influence on breast tissue is decreased, so fluid retention and tenderness are reduced. Teach women whose breast tissue is no longer influenced by hormonal fluctuations, such as after a total hysterectomy or menopause, to pick a day each month to do BSE, such as the first day of the month.

Ensure that the setting in which you demonstrate BSE is private and comfortable. Ask the woman to undress from the waist up, and provide a gown and sheet. Teach the woman to stand in front of a mirror to inspect the breast for abnormalities. She should raise her arms above her head and press her hands on her hips to emphasize any changes in the shape of the breasts. Palpation should be performed in a lying position and while bathing or showering. Before teaching breast palpation, ask the woman to demonstrate her own method. If she is unsure or has not performed BSE before, slowly lead her through the examination while explaining the rationale for the technique and answering questions. Demonstrate the correct technique of examining the breasts with the arm overhead instead of having the arm by her side. Showing the difference in the two positions, especially in large-breasted women, reveals the advantage of using the correct method, which spreads the tissue over the chest wall for more effective palpation (Fig. 73-4).

It is also helpful to point out different findings at this time, especially those that the woman might perceive as abnormal. Placing the woman's hand directly on the involved area and showing her precisely what is normal for her can build self-confidence. Teach her that nodular breast tissue may normally feel lumpy, which may be interpreted as widespread cancer. Indicate the *inframammary ridge,* the area of the breast where the skin folds under the breast. This thickened area may be perceived as a lump instead of a normal finding. In thin or small-breasted women, the ribs may be mistaken for masses. Demonstrate how to follow the rib to the sternum to be sure that what she is feeling is bone and not breast tissue.

Any one of three palpation methods can be used to examine the breast tissue (Fig. 73-5). Teach the importance of covering all tissue during palpation. Demonstrate the proper amount of pressure needed to palpate the breast tissue and the correct position of the hands. The finger pads, which are more sensitive than the fingertips, are used when palpating the breasts. Teach the woman to press firmly enough to detect the underlying tissue.

Clinical Breast Examination

Clinical breast examination (CBE) is typically performed by advanced practice nurses and other health care providers. However, nurses in general practice who are skilled in the technique can also perform the procedure. It is recommended that the CBE be part of a periodic health assessment, at least every 3 years for women in their 20s and 30s and every year for asymptomatic women at least 40 years of age (ACS, 2010a). Provide a private and comfortable setting, protect the patient's dignity, and allow time for discussion.

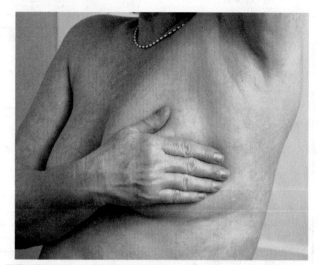

FIG. 73-4 A woman performing breast self-examination (BSE).

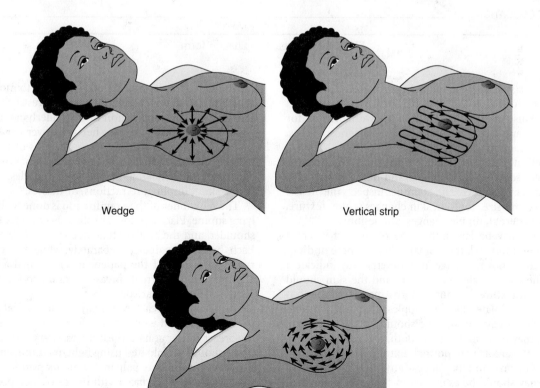

Wedge

Vertical strip

Circular

FIG. 73-5 Breast palpation techniques.

PATIENT'S NAME _____ Gender _____ Ethnicity/Race _____ Age _____

Weight _____ Ideal Weight _____ Marital Status _____

HISTORY   Yes   No   Comments

    Family history of breast cancer   _____   _____   _____
    Personal history of breast cancer   _____   _____   _____
    Previous mammograms   _____   _____   _____
    Previous biopsy (findings)   _____   _____   _____
    Nipple discharge   _____   _____   _____
    Hormone use (specify)   _____   _____   _____
    BSE Practice   _____   _____   _____
    High-fat diet   _____   _____   _____
    ETOH/smoking   _____   _____   _____
    Current medications (list)   _____   _____   _____
    Age at menses _____ Age at menopause _____
    Number of pregnancies _____

COMMENTS _____
_____

PHYSICAL FINDINGS

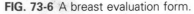

Mammogram Results _____
Ultrasound Results _____
Other Imaging Tests _____
Biopsy/Cytology Results _____
BSE Return Demonstration _____
Plan _____
_____
PATIENT EDUCATION _____

FIG. 73-6 A breast evaluation form.

Taking a breast history is vital. Results may be recorded on a breast evaluation form, which is a part of the medical record (Fig. 73-6). This record helps establish the woman's risk for breast disease and the need for follow-up diagnostic tests, such as mammograms, and teaching.

The physical assessment begins with inspection. The woman undresses from the waist up and first sits or stands with her hands by her sides. The examiner inspects the breasts for symmetry and size, contour, skin changes (color, texture, and venous patterns), nipple changes, and lesions.

One breast may be larger than the other, and inverted nipples are common. Ask the woman whether these findings are normal for her. Any change in symmetry may indicate a problem. The contour should be even, and the skin should have a smooth texture. Venous patterns may be visible but should be similar bilaterally. The nipples and areolae should be equal or nearly equal in size and should be a similar color. The nipples may be wrinkled or smooth, and Montgomery's tubercles on the areolae are normal. Extra nipples, although rare, are also normal and may appear anywhere on the chest. If present, they should be examined in the same manner as the normal nipples.

While the arms are by the side and relaxed, palpate the axillae (underarms) and the area above and below the clavicle for enlarged lymph nodes. If it is necessary to move the arms away from the body, the woman should rest her arm on the examiner's to prevent flexion of the underlying muscles. The woman is then asked to raise her arms over her head, which exposes the sides and underneath portions of the breast for inspection. Finally, she is asked to place her hands on her hips and press, thus flexing the pectoral muscles. This action shows skin dimpling, retractions, or masses.

The remainder of the examination is done with the patient lying supine. Place a pillow or rolled sheet under the patient's shoulder, and the arm on that side is raised above the head. Each breast is palpated separately while the other breast remains covered. If the patient has identified a problem in one breast, the "normal" breast is examined first to establish a baseline for comparison.

For a clinical breast examination, the vertical strip, three-pressured method is the most effective technique for detecting breast cancer at its earliest stages. Every inch of the breast tissue should be palpated using light, medium, and then deep pressure. If a mass is palpated, note its position by viewing the breast as a clock face (with the 12 o'clock position being toward the woman's head) and noting the "area of the clock" where the mass is located. Palpate the tail of Spence, which extends from the upper outer quadrant of the breast into the axilla. The supraclavicular lymph nodes are palpated for the presence of any enlarged nodes by hooking the fingers over the clavicle.

Finally, the nipple is gently compressed to detect the presence of a discharge. If a discharge is produced, note the "area of the clock" where the breast was compressed when the discharge was released. If there is a history of discharge, the woman may be able to express the discharge more successfully than the examiner can and should be asked to do so.

Discovery of a suspicious lesion or discharge during the examination requires referral to a health care provider who specializes in caring for breast disorders. Follow-up usually involves mammography and possibly ultrasound. If there is a dominant mass or high genetic risk, the woman should be referred for biopsy even if the mammogram is negative.

CONSIDERATIONS FOR OLDER ADULTS

As women age, the breast tissue becomes flattened and elongated and is suspended loosely from the chest wall. On palpation, the breast tissue of the older woman has a finer, more granular feel than the lobular feel in a younger woman. The inframammary ridge may be more prominent as a result of atrophy of the breast tissue. Breast examination in older adults may be easier because of tissue atrophy and relaxation of the suspensory ligaments.

Women in nursing homes and other chronic care facilities often do not have clinical breast examinations and may not be deliberately aware of the normal appearance and feel of their breasts. Teach the importance of breast self-awareness and reporting any breast changes the woman may notice. Teach BSE as an option for older women who are comfortable with and able to perform this method. Collaborate with the health care provider to ensure that residents have clinical breast examinations.

Options for High-Risk Women

Women with a personal history of breast cancer are at risk for developing a recurrence or a new breast cancer. Those with known *BRCA1* and *BRCA2* genetic mutations, strong family history, or other high risk factors are also considered high-risk. Women in this category usually practice *close surveillance* as a prevention option. It is referred to as "secondary prevention" and is used to detect cancer early in the initial stages. In addition to annual mammography and clinical breast examination, high-risk women are recommended to have an annual breast MRI screening (ACS, 2010a). Close surveillance may begin as early as age 30, but evidence is limited regarding the best age at which to start screening. Encourage high-risk women to discuss their personal preferences for close surveillance with their health care providers.

Options currently available for reducing a woman's breast cancer risk are prophylactic mastectomy (preventive surgical removal of one or both breasts), prophylactic oophorectomy (removal of the ovaries), and anti-estrogen chemopreventive drugs. Although each option significantly reduces the risk for breast cancer, no option completely eliminates it. Each option has its own risks and potentially serious complications.

Even though a woman may decide to have a prophylactic mastectomy, there is a small risk that breast cancer will develop in residual breast glandular tissue because no mastectomy reliably removes all mammary tissue. Women must also understand that breast reconstruction after a prophylactic mastectomy is very different from breast augmentation. It

is a more complex surgical procedure with a greater potential for complications.

Women undergoing oophorectomy will likely experience menopausal symptoms, and they will still have some estrogen stored in body fat tissue. Antiestrogen drugs reduce breast cancer recurrence but carry other risks such as blood clots and endometrial cancer. Encourage women to carefully consider the benefits and risks of breast cancer–risk-reducing options and discuss them with their health care provider.

PATIENT-CENTERED COLLABORATIVE CARE

■ ASSESSMENT

History

Often the history is taken after a mass has been discovered but before a diagnosis has been made for a woman or man with breast cancer. For some patients, the history may be obtained at the time they are seen for treatment of an identified cancer. The interview should focus on three major areas: risk factors, the breast mass, and health maintenance practices.

Record age, gender, marital status, weight, and height. Marital status and identifying the patient's primary support person provide information about who should be included in the patient's care, teaching, and support.

🌐 CULTURAL AWARENESS

Remember that some cultures do not allow the man to be part of a woman's care or only women are allowed to care for her (e.g., Arab Muslim women). Other cultures are male-predominant, and all decisions about female care are made by the man (e.g., Nigerian women). Chapter 4 describes additional general cultural considerations related to health care.

Ask specific information on personal and family histories of breast cancer. In addition to increasing the woman's own risk, these factors also affect any sisters' or daughters' risk and should be part of later counseling.

Ask about the woman's gynecologic and obstetric history, including:

- Age at menarche
- Age at menopause
- Symptoms of menopause
- Age at first child's birth
- Number of children/pregnancies

Prolonged hormonal stimulation (e.g., early menses, late menopause) increases a woman's risk, as do birth of the first child after 30 years of age and nulliparity (having no children).

A history of the breast mass or lump reveals not only the course of the disease but also information related to health care–seeking practices and health-promoting behaviors. Ask the patient about how, when, and by whom the mass was discovered and the time between discovery and seeking care. If the patient found the mass, ask how it was discovered. The answer to this question reveals the need for discussion and teaching about health promotion practices, regardless of whether the mass proves to be cancerous. If there was a delay between discovery and seeing the health care provider, ask

Assessing a Breast Mass

- Identify the location of the mass by using the "face of the clock" method.
- Describe the shape, size, and consistency of the mass.
- Assess whether the mass is fixed or movable.
- Note any skin changes around the mass, such as dimpling (peau d'orange), increased vascularity, nipple retraction, and ulceration.
- Assess the adjacent lymph nodes, both axillary and supraclavicular nodes.
- Ask patients if they experience pain or soreness in the area around the mass.

what caused the delay. These questions are linked to the psychosocial assessment but also reveal the length of time that the tumor has been present. Ask what procedures have been performed to diagnose the problem. Also, ask patients if they have noticed any other changes in their body within the past year. This information can help determine whether there has been obvious cancer spread. Ask especially about the presence of joint or bone pain.

Ask about the use of alcohol intake, because this is a factor that may increase breast cancer risk. Ask what prescribed and over-the-counter (OTC) drugs are used, specifically, hormonal supplements such as estrogen and natural or herbal substances that stimulate hormones. Estrogen can be taken orally, intravaginally, or via a transdermal patch. Document the type and form of hormones (birth control pills or patches, supplements) and length of use.

Physical Assessment/Clinical Manifestations

Document in the medical record any abnormal findings from the clinical breast examination. Describe specific information about a breast mass (Chart 73-1) such as location, using the "face of the clock" method; shape; size; consistency; and whether the mass is mobile or fixed to the surrounding tissue. Note any skin change, such as peau d'orange (dimpling, orange peel appearance), redness and warmth, nipple retraction, or ulceration, which can indicate advanced disease. Document the location of any enlargements of axillary and supraclavicular lymph nodes. Evaluate the presence of pain or soreness in the affected breast.

Psychosocial Assessment

A breast cancer diagnosis is usually an unanticipated event in the life of a woman who feels physically well. It initiates a sudden and distressing transition into a potentially life-threatening illness. Feelings of fear, shock, and disbelief are predominant as a woman learns about her disease and faces numerous treatment decisions. As a result, the period between diagnosis and treatment is one of the most demanding and stressful times for women with breast cancer (Lally, 2010). Use psychosocial interventions and appropriate therapeutic communication skills to assist women to cope effectively during this time.

Assess the patient's need for information. Some people may not be ready for a lot of information at first. Most want to know how advanced the disease is, the likelihood of cure, treatment options and side effects, how treatment will affect their life and self-image, how family or partners will be affected, and what is required for home self-management. A previous experience with cancer, especially with other people who had breast cancer, influences the reactions to the disease. Ask patients and family members whether they have known anyone with breast cancer, and explore their feelings about the disease. Provide current information about the stage of the disease and treatment options. Determine if a referral to a breast cancer support group would be helpful. Talking with someone who has been through the experience is particularly helpful in dealing with the emotional aspects of the disease.

Also assess the patient for problems related to *sexuality*. Sexual dysfunction affects up to 90% of women treated for breast cancer, although it is an issue seldom discussed between patients and health care providers (Dizon, 2009). Lack of libido (sexual desire) related to hormonal changes, psychological distress, and severe anxiety are commonly experienced by women with breast cancer. If the patient does not discuss sexual concerns voluntarily, ask about the frequency of and satisfaction with sexual relations with her partner. Use resources that provide education about alternative expressions of intimacy and a focus on pleasure rather than performance. Refer the patient and her partner to counseling if appropriate.

Laboratory Assessment

The diagnosis of breast cancer relies on pathologic examination of tissue from the breast mass. After the diagnosis of cancer is established, laboratory tests, including pathologic study of the lymph nodes, help detect possible metastases. Elevated liver enzyme levels indicate possible liver metastases, and increased serum calcium and alkaline phosphatase levels suggest bone metastases.

Imaging Assessment

Mammography is a sensitive screening tool for breast cancer. The uniqueness of this test results from its ability to reveal preclinical lesions (masses too small to be palpated manually). Traditional film mammography is increasingly being replaced by *digital mammography* in most Western countries (Skaane, 2009). *Digital mammography* has the advantage of being able to read, file, and transmit mammograms electronically. Studies have shown a slightly greater benefit from digital mammography in women who have dense breasts, such as those younger than 50 years. Patient preparation and the procedure for mammography are discussed in Chapter 72.

Ultrasonography of the breast is an additional diagnostic tool used to clarify findings on mammography. If the mammogram reveals a lesion, ultrasonography is helpful in differentiating a fluid-filled cyst from a solid mass. Mammography screening combined with ultrasound is also more effective for detecting cancers in women with dense breasts (Nothacker et al., 2009).

Magnetic resonance imaging (MRI) may be used to better examine suspicious areas found by a mammogram or for women with dense breasts. It can help determine the actual size of the cancer and look for any other cancers in the breast (ACS, 2010b). Some facilities may offer other types of imaging tests such as *breast-specific gamma imaging (BSGI) and positron emission mammography (PEM)*. These tests require the patient to be injected with a small amount of tracing agent that concentrates in the tumor area if present. The agent emits x-rays that the imaging system can detect. In some cases, these tests detect cancers not seen with traditional imaging.

If the patient has an invasive breast cancer, other imaging tests may be done to rule out metastases. A chest x-ray is done to screen for lung metastases. Bone, liver, and brain scans and computed tomography (CT) scans of the chest and abdomen can reveal distant metastases.

Other Diagnostic Assessment

Whereas imaging techniques serve as tools for screening and more precise visualization of potential breast cancers, *breast biopsy (pathologic examination of the breast tissue) is the only definitive way to diagnose breast cancer.* Breast tissue is obtained by one of several types of biopsies (see Chapter 72). Tissue samples are analyzed by a pathologist to determine the presence of breast cancer. If breast cancer is identified, it is classified according to the size and type of breast cancer, the histologic grade, and the type of receptors on the cells. These characteristics are used to guide treatment. For example, a small, noninvasive breast cancer may be treated only with lumpectomy and radiation, whereas a larger, aggressive tumor (one with a high histologic grade) may be treated with a mastectomy and chemotherapy, followed by radiation. Cancer cells that contain estrogen receptors (*ER positive*) or progesterone receptors (*PR positive)* have a better prognosis and usually respond to hormonal therapy. If the type of breast cancer is *HER2,* or one in which the *neu* gene product is overexpressed, it may be treated successfully with trastuzumab (Herceptin), which is a breast cancer *targeted therapy* for this specific type.

Most women, even those with very small tumors, receive some sort of treatment in addition to surgery for breast cancer. Research has focused on ways to predict clinical outcomes so that low-risk women may avoid unnecessary treatments. Gene expression profiling systems, such as Oncotype DX and MammaPrint, have been developed to help predict clinical outcomes by analyzing genes in breast cancer tissue. Some clinicians use this information in addition to the pathologic analysis for guiding treatment decisions. However, appropriate treatment recommendations are often made without using these tests (Sotiriou & Pusztai, 2009). More research is underway to develop new systems for predicting outcomes that focus on molecular subgroups in breast cancer.

ANALYSIS

The priority problems for breast cancer include:
1. Ineffective Coping related to unanticipated breast cancer diagnosis
2. Potential for metastasis of cancer to other parts of the body

PLANNING AND IMPLEMENTATION

Developing Coping Strategies

Planning: Expected Outcomes. The patient with breast cancer is expected to report the use of methods to help increase coping ability and reduce anxiety. The patient will maintain relationships and participate as an active partner in management of her disease.

Interventions. The anxiety and uncertainty for the patient with breast cancer begin the moment a lump is discovered or when a mammogram reveals an abnormality. These feelings may be related to past experiences and personal associations with the disease. Assess the patient's perceptions of his or her own situation. Allow the patient to ventilate these feelings even if a diagnosis has not been established.

If the mass has been diagnosed as cancer, many people feel a partial sense of relief to be dealing with a known entity. A feeling of shock or disbelief usually occurs. It is difficult to accept a diagnosis of cancer when one feels basically well. Patients and their families or significant others deal in individual ways with the mix of feelings. Flexibility is the key to nursing care. Adjust your approach to care as the patient's emotional state changes. Those who have an interval between the diagnosis and treatment, during which they actively participate in the choice of treatment, cope more effectively after surgery, no matter which treatment is chosen.

An integral part of the plan to meet these emotional needs is the use of outside resources. Health care providers working with breast cancer may know other patients willing to make a preoperative visit. For example, the patient who is worried in particular about the side effects of radiation therapy may benefit more from talking to someone who has undergone radiation than from talking to the nurse or health care provider. Be sure to assess his or her preference.

Assess the patient's need for knowledge. Some may want to read and discuss any available information. Provide accurate information, and clarify any misinformation the patient may have received by the media, on the Internet, or from family and friends. The American Cancer Society (www.cancer.org) and Breastcancer.org (www.breastcancer.org) are two Internet sources that provide evidence-based information in language a lay person can understand.

> ### ! NURSING SAFETY PRIORITY
> **Action Alert**
>
> Women are exposed to many misconceptions and much misinformation about breast cancer through various media. Clarify misconceptions and provide current information regarding risk factors, screening recommendations, and treatment for breast cancer.

Decreasing the Risk for Metastasis

Planning: Expected Outcomes. The patient with breast cancer is expected to remain free of metastases or recurrence of disease, if possible. If cancer recurs, the patient will experience optimal health outcomes, including potential palliation and end-of-life care.

Interventions. There are many surgical and nonsurgical options for breast cancer treatment. Because of the various options, the patient with breast cancer often faces difficult decisions. Although patients are living longer with metastatic disease, the 5-year survival rate remains low. Newer therapeutic regimens are needed to improve outcomes for these patients (Liu et al., 2010). Once cancer is diagnosed, the extent and location of metastases determine the overall therapeutic strategy. The emphasis of breast cancer treatment is on preventing or stopping the spread of tumor cells that leads to distant metastasis. Treatment is tailored specifically to each patient, taking into account other health problems and the patient's ability to tolerate a particular therapy.

Nonsurgical Management. For patients with breast cancer at a stage for which surgery is the main treatment, follow-up with adjuvant (in addition to surgery) radiation, chemotherapy, hormone therapy, or targeted therapy is commonly prescribed. For those who cannot have surgery or whose cancer is too advanced, these therapies are used to promote comfort (palliation). These options are discussed in the Adjuvant Therapy section on p. 1605.

Complementary and Alternative Therapies. Women with breast cancer often cope with distressing symptoms related to the disease itself or the side effects of chemotherapy, radiation, and hormonal therapy. Common symptoms associated with these therapies include pain, nausea, hot flashes, anxiety, depression, and fatigue. Physical and emotional symptoms associated with breast cancer may be eased with the use of complementary and alternative medicine (CAM). Up to 80% of women use some form of CAM during breast cancer treatment (Wyatt et al., 2010). The most frequently used types of CAM are biologically based therapies such as vitamins, special cancer diets, and herbal therapy. Prayer is also widely used. Other types of CAM are mind-body or body-based such as guided imagery and massage. Encourage women to seek a practitioner with a certification or license for the specific type of CAM therapy. In some states, a certification or license is required for acupuncture, chiropractic therapy, massage, and shiatsu. Some types of CAM can be self-taught or done alone after a few sessions of instruction. Table 73-3 lists complementary therapies for specific symptoms associated with breast cancer and its treatments.

There is no proven benefit to using CAM alone as a cure for breast cancer. Therefore *nurses must ensure that patient choices can be safely integrated with conventional treatment for breast cancer* (Wyatt et al., 2010). Encourage patients who are interested in trying CAM therapies to check with their health care provider before using them. Refer patients to reliable resources for information about CAM. The website *breast-cancer.org* provides accurate information about complementary therapies and the extent to which they have been researched in breast cancer patients. Cost may be a factor in decision making, since not all insurances provide coverage for CAMs. Teach the patient that all ingested CAM agents potentially risk interaction with conventional drugs.

Surgical Management. The most common types of breast surgeries are shown in Fig. 73-7. Although controversy exists concerning the best treatment for breast cancer, experts agree that the mass itself should be removed to reduce the risk for local recurrence. A large tumor is sometimes treated with chemotherapy, called neoadjuvant therapy, to shrink the tumor before it is surgically removed. An advantage of this therapy is that cancers can be removed by lumpectomy rather than mastectomy.

Axillary lymph nodes are analyzed for the presence of cancer and staging purposes. Axillary lymph node dissection (ALND) is usually done when there are palpable axillary lymph nodes or when cancer is suspected to be at a later stage. Sentinel lymph node biopsy (SLNB) is a much less invasive approach now preferred by most surgeons for analyzing lymph nodes in early-stage breast cancers with low to moderate risk for lymph node involvement. In this method, the sentinel lymph node is identified during breast surgery by injecting the breast with radioisotope and/or dye that travels via lymphatic pathways to the sentinel lymph node. The nodes that take up the dye (or give off a certain level of radiation picked up by a handheld counter) are removed and examined for the presence of cancer cells. It is believed that

TABLE 73-3	COMPLEMENTARY AND ALTERNATIVE MEDICINE (CAM) FOR BREAST CANCER	
SYMPTOM	**CAM**
Physical	
Pain	Acupuncture, chiropractic therapy, hypnosis, massage, music, reiki, shiatsu
Nausea/vomiting	Acupuncture, aromatherapy, ginger, hypnosis, progressive muscle relaxation, shiatsu
Fatigue	Acupuncture, massage, meditation, reiki, tai chi, yoga
Hot flashes	Acupuncture, black cohosh, flaxseed
Muscle tension	Aromatherapy, massage, shiatsu
Emotional	
Anxiety/stress/fear	Aromatherapy, guided imagery, hypnosis, journaling, massage, meditation, music therapy, progressive muscle relaxation, prayer, support groups, tai chi, yoga
Depression	Aromatherapy, yoga, journaling, progressive muscle relaxation

if cancer cells have traveled through the lymph channels, the cells will lodge in the sentinel nodes. Travel beyond these nodes to higher-level nodes may occur as a secondary event. Therefore the absence of cancer cells in the sentinel nodes is an indicator that no other nodes in the regional area are involved.

Preoperative Care. Care of the patient facing surgery for breast cancer focuses on psychological preparation and preoperative teaching. Priority nursing interventions are directed toward relieving anxiety and providing information to increase patient knowledge. *Include the spouse or partner, who may be experiencing similar stress and confusion, in the health teaching, unless the patient's culture does not permit this approach.*

Review the type of procedure planned. Use open-ended questions (e.g., "What type of surgery are you having? Can

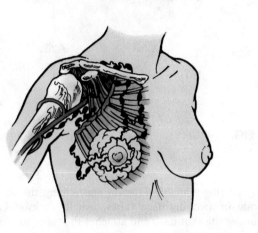

NORMAL ANATOMY

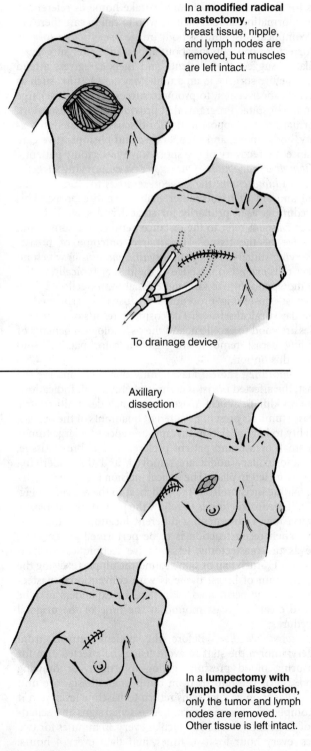

In a **modified radical mastectomy**, breast tissue, nipple, and lymph nodes are removed, but muscles are left intact.

To drainage device

Axillary dissection

In a **simple mastectomy**, breast tissue and (usually) nipple are removed, but lymph nodes are left intact.

In a **lumpectomy with lymph node dissection**, only the tumor and lymph nodes are removed. Other tissue is left intact.

FIG. 73-7 Surgical management of breast cancer.

you explain what will happen?") to assess the current level of knowledge. Provide postoperative information, including:

- The need for a drainage tube
- The location of the incision
- Mobility restrictions
- The length of the hospital stay (if any)
- The possibility of adjuvant therapy
- General preoperative and postoperative information needed by any surgical patient (see Chapters 16 and 18)

Supplement teaching with written or electronic (DVD) materials for the patient and family to take home as references. This information should include who to call in case there are any complications. Address body image issues before surgery to correct misconceptions about appearance after surgery. If available, suggest that patients and their caregivers attend classes before surgery in an ambulatory care setting, such as a breast cancer center, to promote successful early discharge from the hospital. Programs that provide emotional support, information, and opportunities for discussion related to sexuality, body image, and preoperative and postoperative care enhance the recovery of the short-stay mastectomy patient.

Operative Procedures. During breast-conserving surgery, such as a *lumpectomy,* the surgeon removes the tumor and a small amount of tissue rather than the entire breast. This procedure is used primarily for stage I and stage II breast cancer. *Margins* refer to the distance between the tumor and the edge of the tissue. The desired outcome of breast-conserving surgery is to obtain *negative margins* in which no cancer cells extend to the edge of the tissue. Typically, radiation therapy follows to kill any residual tumor cells.

Breast-conserving procedures are usually performed in same-day surgical settings. The cosmetic results of these surgeries are good to excellent, and the psychological benefits of avoiding breast removal are significant for patients who choose this option.

The modified radical mastectomy does *not* conserve the breast; the affected breast is completely removed. Indications for a modified radical mastectomy include multi-centric disease (tumor is present in different quadrants of the breast), inability to have radiation therapy, presence of a large tumor in a small breast, and patient preference. The breast tissue, skin, and axillary nodes are removed, and the underlying muscles are left in place. The typical incision is a 4- to 5-inch–long elliptic incision from the midchest to the axilla (see Fig. 73-7). If reconstruction is to follow the procedure, the plastic surgeon may recommend a different location for the incision. When reconstruction is to be performed at the same time as the mastectomy, less-invasive techniques, such as incising a 1½-inch flap of skin around the nipple (excising the same amount of breast tissue as with conventional mastectomy), may be performed. Skin flaps or expanders may be used to create a breast mound at the time of the original procedure.

Postoperative Care. Before the patient returns from surgery, inform the staff to avoid using the affected arm for measuring blood pressure, giving injections, or drawing blood. He or she returns from the postanesthesia care unit (PACU) as soon as vital signs return to baseline levels and if no complications have occurred. Assess vital signs on a schedule of decreasing frequency, such as every 30 minutes for two times, every hour for two times, and then every 4 hours. During these checks, assess the dressing for bleeding.

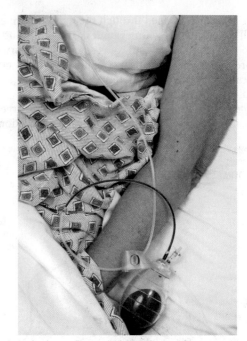

FIG. 73-8 Jackson-Pratt drain in place after a mastectomy.

During a *modified radical mastectomy,* the surgeon places one or two drainage tubes, usually Jackson-Pratt drains, under the skin flaps and attaches the tubes to a small collection chamber (Fig. 73-8). Gentle suction is exerted, and fluid that would accumulate under the flaps and delay healing is collected. Various drains are available, but all allow the drainage to be seen and measured. When taking vital signs, monitor for the amount and color of drainage. Add this information to the intake and output record. Patients undergoing a *lumpectomy* may also have drainage tubes (usually Jackson-Pratt drains) placed if the lump is large or if axillary node dissection is performed.

> **! NURSING SAFETY PRIORITY**
>
> ***Action Alert***
>
> After breast surgery, observe the surgical wound for signs of swelling and infection throughout recovery. With short hospital stays, drainage tubes are usually removed about 1 to 3 weeks after hospital discharge when the patient returns for an office visit. The drainage amount should be less than 25 mL in a 24-hour period. Inform the patient that tube removal may be uncomfortable although these tubes lie just under the skin. Provide or suggest analgesia before they are removed.

Assess the patient's position to ensure that the drainage tubes or collection device is not pulled or kinked. The patient should have the head of the bed up at least 30 degrees with the affected arm (the arm on the same side as the axillary dissection) elevated on a pillow while awake. Keeping the affected arm elevated promotes lymphatic fluid return after removal of lymph nodes and channels. Provide other basic comfort measures, such as repositioning and analgesics as prescribed on a regular basis until pain ceases. Patient-controlled analgesia may be used for some patients for a short time depending on the type of surgery that was performed.

CHART 73-2   PATIENT AND FAMILY EDUCATION: PREPARING FOR SELF-MANAGEMENT

Postmastectomy Exercises

Hand Wall Climbing
- Face the wall, and put the palms of your hands flat against the wall at shoulder level.
- Flex your fingers so that your hands slowly "walk" up the wall.
- Stop when your arms are fully extended.
- Slowly "walk" your hands back down the wall until they return to shoulder level.

Pulley Exercise
- Drape a 6-foot-long rope over a shower curtain rod or over the top of a door. If you use a door for this exercise, have someone put a nail or hook at the top of the door so that the rope does not slip off.
- Grab the ends of the rope, one in each hand, and extend your arms out to your sides until they are straight.
- Keeping your arms straight, pull down with your left arm to raise your right arm as high as you can.
- Pull down with your right arm to raise your left arm as high as you can.

Rope Turning
- Tie a rope to the knob of a closed door.
- Hold the other end of the rope and step back from the door until your arm is almost straight out in front of you.
- Swing the rope in a circle. Start with small circles, and gradually increase to larger circles as you become more flexible.

! NURSING SAFETY PRIORITY

Action Alert

Assess the incision and flap of the post-mastectomy patient for signs of bleeding, infection, and poor tissue perfusion. Document and report abnormal findings to the surgeon immediately!

The hospital stay after breast surgery is short, often same-day or just overnight, and recovery is usually not complicated. Because some managed care plans will not authorize an overnight stay in the hospital after a mastectomy, several states have enacted legislation mandating inpatient benefits. The patient who chooses an early discharge should have a home care visit within 24 hours of the discharge.

Ambulation and a regular diet are resumed by the day after surgery. While the patient is walking, the arm on the affected side may need to be supported at first. Gradually, the arm should be allowed to hang straight by the side. Instruct the patient to avoid the hunched-back position with the arm flexed because of the risk for elbow contracture. Beginning exercises that do not stress the incision can usually be started on the first day after surgery. These exercises include squeezing the affected hand around a soft, round object (a ball or rolled washcloth) and flexion/extension of the elbow. The progression to more strenuous exercises depends on the subsequent procedures planned (e.g., reconstruction) and the surgeon's prescription.

As soon as the patient is ambulatory and surgical pain is under control, he or she is discharged to home. Common instructions for exercises after mastectomy are listed in Chart 73-2.

? NCLEX EXAMINATION CHALLENGE

Physiological Integrity

The nurse is assigned to care for a client immediately after breast-conserving surgery for cancer. What is the priority for care of the client at this time?
A. Teach the client to sleep in the prone position each night.
B. Empty wound drains and record the output amount.
C. Remind the client how to perform breast self-examination.
D. Monitor the incision and flap for adequate tissue perfusion.

Breast Reconstruction. Breast reconstruction after or during mastectomy for women is common with few complications. Patients consult with the plastic surgeon to discuss the type of reconstruction, timing of the procedure, and technique desired. Many women prefer reconstruction immediately after mastectomy using their own tissue (autogenous reconstruction). Breast reconstruction at the time of mastectomy, both autogenous and prosthetic, may lessen the psychological strain associated with undergoing a mastectomy.

The surgeon should offer the option of breast reconstruction before surgery is performed. If the woman does not choose immediate reconstructive surgery, a temporary prosthesis can be used. Refer the patient to the American Cancer Society's Reach to Recovery program (www.cancer.org). In this program, a volunteer who has had breast cancer surgery visits the woman at home, offering information on breast forms, clothing, coping with breast cancer, and possible reconstructive options. For this intervention to be as helpful as possible, the volunteer should be about the same age as the patient and have experienced the same surgical procedure.

Evaluate the woman's level of satisfaction with her prosthesis several weeks after surgery. Assess her attitude by asking about future plans for restoring appearance. Although reconstruction is not appropriate for some women and others may not be interested in it, the surgeon should discuss the indications and contraindications, advantages and disadvantages, and typical recovery. If immediate reconstruction is chosen, the surgeon should be aware of this before surgery so that plans can be coordinated with those of the plastic surgeon.

Several procedures are available for restoring the appearance of the breast (Table 73-4). Reconstruction may begin during the original operative procedure or later in one to several stages. Common types of breast reconstruction are:
- Breast expanders (saline or gel)
- Autologous reconstruction using the patient's own skin, fat, and muscle

Breast expanders are the most common method of breast reconstruction used today in the United States. A tissue expander is a balloon-like device with a resealable metal port that is placed under the pectoralis muscle. A small amount of normal saline is injected intraoperatively into the expander to partially inflate it. The patient then receives additional weekly saline injections for about 6 to 8 weeks until the expander is fully inflated. When full expansion is achieved, the tissue expander is then exchanged for a permanent implant during outpatient surgery. The permanent implant is filled with either saline or silicone gel. Despite earlier claims that silicone gel caused autoimmune diseases like lupus and arthritis, silicone implants have been safely used in the majority of women who choose this type of breast implant.

TABLE 73-4	EXAMPLES OF BREAST RECONSTRUCTION PROCEDURES		
PROCEDURE	**DESCRIPTION**	**PROCEDURE**	**DESCRIPTION**
Implantation	An implant matching the size of the other breast is placed under the muscle on the operative side to create a breast mound.	Myocutaneous flaps	A flap of skin, fat, and muscle is transferred from the donor site to the operative area. The flap contains an appropriate amount of fat to match the other breast and is similar in appearance to breast tissue. A blood supply is established by reanastomosis of vessels from the operative area to those with the flap when possible. A new nipple may be created with tissue from areas such as the labia or upper, inner thigh. Nipples can also be created by tattooing.
Tissue expansion	A tissue expander is placed under the muscle and gradually expanded with saline to stretch the overlying skin and create a pocket. After several weeks, the tissue expander is exchanged for an implant.		

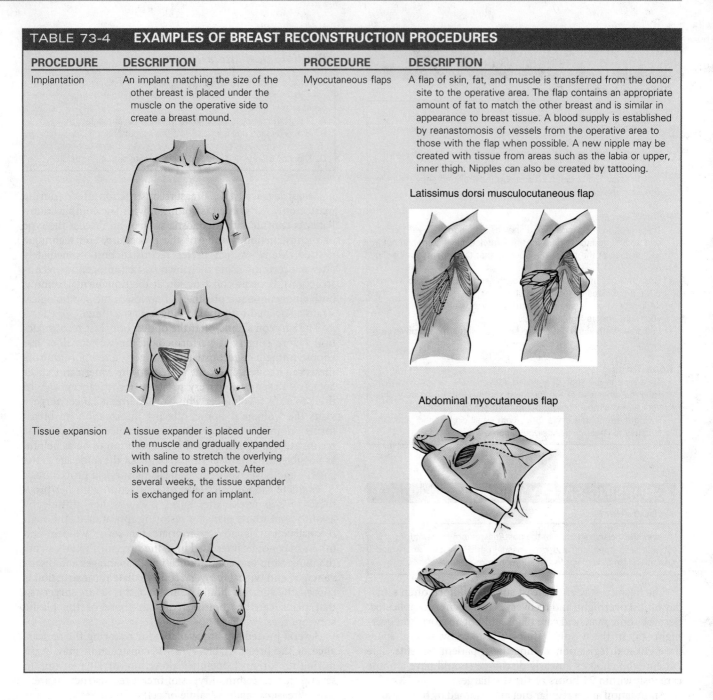

Latissimus dorsi musculocutaneous flap

Abdominal myocutaneous flap

Autologous reconstruction using the patient's own skin, fat, and muscle is advantageous because the donor site tissue is similar in consistency to the natural breast. Therefore the results more closely resemble a real breast as compared with implant reconstruction. Flap donor sites include the latissimus dorsi flap (back muscle); transverse rectus abdominis myocutaneous flap, known as the *TRAM flap* (abdominal muscle); and the gluteal flap (buttock muscle). Reconstruction of the nipple-areola complex is the last stage in the reconstruction of the breast. If necessary, a new nipple may be created with other body tissue, such as from the labia, abdomen, or inner thigh.

Women who have had a mastectomy and breast reconstruction in one breast should have close surveillance breast cancer screening in the contralateral (opposite) breast, including imaging with mammography or mammography and MRI. Mammography and MRI are not recommended to be routinely done in reconstructed breasts because most local recurrences of breast cancer in the residual tissue are palpable during clinical breast examination (Zakhireh et al., 2010). Nursing care of the woman who has undergone breast reconstruction is outlined in Chart 73-3.

Adjuvant Therapy. The decision to follow the original surgical procedure with adjuvant therapy (in addition to surgery) for breast cancer is based on:
- The stage of the disease
- The patient's age and menopausal status
- Patient preferences

- Pathologic examination
- Hormone receptor status
- Presence of a known genetic predisposition

Adjuvant therapy for breast cancer consists of radiation therapy and drug therapy. The purpose of radiation therapy is to reduce the risk for local recurrence of breast cancer. Drug therapy includes chemotherapy, targeted therapy, and/or hormonal therapy. These drugs destroy breast cancer cells that may be present anywhere in the body. They are typically delivered after surgery for breast cancer, although neoadjuvant chemotherapy may be given to reduce the size of a tumor before surgery. Hormonal therapy is a chemoprevention option for high-risk women with a personal history of breast cancer.

Radiation Therapy. Radiation therapy is administered after breast-conserving surgery to kill breast cancer cells that may remain near the site of the original tumor. This therapy can be delivered to the whole breast or to only part of the breast. Until recently, the traditional method has been whole-breast irradiation delivered by external beam radiation over a period of 5 to 6 weeks. More recently, partial breast irradiation (PBI) has become an option for women with early-stage breast cancer. The use of brachytherapy (radioactive implants) has been increasing steadily, accounting for approximately 10% of radiation therapy administered to breast cancer patients (Smith et al., 2009). The advantage of this type of radiation is that it is delivered over a much shorter time interval, eliminating the need for daily trips for treatment. However, few long-term studies exist showing the effectiveness of brachytherapy compared with traditional radiation therapy. The

types of methods available for delivering *partial-breast irradiation* include:

- Interstitial brachytherapy, in which several catheters loaded with a radioactive source are inserted at the lumpectomy cavity and surrounding margin, is given over a period of 4 to 5 days.
- Balloon brachytherapy, also known as *MammoSite*, involves the use of a single balloon-tipped catheter that is surgically placed near the tumor bed. The catheter is loaded with a radiation source and inflated to conform to the total cavity. Ten total treatments are given, with at least 6 hours between each treatment.
- Intraoperative radiation therapy is the most accelerated form of partial breast irradiation. It utilizes a high single dose of radiation delivered during the lumpectomy surgery.

Nursing care for the patient undergoing radiation therapy includes patient education and side effect management. Skin changes are a major side effect during this therapy (see Chapter 24). If brachytherapy is planned, instruct patients about the procedure. Assure them that they will be radioactive only while the radiation source is dwelling inside the breast tissue.

! NURSING SAFETY PRIORITY
Action Alert

Teach women undergoing brachytherapy for breast cancer that radiation is contained in the temporary implant. The risk for others to be exposed to radiation is very small. Body fluids and items contacted by patients with brachytherapy are not radioactive. However, during the time the radiation is delivered, it is recommended they limit visitors, including pregnant women and children.

Chemotherapy. Chemotherapy for breast cancer is delivered systemically. Its purpose is to kill breast cancer cells that may have left the original tumor and moved to more distant sites. Chemotherapy is the standard of care for women with node-positive cancer or with a tumor larger than 1 cm (Maughan et al., 2010). As more scientific evidence emerges about the biology of tumors, it is hoped that the need for chemotherapy may be more specifically determined. Chemotherapy may be given before surgery to reduce the size of the tumor. Table 73-5 lists common agents used in breast cancer and their mechanism of action. They are usually delivered in four to six courses of treatment. Combination regimens of chemotherapy have been demonstrated to be more effective than single-agent treatments. A common chemotherapy regimen for breast cancer treatment is Cytoxan, Adriamycin, and 5-FU (CAF), but several other types and combinations may be given. In early-stage breast cancer, chemotherapy regimens lower the risk for breast cancer recurrence. In advanced breast cancer, chemotherapy regimens reduce cancer size in many patients. Regimens that contain anthracyclines and taxanes have a small benefit over other chemotherapies for some types of breast cancer (Maughan et al., 2010).

Most chemotherapy for breast cancer is delivered via the central IV route such as an implantable venous access device (port-a-cath). Nurses must be very proficient in the preparation and administration of chemotherapy drugs and knowledgeable about various venous access devices. They must also be able to manage the distressing symptoms associated with side effects of chemotherapy. Chapter 24 discusses general nursing management of alopecia, nausea and vomiting, mucositis, and bone marrow suppression. Fatigue and sleep disturbance are often major concerns as side effects of chemotherapy.

! NURSING SAFETY PRIORITY

Action Alert

Teach patients undergoing chemotherapy with anthracyclines such as doxorubicin (Adriamycin) to be aware of cardiotoxic effects. Instruct them to report excessive fatigue, shortness of breath, chronic cough, and edema to the health care provider.

TABLE 73-5   DRUG THERAPY FOR BREAST CANCER

CATEGORY	MECHANISM OF ACTION	AGENTS
Chemotherapy		
Anthracyclines	Inhibit DNA synthesis in susceptible cells	Doxorubicin (Adriamycin) (A) Epirubicin (Ellence) (E)
Taxanes	Inhibit microtubule network in rapidly dividing cells	Docetaxel (Taxotere) (D) Paclitaxel (Taxol) (P) Paclitaxel, protein-bound (Abraxane)
Alkylating agents	Interfere with the replication of susceptible cells	Cyclophosphamide (Cytoxan) (C)
Antimetabolites	Inhibit DNA synthesis and cellular replication in rapidly dividing cells	Methotrexate (Mexate) (M) Fluorouracil (5-FU) (F) Capecitabine (Xeloda)
Targeted Therapy	Selectively target critical steps in the processes required for tumor growth, viability, or invasion	Trastuzumab (Herceptin)
Hormonal Therapy		
LH-RH agonists	Block release of LH and FSH, thereby preventing ovarian production of estrogen	Goserelin (Zoladex) Leuprolide (Lupron)
Selective estrogen receptor modulators (SERMs)	Bind to estrogen receptors; have both agonist and antagonist properties (selectively block action of estrogen in the breast but not in other organs)	Tamoxifen (Nolvadex) Raloxifene (Evista)
Aromatase inhibitors	Prevent conversion of adrenal and ovarian androgens to estrogens by inhibiting the aromatase enzyme	Anastrozole (Arimidex) Letrozole (Femara) Exemestane (Aromasin)
Estrogen receptor down-regulators	Induce degradation of estrogen receptor	Fulvestrant (Faslodex)

FSH, Follicle-stimulating hormone; *LH,* luteinizing hormone; *LH-RH,* luteinizing hormone–releasing hormone.

Chemotherapy is unpleasant and expensive and can have life-threatening short-term and long-term side effects. Because more women are living longer with breast cancer, long-term effects are increasingly emerging. Although targeted therapy is effective with fewer side effects, some side effects are nevertheless life threatening. For example, cardiac toxicity is a risk associated with the use of Herceptin, particularly when it is combined with other chemotherapy. Chemotherapy and ovarian suppression can result in infertility, a devastating effect for women of childbearing age. Hormonal therapy can result in long-term ill effects from bone loss. Discuss patient concerns, provide accurate information, and assist him or her in decision making.

Targeted Therapy. Targeted cancer therapies are drugs that target specific characteristics of cancer cells, such as a protein, an enzyme, or the formation of new blood vessels. The advantage of targeted therapy over traditional chemotherapy is that targeted therapy does not harm normal, healthy cells and therefore it has fewer side effects. The best known targeted therapy for breast cancer is the monoclonal antibody *trastuzumab* (Herceptin). This drug targets the *HER2/neu* gene product in breast cancer cells. The combination of trastuzumab and anthracyclines increases the risk for cardiotoxicity and must be used with caution (Maughan et al., 2010).

Bevacizumab (Avastin) inhibits tumor growth by targeting the growth factor *VEGF* and stopping the formation of new blood vessels that are needed to nourish the tumor. It is a drug used in several types of cancer. However, a recent review of bevacizumab by a panel of the Food and Drug Administration (FDA) showed there was no significant improvement in life span for patients with metastatic breast cancer and recommended against the use of bevacizumab in metastatic breast cancer (Food and Drug Administration [FDA], 2010).

Hormonal Therapy. The purpose of hormonal therapy is to reduce the estrogen available to breast tumors to stop or prevent their growth. *Premenopausal* women whose main estrogen source is the ovaries may benefit from *LH-RH agonists* that inhibit estrogen synthesis. These drugs include leuprolide (Lupron) and goserelin (Zoladex), which suppress the hypothalamus from making luteinizing hormone–releasing hormone (LH-RH). When LH-RH is inhibited, the ovaries do not produce estrogen. Although the suppression of ovarian function decreases breast cancer risk, the drastic drop in estrogen causes significant menopausal symptoms. Therefore the decision to use these drugs is not made lightly.

Selective estrogen receptor modulators (SERMs), on the other hand, do not affect ovarian function. Rather, they block the effect of estrogen in women who have estrogen receptor (ER)–positive breast cancer. SERMs are also used as chemoprevention in women at high risk for breast cancer and in women with advanced breast cancer. Tamoxifen is recommended to be taken for 5 years to achieve the best benefit for risk reduction. Common side effects of SERMs include hot flashes and weight gain. Rare but serious side effects of these drugs include endometrial cancer and thromboembolic events.

Aromatase inhibitors (AIs) are used in *postmenopausal* women whose main source of estrogen is not the ovaries but, rather, body fat. AIs reduce estrogen levels by inhibiting the conversion of androgen to estrogen through the action of the enzyme *aromatase*. AIs are beneficial when given to post-menopausal women after 5 years of treatment with tamoxifen. A major side effect of the AIs, not seen with tamoxifen, is loss of bone density. Women taking AIs are candidates for bone-strengthening drugs and must be closely monitored for osteoporosis. Fulvestrant (Faslodex), a second-line hormonal therapy for postmenopausal women with advanced breast cancer, is used after other hormonal treatments have stopped working.

Stem Cell Transplantation. Autologous or allogeneic stem cell transplantation is an option for patients with a high risk for recurrence or who have advanced disease. Autologous bone marrow transplantation (taken from the patient's bone marrow), peripheral blood stem cell transplantation (taken from circulating blood), or allogeneic bone marrow transplantation (taken from a healthy donor's bone marrow or peripheral blood) is performed as a means of rescue therapy after very high doses of chemotherapy. The general care of the patient undergoing bone marrow or stem cell transplantation is discussed in Chapter 42.

? DECISION-MAKING CHALLENGE

Patient-Centered Care; Safety

A 39-year-old African-American woman who is an executive for a major technology business is diagnosed with breast cancer and scheduled for a lumpectomy and radiation therapy. She tells you that she regrets that her life has not allowed time for having children. She is currently single but has a male partner whom she has been dating for 3 years. After surgery, she tells the nurse that she plans on going back to work in a week or two but that she is very anxious about her future.

1. What evidence-based risk factors does this patient have?
2. What discharge instructions will you provide for her and why?
3. What will you teach the patient about radiation therapy to maintain her safety?
4. How might you help allay the patient's anxiety?

Community-Based Care
Home Care Management

In collaboration with the case manager, make the appropriate referrals for care after discharge. Preoperative teaching and arrangements for home care management and referrals (Reach to Recovery, social services, home care) can be started before surgery or other treatment.

The patient who has undergone breast surgery can be discharged to the home setting unless other physical disabilities exist. Some are discharged the day after surgery with Jackson-Pratt or other types of drains in place. Many patients are discharged to home on the day of surgery. Older adults should not be sent home without a family member or friend who can stay with them for 1 to 2 days. These patients may need some assistance at home with drain care, dressings, and ADLs because of pain and impaired range of motion of the affected arm. Summaries of continuing care instructions are given in Charts 73-4 and 73-5.

Teach patients that activities involving stretching or reaching for heavy objects should be avoided temporarily. This restriction can be discussed with a family member or significant other who can perform these tasks or place the objects within easy reach.

Teaching for Self-Management

The teaching plan for the patient after surgery includes:

- Measures to improve body image
- Information about interpersonal relationships and roles
- Exercises to regain full range of motion
- Measures to prevent infection of the incision
- Measures to avoid lymphedema
- Measures to avoid injury, infection, and swelling of the affected arm
- Care of the incision and drainage device

Teach incisional care to the patient, family, and/or other caregiver. The patient may wear a light dressing to prevent irritation. Explain that no lotions or ointments should be used on the area and that the use of deodorant under the affected arm should be avoided until healing is complete. Although swelling and redness of the scar itself are normal for the first few weeks, swelling, redness, increased heat, and tenderness of the

CHART 73-4 PATIENT AND FAMILY EDUCATION: PREPARING FOR SELF-MANAGEMENT

Recovery from Breast Cancer Surgery

- There may be a dry gauze dressing over the incision when you leave the hospital. You may change this dressing if it becomes soiled.
- A small, dry dressing will be around the site where a drain is placed. Often there is some leakage of fluid around the drain. Check the gauze dressing for drainage, and change it if it becomes soiled. Some leakage is normal, but if the dressing becomes soaked more than once a day, call your health care provider.
- You have been taught how to empty the reservoir from your drain and how to measure the volume of drainage. You should empty the drain twice a day and record the measurements.
- Drains are generally removed when drainage is less than 25 mL in 24 hours.
- Drains are often removed at the same time as the stitches or staples, generally 7 to 10 days (could be as long as 3 weeks if needed) after surgery.
- You may take sponge baths or tub baths, making certain that the area of the drain and incision stays dry. You may shower after the stitches, staples, and drains are removed.
- You can begin using your arm for normal activities, such as eating or combing your hair. Exercises involving the wrist, hand, and elbow, such as flexing your fingers, circular wrist motions, and touching your hand to your shoulder, are very good. You can usually resume more strenuous exercises after the drains have been removed.
- You can expect some discomfort or mild pain after surgery, but within 4 to 5 days, most women have no need for pain medication or require medication only at bedtime.
- Numbness in the area of the surgery and along the inner side of the arm from the armpit to the elbow occurs in almost all women. It is the injury to the nerves that causes sensation to the skin in those areas. Women have described sensations of heaviness, pain, tingling, burning, and "pins and needles." Neuropathic pain is sometimes relieved by gabapentin (Neurontin). These sensations change over the months and usually resolve by 1 year.
- Pamphlets on exercises, hand and arm care, and general facts about breast cancer are available from us or from a volunteer visitor. The American Cancer Society has volunteers who have had surgery similar to yours and are available to visit you.

CHART 73-5 **HOME CARE ASSESSMENT**

Patients Recovering from Breast Cancer Surgery

Assess cardiovascular, respiratory, and urinary status:
- Vital signs
- Lung sounds
- Urine output patterns

Assess for pain and effectiveness of analgesics.

Assess dressing and incision site:
- Excess drainage
- Manifestations of infection
- Wound healing
- Intact staples

Assess drain and site:
- Drainage around drain site and in drain
- Color and amount of drainage
- Manifestations of infection

Review patient's recordings of drainage.

Evaluate patient's ability to care for and empty drain.

Assess status of affected extremity:
- Range of motion
- Ability to perform exercise regimen
- Lymphedema

Assess nutritional status:
- Food and fluid intake
- Presence of nausea and vomiting
- Bowel sounds

Assess functional ability:
- Activities of daily living
- Mobility and ambulation

Assess home environment:
- Safety
- Structural barriers

Assess patient's compliance and knowledge of illness and treatment plan:
- Follow-up appointment with surgeon
- Manifestations to report to health care provider
- Hand and arm care guidelines
- Referral to Reach to Recovery

Assess patient and caregiver coping skills:
- Determine if patient and/or caregiver has looked at incision site.
- Assess their reaction to incision site.

surrounding area indicate infection and should be reported to the surgeon immediately. If a lymph node dissection was performed, instruct the patient to elevate the affected arm on a pillow for at least 30 minutes a day for the first 6 months. Ask the patient to have someone bring a loose-fitting, non-wire bra or camisole for her to try before discharge with a soft, cotton-filled or polyester fiber–filled form supplied by the hospital or by Reach to Recovery. The patient wears this form until the incision is completely healed and the health care provider approves the fitting of a more sophisticated prosthesis, usually 6 to 8 weeks after discharge. Encourage the patient to dress in loose-fitting street clothes at home, not pajamas, to further enhance a positive self-image.

Teach the patient to continue performing the exercises that began in the hospital. Active range-of-motion exercises should begin 1 week after surgery or when sutures and drains are removed. Emphasize that reaching and stretching exercises should continue only to the point of pain or pulling, never beyond that. ENCORE, a YWCA program, is appropriate for women as early as 3 weeks after surgery and includes exercise to music, exercise in water, and psychological support. Before discharge, the surgeon may prescribe precautions or

limitations specific to plans for future procedures, such as reconstruction.

Lymphedema, an abnormal accumulation of protein fluid in the subcutaneous tissue of the affected limb after a mastectomy, is a commonly overlooked topic in health teaching. Risk factors include injury or infection of the extremity, obesity, presence of extensive axillary disease, and radiation treatment. Once it develops, it can be very difficult to manage, and *lifelong measures must be taken to prevent it.* Nurses play a vital role in educating patients about this complication (Fu et al., 2008).

! **NURSING SAFETY PRIORITY**

Action Alert

Provide information needed to help the patient avoid infection and subsequent lymphedema of the affected arm after the mastectomy. Teach the importance of avoiding having blood pressure measurements taken on, having injections in, or having blood drawn from the arm on the side of the mastectomy. Instruct the patient to wear a mitt when using the oven, wear gloves when gardening, and treat cuts and scrapes appropriately. If lymphedema occurs, early intervention provides the best chance for control. The arm should be elevated when possible and special attention paid to the special precautions. A referral to a lymphedema specialist may be necessary for the patient to be fitted for a compression sleeve and/or glove, to be taught exercises and manual lymph drainage, and to discuss ways to modify daily activities to avoid worsening the problem. Management is directed toward measures that promote drainage of the affected arm. Teach patients, especially those who have had axillary lymph nodes removed, that measures to prevent lymphedema are lifelong and include avoiding trauma to the arm on the side of the mastectomy.

Psychosocial Preparation

Concerns about appearance after surgery are common and are often a threat to the patient's self-concept as a woman. Before breast surgery, the woman and her partner can benefit from an explanation of the expected postoperative appearance. After a modified radical mastectomy, the chest wall is fairly smooth and has a horizontal incision from the axilla to the midchest area. After breast-conserving surgery, scars vary according to the amount of breast tissue removed. Women are sometimes shown pictures of post-mastectomy reconstruction but are disappointed with their own results. Emphasize that scars will fade and edema will lessen with time. Scars may be red and raised at first, but these features lessen in the first few months. After surgery, encourage the woman to look at her incision when she is ready. Do not push her to accept this body image change immediately.

Much of one's body image is a reflection of how others respond. Therefore the response of the patient's family or partner to the surgery is crucial in determining the effect on self-concept. These people may also need the support of the nurse. They may have concerns about their ability to accept the changes and need to discuss these feelings with an objective listener. They may also need help with communicating their feelings, both negative and positive, with their loved one. Involving them in teaching may also help reinforce learning and increase retention.

Discuss sexual concerns before discharge. Most surgeons recommend avoiding sexual intercourse for 4 to 6 weeks. Patients may prefer to lay a pillow over the surgical site or to wear a bra, camisole, or T-shirt to prevent contact with the surgical site during intercourse. He or she may be embarrassed to discuss the topic of *sexuality*. Be sensitive to possible concerns, and approach the subject first.

For young women, issues related to childbearing may be a concern. Chemotherapy and radiation are considered serious teratogenic (birth defect–causing) agents. Advise sexually active patients receiving chemotherapy or radiotherapy to use birth control during therapy. The method and length of birth control should be discussed with the health care provider.

Health Care Resources

Resources available to the patient after discharge include personal support and community programs. After discharge, the spouse or partner may need help in planning support for home responsibilities. For example, a partner who may be assuming additional duties at home and work may feel stressed. Discussing the need for ongoing emotional support is also beneficial to both the patient and partner. Leaving the hospital and appearing normal do not end the anxiety and fear. Identifying a support person with whom the patient or couple can explore these feelings and discussing the need to ventilate feelings enhance personal and family recovery.

Numerous support and educational resources are available to those diagnosed with breast cancer. Nurses must provide accurate and current information to patients who may have obtained inaccurate information from various media. There are over two million breast cancer survivors in the United States, and many men and women are active in breast cancer support and advocacy organizations. National breast cancer organizations are accessible online, and many of them have local affiliates. Examples of such organizations are Susan G. Komen for the Cure, the National Breast Cancer Coalition, Y-Me, Sisters Network, Young Survival Coalition, and Pink Ribbon Girls. Also, local support groups can be accessed through the health care provider, the local hospital, wellness centers, home care agencies, or by word of mouth. The American Cancer Society (ACS) (www.cancer.org) is a good resource for information and support.

▌EVALUATION: OUTCOMES

Evaluate the care of the patient with breast cancer based on the identified priority patient problems. The expected outcomes include that he or she will:

- Be able to cope with the diagnosis by being knowledgeable, supported, and actively involved in decision making
- Remain free of metastasis

NURSING CONCEPT REVIEW

What might you NOTICE if a patient is experiencing impaired sexuality as a result of breast cancer or other disorder?

- Breast swelling or lump (with or without pain)
- Discharge from nipple(s)
- Skin dimpling or orange peel appearance
- Asymmetric breast tissue
- Very large or very small breasts
- Skin redness and warmth

What should you INTERPRET and how should you RESPOND to a patient having impaired sexuality as a result of breast cancer or other disorder?

Perform and interpret physical assessment, including:

- Take a thorough patient and family history.
- Examine each breast, comparing sides, and document.
- Assess pain, and document.
- Assess psychosocial reaction to the breast changes.

Respond by:

- Checking recent mammogram test or other imaging assessment results
- Acknowledging patient's concerns about body image and sexuality changes
- Asking the patient about resources for support that have been used in the past for coping with crisis
- Preparing the patient for testing and possible biopsy
- Listening to the patient's concerns in a nonjudgmental manner

On what should you REFLECT?

- Consider what health care resources (team members) the patient and family will need throughout disease management.
- Think about what other community resources the patient and family will need.
- Observe the patient's progress in adapting to body image changes.

GET READY FOR THE NCLEX® EXAMINATION!

KEY POINTS

Review these Key Points for each NCLEX Examination Client Needs Category.

Safe and Effective Care Environment

- In collaboration with the health care team, identify community resources for patients with breast cancer, including Reach to Recovery of the American Cancer Society.

Health Promotion and Maintenance

- Identify patients at high risk for breast cancer, especially women with family history of breast cancer; those who have had early menarche, late menopause, or first pregnancy after 30 years of age; or those who are nullipara.
- Reinforce options available to women who are high risk for breast cancer, including close surveillance and prophylactic surgery.
- Teach women to become self-aware of breasts and any breast changes; teach breast self-examination (BSE) to women who choose this method of breast self-awareness.
- Encourage women to have screening mammography according to recommended guidelines. Baseline screening should begin at 40 years of age and continue yearly. In high-risk women, screening should be started earlier.
- Encourage women to have clinical breast examination (CBE) according to recommended guidelines.

Psychosocial Integrity

- Assess patients' reactions to the diagnosis of breast cancer and the effect of breast cancer treatment on their body image and sexuality.
- Identify resources that facilitate their grief work and coping skills.
- Allow patients opportunities to express feelings of grief, fear, and anxiety.

- Teach women ways to minimize surgical area deformity and enhance body image, such as use of a breast prosthesis or the option of breast reconstruction.
- Address the reactions of family and significant others to the diagnosis of breast cancer; provide support and education.

Physiological Integrity

- Assess benign lumps as mobile and round or oval; assess possible malignant lumps as fixed and irregularly shaped, often in the upper outer breast quadrant.
- A breast reduction is an option for women with very large, heavy breasts to promote comfort.
- A breast augmentation is done for either small breasts or for reconstruction after breast removal.
- After breast cancer surgery, assess vital signs, dressings, drainage tubes, and amount of drainage.
- Notify the health care team that the arm of the surgical mastectomy side should not be used for blood pressures, blood drawing, or injections.
- Assess the return of arm and shoulder mobility after breast surgery and axillary dissection.
- Assess for the presence of lymphedema, and assist the patient to perform therapeutic measures to reduce lymphedema in the affected arm.
- Teach the patient measures to prevent lymphedema after axillary node dissection.
- Observe for and report other complications of breast cancer surgery or breast reconstruction, especially infection and inadequate vascular perfusion.
- After an axillary lymph node dissection, elevate the affected arm on a pillow.
- Radiation and drug therapy are used most often as adjuvant therapy after breast surgery but may be used before surgery to shrink the tumor.

Care of Patients with Gynecologic Problems

Donna D. Ignatavicius

LEARNING OUTCOMES

Safe and Effective Care Environment

1. Collaborate with members of the health care team when caring for patients with gynecologic cancers.

Health Promotion and Maintenance

2. Identify the risk factors for gynecologic cancers.
3. Provide health teaching on community resources for patients with gynecologic health problems.
4. Describe evidence-based health promotion and maintenance measures to help prevent or early-detect gynecologic cancers.

Psychosocial Integrity

5. Explain the psychosocial needs of patients with gynecologic health problems, including their effect on sexuality.
6. Discuss ways to help patients adapt to physical changes, including impaired sexuality, caused by gynecologic problems and their treatment.

Physiological Integrity

7. Compare the pathophysiology, manifestations, and treatments of common menstrual cycle disorders.
8. Describe the mechanisms of action, side effects, and nursing implications of drug therapy for endometriosis.
9. Develop a teaching plan for a patient with a vaginal inflammation or infection.
10. Discuss common assessment findings associated with menopause.
11. Prioritize care after surgery for the woman undergoing an anterior and/or posterior repair.
12. Develop a plan of care for a patient undergoing a hysterectomy.
13. Explain the purpose of radiation and chemotherapy for patients with gynecologic cancers.
14. Provide information about complementary and alternative therapies.
15. Develop a community-based plan of care for patients with gynecologic cancers.

The most common gynecologic manifestations are pain, vaginal discharge, and bleeding. Some patients also have urinary symptoms associated with their gynecologic problem. Women are often hesitant to seek medical attention for these problems because of fear of a life-threatening disease diagnosis or concern about privacy and dignity. Be sensitive to the woman's concerns and encourage discussion about menstrual or other reproductive problems. Teach women about their bodies, and help them recognize when professional help should be sought. Teach them how to make informed decisions about treatments. Assess the effects of gynecologic

disorders on *sexuality* in any setting. These health problems often impair sexual function and therefore can affect the woman's relationship with her partner. Remember that *sexuality* affects a woman's sense of being, self-esteem, and body image.

ENDOMETRIOSIS

Pathophysiology

Endometriosis is endometrial (inner uterine) tissue implantation *outside* the uterine cavity. The tissue typically appears

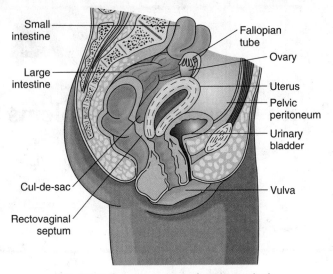

FIG. 74-1 Common sites of endometriosis.

on the ovaries and the cul-de-sac (posterior rectovaginal wall) and less commonly on other pelvic organs and structures (Fig. 74-1). A "chocolate" cyst is an area of endometriosis on an ovary. The disease affects millions of women in the United States and Canada.

Endometriosis responds to cyclic hormonal stimulation just as if it were in the uterus. Monthly cyclic bleeding occurs at the ectopic (out of place) site of implantation, which irritates and scars the surrounding tissue. Scarring can lead to adhesions, causing infertility (inability to become pregnant). Endometriosis progresses slowly and regresses during pregnancy and at menopause. Rarely does it become cancerous.

The cause of endometriosis is unknown. One theory is that the endometrial tissue migrates directly through the fallopian tubes during menses. The tissue then implants on pelvic structures or distant organs such as lungs or heart. The formation theory suggests that endometrial tissue develops outside the uterus as a birth defect. Other theories focus on immune, genetic, and environmental factors (e.g., exposure to dioxin, a toxic chemical). Many women with endometriosis have allergies and chemical sensitivities.

The disorder is most often found in women during their reproductive years, but it can affect women into their 80s. The prevalence among infertile women is higher than it is for women who are fertile. It is also common in those whose mothers had endometriosis.

PATIENT-CENTERED COLLABORATIVE CARE

ASSESSMENT

Collect a detailed history, including the woman's menstrual history, sexual history, and bleeding characteristics. *Pain is the most common symptom of endometriosis.* The pain usually peaks just before the menstrual flow. It is usually located in the lower abdomen, causing many women to feel a sense of rectal pressure. The degree of pain is not related to the extent of the endometriosis but to the site. Often, women with minimal disease have more severe pain than do women with extensive disease. Other manifestations include dyspareunia

(painful sexual intercourse), painful defecation, low backache, and infertility. GI disturbances such as nausea and diarrhea are also common. Always ask about current or past physical or sexual abuse.

A pelvic examination may reveal pelvic tenderness, tender nodules in the posterior vagina, and limited movement of the uterus. Psychosocial assessment may reveal anxiety because of uncertainty about the diagnosis. The woman may also have concerns about her self-concept if she is infertile but wants to become pregnant.

Diagnostic studies include tests to rule out pelvic inflammatory disease caused by chlamydia or gonorrhea. Serum cancer antigen *CA-125* helps screen for ovarian cancer but also may be positive in women with endometriosis. Transvaginal ultrasound is used to differentiate pelvic masses that might be mistaken for endometriosis.

INTERVENTIONS

Hormonal and surgical management may be used, depending on the symptoms, the extent of disease, and the woman's desire for childbearing. Collaborative care is aimed at:

- Reducing pain
- Restoring sexual function
- Alleviating anxiety related to the disease and the uncertainty of the diagnosis
- Educating the patient about the disease and its treatment
- Alleviating fear related to the possibility of laparoscopy or surgery
- Preventing self-esteem disturbance related to infertility

Nonsurgical Management

Several resources, such as the Endometriosis Association (www.endometriosisassn.org) and RESOLVE (an organization for infertile couples) (www.resolve.org), offer information on endometriosis that is helpful for patients and caregivers.

Disease management depends of the patient's symptoms, severity, and preference for treatment. Menstrual cycle control using oral contraceptives or progestins, such as oral medroxyprogesterone acetate (Provera, Medroxyhexal, Alti-MPA ✦ Novo-Medrone ✦) and norethindrone acetate (Aygestin, Norlutate ✦), may be prescribed. Injectable forms of progestins, such as medroxyprogesterone (Depo-Provera), may be more convenient because these drugs are taken every 2 weeks or monthly.

Continuous low-level heat using wearable heat packs may provide temporary pain relief. Relaxation techniques, yoga, massage, and biofeedback may decrease muscle tissue hypoxia and hypertonicity and relieve ischemia by increasing blood flow to the affected areas. Calcium and magnesium may also relieve muscle cramping for some patients.

Surgical Management

Surgical management of endometriosis for a woman who wants to remain fertile is the laparoscopic removal of endometrial implants and adhesions in a same-day surgical setting. Chapter 18 describes the general postoperative care for patients having surgery. The surgeon may use a laser to treat endometriosis by vaporizing adhesions and endometrial implants. Teach patients that temporary postoperative pain from carbon dioxide can occur in the shoulders and chest.

TABLE 74-1	RISK FACTORS FOR DYSFUNCTIONAL UTERINE BLEEDING
• Obesity	• Polycystic ovary disease
• Extreme weight loss or gain	• Long-term drug use
• Age older than 40 years	(e.g., oral contraceptives)
• High stress levels	• Excessive exercise

DYSFUNCTIONAL UTERINE BLEEDING

Pathophysiology

Dysfunctional uterine bleeding (DUB) is excessive and frequent bleeding (more than every 21 days). It is a diagnosis of exclusion, made after ruling out anatomic or systemic conditions such as drug therapy or disease. DUB occurs most often at the beginning or end of a woman's reproductive years—when ovulation is becoming established or when it is becoming irregular at or after menopause.

Normally the menstrual cycle is a series of delicately timed hormonal events regulated by hypothalamic, pituitary, ovarian, and uterine functions. Menses, the sloughing of the endometrial lining, is an expected result. DUB occurs when there is a hormonal imbalance. Generally, it happens when the ovaries fail to ovulate. This decreases progesterone production, which is needed to mature the uterine lining and prevent overgrowth. Without progesterone, prolonged estrogen stimulation causes the endometrium to grow past its hormonal support, causing disordered shedding of uterine lining. Most cases of DUB are classified into two types: anovulatory DUB (most common) and ovulatory DUB (Ayers & Montgomery, 2009). Common risk factors for DUB during the reproductive years are listed in Table 74-1.

PATIENT-CENTERED COLLABORATIVE CARE

ASSESSMENT

When interviewing a woman with DUB, take a complete menstrual history. Ask about illnesses, changes in weight or nutritional intake, exercise, drug ingestion, and whether she has pain.

Assess for symptoms of anemia or systemic disease, such as:

- Renal or hepatic disease
- Abnormal weight
- Signs of hormonal dysfunction, such as thyroid enlargement or male hair pattern
- Evidence of abdominal pain or masses

The health care provider inspects the external genitalia and does a bimanual pelvic examination, Papanicolaou test, and rectal examination to identify infections, lesions, or tenderness. Vaginal specimens are also tested for sexually transmitted diseases (STDs), such as that caused by chlamydia. Women at high risk for endometrial cancer should also have an endometrial biopsy. Risk factors are described later in this chapter.

A complete blood count determines if the patient is anemic. Depending on the patient's history and physical examination, thyroid-stimulating hormone and reproductive hormone levels may be evaluated.

Transvaginal ultrasound may reveal leiomyomas (fibroids) and measure an excessively thick endometrium. *Sonohysterography* uses vaginal ultrasound to visualize the uterus after 5 to 10 mL of sterile saline is infused through the cervix, thus outlining the inner uterine cavity.

INTERVENTIONS

Management of the patient often includes nonsurgical and surgical interventions. When nonsurgical treatment is not effective, surgery may be performed.

Nonsurgical Management

As with endometriosis, hormone manipulation is usually the treatment of choice for women with anovulatory DUB. The drugs used depend on the severity of bleeding and age of the patient. Progestin or combination hormone therapy (estrogen and progestin) is indicated when bleeding is heavy and acute. For nonemergent bleeding, contraceptives (oral or patch) provide the progestin (artificial progesterone) needed to stabilize the endometrial lining. Progestin-only pills (e.g., norethindrone [Aygestin, Norlutate ✦]) or long-acting progestins (e.g., injectable medroxyprogesterone acetate [Depo-Provera]) are preferable for women older than 35 years who smoke or are at risk for thrombophlebitis. Some cases are managed with injectable leuprolide (Lupron), a gonadotropin-releasing (GR) hormone analog, to reduce the follicle-stimulating and luteinizing hormone levels to cause amenorrhea. This drug has many potent side and adverse effects and is not used as frequently today.

Explain the desired effects and the side effects of these drugs, and evaluate the woman's knowledge of the effects, dosage, and schedule. Be sure to remind her to take the drug exactly as prescribed and to not skip a dose or run out of it. If bleeding worsens, teach the patient to call her health care provider immediately.

Surgical Management

Removal of the built-up uterine lining, called endometrial ablation, stops the blood flow to fibroids that are causing excessive bleeding. This is a safe alternative for women who do not respond to medical management. Other invasive options include uterine artery embolization, dilation and curettage, and hysterectomy. A hysterectomy is performed only after other treatments have failed. (Hysterectomy is discussed under Surgical Management on p. 1619 of the Uterine Leiomyoma section.)

VULVOVAGINITIS

Pathophysiology

Vaginal discharge and itching are two problems experienced by most women at some time in their lives. Women can suffer vaginal infections from both sexually and non–sexually transmitted sources. Gonorrhea, syphilis, chlamydia, and herpes simplex virus are sexually transmitted diseases (STDs) discussed in Chapter 76.

Vulvovaginitis is inflammation of the lower genital tract resulting from a disturbance of the balance of hormones and flora in the vagina and vulva. It may be characterized by itching, change in vaginal discharge, odor, or lesions. The most common causes include:

- Fungal (yeast) infections (*Candida albicans*)
- Bacterial vaginosis
- STDs (*Trichomonas vaginalis*)
- Postmenopausal vaginal atrophy
- Changes in the normal flora or pH (from douching)
- Chemical irritant or allergens (vaginal spray, fabric dyes, detergent) or foreign body (tampon)
- Drugs, especially antibiotics
- Immunosuppression from diabetes or human immune deficiency virus (HIV)

Primary infections that affect the vulva include *herpes genitalis* and *condylomata acuminata* (human papilloma virus, venereal warts) (see Chapter 76). Secondary infections of the vulva are caused by organisms responsible for the many types of vaginitis, including *candidiasis*. Pediculosis pubis (crab lice) and scabies (itch mite) are common parasitic infestations of the skin of the vulva. Other causes of vulvitis include:

- Atrophic vaginitis
- Lichen planus (thickened, leathery skin from scratching)
- Vulvar leukoplakia (postmenopausal atrophy and thickening of vulvar tissues)
- Vulvar cancer
- Urinary incontinence

Some women may have an *itch-scratch-itch cycle,* in which the itching leads to scratching, which causes excoriation that then must heal. As healing takes place, itching occurs again. If the cycle is not interrupted, the chronic scratching may lead to the white, thickened skin of lichen planus. This dry, leathery skin cracks easily, increasing the woman's risk for infection.

PATIENT-CENTERED COLLABORATIVE CARE

Assess for vulvovaginitis by asking questions about the symptoms, assisting with a pelvic examination, and obtaining vaginal smears for laboratory testing. Inquire about symptoms of itching and burning sensation. Erythema (redness), edema, and superficial skin ulcers also may be present. Use a nonjudgmental approach and provide reassurance during the assessment because the patient may be embarrassed or afraid to discuss her symptoms. Encourage her to talk about her problem and its effect on her sexual health.

Interventions for vulvovaginitis depend on the causes and the specific vaginal infection. Proper health habits can benefit treatment. Instruct the patient to get enough rest and sleep, observe good dietary habits, exercise regularly, and use good personal hygiene. Teach her about how to manage her infection (Chart 74-1). Chart 74-2 outlines measures to help prevent further infections.

Nursing interventions to relieve itching include applying wet compresses, sitz baths for 30 minutes several times a day, and using topical drugs such as estrogens and lidocaine. Encourage the removal of any irritant or allergen, such as changing detergents.

Treatment of pediculosis and scabies is used if needed and includes:

- Applying lindane (Kwell, Kwellada ♦) lotion, shampoo, or cream to the affected area as directed
- Cleaning affected clothes, bedding, and towels
- Disinfecting the home environment (lice cannot live for more than 24 hours away from the body)

CHART 74-1 PATIENT AND FAMILY EDUCATION: PREPARING FOR SELF-MANAGEMENT

Vaginal Infections

- Your risk for getting vaginal infections increases if you have sex with more than one person.
- When you have a vaginal infection, do not have sexual intercourse, if possible, or at least make sure that your partner wears a condom.
- Sexual partners may need to be treated for infection.
- The only way to identify what infection you have is to be examined by a health care provider and to get the results of laboratory tests.
- Take your medicine as prescribed, not just until your symptoms go away.

CHART 74-2 PATIENT AND FAMILY EDUCATION: PREPARING FOR SELF-MANAGEMENT

Prevention of Vulvovaginitis

- Wear cotton underwear.
- Avoid wearing tight clothing, such as pantyhose or tight jeans, because they can cause chafing. You can also get hot and sweaty, which can cause an infection.
- Always wipe front to back after having a bowel movement or urinating.
- During bath or shower, cleanse inner labial mucosa with water, not soap.
- Do not douche or use feminine hygiene sprays.
- If your sexual partner has an infection of the sex organs, do not have intercourse with him or her until he or she has been treated.
- You are more likely to get an infection if you are pregnant, have diabetes, take oral contraceptive drugs, or are menopausal.
- Practice vulvar self-examination monthly.

❓ NCLEX EXAMINATION CHALLENGE

Health Promotion and Maintenance

A client reports new onset of vulvar burning, redness, and pruritus. Which of these questions by the nurse would be the most appropriate?
A. "Have you recently changed clothes detergents?"
B. "Have you seen your health care provider about this problem?"
C. "Have you had your HPV vaccine yet?"
D. "Does this problem run in your family?"

TOXIC SHOCK SYNDROME

Pathophysiology

Toxic shock syndrome (TSS) was first recognized in 1980 when it was found to be related to menstruation and tampon use. Other conditions associated with TSS include surgical wound infection, nonsurgical infections, and gynecologic surgeries. Use of internal contraceptives has also been linked to this health problem.

In infection related to menstruation, menstrual blood provides a growth medium for *Staphylococcus aureus* (or, less frequently, *Streptococcus*). Exotoxins produced from the bacteria cross the vaginal mucosa to the bloodstream via microabrasions from tampon insertion or prolonged use. A small number of TSS cases are fatal. Extensive public education

---

CHART 74-3   KEY FEATURES

Toxic Shock Syndrome

- Fever (temperature >102° F [38.9° C])
- Diffuse rash resembling sunburn
- Peeling of skin—primarily the soles of the feet and the palms of the hands—1 to 2 wk after onset of the illness
- Hypotension (systolic blood pressure <90 mm Hg or orthostatic syncope)
- Involvement of three or more of these:
  - Gastrointestinal system: vomiting, diarrhea at the onset of the syndrome
  - Musculoskeletal system: severe aching or a serum creatinine phosphatase level twice the normal level
  - Respiratory system: acute respiratory distress syndrome (ARDS)
  - Renal/urinary system: decreased urine output, pyuria
  - Cardiovascular system: decreased left ventricular contractility; ischemic changes shown on the electrocardiogram
  - Liver: total bilirubin, aspartate aminotransferase (serum glutamic–oxaloacetic transaminase), and alanine amino–transferase (serum glutamic–pyruvic transaminase) levels elevated; jaundice; disseminated intravascular coagulation (DIC)
  - Hematologic system: platelet levels below normal
  - Central nervous system: disorientation, altered consciousness in the absence of fever or hypertension
  - Mucous membranes: hyperemia of the vaginal walls, the throat, or the conjunctiva of the eye
- Negative results for Rocky Mountain spotted fever, measles, and scarlet fever and for throat, blood, and cerebrospinal fluid cultures
- Positive culture for *Staphylococcus aureus* from blood, urine, or stool

---

CHART 74-4   PATIENT AND FAMILY EDUCATION: PREPARING FOR SELF-MANAGEMENT

Prevention of Toxic Shock Syndrome

- Wash your hands before inserting a tampon.
- Do not use a tampon if it is dirty.
- Insert the tampon carefully to avoid injuring the delicate tissue in your vagina.
- Change your tampon every 3 to 6 hours.
- Do not use superabsorbent tampons.
- Use sanitary napkins at night.
- Call your health care provider if you suddenly experience a high temperature, vomiting, or diarrhea.
- Do not use tampons at all if you have had toxic shock syndrome.
- Not using tampons almost guarantees that you will not get toxic shock syndrome.

---

has led to a decreased number of women having the infection.

PATIENT-CENTERED COLLABORATIVE CARE

Within 24 hours of contact with the causative agent, the abrupt onset of a high fever, along with headache, flu-like symptoms, and severe hypotension with fainting, is often present. A sunburn-like rash with broken capillaries in the eyes and skin is another warning sign of TSS. Because not all women have all these manifestations, the criteria established by the Centers for Disease Control and Prevention (CDC) are used to verify cases (Chart 74-3). Educate all women on the prevention of TSS (Chart 74-4).

Treatment includes removal of the infection source, such as a tampon; restoring fluid and electrolyte balance; drugs to manage hypotension; and IV antibiotics. Other measures may include transfusions to reverse low platelet counts and corticosteroids to treat skin changes.

PELVIC ORGAN PROLAPSE

Pathophysiology

The pelvic organs are supported by a sling of muscles and tendons, which sometimes become weak and no longer able to hold an organ in place. Uterine prolapse, the most common type of pelvic organ prolapse (POP), can be caused by neuromuscular damage of childbirth; increased intra-abdominal

pressure related to pregnancy, obesity, or physical exertion; or weakening of pelvic support due to decreased estrogen. The stages of uterine prolapse are described by the degree of descent of the uterus (Fig. 74-2) through the pelvic floor.

Whenever the uterus is displaced, other structures such as the bladder, rectum, and small intestine can protrude through the vaginal walls (Fig. 74-3). A cystocele is a protrusion of the bladder through the vaginal wall (urinary bladder prolapse), which can lead to stress urinary incontinence (SUI) and urinary tract infections (UTIs). A rectocele is a protrusion of the rectum through a weakened vaginal wall (rectal prolapse).

PATIENT-CENTERED COLLABORATIVE CARE

ASSESSMENT

Assessment findings for patients with a suspected uterine prolapse include the patient's feeling as if "something is falling out," dyspareunia (painful intercourse), backache, and a feeling of heaviness or pressure in the pelvis. A pelvic examination may reveal a protrusion of the cervix when the woman is asked to bear down. Listen to her concerns, and note signs of depression from having long-term symptoms.

Ask the patient about manifestations that may indicate that she has a *cystocele*. These signs and symptoms may include:

- Difficulty in emptying the bladder
- Urinary frequency and urgency
- Urinary tract infection
- Stress urinary incontinence (SUI) (loss of urine during activities that increase intra-abdominal pressure, such as laughing, coughing, sneezing, or lifting heavy objects)

A pelvic examination reveals a large bulge of the anterior vaginal wall when the woman is asked to bear down. Diagnostic tests include cystography (to show the presence of bladder herniation), measurement of residual urine by bladder ultrasound, and urine culture and sensitivity testing. Radiographic imaging of urinary anatomy and voiding function is useful in determining the degree of cystocele.

Rectocele assessment usually includes symptoms of constipation, hemorrhoids, fecal impaction, and feelings of rectal or vaginal fullness. A vaginal and rectal examination may show a bulge of the posterior vaginal wall when the woman is asked to bear down.

INTERVENTIONS

Interventions are based on the degree of the POP. Conservative treatment is preferred over surgical treatment when possible.

Nonsurgical Management

Teach women to improve pelvic support and tone via pelvic floor muscle exercises (PFMEs, or Kegel exercises). Space-filling devices such as pessaries or spheres can be worn in the vagina to elevate the uterine prolapse. Intravaginal estrogen therapy may be prescribed for the postmenopausal woman to prevent atrophy and weakening of vaginal walls. Women with bladder symptoms may benefit from bladder training and attention to complete emptying. Management of a rectocele focuses on promoting bowel elimination. The health care provider usually prescribes a high-fiber diet, stool softeners, and laxatives.

Surgical Management

Surgery may be recommended for severe symptoms. Address the fears and concerns of the patient and her family. The least invasive procedure is usually used.

Transvaginal repair for pelvic organ prolapse (POP) using surgical vaginal mesh or tape is a commonly performed minimally invasive technique. It is particularly useful for women who are very obese. Depending on the procedure that is planned, the patient has either local or general anesthesia. The surgeon creates a sling with the mesh or tape, and the woman is discharged the same day. Procedures done under local anesthesia can be done in the surgeon's office. Over the past several years, patient report of several rare complications associated with the use of transvaginal mesh has required the U.S. Food and Drug Administration to recall at least one company's product. These complications include vaginal erosion and severe infection (Mirsaidi, 2009).

Patients who choose to have the procedure may return to usual activities, including driving, 2 weeks after surgery. Teach them to avoid sexual intercourse for at least 6 weeks or as the surgeon recommends.

Alternatives to minimally invasive surgery are open surgical techniques. An anterior colporrhaphy (anterior repair)

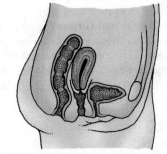
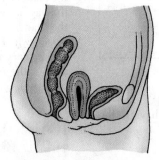
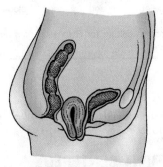

In **grade I uterine prolapse**, the uterus bulges into the vagina, but the cervix does not protrude through the entrance to the vagina.

In **grade II uterine prolapse**, the uterus bulges farther into the vagina, and the cervix protrudes through the entrance to the vagina.

In **grade III uterine prolapse**, the body of the uterus and the cervix protrude through the entrance to the vagina. The vagina is turned inside out.

FIG. 74-2 Types of uterine prolapse.

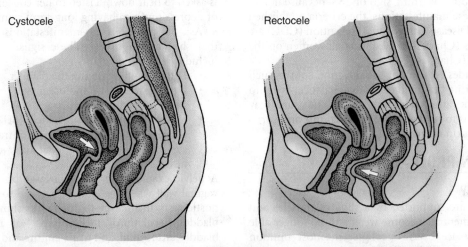

FIG. 74-3 In cystocele, the urinary bladder is displaced downward, causing bulging of the anterior vaginal wall. In rectocele, the rectum is displaced, causing bulging of the posterior vaginal wall.

! NURSING SAFETY PRIORITY

Action Alert

To help patients decide if she should decide on any surgical procedure using mesh or tape, be sure that the patient has received informed consent prior to surgery. Teach the patient about these possible adverse events, the signs and symptoms of infection, and when she should contact her surgeon. If possible, provide the patient with the manufacturer's labeling and written information.

tightens the pelvic muscles for better *bladder* support. A vaginal surgical approach is used and may be done as a laparoscopic-assisted procedure. Nursing care for a woman undergoing an anterior repair is similar to that for a woman undergoing a vaginal hysterectomy.

After surgery, instruct the patient to limit her activities. *Teach her to avoid lifting anything heavier than 5 pounds, strenuous exercises, and sexual intercourse for 6 weeks.* For discomfort, tell her to use heat either as a moist heating pad or warm compresses applied to the abdomen. A hot bath may also be helpful. Sutures do not need to be removed because some are absorbable and others will fall out as healing occurs. Tell the woman to notify her health care provider if she has signs of infection, such as fever, persistent pain, or purulent, foul-smelling discharge. Encourage her to keep her follow-up appointment after surgery.

Posterior colporrhaphy (posterior repair) reduces *rectal* bulging. If both a cystocele and a rectocele are present, an *anterior and posterior colporrhaphy (A&P repair)* is performed.

The nursing care after a posterior repair is similar to that after any rectal surgery. After surgery, a low-residue (low-fiber) diet is usually prescribed to decrease bowel movements and allow time for the incision to heal. Instruct the patient to avoid straining when she does have a bowel movement so that she does not put pressure on the suture line. Bowel movements are often painful, and she may need pain medication before having a stool. Provide sitz baths or delegate this activity to unlicensed nursing personnel to relieve the

woman's discomfort. Health teaching for the patient undergoing a posterior repair is similar to that for the patient undergoing an anterior repair.

Vaginal hysterectomy may accompany any uterine prolapse repair surgery unless the woman wants children or more children. This procedure is described on p. 1619.

BENIGN NEOPLASMS

OVARIAN CYST

Functional ovarian cysts can occur in a woman of any age but are rare after menopause. Other cysts and tumors of the ovaries are not related to the menstrual cycle but arise from ovarian tissue. Primary assessment involves pelvic examination and transvaginal ultrasound. Further testing with computerized tomography (CT), magnetic resonance imaging (MRI), or laparoscopic biopsy to rule out cancer may be indicated. Some ovarian cysts disappear over time, and others cause discomfort for a prolonged period. Laparoscopic surgery to remove the cyst or ovary may be needed.

UTERINE LEIOMYOMA

Pathophysiology

Leiomyomas, also called fibroids or myomas, are benign, slow-growing solid tumors of the uterine myometrium (muscle layer). They are classified according to their position in the layers of the uterus. The most common types are intramural, submucosal, and subserosal (Fig. 74-4).

Intramural leiomyomas are contained in the uterine wall within the myometrium. *Submucosal* leiomyomas protrude into the cavity of the uterus and can cause bleeding and disrupt pregnancy. *Subserosal* leiomyomas protrude through the outer surface of the uterine wall and may extend to the broad ligament, pressing other organs.

Although most fibroids develop within the uterine wall, a few may appear in the cervix. Pedunculated leiomyomas are attached by a pedicle (stalk) to the outside of the uterus and

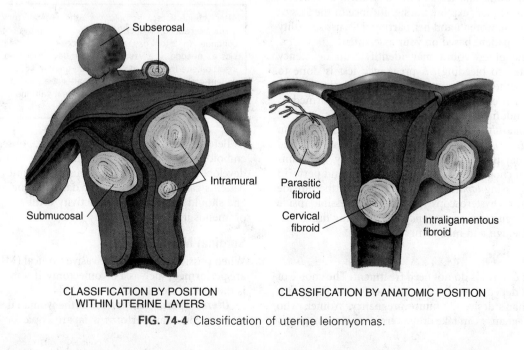

CLASSIFICATION BY POSITION
WITHIN UTERINE LAYERS

CLASSIFICATION BY ANATOMIC POSITION

FIG. 74-4 Classification of uterine leiomyomas.

occasionally break off and attach to other tissues (parasitic fibroids).

Although the cause is not known, leiomyomas develop from excessive local growth of smooth muscle cells. This may be a genetic error causing a lack of ability to halt growth. The growth of leiomyomas may be related to stimulation by estrogen, progesterone, and growth hormone. This explains why fibroids sometimes enlarge during pregnancy and diminish in size after menopause.

The incidence of leiomyomas increases as women get older. Women who have never been pregnant also are at a high risk. Many women have asymptomatic fibroids, whereas others have severe symptoms.

PATIENT-CENTERED COLLABORATIVE CARE

ASSESSMENT

Women with fibroids do not usually have pain, although acute pain may occur with twisting of the fibroid on its stalk. *The patient often seeks medical attention because of heavy vaginal bleeding.* Ask about how many tampons or menstrual pads she uses a day. The woman may report a feeling of pelvic pressure, constipation, or urinary frequency or retention. These symptoms result when an enlarged fibroid presses on other organs. The patient may notice that her abdomen has increased in size. Assess the woman's abdomen for distention or enlargement. Ask if she has dyspareunia (painful intercourse) and infertility (inability to become pregnant).

Abdominal, vaginal, and rectal examinations usually reveal the presence of a uterine enlargement. Further diagnostic procedures are needed to differentiate benign tumors from cancerous ones.

Symptoms such as dyspareunia may significantly lower the patient's quality of life. A woman who is symptomatic may fear that she has cancer. She may be anxious about abnormal bleeding or her failure to conceive. She may also be concerned if surgery is recommended if she wants to have children or more children. Assess the woman's feelings and concerns about her symptoms and fears of the unknown. If hysterectomy is recommended, explore the significance of the loss of the uterus for the woman and her partner. Discuss sexuality issues with the patient based on your assessment.

A complete blood count may identify iron deficiency anemia (related to bleeding). A pregnancy test is done to determine whether pregnancy is the cause of the uterine enlargement. An endometrial biopsy may be performed to evaluate for endometrial cancer.

Transvaginal ultrasound alone or with saline infusion (saline sonogram) provides a good picture of a submucosal fibroid that may protrude into the uterine cavity. The clinician may then choose to directly view a tumor and perform a biopsy of it, using *laparoscopy* (for tumors on the outside of the uterus) or hysteroscopy (for tumors accessible inside the uterus). *Magnetic resonance imaging (MRI)* can differentiate between benign and malignant lesions.

INTERVENTIONS

Asymptomatic fibroids do not need treatment. The choice of management depends on the size and location of the tumor and the woman's desire for future pregnancy. Women who still desire pregnancy can take drug therapy or have magnetic resonance–guided focused ultrasound surgery or laparoscopic myomectomy to remove the tumor. Uterine artery embolization and hysterectomy are choices for women who no longer desire pregnancy.

Nonsurgical Management

If the woman is menopausal, the fibroids usually shrink and surgery may not be necessary. *Teach the patient who is receiving hormone replacement therapy for menopausal symptoms that the fibroids may continue to grow because of estrogen stimulation.*

If the woman has few symptoms or desires childbearing, the health care provider may recommend observation and examination every 4 to 6 months. As with dysfunctional uterine bleeding, mild leiomyoma symptoms can be managed with oral contraception. *Gonadotropin-releasing hormone (GnRH) agonists* such as goserelin (Zoladex) and leuprolide (Lupron Depot) induce artificial menopause but are less commonly used in the past few years due to side and adverse effects. These drugs decrease hormone exposure and may give the tumor time to shrink temporarily. This may also be done before surgery.

Magnetic resonance–guided focused ultrasound is a noninvasive, painless technique for women with few smaller fibroids who wish to preserve their fertility. The woman lies prone on an MRI scanner, which provides a three-dimensional image of the pelvis. The radiologic clinician then guides a focused pulse of ultrasound to heat the tumor to destroy it.

An alternative to surgery for the woman who does not desire pregnancy is uterine artery embolization (also called *uterine fibroid embolization [UFE]*) under moderate sedation. The interventional radiologist uses a percutaneous catheter inserted through the femoral artery to inject polyvinyl alcohol pellets into the uterine artery. The resulting blockage starves the tumor of circulation, allowing it (or them) to shrink. The patient stays overnight in the hospital.

! NURSING SAFETY PRIORITY

Action Alert

After uterine artery embolization, the woman may have severe cramping caused by decreased blood flow to the uterus. Cramping continues for 2 to 4 days. Assess her pain level, and provide analgesics as needed. If a vascular closure device is used at the arterial insertion site (most commonly), raise the head of the bed. Help the patient ambulate in about 2 hours after the procedure. If a closure device was not used, keep her on bedrest with the legs immobilized for 4 hours before ambulating to prevent bleeding.

Before discharge, tell the patient to observe for post-embolectomy syndrome, a flu-like illness that some women develop. Teach her to resume usual activities slowly. Most patients can return to work or daily routine within a week. She should avoid strenuous activity until the physician recommends it.

Surgical Management

When possible, minimally invasive surgical (MIS) techniques are performed, such as a myomectomy. If not, a hysterectomy is the procedure of choice.

Uterus-Sparing Surgeries. If the woman desires children, the surgeon may perform a laparoscopic or hysteroscopic myomectomy (the removal of leiomyomas from the uterus). During this procedure, a laser may be used to remove the tumors. This minimally invasive procedure is usually performed in the early phase of the menstrual cycle to minimize blood loss and to avoid the possibility of interrupting an unsuspected pregnancy. A small percentage of leiomyomas recur after surgery. Scarring makes the uterus more likely to rupture during labor, so future deliveries will be planned cesarean deliveries. Nursing care is similar to that for a woman undergoing a hysterectomy (see below).

In selected cases (e.g., submucous fibroids, menorrhagia), a *transcervical endometrial resection (TCER)* is performed via hysteroscopy. A hysteroscope (endoscope) is inserted into the uterus, and the endometrium is destroyed using diathermy (heat) or radioablation.

! NURSING SAFETY PRIORITY

Critical Rescue

Monitor for rare but potential complications of hysteroscopic surgery, which include:

- Fluid overload (fluid used to distend the uterine cavity can be absorbed)
- Embolism
- Hemorrhage
- Perforation of the uterus, bowel, or bladder and ureter injury
- Persistent increased menstrual bleeding
- Incomplete suppression of menstruation

Monitor for any indications of these problems, and report signs and symptoms, such as severe pain and heavy bleeding, to the surgeon immediately. Scarring may cause a small risk for complications in future pregnancies.

Hysterectomy. Leiomyomas are the most common reason for hysterectomies. A uterus that has smaller fibroids may be removed via a *total vaginal hysterectomy (TVH)*. The surgeon may perform a laparoscopic-assisted vaginal hysterectomy (LAVH) or use a robotic-assisted operative system (Everett & Crawford, 2010). The surgeon removes the uterus and cervix, sometimes in pieces, through the vagina without an external surgical incision.

A *total abdominal hysterectomy (TAH)* is usually performed for leiomyomas larger than the size of a 16-week pregnancy. The uterus and cervix are removed by laparoscopic-assisted minimally invasive surgery (MIS), which requires one or more very small umbilical incisions through a horizontal bikini incision (traditional open procedure). Some surgeons use robotic technology to assist in performing a TAH (Matthews et al., 2010). Robotic surgery is especially helpful when performing hysterectomies on patients who are extremely obese (Stone et al., 2010). In both vaginal and abdominal hysterectomies, the surgeon removes the uterus from the five supporting ligaments, which are then attached to the vaginal cuff so that normal depth of the vagina is maintained (Table 74-2).

Preoperative teaching by the health care team begins in the surgeon's office. Explain procedures that routinely take place before surgery, including laboratory tests and expected drugs such as a prophylactic antibiotic. Depending on the type of surgical technique planned, teach about the need for turning, coughing, and deep-breathing exercises; incentive spirometry; early ambulation; and pain relief (see Chapter 16 for a discussion of general patient care before surgery).

TABLE 74-2	COMMON GYNECOLOGIC SURGERIES

Total Hysterectomy
All the uterus, including the cervix, is removed. The procedure may be vaginal or abdominal, with laparoscopic or robotic assistance.

Bilateral Salpingo-Oophorectomy (BSO)
Fallopian tubes and ovaries are removed.

Panhysterectomy
Total abdominal hysterectomy and BSO: The uterus, ovaries, and fallopian tubes are removed.

Radical Hysterectomy
The uterus, cervix, adjacent lymph nodes, the upper third of the vagina, and the surrounding tissues (parametrium) are removed.

Psychological assessment is essential. Assess the significance of the surgery for the woman and her partner. If it involves loss of the uterus, she may feel a great loss if she wishes to retain her childbearing ability. Many women relate their uterus to self-image and femininity or believe that their sexual function is related to their uterus. Although surgical menopause by hysterectomy can create loss of libido and vaginal changes, teach the patient that vaginal estrogen cream and gentle dilation can help correct that. Reassure her regarding any misperceptions about the effects of hysterectomy, such as association with masculinization and weight gain. Assess the patient's support system. She may fear rejection by her sexual partner. Include the partner in all teaching sessions, unless this practice is not culturally acceptable.

Patients who have *uterus-sparing surgeries* usually go home the same day of surgery. They often experience less postoperative pain and fewer complications when compared with patients who have their uterus and cervix removed. Teach patients that they usually return to usual daily activities in 2 weeks, but sexual intercourse should be avoided for at least 6 weeks.

Postoperative care of the woman who has undergone a TAH is similar to that of any patient who has had laparoscopic or traditional open abdominal surgery (see Chapter 18). Assess (Chart 74-5):

- Vaginal bleeding (there should be less than one saturated perineal pad in 4 hours)
- Abdominal bleeding at the incision site(s) (a small amount is normal)
- Intactness of the incision(s)
- Urine output per urinary catheter for 24 hours or less (for open surgery)
- Pain

Specific postoperative interventions for a *vaginal hysterectomy* include:

- Assessment of vaginal bleeding (there should be less than one saturated pad in 4 hours)
- Urinary catheter care
- Perineal care

Community-Based Care

The patient with uterine leiomyomas is managed on an ambulatory care basis unless surgery is performed. After discharge, she usually returns to her home.

Postoperative Nursing Care of the Patient After Total Abdominal Hysterectomy

Assess cardiovascular, respiratory, renal, and gastrointestinal status, including:
- Vital signs
- Heart, lung, and bowel sounds
- Urine output
- Temperature and color of the skin
- Red blood cell, hemoglobin, and hematocrit levels
- Activity tolerance
- Dressing and drains for color and amount of drainage
- Peripads for vaginal bleeding and clots
- Fluid intake (IVs until peristalsis returns and patient is tolerating oral intake)

Teach the patient to use these interventions to prevent postoperative complications:
- Cough and deep-breathing exercises
- Incentive spirometry
- Sequential compression devices
- Ambulation
- Avoidance of heavy lifting or strenuous activity
- Adequate hydration

Assess the home care teaching needs of the patient related to the illness and surgery, including:
- Physiologic effects of the surgery
- Signs or symptoms to report
- Side or toxic effects of medications
- Activity limitations related to driving and use of stairs
- Follow-up care
- Postoperative restrictions related to sexual activity, use of tampons, and bathing
- Care of wound and/or drains

Assess the patient's coping skills and reaction to the diagnosis and surgical procedure.

❓ NCLEX EXAMINATION CHALLENGE

Physiological Integrity

A client returns from surgery after a total vaginal hysterectomy. What is the nurse's priority action immediately after surgery?
A. Assess for excessive vaginal bleeding.
B. Monitor temperature for infection.
C. Assess for deep vein thrombosis.
D. Check dressing for intactness.

If the patient had a hysterectomy, teach her to limit stair climbing for several weeks. If she lives alone and is not permitted to drive for 2 to 6 weeks, she will need to arrange for transportation for follow-up surgical visits.

Teach the woman who has undergone an abdominal hysterectomy about the expected physical changes, any activity restrictions, diet, sexual activity, wound care, complications, and the need for follow-up care. Chart 74-6 lists areas to include for health teaching.

Generally, women adjust well to surgery if they have completed childbearing, have interests outside the home, work, have no misconceptions about the effects of hysterectomy, and have support from the family, especially their sexual partner. Psychological reactions can occur months to years after surgery, particularly if sexual functioning and libido are diminished. Women identified as being at high risk for psychological problems may need long-term follow-up care or referral. They may need to be counseled about signs of

Care After a Total Vaginal or Abdominal Hysterectomy

Expected Physical Changes
- You will no longer have a period, although you may have some vaginal discharge for a few days after you go home.
- It will not be possible for you to become pregnant, and birth control methods are no longer needed.
- If your ovaries were removed, you may have some menopause symptoms such as hot flushes, night sweats, and vaginal dryness.
- It is normal to tire more easily and require more sleep and rest during the first few weeks after surgery.

Activity
- Limit stair climbing to fewer than five times per day.
- Do not lift anything heavier than 5 to 10 lbs.
- Gradually increase walking as exercise, but stop before you become fatigued.
- Avoid the sitting position for any extended period. When you sit, do not cross your legs at the knees.
- Avoid jogging, aerobic exercise, participating in sports, and any strenuous activity for 2 to 6 weeks, depending on what type of surgical procedure was performed.
- Do not drive until your surgeon has told you it is alright.

Sexual Activity
- Do not engage in sexual intercourse for 4 to 6 weeks, or as prescribed by your surgeon.
- If you had a vaginal "repair" as part of your surgery, the first time you have intercourse you may have some tenderness or pain because the vaginal walls are tighter. Careful intercourse and the use of water-based lubricants can help reduce this discomfort. This discomfort usually goes away with time and stretching of the vagina.

Complications
- Take your temperature twice each day for the first 3 days after surgery.
- Check your incision, if you have any, daily for signs of infection (increasing redness, open areas, drainage that is thick or foul-smelling, incision pain).

Report Any of the Following to Your Surgeon
- Increased vaginal drainage or change in drainage (bloodier, thicker, foul-smelling)
- Temperature over 100° F
- Pain, tenderness, redness, or swelling in your calves
- Pain or burning on urination

depression. Intermittent sadness is normal, but continued feelings of low self-esteem or loss of interest or pleasure in usual activities and pastimes is not normal and should be evaluated. Provide written materials, and focus on the positive aspects of the woman's life to help decrease adverse psychological reactions.

BARTHOLIN CYST

Pathophysiology

Bartholin cyst is a common disorder of the vulva. It results from obstruction of the duct of the Bartholin gland. The secretory function of the gland continues, and the fluid fills the obstructed duct. The main causes of the obstruction are infection, thickened mucus near the ductal opening, or trauma, such as lacerations.

PATIENT-CENTERED COLLABORATIVE CARE

The patient may be asymptomatic if the cyst is small. Ask if she has dyspareunia (painful intercourse) or inadequate genital lubrication. Assess for swelling in the perineal area. A large cyst usually causes constant local pain and may cause difficulty walking or sitting. Physical examination of the vulva reveals a swelling immediately beneath the skin in the posterior portion of the vulva. The cyst may appear brown or bloody, depending on its contents. Usually it is present on only one side and ranges from ⅜ to 4 inches (1 to 10 cm) in size.

If the cyst is draining, a fluid sample is sent to the laboratory for culture (for gonorrhea and aerobic and anaerobic organisms) and sensitivity testing. If the woman is older than 40 years, a biopsy of the cyst is done to identify possible cancer.

If the woman is asymptomatic, no intervention is needed. An abscess usually ruptures spontaneously within 72 hours of forming. Teach the woman with an abscess to take over-the-counter or prescribed analgesics and apply moist heat (sitz baths or hot wet packs) to the vulva. Cultures most often reveal *Escherichia coli* or *Staphylococcus aureus,* for which antibiotics are prescribed.

Simple incision and drainage (I&D) may provide temporary relief. However, cysts tend to recur when the opening of the duct re-obstructs. Usually the surgeon establishes a permanent opening for drainage. Marsupialization (formation of a pouch that is a new duct opening) is performed using local, regional, or general anesthesia. Discomfort after surgery may be relieved with analgesics and sitz baths. Prophylactic antibiotics may be prescribed.

The Bartholin glands may be totally removed in older women when cancer is suspected or if infections with abscess formation recur. Care after surgery includes:

- Application of ice packs or sitz baths several times a day for comfort and promotion of healing
- Analgesics for pain
- Prophylactic antibiotics
- Assessment of the incision for signs of healing or infection

CERVICAL POLYP

Cervical polyps are *pedunculated* (on stalks) tumors that arise from the mucosa and extend through the opening of the cervical os. They result from a hyperplasia (overgrowth) of the endocervical epithelium in response to hormonal stimulation. Polyps may also be due to inflammation or to localized vascular congestion of the cervical blood vessels. They are the most common benign growth of the cervix and occur most often in women older than 40 years who have had several children.

A woman may be asymptomatic, have premenstrual or postmenstrual bleeding, or have bleeding after intercourse. A speculum examination may reveal a small single polyp or multiple polyps. They are bright red, are soft and fragile, and may bleed when touched.

Polyp removal is a simple office procedure. The base of the polyp is grasped with a clamp, and the polyp is twisted off and sent to the pathology laboratory for evaluation. Cautery usually stops any bleeding at the site of removal. The woman does not feel any pain during the procedure. Instruct her to avoid tampon use, douches, and sexual intercourse for a week or until healing has taken place.

GYNECOLOGIC CANCERS

ENDOMETRIAL (UTERINE) CANCER

Pathophysiology

Endometrial cancer (cancer of the inner uterine lining) is the most common gynecologic malignancy in the United States. This chapter includes two other common gynecologic cancers, but the disease can affect any organ in the reproductive tract.

Endometrial cancer grows slowly in most cases, and early symptoms of vaginal bleeding generally lead to prompt evaluation and treatment. As a result, this type of cancer has a good prognosis. *Adenocarcinoma* is the most common type, accounting for 80% of all cases. The tumor arises from the glandular part of the endometrium and usually follows endometrial hyperplasia (overgrowth).

The initial growth of the cancer is within the uterine cavity, followed by extension into the myometrium and the cervix. Stage I endometrial cancer is confined to the endometrium. Stage II cancer also involves the cervix, and stage III reaches the vagina or lymph nodes. Stage IV endometrial cancer has spread beyond the pelvis.

Metastasis outside the uterus occurs in these ways:

- Through lymphatic spread to the ovaries and parametrial, pelvic, inguinal, and para-aortic lymph nodes
- By blood, to the lungs, liver, or bone
- By transtubal or intra-abdominal spread to the peritoneal cavity

Etiology and Genetic Risk

Endometrial cancer is strongly associated with conditions causing prolonged exposure to estrogen without the protective effects of progesterone. Risk factors for endometrial cancer are listed in Table 74-3. Although most cases of endometrial cancer do not have a genetic predisposition, it is more common in families who have gene mutations for hereditary nonpolyposis colon cancer (HNPCC) (Nussbaum et al., 2007).

Incidence and Prevalence

About 44,000 new cases of endometrial cancer occur annually in the United States. White women get the disease more often than African-American women, but African-American women die more often from the disease (American Cancer Society [ACS], 2010). Factors accounting for the differences in these death rates may include access to care and patient education opportunities.

PATIENT-CENTERED COLLABORATIVE CARE

ASSESSMENT

Physical Assessment/Clinical Manifestations

The main symptom of endometrial cancer is postmenopausal bleeding. Ask the patient how many tampons or menstrual pads she uses each day. Some women also have a watery, bloody vaginal discharge, low back or abdominal pain, and low pelvic

TABLE 74-3 RISK FACTORS FOR ENDOMETRIAL (UTERINE) CANCER AND CERVICAL CANCER	
ENDOMETRIAL (UTERINE) CANCER	**CERVICAL CANCER**
• Women in reproductive years	• Girls and young women
• Family history of endometrial cancer or HNPCC	• Infection with HPV
• Diabetes mellitus	• Multiparity (multiple births)
• Hypertension	• Smoking
• Obesity	• Younger than 18 years at first intercourse
• Uterine polyps	• Multiple sex partners
• Late menopause	• African American
• Nulliparity (no childbirths)	• Oral contraceptive use
• Smoking	• History of STDs
• Tamoxifen (Nolvadex) given for breast cancer	• Obesity or poor diet
	• Family history of cervical cancer
	• HIV/AIDS
	• Lower socioeconomic status
	• Sexual partner had a previous partner who developed cervical cancer
	• Intrauterine exposure to DES

AIDS, Acquired immune deficiency syndrome; *DES,* diethylstilbestrol; *HIV,* human immune deficiency virus; *HNPCC,* hereditary nonpolyposis colon cancer; *HPV,* human papilloma virus; *STDs,* sexually transmitted diseases.

pain (caused by pressure of the enlarged uterus). Ask the patient to describe the exact location and intensity of her discomfort. A pelvic examination may reveal the presence of a palpable uterine mass or uterine polyp. The uterus is enlarged if the cancer is advanced.

Laboratory Assessment

Several laboratory tests are used to determine the overall condition of the woman with possible or confirmed endometrial cancer. For example, the complete blood count typically shows anemia because the patient has heavy bleeding. Serum tumor markers to assess for metastasis include CA-125 (cancer antigen–125) and alpha-fetoprotein (AFP), both of which may be elevated when ovarian cancer is present (Pagana & Pagana, 2010). A human chorionic gonadotropin (hCG) level may be taken to rule out pregnancy before treatment for cancer begins. Genetic testing may be done for the mutation causing HNPCC, if there is a family history of this disease.

Other Diagnostic Assessment

Transvaginal ultrasound and *endometrial biopsy* are the gold standard tests to determine the presence of endometrial thickening and cancer. Saline may be infused during the ultrasound to improve the image of the uterine cavity. The clinician then collects an endometrial biopsy from inside the uterus via a thin, flexible suction curette through the cervix (Pagana & Pagana, 2010).

Other diagnostic tests to determine the patient's overall health status and the presence of metastasis (cancer spread) include:

• Chest x-ray
• Intravenous pyelography (IVP), or excretory urography, to assess renal function and to assess for renal metastasis
• Abdominal ultrasound

• Computed tomography (CT) of the pelvis
• Magnetic resonance imaging (MRI) of the abdomen and pelvis
• Liver and bone scans to assess for distant metastasis

Some women also have a hysteroscopic examination of the uterus and proctosigmoidoscopy depending on the stage of their cancer.

Psychosocial Assessment

Before a diagnosis is made, the woman may deny that the symptoms are related to cancer. During the diagnostic phase, the woman may express fears and concerns about having the disease. After the diagnosis is confirmed, she may express disbelief, anger, depression, anxiety, or withdrawal behaviors. Assess these emotional reactions, and encourage the patient to discuss them. Ask her about how she copes with other stressful events, and assess her support systems.

■ ANALYSIS

The priority problems for patients with endometrial cancer are:

1. Potential for disease metastasis
2. Ineffective Coping related to the diagnosis of cancer and fear of dying

■ PLANNING AND IMPLEMENTATION

Reducing the Risk for Metastasis

Planning: Expect Outcomes. The patient is expected to be free of metastatic disease if she has been diagnosed without obvious metastasis. For patients whose cancer has already spread, the expected outcomes are to have the highest quality life for as long as possible. In some cases, palliation and end-of-life care are desired.

Interventions. Surgical removal and cancer staging of the tumor with adjacent lymph nodes are the most important interventions for endometrial cancer. Cancer staging is often done using minimally invasive techniques, such as laparoscopic or robotic-assisted procedures.

Surgical Management. For stage I disease, the gynecology oncologist usually removes the uterus, fallopian tubes, and ovaries (total hysterectomy and bilateral salpingectomy/oophorectomy [BSO]), as well as peritoneum fluid or washings for cytologic examination. Laparoscopic surgery has fewer complications, shorter hospital stay, and less cost. A radical hysterectomy with bilateral pelvic lymph node dissection and removal of the upper third of the vagina is performed for stage II cancer. Nursing care for a radical hysterectomy is the same as that for a simple hysterectomy except that the woman's hospitalization is usually longer and her convalescence may be extended. Radical surgery and node dissection can also be done as a minimally invasive procedure using laparoscopic or robotic-assisted technology.

Nonsurgical Management. Nonsurgical interventions (radiation therapy and chemotherapy) are used postoperatively and depend on the surgical staging.

Radiation Therapy. The oncologist prescribes radiation therapy to be delivered by external beam and/or brachytherapy for stage II and stage III cancers. Women with stage II disease may use brachytherapy (internal) radiation to prevent recurrence of vaginal cancer and improve survival.

The purpose of *brachytherapy* is to prevent disease recurrence. This treatment no longer requires a hospital stay and

Health Teaching for the Patient Having Brachytherapy for Gynecologic Cancer

Teach the patient to report any of these signs and symptoms to the health care provider immediately:
* Heavy vaginal bleeding
* Urethral burning for more than 24 hours
* Blood in the urine
* Extreme fatigue
* Severe diarrhea
* Fever over 100° F (38° C)
* Abdominal pain

Teach the patient that she is not radioactive between treatments and there are no restrictions on her interactions with others.

is done on an ambulatory care basis. The radiologist places an applicator within the woman's uterus through the vagina. After the correct position of the applicator is confirmed by x-ray, the radioactive isotope is placed in the applicator and remains for several minutes. This procedure may be repeated between 2 and 5 times once or twice a week. Some patients also have external beam radiation while having brachytherapy treatment sessions. There are no restrictions for the woman to stay away from her family or the public between treatments.

While the radioactive implant is in place, radiation is emitted that can affect other people. The amount of time needed for the therapy depends on the amount of radiation emitted from the source. The radiologist calculates the time needed for a specific dose of radiation.

Inform the patient that she is restricted to bedrest during the treatment session. Excessive movement in bed is restricted to prevent dislodgment of the radioactive source.

Chart 74-7 lists the best practices for radiation precautions while caring for the patient receiving brachytherapy. Teach patients about when to call the health care provider after each treatment session.

External *beam radiation therapy (EBRT)* may be used to treat any stage of endometrial cancer in combination with surgery, brachytherapy, and/or chemotherapy. Depending on the extent of the tumor, the treatment is given on an ambulatory care basis for 4 to 6 weeks. Tissue around the tumor and pelvic wall nodes also are treated. *Teach the patient to monitor for signs of skin breakdown, especially in the perineal area; to avoid sunbathing; and to avoid washing the markings outlining the treatment site.*

Drug Therapy. Chemotherapy is used as palliative treatment in advanced and recurrent disease when it has spread to distant parts of the body, but it is not always effective. Although the combination can vary, three of the most common agents used for endometrial cancer are doxorubicin (Adriamycin), cisplatin (Platinol), and paclitaxel (Taxol). Chapter 24 describes chemotherapy and general nursing care during treatment.

Every woman experiences cancer differently. Many complementary therapies have evidence of benefit in decreasing the side effects of drug therapy and boosting the immune system. Help her make informed, evidence-based decisions.

Encourage her to check with her oncologist and/or pharmacist because some alternative therapies can be harmful or interfere with cancer treatment. Current evidence-based information is available about mind-body therapies, healing touch, herbs, vitamins, nutrition, and biologic therapies at the American Cancer Society website (www.cancer.org).

Helping the Patient Develop Coping Strategies

Planning: Expected Outcomes. The patient is expected to develop coping strategies that will help her deal with the diagnosis and collaborative care for endometrial cancer.

Interventions. Women need to discuss their concerns about the presence of cancer and the potential for recurrence. Provide emotional support, and create an atmosphere that encourages them to ask questions or express their fears and concerns. Include family members or significant others in discussions when possible.

Reactions to radiation therapy vary. Some women feel radioactive or "unclean" after treatments and may exhibit withdrawal behaviors. Reassure them by correcting any misconceptions. Patients who have chemotherapy may be upset if alopecia (hair loss) occurs. Warn them of this possibility before treatment starts. Wigs, scarves, or turbans can be worn until the hair grows back. Many women select these replacements before they lose their hair. Others shave their heads and begin wearing them immediately as the treatment begins. Tell women about these options so that they can make the best decision for them.

Often patients experience emotional crises because of the physical effects of cancer treatments. Radical hysterectomy may be seen as mutilating. Both radiation and chemotherapy have side effects that change physical appearance and body image. Women often may have a grief reaction to these changes. The feelings of loss depend on the visibility of the loss and the loss of function. Help the patient adapt to the body changes. One way to do this is to encourage self-management as soon as her physical condition is stable. Use a calm and accepting attitude.

Death can occur with or without treatment. The patient and family want the woman to pass the 5-year survival mark without a recurrence of disease. If there is a recurrence, they may be hostile and have manifestations of a grief reaction. Encourage patients and their families to discuss their feelings. Refer to support services such as certified hospital chaplain or other spiritual leader, social worker, or counselor. Response to loss and grieving is discussed in Chapter 9.

Community-Based Care
Home Care Management

The woman with endometrial cancer is managed at home unless surgery is indicated. After surgery, she is usually discharged to her home. Home care after surgery for endometrial cancer is the same as that after a hysterectomy. (See discussion of Hysterectomy on p. 1619 in the Uterine Leiomyoma section.) Patients who are receiving chemotherapy or radiation therapy are treated on an ambulatory care basis. Most women are surprised by the fatigue caused by radiation and chemotherapy. Help the patient and her family plan daily activities around trips to the clinic or the health care provider's office. If the tumor recurs and cure is not likely, the woman and her family need to think about hospice care and whether she can be cared for in the home.

Teaching for Self-Management

Teach the patient to report vaginal or rectal bleeding, foul-smelling discharge, abdominal pain or distention, and hematuria to the health care provider. These symptoms may be the result of the disease or its treatment.

The high dose of radiation causes sterility, and vaginal shrinkage can occur. Vaginal dilators can be used with water-soluble lubricants for 10 minutes each day until sexual activity resumes (in 10 days to 6 weeks). Reassure the woman that she is not radioactive and that her partner will not "catch" cancer by engaging in sexual intercourse.

Review all prescribed drugs, including the dosage and schedule, effects, and side effects. Emphasize the importance of keeping appointments for follow-up care.

Health Care Resources

In the United States, local American Cancer Society chapters provide written materials about endometrial cancer and information about local support groups. Each province in Canada also has a division of the Canadian Cancer Society (www.cancer.ca). If the patient is in the terminal stages of cancer, hospice care may be appropriate (see Chapter 9). If nursing care is needed at home, the hospital nurse or case manager makes referrals to a home health care agency. A referral to a social services agency may be needed if the patient cannot meet the financial demands of treatment and long-term follow-up.

❓ DECISION-MAKING CHALLENGE

Patient-Centered Care; Evidence-Based Practice; Informatics; Teamwork and Collaboration

A 58-year-old woman is diagnosed with ovarian cancer today. She begins to cry and tells you that she "had a feeling all along" that she had the disease. No one in her family has had ovarian cancer, but she has two friends who recently died of the disease. She is scheduled for an exploratory laparotomy and tumor debulking in 3 days. Her oncologist told her that after she recovers from surgery, she will have brachytherapy and external beam radiation therapy (EBRT).

1. What preoperative teaching will you provide for this patient and why?
2. What will you tell her about restrictions associated with brachytherapy and EBRT?
3. Where would you search for evidence about her expected quality of life and prognosis?
4. What members may need to be involved in her care?

CERVICAL CANCER

Pathophysiology

The uterine cervix is covered with squamous cells on the outer cervix and columnar (glandular) cells that line the endocervical canal. Papanicolaou (Pap) tests sample cells from both areas as a screening test for cervical cancer. The squamo-columnar junction is the *transformation zone* where most cell abnormalities occur. The adolescent has more columnar cells exposed on the outer cervix, which may be one reason she is more vulnerable to sexually transmitted diseases (STDs) and human immune deficiency virus (HIV). In contrast, in the menopausal woman, the squamo-columnar junction may be higher up in the endocervical canal, making it difficult to sample for a Pap test.

Premalignant changes are described on a continuum from atypia (suspicious) to *cervical intraepithelial neoplasia (CIN 1)* to *carcinoma in situ (CIS)*, which is the most advanced premalignant change. It generally takes years for the cervical cells to transform from normal to premalignant to invasive cancer. Many CIN 2 lesions progress to high-grade dysplasia. CIN 3 lesions can progress to squamous cell carcinoma or adenocarcinoma in situ (AIS).

Most cervical cancers arise from the squamous cells on the outside of the cervix. The other cancers arise from the mucus-secreting glandular cells (adenocarcinoma) in the endocervical canal. The disease spreads by direct extension to the vaginal mucosa, lower uterine segment, parametrium, pelvic wall, bladder, and bowel. Metastasis is usually confined to the pelvis, but distant spread can occur through lymphatic spread and the circulation to the liver, lungs, or bones.

Etiology

Human papilloma virus (HPV) is the most common STD in the United States. Almost all women will have HPV sometime in their life, but not all types lead to cancer. Most cases of cervical cancer are caused by certain types of HPV. Women at the highest risk are those who have a long-standing high-risk HPV strain (Wells, 2008). The high-risk HPV types, especially strains 16 and 18, impair the tumor-suppressor gene and cause most of the cervical cancers. The unrestricted tissue growth can spread, becoming invasive and metastatic. Strains 6 and 11 are associated with genital warts. Risk factors for cervical cancer are listed in Table 74-3.

Incidence/Prevalence

Invasive cancer of the cervix is the third most common cancer of the female genital system, after ovarian and uterine cancer. Although much less common than breast cancer, cervical cancer has a lower 5-year survival rate (ACS, 2010).

The peak incidence occurs in patients in their mid-20s. It usually resolves spontaneously within a year. Carcinoma in situ (CIS)) occurs in women about 30 years old, and invasive cancer occurs most commonly in the late 40s (ACS, 2010).

Health Promotion and Maintenance

Girls and young women should receive one of the two currently used HPV vaccines, Gardasil and Cervarix, ideally before their first sexual contact to receive protection against the highest-risk HPV types that are responsible for most cervical cancers. Gardasil is indicated for ages 9 through 26 years. It is also given for boys and men (ages 9 through 26 years) to prevent genital warts because it protects against the 6 and 11 HPV strains.

Cervarix protects girls and women ages 10 through 25 years against infection for HPV strains 16 and 18 to prevent cervical cancer. It allows for longer-lasting protection when compared with Gardasil.

Teach all young patients about the importance of receiving the vaccine and the need to have the entire series (3 injections over 6 months). Tell them that the most frequent side effects are related to local irritation from the injections (e.g., pain, redness). Other common side effects include nausea, vomiting, dizziness, headache, and diarrhea.

The American Cancer Society (ACS) recommends that women have periodic pelvic examinations and Pap tests to screen for cervical cancer early. Teach women that they should begin these screening precautions within 3 years after having sexual intercourse or by the age of 21. Some health care providers, however, recommend the first examination and Pap test by age 18. For conventional Pap testing, *annual* screening is recommended by most experts. If the liquid test is used and the woman has no other risk factors (e.g., weakened immune system, HIV), it may be done *every 2 or 3 years* if she has three consecutive normal Pap smears and depending on the health care provider's recommendations. Teach women that if they have a hysterectomy and have no other health risk factors, a Pap test is no longer needed.

Instruct women ages 70 years and older who have had three consecutive normal Pap smears and no abnormal results that they can stop having Pap tests after a discussion with their health care provider. As women age, the usefulness of testing is questionable. The evidence about precise screening frequency remains conflicting (Wells, 2008).

PATIENT-CENTERED COLLABORATIVE CARE

ASSESSMENT

Physical Assessment/Clinical Manifestations

The patient who has preinvasive cancer is often asymptomatic. *The classic symptom of invasive cancer is painless vaginal bleeding.* Ask the patient if she has had or now has bleeding. It may start as spotting between menstrual periods or after sexual intercourse or douching. As the cancer grows, bleeding increases in frequency, duration, and amount and may become continuous.

Ask the woman if she has a watery, blood-tinged vaginal discharge that becomes dark and foul-smelling (occurs as the disease progresses). Leg pain (along the sciatic nerve) or swelling of one leg may be a late symptom or may indicate recurrent disease. Flank pain may be a late symptom of hydronephrosis, indicating advanced cancer pressing on the ureters, backing up the urine into the kidney. Ask the patient if she has had other signs of recurrence or metastasis such as:

- Unexplained weight loss
- Dysuria (painful urination)
- Pelvic pain (caused by pressure of the tumor on the bladder or the bowel)
- Hematuria (bloody urine)
- Rectal bleeding
- Chest pain
- Coughing

A physical examination may not reveal any abnormalities in early preinvasive cervical cancer. The internal pelvic examination may identify late-stage disease.

Diagnostic Assessment

If Pap results are abnormal, an *HPV-typing DNA test* of the cervical sample can determine the presence of one or more high-risk types. The health care provider may perform a colposcopic examination to view the transformation zone. Colposcopy is a procedure in which application of a 3% acetic acid solution is applied to the cervix. The cervix is then examined under magnification with a bright filter light that enhances the visualization of the characteristics of dysplasia or cancer. If abnormal tissue is recognized, multiple biopsies of the cervical tissue are performed.

If atypical glandular cells are suspected, the health care provider may perform an *endocervical curettage* (scraping of the endocervix wall) as well. Inform her that a small amount of bleeding is expected for up to 2 weeks after the biopsies.

INTERVENTIONS

Interventions for the woman with cervical cancer are similar to those for endometrial cancer: surgery, which is possibly followed by radiation and chemotherapy for later-stage disease.

Surgical Management

Early stage I management techniques include local cervical ablation therapies of electrosurgical excision, laser therapy, or cryosurgery. Small tumors that are only microinvasive are managed with excisional conization or hysterectomy. Early-stage *invasive* cancers are managed with radical surgery and radiation. Advanced inoperable cancers are treated with radiation. Factors that influence the choice of localized treatment versus surgical intervention include patient overall health, desire for future childbearing, tumor size, stage, cancer cell type, degree of lymph node involvement, and patient preference.

Early Surgical Procedures. The loop electrosurgical excision procedure (LEEP) is short (10 to 30 minutes) and is performed in a physician's office or in an ambulatory care setting with a local anesthetic injected into the cervix. A thin loop-wire electrode that transmits a painless electrical current is used to cut away affected tissue. LEEP is both a diagnostic procedure and a treatment, because it provides a specimen that can be examined by a pathologist to ensure the lesion was completely removed. Little discomfort is associated with this procedure. Spotting after the procedure is common. Teach patients to adhere for 3 weeks to the restrictions listed in Chart 74-8.

Laser therapy is also an office procedure used for early cancers. A laser beam is directed to the abnormal tissues, where energy from the beam is absorbed by the fluid in the tissues, causing them to vaporize. A small amount of bleeding occurs with the procedure, and the woman may have a slight vaginal discharge. Healing occurs in 6 to 12 weeks. A disadvantage of this procedure is that no specimen is available for study.

Cryotherapy involves freezing of the cancer, causing subsequent necrosis. The procedure is often painless, although

---

CHART 74-8 **PATIENT AND FAMILY EDUCATION: PREPARING FOR SELF-MANAGEMENT**

Care After Local Cervical Ablation Therapies

- Refrain from sexual intercourse.
- Do not use tampons.
- Do not douche.
- Take showers rather than tub baths.
- Avoid lifting heavy objects.
- Report any heavy vaginal bleeding, foul-smelling drainage, or fever.

The usual time period for these restrictions is 3 weeks. Your health care provider may prescribe a different (longer or shorter) time frame for you.

some women have slight cramping after the procedure. The patient has a heavy watery discharge for several weeks after the procedure. Instruct her to follow the restrictions in Chart 74-8.

In cases of microinvasive cancer, a *conization* can remove the affected tissue while still preserving fertility. This procedure is done when the lesion cannot be visualized by colposcopic examination. A cone-shaped area of cervix is removed surgically and sent to the laboratory to determine the extent of the cancer. Potential complications from this procedure include hemorrhage and uterine perforation. Long-term follow-up care is needed because new cancers can develop.

Hysterectomy. A total hysterectomy may be performed as treatment of microinvasive cancer if the woman does not want children or more children. A laparoscopic vaginal approach is commonly used. A radical hysterectomy and bilateral pelvic lymph node dissection may be as effective as radiation is for treating cancer that has extended beyond the cervix but not to the pelvic wall. Care for patients undergoing hysterectomy is found in the Uterine Leiomyoma section on p. 1619.

Nonsurgical Management

Radiation therapy is reserved for invasive cervical cancer. Brachytherapy and external beam radiation therapy are used in combination, depending on the extent and location of the lesion. The procedure is similar to that described on pp. 1622-1623 for endometrial cancer.

A combination of chemotherapy with cisplatin (Platinol) and radiation may also be used. This treatment modality shows increased survival times but increased toxicity for many patients. Examples of other drugs used alone or in combination include paclitaxel (Taxol), carboplatin, fluorouracil (5-FU), and mitomycin. See Chapter 24 for more information about the general nursing care for the patient on chemotherapy and radiation.

OVARIAN CANCER

Pathophysiology

Most ovarian cancers are epithelial tumors that grow on the surface of the ovaries. These tumors grow rapidly, spread quickly, and are often bilateral. Tumor cells spread by direct extension into nearby organs and through blood and lymph circulation to distant sites. Free-floating cancer cells also spread through the abdomen to seed new sites, usually accompanied by ascites (abdominal fluid).

Ovarian cancer seems to be disordered growth in response to excessive exposure to estrogen. This would explain the protective effects of pregnancies and oral contraceptive use, both of which interrupt the monthly estrogen exposure. Table 74-4 lists known and suspected risk factors for ovarian cancer.

Ovarian cancer is the leading cause of death from female reproductive cancers, but it is not the most common type of cancer. About 22,000 new cases are diagnosed each year, with 14,000 annual deaths (ACS, 2010). The incidence increases in women older than 50 years, and most are diagnosed after menopause. Family history accounts for a small percentage of cases. These women carry *BCRA1* or *BCRA2* genetic mutations. Of these, some choose to have a bilateral salpingo-oophorectomy (BSO) (removal of both ovaries and fallopian

TABLE 74-4	RISK FACTORS FOR OVARIAN CANCER
• Older than 40 years	• Colorectal cancer
• Family history of ovarian or breast cancer or HNPCC	• Infertility
• Diabetes mellitus	• *BRCA1* or *BRCA2* gene mutations
• Nulliparity	• Early menarche/late menopause
• Older than 30 years at first pregnancy	• Endometriosis
• Breast cancer	• Obesity/high-fat diet

HNPCC, Hereditary nonpolyposis colon cancer.

tubes). This surgery may reduce the risk for ovarian cancer by more than 90% in these patients (Nussbaum et al., 2007).

Survival rates are low because ovarian cancer is often not detected until its late stages. The aging of the population makes it important for nurses to teach women to "*think ovarian*" if they have vague abdominal and GI symptoms.

Health Promotion and Maintenance

Health promotion measures to help prevent ovarian cancer include maintaining a normal weight and eating a well-balanced diet. Women who have had children, used oral contraception for at least 5 years, and breast-fed their children also have less risk for having the disease (Bohnenkamp et al., 2007a).

PATIENT-CENTERED COLLABORATIVE CARE

ASSESSMENT

Most women with ovarian cancer have had mild symptoms for several months but may have thought they were due to normal perimenopausal changes or stress. They may report abdominal pain or swelling or have vague GI disturbances such as dyspepsia (indigestion) and gas. Ask the patient if she has had urinary frequency or incontinence, unexpected weight loss, and/or vaginal bleeding.

Complications of advanced metastatic cancer include:
- Pleural effusion
- Ascites
- Lymphedema
- Intestinal obstruction
- Malnutrition

On pelvic examination, an abdominal mass may not be palpable until it reaches a size of 4 to 6 inches (10 to 15 cm). Any enlarged ovary found after menopause should be evaluated as though it were malignant. A Pap smear is of limited value for detecting ovarian cancer.

A cancer antigen test, *CA-125,* measures the presence of damaged endometrial and uterine tissue in the blood. It may be elevated if ovarian cancer is present, but it can also be elevated in patients with endometriosis, fibroids, pelvic inflammatory disease, pregnancy, and even menses. It is also useful for monitoring a patient's progress during and after treatment. Transvaginal ultrasonography, chest radiography, and computed tomography (CT) are part of a complete workup to evaluate for metastasis. Complete blood work includes a liver profile if there is ascites.

The woman with ovarian cancer has concerns similar to those described for the patient with endometrial cancer.

Because the cancer is often diagnosed in an advanced stage, thoughts of death and dying, menopause, and loss of fertility come as a shock.

INTERVENTIONS

Nursing care of the patient with ovarian cancer is similar to that for endometrial or cervical cancer. The options for treatment depend on the extent of the cancer and usually include surgery first, followed by chemotherapy. Radiation is used for more widespread cancers.

Surgical Management

Diagnosis depends on surgical exploration. Exploratory laparotomy (abdominal surgery) is performed to diagnose, treat, and stage ovarian tumors. A total abdominal hysterectomy, bilateral salpingo-oophorectomy (removal of the ovaries and fallopian tubes), and pelvic and para-aortic lymph node dissection are usually performed. Very large tumors that cannot be removed are debulked (cytoreduction). These procedures can be performed via laparoscopic technique to decrease recovery time, minimize pain, and reduce postoperative complications. Ovarian cancer is staged during surgery.

Nursing care of the patient is similar to that for any patient having abdominal surgery (see Chapter 18). As for any patient after abdominal surgery, assess vital signs and pain and maintain catheters and drains. Teach her the importance of anti-embolism stockings, incentive spirometry, and early ambulation. Infections after ovarian cancer surgery commonly affect the respiratory and urinary tract. Assess vital signs, and monitor the quantity and quality of urine output.

Nonsurgical Management

After cytoreduction and staging of ovarian cancer, chemotherapy is the treatment that is used the most often. For all stages of ovarian cancer, cisplatin (Platinol), carboplatin, and taxanes of all types are the most common postoperative *drugs* used for treating ovarian cancer. They may be given IV and/or intraperitoneally. Intraperitoneal (IP) therapy is described in Chapter 15. The drugs are usually given every 3 to 4 weeks for six cycles in an inpatient or ambulatory care setting (Blewitt, 2010). New drugs are being tested that use monoclonal antibodies, hormones, and agents that target cell growth and tumor blood supply.

Community-Based Care

Patients having surgery usually return to their home. Teach them to avoid tampons, douches, and sexual intercourse for at least 6 weeks or as instructed by the health care provider. Remind them to keep their follow-up surgical appointment and talk with the health care provider about resuming usual activities. Refer patients and their families to Gilda's Club (www.gildasclub.org) and the National Ovarian Cancer Coalition (NOCC) (www.ovarian.org) for more information and support groups. In Canada, the National Ovarian Cancer Association (www.ovariancanada.org) is available for the same purpose.

For patients with advanced metastatic disease, collaborate with the case manager, patient, and family for possible referral to hospice. Chapter 9 discusses end-of-life care and hospice in detail. The woman who is faced with the diagnosis of advanced ovarian cancer is usually very anxious about dying. Encourage her to discuss her feelings. Provide realistic assurance, as well as accurate information about treatments. Patients report their most distressing moments in the hospital were when they thought they were not getting adequate information. Encourage them to use their support systems of family members, friends, and clergy, including the hospital chaplain. Grief counseling is very appropriate. A visit from another woman who has survived a similar disease or referral to a support group may decrease fears. Refer the patient who fears passing the *BRCA1* or *BRCA2* gene to her daughter for genetic counseling and testing.

Ovarian cancer has a high recurrence rate. After recurrence, the cancer is treatable but no longer curable. If this occurs, the patient may deny symptoms at first or express feelings of anger and grief. The family is often fearful of the outcome. Provide encouragement and support during this difficult time, and help the patient and her family work through their grief and prepare for death.

NURSING CONCEPT REVIEW

What might you NOTICE if the patient is experiencing impaired sexuality as a result of gynecologic problems?

- Irregular or abnormal vaginal bleeding
- Vaginal discharge
- Report of perineal itching or burning
- Report of painful intercourse
- Abdominal distention and discomfort
- Report of irritability, anxiety, or depression
- Report of decreased libido

What should you INTERPRET and how should you RESPOND to the patient experiencing impaired sexuality as a result of gynecologic problems?

Perform and interpret physical assessment, including:
- Conducting an abdominal assessment
- Conducting a thorough pain assessment
- Checking for bleeding and amount (number of pads or tampons)
- Listening to patient's concerns about her sexuality

Respond by:
- Helping the patient into a sitting position
- Providing pain relief measures, such as heat and analgesia
- Referring the patient to a sexual or intimacy counselor (including the patient's partner if desired)

On what should you REFLECT?
- Think about what else you can do to help provide psychosocial support.
- Prepare for complications, such as hemorrhage, if the patient is bleeding.
- Evaluate pain level after interventions.

GET READY FOR THE NCLEX® EXAMINATION!

KEY POINTS

Review these Key Points for each NCLEX Examination Client Needs Category.

Safe and Effective Care Environment
- Refer patients with gynecologic problems to appropriate community resources such as the American Cancer Society and the Endometriosis Association.
- Collaborate with the case manager when planning care for patients with gynecologic cancers.

Health Promotion and Maintenance
- Teach women to follow the American Cancer Society's screening guidelines to prevent and early-detect for gynecologic cancers.
- Teach all women to have regular Pap tests based on their risk factors.
- Teach women to practice safe sex to prevent infections of the reproductive organs.
- Teach women about risk factors for gynecologic cancers as described in Tables 74-3 and 74-4.
- Teach women how to prevent toxic shock syndrome (TSS) as listed in Chart 74-4.

Psychosocial Integrity
- Explain all tests, procedures, and treatments, especially if they cause discomfort during or after the procedures.

- Assess the patient's anxiety before any gynecologic surgery.
- Encourage women who are having procedures that may interfere with fertility to express feelings of fear or grief.
- Encourage women with chronic or serious health problems to consider using support groups or counseling.

Physiological Integrity
- Urge any woman who experiences postmenopausal vaginal bleeding to consult with her gynecologic health care provider as soon as possible.
- Assess for clinical manifestations of TSS as listed in Chart 74-3.
- Teach patients about specific restrictions after local cervical ablation therapy (see Chart 74-8).
- When caring for a patient who has a radioactive implant, use best practices as described in Chart 74-7.
- Teach the patient who is going home after a hysterectomy how to monitor for infection or other complications.
- Instruct patients receiving external beam radiation to the abdomen to gently wash the area; to not apply creams or lotions (unless prescribed by the radiologist); to not wash off marking; to avoid exposing the area to sunlight or temperature extremes; and to wear soft, nonirritating clothing.

Care of Male Patients with Reproductive Problems

Donna D. Ignatavicius

ꂠvolve WEBSITE

http://evolve.elsevier.com/Iggy/

Answer Key for NCLEX Examination Challenges and
   Decision-Making Challenges
Audio Glossary
Concept Map Creator

Concept Map: Benign Prostatic Hyperplasia (BPH)
Key Points
Review Questions for the NCLEX® Examination

LEARNING OUTCOMES

Safe and Effective Care Environment

1. Identify health care team members to provide collaborative care and discharge planning for patients with male reproductive problems.

Health Promotion and Maintenance

2. Teach men and their partners about community resources for reproductive cancers.
3. Evaluate patient risk factors for male reproductive cancers.
4. Develop a health teaching plan for men to prevent or detect early male reproductive cancers.

Psychosocial Integrity

5. Assess the patient's acceptance of body image changes that may result from male reproductive surgery.
6. Explain the psychosocial needs of men who have male reproductive problems.

Physiological Integrity

7. Perform a focused physical assessment of the man's reproductive system.
8. Describe the mechanisms of action, side effects, and nursing implications for pharmacologic management of benign prostatic hyperplasia (BPH).

9. Develop a postoperative plan of care for a patient undergoing surgery for benign prostatic hyperplasia.
10. Incorporate complementary and alternative therapies into the patient's plan of care.
11. Discuss treatment options for prostate cancer with patients, partners, and/or families.
12. Provide preoperative teaching for patients having a radical prostatectomy.
13. Develop a teaching plan for the patient and family about the role of drug therapy in treating prostate cancer.
14. Identify adverse effects of radiation therapy for reproductive cancers.
15. Develop a community-based plan of care for a man with prostate cancer.
16. Describe the options for treating erectile dysfunction.
17. Discuss cultural considerations related to male reproductive problems.
18. Develop a plan of care for a patient with testicular cancer, including fertility issues.
19. Compare the assessment and treatment for hydrocele, spermatocele, and varicocele.

Male reproductive problems can range from short-term infections to long-term health care problems that may require end-of-life care. Any health issue that affects the male reproductive system can affect the human need for *sexuality.* For example, some patients have surgeries that damage essential nerves that are needed to have an erection. Others have disorders that psychologically prevent the patient from engaging in his usual sexual activity.

The role of the nurse and other health care team members is to be open, supportive, and nonjudgmental when caring

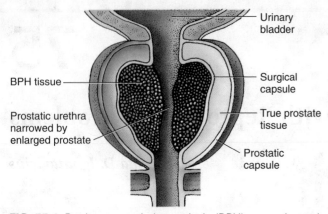

FIG. 75-1 Benign prostatic hyperplasia (BPH) grows inward, causing narrowing of the urethra.

for men with reproductive problems. Respect the man's privacy at all times.

BENIGN PROSTATIC HYPERPLASIA

Pathophysiology

Benign prostatic hyperplasia (BPH) is a very common health problem, but the exact cause is unclear. It is likely the result of a combination of aging and the influence of androgens that are present in prostate tissue, such as dihydrotestosterone (DHT) (McCance et al., 2010). With aging and increased DHT levels, the glandular units in the prostate undergo nodular tissue hyperplasia (an increase in the number of cells). This altered tissue promotes local inflammation by attracting cytokines and other substances (McCance et al., 2010).

As the prostate gland enlarges, it extends upward into the bladder and inward, causing *bladder outlet obstruction* (Fig. 75-1). In response, the urinary system is affected in several ways. First, the detrusor (bladder) muscle thickens to help urine push past the enlarged prostate gland (McCance et al., 2010). In spite of the bladder muscle change, the patient has increased residual urine (stasis) and chronic urinary retention. The increased volume of residual urine often causes overflow urinary incontinence, in which the urine "leaks" around the enlarged prostate causing dribbling. Urinary stasis can also result in urinary tract infections and bladder calculi (stones).

In a few patients, the prostate becomes very large and the man cannot void (acute urinary retention [AUR]). The patient with this problem requires emergent care. In other patients, chronic urinary retention may result in a backup of urine and cause a gradual dilation of the ureters (hydroureter) and kidneys (hydronephrosis) if BPH is not treated. These problems can lead to chronic kidney disease as described in Chapter 71.

PATIENT-CENTERED COLLABORATIVE CARE

❚ ASSESSMENT

❚ History

When taking a history, several standardized assessment tools are used to help the health care provider determine the severity of lower urinary tract symptoms (LUTS) associated with prostatic enlargement. One of the most commonly used assessments is the International Prostate Symptom Score (I-PSS), which incorporates the American Urological Association Symptom Index (AUA-SI) (Fig. 75-2) as questions 1 through 7. The additional question included on the I-PSS is the effect of the patient's urinary symptoms on quality of life. Most patients complete the questions as a self-administered tool because it is available in many languages. If the patient is illiterate or does not feel like reading the questions, the nurse or health care provider can ask them. Be sure that older men wear their glasses or contact lenses, if needed.

Physical Assessment/Clinical Manifestations

Ask about the patient's current urinary pattern. Assess for urinary frequency and urgency. Determine the number of times the patient awakens during the night to void (nocturia). Other symptoms of LUTS include:
- Difficulty in starting (hesitancy) and continuing urination
- Reduced force and size of the urinary stream ("weak" stream)
- Sensation of incomplete bladder emptying
- Straining to begin urination
- Post-void (after voiding) dribbling or leaking

If frequency and nocturia do not occur with restricted urinary flow, the patient may have an infection or other bladder problem. Ask whether the patient has had hematuria (blood in the urine) when starting the urine stream or at the end of voiding. BPH is a common cause of hematuria in older men.

The advanced practice nurse or other health care provider examines the patient for physical changes of the prostate gland. Remind the patient to void before the physical examination. Inspect and palpate the abdomen for a distended bladder. The health care provider may percuss the bladder. If the patient has a sense of urgency when gentle pressure is applied, the bladder may be distended. Obese patients are best assessed by percussion or bedside ultrasound bladder scanner rather than by inspection or palpation.

Prepare the patient for the prostate gland examination. Tell him that he may feel the urge to urinate as the prostate is palpated. Because the prostate is close to the rectal wall, it is easily examined by digital rectal examination (DRE). Help the patient bend over the examination table or assume a side-lying fetal position, whichever is the easiest position for him. The health care provider examines the prostate for size and consistency. BPH presents as a uniform, elastic, nontender enlargement, whereas cancer of the prostate gland feels like a stony-hard nodule. Advise the patient that after the prostate gland is palpated, it may be massaged to obtain a fluid sample for examination to rule out prostatitis (inflammation and possible infection of the prostate), a common problem that can occur with BPH. If the patient has bacterial prostatitis, he is treated with broad-spectrum antibiotic therapy for at least 30 days to prevent the spread of infection (McCance et al., 2010).

Psychosocial Assessment

Patients who have nocturia and other LUTS may be irritable or depressed as a result of interrupted sleep and annoying visits to the bathroom. Assess the effect of sleep interruptions on the patient's mood and mental status.

[Figure labels: Urinary bladder; BPH tissue; Surgical capsule; Prostatic urethra narrowed by enlarged prostate; True prostate tissue; Prostatic capsule]

International Prostate Symptom Score (I-PSS)

Patient Name:_____ Date of Birth:_____ Date Completed_____

In the past month:	Not at All	Less Than 1 in 5 Times	Less Than Half the Time	About Half the Time	More Than Half the Time	Almost Always	Your Score
1. Incomplete Emptying How often have you had the sensation of not emptying your bladder?	0	1	2	3	4	5	
2. Frequency How often have you had to urinate less than every 2 hours?	0	1	2	3	4	5	
3. Intermittency How often have you found you stopped and started again several times when you urinated?	0	1	2	3	4	5	
4. Urgency How often have you found it difficult to postpone urination?	0	1	2	3	4	5	
5. Weak Stream How often have you had a weak urinary stream?	0	1	2	3	4	5	
6. Straining How often have you had to strain to start urination?	0	1	2	3	4	5	
	None	1 Time	2 Times	3 Times	4 Times	5 Times	
7. Nocturia How many times do you typically get up at night to urinate?	0	1	2	3	4	5	
Total I-PSS Score							

Score: 1-7: Mild   8-19: Moderate   20-35: Severe

Quality of Life Due to Urinary Symptoms	Delighted	Pleased	Mostly Satisfied	Mixed	Mostly Dissatisfied	Unhappy	Terrible
If you were to spend the rest of your life with your urinary condition just the way it is now, how would you feel about that?	0	1	2	3	4	5	6

FIG. 75-2 The International Prostate Symptom Score (I-PSS). *Continued*

About the I-PSS

The International Prostate Symptom Score (I-PSS) is based on the answers to seven questions concerning urinary symptoms and one question concerning quality of life. Each question concerning urinary symptoms allows the patient to choose one out of six answers indicating increasing severity of the particular symptom. The answers are assigned points from 0 to 5. The total score can therefore range from 0 to 35 (asymptomatic to very symptomatic).

The questions refer to the following urinary symptoms:

Questions	Symptom
1	Incomplete emptying
2	Frequency
3	Intermittency
4	Urgency
5	Weak Stream
6	Straining
7	Nocturia

Question 8 refers to the patient's perceived quality of life.

The first seven questions of the I-PSS are identical to the questions appearing on the American Urological Association (AUA) Symptom Index, which currently categorizes symptoms as follows:

Mild (symptom score less than or equal to 7)
Moderate (symptom score range 8 to 19)
Severe (symptom score range 20 to 35)

The International Scientific Committee (SCI), under the patronage of the World Health Organization (WHO) and the International Union Against Cancer (UICC), recommends the use of only a single question to assess the quality of life. The answers to this question range from "delighted" to "terrible," or 0 to 6. Although this single question may or may not capture the global impact of benign prostatic hyperplasia (BPH) symptoms or quality of life, it may serve as a valuable starting point for a doctor-patient conversation.

The SCI has agreed to use the symptom index for BPH, which has been developed by the AUA Measurement Committee, as the official worldwide symptoms assessment tool for patients suffering from prostatism.

The SCI recommends that physicians consider the following components for a basic diagnostic workup: history; physical examination; appropriate labs such as U/A, creatinine, etc.; and DRE or other evaluation to rule out prostate cancer.

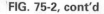

FIG. 75-2, cont'd

Post-void dribbling and overflow incontinence may cause embarrassment and prevent the patient from socializing or leaving his home. For some patients, this social isolation can affect quality of life and lead to clinical depression and/or severe anxiety. Johnson et al. (2010) found a strong correlation between depression and BPH in older men. Depressed patients were three times more likely to have severe symptoms.

Laboratory Assessment

A urinalysis and culture are typically obtained to diagnose urinary tract infection and microscopic hematuria. If infection is present, the urinalysis measures the number of white blood cells (WBCs).

Other laboratory studies that may be performed include:
- A complete blood count (CBC) to evaluate any evidence of systemic infection (elevated WBCs) or anemia (decreased red blood cells [RBCs]) from hematuria
- Blood urea nitrogen (BUN) and serum creatinine levels to evaluate renal function (both are usually elevated with kidney disease)
- A prostate-specific antigen (PSA) and a serum acid phosphatase level if prostate cancer is suspected (both are typically elevated in patients who have prostate cancer)
- Culture and sensitivity of prostatic fluid (if expressed during the examination)

Other Diagnostic Assessment

Imaging studies that are typically performed are *transabdominal ultrasound* and *transrectal ultrasound (TRUS)*. The patient having a TRUS lies on his side while the transducer is inserted into the rectum for viewing the prostate and surrounding structures. A tissue biopsy may also be done if the health care provider is uncertain whether the prostatic problem is benign or malignant.

In some cases, the physician uses a cystoscope to view the interior of the bladder, the bladder neck, and the urethra. This examination is used to study the presence and effect of bladder neck obstruction. The procedure is usually done in an ambulatory care setting. See Chapter 69 for a detailed description of *cystoscopy* and the nursing care needed for patients having this procedure.

Residual urine may be determined by *bladder ultrasound* immediately after the patient voids. As an alternative, because the patient voids before cystoscopy, residual urine may be measured when the cystoscope is inserted. *Urodynamic pressure-flow studies* may help diagnose and grade bladder outlet obstruction and detrusor muscle function.

ANALYSIS

The priority problem for the patient with benign prostatic hyperplasia (BPH) is Impaired Urinary Elimination related to bladder outlet obstruction.

PLANNING AND IMPLEMENTATION

Improving Urinary Elimination

Planning: Expected Outcomes. The patient with BPH is expected to have a normal urinary elimination pattern without urinary hesitancy, urgency, or infection.

Interventions. Patients with symptomatic BPH are first treated with nonsurgical interventions, such as drug therapy. The Concept Map on p. 1634 shows nursing assessment and collaborative interventions for the patient with BPH.

Nonsurgical Management. Drug therapy is a popular option for treating BPH. For patients with AUR or for those who do not respond or cannot tolerate drug therapy, noninvasive procedures or surgery is the treatment of choice.

Drug Therapy. Drugs from two major categories may be used alone, but most commonly they are given in combination. The health care provider usually prescribes a *5-alpha reductase inhibitor (5-ARI) as first-line drug therapy.* Examples of these drugs are finasteride (Proscar) and dutasteride (Avodart). Normally, testosterone is converted to DHT in the prostate gland by the enzyme *5-alpha reductase.* By taking an enzyme-inhibiting agent, the patient's DHT levels decrease, which results in reducing the enlarged prostate.

! NURSING SAFETY PRIORITY

Drug Alert

Remind patients who are being treated with a 5-ARI for BPH that they may need to take it for as long as 6 months before improvement is noticed. Teach them about possible side effects, which include erectile dysfunction (ED), decreased libido (sexual desire), and dizziness due to orthostatic hypotension. Remind them to change positions carefully and slowly.

The alpha-adrenergic receptors in prostatic smooth muscle enable the prostate gland to respond to *alpha-1 selective blocking agents,* such as tamsulosin (Flomax), alfuzosin (Uroxatral), doxazosin (Cardura, Cardura-1 ✦), terazosin (Hytrin), and silodosin (Rapaflo). Tamsulosin is also available as an over-the-counter (OTC) drug. These drugs relax smooth muscles in the prostate gland, creating less urinary resistance and improved urinary flow. They also cause peripheral vasodilation and reduced peripheral vascular resistance.

! NURSING SAFETY PRIORITY

Drug Alert

If giving alpha blockers in an inpatient setting, assess for orthostatic (postural) hypotension, tachycardia, and syncope ("blackout"), especially after the first dose is given to older men. If the patient is taking the drug at home, teach him to be careful when changing position and to report any weakness, lightheadedness, or dizziness to the health care provider immediately. Bedtime dosing may decrease the risk for problems related to hypotension. Drugs used to treat erection problems (e.g., Viagra) can worsen these side effects. Teach patients taking a 5-ARI or alpha blocking drug to keep all appointments for follow-up laboratory testing because both drug classes can cause liver dysfunction.

The most effective drug therapy approach for many patients is a combination of a 5-ARI drug and an alpha-1 selective blocking agent. A commonly prescribed drug regimen is finasteride and doxazosin. Newer drugs, such as Jalyn, provide a combination of dutasteride and tamsulosin in a once-a-day capsule.

Other drugs may be helpful in managing specific urinary symptoms. For example, low-dose oral desmopressin, a synthetic antidiuretic analog, has been used successfully for nocturia (Wang et al., 2011). Drugs being tested for their effectiveness in treating BPH include bisphosphonates, ezetimibe (Zetia), Botox, and Nymox.

Complementary and Alternative Therapies. Although many men use *Serenoa repens* (saw palmetto extract), a plant extract, to help manage the urinary symptoms associated with BPH, studies on the effectiveness of this herb have not shown that it is effective (Tackland et al., 2009). Teach patients who want to try these herbs and other natural substances that scientific evidence to prove they are useful is lacking. However, if they choose to take them, remind them to check with their health care provider before taking any OTC natural substance. Some herbs interfere with prescription drugs the patient may be taking for other health problems. Side effects, such as abdominal pain, nausea, and vomiting, are mild, reversible, and infrequent (Agbabiaka et al., 2009).

Other Nonsurgical Interventions. Other interventions that may reduce obstructive symptoms include those that cause the release of prostatic fluid such as frequent sexual intercourse. This approach is helpful for the man whose obstructive symptoms result from an enlarged prostate with a large amount of retained prostatic fluid.

Teach patients with BPH to avoid drinking large amounts of fluid in a short time; to avoid alcohol, diuretics, and caffeine; and to void as soon as they feel the urge. These measures are aimed at preventing overdistention of the bladder, which may result in loss of detrusor muscle tone. Teach patients to avoid any drugs that can cause urinary retention, especially anticholinergics, antihistamines, and decongestants. Emphasize the importance of telling any health care

Concept Map: Benign Prostatic Hyperplasia (BPH)

INTERVENTIONS

1 Nonjudgment

Respect privacy at all times.
Being open, supportive, and nonjudgmental when caring for the patient with reproductive problems facilitates trust.

2 Physical Assessment

Perform focused assessment of urinary pattern: frequency, hesitancy, urgency, presence of weak stream, nocturia, sensation of incomplete emptying, straining, hematuria, and postvoid dribbling.
Evaluates whether BPH is causing hematuria. If frequency and nocturia do not occur with restricted urinary flow, it may be from infection or other bladder problem.

3 Medications

Explain the mechanisms of action, side effects, and implications for drug therapy for BPH.
Minimizes side effects and the potential for injury.

4 Nursing Safety Priority: Drug Alert!

- Assess for orthostatic hypotension, tachycardia, and syncope from alpha-blockers.
  Minimizes potential for injury from falls from orthostatic hypotension.
- Instruct the patient to report weakness, light-headedness, or dizziness; monitor liver function, and side effects, including ED and decreased libido.
  Providing accurate discharge information prevents serious complications.

5 Lab Findings

- Obtain U/A and culture and CBC.
  U/A and culture detects UTI and hematuria; ↑ WBC is a sign of infection, ↓ RBC indicates anemia from hematuria.
- Obtain BUN and serum creatinine, PSA, and serum acid phosphatase level.
  BUN and serum creatinine increase detects renal dysfunction; increased PSA and serum phosphatase detects prostate cancer.
- Obtain C/S of prostatic fluid if expressed during the exam.

6 Teach/Reduce Obstructive Symptoms

- Instruct to avoid large amounts of fluid, alcohol, diuretics, caffeine; void as soon as the urge is felt.
  Prevents bladder overdistention.
- Instruct to avoid frequent sexual intercourse.
  Releases prostatic fluid.
- Teach to avoid anticholinergics, antihistamines, and decongestants.
  These medications cause urine retention.

7 Psychosocial Integrity

Assess the patient's acceptance of body image related to BPH and impact of sleep interruptions on mood and mental status.
Evaluates irritability or depression that may occur with nocturia. Evaluates embarrassment of postvoid incontinence that can prevent socialization. Evaluates effect on sexuality.

8 Herbal Remedies

Remind the patient to check with their provider before taking complementary therapies.
Teaches patients that scientific evidence is lacking. Some herbs such as saw palmetto used for urinary symptoms can interfere with prescription drugs.

9 Treatment Options – TURP

If surgery is a chosen treatment option, consider the patient's general physical condition, size of prostate, patient preferences, anxiety, and misconceptions.
Assists with options for treatment of BPH and prevents postoperative complications.

Concept Map by Deanne A. Blach, MSN, RN

EXPECTED OUTCOMES

Normal urinary elimination pattern without urinary hesitancy, urgency, or infection.

Planning

Priority Patient Problem

Impaired Urinary Elimination related to bladder outlet obstruction

Analysis

HISTORY

Kevin Waller, a 63-year-old with BPH, is admitted with a UTI, hematuria, and hydronephrosis. His wife says their sexual relationship has been nonexistent due to her husband's BPH. He has used saw palmetto extract for his urinary symptoms with some relief.

As the prostate gland enlarges, bladder outlet obstruction occurs and the patient develops urinary stasis and retention.

- Increased volume of residual → overflow incontinence → urine "leaks" around enlarged prostate → dribbling
- Urinary stasis → UTI and bladder calculi
- Chronic retention → backup of urine causes gradual dilation of ureters, hydronephrosis if not treated

provider about the diagnosis of BPH so that these drugs are not prescribed.

If drug therapy or other measures are not helpful in relieving urinary symptoms, several noninvasive techniques are available to destroy excess prostate tissue using a variety of heat methods (thermotherapy). These procedures are often done in a physician's office or another ambulatory care setting. Examples include:

- Transurethral needle ablation (TUNA) (low radio-frequency energy shrinks the prostate)
- Transurethral microwave therapy (TUMT) (high temperatures heat and destroy excess tissue)
- Interstitial laser coagulation (ILC), also called contact laser prostatectomy (CLP) (laser energy coagulates excess tissue)
- Electrovaporization of the prostate (EVAP) (high-frequency electrical current cuts and vaporizes excess tissue)

Prostatic stents may be placed into the urethra to maintain permanent patency after a procedure for destroying or removing prostatic tissue. All of these highly technical treatments use local or regional anesthesia and do not require an indwelling urinary catheter. They are also associated with less risk for complications such as intraoperative bleeding and erectile dysfunction when compared with traditional surgical approaches. Patients can return to their usual activities in a day or two.

Surgical Management. For patients who are not candidates for nonsurgical management or do not want to take drugs or have other treatment options, surgery may be performed. The gold standard continues to be a transurethral resection of the prostate (TURP) in which the enlarged portion of the prostate is removed through an endoscopic instrument. The newer holmium laser enucleation of the prostate (HoLEP) procedure is a minimally invasive surgical technique that is gaining popularity. For a few men, an open prostatectomy (entire prostate removal) may be performed (see discussion of Surgical Management on p. 1639 in the Prostate Cancer section). Some or all of these criteria indicate the need for surgery:

- Acute urinary retention (AUR)
- Chronic urinary tract infections secondary to residual urine in the bladder
- Hematuria
- Hydronephrosis

Preoperative Care. When planning surgical interventions, the patient's general physical condition, the size of the prostate gland, and the man's preferences are considered. The patient may have many fears and misconceptions about prostate surgery, such as believing that automatic loss of sexual functioning or permanent incontinence will occur. Assess the patient's anxiety, correct any misconceptions about the surgery, and provide accurate information to him and his family. Regardless of the type of surgery to be performed, provide information about anesthesia (see Chapter 17). The patient may have other medical problems that increase the risk for complications of general anesthesia and may be advised to have regional anesthesia. Epidural and spinal anesthesia are the most common types of anesthesia used for a TURP. Because the patient is awake, it is easier to assess for hyponatremia (low serum sodium), fluid overload, and water intoxication, which can result from large bladder irrigations.

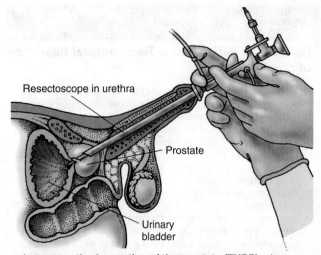

Resectoscope in urethra

Prostate

Urinary bladder

In **transurethral resection of the prostate (TURP),** the surgeon inserts a resectoscope through the urethra and into the bladder and removes pieces of tissue from the prostate gland.

FIG. 75-3 Transurethral resection of the prostate procedure used for benign prostatic hyperplasia.

After a TURP, all patients have an indwelling urethral catheter for at least a day. *Be sure that they know that they will feel the urge to void while the catheter is in place.* Tell the patient that he will likely have traction on the catheter that may cause discomfort. However, reassure him that analgesics will be prescribed to relieve his pain. Explain that it is normal for the urine to be blood-tinged after surgery. Small blood clots and tissue debris may pass while the catheter is in place and immediately after it is removed.

Operative Procedures. The traditional TURP is a "closed" surgery. To perform the procedure, the surgeon inserts a resectoscope (an instrument similar to a cystoscope, but with a cutting and cauterizing loop) through the urethra (Fig. 75-3). The enlarged portion of the prostate gland is then removed in small pieces (prostate chips). A similar procedure is the transurethral incision of the prostate (TUIP), in which small cuts are made into the prostate to relieve pressure on the urethra. This alternate technique is used for smaller prostates. To prevent bleeding and excess clotting, a fibrinolytic inhibitor like tranexamic acid (Cyklokapron) may be used during surgery.

The disadvantage of a TURP is that, because only small pieces of the gland are removed, remaining prostate tissue may continue to grow and cause urinary obstruction, requiring additional TURPs. Also, urethral trauma from the resectoscope with resulting urethral strictures is possible.

In many large medical centers around the world, specialists can perform newer surgical treatments, such as the *holmium laser enucleation of the prostate (HoLEP)* (Eltabey et al., 2010). For this procedure, the surgeon uses the laser to remove the obstructive prostatic tissue and push it into the bladder for removal and seals all blood vessels. Very little blood is lost during the short procedure and is therefore safe for patients taking anticoagulants.

Postoperative Care. After both the TURP and HoLEP procedures, a urinary catheter is placed into the bladder. Traction is often applied on the catheter for the patient having a TURP by pulling it taut and taping it to the patient's abdomen or

CHART 75-1 BEST PRACTICE FOR PATIENT SAFETY & QUALITY CARE

Care of the Patient After Transurethral Resection of the Prostate

- Monitor the patient closely for signs of infection. Older men undergoing prostate surgery often also have underlying chronic diseases (e.g., cardiovascular disease, chronic lung disease, diabetes).
- Help the patient out of the bed to the chair as soon as permitted to prevent complications of immobility. Older men may need assistance because of underlying changes in the musculoskeletal system (e.g., decreased range of motion, stiffness in joints). These patients are at *high risk* for falls.
- Assess the patient's pain every 2 to 4 hours, and intervene as needed to control pain.
- Provide a safe environment for the patient. Anticipate a temporary change in mental status for the older patient in the immediate postoperative period as a result of anesthetics and unfamiliar surroundings. Reorient the patient frequently. Keep catheter tubes secure.
- Use normal saline solution for the bladder irrigant unless otherwise prescribed. Normal saline solution is isotonic.
- Monitor the color, consistency, and amount of urine output.
- Check the drainage tubing frequently for external obstructions (e.g., kinks) and internal obstructions (e.g., blood clots, decreased output).
- Assess the patient for reports of severe bladder spasms with decreased urinary output, which may indicate obstruction.
- If the urinary catheter is obstructed, irrigate the catheter per agency or surgeon protocol.
- Notify the physician immediately if the obstruction does not resolve by hand irrigation or if the urinary return becomes ketchup-like.

thigh. If the catheter is taped to the patient's thigh, instruct him to keep his leg straight. The patient having the HoLEP procedure has a urinary catheter overnight, but the patient with a TURP has a catheter in place for several days. In some cases, the patient is discharged with the catheter in place.

CONSIDERATIONS FOR OLDER ADULTS

When caring for older men who may become confused after surgery, reorient them frequently and remind them not to pull on the catheter. If the patient is restless or "picks" at tubes, provide a familiar object such as a family picture for him to hold for distraction and a feeling of security. Do not restrain the patient unless all other alternatives have failed.

Remind the patient that because of the urinary catheter's large diameter and the pressure of the retention balloon on the internal sphincter of the bladder, he will feel the urge to void continuously. This is a normal sensation, not a surgical complication. Advise the patient not to try to void around the catheter, which causes the bladder muscles to contract and may result in painful spasms. Chart 75-1 summarizes the nursing care for patients having a TURP.

When the urinary catheter is removed, the patient may experience burning on urination and some urinary frequency, dribbling, and leakage. Reassure him that these symptoms are normal and will decrease. The patient may also pass small clots and tissue debris for several days after the TURP. *Instruct him to increase fluid intake to at least 2000 to 2500 mL daily, which helps decrease dysuria and keep the urine clear.* An older

! NURSING SAFETY PRIORITY

Critical Rescue

After a TURP, monitor the patient's urine output every 2 hours and vital signs, including pain assessment, every 4 hours for the first postoperative day. Assess for postoperative bleeding. *Patients who undergo a TURP or open prostatectomy are at risk for severe bleeding or hemorrhage after surgery. Although rare, bleeding is most likely within the first 24 hours.* Blood transfusions are commonly given after a TURP surgery but are not needed after the HoLEP procedure. Bladder spasms or movement may trigger fresh bleeding from previously controlled vessels. This bleeding may be arterial or venous, but venous bleeding is more common.

If the bleeding is arterial, the urinary drainage is bright red or ketchup-like with numerous clots. If arterial bleeding occurs, notify the surgeon immediately, and irrigate the catheter with normal saline solution per physician or hospital protocol. In rare instances, the surgeon may prescribe aminocaproic acid (Amicar) to control bleeding. If this drug does not work, surgical intervention may be needed to clear the bladder of clots and to stop bleeding.

If the bleeding is venous, *the urine output is burgundy, with or without any change in vital signs. Inform the surgeon of any bleeding.* Closely monitor the patient's hemoglobin (Hgb) and hematocrit (Hct) levels for anemia as a result of blood loss.

patient who has renal disease or who is at risk for heart failure may not be able to tolerate this much fluid. By the time of discharge (usually 2 to 3 days after surgery), he should be voiding 150 to 200 mL of clear yellow urine every 3 to 4 hours. By discharge, pain is minimal and analgesics may not be required.

Observe for other possible but uncommon complications of TURP, such as infection and incontinence. Teach the patient that sexual function should not be affected after surgery but that retrograde ejaculation is possible. In this case, most of the semen flows backwards into the bladder so only a small amount will be ejaculated from the penis.

Community-Based Care

The patient with benign prostatic hyperplasia (BPH) is typically managed at home. Patients who have surgery are also discharged to their home or other setting from where they were admitted. Some patients, especially those who have had a TURP, may have temporary loss of control of urination or a dribbling of the urine. Reassure the patient that these symptoms are almost always temporary and will resolve. Assist the patient and his family in finding ways to keep his clothing dry until sphincter control returns. Instruct him to contract and relax his sphincter frequently to re-establish urinary control (Kegel exercises). External urinary (condom) catheters are not used except in extreme cases because they may give the patient a false sense of security and delay urinary control.

? NCLEX EXAMINATION CHALLENGE

Physiological Integrity

A client had a transurethral resection of the prostate (TURP) yesterday. The staff nurse notes that the hemoglobin is 8.2 g/dL. What is the nurse's best action?

A. Notify the charge nurse as soon as possible.
B. Irrigate the catheter with 30 mL normal saline.
C. Document the assessment in the medical record.
D. Prepare for a blood transfusion.

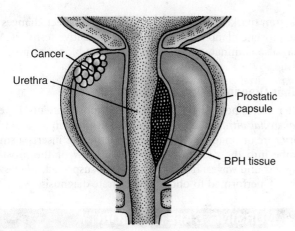

FIG. 75-4 The prostate gland with cancer and benign prostatic hyperplasia (BPH). Note that cancer normally arises in the periphery of the gland, whereas BPH occurs in the center of the gland.

Patients having the HoLEP procedure typically stay in the hospital overnight and usually have no urinary symptoms after surgery. This procedure may soon replace the TURP as the gold standard for surgical management of the patient with BPH.

PROSTATE CANCER

Pathophysiology

Prostate cancer is one of the most common types of cancer in men in the world. Men older than 65 years have the greatest risk for the disease. In the United States, it affects African-American men more commonly than Euro-American men and at an earlier age. The exact cause for this difference is not known.

Testosterone and dihydrotestosterone (DHT) are the major androgens (male hormones) in the adult male. Testosterone is produced by the testis and circulates in the blood. DHT is a testosterone derivative in the prostate gland. In some patients, the prostate grows very rapidly, leading to noncancerous high-grade prostatic intraepithelial neoplasia (PIN). Patients with PIN are at a higher risk for developing prostate cancer than men who do not have that growth pattern.

Many prostate tumors are androgen sensitive (McCance et al., 2010). Most are adenocarcinomas and arise from epithelial cells located in the posterior lobe or outer portion of the gland (Fig. 75-4).

Of all malignancies, prostate cancer is one of the slowest growing, and it metastasizes (spreads) in a predictable pattern. Common sites of metastasis are the nearby lymph nodes, bones, lungs, and liver (McCance et al., 2010). The bones of the pelvis, sacrum, and lumbar spine are most often affected. Chapter 23 describes staging categories of localized and advanced cancers.

Prostate cancer is likely caused by a number of factors, including androgens. Dietary factors, such as eating a diet high in animal fat (e.g., red meat) and complex carbohydrates or having a low fiber intake, increase the risk for prostate cancer. Men who have had a vasectomy or those who were exposed to environmental toxins, such as arsenic, may also be at increased risk for the disease (Held-Warmkessel, 2008; McCance et al., 2010).

GENETIC/GENOMIC CONSIDERATIONS

Many gene mutations play a role in various types of prostate cancer. Some men with the most aggressive prostate cancers have *BRCA2* mutations similar to those women who have *BRCA2*-associated breast and ovarian cancers. The most common genetic factor that increases the risk for prostate cancer is a mutation in the glutathione S-transferase (*GST P1*) gene. This gene is normally part of the pathway that helps prevent cancer (McCance et al., 2010).

Health Promotion and Maintenance

Teach men about the most recent American Cancer Society (ACS) guidelines for prostate cancer screening and early detection (ACS, 2011). The current recommendations are that men should make an informed decision about whether to have prostate cancer screening. Starting at the age of 50, men should discuss the options of having prostate-specific antigen testing with their health care provider. Men at a higher risk for prostate cancer, including African Americans or men who have a first-degree relative with prostate cancer before the age of 65, should have this discussion at age 45. Men who have multiple first-degree relatives with prostate cancer at an early age should discuss screening at age 40.

Although a family history of prostate cancer cannot be changed, certain nutritional habits can be altered to possibly decrease the risk for the disease. First, teach men to eat a healthy, balanced diet, including decreasing animal fat (e.g., red meat). Instead of red meat, remind them to eat more fish and other foods high in *omega-3 fatty acids* because they are thought to be helpful in preventing cancer. Also reinforce the need to increase fruits, vegetables, soy, and high-fiber foods.

PATIENT-CENTERED COLLABORATIVE CARE

ASSESSMENT

History

Assess the patient's age, race/ethnicity, and family history of prostate cancer. Ask about his nutritional habits, especially focusing on the intake of red meat, fish, and fruits and vegetables. Assess whether the patient has any problems with urination. Take a drug history to determine if he is taking any medication that could affect voiding. The first symptoms that the man may report are related to bladder outlet obstruction, such as difficulty in starting urination, frequent bladder infections, and urinary retention. Ask about urinary frequency, hematuria (blood in the urine), and nocturia (voiding during the night). Ask if he has had any pain during intercourse, especially when ejaculating. Inquire if the patient has had or currently has any other pain (particularly bone pain), a symptom associated with advanced prostate cancer. Ask him if he has had any recent unexpected weight loss.

Take a sexual history for recent changes in desire or function. Ask about current or previous sexually transmitted diseases, penile discharge, or scrotal pain or swelling.

Physical Assessment/Clinical Manifestations

Most *early* cancers are diagnosed while the patient is having a routine physical examination or is being treated for benign prostatic hyperplasia (BPH). Gross blood in the urine (hematuria) is a common clinical manifestation of *late* prostate cancer. Assess for pain in the pelvis, spine, hips, or ribs. Complete a thorough pain assessment. Palpate for swollen lymph nodes, especially in the groin areas. Pain and swollen nodes also indicate advanced disease that has spread. Take and record the patient's weight because unexpected weight loss is also common when the disease is advanced.

Prepare the patient for a digital rectal examination (DRE). On rectal examination, a prostate that is found to be stony hard and with palpable irregularities or indurations is suspected to be malignant.

Psychosocial Assessment

A diagnosis of any type of cancer causes fear and anxiety for most people. Some men, particularly African Americans, develop the disease in their 40s and 50s when they are perhaps planning their retirements, putting their children through college, and/or enjoying their middle years. Assess the reaction of the patient to the diagnosis, and observe how his family reacts to the illness. Men may describe their feelings as shock, fear, anger, and "roller coaster" (Wallace & Storms, 2007). Expect that patients will go through the grieving process and may be in denial or depressed. Determine what support systems they have, such as spiritual leaders or community group support, to help them through diagnosis, treatment, and recovery.

One of the biggest concerns for the man may be his ability for sexual function after cancer treatment. Tell him that function will depend on the type of treatment he has. Most surgical techniques used today do not involve cutting the perineal nerves that are needed for an erection. A dry climax may occur if the prostate is removed because it produces most of the fluid in the ejaculate. Refer the patient to his surgeon (urologist), sex therapist, or intimacy counselor if available.

Laboratory Assessment

Prostate-specific antigen (PSA) is a glycoprotein produced by the prostate. *PSA analysis is used as a screening test for prostate cancer.* If the test is performed, it should be drawn before the DRE because the examination can cause an increase in PSA due to prostate irritation.

The normal blood level of PSA in men younger than 50 years is less than 2.5 ng/mL. PSA levels increase to as high as 6.5 ng/mL when men reach their 70s. *African-American men have a slighter higher normal value, but the reason for this difference is not known. Because other prostate problems also increase the PSA level, it is not specifically diagnostic for cancer.* The level associated with prostate cancer, however, is usually much higher than those occurring with problems such as prostatitis and benign prostatic hyperplasia (Pagana & Pagana, 2010).

An elevated PSA level should decrease a few days after a prostatectomy for cancer. An increase in the PSA level several weeks after surgery usually indicates that the disease has recurred.

Because PSA is not absolutely specific to prostate cancer, another test, *early prostate cancer antigen (EPCA-2)*, may be a serum marker for prostate cancer. It can detect changes in the prostate gland early and is a very sensitive test. EPCA-2 may also eliminate the need to perform a biopsy of prostate tissue.

Other Diagnostic Assessment

After assessments by DRE and PSA, most patients have a *transrectal ultrasound (TRUS)* of the prostate in an ambulatory care or imaging setting. The practitioner inserts a small probe into the rectum and obtains a view of the prostate using sound waves. If prostate cancer is suspected, a *biopsy* is usually performed to obtain an accurate diagnosis.

> ## ! NURSING SAFETY PRIORITY
> ### Action Alert
>
> After a *transrectal ultrasound with biopsy*, instruct the patient about possible complications, although rare, including hematuria with clots, signs of infection, and perineal pain. Teach him to report fever, chills, bloody urine, and any difficulty voiding. Advise him to avoid strenuous physical activity and to drink plenty of fluids, especially in the first 24 hours after the procedure. Teach him that a small amount of bleeding turning the urine pink is expected during this time.

After prostate cancer is diagnosed, the patient has additional imaging and blood studies to determine the extent of the disease. Common tests include lymph node biopsy, computed tomography (CT) of the pelvis and abdomen, and magnetic resonance imaging (MRI) to assess the status of the pelvic and para-aortic lymph nodes. A radionuclide bone scan may be performed to detect metastatic bone disease. An enlarged liver or abnormal liver function study results indicate possible liver metastasis.

Patients with advanced prostate cancer often have *elevated levels of serum acid phosphatase*. Most men with bone metastasis have *elevated serum alkaline phosphatase* levels.

INTERVENTIONS

As with any cancer, accurate staging and grading of prostate tumors guide treatment planning and monitoring during the course of the disease. Patients are faced with several treatment options. A urologist and oncologist are needed to help patients make the best decision. Because prostate cancer is slow growing with late metastasis, older men who are asymptomatic and have other illnesses may choose observation without immediate active treatment, especially if the cancer is early stage. This option is known as "watchful waiting," or *expectant therapy*. This form of treatment involves initial surveillance with active treatment if the symptoms become bothersome. The average time from diagnosis to start of treatment is up to 10 years. During the watchful waiting period, men are monitored at regular intervals through DRE and PSA testing. Factors that are considered in choosing watchful waiting include potential side effects of treatment (e.g., urinary incontinence, erectile dysfunction), estimated life expectancy, and the risk for increased morbidity and mortality from not seeking active treatment.

Patients who have very early–stage cancer of the prostate who choose watchful waiting require close follow-up by their health care provider. If obstruction occurs, a transurethral resection of the prostate (TURP) may be done. The care of patients having this procedure is described in the discussion of Surgical Management on p. 1635 in the Benign Prostatic Hyperplasia section.

Specific management is based on the extent of the disease and the patient's physical condition. The patient may undergo surgery for a biopsy, staging and removal of the tumor, or palliation to control the spread of disease or relieve distressing symptoms. As with watchful waiting, the health care provider and patient must weigh the benefits of treatment against potential adverse effects such as incontinence and erectile dysfunction (ED).

Surgical Management

Surgery is the most common intervention for a cure. Minimally invasive surgery (MIS) or an open surgical technique for radical prostatectomy (prostate removal) is most often performed. A **bilateral orchiectomy** (removal of both testicles) is another palliative surgery that slows the spread of cancer by removing the main source of testosterone.

Preoperative Care. Preoperative care depends on the type of surgery that will be done. Minimally invasive surgery (MIS) is most appropriate for localized prostate cancer and is used as a curative intervention. The most common procedure is the *laparoscopic radical prostatectomy (LRP)*, with or without robotic assistance (Strief, 2008). Other newer procedures include transrectal high-intensity focused ultrasound (HIFU) and cryosurgery. Patients who qualify for LRP must have a PSA less than 10 ng/mL and have no previous hormone therapy or abdominal surgeries. Remind the patient that the advantages of this procedure over open surgery are:

- Decreased hospital stay (1 to 2 days)
- Minimal bleeding
- Smaller or no incisions and less scarring
- Less postoperative discomfort
- Decreased time for urinary catheter placement
- Fewer complications
- Faster recovery and return to usual activities
- Nerve-sparing advantages

For the patient undergoing an *open* radical prostatectomy, provide preoperative care as for any patient having surgery (see Chapter 16).

Operative Procedures. For the *LRP procedure,* the urologist makes one or more small punctures or incisions into the abdomen. A laparoscope with a camera on the end is inserted through one of the incisions while other instruments are inserted into the other incisions. The robotic system may be used to control the movement of the instruments by a remote device. The prostate is removed along with nearby lymph nodes.

The *open* radical prostatectomy can be performed via several surgical approaches, depending on the patient's desired outcomes and the staging of the disease. The transperineal and retropubic (nerve-sparing) approaches are most commonly used. The surgeon removes the entire prostate gland along with the prostatic capsule, the cuff at the bladder neck, the seminal vesicles, and the regional lymph nodes. The remaining urethra is connected to the bladder neck. The removal of tissue at the bladder neck allows the seminal fluid to travel upward into the bladder rather than down the urethral tract, resulting in retrograde ejaculations. The patient is sterile and has little ejaculate fluid. If the surgery spares the perineal nerves, the patient often experiences temporary erectile dysfunction (ED) for many months. For men who do not

---

CHART 75-2 **BEST PRACTICE FOR PATIENT SAFETY & QUALITY CARE**

Care of the Patient After an Open Radical Prostatectomy

- Encourage the patient to use patient-controlled analgesia (PCA) as needed.
- Help the patient get out of bed into a chair on the night of surgery and ambulate by the next day.
- Maintain the sequential compression device until the patient begins to ambulate.
- Monitor the patient for deep vein thrombosis and pulmonary embolus.
- Keep an accurate record of intake and output, including Jackson-Pratt or other drainage device drainage.
- Keep the urinary meatus clean using soap and water.
- Avoid rectal procedures or treatments.
- Teach the patient how to care for the urinary catheter because he may be discharged with the catheter in place.
- Teach the patient how to use a leg bag.
- Emphasize the importance of not straining during bowel movement. Advise the patient to avoid suppositories or enemas.
- Remind the patient about the importance of follow-up appointments with the physician to monitor progress.

---

regain sexual potency but had a nerve-sparing procedure, a drug such as sildenafil (Viagra) may be helpful. ED is discussed later in this chapter.

Postoperative Care. Provide postoperative care of the patient after *open* radical prostatectomy as summarized in Chart 75-2. Nursing interventions include all the typical care for a patient undergoing major surgery. Maintaining hydration, caring for wound drains (open procedure), managing pain, and preventing pulmonary complications are important aspects of nursing care (see Chapter 18).

Assess the patient's pain level, and monitor the effectiveness of pain management with opioids given as patient-controlled analgesia (PCA), a common method of delivery during the first 24 hours after surgery. Administer a stool softener if needed to prevent possible constipation from the drugs. Patients having the minimally invasive surgery have much less pain and fewer complications.

The patient has an indwelling urinary catheter to straight drainage. Monitor intake and output every shift and record, or delegate this activity to and supervise unlicensed assistive personnel (UAP). An antispasmodic may be prescribed to decrease bladder spasm induced by the indwelling urinary catheter. The time for catheter removal depends on the type of procedure that is performed and overall patient condition. Those with open surgical procedures use the catheter for 7 to 10 days or longer.

Ambulation should begin no later than the day after surgery. Provide assistance in walking the patient when he first gets out of bed. Assess for scrotal or penile swelling from the disrupted pelvic lymph flow. If this occurs, elevate the scrotum and penis and apply ice to the area intermittently for the first 24 to 48 hours.

Many patients who have the minimally invasive techniques are discharged in 1 to 3 days after surgery and can resume usual activities in about a week or two. Those who have open procedures are discharged in 2 to 3 days or longer, depending on their progress.

Remind patients that common potential long-term complications of open radical prostatectomy are urinary incontinence and erectile dysfunction (ED). *Urge incontinence* may occur because the internal and external sphincters of the bladder lie close to the prostate gland and are often damaged during the surgery. Kegel perineal exercises may reduce the severity of urinary incontinence after radical prostatectomy. Teach the patient to contract and relax the perineal and gluteal muscles in several ways. For one of the exercises, teach him to:

1. Tighten the perineal muscles for 3 to 5 seconds as if to prevent voiding, and then relax.
2. Bear down as if having a bowel movement.
3. Relax and repeat the exercise.

Show him how to inhale through pursed lips while tightening the perineal muscles and how to exhale when he relaxes. To regain urinary control, teach the patient to practice holding an object, such as a pencil, in the fold between the buttock and the thigh. He may also sit on the toilet with the knees apart while voiding and start and stop the stream several times.

Nonsurgical Management

Nonsurgical management may be an adjunct to surgery or alternative intervention if the cancer is widespread or the patient's condition or age prevents surgery. Available modalities include radiation therapy, hormonal therapy, and chemotherapy (less often).

Radiation Therapy. External or internal radiation therapy may be used in the treatment of prostate cancer or as "salvage" treatments when cancer recurs. It may also be done for palliation of the patient's symptoms.

External beam radiation therapy (EBRT) comes from a source outside the body. Patients are usually treated 5 days a week for 4 to 6 weeks. Three-dimensional conformal radiation therapy (3D-CRT) can more accurately target prostate tissue and can reduce side effects such as damage to the rectum. An advanced type of this radiation called *intensity-modulated radiation therapy* provides very high doses to the prostate. EBRT can also be used to relieve pain from bone metastasis. Teach patients that external beam radiation causes ED in many men well after the treatment is completed.

Other complications from EBRT include *acute radiation cystitis* causing persistent pain and hematuria. Symptoms are usually mild to moderate and subside in 6 weeks after treatment. Drugs to prevent urinary urgency such as tolterodine (Detrol LA) may be prescribed. Teach the patient to avoid caffeine and continue drinking plenty of water and other fluids.

Radiation proctitis (rectal mucosa inflammation) may also develop but is less likely with 3D-CRT. The man reports rectal urgency and cramping and passes mucus and blood. Teach him to report these symptoms to the health care provider. Like cystitis, this problem usually resolves in 4 to 6 weeks after the treatment stops. If proctitis occurs, teach patients to limit spicy or fatty foods, caffeine, and dairy products.

Low-dose brachytherapy (internal radiation) can be delivered by implanting low-dose radiation seeds directly into and around the prostate gland. This treatment includes ultrasonically guided interstitial or radioactive seed implantation. These procedures are done on an ambulatory care basis and

are the most cost-effective treatment for early-stage prostate cancer. Reassure the patient that the dose of radiation is low and that the radiation will not pose a hazard to himself or others. Teach him that ED, urinary incontinence, and rectal problems do occur in a small percentage of cases. Fatigue is also common and may last for several months after the treatment stops. Chapter 24 describes general nursing care for patients having radiation therapy.

Drug Therapy. Drug therapy may consist of either hormonal therapy (androgen deprivation therapy [ADT]) or chemotherapy. Several vaccines to locate and destroy prostate cancer cells are being studied (Slovin, 2008).

Hormone Therapy. Because most prostate tumors are hormone dependent, patients with extensive tumors or those with metastatic disease may be managed by androgen deprivation. Luteinizing hormone–releasing hormone (LH-RH) agonists or anti-androgens can be used.

Examples of *LH-RH agonists* are leuprolide (Lupron), goserelin (Zoladex), and triptorelin (Trelstar). These drugs first stimulate the pituitary gland to release the luteinizing hormone (LH). After about 3 weeks, the pituitary gland "runs out" of LH, which reduces testosterone production by the testes.

> ### ❗ NURSING SAFETY PRIORITY
> #### *Drug Alert*
>
> Teach patients taking LH-RH agonists that side effects include "hot flashes," erectile dysfunction, and decreased libido (desire to have sex). Some men also have gynecomastia (breast tenderness and growth). These drugs can also cause osteoporosis. Bisphosphonates like pamidronate (Aredia) are prescribed to prevent bone fractures. They can also be used to slow the damage caused by bone metastasis.

Anti-androgen drugs, also known as *androgen deprivation therapy (ADT),* work differently in that they block the body's ability to use the available androgens (National Comprehensive Cancer Network [NCCN], 2007). These drugs are the major treatment for metastatic disease. Examples include flutamide (Eulexin, Euflex ✦), bicalutamide (Casodex), and nilutamide (Nilandron). These drugs inhibit tumor progression by blocking the uptake of testicular and adrenal androgens at the prostate tumor site.

Anti-androgens may be used alone or in combination with LH-RH agonists for a total or maximal androgen blockade (hormone ablation). Patients who have this drug combination often have "hot flashes" similar to those experienced by menopausal women, and they can decrease the patient's perceived quality of life. Ask the patient if he has been experiencing this problem. Megestrol acetate may be prescribed for this uncomfortable condition.

Chemotherapy. Systemic chemotherapy may be an option for patients whose cancer has spread and for whom other therapies have not worked. For example, small cell prostate cancer is rare and is more responsive to chemotherapy than to hormone therapy (NCCN, 2007). Cisplatin (Platinol) and etoposide (VP-16, VePesid) often work for this type of cancer. Chapter 24 describes general nursing care for patients receiving chemotherapy.

Other Drugs. Other less commonly used drugs that are available if other drugs have failed or stopped working include high doses of ketoconazole (Nizoral), an antifungal drug that blocks androgen production, and the female hormone *estrogen* (diethylstilbestrol or DES). Teach patients taking ketoconazole that it can cause liver and adrenal problems. Teach them to take the drug on an empty stomach and to avoid drugs such as histamine blockers and antacids, which can interfere with drug absorption (Held-Warmkessel, 2008). Patients are followed closely and have frequent laboratory tests to detect any early organ damage. The drug also interacts with many other drugs, including warfarin (Coumadin), phenytoin (Dilantin), and prednisone (Deltasone). Corticosteroids such as prednisone may be given alone as palliation to reduce pain and improve the quality of life (Held-Warmkessel, 2008).

Community-Based Care

Patient-centered collaborative care of the man with prostate cancer should include his partner, if any, and family. Recognize that the patient has specific physical and psychosocial needs that should be addressed before hospital discharge and management should continue in the community setting.

Patients with prostate cancer may require care in a wide variety of settings: at the hospital, the radiation therapy department, the oncologist's office, or home at any stage of the disease process. Specific interventions depend on which treatment the patient had or if he had a combination of treatments. This section focuses on the needs of those who had a radical prostatectomy.

Home Care Management

Discharge planning and health teaching start early, even before surgery. A patient can better plan home care management when he knows what to expect. Collaborate with the case manager to coordinate the efforts of various health care providers, surgical unit nursing staff, and possibly a home care nurse. As specified by The Joint Commission and other accrediting agencies, continuity of care is essential when caring for this patient because he may need weeks or months of therapies.

Teaching for Self-Management

An important area of teaching for the patient going home after an *open* radical prostatectomy may be urinary catheter care. An indwelling urinary catheter may be in place for up to several weeks, depending on the surgical technique that was used. Teach him and his family how to care for the catheter, use a leg bag, and identify manifestations of infection and other complications. See Chart 75-3 for patient and family education.

Encourage the patient to walk short distances. Lifting may be restricted to no more than 15 pounds for up to 6 weeks, depending on the type of surgery that was done. Remind him to maintain an upright position and not walk bent or flexed. Vigorous exercise such as running or jumping should be avoided for at least 12 weeks and then gradually introduced.

Teach the patient to not strain to defecate. A stool softener may be prescribed to reduce the need for straining. If an opioid is prescribed for pain management, encourage the patient to drink adequate water to prevent constipation.

If the patient had an *open* radical prostatectomy, teach him to shower for the first 2 to 3 weeks rather than soak in a bathtub. Show patients how to inspect the incision or

---

Urinary Catheter Care at Home

- Once a day, gently wash the first few inches of the catheter starting at the penis and washing outward with mild soap and water.
- Rinse and dry the catheter well.
- If you have not been circumcised, push the foreskin back to clean the catheter site; when finished, push the foreskin forward.
- Change the drainage bag at least once a week as needed:
  - Hold the catheter with one hand and the tubing with the other hand, and twist in opposite directions to disconnect.
  - Place the end of the catheter in a clean container to catch leakage of urine.
  - Remove the rubber cap from the tubing of the leg bag or clean drainage bag.
  - Clean the end of the new tubing with alcohol swabs.
  - Insert the end of the new tubing into the catheter, and twist to connect securely.
- Clean the drainage bag just removed by pouring a solution of one part vinegar to two parts water through the tubing and bag. Rinse well with water, and allow the bag to dry.

---

puncture site(s) daily for signs of infection. Remind them to keep all follow-up appointments. PSA blood tests are taken 6 weeks after surgery and then every 4 to 6 months to monitor progress.

Health Care Resources

Refer the patient and partner to agencies or support groups such as the American Cancer Society's Man to Man program to help cope with prostate cancer. This program provides one-on-one education, personal visits, educational presentations, and the opportunity to engage in open and candid discussions. Another prostate cancer support group is Us TOO International (www.ustoo.com) sponsored by the Prostate Cancer Education and Support Network. This group provides education and support with national and international chapters. Information can also be obtained from the Prostate Cancer Foundation (www.prostatecancerfoundation.org) or the National Prostate Cancer Coalition (www.fight prostatecancer.org). Other personal and community support

---

❓ DECISION-MAKING CHALLENGE

Patient-Centered Care; Teamwork and Collaboration

An 82-year-old man is diagnosed with advanced-stage prostate cancer. His health care provider suspects bone metastasis based on the patient's report of pain in his ribs and pelvis. The patient works as a farmer in a rural community and tells you that he doesn't "care about much" since his wife died a year ago. The health care provider wants to admit him to the hospital immediately for treatment and further diagnostic testing.

1. What is your best response to the patient at this time?
2. What diagnostic testing would be appropriate for the patient at this time?
3. What possible interventions might help this patient be more comfortable?
4. With what members of the health care team might you need to collaborate?

services such as spiritual leaders or churches and synagogues are also important to many patients.

Many men have erectile dysfunction (ED) for the first 3 to 18 months after a prostatectomy. Refer them to a specialist who can help with this problem. ED is discussed in the next section (Erectile Disfunction). Refer patients with urinary incontinence to a urologist who specializes in this area. Drug therapy and other strategies may be used. Chapter 69 discusses incontinence management in detail.

ERECTILE DYSFUNCTION

Pathophysiology

Erectile dysfunction (ED), also known as *impotence,* is the inability to achieve or maintain an erection for sexual intercourse. It affects millions of men in the United States. There are two major types of ED: organic and functional.

Organic ED is a gradual deterioration of function. The man first notices diminishing firmness and a decrease in frequency of erections. Causes include:

- Inflammation of the prostate, urethra, or seminal vesicles
- Surgical procedures such as prostatectomy
- Pelvic fractures
- Lumbosacral injuries
- Vascular disease, including hypertension
- Chronic neurologic conditions, such as Parkinson disease or multiple sclerosis
- Endocrine disorders, such as diabetes mellitus (a major cause) or thyroid disorders
- Smoking and alcohol consumption
- Drugs, such as antihypertensives
- Poor overall health that prevents sexual intercourse

If the patient has episodes of ED, it usually has a *functional* (psychological) cause. Men with functional ED usually have normal nocturnal (nighttime) and morning erections. Onset is usually sudden and follows a period of high stress.

PATIENT-CENTERED COLLABORATIVE CARE

ASSESSMENT

For a man to have an erection, he must have normal innervation and a normal libido (sex drive). Therefore a medical, social, and sexual history and a complete physical examination are needed. The first step is to determine whether the cause is organic. Diagnostic testing is done to rule out possible organic causes.

If test results are negative, the evaluation then focuses on the specific causes that may have been indicated in the medical history. For example, hormone testing is used for patients who have a poor libido, small testicles, or sparse beard growth. Serum levels of *testosterone* and *gonadotropins* such as luteinizing hormone (LH) and follicle-stimulating hormone (FSH) are measured. LH stimulates the Leydig cells in the testicles to produce testosterone.

Duplex Doppler ultrasonography is another test to evaluate ED. It provides information about arterial and venous blood flow to the penis. It can also be used to determine the best treatment for ED. A *nocturnal penile tumescence test* that measures nighttime erections is done in a sleep laboratory. Usually an erection is expected with each rapid eye movement (REM)

episode. This study can determine whether ED is caused by an organic or functional problem. If the man has nocturnal erections, the ED is functional. Sex or intimacy counseling is needed in this case, and the patient is referred to a certified sex therapist or other qualified specialist.

INTERVENTIONS

The most common intervention for ED is drug therapy. Other interventions include vacuum devices, intracorporal injections, intraurethral applications, and prostheses (implants).

Drug Therapy

First-line oral drugs used to manage ED, phosphodiesterace-5 (PDE-5) inhibitors, work by relaxing the smooth muscles in the corpora cavernosa so blood flow to the penis is increased. The veins exiting the corpora are compressed, limiting outward blood flow and resulting in penile **tumescence** (swelling). Teach patients to take the pill 1 hour before sexual intercourse. For some drugs, such as sildenafil (Viagra) and vardenafil (Levitra), sexual stimulation is needed within $\frac{1}{2}$ to 1 hour to promote the erection. With other drugs, such as tadalafil (Cialis), erection can be stimulated over a longer period. Because the erection occurs more naturally compared with other treatment options, most men and their partners prefer this option.

! NURSING SAFETY PRIORITY

Drug Alert

Instruct patients taking PDE-5 inhibitors to abstain from alcohol before sexual intercourse because it may impair the ability to have an erection. Common side effects of these drugs include dyspepsia (heartburn), headaches, facial flushing, and stuffy nose. If more than one pill a day is being taken, leg and back cramps, nausea, and vomiting also may occur. *Teach men who take nitrates to avoid PDE-5 inhibitors because the vasodilation effects can cause a profound hypotension and reduce blood flow to vital organs.* For patients who cannot take these drugs or do not respond to them, other methods are available to achieve an erection.

Other Interventions

The basic design of a *vacuum constriction device (VCD)* is a cylinder that fits over the penis and sits firmly against the body. Using a pump, a vacuum is created to draw blood into the penis to maintain an erection. A rubber ring (tension band) is placed around the base of the penis to maintain the erection, and the cylinder is removed.

The advantage of this procedure is that the device is easy and safe to use. The disadvantage is its clumsiness and lack of spontaneity. In addition, the man may experience pain from the rubber ring or from pumping the device too quickly. The ring should be removed after an hour, or tissue could be damaged.

Injecting the penis with vasodilating drugs can make the penis erect by engorging it with blood. The most common agents used for this purpose include):

- Alprostadil (Caverject), a synthetic vasodilator identical to prostaglandin E_1 produced in the body
- Paverine, also a vasodilator
- Phentolamine (Regitine), an alpha-1, alpha-2 selective adrenergic receptor antagonist
- A combination of any or all of these drugs

TABLE 75-1   CLASSIFICATION OF TESTICULAR TUMORS

Germ Cell (Germinal) Tumors	Non–Germ Cell (Nongerminal) Tumors

• Seminoma
• Nonseminoma:
  • Embryonal carcinoma
  • Teratoma
  • Choriocarcinoma
	• Interstitial cell tumor
	• Androblastoma

These drugs may be injected into the side of the penis using a 27- or 30-gauge needle. Adverse effects include priapism (prolonged erection), penile scarring, fibrosis, bleeding, bruising at the injection site, pain, infection, and vasovagal responses.

Penile implants (prostheses) are used when other modalities fail. Devices include semirigid, flexible, or hydraulic inflatable and multi-component or one-piece instruments. The three-piece inflatable device is the most commonly implanted prosthesis. A reservoir is placed in the scrotum. Tubes carry the fluid into the inflatable pieces that are placed in the penis. To inflate the prosthesis, the man squeezes the pump located in the scrotum. To deflate the prosthesis, a release button is activated. Advantages include the man's ability to control his erections. The major disadvantages include device failure and infection. The device is implanted as an ambulatory surgical procedure. Teach the patient to observe the surgical site for bleeding and infection.

TESTICULAR CANCER

Pathophysiology

Testicular cancer is a rare cancer that most often affects men between 20 and 54 years of age but can affect men of any age (American Cancer Society [ACS], 2011). It usually strikes men at a productive time of life and thus has significant economic, social, and psychological impact on the patient and his family and/or partner. With early detection by testicular self-examination (TSE) (Chart 75-4) and treatment, testicular cancer can be cured. It can occur in one testicle or both.

Primary testicular cancers fall into two major groups:
- Germ cell tumors arising from the sperm-producing cells (account for most testicular cancers)
- Non–germ cell tumors arising from the stroma, interstitial, or Leydig cells that produce testosterone (account for a very small percentage of testicular cancers)

Testicular germ cell tumors are classified into two broad categories: seminomas and nonseminomas (Table 75-1). The most common type of testicular tumor is *seminoma*. Patients with seminomas have the most favorable prognoses because the tumors are usually localized, metastasize late, and respond to treatment (Bohenkamp & Yoder, 2009). They often are diagnosed when they are still confined to the testicles and retroperitoneal lymph nodes.

Non–germ cell tumors are classified as either *interstitial cell tumors* or *androblastomas* (testicular adenomas). Most of these tumors do not metastasize. Interstitial cell tumors arise from the Leydig cells, which secrete testosterone into the bloodstream. Androblastomas sometimes secrete estrogen, which accounts for the feminization and gynecomastia (breast enlargement) occasionally seen in these men.

The risk for testicular tumors is higher in males who have an undescended testis (cryptorchidism) or have human immune deficiency virus (HIV) infection.

GENETIC/GENOMIC CONSIDERATIONS

Men are at a higher risk for testicular cancer if they have a family history of the disease (Hemminki et al., 2008). The incidence is higher among identical twins, brothers, and other close male relatives. Euro-American men are at a higher risk for testicular cancer than men of other races or ethnicities (Bohenkamp & Yoder, 2009). The reason for these differences is not known.

Primary testicular cancer is rarely bilateral. Other cancers such as leukemia, lymphoma, and metastatic carcinomas may invade the testes. A man with bilateral testicular tumors is more likely to have metastatic disease to the testes than primary cancer.

PATIENT-CENTERED COLLABORATIVE CARE

ASSESSMENT

Physical Assessment/Clinical Manifestations

When taking a history from a patient with a suspected testicular tumor, consider the risk factors. Assess for other risk factors, including a history or presence of an undescended testis and a family history of testicular cancer.

Ask the patient whether he has noticed a discomfort such as heaviness or aching in the lower abdomen or the scrotum. Determine how long any manifestations have been present.

Assess the patient's family situation. Is the patient sexually active? If so, what is his sexual preference? Does he have children? Does he want children in the future? Depending on the treatment plan chosen, would he be interested in sperm storage in a sperm bank?

If the man has one healthy testis, he can function sexually and may not have any reproductive dysfunction. If he has a retroperitoneal lymph node dissection or chemotherapy, he may become sterile because of treatment effects on the sperm-producing cells or surgical trauma to the sympathetic nervous system resulting in retrograde ejaculations.

The testes, lymph nodes, and abdomen should be thoroughly examined. Patients may feel embarrassed about having this examination. Provide privacy, and explain the

---

A Patient with a Testicular Lump

Obtain a medical history from the patient:
- When was the lump discovered?
- Are there any other symptoms (sensation of heaviness, dragging in testicle, pain, discharge from penis)?
- Is there a history of cryptorchidism?

Assess the genital system; always wear gloves during the examination of the male genitalia:
- Inspect and palpate the scrotal contents. Have the patient perform a Valsalva maneuver, and palpate for a varicocele.
- Any lump or enlargement that does not transilluminate should be suspected as malignant.

Palpate for any enlarged lymph nodes. The most common areas for lymphadenopathy are in the inguinal or supraclavicular regions.

Assess the abdomen for a possible mass or hepatomegaly.

Sperm Banking

- You may want to investigate sperm storage in a sperm bank as a way to preserve your sperm for future use.
- No one knows how long sperm can be stored successfully, but pregnancies have resulted from sperm stored for longer than 10 years.
- Check with the sperm bank to see how much it charges to process and store your sperm and to see whether you must pay when the service is provided.
- Investigate whether your health insurance company will reimburse you for sperm collection and storage.

---

procedure to the patient. *Inspect the testicles for swelling or a lump that the patient reports is painless. This is the most common manifestation of testicular cancer.* An advanced practice nurse or other health care provider palpates the testes for lumps and swelling that are not visible (Chart 75-5). The presence of any testicular pain, lymph node swelling, bone pain, abdominal masses, sudden hydrocele (fluid in the scrotum), or gynecomastia often indicates metastatic disease.

Psychosocial Assessment

Because testicular cancer and its treatment often lead to sexual dysfunction, pay close attention to the psychosocial aspects of the disease. *Sexuality* is an issue for men of any age, but it may be even more of an issue for younger men. Even if the cancer is detected at an early stage and the patient is cured after surgery, he may be afraid that he will be sexually deficient. He may also think of himself as "less than a whole person." These fears can disrupt the psychosocial and sexual development of young males and can threaten their identity. The patient may be afraid that he will be unable to perform sexually, will no longer be sexually attractive or desirable, and will face rejection. Feelings of sexual inadequacy may be denied, repressed, or displaced, causing increased stress on the man's personal and work relationships.

Assess the man's support systems, including his partner, family members, and friends. Ask him where he feels that he can be supported, such as a religious or spiritual group, community club, or social group. Friends are often very helpful during this difficult time.

Laboratory Assessment

Common serum tumor markers that confirm a diagnosis of testicular cancer are:
- Alpha-fetoprotein (AFP)
- Beta human chorionic gonadotropin (hCG)
- Lactate dehydrogenase (LDH)

Serum tumor marker levels are also used to evaluate responses to therapy for testicular cancer and to document the presence of residual or recurrent disease. With effective treatment, the levels of abnormal markers fall. The persistence of elevated levels of markers after orchiectomy (testicle removal) is evidence that the patient has metastatic disease, even if x-rays and scans do not show a tumor presence. The reappearance

of the tumor markers indicates recurrence of the cancer. Therefore marker levels must be monitored regularly during the follow-up of patients treated for testicular cancer.

Serum testosterone levels are increased when the tumor affects the Leydig cells, which produce this hormone. Drugs such as alcohol and antiepileptic drugs can also cause an increase in testosterone (Pagana & Pagana, 2010).

Other Diagnostic Assessment

When a patient has a change in testis size, shape, or texture, *ultrasonography* can determine whether the mass is solid or fluid filled. It also can help differentiate benign masses from malignant ones.

After the diagnosis of testicular cancer, the patient should have a *computed tomography (CT)* scan of the abdomen and the chest to identify small metastatic lesions. *Lymphangiography* shows a view of the body's lymph system to look for spread to other areas.

Magnetic resonance imaging (MRI) is used to detect enlarged lymph nodes and abnormal nodules in certain organs that may indicate metastasis from the testicles. Chest x-rays and bone scans may also be performed if metastasis is suspected.

INTERVENTIONS

At diagnosis, the incidence of oligospermia (low sperm count) and azoospermia (absence of living sperm) is common in patients with testicular cancer. This problem is thought to be related to higher testicular temperatures created by cancer cell metabolism. The man may not discover that he has reduced sperm count until he has a sperm count performed before surgery.

Health teaching about reproduction, fertility, and sexuality is started in the pretreatment phase. Review the normal reproductive function, as well as the possible effects of cancer and its treatment on reproductive function. Explore with the patient various reproductive options, if desired (Chart 75-6). A sperm bank facility provides comprehensive information on semen collection, storage of semen, the storage contract, costs, and the insemination process.

When preparing the patient for the collection and storage of sperm, assume the role of patient advocate and keep in mind the effect of the cancer diagnosis. The psychological benefit of having stored sperm may be important for the man and may influence his response to treatment. For some men, knowing that the potential for being a father still exists may help them cope with other fears, such as alopecia or erectile dysfunction (ED).

Suggest that the patient arrange for semen storage, if desired, as soon as possible after diagnosis. Sperm collection should be completed before he begins radiation therapy or chemotherapy or undergoes a radical lymph node dissection. After radiation therapy or chemotherapy has been started, the patient is at increased risk for producing mutagenic sperm, which may not be viable or may result in fetal abnormalities.

The patient's diagnosis and his physical condition may not allow treatment to be postponed, thus making sperm storage impossible. Also, some men may have personal or religious beliefs that do not allow sperm storage. For those who are not candidates for sperm storage in a sperm bank and for those who choose not to bank, discuss other reproductive options such as donor insemination or adoption.

Surgical Management

Surgery is the main treatment for testicular cancer. For Stage 0 or 1 (localized disease), the surgeon performs a radical unilateral orchiectomy to remove the affected testicle. Every effort is made to remove the cancerous testis as an intact organ to prevent releasing cancer cells into the surgical site. Depending on the type and stage of the cancer, radical retroperitoneal lymph node dissection (RPLND) may also be done.

Preoperative Care. Like most patients with cancer, the man with testicular cancer is very apprehensive. Offer support, and reinforce the teaching provided by the surgeon. Teach the patient and his family or partner about what to expect after surgery. Depending on the extent of the lymph node dissection and the need for surgical exploration, the surgeon often makes a midline incision. For patients with very early disease, minimally invasive surgery (MIS) using a laparoscope does not require a midline incision. For patients having MIS, teach them that carbon dioxide may be used as part of the surgery. Carbon dioxide can cause chest or shoulder pain from diaphragmatic irritation after the procedure.

Inform the patient and family that traditional open radical retroperitoneal lymph node dissections are long operations. In some cases, the patient may require care in a critical care unit after surgery for close observation.

Operative Procedures. Most patients with seminoma have only one surgery to remove the diseased testicle through the groin (inguinal) for a cure. A frozen section of the tumor is examined to confirm the type and stage of the cancer. A gel-filled silicone prosthesis may be surgically implanted into the scrotum at the time of the orchiectomy or later if the patient desires. Reassure the patient that this procedure does not impair fertility or sexual function. He cosmetically appears to have two testes (reconstructive surgery).

Some men have more advanced disease or tumor types that are more aggressive. These patients require several surgeries to remove both testicles and lymph nodes. Two options are available for the lymph node dissection: a traditional open approach and minimally invasive surgery (MIS) using a laparoscope. To perform the *open* approach, the surgeon removes the retroperitoneal nodes in the iliac and lumbar regions. Because the blood supply and the lymphatic vessels of the testes and kidneys are directly related, an extensive midline incision from the xiphoid process to the pubis is necessary. Removal of the sympathetic ganglia eliminates peristalsis in the vas deferens and contractions of the seminal vesicles. This disruption results in sterility because the man's ejaculate no longer contains sperm. However, having a normal erection and experiencing orgasm usually are not affected.

The MIS procedure involves using a laparoscope through several small "keyhole" incisions through which the nodes are dissected for examination. This technique shortens the time the patient is in the operating suite, minimizes bleeding, and causes less pain after surgery. The patient has fewer postoperative complications and a shorter hospital stay.

Postoperative Care. Nursing care for the patient after surgery depends on the type of surgical procedure that was performed and the extent of the disease process.

! NURSING SAFETY PRIORITY

Action Alert

Because of the length of the *open* orchiectomy and lymph node dissection approach, manipulation of the abdominal and retroperitoneal viscera, and the loss of lymphatic fluid, observe, assess, and report any complications of this major abdominal surgery (e.g., paralytic ileus) (see Chapter 18). Monitor vital signs (including pain), hydration, and pulmonary function carefully for the first 24 to 48 hours. Ambulate the patient as soon as possible, and teach him how to use the incentive spirometer. Assess the patency of the nasogastric tube (NGT) (if in place) and the urinary catheter. Be sure the patient wears antiembolism stockings or devices, and provide care for surgical incisions and wound drains.

The patient having the *laparoscopic* procedure does not typically have an NGT but may have a urinary catheter in place for 1 to 2 days. The other advantages of the MIS procedure are that patients have less pain and fewer complications than those who had the open surgery. Chapter 17 describes laparoscopic surgery in detail.

? NCLEX EXAMINATION CHALLENGE

Physiological Integrity

A client who had an orchiectomy and laparoscopic radical retroperitoneal lymph node dissection this morning states that he does not understand why he is having shoulder pain. What is the nurse's best response?
A. "The pain is from the carbon dioxide that was used during surgery."
B. "You are having pain because of the way you were positioned during surgery."
C. "What is your level of pain on a scale of 0 to 10, with 10 being the worst pain?"
D. "Your shoulder should not be hurting because you had a minimally invasive surgery."

Nonsurgical Management

Combination *chemotherapy* may be used as adjuvant therapy for nonseminomatous testicular tumors or as primary treatment when there is evidence of metastatic disease. Many drug regimens are used, including varying combinations of bleomycin, cisplatin, etoposide, and/or vinblastine.

The specific combination of drugs and the frequency, cycling, and duration of treatment vary from patient to patient, depending on the extent of the disease and the protocol being followed. Chapter 24 discusses the general nursing care for the patient receiving chemotherapy.

Patients having chemotherapy are at risk for certain health problems that are associated with these drugs. Examples of these problems include hypertension, hyperlipidemia, coronary artery disease, anemia, and leukemia (Bohenkamp & Yoder, 2009). Teach patients taking these drugs about the long-term effects for which they should be continually and carefully monitored by their health care providers.

After orchiectomy for localized disease, *external beam radiation therapy* (EBRT) is commonly used. The remaining testis is shielded with a lead cup to preserve reproductive function. Even with these precautions, the patient may have a temporary decreased sperm count as a result of radiation scatter. Normally the sperm count returns to the pretreatment level within 24 to 30 months after the radiation treatment is completed. If metastases develop outside the lymphatic system, the man may still be cured with radiation therapy if the area of involvement is limited. If lymphatic involvement is extensive or if the visceral organs are involved, combination chemotherapy is used.

Community-Based Care

The patient is usually hospitalized for multiple days after an *open* radical retroperitoneal lymph node dissection but for just 1 to 2 days for the *MIS* procedure. This period may need to be extended if he must undergo additional surgery or chemotherapy. Because it may not be known until after the orchiectomy what type of testicular cancer he has or whether he needs additional surgery or treatment, specific discharge planning may need to be delayed until after surgery.

After an *orchiectomy*, unless the patient has a wound complication, he is discharged without a dressing on the inguinal incision. A scrotal support may be needed for several days. He may want to wear a dry dressing to prevent clothing from rubbing on the sutures and causing irritation. Tell him that the sutures will be removed in the physician's office 7 to 10 days after surgery. Patients who also had an *open retroperitoneal lymph node dissection* recover more slowly. They should not lift anything over 15 pounds, should avoid stair climbing, and should not drive a car for several weeks. Be sure that bathroom facilities are on the first floor of the house where he can easily access them.

> **! NURSING SAFETY PRIORITY**
>
> **Action Alert**
>
> For the patient who has undergone testicular surgery, emphasize the importance of scheduling a follow-up visit with the surgeon to examine the incision for healing and complications. Instruct him to notify the surgeon if chills, fever, increasing tenderness or pain around the incision, drainage, or dehiscence of the incision occurs. These manifestations may indicate infection for which antibiotics are needed. Instruct the patient who had an orchiectomy that he will be able to resume most of his usual activities within 1 week after discharge, except for lifting heavy objects (objects weighing more than 15 pounds [6.8 kg]) and stair climbing. Remind him to ask his surgeon when strenuous activities may be resumed.

Inform the patient that he may make arrangements to have a silicone prosthesis inserted into the scrotum if one was not inserted during the orchiectomy. Explain the importance of performing monthly testicular self-examination (TSE) on the remaining testis and scheduling follow-up examinations with the physician. The patient who has had testicular cancer should schedule tests for urinary and serum levels of tumor markers and CT or MRI studies as part of his routine follow-up for at least 3 years.

Depending on the pathologic findings and the stage of the cancer, the patient may need further treatment. This information may not be known at the time of discharge. If it is known that the patient needs further surgery, he and his family need information about the future surgery. If it is known that he must undergo radiation therapy or chemotherapy, he needs education about these treatments as soon as possible.

The man who has testicular cancer needs emotional support. If permanent sterility occurs and sperm storage has not been feasible, he may desire counseling about other reproductive options. Refer the patient to agencies or support groups, such as the American Fertility Society (www.theafa.org) or RESOLVE: The National Infertility Association (www.resolve.org) (organizations for infertile couples).

OTHER PROBLEMS AFFECTING THE TESTES AND ADJACENT STRUCTURES

Problems that develop inside the scrotum usually occur as a mass or as scrotal edema. Some problems produce pain, but others do not. Fig. 75-5 shows some of the most common conditions found in men, including hydrocele, spermatocele, varicocele, and scrotal torsion.

HYDROCELE

A hydrocele is a cystic mass, usually filled with straw-colored fluid that forms around the testis (see Fig. 75-5). It results from impaired lymphatic drainage of the scrotum causing a swelling of the tissue surrounding the testis. Unless the swelling becomes large and uncomfortable or begins to impair blood flow to the testis, no treatment is necessary. Hydroceles are usually painless. It is important that the cause of the hydrocele is investigated to rule out a serious condition. The cause may be determined by examination and ultrasound. A small hydrocele may go untreated with no further problems. However, a hydrocele may become very large, which makes clothing uncomfortable and may be cosmetically unacceptable.

A hydrocele may be drained via a needle and syringe, or it may be removed surgically in an ambulatory care setting. The patient may or may not have a drain at the incision site. Teach the man that if an incision drain is present, some serosanguineous drainage may be present for the first 24 to 48 hours after surgery. Explain the importance of wearing a scrotal support (jock strap). This device keeps the dressing in place and the scrotum elevated, which helps prevent edema.

The degree of pain experienced after this surgery varies. Assess and observe the patient for pain every 2 to 3 hours immediately after surgery. Moderate incision pain is expected for the first 24 hours after surgery and should markedly decrease within 1 or 2 days. If the pain does not resolve within this time, assess for wound complications, such as infection or bleeding.

Instruct the man to schedule a follow-up visit with the surgeon to have the wound evaluated for healing. Stress the importance of continuing to wear a scrotal support to promote drainage and comfort. The scrotum can remain swollen from residual inflammation and edema for as long as several weeks. Remind the patient to stay off his feet for

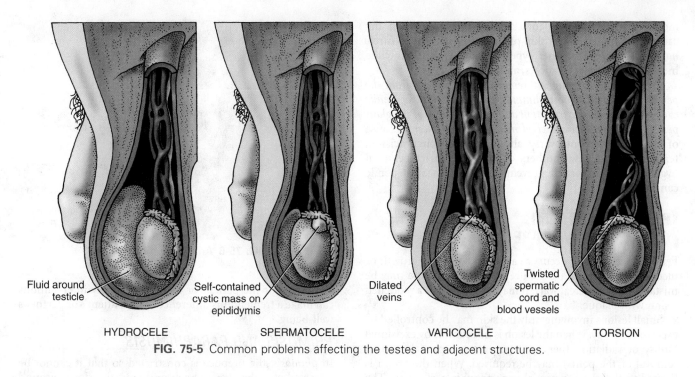

Fluid around testicle

Self-contained cystic mass on epididymis

Dilated veins

Twisted spermatic cord and blood vessels

HYDROCELE   SPERMATOCELE   VARICOCELE   TORSION

FIG. 75-5 Common problems affecting the testes and adjacent structures.

several days and to limit physical activity for a week. Reassure him that this swelling is normal and eventually subsides.

SPERMATOCELE

A spermatocele is a sperm-containing cyst that develops on the epididymis alongside the testicle (see Fig. 75-5). Trauma, infection, congenital abnormalities, or often for no identifiable reason results in the widening of a portion of the epididymis, creating a small cavity where sperm collects.

Normally, spermatoceles are small and asymptomatic and no interventions are needed. If they become large enough to cause discomfort, a spermatocelectomy is performed. In this simple procedure, the spermatocele is removed through a small scrotal incision. Routinely, no incision drain is used because drainage and swelling are minimal. A few patients have recurrence.

VARICOCELE

A varicocele is a cluster of dilated veins behind and above the testis (see Fig. 75-5). Varicosity of the testicles may result from the increased fluid secondary to damaged or incompetent valves in the testicular veins. The diagnosis is made by scrotal palpation, particularly when the patient performs a Valsalva maneuver, creating additional pressure in the varicose veins. The scrotum feels "wormlike" when palpated. If the varicocele is very small and cannot be palpated, thermography, which detects pockets of heat, or a Doppler, which magnifies the sound of the blood flowing through the veins, is used.

Varicoceles can be either unilateral or bilateral, but most are unilateral. They occur most often on the left side of the scrotum. In many cases, they are asymptomatic and no treatment is required. In a few men, varicoceles are painful and must be removed surgically.

Varicoceles can also cause infertility. It is thought that they increase scrotal temperature from the venous stasis near the testis, altering spermatogenesis. Surgical correction may

resolve the infertility. As an alternative, an interventional radiology procedure may be done to embolize the vein that drains the varicocele.

A varicocelectomy (surgical removal of the varicocele) is usually performed through an inguinal incision, in which the spermatic veins are ligated in the cord. It can also be performed through an incision near the superior iliac spine, in which the spermatic veins are ligated in the retroperitoneal space. A varicocelectomy may be done on an ambulatory care basis.

Before surgery, explain to the patient that persistent venous congestion of the scrotum is common after this type of surgery because of the changed circulation in the area. To promote drainage of the scrotum, place a rolled towel under the scrotum while he is in bed. Ice may be applied to the scrotum if needed. Any intervention that facilitates drainage and decreases swelling from the area promotes relief. Instruct the patient about the importance of wearing a scrotal support while ambulating. Usually he can resume normal activities, including sexual activities, within a week.

At discharge, instruct the patient to make a follow-up appointment with the surgeon to have the sutures removed. Remind him to notify the surgeon of any increasing discomfort at the incision site or in the scrotum, which might indicate an infection. Increasing scrotal discomfort can mean that the circulation to the testis has been impaired. Testicular atrophy, a rare complication of a varicocelectomy, may occur if the blood supply to the testis becomes insufficient.

CANCER OF THE PENIS
Pathophysiology

Cancer of the penis is rare among men in the United States. Most penile cancers are epidermoid (squamous) carcinomas developing from the squamous cells. These tumors tend to grow slowly and can develop anywhere on the penis but occur most commonly on the foreskin or the glans. When the cancer is confined to the skin of the penis, it is called *carcinoma in situ (CIS)*. Other types of penile cancers include melanomas, basal cell cancers, and sarcomas.

Circumcision (the surgical removal of the prepuce from the penis) in infancy almost eliminates the possibility of penile cancer in that chronic irritation and inflammation of the glans penis predispose uncircumcised men to penile cancer. Because of the ongoing controversy about neonatal circumcision, teach men and new mothers of boys that strict personal hygiene is an important preventive measure against penile cancer.

PATIENT-CENTERED COLLABORATIVE CARE

Penile cancer usually occurs as a painless, wartlike growth or ulcer on the glans under the prepuce (foreskin) and may be mistaken for a venereal wart. It may also appear as a reddened lesion with plaque.

Small lesions involving only the skin may be controlled by excisional biopsy. When the lesion is not curable by excisional biopsy or radiation therapy, a penectomy (partial or total removal of the penis) may be required. When the lesion is limited to the glans, a partial penectomy is performed. The distal portion of the corpus cavernosum and the corpus spongiosum is amputated. The urethra is connected to the skin, and a dressing is applied. A retention catheter is in place for 3 to 5 days after surgery until the edema surrounding the urethra subsides. Assess the dressing for drainage, which should be minimal. Check the urinary catheter for patency every 4 hours for the first 24 hours.

A total penectomy is required when the lesion has penetrated the shaft of the penis or when the tumor has recurred after a partial penectomy or radiation therapy. An incision is made from the pubic bone, which encircles the penis and extends into the perineum. The bases of both corpora cavernosa are exposed and excised, and the penis is amputated. An incision drain is placed in the wound before it is sutured. Patients who undergo a total penectomy also have a perineal urethrotomy (connecting the urethra to the skin in the perineum) for urinary drainage.

After a total penectomy, observe the incision dressing every 2 to 4 hours during the first 24 hours. A moderate amount of serosanguineous drainage from the incision drains is expected.

Be aware that regardless of how accepting the patient may appear before surgery, he may experience severe emotional problems after surgery. After a partial penectomy, he must adjust to considerable changes in body image and sexuality. Encourage him to verbalize his feelings about the loss of his penis. After a total penectomy, the patient can no longer have penile-vaginal or penile-anal intercourse and cannot urinate in a standing position. It is difficult for most men to accept the possibility that they might die because of a lesion on the penis, especially because they rarely experience any systemic cancer symptoms and are otherwise healthy. Help the patient realize that removal of his penis may save his life. Be aware of the possibility of suicide attempts because his penis may be more important to him than his life. The nurse may be the one to detect the need for professional psychological

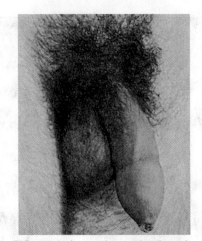

FIG. 75-6 An uncircumcised penis.

assistance for the patient or his partner. Early interventions can make a tremendous difference in the patient's or partner's well-being.

PHIMOSIS AND PARAPHIMOSIS

In *phimosis,* the prepuce is constricted so that it cannot be retracted over the glans. The prepuce remains down, around the tip of the penis. Teach uncircumcised men about the importance of cleaning the prepuce (Fig. 75-6).

In *paraphimosis,* the prepuce has not been returned to its normal position after being retracted and forms a constricting band around the glans. This constricts lymph drainage, causing the penis to swell. Blood flow becomes impeded, and tissue death can occur. *This problem is an emergency requiring immediate treatment. Uncircumcised males are at risk.* Causes include infection, not returning the foreskin to the original position, poor hygiene, vigorous sexual intercourse, and penile piercing. *When caring for a man who is not circumcised, be sure to replace the foreskin over the penis after bathing or catheterizing him to prevent this paraphimosis!*

Phimosis is corrected by circumcision (surgical removal of the prepuce or foreskin). This procedure also may be performed for other medical reasons or for aesthetic reasons. Circumcision in the adult male is usually performed in a same-day surgical setting. If the patient has a dressing, instruct him to soak in a warm bath that evening to allow the dressing to loosen. If the dressing falls off before the next day, caution him to not replace it. Explain that the sutures will be absorbed and need not be removed. No residual or side effects result from this surgery, and the patient should be able to resume normal activities within 1 week. Sexual intercourse may be resumed after 1 to 2 weeks when pain has subsided. Advise the man to notify his physician if he has any wound complications, such as swelling at the incision area or drainage, and to schedule a postoperative office visit.

PRIAPISM

Priapism is an uncontrolled, long-maintained erection without sexual desire, which causes the penis to become large, hard, and painful. It affects the two corpora cavernosa. The corpus spongiosum and glans penis are not affected.

Priapism can occur from neural, vascular, or pharmacologic causes, including:

- Thrombosis of the veins of the corpora cavernosa (usually resulting from trauma)
- Leukemia
- Sickle cell disease
- Diabetes mellitus
- Malignancies

Sickle cell disease causes priapism through the collection of erythrocytes within the corporal bodies. Leukemia may cause priapism because the increased number of white blood cells (WBCs) permits persistent engorgement of the corporal bodies. Cancer may also infiltrate the corporal bodies causing persistent engorgement. Priapism can also result from an abnormal neurogenic reflex, psychotropic drugs, antidepressants, antihypertensive drugs, and drugs used to treat erectile dysfunction. Other risk factors include recreational drugs (cocaine, ecstasy, marijuana), overdose of injectable drugs for erectile dysfunction, and prolonged sexual activity.

Priapism is a urologic emergency because the circulation to the penis may be compromised and the patient may not be able to void with an erect penis. The desired outcome for intervention is to improve the venous drainage of the corpora cavernosa. Conservative measures involve prostatic massage, sedation, ice packs, and bedrest. Meperidine (Demerol) is usually given immediately because of its hypotensive effect. Urinary catheterization is required if the man cannot void.

If conservative therapy is unsuccessful, treatment may proceed to aspiration of the corpora cavernosa with a large-bore needle or surgical intervention. The priapism should be resolved within the first 24 to 30 hours to prevent penile ischemia, gangrene, fibrosis, and erectile dysfunction. If a cause is identified, treatment is directed toward that underlying cause.

When caring for the patient with priapism, be sensitive to his emotional needs. He may be uncomfortable and in crisis but at the same time embarrassed by his erection and loss of control. Reassure the patient that it is understood that he is not in control of his erection, and provide him with privacy.

PROSTATITIS

Pathophysiology

Prostatitis is an inflammation of the prostate gland. The four types of prostatitis are acute bacterial (ABP), chronic bacterial (CBP), nonbacterial (NBP)/chronic pelvic pain syndrome (CPPS), and asymptomatic inflammatory prostatitis. Duration of symptoms, presence or absence of WBCs in the urine, and urinary culture results determine the classification.

Bacterial prostatitis often occurs with urethritis or an infection of the lower urinary tract. Organisms may reach the prostate via the bloodstream or the urethra. The most common organisms are *Escherichia coli, Enterobacter, Proteus,* and group D streptococci. Acute bacterial prostatitis may be manifested by fever, chills, dysuria (painful urination), urethral discharge, and a boggy, tender prostate. Gentle palpation of the prostate usually results in a urethral discharge, which has WBCs in the prostatic secretions.

Chronic bacterial prostatitis generally occurs in older men and has a less dramatic presentation than acute bacterial prostatitis and without the systemic manifestations. The patient reports experiencing hesitancy, urgency, dysuria, difficulty initiating and terminating the flow of urine, and decreased strength and volume of urine. Also, there may be discomfort in the perineum, scrotum, and penis.

Prostatitis can occur after a viral illness or may be associated with sexually transmitted diseases (STDs), especially in young males. Other causes may be autoimmune disorders, neuromuscular etiologies, allergy-mediated reactions, and psychosexual problems. In many instances, an exact cause of the perineal discomfort cannot be found. The patient reports mild urgency and dysuria. Rectal, perineal, and ejaculatory pain may be present. Decreased libido (sexual desire) may also be present.

Prostatodynia (pelvic floor pain) is a related condition in which manifestations of prostatitis are present but there is no inflammation of the prostate and the urine culture is negative. Also, the patient has low back pain with unilateral testicular pain, narrowed urinary stream with diminished force, and post-void dribbling.

▌ PATIENT-CENTERED COLLABORATIVE CARE

The patient with chronic prostatitis usually reports backache, perineal pain, mild dysuria, and urinary frequency. Hematuria may be present. The prostate may feel irregularly enlarged, firm, and slightly tender when palpated. The patient often has an elevated serum WBC count and prostate-specific antigen (PSA) level.

Complications of prostatitis are epididymitis (inflammation of the epididymis) and cystitis (inflammation of the bladder). A rare complication is a prostatic abscess. The patient with either acute or chronic bacterial prostatitis is likely to develop urinary tract infections. Sexual functioning may be reduced because of discomfort.

Early diagnosis and treatment of prostatitis with antimicrobials are important. Treatment may last from weeks to many months because there is poor penetration of antibiotics into prostatic tissue. Acute bacterial prostatitis may require hospitalization with aggressive IV antibiotics.

Emphasize the importance of comfort measures, such as sitz baths, muscle relaxants, and NSAIDs. Stool softeners are prescribed to prevent straining and rectal irritation of the prostate during a bowel movement. Alpha blockers such as tamsulosin (Flomax) may be given to promote voiding. Teach patients to avoid alcohol, coffee, tea, and spicy foods that irritate symptoms. Instruct them to avoid over-the-counter cold preparations containing decongestants or antihistamines that may cause urinary retention.

Teach the patient with chronic prostatitis about the long-term nature of the problem. Because prostatitis can cause other urinary tract infections, explain the importance of long-term antibiotic therapy and increasing fluid intake. Remind him to take the prescribed antibiotics on schedule. Because sulfamethoxazole-trimethoprim (Bactrim, Septra) diffuses into the prostatic fluid, it is often the antibiotic of choice. Before drug administration, be sure that the patient does not have any allergy to sulfa drugs.

Teach the patient about activities that drain the prostate (sexual intercourse, masturbation), which may help in the management of chronic prostatitis. Inform him that prostatitis is not infectious or contagious.

EPIDIDYMITIS

Pathophysiology

Epididymitis is an inflammation of the epididymis and may be a result of an infection or noninfectious source such as trauma. Bacterial infection is the most common cause. The infection may spread from other structures such as the prostate, bladder, or urethra. It can be a complication of an STD, such as gonorrhea or chlamydia. Although not common, epididymitis can also be a complication of long-term use of an indwelling urinary catheter, prostatic surgery, or a cystoscopic examination.

Organisms such as *Staphylococcus* and *E. coli* commonly cause epididymitis. Some men have *Chlamydia trachomatis*, which is transmitted sexually (see Chapter 76). The infective organism passes upward through the urethra and the ejaculatory duct and then along the vas deferens to the epididymis.

The man with epididymitis usually reports pain along the inguinal canal and along the vas deferens, followed by pain and swelling in the scrotum and the groin. If untreated, the epididymis becomes swollen and painful and fever may be present. Pyuria and bacteriuria may develop with resultant chills and fever. An abscess may form, requiring an orchiectomy (removal of one or both testes).

PATIENT-CENTERED COLLABORATIVE CARE

Instruct the patient with epididymitis to remain in bed with his scrotum elevated to prevent traction on the spermatic cord, to facilitate venous drainage, and to relieve pain. The man should wear a scrotal support when ambulating. A smear or culture of the urine or prostate secretions may be obtained to identify the causative organism. Antibiotics appropriate to the specific organism can then be prescribed. These antibiotics are taken until all acute manifestations are gone. If the epididymitis is chlamydial or gonorrheal in origin, the patient's sexual partners are also treated with antibiotics. NSAIDs such as ibuprofen or naproxen (Naprosyn) may be used to decrease inflammation and promote comfort.

The patient may find other comfort measures effective, such as applying cold compresses or ice to the scrotum intermittently and taking sitz baths. Advise him to avoid lifting, straining, or sexual activity until the infection is under control (which may take as long as 4 weeks).

In men with epididymitis, a testicular tumor must always be suspected, especially if the condition does not resolve in a week or two. Ultrasound study is often done to rule out an abscess or tumor. Patients with recurrent or chronic painful conditions may require an epididymectomy (excision of the epididymis from the testicle).

ORCHITIS

Orchitis is an acute testicular inflammation resulting from trauma or infection. The infection may be caused by the direct spread of bacteria through the urethra or by an infection elsewhere in the body, such as pneumonia, tuberculosis, gonorrhea, syphilis, or mumps. Usually both the testes and the epididymides are involved (epididymo-orchitis). Risk factors for orchitis include recurrent urinary tract infections, recurrent STDs, congenital abnormalities of the urogenital tract, instrumentation, and chronic indwelling urethral urinary catheter.

Orchitis may be unilateral or bilateral. If it is bilateral, the patient is at increased risk for sterility because of the testicular atrophy and fibrosis that occur during healing.

The manifestations of orchitis are the same as those of epididymitis and include scrotal pain, edema, reports of heavy feelings in the involved testicle(s), dysuria, pain on ejaculation, blood in the semen, and discharge from the penis. In addition, the patient may experience nausea and vomiting and pain radiating to the inguinal canal.

The treatment of orchitis is the same as for epididymitis and includes:
- Bedrest with scrotal elevation
- Application of ice
- Administration of analgesics and antibiotics

NURSING CONCEPT REVIEW

What might you NOTICE if the patient is experiencing impaired sexuality as a result of male reproductive problems?
- Lump or swelling in prostate or scrotum
- Report of pain in scrotum or during ejaculation
- Report of difficulty voiding (e.g., starting urine stream)
- Hematuria
- Report of dribbling of urine (incontinence)
- Report of inability to have a penile erection
- Report of decreased libido

What should you INTERPRET and how should you RESPOND to a patient experiencing impaired sexuality as a result of male reproductive problems?

Perform and interpret physical assessment, including:
- Conducting a complete pain assessment
- Inspecting and palpating bladder for distention
- Inspecting and palpating scrotum for swelling or masses
- Palpating lymph nodes for swelling, especially in the inguinal areas
- Sending urine sample for urinalysis and culture
- Checking most recent laboratory values for PSA, CBC, and serum tumor markers

Respond by:
- Catheterizing patient if retaining urine
- Providing pain relief measures, such as ice or medication as prescribed

NURSING CONCEPT REVIEW—cont'd

- Elevating scrotum if swollen
- Arranging for consultation with sex or intimacy therapist, if patient desires

On what should you REFLECT?
- Evaluate patient for need for indwelling urinary catheter.

- Evaluate effectiveness of actions to control pain and swelling.
- Think about what additional resources the patient will need to cope with his problem.

GET READY FOR THE NCLEX® EXAMINATION!

KEY POINTS

Review these Key Points for each NCLEX Examination Client Needs Category.

Safe and Effective Care Environment
- Teach patients with prostate cancer about American Cancer Society's Man to Man program and the American Foundation for Urologic Disease's Us TOO program to help men and their partners cope with prostate cancer.
- Have patients report signs of infection when caring for a urinary catheter in the home.

Health Promotion and Maintenance
- Teach men at risk for prostate cancer to follow the current American Cancer Society's screening and early detection guidelines.
- Teach men how to perform testicular self-examination as described in Chart 75-4.
- Teach uncircumcised men the importance of keeping the penis clean to prevent penile cancer.

Psychosocial Integrity
- Because most patients with testicular cancer are young and middle-aged adults, assess their reaction to the possible loss of reproductive ability.
- Because of the high incidence of erectile dysfunction after radical prostatectomy, assess the patient's adjustment to these changes in body function.
- Assess the patient's anxiety before prostate surgery, and allow him to express feelings of fear or grief.

Physiological Integrity
- Perform a focused physical assessment for patients reporting lumps or swelling in their genital area; inspect and palpate bladder and scrotum.
- Observe for and report complications after radical prostatectomy.

- Observe for and report bloody urine with clots after TURP; irrigate the bladder per agency or surgeon protocol.
- Maintain traction on the urinary catheter after a TURP.
- Teach patients about drug therapies (5-ARIs and alpha blocking agents) used to treat BPH, including side effects.
- Teach patients to avoid any drugs that can cause urinary retention, especially anticholinergics, antihistamines, and decongestants if BPH is present.
- Remind patients wanting to use complementary and alternative therapies to check with their health care providers before using them.
- Eating a well-balanced diet with plenty of fish and fruits and vegetables may help prevent prostate cancer.
- Reinforce the man's option for managing prostate cancer; some procedures and drugs cause erectile dysfunction and incontinence either temporarily or permanently.
- Use the information listed in Chart 75-3 to teach patients urinary catheter care after prostate cancer surgery.
- Teach patients about not lifting more than 15 lb (6.8 kg) after prostate surgery.
- Options for erectile dysfunction (ED) include drug therapy (most common), vacuum assist devices, penile injections, transurethral suppositories, or penile implants.
- Be aware that African-American middle-aged men are the most at risk for prostate cancer; Euro-American young men are the most at risk for testicular cancer.
- Teach patients to report symptoms of radiation cystitis or proctitis to their health care provider as soon as possible; these complications resolve in 4 to 6 weeks after the end of radiation therapy.
- Teach patients and their partners about hormonal therapy used to manage prostate cancer: LH-RH agonists and anti-androgen drugs.
- Be aware that sexually transmitted diseases (STDs) are a major cause of male reproductive system infections.

CHAPTER 76

Care of Patients with Sexually Transmitted Disease

Shirley E. Van Zandt

evolve WEBSITE

http://evolve.elsevier.com/Iggy/

Answer Key for NCLEX Examination Challenges and
   Decision-Making Challenges
Audio Glossary

Concept Map Creator
Key Points
Self-Assessment Questions for the NCLEX® Examination

LEARNING OUTCOMES

Safe and Effective Care Environment

1. Maintain patient confidentiality and privacy related to sexually transmitted diseases (STDs).
2. Educate patients with STDs and their sexual partners on self-care measures.

Health Promotion and Maintenance

3. Describe the role of expedited partner treatment in reducing STD recurrence.
4. Develop a health teaching plan for young adults and other at-risk people about risk factors, prevention, and treatment for STDs.

Psychosocial Integrity

5. Assess patients' and their partners' responses to a diagnosis of STD.

6. Explain the need to respect patients' personal values and beliefs regarding sexual practices.

Physiological Integrity

7. Compare the stages of syphilis.
8. Identify the role of drug therapy in managing patients with STDs.
9. Develop a health teaching plan for patients on how to self-manage their STD, including antibiotic therapy.
10. Describe the assessment findings that are typical in patients with STDs.
11. Develop a collaborative plan of care for a patient with pelvic inflammatory disease (PID).
12. Identify three sexually transmitted vaginal infections.

OVERVIEW

Sexually transmitted diseases (STDs) are caused by infectious organisms that have been passed from one person to another through intimate contact, usually oral, vaginal, or anal intercourse. Some organisms that cause these diseases are transmitted only through sexual contact. Other organisms are transmitted also by parenteral exposure to infected blood, fecal-oral transmission, intrauterine transmission to the fetus, and perinatal transmission from mother to neonate (Table 76-1). *Sexually transmitted infections (STIs)* is another term that has been used to describe the same group of health problems. This terminology was intended to focus on the management of these infections and to decrease the social stigma of labeling them as diseases. Though used in the literature, *STI* is the less common terminology. *STD continues to be the most acceptable term used by the Centers for Disease Control and Prevention (CDC).*

In spite of improved diagnostic techniques, increased knowledge about organisms that can be sexually transmitted, and changes in sexual attitudes and practices, the number of cases of STDs continues to increase. *Sexual issues are often sensitive, personal, and controversial, and nurses must respect the patients' lifestyle. Providing confidentiality is essential for patients to receive correct information, make informed decisions, and obtain appropriate care.*

The prevalence of STDs is a major health concern worldwide. Populations at greatest risk for acquiring STDs are

TABLE 76-1 SEXUALLY TRANSMITTED DISEASES

- Human immune deficiency virus infection
- Chancroid
- Syphilis
- Lymphogranuloma venereum
- Genital herpes simplex virus infection
- Genital warts
- Gonococcal infection
- Chlamydia infection
- Nongonococcal urethritis
- Mucopurulent cervicitis
- Epididymitis
- Pelvic inflammatory disease
- Sexually transmitted enteritis
- Sexually transmitted proctitis
- Trichomoniasis
- Candidal infection
- Bacterial vaginosis
- Viral hepatitis
- Cytomegalovirus infection
- Ectoparasitic infection:
  - Pediculosis pubis
  - Scabies

From Centers for Disease Control and Prevention (CDC). (2010). Sexually transmitted diseases treatment guidelines, 2010. *Morbidity and Mortality Weekly Report, 59* (RR-12), 1-110.

pregnant women, adolescents, and men who have sex with men (MSM). External factors such as an increasing population, cultural factors (e.g., earlier first intercourse), political and economic policies, and international travel and migration affect the prevalence of STDs. It is also affected by changing human physiology patterns such as earlier menarche, comorbidities leading to immunosuppression such as from human immune deficiency virus (HIV), or treatments for cancer or organ transplantation. Access to care plays a major role in the risk for acquiring an STD.

WOMEN'S HEALTH CONSIDERATIONS

Because of the very vascular mucous membranes of the vagina, women are more easily infected with STDs than are men and are at greater risk for health problems caused by STDs. Young women who are sexually active with men have an increased risk for contracting an STD for several reasons including increased rates of sexual activity that may be unprotected and exposure of cervical basal epithelium cells to infections. Lesbian women have a decreased risk for STDs, although many have or have had sex with men.

Some young women may also be at high risk because they:
- Lack knowledge about the risk for disease
- Believe that they are not vulnerable to disease
- Mistakenly believe that oral contraceptives; contraceptive patches, sponges, and foams; and intrauterine devices also protect them from STDs
- Consume large amounts of alcohol, which promotes risky sexual behavior

Postmenopausal women also may be at risk for STDs because many perceive that pregnancy is no longer likely and thus do not use barrier protection. Mucosal tears from vaginal atrophy in postmenopausal women may also place them at risk.

Women have more asymptomatic infections that may delay diagnosis and treatment. Many STDs reside in the cervical os and cause little change in vaginal discharge or vulvar tissue. This delay increases the likelihood of complications from STDs, including ascending infections that may cause reproductive organ damage and illness. Embarrassment, denial, or fear about STDs may further delay treatment, increasing the potential for serious complications.

STDs cause complications that can contribute to severe physical and emotional suffering, including infertility, ectopic pregnancy, cancer, and death. Some of the most common complications caused by sexually transmitted organisms are listed in Table 76-2.

TABLE 76-2 COMPLICATIONS CAUSED BY SEXUALLY TRANSMITTED ORGANISMS

COMPLICATION	CAUSATIVE ORGANISMS
Salpingitis, infertility, and ectopic pregnancy	*Neisseria gonorrhoeae* *Chlamydia trachomatis* *Mycoplasma hominis* *Ureaplasma urealyticum*
Reproductive loss (abortion/miscarriage)	*N. gonorrhoeae* *C. trachomatis* Herpes simplex virus *M. hominis* *U. urealyticum* *Treponema pallidum*
Puerperal infection	*N. gonorrhoeae* *C. trachomatis*
Perinatal infection	Hepatitis B virus Human immune deficiency virus Human papilloma virus *N. gonorrhoeae* *C. trachomatis* Herpes simplex virus *T. pallidum* Cytomegalovirus Group B streptococcus
Cancer of genital area	Human papilloma virus
Male urethritis	*M. hominis* Herpes simplex virus *N. gonorrhoeae* *C. trachomatis* *U. urealyticum*
Vulvovaginitis	Herpes simplex virus *Trichomonas vaginalis* Bacterial vaginosis *Candida albicans*
Cervicitis	*N. gonorrhoeae* *C. trachomatis* Herpes simplex virus
Proctitis	*N. gonorrhoeae* *C. trachomatis* Herpes simplex virus *Campylobacter jejuni* *Shigella species* *Entamoeba histolytica*
Hepatitis	*T. pallidum* Hepatitis A, hepatitis B, and hepatitis C viruses
Dermatitis	*Sarcoptes scabiei* *Phthirus pubis*
Genital ulceration or warts	*C. trachomatis* Herpes simplex virus Human papilloma virus *T. pallidum* *Haemophilus ducreyi* *Calymmatobacterium granulomatis*

Chlamydia infection, gonorrhea, syphilis, chancroid, human immune deficiency virus (HIV) infection, and acquired immune deficiency syndrome (AIDS) are reportable to local health authorities in every state (Centers for Disease Control and Prevention [CDC], 2008). Other STDs such as genital herpes (GH) may or may not be reported, depending on local legal requirements. Positive results can be reported by clinicians and laboratories. Reports are kept strictly confidential.

Nurses in a variety of settings are responsible for identifying people at risk for STDs, caring for patients with diagnosed STDs, and preventing further cases through education and case finding. Nurses in secondary and tertiary care settings, such as acute care hospitals, have a responsibility to recognize patients who are at risk for or who have STDs, possibly while being treated for another unrelated health problem.

The CDC provides regularly updated guidelines for treatment of STDs. These best practice guidelines provide information, treatment standards, and counseling advice to help decrease the spread of these diseases (CDC, 2010a).

INFECTIONS ASSOCIATED WITH ULCERS

SYPHILIS

Pathophysiology

Syphilis is a complex sexually transmitted disease (STD) that can become systemic and cause serious complications, including death. The causative organism is a spirochete called *Treponema pallidum*. Although the organism can be seen only with a darkfield microscope, several serologic tests may be used to screen for the presence of syphilis antibody. *T. pallidum* is damaged by dry air or any known disinfectant. The organisms die within hours at temperatures of 105.8° to 107.6° F (41° to 42° C) and are not airborne. *The infection is usually transmitted by sexual contact and blood exposure, but transmission can occur through close body contact such as kissing.*

Syphilis progresses through four stages: primary, secondary, latent, and tertiary. The appearance of an ulcer called a chancre is the first sign of *primary* syphilis. It develops at the site of entry (inoculation) of the organism from 10 to 90 days after exposure (3 weeks is average). Chancres may be found on any area of the skin or mucous membranes but occur most often on the genitalia, lips, nipples, and hands and in the mouth, anus, and rectum.

During this highly infectious stage, the chancre begins as a small papule. Within 3 to 7 days, it breaks down into its typical appearance: a painless, indurated (hard), smooth, weeping lesion. Regional lymph nodes enlarge, feel firm, and are not painful. Without treatment, the chancre usually disappears within 6 weeks. However, the organism spreads throughout the body and the patient is still infectious.

Secondary syphilis develops 6 weeks to 6 months after the onset of primary syphilis. During this stage, syphilis is a systemic disease because the spirochetes circulate throughout the bloodstream. Common manifestations include:
- Malaise
- Low-grade fever
- Headache
- Muscular aches and pains
- Sore throat
- Generalized rash

These symptoms are often mistaken for those of influenza. The rash, the most commonly presenting symptom, usually involves the palms and soles of the feet. Although it has no typical appearance, the rash tends to change from papules to squamous papules to pustules. Other skin lesions include psoriasis-like rashes (Fig. 76-1), wartlike lesions (condylomata lata), and mucous patches. *These lesions are highly*

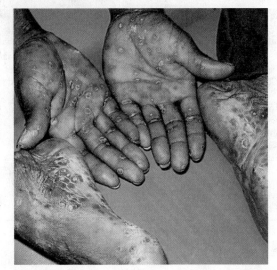

FIG. 76-1 Palmar and plantar secondary syphilis.

contagious and should not be touched without gloves. The rash subsides without treatment in 4 to 12 weeks.

After the second stage of syphilis, there is a period of latency. *Early latent* syphilis occurs during the first year after infection, and infectious lesions can recur. *Late latent* syphilis is a disease of more than 1 year's duration after infection. This stage is not infectious except to the fetus of a pregnant woman. Patients with latent syphilis may or may not have reactive serologic test (e.g., Venereal Disease Research Laboratory [VDRL]) findings.

Tertiary, or late, syphilis occurs after a highly variable period, from 4 to 20 years. This stage develops in untreated cases and can mimic other conditions because any organ system can be affected. Manifestations of late syphilis include:
- Benign lesions (gummas) of the skin, mucous membranes, and bones
- Cardiovascular syphilis, usually in the form of aortic valvular disease and aortic aneurysms
- Neurosyphilis, causing central nervous system problems (e.g., meningitis, hearing loss, generalized paresis [weakness])

Because of strong U.S. public health efforts between 1990 and 1996, there was a 90% decrease in syphilis cases to an all-time low in 2000. Since 2001, there has been a steady increase in cases of primary and secondary syphilis with the majority among men having sex with men (MSM) (CDC, 2009).

⊕ CULTURAL AWARENESS

African Americans have an 8 times greater rate of acquiring syphilis than whites. Compared with whites, the 2008 rate for Hispanics was 2 times higher (CDC, 2009). The reason for these differences is unclear, but lack of access to health care may be a factor.

Health Promotion and Maintenance

One of the *Healthy People 2020* objectives is to completely eliminate syphilis in the United States (U.S. Department of Health and Human Services [USDHHS], 2010) (Table 76-3). The most important tool for prevention of sexually transmitted diseases (STDs), including syphilis, is education. All people, regardless of age, gender, ethnicity, socioeconomic

TABLE 76-3	MEETING *HEALTHY PEOPLE 2020* OBJECTIVES AND TARGETS FOR IMPROVEMENT: SEXUALLY TRANSMITTED DISEASES

- Reduce the proportion of adolescents and young adults with Chlamydia trachomatis infections (by 10%).
- Reduce the proportion of females ages 15 to 44 years who have ever required treatment for pelvic inflammatory disease (by 10%).
- Reduce gonorrhea rates (by 10%).
- Reduce sustained domestic transmission of primary and secondary syphilis (by 10%).
- Reduce the proportion of females with human papilloma virus (HPV) infection (no specific target).
- Reduce the proportion of young adults with genital herpes due to herpes simplex type 2 (by 10%).

status, education, or sexual orientation, are susceptible to these diseases. STDs are largely preventable through safer sex practices. *Do not assume that a person is not sexually active because of his or her age, education, marital status, profession, or religion.* Discuss prevention methods, including safe sex, with all patients who are or may become sexually active.

Safe sex practices are those that reduce the risk for nonintact skin or mucous membranes coming in contact with infected body fluids and blood. These practices include using:

- A latex or polyurethane condom for genital and anal intercourse
- A condom or latex barrier (dental dam) over the genitals or anus during oral-genital or oral-anal sexual contact
- Gloves for finger or hand contact with the vagina or rectum

Abstinence, mutual monogamy, and decreasing the number of sexual partners also decrease the risk for acquiring an STD.

PATIENT-CENTERED COLLABORATIVE CARE

ASSESSMENT

Assessment of the patient who has manifestations of syphilis begins with a history to gather information about any ulcers or rash. Take a sexual history and conduct a risk assessment to include whether previous testing or treatment for syphilis or other STDs has ever been done (Chart 76-1). Ask about allergic reactions to drugs, especially penicillin. A woman may report inguinal lymph node enlargement resulting from a chancre in the vagina or cervix that is not easily visible to her. She may state a history of sexual contact with a male partner who had an ulcer that she noticed during the encounter. Men usually discover the chancre on the penis or scrotum.

Conduct a physical examination, including inspection and palpation, to identify manifestations of syphilis. *Wear gloves while palpating any lesions because of the highly contagious treponemes that are present.* Observe for and document rashes of any type because of the variable presentation of secondary syphilis.

After the physical examination, the health care provider obtains a *specimen of the chancre* for examination under a darkfield microscope. Diagnosis of primary or secondary syphilis is confirmed if *T. pallidum* is present.

CHART 76-1	FOCUSED ASSESSMENT

The Patient with a Sexually Transmitted Disease

Assess history of present illness:
- Chief concern
- Symptoms by quality and quantity, precipitating and palliative factors
- Any treatments taken (self-prescribed or over-the-counter products)

Assess past medical history:
- Major health problems—including any history of STDs/PID or immunosuppression
- Surgeries—obstetric and gynecologic, circumcision

Assess current health status:
- Menstrual history for irregularities
- Sexual history:
  - Type and frequency of sexual activity
  - Number of sexual contacts/partners
  - Sexual orientation
- Contraceptive history
- Medications
- Allergies
- Lifestyle risks—drugs, alcohol, tobacco

Assess preventive health care practices:
- Papanicolaou (Pap) tests
- Regular STD screening
- Use of barrier contraceptives to prevent STDs and pregnancy

Assess physical examination findings:
- Vital signs
- Oropharyngeal findings
- Abdominal findings
- Genital or pelvic findings
- Anorectal findings

Assess laboratory data:
- Urinalysis
- Hematology
- ESR or CRP if PID is being considered
- Cervical, urethral, oral, rectal specimens
- Lesion samples for microbiology and virology
- Pregnancy testing

CRP, C-reactive protein; *ESR,* erythrocyte sedimentation rate; *PID,* pelvic inflammatory disease; *STDs,* sexually transmitted diseases.

Blood tests are also used to diagnose syphilis. The usual screening and/or diagnostic nontreponemal tests are the *Venereal Disease Research Laboratory (VDRL)* serum test and the more sensitive *rapid plasma reagin (RPR).* These tests are based on an antibody-antigen reaction that determines the presence and amount of antibodies produced by the body in response to an infection by *T. pallidum.* They become reactive 2 to 6 weeks after infection. VDRL titers are also used to monitor treatment effectiveness. The antibodies are not specific to *T. pallidum,* and false-positive reactions often occur from such conditions as viral infections, hepatitis, and systemic lupus erythematosus (SLE) (Pagana & Pagana, 2010).

If a VDRL result is positive, the health care provider requests or the laboratory may automatically perform a more specific treponemal test, such as the *fluorescent treponemal antibody absorption (FTA-ABS)* test or the *microhemagglutination assay for T. palladium (MHA-TP),* to confirm the infection. These tests are more sensitive for all stages of syphilis, although false-positive results may still occur. Patients who have a reactive test will have this positive result for their entire life, even after sufficient treatment. This poses a challenge when receiving a positive result for a patient who denies a history of or does not know he or she had syphilis.

INTERVENTIONS

Patient-centered collaborative care includes drug therapy and health teaching to resolve the infection and prevent infection transmission to others.

Drug Therapy

Benzathine penicillin G given IM as a single 2.4 million-unit dose is the evidence-based treatment for primary, secondary, and early latent syphilis (CDC, 2010a). Patients in the late latent stage receive the same dose every week for 3 weeks (CDC, 2010a).

! NURSING SAFETY PRIORITY

Drug Alert

Allergic reactions to benzathine pencillin G can occur. Therefore monitor for allergic manifestations (e.g., rash, edema, shortness of breath, chest tightness, anxiety). Be sure that the patient who has never had penicillin has a skin test before receiving the injection. Penicillin desensitization is recommended for penicillin-allergic patients. Keep all patients at the health care agency for at least 30 minutes after they have received the antibiotic so that manifestations of an allergic reaction can be detected and treated. The most severe reaction is anaphylaxis. Treatment should be available and implemented immediately if symptoms occur. Chapter 19 describes the management of drug allergies in detail.

After treatment, the CDC recommends follow-up evaluation including blood tests at 6, 12, and 24 months. Repeat treatment may be needed if the patient does not respond to the initial antibiotic.

The *Jarisch-Herxheimer reaction* may also follow antibiotic therapy for syphilis. This reaction is caused by the rapid release of products from the disruption of the cells of the organism. Symptoms include generalized aches, pain at the injection site, vasodilation, hypotension, and fever. They are usually benign and begin within 2 hours after therapy with a peak at 4 to 8 hours. This reaction may be treated symptomatically with analgesics and antipyretics.

Teaching for Self-Management

Reinforce teaching about the cause of infection (sexual transmission); treatment, including side effects; possible complications of untreated or incompletely treated disease; and the need for follow-up care.

! NURSING SAFETY PRIORITY

Drug Alert

Discuss with the patient with syphilis the importance of partner notification and treatment, including the risk for re-infection if the partner goes untreated. All sexual partners must be prophylactically treated as soon as possible, preferably within 90 days of the syphilis diagnosis.

Inform the patient that the disease will be reported to the local health authority and that all information will be held in strict confidence. Encourage the patient to provide accurate information for this follow-up to ensure that all at-risk partners are treated appropriately. Provide a setting that offers privacy and encourages open discussion. Urge the patient to adhere to the treatment regimen, which includes follow-up visits. Also recommend sexual abstinence until the treatment of both the patient and partner(s) is completed.

The emotional responses to syphilis vary and may include feelings of fear, depression, guilt, and anxiety. Patients may experience guilt if they have infected others or anger if they have been infected by a partner. If further psychosocial interventions are needed, encourage the patient to discuss these feelings or refer him or her to other resources such as psychotherapy groups, self-help support groups, or STD clinics.

? NCLEX EXAMINATION CHALLENGE

Physiological Integrity

The nurse gives a client an IM dose of penicillin G for syphilis. What is the priority action for the nurse after giving the drug?
A. Monitor the client for at least 30 minutes for any reaction to the drug.
B. Rub the site with an alcohol prep to ensure even distribution of the drug.
C. Teach the client the importance of not having sexual intercourse for 7 days.
D. Ask the client if she is allergic to any drugs, especially penicillin.

GENITAL HERPES

Pathophysiology

Genital herpes (GH) is an acute, recurring, incurable viral disease. It is the most common STD in the United States, with 16.2% of Americans currently infected with herpes simplex virus type 2 (HSV-2). The prevalence among African Americans is 39.2%, disproportionately affecting African-American women (48.0%) (CDC, 2010b). These rates are based on the presence of HSV-2 antibodies in the blood of those tested, the majority of whom have had no symptoms and most have never received a diagnosis of GH infection (CDC, 2010b).

Two serotypes of herpes simplex virus (HSV) affect the genitalia: type 1 (HSV-1) and type 2 (HSV-2). Most *nongenital* lesions such as cold sores are caused by HSV-1. Historically, HSV-2 caused most of the genital lesions. However, this distinction is academic because the transmission, symptoms, diagnosis, and treatment are nearly identical for the two types. Either type can produce oral or genital lesions through oral-genital contact with an infected person. HSV-2 has been thought to cause the majority of the primary episodes of GH, though up to one-third are caused by HSV-1 (Drugge & Allen, 2008). HSV-2 recurs and sheds asymptomatically more often than HSV-1. Most people with GH have not been diagnosed because they have mild symptoms and shed virus intermittently (CDC, 2010a).

The incubation period of genital herpes is 2 to 20 days, with the average period being 1 week. Many people do not have symptoms during the primary outbreak. When outbreaks occur, they are usually more severe than in recurrent outbreaks and occasionally require hospitalization.

Recurrences are not caused by re-infection. Additional episodes are usually less severe and of shorter duration than the primary infection episode. Some patients have no symptoms at all during recurrence or viral reactivation. *However, there is viral shedding and the patient is infectious.* Long-term complications of GH include the risk for neonatal transmission and an increased risk for acquiring HIV infection.

PATIENT-CENTERED COLLABORATIVE CARE

ASSESSMENT

The diagnosis of GH is usually based on the patient's history and physical examination (see Chart 76-1). Ask the patient if he or she felt itching or a tingling sensation in the skin 1 to 2 days before the outbreak. These sensations are usually followed by the appearance of vesicles (blisters) in a typical cluster on the penis, scrotum, vulva, vagina, cervix, or perianal region. The blisters rupture spontaneously in a day or two and leave painful erosions that can become extensive. Assess for other symptoms such as headaches, fever, general malaise, and swelling of inguinal lymph nodes. Ask if urination is painful. Patients with urinary retention may need to be catheterized. Lesions resolve within 2 to 6 weeks.

After the lesions heal, the virus remains in a dormant state in the nerve ganglia (specifically, the sacral ganglia). Periodically, the virus may activate and symptoms recur. These recurrences may be triggered by many factors, including stress, fever, sunburn, poor nutrition, menses, and sexual activity. Assess the patient for these risk factors.

GH is confirmed through a viral culture or polymerase chain reaction (PCR) assays of the lesions. PCR is the more sensitive test. Fluid from inside the blister should be obtained within 48 hours of the first outbreak of the blisters, since accuracy decreases as they begin to heal. Serology testing, which is glycoprotein G antibody-based, can identify the HSV type, either 1 or 2. Serologic tests are used to identify infection in high-risk groups such as HIV-positive patients, patients who have partners with HSV, or MSM (CDC, 2010a). The POCkit HSV-2 Rapid Test is a point-of-care test with results in 6 minutes. The HerpeSelect Immunoblot IgG test, HerpeSelect ELISA, and the Western Blot are qualitative assays that can differentiate between HSV-1 and HSV-2. All of these tests are highly specific and sensitive (Bavis et al., 2009).

INTERVENTIONS

The desired outcomes of treatment for HSV-infected patients are to decrease the discomfort from painful ulcerations, promote healing without secondary infection, decrease viral shedding, and prevent infection transmission (Chart 76-2).

Drug Therapy

Antiviral drugs are used to treat GH. *The drugs do not cure the infection but do decrease the severity, promote healing, and decrease the frequency of recurrent outbreaks while they are being used.*

Drug therapy should be offered to anyone with an initial outbreak of GH. Though the initial symptoms may be mild, they may become more severe. Topical therapy is not recommended. Acyclovir (Zovirax, Avirax ✤), famciclovir (Famvir), or valacyclovir (Valtrex) may be prescribed. The main differences in these drugs are cost and frequency of use. Dosage and length of treatment differ for primary outbreaks (lasting 7 to 10 days) and recurrent outbreaks (lasting 1 to 5 days). Intermittent or continuous suppressive antiviral therapy is offered to patients to lessen or prevent outbreaks, even for

---

CHART 76-2	BEST PRACTICE FOR PATIENT SAFETY & QUALITY CARE

Care of or Self-Management for the Patient with Genital Herpes

- Administer oral analgesics as prescribed.
- Apply local anesthetic sprays or ointments as prescribed.
- Apply ice packs or warm compresses to the patient's lesions.
- Administer sitz baths three or four times a day.
- Encourage an increase in fluid intake to replace fluid lost through open lesions.
- Encourage frequent urination.
- Pour water over the patient's genitalia while voiding, or encourage voiding while the patient is sitting in a tub of water or standing in a shower.
- Catheterize the patient as necessary.
- Encourage genital hygiene, and encourage keeping the skin clean and dry.
- Wash hands thoroughly after contact with lesions, and launder towels that have had direct contact with lesions.
- Wear gloves when applying ointments or making any direct contact with lesions.
- Advise the patient to avoid sexual activity when lesions are present.
- Advise the patient to use latex or polyurethane condoms during all sexual exposures.
- Instruct the patient in the use, side effects, and risks versus benefits of antiviral agents.
- Advise the patient to discuss the diagnosis of genital herpes (GH) with current and new partners.

---

those with infrequent recurrent episodes. Therapy for severe recurrent outbreaks is most beneficial if it is started within 1 day of the appearance of lesions or during the period of itching or tingling before lesions appear.

Patients who have recurrences, regardless of frequency, may benefit from daily suppressive treatment. Suppression reduces recurrences in most patients, but it does not prevent viral shedding, even when symptoms are absent (CDC, 2010a). Patients receiving continuous therapy should periodically (possibly once a year) be reassessed for recurrences, usually by stopping the antiviral drug temporarily.

IV acyclovir and hospitalization may be indicated for patients with severe HSV infections, such as disseminated disease or encephalitis. These are severe complications of genital herpes and may be fatal.

Teaching for Self-Management

Nursing interventions focus on patient counseling and education about the infection, the potential for recurrent episodes, the correct use and possible side effects of antiviral therapy, and sexual transmission. Discussion about sexual activity is extremely important.

! NURSING SAFETY PRIORITY

Action Alert

Remind patients to abstain from sexual activity while GH lesions are present. Urge condom use during all sexual exposures because of the increased risk for HSV transmission. Viral shedding can occur even when lesions are not present. Teach the patient about how and when to use condoms (Chart 76-3).

CHART 76-3   PATIENT AND FAMILY EDUCATION: PREPARING FOR SELF-MANAGEMENT

Use of Condoms

- Use latex or polyurethane condoms rather than natural membrane condoms.
- Use a condom with every sexual encounter (including oral, vaginal, and anal).
- Female condoms (Reality)—polyurethane or nitrile sheaths in the vagina—are effective in preventing transmission of viruses, including HIV.
- Condoms infrequently (2 per 100) break during sexual intercourse.
- Keep condoms (especially latex) in a cool, dry place, out of direct sunlight.
- Do not use condoms that are in damaged packages or that are brittle or discolored.
- Always handle a condom with care to avoid damaging it with fingernails, teeth, or other sharp objects.
- Put condoms on before any genital contact. Hold the condom by the tip and unroll it on the penis. Leave a space at the tip to collect semen.
- If you use a lubricant with condoms, make sure that the lubricant is water based and washes away with water. Oil-based products damage latex condoms.
- Use of spermicide (nonoxynol-9) with condoms, either lubricated condoms or vaginal application, has *not* been proven to be more or less effective against STDs than use without spermicide. *Spermicide-coated condoms have been associated with Escherichia coli urinary tract infections in women. Nonoxynol-9 may increase risk for transmission of HIV during vaginal intercourse and anal intercourse. Its use is discouraged for anal intercourse.*
- If a condom breaks, replace it immediately.
- After ejaculation, withdraw the erect penis carefully, holding the condom at the base of the penis to prevent the condom from slipping off.
- Never use a condom more than once.

Modified from Centers for Disease Control and Prevention (CDC). (2010a). Sexually transmitted diseases treatment guidelines, 2010. *Morbidity and Mortality Weekly Report, 59*(RR-12), 4-5.
HIV, Human immune deficiency virus; *STDs,* sexually transmitted diseases.

Assess the patient's and partner's emotional responses to the diagnosis of genital herpes. Many people are initially shocked and need reassurance that they can manage the disease. Infected patients may have feelings of disbelief, uncleanness, isolation, and loneliness. They may also be angry at their partners for transmitting the infection or fear rejection by partners because they have the infection. Help patients cope with the diagnosis by being sensitive and supportive during assessments and interventions. Encourage social support, and refer patients to support groups (e.g., local support groups of the National Herpes Resource Center [www.ashastd.org/herpes/herpes_comm_support.cfm]). Symptomatic care may include oral analgesics, topical anesthetics, sitz baths, and increased oral fluid intake (Bavis et al., 2009).

Emphasize the risk for neonatal infection to all patients, both male and female. Men and women who have genital herpes need to inform the pregnancy care provider of their history. Infected male partners will be advised to avoid intercourse during pregnancy if the pregnant partner is not infected. This avoids the risk for a new primary infection and outbreak during pregnancy. People who have tested serology positive to HSV-1 or HSV-2 but have never had GH symptoms should be counseled with the same information as those who have symptoms (CDC, 2010a).

INFECTIONS OF THE EPITHELIAL STRUCTURES

CONDYLOMATA ACUMINATA (GENITAL WARTS)

Pathophysiology

Condylomata acuminata (also known as *genital warts*) are caused by certain types of *human papilloma virus (HPV)*, 90% of which are types 6 and 11 or low-risk HPV (Winer & Koutsky, 2008). These types *rarely* result in invasive cancer of the genital tract such as cervical cancer. *However, HPV types 16, 18, 31, 33, and 35, considered high-risk HPV, can be found on the skin of the genitalia and increase the risk for genital cancers, especially cervical cancer.* Infection with several HPV types can occur at the same time. The presence of one strain increases the risk for acquiring a higher-risk strain. Genital warts are the most common viral disease that is sexually transmitted and are often seen with other infections. Many American women, ages 14 to 59 years, are infected with either high- or low-risk HPV (Dunne et al., 2007).

HPV infection is thought to be the primary risk factor for development of cervical cancer (Winer & Koutsky, 2008). Sites commonly affected by infection include the urinary meatus, labia, vagina, cervix, penis, scrotum, anus, and perineal area. The incubation period is usually 2 to 3 months. There is growing evidence that HPV infection through oral and anal sex, especially in men who have sex with men (MSM), may be a risk factor for developing oral and anal cancers (Chaturvedi et al., 2008; Kim, 2010).

PATIENT-CENTERED COLLABORATIVE CARE

ASSESSMENT

The diagnosis of condylomata acuminata is made by examination of the lesions. They are initially small, white or flesh-colored papillary growths that may grow into large cauliflower-like masses (Fig. 76-2). Multiple warts usually occur in the same area. Bleeding may occur if the wart is disturbed. Warts may disappear or resolve on their own without treatment. They may occur once or recur at the original site.

A Papanicolaou (Pap) test and HPV DNA probe are used to obtain cervical specimens to assess for dysplasia and isolate and diagnose HPV of the cervix. High-risk strains of HPV can be identified and correlated with an abnormal Pap smear finding. High-risk HPV may co-exist with low-risk HPV, the likely cause of the warts. To rule out the presence of other STDs, a VDRL test, HIV test, and cultures for chlamydia and gonorrhea infections are done. If a wartlike lesion bleeds easily, appears infected, is atypical, or persists, a biopsy of the lesion is performed to rule out other pathologic problems such as cancer.

INTERVENTIONS

The desired outcomes of management are to remove the warts and treat the symptoms. No current therapy eliminates HPV. Therefore recurrences after treatment are likely. It is not

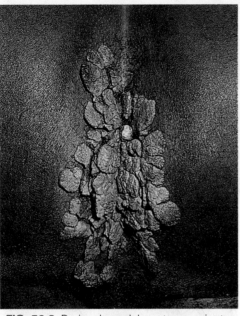

FIG. 76-2 Perianal condylomata acuminata.

known whether removal of visible warts decreases the risk for disease transmission (CDC, 2010a).

Drug Therapy

Patients may apply podofilox (Condylox) 0.5% cream or gel twice daily for 3 days with no treatment for the next 4 days. This regimen should be repeated for four cycles. Other options are imiquimod (Aldara) 5% cream applied topically at bedtime three times a week and sinecatechins 15% ointment applied three times a day, both until the warts disappear or for up to 16 weeks. Imiquimod boosts the immune system rather than simply destroying the warts. These self-treatments are less expensive than those performed in the health care provider's office, but they take longer for healing. *Teach patients that over-the-counter (OTC) wart treatments should not be used on genital tissue* (CDC, 2010a).

Cryotherapy, trichloroacetic acid (TCA) or bichloroacetic acid (BCA), and podophyllin (Pododerm) are provider-applied treatments. Cryotherapy (freezing), usually with liquid nitrogen, can be used every 1 to 2 weeks until lesions are resolved. TCA/BCA (80% to 90%) can be applied weekly. Podophyllin resin can be applied weekly but needs to be washed off 1 to 4 hours after application. Extensive warts have been treated with the carbon dioxide laser, intra-lesion interferon injections, and surgical removal (CDC, 2010a).

Teaching for Self-Management

The priority for nursing management is patient and sexual partner education about the mode of transmission, incubation period, treatment, and complications, especially the association with cervical cancer. Reinforce instructions about local care of the lesions or patient-applied treatment for self-management.

Inform patients that recurrence is likely, especially in the first 3 months, and that repeated treatments may be needed. Urge all patients to have complete STD testing, since exposure to one may increase risk for contracting another.

> **! NURSING SAFETY PRIORITY**
> *Drug Alert*
>
> Teach patients that after treatment with cryotherapy, podophyllin, or TCA, they may experience discomfort, bleeding, or discharge from the site or sloughing of parts of warts. Instruct patients to keep the area clean (shower or bath) and dry. Teach them to be alert for any signs or symptoms of infection or side effects of the treatment.

Condylomata lata (secondary syphilis) can resemble condylomata acuminata (genital warts). Sexual partners should also be evaluated and offered treatment if warts are present. Teach patients to avoid intimate sexual contact until external lesions are healed. Recommend condoms to help reduce transmission even after warts have been treated (see Chart 76-3). Encourage women to have an annual Pap test. The presence of warts requires HPV testing of the patient and partner.

In 2006, the U.S. Food and Drug Administration (FDA) approved an HPV vaccine *Gardasil®* (Merck) that provides almost 100% immunity for HPV types 6 and 11 (predominantly types causing warts, low risk for cervical cancer) and 16 and 18 (high risk for cervical cancer). The vaccine was approved for females initially. In 2010, it was approved for males ages 9 to 26 years as a method for reducing cervical cancer. In 2009, CERVARIX® (GSK) was approved for 10- to 25-year-old females and protects only against HPV types 16 and 18. Both vaccines are recommended to be given before onset of sexual activity before there may be contact with HPV. They are also effective in protecting against infection if exposed to a second strain later. Early results have suggested that rates of genital warts and cervical cancer will be significantly lowered by these vaccines (Muñoz et al., 2010).

GONORRHEA

Pathophysiology

Gonorrhea is a sexually transmitted bacterial infection that occurs in both men and women. The causative organism is *Neisseria gonorrhoeae*, a gram-negative intracellular diplococcus. It is transmitted by direct sexual contact with mucosal surfaces (vaginal intercourse, orogenital contact, or anogenital contact).

The first symptoms of gonorrhea may appear 3 to 10 days after sexual contact with an infected person. The disease can be present without symptoms and can be transmitted or progress without warning. In women, ascending spread of the organism can cause pelvic infection (pelvic inflammatory disease [PID]), endometritis (endometrial infection), salpingitis (fallopian tube infection), and pelvic peritonitis. Rare complications of gonorrhea in adults include arthritis, meningitis, hepatitis, and disseminated infection.

An estimated 700,000 new infections occur each year, only half of which are diagnosed or reported (CDC, 2010a). Significant disparity exists between age and racial groups. In 2008, young African-American women had the highest gonorrhea rate, followed by young African-American men (CDC, 2009). The reasons for these differences are not known, although lack of access to health care may be a factor.

Over the years, gonorrhea has become resistant to penicillin, tetracycline, and ciprofloxacin. Ciprofloxacin is no longer the drug of choice because of the development of fluoroquinolone-resistant *N. gonorrhoeae* (CDC, 2007a).

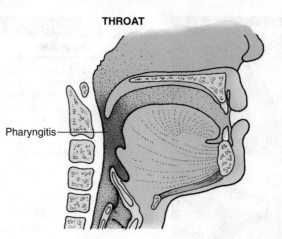

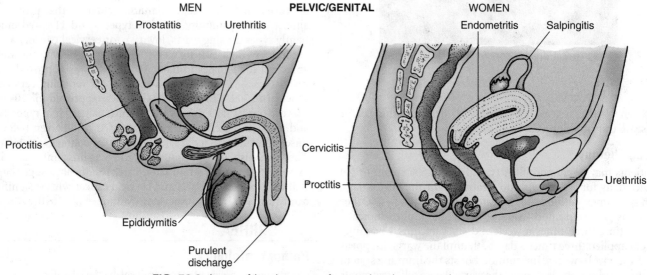

FIG. 76-3 Areas of involvement of gonorrhea in men and women.

Cephalosporins are currently the only class of antibiotics that have not developed gonorrhea resistance (CDC, 2010c).

PATIENT-CENTERED COLLABORATIVE CARE

ASSESSMENT

A complete history includes reviewing possible symptoms of gonorrhea and taking a sexual history that includes sexual orientation and sites of sexual exposure or intercourse. Assess for allergies to antibiotics (see Chart 76-1). Establish a trusting relationship and use a nonjudgmental approach to gather more complete information. This approach may decrease the patient's anxiety and fear about having an STD.

The infection can be asymptomatic in both men and women, but women have asymptomatic, or "silent," infections more often than do men. If symptoms are present, men usually notice dysuria and a penile discharge that can be either profuse yellowish green fluid or scant clear fluid. The urethra is most commonly affected, but infection can extend to the prostate, the seminal vesicles, and the epididymis. Men seek curative treatment sooner, usually because they have

symptoms, and thereby avoid some of the serious complications.

Women may report a change in vaginal discharge (yellow, green, profuse, odorous), urinary frequency, or dysuria. The cervix and urethra are the most common sites of infection.

Anal manifestations may include itching and irritation, rectal bleeding or diarrhea, and painful defecation. Assess the mouth for a reddened throat, ulcerated lips, tender gingivae, and blisters in the throat. Fig. 76-3 shows common sites of gonococcal infections.

Inspect for discharge from the urethra, cervix, and rectum. Palpation of the lower abdomen may reveal tenderness. Fever may be present, especially if an ascending or systemic infection has occurred. Gonorrheal infections that have become systemic may develop quickly. Manifestations of disseminated gonococcal infection (DGI) include fever, chills, skin lesions on distal extremities, and joint pain, with or without swelling, heat, or redness.

Clinical symptoms of gonorrhea can resemble those of chlamydia infection and therefore need to be differentiated. *Molecular testing for N. gonorrhoeae is currently the most widely used standard and preferred over cultures or microscopic examinations.* These nucleic acid amplification tests (NAATs) are highly sensitive and specific. During examination, providers can swab the male urethra or female cervix to obtain specimens. These specimens can be cultured on chocolate agar (gold standard), viewed microscopically after Gram staining (male urethral specimens only), or placed in medium for molecular testing. Patient-collected urine or vaginal swabs can also be used to diagnose both gonorrhea and chlamydia infections, allowing for screening without a full examination.

In men, gonorrhea can be diagnosed by Gram staining smears of urethral discharge that has been swabbed onto a glass slide, dried, and stained. The presence of gram-negative diplococci is diagnostic for gonococcal urethritis in men. If the man has symptoms, Gram stains are very sensitive and specific for gonorrhea and allow for immediate diagnosis and treatment in the clinical setting. Without symptoms, Gram stains are less reliable. Smears do not confirm the diagnosis in women because the female genital tract normally harbors organisms that resemble *N. gonorrhoeae.*

All patients with gonorrhea should be tested for HPV, syphilis, chlamydia, hepatitis B and hepatitis C, and HIV infection because they may have been exposed to these STDs as well. Sexual partners who have been exposed in the past 30 days should be examined, and specimens should be obtained.

▌INTERVENTIONS

Uncomplicated gonorrhea is treated with antibiotics. Chlamydia infections are frequently found in patients with gonorrhea. Patients treated for gonorrhea should also be managed with drugs that treat chlamydia infections.

Drug Therapy

Drug therapy recommended by the CDC is ceftriaxone (Rocephin) 250 mg IM or cefixime (Suprax) 400 mg orally in a single dose, *plus* azithromycin (Zithromax) 1 g orally in a single dose *or* doxycycline (Monodox, Doxy-Caps, Doxycin ✤) 100 mg orally twice daily for 1 week to treat a presumed co-infection with *Chlamydia,* unless a negative *Chlamydia* result has been obtained. These combinations seem to be effective for all mucosal gonorrheal infections; treatment failure is rare (CDC, 2010a). The CDC recommends the ceftriaxone injection because the treatment is given at the point of care, which increases drug adherence and is slightly more effective than cefixime (CDC, 2010a). A test of cure is not required. Advise the patient to return for a follow-up examination if symptoms persist after treatment. Re-infection is often the cause of these symptoms.

Sexual partners must be treated, not only evaluated, to prevent re-infection. Sexual partners also need to receive education about the infection.

A newer approach to preventing recurrence or persistent infections of STDs is expedited partner therapy (EPT), which is providing patients with newly diagnosed gonorrhea or other STD treatment for their partners. Patients are given the antibiotic or a prescription with specific instructions for administration to their partners without direct evaluation by a health care provider (CDC, 2010a). Legal questions have arisen about whether a drug can be prescribed without a relationship between the health care provider and the patient (CDC, 2010e). When patients have been given the drug to give to their partner, rates of infection have decreased and

more partners have reported receiving treatment (Trelle et al., 2007).

Gonorrhea infection can become disseminated (DGI) requiring hospitalization and IV or IM ceftriaxone 1 g every 24 hours. If symptoms resolve within 24 to 48 hours, the patient may be discharged to home to continue oral antibiotic therapy (cefixime 400 mg twice a day) for at least a week (CDC, 2010a).

Meningitis and endocarditis occur rarely. Hospitalization of patients with these problems is recommended for the initial treatment. Treatment includes IV antibiotic therapy, usually ceftriaxone 1 to 2 g every 12 hours. If meningitis or endocarditis is present, therapy is continued for 10 to 14 days for meningitis and at least 4 weeks for endocarditis. Collaborate with the infectious disease specialist for management of these infections.

Teaching for Self-Management

Teach the patient about transmission and treatment of gonorrhea. Patients must understand the need for drugs to be taken for the prescribed time for maximum effectiveness and to prevent drug resistance. Discuss the possibility of re-infection, including the risk for pelvic inflammatory disease (PID), and resultant problems such as ectopic pregnancy, infertility, and chronic pelvic pain. Instruct patients to cease sexual activity until the antibiotic therapy is completed and they no longer have symptoms; but if abstinence is not possible, urge men and women to use condoms. Explain that gonorrhea is a *reportable disease.*

When a diagnosis of gonorrhea is made, patients may have feelings of fear or guilt. They may be concerned that they have contracted other STDs or see the disease as a punishment for promiscuity or "unnatural" sex acts. They may believe that

---

❓ DECISION-MAKING CHALLENGE

Patient-Centered Care; Teamwork and Collaboration

A 49-year-old woman develops a heavy greenish vaginal discharge with a very foul odor. She visits her gynecologist, who tells her that she has gonorrhea. When the patient learns how the infection is transmitted, she tells her physician that she has not "slept with any other man" since she was married 29 years ago and that the diagnosis cannot be correct. When her husband returns home from work, she confronts him about her diagnosis. He initially denies that he has had sex with any other woman but then confesses that he has been "seeing" a young woman who works at his store for about 3 months. He admits that he has symptoms of the infection, too. The patient is very upset and returns to her gynecologist in 1 week. Her husband refuses to come with her. She tells you, the office nurse, that she just can't understand how her husband can be so unfaithful after all the years they have had together. She is considering filing for a divorce, but she is worried about her three children, ranging in age from 28 to 15.

1. What is the most appropriate way for you to respond to the patient at this time?
2. You tell the patient that her husband and the young woman involved need to be treated for the disease, and suggest expedited partner therapy. How will you explain this treatment method?
3. The patient tells you that she "never wants to meet that slut who stole my husband." How will you respond to this statement?
4. What emotional feelings is this patient experiencing? Develop a collaborative plan of care for this patient to ensure that desired patient and family outcomes will be met.

acquiring gonorrhea (or any STD) is a risk that they must take to pursue their desired lifestyle. Such feelings can impair relationships with sexual partners. Encourage patients to express their feelings during assessments and teaching sessions. Ensuring privacy for teaching and maintaining confidentiality of medical records are essential in meeting psychosocial needs.

CHLAMYDIA INFECTION

Pathophysiology

Chlamydia trachomatis is an intracellular bacterium and the causative agent of genital chlamydia infections. It invades the epithelial tissues in the reproductive tract. The incubation period ranges from 1 to 3 weeks, but the pathogen may be present in the genital tract for months without producing symptoms (Stamm, 2008a).

C. trachomatis is reportable to local health departments in all states. Diagnosed cases continue to increase yearly, which reflects more sensitive screening tests and increased public health efforts to screen high-risk people. Each year there are an estimated 2.8 million new cases in the United States (CDC, 2009). African-American women between 16 and 24 years of age are at the highest risk for the disease (CDC, 2009).

The rate of chlamydia infections in men has increased faster than the rate of increase in women (CDC, 2009). In women, 20% to 40% of those infected develop pelvic inflammatory disease (PID), discussed later in this chapter on p. 1663.

PATIENT-CENTERED COLLABORATIVE CARE

ASSESSMENT

Obtain a complete history including medical, menstrual, and sexual information (see Chart 76-1). In particular, ask about:
- Presence of symptoms, including vaginal or urethral discharge, dysuria (painful urination), pelvic pain, irregular bleeding
- Any history of sexually transmitted diseases (STDs)
- Whether sexual partners have had symptoms or a history of STDs
- Whether patient or partner has had unprotected intercourse

Many women with chlamydia infections are asymptomatic. For men and women, their history may reveal only risk factors associated with *C. trachomatis*, such as new or multiple sexual partners, age younger than 26 years and female, or a male having sex with a male (MSM). As with all interviews concerning sexual behavior, use a nonjudgmental approach and provide privacy and confidentiality.

> **! NURSING SAFETY PRIORITY**
>
> **Action Alert**
>
> For men, ask about dysuria, frequent urination, and a mucoid discharge that is more watery and less copious than a gonorrheal discharge. *These manifestations indicate urethritis, the main symptom of chlamydia infection in men.* Some men have the discharge only in the morning on arising. Complications include epididymitis, prostatitis, infertility, and Reiter's syndrome, a type of connective tissue disease discussed in Chapter 20.

In contrast, many women have no symptoms. Those with symptoms have a mucopurulent cervicitis with a change in vaginal discharge, easily induced cervical bleeding presenting as spotting or bleeding between menses, urinary frequency, and abdominal discomfort or pain. The vaginal discharge typically becomes yellow and more opaque. Complications of infection with *C. trachomatis* include salpingitis (inflammation of the fallopian tubes), PID, ectopic pregnancy, and infertility. These health problems are discussed in detail in maternal-child textbooks.

Diagnosis is made by sampling cells from the endocervix, urethra, or both, easily obtained with a swab. Because chlamydiae can reproduce only inside cells, host cells that harbor the organism (or parts of it) are required in the sample. Diagnosis is made definitively with a tissue culture (gold standard) obtained from the cervical os during the female pelvic examination or male urethral examination.

As with gonorrhea, the nucleic acid amplification tests (NAATs) and gene amplification tests (ligand chain reaction [LCR] and polymerase chain reaction [PCR] transcription-mediated amplification) are the newest methods of detecting *Chlamydia* in endocervical samples, urethral swabs, and urine. Samples can be obtained by swab by the examining clinician or by a patient-collected urine specimen. This urine self-collection method has been found to be more acceptable and highly sensitive and specific. The acceptability of urine testing has resulted in increased identification of asymptomatic people.

All sexually active women 25 years old or younger and all women older than 25 years with new or multiple partners should be screened annually for *Chlamydia* (CDC, 2010a). There is no recommendation for or against screening asymptomatic men, regardless of age or other risk, and low-risk asymptomatic women.

INTERVENTIONS

The treatment of choice for chlamydia infections is azithromycin (Zithromax) 1 g orally in a single dose or doxycycline (Monodox, Doxy-Caps, Doxycin ♣) 100 mg orally twice daily for 7 days. The one-dose course, although more expensive, is preferred because of the ease in completing the treatment. Drugs that are prescribed for patients with allergies to these drugs include erythromycin, ofloxacin, and levofloxacin, all for 7 days (CDC, 2010a).

Giving the drug while the patient is in the health care agency helps ensure adherence. Sexual partners should be treated and tested for other STDs. Expedited partner therapy (EPT), or patient-delivered partner therapy, shows signs of reducing chlamydia infection rates (CDC, 2010a).

Patient and partner education is an important nursing intervention. Explain:
- The mode of disease transmission
- The incubation period
- Manifestations, including the high possibility of asymptomatic infections
- Treatment of infection with antibiotics
- The need for abstinence from sexual intercourse until the patient and partner(s) have completed treatment (7 days from the start of treatment, including a single-dose regimen)
- No test of cure is required, but all women should be re-screened for re-infection 3 to 12 months after

treatment because of the high risk for PID. There is less evidence of the need for re-screening of treated men, but it should be considered
- The need to return for evaluation if symptoms recur or new symptoms develop (most recurrences are re-infections from a new or untreated partner)
- Possible complications of untreated or inadequately treated infection, such as PID, ectopic pregnancy, or infertility

OTHER GYNECOLOGIC CONDITIONS

PELVIC INFLAMMATORY DISEASE

Pathophysiology

Pelvic inflammatory disease (PID) is a complex infectious process in which organisms from the lower genital tract migrate from the endocervix upward through the uterine cavity into the fallopian tubes. The spread of infection to other organs and tissues of the upper genital tract occurs from direct contact with mucosal surfaces or through the fimbriated ends of the tubes to the ovaries, parametrium, and peritoneal cavity (Fig. 76-4). This may involve one or more pelvic structures, including the uterus, fallopian tubes, and adjacent pelvic structures. The most common site is the fallopian tube. Resulting infections include:
- Endometritis (infection of the endometrial cavity)
- Salpingitis (inflammation of the fallopian tubes)
- Oophoritis (ovarian infection)
- Parametritis (infection of the parametrium)
- Peritonitis (infection of the peritoneal cavity)
- Tubal or tubo-ovarian abscess

Many different pathogens are linked to PID. Sexually transmitted organisms are most often responsible, especially *Chlamydia trachomatis* and *Neisseria gonorrhoeae*. Organisms that are part of the vaginal flora can also cause PID. In addition, *Gardnerella vaginalis, Haemophilus influenzae, Staphylococcus, Streptococcus, Escherichia coli*, and other aerobic and anaerobic organisms have been identified in patients with PID. There is increasing evidence that the anaerobes involved in bacterial vaginosis may have a role in the development of PID and increase the risk for infection with HIV, *N. gonorrhea, C. trachomatis*, and HSV (CDC, 2010a).

The organisms invade the pelvis from an infection ascending from the vagina or cervix. Infections are spread during sexual intercourse, during childbirth (including the postpartum period), and after abortion. Rarely do they result from transperitoneal spread from a ruptured appendix or intra-abdominal abscess. *Sepsis and death can occur, especially if treatment is delayed or inadequate.*

Many practitioners use the terms *PID* and *salpingitis* as equal terms for acute infections. PID is one of the leading causes of infertility and is related to the increase in the number of ectopic pregnancies reported in the United States. It is an acute syndrome resulting in tenderness in the tubes and ovaries (adnexa) and low, dull abdominal pain. However, many women experience only mild discomfort or menstrual irregularity. Others experience no symptoms at all—so-called "silent" or "subclinical" PID. The diagnosis and treatment of this disease are challenging. Irreversible scarring or stricture, causing sterility, may occur before it is diagnosed.

Because of variations in patient manifestations, the diagnosis is difficult because women may have subtle symptoms not typical of the disease. Delay in diagnosis and treatment may add to complications of PID in the upper genital tract. The disease is usually diagnosed on the basis of clinical signs and symptoms. The Centers for Disease Control and Prevention (CDC) (2010d) has set minimum criteria for diagnosis, but no laboratory or physical examination techniques alone are both sensitive and specific (Table 76-4).

PATIENT-CENTERED COLLABORATIVE CARE

ASSESSMENT

History

Obtain a complete medical, family, menstrual, obstetric, and sexual history, including a history of previous episodes of pelvic inflammatory disease (PID) or other sexually transmitted diseases (see Chart 76-1). Assess for contraceptive use, a history of reproductive surgery, and other risk factors previously identified. Ask the patient if sexual abuse has occurred. If so, encourage her to discuss what happened and whether she was seen by a health care provider.

Many of the same factors that place women at risk for STDs also place them at risk for PID. Risk factors for sexually active women include:
- Age younger than 26 years
- Multiple sexual partners
- Intrauterine device (IUD) placed within the previous 3 weeks
- Smoking
- A history of PID
- Chlamydial or gonococcal infection; bacterial vaginosis
- A history of sexually transmitted diseases (STDs)

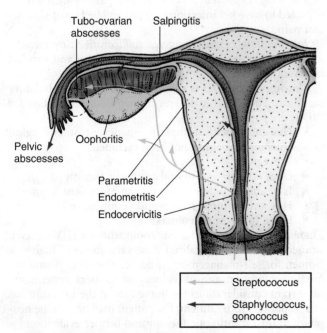

FIG. 76-4 The spread of pelvic inflammatory disease.

Labels in figure:
Tubo-ovarian abscesses
Salpingitis
Pelvic abscesses
Oophoritis
Parametritis
Endometritis
Endocervicitis

→ Streptococcus
→ Staphylococcus, gonococcus

TABLE 76-4	DIAGNOSTIC CRITERIA FOR PELVIC INFLAMMATORY DISEASE

Minimum Criteria for Initiating Empiric Treatment for Pelvic Inflammatory Disease
- Sexually active woman and at risk for STDs
- Pelvic or lower abdominal pain
- No other cause for illness can be found (e.g., appendicitis)

and
- Uterine tenderness *or*
- Adnexal tenderness *or*
- Cervical motion tenderness (chandelier sign)

Additional Criteria to Increase the Specificity of the Diagnosis of PID
- Oral temperature >101° F (>38.3° C)
- Abnormal cervical or vaginal mucopurulent discharge
- Presence of white blood cells on saline microscopy of vaginal secretions
- Elevated erythrocyte sedimentation rate
- Elevated C-reactive protein
- Laboratory documentation of cervical infection with *Neisseria gonorrhoeae* or *Chlamydia trachomatis*

Definitive Criteria for Diagnosing PID, Warranted in Selected Cases
- Histopathologic evidence of endometritis on endometrial biopsy
- Transvaginal sonography or magnetic resonance imaging techniques showing thickened fluid-filled tubes with or without free pelvic fluid or tubo-ovarian complex, or Doppler studies suggesting pelvic infection
- Laparoscopic abnormalities consistent with PID

Modified from Centers for Disease Control and Prevention (CDC). (2010a). *Sexually transmitted diseases treatment guidelines, 2010. Morbidity and Mortality Weekly Report, 59*(RR-12), 63-64.
PID, Pelvic inflammatory disease; *STDs,* sexually transmitted diseases.

Physical Assessment/Clinical Manifestations

One of the most frequent symptoms of PID is lower abdominal pain. Conduct a complete pain assessment. Other symptoms include irregular vaginal bleeding (spotting or bleeding between periods), dysuria (painful urination), an increase or change in vaginal discharge, dyspareunia (painful sexual intercourse), malaise, fever, and chills.

Observe whether the patient has discomfort with movement. Often the patient has a hunched-over gait to protect her abdomen. She may find it difficult to independently get on the examination table or stretcher. Assess for lower abdominal tenderness, possibly with rigidity or rebound tenderness. A pelvic examination by the health care provider may reveal yellow or green cervical discharge and a reddened or friable cervix (a cervix that bleeds easily). Criteria for accurate diagnosis of PID are listed in Table 76-4. The diagnosis of PID is usually based on clinical history, physical examination, and laboratory tests. Imaging studies and laparoscopy are not generally used to make the diagnosis.

Psychosocial Assessment

The woman who has symptoms of PID is usually anxious and fearful of the examination and unknown diagnosis. She may need much reassurance and support during the physical examination because her abdomen may be very tender or painful. Explain what is taking place to help promote comfort during the examination.

Because PID is often associated with an STD, the woman may feel embarrassed or uncomfortable discussing her symptoms or history. Use a nonjudgmental approach, and encourage the patient to express her feelings and concerns. The patient's ability to follow through with the treatment plan is essential in deciding whether ambulatory care treatment is appropriate.

Laboratory Assessment

The health care provider obtains specimens from the cervix, urethra, and rectum to determine the presence of *N. gonorrhoeae* or *C. trachomatis.* The white blood cell (WBC) count, erythrocyte sedimentation rate (ESR) and C-reactive protein may be elevated but are not specific for PID. A sensitive test that detects human chorionic gonadotropin (hCG) in urine or blood should be performed to determine whether the patient is pregnant. Microscopic examination of vaginal discharge should be done to evaluate for the presence of more than 10 WBCs per high-power field, which correlates with infection. Bacterial vaginosis can be found by observing the diagnostic "clue" cells with microscopic examination of vaginal discharge.

Other Diagnostic Assessment

Abdominal *ultrasonography* may be used to determine the presence of appendicitis and tubo-ovarian abscesses that need to be ruled out when the diagnosis of PID is made. Transvaginal ultrasound and *magnetic resonance imaging (MRI)* are used in some cases to detect tubal wall thickening, fluid-filled tubes, and free pelvic fluid or a tubo-ovarian abscess, all associated with PID. *Endometrial biopsy* also has been used to increase the accuracy of the diagnosis.

ANALYSIS

The priority problem for patients with pelvic inflammatory disease (PID) is infection related to invasion of pelvic organs by pathogens.

PLANNING AND IMPLEMENTATION

Managing Infection

Planning: Expected Outcomes. The patient with PID is expected to have her infection resolved and be free of abdominal pain.

Interventions. Patient-centered collaborative care includes antibiotic therapy, self-management measures, and surgical intervention (rarely).

Uncomplicated PID is usually treated on an ambulatory care basis. The CDC (2010d) recommends hospitalization for PID if the patient:
- Has appendicitis, ectopic pregnancy, or other surgical emergency that has not been excluded
- Is pregnant
- Does not respond to oral antibiotic therapy
- Is unable to follow or tolerate an outpatient regimen
- Has severe illness, nausea and vomiting, or high fever
- Has a tubo-ovarian abscess

There are no recommendations about whether HIV-infected women should be hospitalized. Assess the ability of high-risk women for self-management at home. The clinical patient's medical condition and availability of support systems are important considerations for home care. If the infection has not responded to treatment, the patient may need to be hospitalized for IV antibiotic therapy and further evaluation.

The CDC recommends oral and/or parenteral antibiotics for PID (CDC, 2010d). Drug therapy is required for 14 days.

If the woman has not responded to oral antibiotics, she is hospitalized for IV antibiotic therapy and further evaluation. Inpatient therapy involves a combination of several IV antibiotics until the woman shows signs of improvement (e.g., decreased pelvic tenderness for at least 24 hours). Then oral antibiotics are continued until the course of treatment has lasted 14 days.

Antibiotic therapy relieves pain by decreasing the inflammation caused by infection. Other pain relief measures include taking mild analgesics and applying heat to the lower abdomen or back. *Teach the patient to maintain rest in a semi-Fowler's position to promote gravity drainage of the infection that may help relieve pain.*

❗ NURSING SAFETY PRIORITY

Action Alert

Instruct women who are being treated for PID as outpatients to avoid sexual intercourse and to check their temperature twice a day. Teach them to report an increase in temperature to their health care provider. Remind them to be seen by the health care provider within 72 hours from starting the antibiotics and then 1 and 2 weeks from the time of the initial diagnosis.

In a small number of patients, the pain and tenderness may not be relieved by antibiotic therapy. The surgeon may perform a laparoscopy to remove an abscess through one or more sub-umbilical incisions to provide better access to the fallopian tubes. Before surgery, provide information about hospital routines and procedures. After surgery, the care of the woman with PID is similar to that of any patient after laparoscopic abdominal surgery. One difference is that she may have a wound drain for drainage of abscess fluid that may not have been completely removed during surgery. Observe, measure, and record wound drainage every 4 to 8 hours as requested.

Community-Based Care

Collaborate with the case manager or discharge planner before the woman is discharged to home. Teach the patient with PID to have regular follow-up with her health care provider to assess for complications and assess that the infection has resolved. The ongoing role of the nurse is to assess for any continued risk for contracting PID again, signs of persistent or recurrent infection, and education to prevent exposure to and infection with all STDs (e.g., decrease the number of partners, consistently use condoms). Establish an atmosphere of trust that encourages the woman to return frequently, if needed, for education or reassurance.

Home Care Management

Parenteral antibiotic therapy may be given at home, but usually the health care provider changes the treatment regimen to oral antibiotics before hospital discharge.

Teaching for Self-Management

Patient teaching focuses on providing information about PID, identifying recurrences (persistent pelvic pain, dysmenorrhea, low backache, fever), and urging early and complete self-management to prevent complications. Review information for oral antibiotic therapy (Chart 76-4).

Counsel the patient to contact her sexual partner(s) for examination and treatment. Partners should be treated for

CHART 76-4 PATIENT AND FAMILY EDUCATION: PREPARING FOR SELF-MANAGEMENT

Oral Antibiotic Therapy for Sexually Transmitted Diseases

- Take your medicine for the number of times a day it is prescribed and until it is completed.
- Your sexual partner must be treated if you have a sexually transmitted disease (STD). Expedited partner therapy is one way to ensure partners are treated.
- Be sure to return for your follow-up appointment after completing your antibiotic treatment.
- Call if you have any questions or concerns.
- Do not have sex until after you and your partner complete your antibiotic therapy. This should be at least 7 days, even if treatment is one dose.
- Drink at least 8 to 10 glasses of fluid a day while taking your antibiotics.
- Do not take antacids containing calcium, magnesium, or aluminum, such as Tums, Maalox, or Mylanta, with your antibiotics. They may decrease the effectiveness of the antibiotic.
- Take your antibiotics on an empty stomach unless your health care provider instructs you to take them with food.
- If you are taking oral contraceptives, you should discuss with your health care provider whether the antibiotics will decrease the effectiveness of your pills.

gonorrhea and chlamydia infection regardless of their lack of symptoms. Remind the patient about follow-up care, and counsel her about the complications that can occur after an episode of PID. These problems include increased risk for recurrence, ectopic pregnancy, and infertility. Chronic pelvic pain may also develop.

Discuss contraception and the patient's need or desire for it. This discussion includes methods that may decrease the risk for future episodes of PID, such as the use of barrier methods (e.g., condom). Help the patient understand lifestyle factors that increase the risk for recurrent episodes, including sexual intercourse with multiple partners. Douching has also been suggested as a risk behavior for development of PID and/or infection with *Chlamydia* or *N. gonorrhea*.

Psychosocial concerns may require teaching and counseling. A patient who has PID may exhibit a variety of feelings (guilt, disgust, anger) about having a condition that may have been transmitted to her sexually. These feelings may affect her relationship with significant others and future sexual relationships. She may also have concerns about future fertility if PID has damaged or scarred the fallopian tubes and other reproductive organs. Provide nonjudgmental emotional support, and allow time for the woman to discuss her feelings.

❓ NCLEX EXAMINATION CHALLENGE

Physiological Integrity

A client is being treated with oral antibiotics in the clinic for pelvic inflammatory disease. Which of these changes will the nurse teach the client to report immediately to the health care provider?
A. Increased anxiety that her partner may "catch" the disease
B. Mild nausea after taking some doses of the antibiotic
C. One or two diarrheal stools every day since taking the antibiotic
D. Temperature of 102° F after 3 days of taking the antibiotic

Health Care Resources

If infertility is a result of PID, the patient may need referral to a clinic specializing in infertility treatment and counseling. She can also contact support groups for infertile couples, which exist in many local communities.

The costs of antibiotics for care of patients with PID and other STDs may be a concern for those who are uninsured, underinsured, or impoverished. In collaboration with the case manager or social worker, help locate community resources for free or discounted drugs for women who cannot afford them. Ask the patient directly if she has money to pay for the drug therapy including her insurance co-pay, regardless of her apparent financial status.

▌EVALUATION: OUTCOMES

Evaluate the care of the patient with PID based on the identified priority patient problem. The expected outcomes include that the patient should:

- Show evidence that the infection has resolved
- Report or demonstrate that pain is relieved or reduced and that she feels more comfortable

VAGINAL INFECTIONS

Vaginal infection associated with sexual activity may produce vaginal discharge or vulvar irritation. The common causes of vaginal infection that can be but are not always sexually transmitted include:

- *Trichomonas vaginalis*
- *Candida*, primarily *C. albicans*
- Bacteria that produce bacterial vaginosis, including *Gardnerella vaginalis, Mycoplasma hominis* and anaerobes including *Prevotella* and *Mobiluncus* species

Men can also get these infections but are not always symptomatic.

Trichomoniasis and candida infections are limited to the vagina. They can be very irritating and bothersome but do not cause any long-term problems. The partner must also be treated for *trichomoniasis* if the infection is to be resolved. *Candidiasis* does not usually require partner treatment. However, if the male partner is symptomatic (irritation of the genital skin), treatment is indicated. It is important to remember that *Candida* is a normal flora on the skin and can easily be relocated to the vagina. Although it can be transmitted sexually, candidiasis occurs among women who are not sexually active. Also, antibiotics that change the normal flora of the vagina contribute to infection.

Bacterial vaginosis (BV) has been implicated in upper genital tract infections. Women undergoing surgery of the upper genital tract should be evaluated and treated if BV is found. Chapter 74 describes the management of each of these infections.

▌OTHER SEXUALLY TRANSMITTED DISEASES

Less common diseases in the United States that are transmitted by sexual contact are lymphogranuloma venereum, chancroid, and granuloma inguinale. Like syphilis, all of these diseases are associated with ulcers but they are seen most often in less affluent countries. As newcomers migrate into the United States, these STDs may become more common. Ask patients suspected of these infections whether they have traveled out of the United States and whether they had sexual contact with people who live in other countries.

NURSING CONCEPT REVIEW

What might you NOTICE if the patient has altered sexuality as a result of a sexually transmitted disease (STD)?

- Report of heavy and abnormal vaginal discharge
- Report of urinary frequency or dysuria
- Ulcers, blisters, or warts in the genital area
- Low-grade fever
- Report of malaise
- Report of vaginal, penile, or anal itching or irritation
- Report of abdominal pain (pelvic inflammatory disease [PID])
- Anxious behavior

What should you INTERPRET and how should you RESPOND to a patient with altered sexuality as a result of STD?

Perform and interpret focused physical assessment, including:
- Vital signs
- Pain intensity and quality
- Skin inspection (genital area)

Respond by:
- Reporting and documenting all findings

- Helping patient with abdominal pain into a semi-Fowler's position
- Providing pain control measures
- Teaching patient about prescribed antibiotic or antiviral therapy
- Teaching patient to avoid sexual intercourse while being treated
- Teaching patient the importance of treating all sexual partners
- Teaching patient and partner(s) about safe sex practices
- Providing support and listening to the patient and partner(s) without judgment

On what should you REFLECT?

- Examine your feelings about patients who make sexual choices different from your own.
- Think about what else you could do to help patients meet their physical and emotional needs during this time.
- Determine what other health teaching may be needed for this patient.
- Monitor the patient's response to pain control interventions.

GET READY FOR THE NCLEX® EXAMINATION!

KEY POINTS

Review these Key Points for each NCLEX Examination Client Needs Category.

Safe and Effective Care Environment

- Teach patients to not have sexual intercourse during their treatment for sexually transmitted disease (STD).
- Maintain patient and partner confidentiality and privacy at all times.
- Use gloves when examining the patient's genitalia or skin lesions.

Health Promotion and Maintenance

- Teach the patient about the availability of expedited partner treatment; be sure that all doses of the drug are taken by both the patient and the partner.
- Encourage all patients who are sexually active to use condoms during sexual intimacy (see Chart 76-3).
- Urge sexually active people, especially those younger than 25 years or those older than 25 years if at high risk, to have STD screenings at least annually.

Psychosocial Integrity

- Treat all patients, regardless of diagnosis, with respect.

- Provide privacy for patients undergoing examination or testing for STDs.
- Respect the sexual choices of all patients.
- Allow the patient the opportunity to express fear or anxiety regarding a diagnosis of STD.
- Refer patients newly diagnosed with an STD to local resources and support groups as needed based on their response.
- Encourage all patients who have an STD to inform their sexual partner(s) of their health status.

Physiological Integrity

- Encourage patients to adhere to their anti-infective drug regimen (see Chart 76-4).
- Teach patients the expected side effects and possible adverse reactions to prescribed drugs.
- Assess patients with STD using the guidelines in Chart 76-1.
- Teach patients about the complications of STD using the information in Table 76-2.
- Be aware that PID is diagnosed based on the criteria in Table 76-4.

Asterisk indicates a classic or definitive work on this subject.

Chapter 1

*Academy of Medical-Surgical Nursing (AMSN). (2007). *Scope and standards of medical-surgical nursing practice* (4th ed.). Pitman, NJ: Anthony J. Janetti.

Alfaro-LeFevre, R. (2008). *Critical thinking and clinical judgment: A practical approach to outcome-focused thinking* (4th ed.). Philadelphia: Saunders.

Alfaro-LeFevre, R. (2010). *Applying the nursing process: A tool for critical thinking* (7th ed.). Philadelphia: Lippincott Williams & Wilkins.

Benner, P. E., Malloch, K., & Sheets, V. (2010). *Nursing pathways for patient safety*. St. Louis: Mosby.

Bogert, S., Ferrell, C., & Rutledge, D. N. (2010). Experience with family activation of rapid response teams. *MEDSURG Nursing*, 19, 215-222.

Deno, K., & Schaper, J. (2011). Glucose control in the medical patient: Bolus insulin dosing compared to basal-bolus dosing. *MEDSURG Nursing*, 20(5), 217-222, 234.

Donaldson, N., Shapiro, S., Scott, M., Foley, M., & Spetz, J. (2009). Leading successful rapid response teams: A multi-site implementation evaluation. *Journal of Nursing Administration*, 39, 176-181.

Fisher, J. A., & Monahan, T. (2008). Tracking the social dimensions of RFID systems in hospitals. *International Journal of Medical Informatics*, 77, 176-183.

Fowler, M. D. M. (2008). *Guide to the code of ethics for nurses: Interpretation and application*. Washington, DC: American Nurses Association.

Gasarian, P. K., Henneman, E. A., & Chandler, G. E. (2010). Nurse decision making in the pre-arrest period. *Clinical Nursing Research*, 19, 21-37.

*Institute for Healthcare Improvement. (2005). Protecting 5 million lives from harm. Retrieved July 2, 2011, from www.ihi.org.

*Institute of Medicine (IOM). (2000). *To err is human: Building a safer health care system*. Washington, DC: National Academies Press.

*Institute of Medicine (IOM). (2003). *Health professions education: A bridge to quality*. Washington, DC: National Academies Press.

Joint Commission Center for Transforming Healthcare. (2010). Joint Commission Center for Transforming Healthcare tackles miscommunication among caregivers. Retrieved July 2, 2011, from www.centerfortransforminghealthcare.org.

Melnyk, B. M., & Fineout-Overholt, E. (2011). *Evidence-based practice in nursing and healthcare* (2nd ed.). Philadelphia: Lippincott Williams & Wilkins.

*Morse, K. J., Warshawsky, D., Moore, J. M., & Pecora, D. C. (2007). Rapid response teams: Reducers of death. *Nursing2007*, Spring(Suppl.), 2-8.

*National Council of State Boards of Nursing. (1995). Delegation: Concepts and decision making process. Retrieved July 2, 2011, from www.ncsbn.org.

Quality and Safety Education for Nurses. (2011). Competency KSAs (pre-licensure). Retrieved July 2, 2011, from www.qsen.org.

*Schroeder, S. J. (2006). Picking up the PACE: A new template for shift report. *Nursing2006*, 36(10), 22-23.

The Joint Commission. (2011). Speak Up initiatives: The Joint Commission's award-winning patient safety program. Retrieved April 6, 2011 from http://www.jointcommission.org/speakup.aspx.

Tzeng, H.-M. & Yin, C.-Y. (2010). Nurses response time to call lights and fall occurrences. *MEDSURG Nursing*, 19(5), 266-272.

Yoder-Wise, P. S. (2011). Leading and managing in nursing (5th ed.). St. Louis: Mosby.

Chapter 2

Albert, N. M., Gillinov, A. M., Lytle, B. W., Feng, J., Cwynar, R., & Blackstone, E. H. (2009). A randomized trial of massage therapy after heart surgery. *Heart and Lung*, 38(6), 480-490.

Chan, M. F., Chan, E. A., Mok, E., & Tse, F. Y. (2009). Effect of music on depression levels and physiological responses in community-based older adults. *International Journal of Mental Health Nursing*, 18(4), 285-294.

Engberg, S., Cohen, S., & Sereika, S. M. (2009). The efficacy of acupuncture in treating urge and mixed incontinence in women: A pilot study. *Journal of Wound, Ostomy, and Incontinence Nursing*, 36(6), 661-670.

Good, M., Albert, J. M., Anderson, G. C., Wotman, S., Cong, X., Lane, D., et al. (2010). Supplementing relaxation and music for pain after surgery. *Nursing Research*, 59(4), 259-269.

Holliday-Welsh, D. M., Gessert, C. E., & Renier, C. M. (2009). Massage in the management of agitation in nursing home residents with cognitive impairment. *Geriatric Nursing*, 30(2), 108-117.

Kale-Pradhan, P., Jassal, H. K., & Wilhelm, S. M. (2010). Role of *Lactobacillus* in the prevention of antibiotic-associated diarrhea: A meta-analysis. *Pharmacotherapy*, 30, 119-126.

Klemm, P., Waddington, C., Bradley, E., Bucher, L., Collins, M., Lyons, D. L., et al. (2010). Unleashing animal-assisted therapy. *Nursing2010*, 40(10), 12-13.

*Krieger, D. (1976). Healing by laying on of hands as facilitators of bioenergetic change: The response of in-vivo hemoglobin. *Psychoenergetic Systems*, 1, 121-129.

Lee, L. Y., Lee, D. T., & Woo, J. (2009). Tai chi and health-related quality of life in nursing home residents. *Journal of Nursing Scholarship*, 41(1), 35-43.

*Lu, Y. (2003). Herb use in critical care: What to watch for. *Critical Care Nursing Clinics of North America*, 15(3), 313-319.

Moquin, B., Blackman, M. R., Mitty, E., & Flores, S. (2009). Complementary and alternative medicine (CAM). *Geriatric Nursing*, 30(3), 196-203.

National Center for Complementary and Alternative Medicine (NCCAM). (2008). The use of complementary and alternative medicine in the United States. Retrieved July 2, 2011, from http://www.nccam.nih.gov/.

National Center for Complementary and Alternative Medicine (NCCAM). (2011a). Acupuncture. Retrieved April 6, 2011, from http://www.nccam.nih.gov/health/acupuncture/.

National Center for Complementary and Alternative Medicine (NCCAM). (2011b). Aromatherapy. Retrieved July 2, 2011, from http://www.nccam.nih.gov/health/aromatherapy/.

National Center for Complementary and Alternative Medicine (NCCAM). (2011c). Ayurvedic medicine. Retrieved July 2, 2011, from http://www.nccam.nih.gov/health/ayurvedicmedicine/.

National Center for Complementary and Alternative Medicine (NCCAM). (2011d). Meditation. Retrieved July 2, 2011, from http://www.nccam.nih.gov/health/meditation/.

National Center for Complementary and Alternative Medicine (NCCAM). (2011e). Probiotics. Retrieved April 6, 2011, from http://www.nccam.nih.gov/health/probiotics/.

National Center for Complementary and Alternative Medicine (NCCAM). (2011f). Yoga. Retrieved April 6, 2011, from http://www.nccam.nih.gov/health/yoga/.

*Pierce, B. (2007). The use of biofield therapies in cancer care. *Clinical Journal of Oncology Nursing, 11*(2), 253-258.

*Richards, T., Johnson, J., Sparks, A., & Emerson, H. (2007). The effect of music therapy on patients' perception and manifestation of pain, anxiety, and patient satisfaction. *MEDSURG Nursing, 16*(1), 7-15.

*Snyder, M., & Lindquist, R. (Eds.). (2006). *Complementary/ alternative therapies in nursing* (5th ed.). New York: Springer.

Tsai, P. F., Beck, C., Chang, J. Y., Hagen, J., Kuo, Y. F., Roberson, P. K., et al. (2009). The effect of tai chi on knee osteoarthritis pain in cognitively impaired elders: Pilot study. *Geriatric Nursing, 30*(2), 132-139.

Wall, M., & Duffy, A. (2010). The effects of music therapy for older people with dementia. *British Journal of Nursing, 19*(2), 108-113.

*Wardell, D. W., & Weymouth, K. F. (2004). Review of studies of Healing Touch. *Journal of Nursing Scholarship, 36*, 147-154.

Zarowitz, B. J. (2010). Complementary and alternative medicines: Clinical pearls for commonly used dietary supplements. *Geriatric Nursing, 31*(4), 281-287.

Chapter 3

Abdallah, L. M., Remington, R., Melillo, K. D., & Flanagan, J. (2008). Using antipsychotic drugs safely in older patients. *Nursing2008, 38*(10), 28-31.

*Cole, C., & Richards, K. (2007). Sleep disruption in older adults. *AJN, 107*(5), 40-48.

Dacenko-Grave, L., & Holm, K. (2008). Evidence-based practice: A fall prevention program that continues to work. *MEDSURG Nursing, 17*(4), 223-228.

*DiMaria-Ghalili, R. A., & Amella, E. (2005). Nutrition in older adults. *AJN, 105*(3), 40-50.

*Fink, A., Tsai, M. C., Hays, R. D., Moore, A. A., Morton, S. C., Spritzer, K., et al. (2002). Comparing the alcohol-related problems survey (ARPS) to traditional alcohol screening measures in elderly outpatients. *Archives of Gerontology and Geriatrics, 34*(1), 55-78.

*Forrest, J., Willis, L., Holm, K., Kwon, M. S., Anderson, M. A., & Foreman, M. D. (2007). Recognizing quiet delirium. *AJN, 107*(4), 35-39.

*Fulmer, T. (2007). How to try this: Fulmer SPICES. *AJN, 107*(10), 40-48.

Fulmer, T. (2008). How to try this: Elder mistreatment assessment. *AJN, 108*(12), 57-58.

Gerber, L. (2009). Putting older patients' sleep concerns to rest. *Nursing2009, 39*(4), 60-61.

Greenawalt, K. L. (2009). How are all those medications affecting your older patient? *Nursing2009, 39*(5), 56hn1-56hn2.

*Greenberg, S. A. (2007). How to try this: The Geriatric Depression Scale—Short Form. *AJN, 107*(10), 60-69.

*Hendrich, A. (2007). Predicting patient falls: Using the Hendrich II Fall Risk Model in clinical practice. *AJN, 107*(11), 50-59.

Janelli, L. M., & Quiones-Ramos, E. (2009). Can an exercise program enhance mood among Hispanic elders? *MEDSURG Nursing, 18*(6), 356-360.

*King, B. D. (2006). Functional decline in hospitalized elders. *MEDSURG Nursing, 15*(5), 265-270.

Lee, L. Y., Lee, D. T., & Woo, J. (2010). The psychosocial effect of Tai Chi on nursing home residents. *Journal of Clinical Nursing, 19*(7-8), 927-938.

Lyons, D. L., Grimley, S. M., & Snydor, L. (2008). Double trouble: When delirium complicates dementia. *Nursing2008, 38*(9), 48-54.

McCaffrey, R., Hanson, C., & McCaffrey, W. (2010). Garden walking for depression: A research report. *Holistic Nursing Practice, 24*(5), 252-259.

*Milisen, K., Braes, T., Fick, T. M., & Foreman, M. D. (2006). Cognitive assessment and differentiating the 3 Ds (dementia, depression, delirium). *Nursing Clinics of North America, 41*(1), 1-22.

Molony, S. L. (2009). Monitoring medication use in older adults. *AJN, 109*(1), 68-78.

Naegle, M. A. (2008). How to try this: Screening for alcohol use and misuse in older adults. *AJN, 108*(11), 50-56.

National Institute on Alcohol Abuse and Alcoholism (NIAAA). (2011). Older adults and alcohol problems. Retrieved July 3, 2011, from www.pubs.niaaa.nih.gov/publications/ socialworkeducationmodule.

National Institute of Mental Health (NIMH). (2011). Older adults and depression. Retrieved July 3, 2011, from www.nimh.nih. gov/health/topics/depression.

*Odenheimer, G. L. (2006). Driver safety in older adults: The physician's role in assessing driving skills in older patients. *Geriatrics, 61*(10), 14-21.

Pagana, P. D., & Pagana, T. J. (2010). *Mosby's manual of diagnostic and laboratory tests.* St. Louis: Mosby.

Planton, J., & Edlund, B. J. (2010). Strategies for reducing polypharmacy in older adults. *Journal of Gerontological Nursing, 36*(1), 8-12.

Rocchiccioli, J. T., & Sanford, J. T. (2009). Revisiting geriatric failure to thrive. *Journal of Gerontological Nursing, 35*(1), 18-24.

Rogers, C., Keller, C., & Larkey, L. K. (2010). Perceived benefits of meditative movement in older adults. *Geriatric Nursing, 31*(1), 37-51.

*Rigney, T. S. (2006). Delirium in the hospitalized elder and recommendations for practice. *Geriatric Nursing, 27*(3), 151-157.

Sendelbach, S., & Guthrie, P. F. (2009). Evidence-based guideline— Acute confusion/delirium: Identification, assessment, treatment, and prevention. *Journal of Gerontological Nursing, 35*(11), 11-17.

Sweeny, S. J., Bridges, E. J., Wild, L. M., & Sayre, C. A. (2008). Care of the patient with delirium. *AJN, 108*(5), 72CC-72GG.

Tseng, H. M., & Yin, C.-Y. (2010). Nurses response time to call lights and fall occurrences. *MEDSURG Nursing, 19*(5), 266-272.

Volkert, D., Saegitz, C., Gueldenzoph, H., Sieber, C. C., & Stehle, P. (2010). Underdiagnosed malnutrition and nutrition-related problems in geriatric patients. *Journal of Nutrition, Health and Aging, 14*(5), 387-392.

Weeks, L. E., Campbell, B., Graham, H., Chircop, A., & Sheppard-LeMoine, D. (2008). Participation in physical activity: Influences reported by seniors in the community and long-term care facilities. *Journal of Gerontological Nursing, 34*(7), 36-43.

Weierbach, F. M., & Click, D. F. (2009). Community resources for older adults with chronic illness. *Holistic Nursing Practice, 23*(6), 355-360.

Williams, K. N., & Kemper, S.. (2010). Interventions to reduce cognitive decline in aging. *Journal of Psychosocial Nursing and Mental Health Services, 48*(5), 42-51.

Wooten, A. C. (2010). An integrative review of Tai Chi research: An alternative form of physical activity to improve balance and prevent falls in older adults. *Orthopedic Nursing, 29*(2), 108-118.

Chapter 4

Badiaga, S., Raoult, D., & Brouqui, P. (2008). Preventing and controlling emerging and reemerging transmissible diseases in the homeless. *Emerging Infectious Diseases, 14*(9), 1353-1359.

*Campinha-Bacote, J. (2003). Many faces: Addressing diversity in health care. *Online Journal of Issues in Nursing, 8*(1). Retrieved January 15, 2008, from www.nursingworld.com.

Drury, L. J. (2008). Increasing competency in the care of homeless patients. *Journal of Continuing Education in Nursing, 39*(4), 153-154.

*Giger, J., Davidhizar, R. E., Purnell, L., Harden, J. T., Phillips, J., & Strickland, O., American Academy of Nursing. (2007). American Academy of Nursing Expert Panel Report: Developing cultural competence to eliminate health disparities in ethnic minorities and other vulnerable populations. *Journal of Transcultural Nursing, 18*(2), 95-102.

Hamilton, C. J., & Mahalik, J. R. (2009). Minority stress, masculinity, and social norms predicting gay men's health risk behaviors. *Journal of Counseling Psychology, 56*(1), 132-138.

Jenner, C. O. (2010). Transgender primary care. *Journal of the American Academy of Nurse Practitioners, 22*, 403-408.

Jones, C. A., Perera, A., Chow, M., Ho, I., Nguyen, J., & Davachi, S. (2009). Cardiovascular disease risk among the poor and homeless: What we know so far. *Current Cardiology Review, 5*, 69-77.

*Leininger, M. (2002). Culture care theory: A major contribution to advance transcultural nursing knowledge and practices. *Journal of Transcultural Nursing, 13*(3), 189-192.

Mayer, K. H., Bradford, J. B., Makadon, H. J., Stall, R., Goldhammer, H., & Landers, S. (2008). Sexual and gender minority health: What we know and what needs to be done. *American Journal of Public Health, 98*, 989-994.

*McClung, E., Grossoehme, D. H., & Jacobson, A. F. (2006). Collaborating with chaplains to meet spiritual needs. *MEDSURG Nursing, 15*(3), 147-156.

*MuÑoz, C., & Hilgenberg, C. (2005). Ethnopharmacology. *AJN, 105*(8), 41-48.

National Coalition for the Homeless. (2009). How many people experience homelessness? Retrieved April 6, 2011, from http://www.nationalhomeless.org/factsheets/How_Many.html.

*Pullen, R. L. (2007). Tips for communicating with a patient from another culture. *Nursing2007, 37*(10), 48.

Purnell, L. D., & Paulanka, B. J. (2008). *Transcultural healthcare: A culturally competent approach* (3rd ed.). Philadelphia: Davis.

*Smith, L. S. (2007). Speaking up for medical language interpreters. *Nursing2007, 37*(12), 48-49.

*U.S. Department of Health and Human Services (USDHHS), Office of Disease Prevention and Health Promotion. (2001). *Tracking Healthy People 2010* (2nd ed.). Pittsburgh: U.S. Government Printing Office.

U.S. Interagency Council on Homelessness. (June 2010). Supplemental document to the Federal Strategic Plan to Prevent and End Homelessness. Retrieved November 15, 2011 from www.usich.gov/resources/uploads/asset_library/BkgrdPap_Community.pdf.

Weisz, V. K. (2009). Social justice considerations for lesbian and bisexual women's health care. *Journal of Obstetric, Gynecologic, and Neonatal Nursing, 38*(1), 81-87.

Chapter 5

*American Geriatrics Society (AGS). (2002). The management of persistent pain in older persons. *Journal of the American Geriatrics Society, 50*(56), 205-224.

*American Society for Pain Management Nursing (ASPMN). (2002). *ASPMN position statement: Pain management in patients with addictive disease* (pp. 1-4). Retrieved November 14, 2010, from www.aspmn.org.

American Society for Pain Management Nursing (ASPMN). (2010). *ASPMN position statement: Use of placebos in pain management (revised)*. Retrieved April 6, 2011, from www.aspmn.org.

*American Society for Pain Management Nursing and the American Pain Society. (2004). A position statement on the use of "as-needed" range orders for opioid analgesics in the management of acute pain. Retrieved November 10, 2010, from www.aspmn.org.

Baumann, S. (2009). A nursing approach to pain in older adults. *MEDSURG Nursing, 18*(2), 77-82.

Boyd-Seale, D., Wilkie, D. J., Kim, Y. O., Suarez, M. L., Lee, H., Molokie, R., et al. (2010). Pain barriers: Psychometrics of a 13-item questionnaire. *Nursing Research, 59*, 93-101.

*Cranwell-Bruce, L. (2007). Update on pain management: New methods of opiate delivery. *MEDSURG Nursing, 16*(5), 333-335.

*D'Arcy, Y. (2007a). Managing pain in a patient who's drug dependent. *Nursing2007, 37*(3), 37-40.

*D'Arcy, Y. (2007b). New pain management options: Delivery systems and techniques. *Nursing2007, 372*, 26-27.

D'Arcy, Y. (2009a). Overcoming barriers to pain relief in older adults. *Nursing2009, 39*(10), 32-38.

D'Arcy, Y. (2009b). Putting pain research into practice. *Nursing2009, 39*(8), 58.

Dobbins, E. H. (2010). Where has all the meperidine gone? *Nursing2010, 40*(1), 65-66.

Elliott, A. F., & Horgas, A. L. (2009). Effects of an analgesic trial in reducing pain behaviors in community-dwelling older adults with dementia. *Nursing Research, 58*, 140-145.

Federico, A. (2009). Assessing pain in patients with dementia. *Nursing2009, 39*(12), 64.

Flaherty, E. (2008). Using pain-rating scales with older adults. *AJN, 108*(6), 40-48.

Gevirtz, C. (2009). Cannabinoids: An emerging role in pain management? *Nursing2009, 39*(6), 59-60.

*Herr, K., Coyne, P. J., Key, T., Manworren, R., McCaffery, M., Merkel, S., et al., American Society for Pain Management Nursing. (2006). Pain assessment in the nonverbal patient: Position statement with clinical practice recommendations. *Pain Management Nursing, 7*(2), 44-52.

Jarvis, C. (2012). *Physical examination and health assessment* (6th ed.). Philadelphia: Saunders.

Lilley, L. L., Collins, S. R., Harrington, S., & Snyder, J. S. (2011). *Pharamacology and the nursing process*. St. Louis: Mosby.

*McCaffery, M., & Pasero, C. (1999). Harmful effects of unrelieved pain. In M. McCaffery & C. Pasero (Eds.), *Pain: Clinical manual* (2nd ed., pp. 15-34). St. Louis: Mosby.

*Melzack, R., & Wall, P. D. (1982). *The challenge of pain.* New York: Basic Books.

Mitchell, A. A., Sapienza-Crawford, A. J., Hanley, K. L., Lokey, K. J., & Wells, L. (2008). Using ziconotide for intrathecal infusions. *Nursing2008, 38*(12), 19.

Quality and Safety Education for Nurses. (QSEN). (2011). Competency KSAs (pre-licensure). Retrieved July 3, 2011, from www.qsen.org.

*van Herk, R., van Dijk, M., Baar, F. P. M., Tibboel, D., & de Wit, R. (2007). Observation scales for pain assessment in older adults with cognitive impairments or communication difficulties. *Nursing Research, 56*(1), 34-43.

*Wuhrman, E., Cooney, M. F., Dunwoody, C. J., Eksterowicz, N., Merkel, S., Oakes, L. L., American Society for Pain Management Nursing. (2007). Authorized and unauthorized ("PCA by Proxy") dosing of analgesic infusion pumps: Position statement with clinical practice recommendations. *Pain Management Nursing, 8*(1), 4-11.

Chapter 6

American Association of Colleges of Nursing. (2008). *The essentials of baccalaureate education for nursing practice.* Washington, DC: Author.

American Nurses Association. (2008). *Essentials of genetic and genomic nursing: Competencies, curricula guidelines, and outcome indicators* (2nd ed.). Silver Springs, MD: Author.

Ashcraft, P. F., Coleman, E. A., Lange, U., Enderlin, C., & Stewart, C. B. (2007). Obtaining family histories from patients with cancer. *Clinical Journal of Oncology Nursing, 11*(1), 119-124, 130-134.

Cashion, A. (2009). The importance of genetics education for undergraduate and graduate nursing programs. *Journal of Nursing Education, 48*(10), 535-536.

Conley, Y., & Tinkle, M. (2007). The future of genomic nursing research. *Journal of Nursing Scholarship, 39*(1), 17-24.

Crockett-Maillet, G. (2010). Know the red flags of hereditary cancers. *The Nurse Practitioner Journal, 35*(7), 39-43.

Feero, G., Guttmacher, E., & Collins, F. (2010). Genomic medicine: An updated primer. *New England Journal of Medicine, 362,* 2001-2011.

Gallo, A., Angst, D., & Knafl, K. (2009). Disclosure of genetic information within families. *AJN, 109*(4), 65-69.

Greco, K., & Salveson, C. (2009). Identifying genetics and genomics nursing competencies common among published recommendations. *Journal of Nursing Education, 48*(10), 557-565.

Hamilton, R., & Bowers, B. (2007). The theory of genetic vulnerability: A Roy model exemplar. *Nursing Science Quarterly, 20*(3), 254-265.

Jenkins, J., & Calzone, K. (2007). Establishing the essential nursing competencies for genetics and genomics. *Journal of Nursing Scholarship, 39*(1), 10-16.

Kelly, P. (2008). Understanding genomics: No longer an option for gastroenterology nurses. *Gastroenterology Nursing, 31*(1), 45-54.

Kudzma, E., & Carey, E. (2009). Pharmacogenomics: Personalizing drug therapy. *AJN, 109*(10), 50-57.

Lea, D., Feero, G., & Jenkins, J. (2009). Keeping genetic information confidential: What you should know about the new federal law. *American Nurse Today, 4*(5), 26.

Lea, D., Skirton, H., Read, C., & Williams, K. (2011). Implications for educating the next generation of nurses on genetics and genomics in the 21st century. *Journal of Nursing Scholarship, 43*(1), 3-12.

Monsen, R. (2009). *Genetics and ethics in health care.* Silver Springs, MD: American Nurses Association.

National Coalition for Health Professional Education in Genetics. (2007, September). *Core competencies in genetics for health professionals* (3rd ed.). Retrieved October 2010, from www.nchpeg.org/core/Core_Comps_English2007.pdf.

National Institutes of Health. (2009). NIH Genetics Home Reference: Your guide to understanding genetics conditions. Retrieved August 2010, from http://ghr.nim.nih.gov/condition/.

Nussbaum, R., McInnes, R., & Willard, H. (2007). *Thompson & Thompson: Genetics in medicine* (7th ed.). Philadelphia: Saunders.

Nyrhinen, T., Hietala, M., Puukka, P., & Leino-Kilpi, H. (2007). Privacy and equality in diagnostic genetic testing. *Nursing Ethics, 14*(3), 295-308.

Pestka, E., Burbank, K., & Junglen, L. (2009). Improving nursing practice with genomics. *Nursing2009, 39*(12), 50-53.

*Spahis, J. (2002). Human genetics: Constructing a family pedigree. *AJN, 102*(7), 44-50.

Chapter 7

American Nurses Association. (2010). *Nursing: Scope and standards of practice* (2nd ed.). Silver Spring, MD: Author.

Carlson, C. (2009). Use of three evidence-based postoperative pain assessment practices by registered nurses. *Pain Management Nursing, 10*(4), 174-187.

*Committee on Quality of Health Care in America, Institute of Medicine. (2001). *Crossing the quality chasm: A new health care system for the 21st century.* Washington, DC: National Academies Press.

Cullum, N., Ciliska, D., Haynes, R. B., & Marks, S. (2008). *Evidence-based nursing: An introduction.* Oxford: Blackwell.

Decker, S. (2009). Behavioral indicators of postoperative pain in older adults with delirium. *Clinical Nursing Research, 18*(4), 336-347.

DiCenso, A., Guyatt, G., & Ciliska, D. (2005). *Evidence-based nursing: A guide to clinical practice.* St. Louis: Mosby.

*Ervin, N. E. (2002). Evidence-based nursing practice: Are we there yet? *Journal of the New York State Nurses Association, 33*(2), 11-16.

*Feldt, K. S. (2000). The Checklist of Nonverbal Pain Indicators (CNPI). *Pain Management Nursing, 1*(1), 13-21.

Fineout-Overholt, E., & Stillwell, S. B. (2011). Asking compelling clinical questions. In B. M. Melnyk & E. Fineout-Overholt (Eds.), *Evidence-based practice in nursing and healthcare: A guide to best practice* (2nd ed.). Philadelphia: Lippincott Williams & Wilkins.

*Hall, D. (2007). Evaluation of 3 pain assessment tools for use with critically ill adult patients. *American Journal of Critical Care, 16*(3), 309-310.

Institute of Medicine; Committee on the Health Professions Education Summit. (2003). *Health professions education: A bridge to quality.* Washington, DC: National Academies Press.

Institute of Medicine; Committee on the Robert Wood Johnson Foundation Initiative on the Future of Nursing, at the Institute of Medicine. (2010). *The future of nursing: Leading change, advancing health (Report Brief).* Washington, DC: National Academies Press. Available online at www.nap.edu.

Langley, G. J., Moen, R. G., Nolan, K. M., Nolan, T. W., Norman, C. L., & Provost, L. P. (2009). *The improvement guide: A practical approach to enhancing organizational performance* (2nd ed.). San Francisco: Jossey-Bass.

Levin, R. F. (2008). Translating research evidence for WOCN practice—Evidence levels and quality ratings: What do they mean? *WCET Journal, 28*(1), 30-31.

Levin, R. F. (2009). Evidence-based practice—Implementing practice changes: Walk before you run. *Research and Theory in Nursing Practice, 23*(2), 85-87.

Levin, R. F., Keefer, J. M., Marren, J., Vetter, M., Lauder, B. & Sobolewski, S. (2010). Evidence-based practice: Merging 2 paradigms. *Journal of Nursing Care Quality, 25*(2), 117-126.

*Levin, R. F., & Lane, H. T. (2006). Strategies to teach evidence searching: It takes a library. In R. F. Levin & H.R. Feldman (Eds.), *Teaching evidence-based practice in nursing: A guide for academic and clinical settings*. New York: Springer.

Levin, R. F., Melnyk, B. M., Fineout-Overholt, E., Barnes, M., & Vetter, M. (2011). Fostering evidence-based practice to improve nurse and cost outcomes in a community health setting: A pilot test of the ARCC model. *Nursing Administration Quarterly, 35*(1), 1-13.

*Levin, R. F., Singleton, J. K., & Jacobs, S. K. (2007). Developing and evaluating clinical practice guidelines: A systematic approach. In E. Capezuti, M. Mezey, T. Fulmer, & D. Zwicker (Eds.), *Evidence-based geriatric nursing protocols* (3rd ed.). New York: Springer.

*Melnyk, B. M., & Fineout-Overholt, E. (2005). *Evidence-based practice in nursing and healthcare: A guide to best practice*. Philadelphia: Lippincott Williams & Wilkins.

Melnyk, B. M., & Fineout-Overholt, E. (2010). ARCC (Advancing Research and Clinical Practice through Close Collaboration): A model for system-wide implementation and sustainability of evidence-based practice. In J. Rycroft-Malone & T. Bucknall (Eds.), *Models and frameworks for implementing evidence-based practice: Linking evidence to action*. Oxford: Wiley-Blackwell.

Melnyk, B. M., & Fineout-Overholt, E. (2011). *Evidence-based practice in nursing and healthcare: A guide to best practice* (2nd ed.). Philadelphia: Lippincott Williams & Wilkins.

Reavy, K., & Tavernier, S. (2008). Nurses reclaiming ownership of their practice: Implementation of an evidence-based practice model and process. *Journal of Continuing Education in Nursing, 39*(4), 166-172.

Rycroft-Malone, J., & Bucknall, T. (2010). Using theory and frameworks to facilitate the implementation of evidence into practice. *Worldviews on Evidence-Based Nursing, 7*(2), 57.

*Sackett, D. L., Straus, S. E., Richardson, W. S., Rosenberg, W., & Haynes, R. B. (2000). *Evidence-based medicine: How to practice and teach EBM* (2nd ed.). Edinburgh: Churchill Livingston.

Stetler, C. B. (2010). Stetler model. In J. Rycroft-Malone & T. Bucknall (Eds.), *Models and frameworks for implementing evidence-based practice: Linking evidence to action*. Oxford: Wiley-Blackwell.

The Joint Commission. (2010). *Approaches to pain management* (2nd ed.). Oakbrook Terrace, IL: Author.

Titler, M. (2010). Iowa model of evidence-based practice. In J. Rycroft-Malone & T. Bucknall (Eds.), *Models and frameworks for implementing evidence-based practice: Linking evidence to action*. Oxford: Wiley-Blackwell.

Wilding, J., Manias, E., & McCoy, D. (2009). Pain assessment and management in patients after abdominal surgery from PACU to the postoperative unit. *Journal of Perianesthesia Nursing, 24*(4), 233-240.

Wolosin, R. (2008). Safety and satisfaction: Where are the connections? *Patient Safety & Quality Healthcare,* May/June. Available online at www.psqh.com.

Worral, P. S., Levin, R. F., & Arsenault, D. C. (2009-2010). Documenting an EBP project: Guidelines for what to include and why. *Journal of the New York State Nurses Association, 40*(2), 12-19.

Chapter 8

*Association of Rehabilitation Nurses (ARN). (2002). *Practice guidelines for the management of constipation in adults.* Glenview, IL: Author.

Association of Rehabilitation Nurses (ARN). (2008a). *Standards and scope of rehabilitation nursing practice*. Glenview, IL: Author.

Association of Rehabilitation Nurses (ARN). (2008b). *The specialty practice of rehabilitation nursing: A core curriculum* (5th ed.). Skokie, IL: Author.

Coggrave, M. J., & Norton, C. (2010). The need for manual evacuation and oral laxatives in the management of neurogenic bowel dysfunction after spinal cord injury: A randomized controlled trial of a stepwise protocol. *Spinal Cord, 48*(6), 504-510.

Frisina, P. G., Guellnitz, R., & Alverzo, J. (2010). A time series of falls and injury in the inpatient rehabilitation setting. *Rehabilitation Nursing, 35*(4), 141-146, 166.

*Granger, C. V., & Gresham, G. E. (1984). *Functional assessment in rehabilitation medicine*. Baltimore: Williams & Wilkins.

*Lutz, B. J., Chumbler, N. R., & Roland, K. (2007). Care coordination/home telehealth for veterans with stroke and their caregivers: Addressing an unmet need. *Topics in Stroke Rehabilitation, 14*(2), 32-42.

Nelson, A., Motacki, K., & Menzel, N. (2009). *An illustrated guide to safe patient handling and movement*. New York: Springer.

Poslawsky, I. E., Schuurmans, M. J., Lindeman, E., & Hafsteinsdottir, T. B. (2010). A systematic review of nursing rehabilitation of stroke patients with aphasia. *Journal of Clinical Nursing, 19*(1-2), 17-32.

Pryor, J. (2010). Nurses create a rehabilitation milieu. *Rehabilitation Nursing, 35*(3), 123-128.

Pullen, R. L. (2008). Transferring a patient from bed to wheelchair. *Nursing2008, 38*(2), 46-48.

*Quigley, P. A., Bulat, T., & Hart-Hughes, S. (2007). Strategies to reduce risk of fall-related injuries in rehabilitation nursing. *Rehabilitation Nursing, 32*(3), 120-125.

*Rieg, L. S., Mason, C. H., & Preston, K. (2006). Spiritual care: Practical guidelines for rehabilitation nurses. *Rehabilitation Nursing, 31*(6), 249-256.

Sievert, K. D., Amend, B., Gakis, G., Toomey, P., Badke, A., Kaps, H. P., et al. (2010). Early sacral neuromodulation prevents urinary incontinence after complete spinal cord injury. *Annals of Neurology, 67*(1), 74-84.

U.S. National Library of Medicine (NIH). (2011). Cranberry. Retrieved September 5, 2011, from http://www.nlm.nih.gov/medlineplus/druginfo/natural/958.html.

*Waters, T. R. (2007). When is it safe to manually lift a patient? *AJN, 107*(8), 53-58.

Waters, T. R., & Rockefeller, K. (2010). Safe patient handling for rehabilitation professionals. *Rehabilitation Nursing, 35*(5), 216-222.

*Whipple, K. (2007). Therapeutic use of assistive technology: A clinical perspective. *Rehabilitation Nursing, 32*(2), 48-50.

*World Health Organization (WHO). (2001). International classification of functioning, disability, and health. Geneva: Author.

Chapter 9

*American Association of Colleges of Nursing. (2004). ELNEC core curriculum. Retrieved September 23, 2010, from www.aacn.nche.edu/elnec/curriculum.htm.

Arnstein, P. R., & Robinson, E. M. (2011). Is palliation sedation right for your patient? *Nursing2011*, *41*(8), 50.

Beck, I., Runeson, I., & Blomqvist, K. (2009). To find inner peace: Soft massage as an established and integrated palliative care. *International Journal of Palliative Nursing*, *15*(11), 541-545.

*Carlson, A. L. (2007). Death in the nursing home: Resident, family, and staff perspectives. *Journal of Gerontological Nursing*, *33*(4), 32-41.

Clarke, V., & Holtslander, L. F. (2010). Finding a balanced approach: Incorporating medicine wheel teachings in the care of Aboriginal people at the end of life. *Journal of Palliative Care*, *26*(1), 34-36.

Ferrell, B. (2010). Palliative care research: Nursing response to emergent society needs. *Nursing Science Quarterly*, *23*(3), 221-225.

*Field, M. J., & Cassel, C. K., Committee on Care at the End of Life, Institute of Medicine. (1997). *Approaching death: Improving care at the end of life*. Washington, DC: National Academies Press.

Gillick, M. R. (2010). Reversing the code status of advance directives? *New England Journal of Medicine*, *362*, 1239-1240.

Granda-Cameron, C., Viola, S. R., Lynch, M. P., & Polomano, R. C. (2008). Measuring patient-oriented outcomes in palliative care: Functionality and quality of life. *Clinical Journal of Oncology Nursing*, *12*(1), 65-77.

Heron, M., Hoyert, D., Murphy, S., Xu, J., Kochanek, K., & Tejuda-Veja, B. (2009, April 17). *National Vital Statistics Reports*. Deaths: Final data for 2006.

HPNA 2008 Research Committee. (2008). *Hospice and Palliative Nurses Association: 2009-2010 research agenda*. Pittsburgh: HPNA.

*Kapo, J., Morrison, L. J., & Liao, S. (2007). Palliative care for the older adult. *Journal of Palliative Medicine*, *10*(1), 185-209.

Kirk, T., Coyle, N., Poppito, S., & Bigoney, R. (2010, March 5). *Palliative sedation and existential suffering: A dialogue between medicine, nursing, philosophy, and psychology*. Boston: American Academy of Hospice and Palliative Medicine.

Lachman, V. (2010). Do-not-resuscitate orders: Nurse's role requires moral courage. *MEDSURG Nursing: The Journal of Adult Health*, *19*(4), 249-251.

Lipman, A. G. (2009). Evidence-based palliative care. In A. G. Lipman, K. C. Jackson, & S. Tyler (Eds.), *Evidence-based symptom control in palliative care* (pp. 1-9). New York: Informa Healthcare.

Matzo, M.L., & Sherman, D. W. (Eds.), (2010). *Palliative care nursing: Quality care to the end of life* (3rd ed.). New York: Springer.

Morrell, E. D., Brown, B. P., Qi, R., Drabiak, K., & Helft, P. R. (2008). The do-not-resuscitate order: Associations with advance directives, physician specialty and documentation of discussion 15 years after the Self-Determination Act. *Journal of Medical Ethics*, *34*(9), 642-647.

*National Center for Health Statistics. (2006). *Deaths: Final data for 2004. National Vital Statistics Reports*. Hyattsville, MD: Author.

National Consensus Project for Quality Palliative Care Task Force. (2009*). Clinical practice guidelines for quality palliative care* (2nd ed.). Pittsburgh: Author.

*National Hospice and Palliative Care Organization. (2005). Caring connections. Retrieved July 18, 2010, from www.caringinfo.org.

National Hospice and Palliative Care Organization. (2010). NHPCO position statement and commentary on the use of palliative sedation in imminently dying terminally ill patients. Retrieved March 20, 2011, from www.jpsmjournal.com.

Newshan, G., & Schuller-Citella, D. (2003). Large clinical study shows value of Therapeutic Touch program. *Holistic Nursing Practice*, *17*(4), 189-192.

Oregon Hospice Association. (2009). Hospice FAQ. Retrieved July 18, 2010, from www.oregonhospice.org.

Perrin, K. (2010a). Communicating with seriously ill and dying patients, their families, and their healthcare providers. In M. Matzo & D. W. Sherman (Eds.), *Palliative care nursing* (3rd ed.). New York: Springer.

Perrin, K. (2010b). Legal aspects of end-of-life decision making. In M. Matzo & D. W. Sherman (Eds.), *Palliative care nursing* (3rd ed.). New York: Springer.

Silveira, M. J., Kim, S. Y. H., & Langa, K. M. (2010). Advance directives and outcomes of surrogate decision-making before death. *New England Journal of Medicine*, *362*, 1211-1218.

*Support Study Principal Investigators. (1995). A controlled trial to improve care for seriously ill hospitalized patients: The Study to Understand Prognoses and Preferences for Outcomes and Risks for Treatments (SUPPORT). *Journal of the American Medical Association*, *274*, 1591-1598.

Supportive Care Coalition. (2008, October). Key clinical considerations on tube feeding for guiding policy and decision makers in Catholic medical care. Retrieved June 1, 2010, from www.supportivecarecoalition.org.

Taylor, D. H. (2009). The effect of hospice on Medicare and informal care costs: The U.S. experience. *Journal of Pain and Symptom Management*, *38*(1), 110-114.

Thacker, K. S. (2008). Nurses' advocacy behaviors in end-of-life nursing care. *Nursing Ethics*, *15*(2), 174-185.

Thomas, R., Wilson, D. M., Justice, C., Birch, S., & Sheps, S. (2008). A literature review of preferences for end-of-life care in developed countries by individuals with different cultural affiliations and ethnicity. *Journal of Hospice and Palliative Nursing*, *10*(3), 142-161.

Venneman, S. S., Narnor-Harris, P., Perish, M., & Hamilton, M. (2008). "Allow natural death" versus "do not resuscitate": Three words that can change a life. *Journal of Medical Ethics*, *34*(1), 2-6.

Wijk, H. & Grimby, A. (2008). Needs of elderly patients in palliative care. *American Journal Hospice and Palliative Care*, *25*(2), 106-111.

Chapter 10

*American College of Surgeons Committee on Trauma. (2006). *Resources for optimal care of the injured patient 2006*. Chicago, IL: Author.

American College of Surgeons Committee on Trauma. (2008). *Advanced trauma life support course for doctors student manual* (8th ed.). Chicago, IL: Author.

Barnard, S. (2009). Implementing an SBIRT (Screening, Brief Intervention, and Referral to Treatment) program in the emergency department: Challenges and rewards. *Journal of Emergency Nursing*, *35*(6), 561-563.

Centers for Disease Control and Prevention (CDC). (2010, June 18). FastStats: Emergency department visits. Retrieved

September 12, 2010, from www.cdc.gov/nchs/fastats/ervisits.htm.

Centers for Medicare and Medicaid Services. (2010, June 16). Critical access hospitals. Retrieved September 12, 2010, from www.cms.gov/CertificationandComplianc/04_CAHs.asp.

*Cooper, G., & Laskowski-Jones, L. (2006). Development of trauma care systems. *Prehospital Emergency Care, 10*(3), 328-331.

*Fernandes, C. M., Tanabe, P. L., Gilboy, N., Johnson, L. A., McNair, R. S., Rosenau, A. M., et al. (2005). Five-level triage: A report from the ACEP/ENA five-level triage task force. *Journal of Emergency Nursing, 31*(1), 39-50.

Howard, P. K. (2009). Crowding: A report of the ENA ED crowding work team. *Journal of Emergency Nursing, 35*(1), 55-56.

*Huryk, L. (2006). Is it really an emergency? *AJN, 106*(1), 69-72.

Institute of Medicine (IOM) Board on Health Care Services. (2010). *Regionalizing emergency care workshop summary*. Washington, DC: National Academies Press. Retrieved September 12, 2010, from www.nap.edu/catalog.php?record_id=12872.

Johnson, D., & Parker, D. (2009). Managers Forum—Cutting-edge discussion of management, policy, and program issues in emergency care: Canine security (Solheim, J., & Papa, A. [Eds.]). *Journal of Emergency Nursing, 35*(5), 469-470.

*Laskowski-Jones, L. (2007). Should families be present during resuscitation? *Nursing2007, 37*(5), 44-47.

Laskowski-Jones, L. (2008). Change management at the hospital front door: Integrating automatic patient tracking in a high volume emergency department and Level I trauma center. *Nurse Leader, 6*(2), 52-57.

Laskowski-Jones, L. (2009). Responding to trauma: Your priorities in the first hour. *Nursing2009, Critical Care, 4*(1), 35-41.

*Laskowski-Jones, L., Toulson, K., & McConnell, L. (2005). Assessing and planning for triage redesign. *Journal of Emergency Nursing, 31*(3), 315-318.

Mascioli, S., Laskowski-Jones, L., Urban, S., & Moran, S. (2009). Improving hand-off communication. *Nursing2009, 39*(2), 52-55.

Moskop, J. C., Sklar, D. P., Geiderman, J. M., Schears, R. M., & Bookman, K. J. (2009). Emergency department crowding, Part 1: Concepts, causes and moral consequences. *Annals of Emergency Medicine, 53*(5), 605-611.

Mower-Wade, D., & Pirrung, J. M. (2010). Advanced practice nurses making a difference: Implementation of a formal rounding process. *Journal of Trauma Nursing, 17*(2), 69-71.

National Center for Injury Prevention and Control. (2010, September 10). Injury prevention and control: Data & statistics (WISQARS). Retrieved September 12, 2010, from www.cdc.gov/injury/wisqars/index.html.

Nolan, M. R. (2009). Older adults in the emergency department: What are the risks? *Journal of Gerontological Nursing, 35*(12), 14-18.

Sadowski, L. S., Kee, R. A., VanderWeele, T. J., & Buchanan, D. (2009). Effect of a housing and case management program on emergency department visits and hospitalizations among chronically ill homeless adults. *JAMA: The Journal of the American Medical Association, 301*(17), 1771-1778.

Scales, M. H., Lewchick, J., Bauer, J., & Kiljanski, A. (2007). An informal discussion of emergency nurses' current clinical practice: What's new and what works. *Journal of Emergency Nursing, 33*(5), 480-483.

The Joint Commission. (2010). National Patient Safety Goals. Retrieved September 12, 2010, from www.jointcommission.org/patientsafety/nationalpatientsafetygoals/.

*Toulson, K., Laskowski-Jones, L., & McConnell, L. (2005). Implementation of the five-level Emergency Severity Index in a Level I trauma center emergency department with a three-tiered triage scheme. *Journal of Emergency Nursing, 31*(3), 259-264.

*VanHoy, S., & Laskowski-Jones, L. (2006). Early intervention for the pneumonia patient: An emergency department triage protocol. *Journal of Emergency Nursing, 32*(2), 154-158.

Wolf, L. (2008). Nurse educator: The use of human patient simulation in ED triage training can improve nursing confidence and patient outcomes. *Journal of Emergency Nursing, 34*(2), 169-171.

Chapter 11

*American Heart Association. (2005a). Part 10.3: Drowning. *Supplement to Circulation: Journal of the American Heart Association, 112*(24), IV-133-IV-135.

*American Heart Association. (2005b). Part 10.4: Hypothermia. *Supplement to Circulation: Journal of the American Heart Association, 112*(24), IV-136-IV-137.

*Auerbach, P. S. (2007). *Wilderness medicine* (5th ed.). St. Louis: Mosby.

Auerbach, P. S. (2009). *Medicine for the outdoors: The essential guide to first aid and medical emergencies* (5th ed.). St. Louis: Mosby.

Auerbach, P. S., Donner, H. J., & Weiss, E. A. (2008). *Field guide to wilderness medicine* (3rd ed.). St. Louis: Mosby.

Bledsoe, G. H., Manyak, M. J., & Townes, D. A. (2009). *Expedition & wilderness medicine*. New York: Cambridge University Press.

*Cherington, M. (2005). Spectrum of neurologic complications of lightning injuries. *NeuroRehabilitation, 20*, 3-8.

Choo, K. J. L., Simons, F. E. R., & Sheikh, A. (2010). Glucocorticoids for the treatment of anaphylaxis (Review). *The Cochrane Library 2010*, Issue 3. John Wiley & Sons.

Guoen, J., Shenghua, L., Rili G., Mitchell, A., & Yanping, S. (2009). High altitude disease: Consequences of genetic and environmental interactions. *North American Journal of Medicine and Science, 2*(3), 74-80.

Hausfater, P., Doumenc, B., Chopin, S., Le Manach, Y., Dautheville, S., Hericord, P., et al. (2010a). Elevation of cardiac troponin I during non-exertional heat-related illnesses in the context of a heat wave. *Critical Care, 14*(3), R99.

Hausfater, P., Megarbane, B., Dautheville, S., Patzak, A., Andronikof, M., Andre, S., et al. (2010b). Prognostic factors in non-exertional heatstroke. *Intensive Care Medicine, 36*, 272-280.

Johnson, C., Anderson, S. R., Dallimore, J., Winser, S., & Warrell, D. A. (2008). *Oxford handbook of expedition and wilderness medicine*. New York: Oxford University Press.

Lasater, M. (2008). Treatment of severe hypothermia with intravascular temperature modulation. *Critical Care Nurse, 28*(6), 24-29.

Laskowski-Jones, L. (2009). Winter emergencies: Managing ski and snowboard injuries. *Nursing2009, 39*(11), 24-30.

Laskowski-Jones, L. (2010). Summer emergencies: Can you take the heat? *Nursing2010, 40*(6), 24-32.

Layon, A. J., & Modell, J. H. (2009). Drowning: Update 2009. *Anesthesiology, 110*(6), 1390-1401.

*Lewis, A. M. (2007). Heatstroke in older adults. *AJN, 107*(6), 52-56.

Luks, A. M., & Swenson, E. R. (2008). Medication and dosage considerations in the prophylaxis and treatment of high-altitude illness. *Chest, 133*(3), 744-755.

*Mitchell, A. (2006). Africanized killer bees: A case study. *Critical Care Nurse, 26*(3), 23-32.

Norris, R. (Last updated December 17, 2008). *Snake envenomation, Coral.* e-Medicine. Retrieved June 16, 2010, from WebMD, www.emedicine.com/EMERG/topic542.htm.

Protherics, Inc. (2008). CroFab (Crotalidae Polyvalent Immune Fab [Ovine]). [Prescribing information]. Retrieved January 11, 2011, from www.fda.gov/downloads/biolgicsBloodVaccines/BloodBloodProducts/ApprovedProducts/LicensedProductsBLAs/FractionatedPlasmaProducts/UCM117573.pdf.

Schaeffer, S., & Badillo, R. B. (2009). Poison control therapy: Updates on treating ingested-poison toxicities and snakebites. *AJN, 109*(12), 42-45.

*Suchard, J. R. (2007). Scorpion envenomation. In P. S. Auerbach (Ed.), *Wilderness medicine* (5th ed., pp. 1033-1051). St. Louis: Mosby.

Weinstein, S. A., Dart, R. C., & Staples, A. (2009). Envenomation: An overview of clinical toxinology for the primary care physician. *American Family Physician, 80*, 793-802.

*Wozniak, E. J., Wisser, J., & Schwartz, M. (2006). Venomous adversaries: A reference to snake identification, field safety, and bite-victim first aid for disaster-response personnel deploying into the hurricane-prone regions of North America. *Wilderness and Environmental Medicine, 17*(4), 246-266.

Chapter 12

*American College of Surgeons. (2006). *Resources for optimal care of the injured patient.* Chicago: Author.

*American Nurses Association (ANA). (2001). *Code of ethics for nurses with interpretive statements.* Washington, DC: Author.

*Casani, J. A. P., & Romanosky, A. J. (2006). Surge capacity. In G. R. Ciottone (Ed.), *Disaster medicine* (pp. 193-202). St. Louis: Mosby.

*Chaffee, M. (2006). Making the decision to report to work in a disaster. *AJN, 106*(9), 54-57.

Claudius, I., Behar, S., Ballow, S., Wood, R., Stevenson, K., Blake, N., et al. (2008). Disaster drill exercise documentation and management: Are we drilling to standard? *Journal of Emergency Nursing, 34*(6), 504-508.

DeSimone, C. L. (2009). Response of public health workers to various emergencies. *AAOHN Journal, 57*(1), 17-23.

*Federal Emergency Management Agency (FEMA). (2004). *Are you ready? An in-depth guide to citizen preparedness.* Jessup, MD: Author.

Hyer, K., & Brown, L. M. (2008). The Impact of Event Scale—Revised. *AJN, 108*(11), 60-68.

Hyett, J. M. (2009). How to respond when lightning strikes. *Nursing2009, 39*(7), 32-35.

Landry, L. G., & Stockton, A. (2008). Evaluation of a collaborative project in disaster preparedness. *Nurse Educator, 33*(6), 254-258.

Laskowski-Jones, L. (2008). Change management at the hospital front door: Integrating automatic patient tracking in a high volume emergency department and Level I trauma center. *Nurse Leader, 6*(2), 52-57.

Laskowski-Jones, L. (2010). When disaster strikes: Ready, or not? (Editorial). *Nursing2010, 40*(4), 6.

Merchant, R. M., Leigh, J. E., & Lurie, N. (2010, February 24). Health care volunteers and disaster response: First be prepared.

New England Journal of Medicine. Retrieved April 4, 2011, from www.nejm.org February 24, 2010 (10.1056/NEJMp1001737).

*Mitchell, A. M., Kameg, K., & Sakraida, T. J. (2003a). Post-traumatic stress: Clinical implications. *Disaster Management & Response, 1*(1), 14-18.

*Mitchell, A. M., Sakraida, T. J., & Kameg, K. (2003b). Critical incident stress debriefing: Implications for best practice. *Disaster Management & Response, 1*(2), 46-51.

*Mitchell, A. M., Sakraida, T. J., & Zalice, K. K. (2005). Disaster care: Psychological considerations. *Nursing Clinics of North America, 40*(3), 535-550.

*Olszewski, T. M., & Varrasse, J. F. (2005). The neurobiology of PTSD: Implications for nurses. *Journal of Psychosocial Nursing, 43*(6), 40-47.

*Papp, E. (2005). Preparing for disasters: Helping yourself as you help others. *AJN, 105*(5), 112.

*Rice, K. L., Colletti, L. S., Hartmann, S., Schaubhut, R., & Davis, N. L. (2006). Learning from Katrina. *Nursing2006, 36*(4), 44-47.

Rushing, J. (2008). Responding to mild and moderate unintentional hypothermia. *Nursing2008, 38*(11), 22.

Smith, J. S. (2010). Mass casualty events: Are you prepared? *Nursing2010, 40*(4), 40-45.

Subbarao, I., Lyznicki, J. M., Hsu, E. B., Gebbie, K. M., Markenson, D., Barzansky, B., et al. (2008). A consensus-based educational framework and competency set for the discipline of disaster medicine and public health preparedness. *Disaster Medicine and Public Health Preparedness, 2*(1), 57-68.

*Sutingco, N. (2006). The incident command system. In G. R., Ciottone (Ed.), *Disaster medicine* (pp. 208-214). St. Louis: Mosby.

The Joint Commission. (2008). Standards FAQs: Emergency management. Retrieved July 29, 2010, from www.jointcommission.org/AccreditationPrograms/HomeCare/Standards/09_FAQs/EM/Emergency_Management.htm.

Tomczyk, D., Alvarez, D., Borgman, P., Cartier, M. J., Caulum, L., Galloway, C., et al. (2008). Caring for those who care: The role of the occupational health nurse in disasters. *AAOHN Journal, 56*(6), 243-250.

U.S. Department of Health & Human Services. (2010). National Disaster Medical System helping U.S. hospitals treat survivors of earthquake in Haiti. Retrieved July 29, 2010, from www.hhs.gov/haiti/ndms_ushospitals.html.

*Wielawski, I. M. (2006). The health legacy of September 11. *AJN, 106*(9), 27-28.

Chapter 13

Atassi, K. (2008). Action STAT: Water intoxication. *Nursing2008, 38*(2), 72.

Avent, Y. (2007). Managing calcium imbalance in acute care. *Nurse Practitioner, 32*(10), 7-10.

Collins, M., & Claros, E. (2011). Recognizing the face of dehydration. *Nursing2011, 41*(8), 26-31.

Crawford, A., & Harris, H. (2011). Balancing act: Hypomagnesemia and hypermagnesemia. *Nursing2011, 41*(10), 52-55.

Crawford, A., & Harris, H. (2011). Balancing act: Na+ and K+. *Nursing2011, 41*(7), 44-50.

Crawford, A., & Harris, H. (2011). I.V. Fluids: What nurses need to know. *Nursing2011, 41*(5), 30-38.

David, K. (2007). IV fluids: Do you know what's hanging and why? *RN, 70*(10), 35-40.

*Edwards, N. (2005). Interpreting laboratory values in older adults. *MEDSURG Nursing: The Journal of Adult Health, 14*(4), 220-229.

Given, S. (2010). Hypernatremia. *Nursing2010, 40*(10), 72.

Gordon, M. (2010). *Manual of nursing diagnosis* (12th ed.). Boston: Jones & Bartlett.

Hadaway, L. (2009). Protect patients from IV infiltration. *American Nurse Today, 4*(7), 10-12.

Hankins, J. (2007). The role of albumin in fluid balance. *Nursing2007, 37*(12), 14-15.

Hayes, D. (2007a). When potassium takes dangerous detours. *Nursing2007, 37*(11), 56hn1-56hn4.

Hayes, D. (2007b). How to respond to abnormal serum sodium levels. *Nursing2007, 37*(12), 56hn1-56hn4.

Holcomb, S. (2008). Third-spacing: When body fluid shifts. *Nursing2008, 38*(7), 50-53.

Huber, C., & Augustine, A. (2009). IV infusion alarms: Don't wait for the beep. *AJN, 109*(4), 32-33.

Koo, L., Reedy, S., & Smith, J. (2010). Patient history key to diagnosing peripheral edema. *Nurse Practitioner, 35*(3), 44-52.

Krost, W., Mistovich, J., & Limmer, D. (2009). Beyond the basics: Electrolyte disturbances. *EMS Magazine, 38*(4), 47-53.

Lecko, C. (2008). Improving hydration: An issue of safety. *Nursing & Residential Care, 10*(3), 149-150.

Lien, Y., & Shapiro, J. (2007). Hyponatremia: Clinical diagnosis and management. *American Journal of Medicine, 120*(8), 653-658.

McCance, K., Huether, S., Brashers, V., & Rote, N. (2010). *Pathophysiology: The biologic basis for disease in adults and children* (6th ed.). St. Louis: Mosby.

*Mentes, J. (2006). Oral hydration in older adults. *AJN, 106*(6), 40-49.

Munger, M. (2007). New agents for managing hyponatremia in hospitalized patients. *American Journal of Health-System Pharmacy, 64*(3), 253-265.

O'Neill, P. (2007). Helping your patient to restrict potassium. *Nursing2007, 37*(4), 64hn6, 64hn8.

Pagana, K., & Pagana, T. (2010). *Mosby's manual of diagnostic and laboratory tests* (4th ed.). St. Louis: Mosby.

Reynolds, I. (2007). Discovering and stopping hyperkalemia. *American Nurse Today, 2*(11), 52.

Rushing, J. (2009). Assessing for dehydration in adults. *Nursing2009, 39*(4), 14.

Sweeney, J. (2010). Managing hyponatremia. *Nursing2010, 40*(9), 63.

Tocco, S. (2010). Cerebral salt wasting: An overlooked cause of hyponatremia. *American Nurse Today, 5*(3), 34-36.

Touhy, T., & Jett, K. (2010). *Ebersole and Hess' gerontological nursing & healthy aging* (3rd ed.). St. Louis: Mosby.

Trissel, L. (2009). *Handbook on injectable drugs* (15th ed.). Bethesda, MD: American Society of Hospital-System Pharmacists.

Vacca, V. (2008). Hyperkalemia. *Nursing2008, 38*(7), 72.

Chapter 14

*Casaletto, J. (2005). Differential diagnosis of metabolic acidosis. *Emergency Medicine Clinics of North America, 23*(3), 771-787.

Fornier, M. (2009). Perfecting your acid-base balancing act. *American Nurse Today, 4*(1), 17-21.

Gordon, M. (2010). *Manual of nursing diagnosis* (12th ed.). Boston: Jones & Bartlett.

Jarvis, C. (2012). *Physical examination and health assessment* (6th ed.). Philadelphia: Saunders.

Jones, M. (2010). Basic interpretation of metabolic acidosis. *Critical Care Nurse, 30*(5), 63-69.

Kramer, B. (2009). Arterial blood gases. *RN, 72*(4), 22-24.

Lawes, R. (2009). Body out of balance: Understanding metabolic acidosis and alkalosis. *Nursing2009, 39*(11), 50-54.

McCance, K., Huether, S., Brashers, V., & Rote, N. (2010). *Pathophysiology: The biologic basis for disease in adults and children* (6th ed.). St. Louis: Mosby.

Pagana, K., & Pagana, T. (2010). *Mosby's manual of diagnostic and laboratory tests* (4th ed.). St. Louis: Mosby.

Pruitt, B. (2010). Interpreting ABGs: An inside look at your patient's status. *Nursing2010, 40*(7), 31-35.

Roman, M., Thimothee, S., & Vidal, J. (2008). Arterial blood gases. *MEDSURG Nursing, 17*(4), 268-269.

Swiderski, D., & Byrum, D. (2007). Are you an ABG ace? *American Nurse Today, 2*(4), 18-21.

Touhy, T., & Jett, K. (2010). *Ebersole and Hess' gerontological nursing & healthy aging* (3rd ed.). St. Louis: Mosby.

Vacca, V. (2008). Hyperkalemia. *Nursing2008, 38*(7), 72.

Chapter 15

Aguiar, T. (2010, May). *Intraosseous access: Not just for emergencies anymore.* Presentation at the Infusion Nurses Society annual meeting: Las Vegas, NV.

*Almadrones, L. (2007). Evidence-based research for intraperitoneal chemotherapy in epithelial ovarian cancer. *Clinical Journal of Oncology Nursing, 11*(2), 211-216.

Bard Access Systems. (2011). PowerPICC Solo*[2] Catheter: Overview. Retrieved April 6, 2011, from http://www.bardaccess.com/nurse-powerpiccsolo.php.

Crawford, A., & Harris, H. (2011). I.V. fluids: What nurses need to know. *Nursing2011, 41*(5), 30-39.

Crimlisk, J. T., Johnstone, D. J., & Sanchez, G. M. (2009). Evidence-based practice, clinical simulations workshop, and intravenous medications: Moving toward safer practice. *MEDSURG Nursing, 18*(3), 153-160.

*Earhart, A., & Kaminski, D. (2007). Evidence-based practice in infusion nursing: 2007 NACNS national conference abstracts. *Clinical Nurse Specialist, 21*(2), 107.

Food and Drug Administration (FDA). (2009). FDA public health notification: PVC devices containing plasticizer DEHP. Retrieved October 13, 2010, from www.fda.gov/MedicalDevice/Safety/AlertsandNotices/PublichealthNotifications/UCM062182.

*Fowler, R., Gallagher, J. V., Isaacs, S. M., Ossman, E., Pepe, P., & Wayne, M. (2007). The role of intraosseous vascular access in the out-of-hospital environment. *Prehospital Emergency Care, 11*(1), 63-66.

Garcia, L. S., & Isenberg, H. D. (2010). *Clinical microbiology procedures handbook* (3rd ed.). Washington, DC: ASM Press.

Genentech USA, Inc. (2011). Cathflo(r) Activase (r) (Alteplase). Retrieved April 6, 2011, from http://www.cathflo.com.

*Gillies, D., O'Riordan, L., Wallen, M., Morrison, A., Rankin, K., & Nagy, S. (2005). Optimal timing for intravenous administration set replacement. *Cochrane Database of Systematic Reviews, 4*, CD003588.

*Goldberg, P. A., Kedves, A., Walter, K., Groszmann, A., Belous, A., & Inzucchi, S. E. (2006). Waste not, want not: Determining the optimal priming volume for intravenous insulin infusions. *Diabetes Technology & Therapeutics, 8*(5), 598-601.

*Gorski, L. (2007). Standard 44: Dressings. *Journal of Infusion Nursing, 30*(2), 87-88.

Gorski, L., Perucca, R., & Hunter, M. R. (2010). Central venous access devices: Care, maintenance, and potential complications. In M. Alexander, A. Corrigan, L. Gorski, J. Hankins, & R. Perucca (Eds.), *Infusion nursing: An evidence-based approach* (3rd ed.). St. Louis: Saunders.

*Griffiths, V. (2007). Midline catheters: Indications, complications and maintenance. *Nursing Standard, 22*(11), 48-57.

*Guthrie, D., Dreher, D., & Munson, M. (2007). What you need to know about PICCs, Part 1. *Nursing2007, 37*(8), 18.

*Hadaway, L. (2007). Emergency: Infiltration and extravasation. *AJN, 107*(8), 62-72.

Hadaway, L. C. (2009). Managing vascular access device occlusions, Part 1. *Nursing2009, 39*(1), 10.

Hadaway, L. C. (2010a). Infusion therapy equipment. In M. Alexander, A. Corrigan, L. Gorski, J. Hankins, & R. Perucca (Eds.), *Infusion nursing; An evidence-based approach* (3rd ed.). St. Louis: Saunders.

Hadaway, L. C. (2010b). Preventing and managing peripheral extravasation. *Nursing2009, 39*(10), 26-27.

*Infusion Nurses Society (INS). (2006). Infusion nursing standards of practice. *Journal of Infusion Nursing, 29*(1 Suppl. 6S), S1-S92.

Institute for Healthcare Improvement (IHI). (2008). Implement the central line bundle. *Five Million Lives Campaign.* Retrieved October 13, 2010, from www.ihi.org/IHI/Topics/CriticalCare/IntensiveCare/Changes/ImplementtheCentralLineBundle.htm.

*Jacobs, B. (2006). Using an infusion pump safely. *Nursing2006, 36*(10), 24.

Khalidi, N., Kovacevich, D. S., Papke-O'Donnell, L. F., & Btaiche, I. (2009). Impact of the positive pressure valve on vascular access device occlusions and bloodstream infections. *Journal of the Association for Vascular Access, 14*(2), 84-91.

*Khan, M., & Younger, G. (2007). Promoting safe administration of subcutaneous infusions. *Nursing Standard, 21*(31), 50-56.

Madigan, K. (2008). Now, intraosseous infusions for adults. *American Nurse Today, 3*(1), 11-12.

*Masoorli, S. (2007). Nerve injuries related to vascular access insertion and assessment. *Journal of Infusion Nursing, 30*(6), 346-350.

McGoldrick, M. (2010). Infection prevention and control. In M. Alexander, L. Gorski, J. Hankins, & R. Perucca (Eds.), *Infusion nursing: An evidence-based approach* (3rd ed.). St. Louis: Saunders.

Mitchell, M. D., Anderson, B. J., Williams, K., & Umscheid, C. A. (2009). Heparin flushing and other interventions to maintain patency of central venous catheters: A systematic review. *Journal of Advanced Nursing, 65*(10): 2007-2021.

Moran, J. E., & Ash, S. R. (2010). Locking solutions for hemodialysis catheters: Heparin and citrate—a position paper by ASDIN. *ASDIN Position Papers.* Retrieved June 18, 2010, from http://asdin.affiniscape.com/associations/9795/filesSDI%20466%20Locking%20Solutions.pdf.

Moreau, N. L. (2008a). Tips for inserting an I.V. device in an older adult. *Nursing2008, 38*(12), 12.

Moreau, N. L. (2008b). Using ultrasound to guide PICC and peripheral cannula insertion. *Nursing2008, 38*(10), 20-21.

Moreau, N. L. (2009a). Are your skin-prep and catheter maintenance techniques up-to-date? *Nursing2009, 39*(5), 15-16.

Moreau, N. L. (2009b). Reducing the cost of catheter-related bloodstream infections. *Nursing2009, 39*(7), 14-15.

O'Grady, N. P., Alexander, M., Burns, L. A., Dellinger, E. P., Garland, J., Heard, S. O., et al. (2011). *Guidelines for the prevention of intravascular catheter-related infections.* Atlanta: Centers for Disease Control and Prevention.

Perucca, R. (2010). Peripheral venous access devices. In M. Alexander, A. Corrigan, L. Gorski, J. Hankins, & R. Perucca (Eds.), *Infusion nursing; An evidence-based approach* (3rd ed.). St. Louis: Saunders.

*Rosenthal, K. (2006a). Do needleless connectors increase bloodstream infection risk? *Nursing Management, 37*(4), 78-80.

*Rosenthal, K. (2006b). Guarding against vascular site infection. *Nursing Management, 37*(4), 54-66.

Rosenthal, K. (2008). Bridging the I.V. access gap with midline catheters. *Med/Surg Insider, Fall,* 2-5.

*Swanson, J. M. (2007). Heparin-induced thrombocytopenia: A general review. *Journal of Infusion Nursing, 30*(4), 232-240.

*Winfield, C., Davis, S., Schwaner, S., Conaway, M., & Burns, S. (2007). Evidence: The first word in safe I.V. practice. *American Nurse Today, 2*(5), 31-33.

Chapter 16

Adams, A. (2008). Is hair removal necessary before the surgical incision? *Perioperative Nursing Clinics, 3*(2), 107-113.

*American Society of Anesthesiologists Task Force. (1999). Practice guidelines for preoperative fasting and the use of pharmacologic agents to reduce the risk of pulmonary aspiration: Application to healthy patients undergoing elective procedures. *Anesthesiology, 90*(3), 896-905.

*American Society of PeriAnesthesia Nurses (ASPAN). (2004). *Standards, recommended practices, and guidelines.* Denver: Author.

Association of periOperative Registered Nurses (AORN). (2010a). Position statement on correct site surgery. In *Perioperative standards and recommended practices* (p. 708). Denver: Author.

Association of periOperative Registered Nurses (AORN). (2010b). Perioperative explications for the ANA code of ethics for nurses. In *Perioperative standards and recommended practices* (pp. 30-61). Denver: Author.

Association of periOperative Registered Nurses (AORN). (2010c). Position statement on perioperative care of patients with do-not-resuscitate (DNR) or allow-natural-death orders. In *Perioperative standards and recommended practices* (pp. 740-742). Denver: Author.

Association of periOperative Registered Nurses (AORN). (2010d). Recommended practices for perioperative patient skin antisepsis. In *Perioperative standards and recommended practices* (pp. 351-356). Denver: Author.

*Beyea, S. (2002). Accident prevention in surgical settings: Keeping patients safe. *AORN Journal, 75*(2), 361-363.

*Beyea, S. (2004). Evidence-based practice in perioperative nursing. *American Journal of Infection Control, 32*(2), 97-100.

Beyea, S. (2007). Update on correct site surgery. *AORN Journal, 85*(2), 415-417.

Cawley, Y. (2008). Mechanical thromboprophylaxis in the perioperative setting. *MEDSURG Nursing: Official Journal of the Academy of Medical-Surgical Nurses, 17*(3), 177-182.

Centers for Disease Control and Prevention. (2008). National health statistics report: Ambulatory medical care utilization estimates for 2006. Retrieved July 2010, from www.cdc.gov/nchs/data/nhsr/nhsr008.pdf.

Cheek, D., & Jones, T. (2009). Safe surgery initiative saves lives. *Nursing2009, 39*(8), 14-15.

Crenshaw, J., & Winslow, E. (2008). Preoperative fasting duration and medication instruction: Are we improving? *AORN Journal, 88*(6), 963-976.

Daniels, S. (2007). Protecting patients from harm: Improving hospital care for surgical patients. *Nursing2007, 37*(8), 36-41.

DeLamar, L. (2007). Anesthesia. In J. C. Rothrock & D. McEwen (Eds.), *Alexander's care of the patient in surgery* (13th ed., Chapter 4). St. Louis: Mosby.

Doerflinger, D. (2009). Older adult surgical patients: Presentation and challenges. *AORN Journal, 90*(2), 223-240.

Grebe, R. (2007). Informed consent for patient with cognitive impairment. *Nurse Practitioner, 32*(12), 39-44.

Gupta, A. (2009). Preoperative screening and risk assessment in the ambulatory surgery patient. *Current Opinion in Anaesthesiology, 22*(6), 705-711.

James, A., & Abbott, J. (2009). Preoperative assessment. *British Journal of Hospital Medicine, 70*(11), M170-M172.

Johnson, J. (2011). Preoperative assessment of high-risk orthopedic surgery patients. *Nurse Practitioner, 36*(7), 40-47.

Kruzik, N. (2009). Benefits of preoperative education for adult elective surgery patients. *AORN Journal, 90*(3), 381-387.

Lucas, B. (2008). Total hip and total knee replacement: Preoperative nursing management. *British Journal of Nursing, 17*(21), 1346-1351.

McEwen, D. (2007). Ambulatory surgery. In J. C. Rothrock & D. McEwen (Eds.), *Alexander's care of the patient in surgery* (13th ed.). St. Louis: Mosby.

Morse, K. (2009). Focusing on the surgical patient with cardiac problems. *Nursing2009, 39*(3), 22-27.

Neil, J. A. (2007). Perioperative care of the immunocompromised patient. *AORN Journal, 85*(3), 544-560.

Pagana, K., & Pagana, T. (2010). *Mosby's manual of diagnostic and laboratory tests* (4th ed.). St. Louis: Mosby.

Ridge, R. (2008). Doing right to prevent wrong-site surgery. *Nursing2008, 38*(3), 24-25.

Roesler, R., Halowell, C., Elias, G., & Peters, J. (2010). Chasing zero: Our journey to preventing surgical site infection. *AORN Journal, 91*(2), 224-235.

Rothrock, J. C., & McEwen, D. (2007). *Alexander's care of the patient in surgery* (13th ed.). St. Louis: Mosby.

Scherer, D., & Fitzpatrick, J. (2008). Perceptions of patient safety culture among physicians and RNs in the perioperative area. *AORN Journal, 87*(1), 163-164, 166, 168-174.

Sendelbach, S. (2010). Preoperative fasting doesn't mean nothing after midnight. *AJN, 110*(9), 64-65.

Smith, L. (2007). Speaking up for medical language interpreters. *Nursing2007, 37*(12), 48-49.

The Joint Commission. (2010). National Patient Safety Goals. Retrieved October 2010, from www.jointcommission.org/patientsafety/nationalpatientsafetygoals/.

Touhy, T., & Jett, K. (2010). *Ebersole and Hess' gerontological Nursing & healthy aging* (3rd ed.). St. Louis: Mosby.

Watson, D. (2010). Never events in health care. *AORN Journal, 91*(3), 378-382.

Winkelman, C. (2009). Bed rest in health and critical illness: A body systems approach. *AACN Advanced Critical Care, 20*(3), 254-266.

Woolger, J. (2008). Preoperative testing and medication management. *Clinics in Geriatric Medicine, 24*(4), 573-583.

Chapter 17

*American Society of PeriAnesthesia Nurses. (2000). *Standards of perianesthesia nursing practice.* Cherry Hill, NJ: Author.

Association of periOperative Registered Nurses (AORN). (2010a). Position statement: AORN position statement on RN first assistants. In *Perioperative standards and recommended practices* (pp. 744-745). Denver: Author.

Association of periOperative Registered Nurses (AORN). (2010b). Position statement: Perioperative care of patients with do not resuscitate (DNR) or allow natural death orders. In *Perioperative standards and recommended practices* (pp. 740-742). Denver: Author.

Association of periOperative Registered Nurses (AORN). (2010c). Recommended practices for cleaning and care of surgical instruments and powered equipment. In *Perioperative standards and recommended practices* (pp. 424-445). Denver: Author.

Association of periOperative Registered Nurses (AORN). (2010d). Recommended practices for high-level disinfection. In *Perioperative standards and recommended practices* (pp. 389-404). Denver: Author.

Association of periOperative Registered Nurses (AORN). (2010e). Recommended practices for documentation of perioperative nursing care. In *Perioperative standards and recommended practices* (pp. 289-291). Denver: Author.

Association of periOperative Registered Nurses (AORN). (2010f). Recommended practices for environmental cleaning in the perioperative setting. In *Perioperative standards and recommended practices* (pp. 241-255). Denver: Author.

Association of periOperative Registered Nurses (AORN). (2010g). Recommended practices for safe care through identification of potential hazards in the surgical environment. In *Perioperative standards and recommended practices* (pp. 575-581). Denver: Author.

Association of periOperative Registered Nurses (AORN). (2010h). Recommended practices for laser safety in the practice settings. In *Perioperative standards and recommended practices* (pp. 133-138). Denver: Author.

Association of periOperative Registered Nurses (AORN). (2010i). Recommended practices for managing the patient receiving moderate sedation/analgesia. In *Perioperative standards and recommended practices* (pp. 315-325). Denver: Author.

Association of periOperative Registered Nurses (AORN). (2010j). Recommended practices for positioning the patient in the perioperative practice setting. In *Perioperative standards and recommended practices* (pp. 327-350). Denver: Author.

Association of periOperative Registered Nurses (AORN). (2010k). Recommended practices for perioperative patient skin antisepsis. In *Perioperative standards and recommended practices* (pp. 351-369). Denver: Author.

Association of periOperative Registered Nurses (AORN). (2010l). Recommended practices for sponge, sharp, and instrument counts. In *Perioperative standards and recommended practices* (pp. 207-216). Denver: Author.

Association of periOperative Registered Nurses (AORN). (2010m). Recommended practices for maintaining a sterile field. In *Perioperative standards and recommended practices* (pp. 91-99). Denver: Author.

Association of periOperative Registered Nurses (AORN). (2010n). Recommended practices for sterilization in the perioperative practice setting. In *Perioperative standards and recommended practices* (pp. 457-480). Denver: Author.

Association of periOperative Registered Nurses (AORN). (2010o). Recommended practices for surgical attire. In *Perioperative standards and recommended practices* (pp. 67-73). Denver: Author.

Association of periOperative Registered Nurses (AORN). (2010p). Recommended practices for hand hygiene in the perioperative setting. In *Perioperative standards and recommended practices* (pp. 75-89). Denver: Author.

Association of periOperative Registered Nurses (AORN). (2010q). Recommended practices for traffic patterns in the perioperative practice setting. In *Perioperative standards and recommended practices* (pp. 101-104). Denver: Author.

Association of periOperative Registered Nurses (AORN). (2010r). Recommended practices for selection and use of surgical gowns and drapes. In *Perioperative standards and recommended practices* (pp. 559-563). Denver: Author.

Association of periOperative Registered Nurses (AORN). (2010s). Statement on correct site surgery. In *Perioperative standards and recommended practices* (p. 708). Denver: Author.

Bartely, M. (2006). Preventing venous thromboembolism. *Nursing2006, 36*(1), 64cc1-64cc4.

Birch, D., Asiri, A., & de Gara, C. (2007). The impact of a formal mentoring program for minimally invasive surgery on surgeon practice and patient outcomes. *American Journal of Surgery, 193*(5), 589-591.

Conlon, N., Sullivan, R., Herbison, P., Zacharias, M., & Buggy, D. (2007). The effect of leaving dentures in place on bag-mask ventilation at induction of general anesthesia. *Anesthesia and Analgesia, 105*(2), 370-373.

*DeJonghe, B., Cook, D., Appere-de-Vecchi, C., et al. (2000). Using and understanding sedation scoring systems: A systematic review. *Intensive Care Medicine, 26*(3), 275-285.

DeLamar, L. (2007). Anesthesia. In J. C. Rothrock & D. McEwen (Eds.), *Alexander's care of the patient in surgery* (13th ed.). St. Louis: Mosby.

Dizer, B., Hatipoglu, S., Kaymakcioglu, N., Tufan, T., Yava, A., Iyigun, E., et al. (2009). The effect of nurse-performed preoperative skin preparation on postoperative surgical site infections in abdominal surgery. *Journal of Clinical Nursing, 18*(23), 3325-3332.

Doerflinger, D. (2009). Older adult surgical patients: Presentation and challenges. *AORN Journal, 90*(2), 223-240.

*Dunn, D. (2005). Preventing perioperative complications in special populations. *Nursing2005, 35*(11), 36-43.

Durai, R., & Ng, P. (2010). Surgical vacuum drains: Types, uses, and complications. *AORN Journal, 91*(2), 226-271.

*Hommertzheim, R., & Steinke, E. E. (2006). Malignant hyperthermia: The perioperative nurse's role. *AORN Journal, 83*(1), 149-164.

Hopper, W., & Moss, R. (2010). Common breaks in sterile technique: Clinical perspectives and perioperative implications. *AORN Journal, 91*(3), 350-364.

Jackson, S., & Brady, S. (2008). Counting difficulties: Retained instruments, sponges, and needles. *AORN Journal, 87*(2), 315-321.

Johnson, J. (2011). Preoperative assessment of high-risk orthopedic surgery patients. *Nurse Practitioner, 36*(7), 40-47.

Kaplow, R. (2010). Care of postanesthesia patients. *Critical Care Nurse, 30*(1), 60-62.

McCance, K., Huether, S., Brashers, V., & Rote, N. (2010). *Pathophysiology: The biologic basis for disease in adults and children* (6th ed.). St. Louis: Mosby.

McEwen, D. (2007). Ambulatory surgery. In J. C. Rothrock & D. McEwen (Eds.), *Alexander's care of the patient in surgery* (13th ed.). St. Louis: Mosby.

National Center for Health Statistics. (2007). National survey of ambulatory surgery. Retrieved March 15, 2008, from www.cdc.gov/nchs/nsas.htm.

Nussbaum, R., McInnes, R., & Willard, H. (2007). *Thompson & Thompson: Genetics in medicine* (7th ed.). Philadelphia: Saunders.

Pear, S., & Williamson, T. (2009). The RN first assistant: An expert resource for surgical site infection prevention. *AORN Journal, 89*(6), 1093-1097.

Ridge, R. (2008). Doing right to prevent wrong-site surgery. *Nursing2008, 38*(3), 24-25.

Roesler, R., Halowell, C., Elias, G., & Peters, J. (2010). Chasing zero: Our journey to preventing surgical site infection. *AORN Journal, 91*(2), 224-235.

Rothrock, J. C., & McEwen, D. (2007). *Alexander's care of the patient in surgery* (13th ed.). St. Louis: Mosby.

*Schoonhoven, L., Defloor, T., & Grypdonck, M. (2002). Incidence of pressure ulcers due to surgery. *Journal of Clinical Nursing, 11*(4), 479-487.

The Joint Commission (TJC). (2010). National Patient Safety Goals. Retrieved October 2010, from www.jointcommission.org/patientsafety/nationalpatientsafetygoals/.

Touhy, T., & Jett, K. (2010). *Ebersole and Hess' gerontological nursing & healthy aging* (3rd ed.). St. Louis: Mosby.

Ulmer, B. (2010). Best practices for minimally invasive procedures. *AORN Journal, 91*(5), 558-575.

Watson, D. (2010). Never events in health care. *AORN Journal, 91*(3), 378-382.

Weirich, T. (2008). Hypothermia/warming protocols: Why are they not widely used in the OR? *AORN Journal, 87*(2), 333-344.

Chapter 18

*American Society of PeriAnesthesia Nurses. (2000). *Standards of perianesthesia nursing practice*. Cherry Hill, NJ: Author.

Association of periOperative Registered Nurses (AORN). (2010). Recommended practices for transfer of patient care information. In *Perioperative standards and recommended practices* (pp. 371-377). Denver: Author.

Baugh, N., Zuelzer, H., Meador, J., & Blankenship, J. (2007). Wounds in surgical patients who are obese. *AJN, 107*(6), 40-50.

Beattie, S. (2007). Wound dehiscence. *RN, 70*(6), 34-37.

Blaney-Koen, L. (2007). Safe surgery: A patient's guide. *Journal of Patient Safety, 3*(1), 56.

Bopp, E. J., Estrada, T. J., Kilday, J. M., Spradling, J. C., Daniel, C., & Pellegrini, J. E. (2010). Biphasic dosing regimen of meclizine for prevention of postoperative nausea and vomiting in a high-risk population. *American Association of Nurse Anesthetists Journal, 78*(1), 55-62.

Crainic, C., Erickson, K., Gardner, J., Haberman, S., Patten, P., Thomas, P., et al. (2009). Comparison of methods to facilitate postoperative bowel function. *MEDSURG Nursing, 18*(4), 235-238.

Dizer, B., Hatipoglu, S., Kaymakciolu, N., Tufan, T., Yava, A., Iyigun, E., et al. (2009). The effect of nurse-performed preoperative skin preparation on postoperative surgical site infections in abdominal surgery. *Journal of Clinical Nursing, 18*(23), 3325-3332.

Dunn, D. (2005). Preventing perioperative complications in special populations. *Nursing2005, 35*(11), 36-43.

Fetzer, S. (2008). Putting a stop to postop nausea and vomiting. *American Nurse Today, 3*(8), 10-12.

*Hahler, B. (2006). Surgical wound dehiscence. *MEDSURG Nursing, 15*(5), 296-300.

Johnson, C. (2009). Development of abdominal wound dehiscence after a colectomy: A nursing challenge. *MEDSURG Nursing, 18*(2), 96-102.

Kaplow, R. (2010). Care of postanesthesia patient. *Critical Care Nurse, 30*(1), 60-62.

Lewthwaite, B. (2009). What do nurses know about postoperative nausea and vomiting? *MEDSURG Nursing, 18*(2), 110-113, 133.

Lucas, B. (2008). Total hip and knee replacement: Postoperative nursing management. *British Journal of Nursing, 17*(22), 1410-1414.

McCance, K., Huether, S., Brashers, V., & Rote, N. (2010). *Pathophysiology: The biologic basis for disease in adults and children* (6th ed.). St. Louis: Mosby.

McEwen, D. (2007). Wound healing, dressings, and drains. In J. C. Rothrock & D. McEwen (Eds.), *Alexander's care of the patient in surgery* (13th ed.). St. Louis: Mosby.

Owens, R. (2008). Teaming up to improve the quality of surgical care. *American Nurse Today, 3*(5), 25-26.

Roesler, R., Halowell, C., Elias, G., & Peters, J. (2010). Chasing zero: Our journey to preventing surgical site infection. *AORN Journal, 91*(2), 224-235.

Rothrock, J. C., & McEwen, D. (2007). *Alexander's care of the patient in surgery* (13th ed.). St. Louis: Mosby.

Sullivan, J. M. (2011). Caring for older adults after surgery. *Nursing2011, 41*(4), 48-51.

The Joint Commission. (2010). National Patient Safety Goals. Retrieved October 2010, from www.jointcommission.org/patientsafety/nationalpatientsafetygoals/.

Touhy, T., & Jett, K. (2010). *Ebersole and Hess' gerontological nursing & healthy aging* (3rd ed.). St. Louis: Mosby.

Walker, C., Hogstel, M., & Curry, L. (2007). Hospital discharge of older adults. *AJN, 107*(6), 60-70.

Chapter 19

Abbas, A., Lichtman, A., & Pillai, S. (2010). *Cellular and molecular immunology* (updated 6th ed.). Philadelphia: Saunders.

Borchers, A. T., Selmi, C., Meyers, F. J., Keen, C. L., & Gershwin, M. E. (2009). Probiotics and immunity. *Journal of Gastroenterology, 44*(1), 26-46.

Braun, L. (2010). How inflammatory markers refine CV risk status. *American Nurse Today, 5*(5), 30-31.

*Graham, J., Christian, L., & Kiecolt-Glaser, J. (2006). Stress, age, and immune function: Toward a lifespan approach. *Journal of Behavioral Medicine, 29*(4), 389-400.

Kaufman, C. (2011). The secret life of lymphocytes. *Nursing2011, 41*(6), 50-54.

Harvard Health. (2007). How your immune system works. In *Truth about your immune system: What you need to know* (pp. 5-14). Cambridge: Harvard Health Publications.

Landis, R. C. (2009). Redefining the systemic inflammatory response. *Seminars in Cardiothoracic and Vascular Anesthesia, 13*(2), 87-94.

McCance, K., Huether, S., Brashers, V., & Rote, N. (2010). *Pathophysiology: The biologic basis for disease in adults and children* (6th ed.). St. Louis: Mosby.

Nussbaum, R., McInnes, R., & Willard, H. (2007). *Thompson & Thompson: Genetics in medicine* (7th ed.). Philadelphia: Saunders.

Pagana, K., & Pagana, T. (2010). *Mosby's manual of diagnostic and laboratory tests* (4th ed.). St. Louis: Mosby.

Stevens, C. D. (2009). *Clinical immunology and serology: A laboratory perspective* (3rd ed.). Philadelphia: F.A. Davis.

Storey, M., & Jordan, S. (2008). An overview of the immune system. *Nursing Standard, 23*(15-17), 47-56.

Touhy, T., & Jett, K. (2010). *Ebersole and Hess' gerontological nursing & healthy aging* (3rd ed.), St Louis: Mosby.

Chapter 20

Akyol, O., Karayury, O., & Salmond, S. (2009). Experiences of pain management in patients undergoing total knee replacement. *Orthopaedic Nursing, 28*(2), 79-85.

Almada, P., & Archer, R. (2009). Planning ahead for better outcomes: Preparation for joint replacement surgery begins at home! *Orthopaedic Nursing, 28*(1), 3-8.

Arthritis Foundation. (2011a). Gout. Retrieved September 7, 2011, from http://www.arthritis.org/disease-center.php?disease-id=428df=causes.

Arthritis Foundation. (2011b). Who gets rheumatoid arthritis? Retrieved September 7, 2011, from http://www.arthritis.org/who-gets-rheumatoid-arthritis.php.

Barbay, K. (2009). Research evidence for the use of preoperative exercise in patients preparing for total hip or total knee arthroplasty. *Orthopaedic Nursing, 28*(3), 127-133.

Brown, F. M., Jr. (2008). Nursing care after a shoulder arthroplasty. *Orthopaedic Nursing, 27*(1), 3-9.

*Chen, S. Y., & Wang, H. H. (2007). The relationship between physical function, knowledge of disease, social support and self-care behavior in patients with rheumatoid arthritis. *Journal of Nursing Research, 15*(3), 183-192.

Cranwell-Bruce, L. A. (2011). Biological disease modifying anti-rheumatic drugs. *MEDSURG Nursing, 20*(3), 147-151.

*Ding, C., Cicuttini, F., Blizzard, L., & Jones, G. (2007). Smoking interacts with family history with regard to change in knee cartilage volume and cartilage defect development. *Arthritis and Rheumatology, 56*(5), 1521-1528.

Firestein, G. S., Budd, R. C., Harris, E. D., McInnes, I. B., Ruddy, S., & Sergent, J. S. (2008). *Kelley's textbook of rheumatology* (8th ed.). Philadelphia: Saunders.

*Fonesca, C., & Denton, C. P. (2007). Genetic association studies in systemic sclerosis: More evidence of a complex disease. *The Journal of Rheumatology, 34*(5), 903-905.

Galimba, J. (2009). Promoting the use of periarticular modal drug injection for total knee arthroplasty. *Orthopaedic Nursing, 28*(5), 250-254.

Gevirtz, C. (2008). How chronic pain affects sexuality. *Nursing2008, 38*(1), 17.

*Giaquinto, S., Cacciato, A., Minasi, S., Sostero, E., & Amanda, S. (2006). Effects of music-based therapy on distress following knee arthroplasty. *British Journal of Nursing, 15*(10), 576-579.

Gillaspie, M. (2010). Better pain management after total joint arthroplasty: A quality improvement approach. *Orthopaedic Nursing, 29*(1), 20-24.

*Hathaway, L. (2005). Lyme disease. *Nursing2005, 35*(4), 44-45.

*Hohler, S. E. (2005). Looking into minimally invasive total hip arthroplasty. *Nursing2005, 35*(6), 54-57.

Horse, J. S. (2010). Improving clinical outcomes with continuous passive motion: An interactive educational approach. *Orthopaedic Nursing, 29*(1), 27-33.

*Jakonsson, U., & Hallberg, I. R. (2006). Quality of life among older adults with osteoarthritis: An explorative study. *Journal of Gerontological Nursing, 32*(8), 51-60.

*Klippel, J. H. (2007). *Primer on the rheumatic diseases* (13th ed.). Atlanta: The Arthritis Foundation.

Leach, D., & Bonfe, M. (2009). The effectiveness of femoral/sciatic nerve blocks on postoperative pain management in total knee arthroplasty. *Orthopaedic Nursing, 28*(5), 257-262.

Lupus Foundation of America. (2011). Demographic information on lupus. Retrieved September 8, 2011 from http://www.lupus.org/webmodules/webarticlesnet/templates/new_newsroomstudent.aspx?articleid=524.

McCance, K. L., Huether, S. E., Brashers, V. L., & Rote, N. S. (2010). *Pathophysiology: The biologic basis for disease in adults and children* (6th ed.). St. Louis: Mosby.

*Nussbaum, R. L., McInnes, R., & Willard, H. (2007). *Thompson & Thompson genetics in medicine* (7th ed.). Philadelphia: Saunders.

Pagana, K. D., & Pagana, T. J. (2010). *Mosby's manual of diagnostic and laboratory tests* (4th ed.). St. Louis: Mosby.

Parker, R. J. (2011). Evidence-based practice: Caring for a patient undergoing total knee arthroplasty. *Orthopaedic Nursing, 30*(1), 4-8.

*Pellino, T. A., Gordon, D. B., Engelke, Z. K., Busse, K. L., Collins, M. A., Silver, C. E., et al. (2005). Use of nonpharmacologic interventions for pain and anxiety after total hip and knee arthroplasty. *Orthopaedic Nursing, 24*(3), 182-192.

Pullen, R. L., Jr., Brewer, S., & Ballard, A. (2009). Putting a face on systemic lupus erythematosus. *Nursing2009, 39*(8), 22-28.

Remadevi, R., & Szallisi, A. (2008). Adlea (ALGRX-4975), an injectable capsaicin (TRPV1 receptor agonist) formulation for long-lasting pain relief. *Drugs, 11*(2), 120-132.

Rutledge, D. N., Mouttapa, M., & Wood, P. B. (2009). Symptom clusters in fibromyalgia: Potential utility in patient assessment and treatment evaluation. *Nursing Research, 58*, 359-366.

Schoen, D. C. (2009). Hip and knee arthroplasties. *Orthopaedic Nursing, 28*(6), 323-327.

Scleroderma Foundation. (2011). What is scleroderma? Retrieved September 7, 2011, from http://www.scleroderma.org/medical/overview.shtm.

*Sestak, A. L., Nath, S. K., Sawalha, A. H., & Harley, J. B. (2007). Current status of lupus genetics. *Arthritis Research and Therapy, 9*(3), 210-219.

Smith-Miller, C. A., Harlos, L., Roszell, S. S., & Bechtel, G. A. (2009). A comparison of patient pain responses and medication regimens after hip/knee replacement. *Orthopaedic Nursing, 28*(5), 242-249.

*Sunk, I. G., Bobacz, K., Hofstaetter, J. G., Amoyo, L., Soleiman, A., Smolen, J., et al. (2007). Increased expression of discoidin domain receptor 2 is linked to the degree of cartilage damage in human knee joints: A potential role in osteoarthritis pathogenesis. *Arthritis and Rheumatology, 56*(11), 3685-3692.

*Taggert, H. M., Arslanian, C. L., Bae, S., & Singh, K. (2003). Effects of T'ai Chi exercise on fibromyalgia symptoms and health-related quality of life. *Orthopaedic Nursing, 22*(5), 353-360.

Thomas, K. M., & Sethares, K. A. (2008). An investigation of the effects of preoperative interdisciplinary patient education on understanding postoperative expectations following a total joint arthroplasty. *Orthopaedic Nursing, 27*(6), 374-381.

Thomas, K. M., & Sethares, K. A. (2010). Is guided imagery effective in reducing pain and anxiety in the postoperative total joint arthroplasty patient? *Orthopaedic Nursing, 29*(6), 393-399.

*Turjanica, M. A. (2007). Postoperative continuous peripheral nerve blockade in the lower extremity total joint arthroplasty population. *MEDSURG Nursing, 16*(3), 151-154.

Zhang, W., Moskowitz, R. W., Nuki, G., Abramson, S., Altman, R. D., Arden, N., et al. (2008). OARSI recommendations for the management of hip and knee osteoarthritis, Part II: OARSI evidence-based expert consensus guidelines. *Osteoarthritis and Cartilage, 16*(2), 137-162.

Chapter 21

Abdool Karim, Q., Abdool Karim, S. S., Frohlich, J. A., Grobler, A. C., Baxter, C., Mansoor, L. E., et al. (2010). Effectiveness and safety of tenovir gel, an antiretroviral microbicide, for the prevention of HIV infection in women. *Science, 329*(5996), 1168-1174. Retrieved July 19, 2010, from www.sciencexpress.org.

Alvarez, M. E., Jakhmola, P., Painter, T. M., Taillepierre, J. D., Romaguera, R. A., Herbst, J. H., et al. (2009). Summary of comments and recommendations from the CDC consultation on the HIV/AIDS epidemic and prevention in the Hispanic/Latino community. *AIDS Education and Prevention, 21*(5 Suppl.), 7-18.

Aouizerat, B. E., Miaskowski, C. A., Gay, C., Portillo, C. J., Coggins, T., Davis, H., et al. (2010). Risk factors and symptoms associated with pain in HIV-infected adults. *Journal of the Association of Nurses in AIDS Care, 21*(2), 125-133.

Bradley-Springer, L., Stevens, L., & Webb, A. (2010). Every nurse is an HIV nurse. *AJN, 110*(3), 32-39.

*Centers for Disease Control (CDC). (1987). Public Health Service guidelines for counseling and antibody testing to prevent HIV infection and AIDS. *Morbidity and Mortality Weekly Report, 36*(31), 509-515.

*Centers for Disease Control (CDC). (1991). Recommendations for preventing transmission of human immunodeficiency virus and hepatitis B virus to patients during exposure-prone invasive procedures. *Morbidity and Mortality Weekly Report, 40*(RR-8), 1-9.

*Centers for Disease Control and Prevention (CDC). (2005a). Antiretroviral postexposure prophylaxis after sexual, injection-drug use, or other nonoccupational exposure to HIV in the United States. *Morbidity and Mortality Weekly Report, 54*(RR-2), 1-27.

*Centers for Disease Control and Prevention (CDC). (2005b). Updated Public Health Service guidelines for the management of health-care worker exposure to HIV and recommendations for postexposure prophylaxis. *Morbidity and Mortality Weekly Report, 54*(RR-9), 1-22.

Centers for Disease Control and Prevention (CDC). (2008). Recommendations and reports: Appendix A—AIDS-defining conditions. *Morbidity and Mortality Weekly Report, 57*(RR-10), 9.

Centers for Disease Control and Prevention (CDC). (2009a). Guidelines for prevention and treatment of opportunistic infections in HIV infected adults and adolescents. *Morbidity and Mortality Weekly Report, 58*(RR-4).

Centers for Disease Control and Prevention (CDC). (2009b). Street smart: Prevention of HIV/AIDS and other STDs. Retrieved November 2010, from www.cdc.gov/hiv/topics/prev_prog/AHP/resources/guidelines/pro_guidance/print/street-smart.htm.

Centers for Disease Control and Prevention (CDC). (2011). *HIV surveillance report: Diagnosis of HIV infection and AIDS in the United States and dependent areas, 2009. Volume 21.* Atlanta: Author.

Cohen, B. (2007). Caring for a patient with HIV/AIDS. *MEDSURG Nursing, 16*(1), 53-54.

Coleman, S. M., Rajabiun, S., Cabral, H. J., Bradford, J. B., & Tobias, C. R. (2009). Sexual risk behavior and behavior change among persons newly diagnosed with HIV: The impact of targeted outreach interventions among hard-to-reach populations. *AIDS Patient Care and STDs, 23*(8), 639-645.

Cosby, C. (2007). Hematologic disorders associated with human immunodeficiency virus and AIDS. *Journal of Infusion Nursing, 30*(1), 22-32.

Courtenay-Quirk, C., Horvath, K. J., Ding, H., Fisher, H., McFarlane, M., Kachur, R., et al. (2010). Perceptions among HIV-related websites among persons recently diagnosed with HIV. *AIDS Patient Care and STDs, 24*(2), 105-115.

Davenport, A., & Meyers, F. (2009). How to protect yourself after body fluid exposure. *Nursing2009, 39*(5), 22-28.

De Clercq, E. (2009). Anti-HIV drugs: 25 compounds approved within 25 years after the discovery of HIV. *International Journal of Antimicrobial Agents, 33*(4), 307-320.

Diel, R., Loddenkemper, R., Meywald-Walter, K., Gottschalk, R., & Nienhaus, A. (2009). Comparative performance of tuberculin skin test, QuantiFERON-TB-Gold in Tube Assay, and T-Spot. TB Test in contact investigations for tuberculosis. *Chest, 135*(4), 1010-1018.

Delgado, S., & Dort, K. (2010). HAART and its effects on the heart. *American Nurse Today, 5*(1), 50-53.

Eaton, L., & Kalichman, S. (2009). Changes in transmission risk behaviors across stages of HIV disease among people living with HIV. *Journal of the Association of Nurses in AIDS Care, 20*(1), 39-49.

Higgins, J., Hoffman, S., & Dworkin, S. (2010). Rethinking gender, heterosexual men, and women's vulnerability to HIV/AIDS. *American Journal of Public Health, 100*(3), 435-445.

Holzemer, W., & Marefat, S. (2007). Poverty, development, and PEPFAR: A U.S. strategy for combating the global HIV/AIDS epidemic. *Nursing Outlook, 55*(5), 215-217.

Holzemer, W. L., Human, S., Arudo, J., Rosa, M. E., Hamilton, M. J., Corless, I., et al. (2009). Exploring HIV stigma and quality of life for persons living with HIV infection. *Journal of the Association of Nurses in AIDS Care, 20*(3), 161-168.

Kaufman, C. (2011). The secret life of lymphocytes. *Nursing2011, 41*(6), 50-54.

Kirton, C. (2008). Managing long-term complications of HIV infection. *Nursing2008, 38*(8), 44-50.

Kirton, C. (2011). The changing HIV epidemic. *Nursing2011, 41*(1), 36-43.

McCance, K., Huether, S., Brashers, V., & Rote, N. (2010). *Pathophysiology: The biologic basis for disease in adults and children* (6th ed.). St. Louis: Mosby.

Meyer, M., & Champion, J. (2010). Protective factors for HIV infection among Mexican American men who have sex with men. *Journal of the Association of Nurses in AIDS Care, 21*(1), 53-62.

Nussbaum, R., McInnes, R., & Willard, H. (2007). *Thompson & Thompson: Genetics in medicine* (7th ed.). Philadelphia: Saunders.

O'Leary, C. (2010). Neutropenia and infection. In C. Brown (Ed.), *A guide to oncology symptom management* (pp. 347-362). Pittsburgh: Oncology Nursing Society.

Pagana, K., & Pagana, T. (2010). *Mosby's manual of diagnostic and laboratory tests* (4th ed.). St. Louis: Mosby.

Purcell, D. (2009). Recommendations from a research consultation to address strategies for HIV/AIDS prevention focused on African Americans. *American Journal of Public Health, 99*(11), 1937-1940.

Scherf, R., & White-Reid, K. (2008). Giving intravenous immunoglobulin. *RN, 71*(1), 29-34.

Scordo, K. (2010). Treating antiretroviral-induced dyslipidemia in HIV-infected adults. *The Nurse Practitioner, 35*(7), 32-37.

Stark, S. (2007). The aging face of HIV/AIDS. *American Nurse Today, 2*(6), 30-34.

Swan, A., Daley, A., & Crowley, A. (2007). Contraceptive counseling for adolescents with HIV. *The Nurse Practitioner, 32*(5), 38-44.

Tangredi, L. A., Danvers, K., Molony, S. L., & Williams, A. (2008). New CDC recommendations for HIV testing in older adults. *The Nurse Practitioner, 33*(6), 37-44.

Vance, D. (2010). Aging with HIV: Clinical considerations for an emerging population. *AJN, 110*(3), 42-47.

Volberding, P., Sande, M., Lange, J., & Greene, W. (2008). *Global HIV/AIDS medicine*. Philadelphia: Saunders.

World Health Organization (WHO). (2010). Global epidemic: HIV/AIDS online questions and answers. Retrieved April 2011 from: www.who.int/features/qa/71/en/index.html.

Wright, S., Maree, J., & Sibanyoni, M. (2009). Treatment of oral thrush in HIV/AIDS patients with lemon juice and lemon grass (*Cymbopogon citratus*) and gentian violet. *Phytomedicine, 16*(2), 118-124.

Wyatt, G. (2009). Enhancing cultural and contextual intervention strategies to reduce HIV/AIDS among African Americans. *American Journal of Public Health, 99*(11), 1941-1945.

Chapter 22

Abbas, A., Lichtman, A., & Pillai, S. (2010). *Cellular and molecular immunology* (Updated 6th ed.). Philadelphia: Saunders.

Bryant, H. (2007). Anaphylaxis: Recognition, treatment, and education. *Emergency Nurse, 15*(2), 24-28.

Cain, J., Daly, M., & Powers, J. (2007). Act fast against anaphylaxis. *American Nurse Today, 2*(2), 30.

Conboy-Ellis, K., & Braker-Shaver, S. (2007). Intranasal steroids and allergic rhinitis. *The Nurse Practitioner, 32*(4), 44-49.

Gelpi, C., & Jacob, S. (2008). Instructions for educating patients on ROAT testing in conjunction with patch testing. *Dermatology Nursing, 20*(2), 139, 143.

IV Rounds. (2008). Handling a type I hypersensitivity reaction. *Nursing2008, 38*(4), 60.

Jevon, P. (2010). Recognition and treatment of anaphylaxis in hospital. *British Journal of Nursing, 19*(16), 1015-1020.

Kemp, S. (2007). Office approach to anaphylaxis: Sooner better than later. *American Journal of Medicine, 160*(8), 664-668.

Kruszka, P., & O'Brian, R. (2009). Diagnosis and management of Sjögren syndrome. *American Family Physician, 79*(6), 465-470.

Lehman, J., & Lieberman, P. (2007). Office-based management of allergic rhinitis in adults. *The American Journal of Medicine, 120*(8), 659-663.

McCance, K., Huether, S., Brashers, V., & Rote, N. (2010). *Pathophysiology: The biologic basis for disease in adults and children* (6th ed.). St. Louis: Mosby.

Morris, A. (2009). Defining allergy. *Practice Nurse, 37*(9), 18-22.

Nussbaum, R., McInnes, R., & Willard, H. (2007). *Thompson & Thompson: Genetics in medicine* (7th ed.). Philadelphia: Saunders.

Pagana, K., & Pagana, T. (2010). *Mosby's manual of diagnostic and laboratory tests* (4th ed.). St. Louis: Mosby.

Pullen, R., Brewer, S., & Ballard, A. (2009). Putting a face on systemic lupus erythematosus. *Nursing2009, 39*(8), 22-28.

Rosen, A., & Casciola-Rosen, L. (2009). Autoantigens in systemic autoimmunity: Critical partner in pathogenesis. *Journal of Internal Medicine, 265*, 625-631.

*Sampson, H. A., Muñoz-Furlong, A., Campbell, R. L., Adkinson, N. F., Jr., Bock, S. A., Branum, A., et al. (2006). Second symposium on the definition and management of anaphylaxis: Summary report—Second National Institute of Allergy and Infectious Disease/Food Allergy and Anaphylaxis Network symposium. *Journal of Allergy and Clinical Immunology, 117*(2), 391-397.

Walker, S., Chantrell, J., Clarke, S., McArthur, R., Proudfoot, C., Roberts, J., et al. (2010). Primary care training for adults and children with confirmed anaphylaxis requiring treatment with adrenaline. *Primary Health Care, 20*(7), 33-38.

Watkins, J. (2010). Pruritus, part 2: Urticaria. *Practice Nursing, 21*(1), 33-37.

Watson, L. (2010). Recognition, assessment and management of anaphylaxis. *Nursing Standard, 24*(46), 35-39.

White, E. (2010). Epinephrine administration: An action plan. *Nurse Practitioner Journal, 35*(3), 33-39.

Chapter 23

American Cancer Society (ACS). (2009). *Cancer facts and figures for African Americans—2009-2010.* Report No. 8614.09. Atlanta: Author.

American Cancer Society (ACS). (2010). *Cancer prevention and early detection. Facts & figures—2010.* Report No. 8600.10. Atlanta: Author.

American Cancer Society (ACS). (2011). *Cancer facts and figures—2011.* Report No. 00-300M–No. 5008.11. Atlanta: Author.

Calzone, K., Masny, A., & Jenkins, J. (Eds.). (2010). *Genetics and genomics in oncology nursing practice.* Pittsburgh: Oncology Nursing Society.

Canadian Cancer Society's Steering Committee. (2010). *Canadian Cancer Statistics, 2010.* Toronto: Canadian Cancer Society.

Crockett-Maillet, G. (2010). Know the red flags of hereditary cancers. *Nurse Practitioner, 35*(7), 39-43.

Feero, G., Guttmacher, E., & Collins, F. (2010). Genomic medicine: An updated primer. *New England Journal of Medicine, 362,* 2001-2011.

*Frank-Stromborg, M., & Olsen, S. (2001). *Cancer prevention in diverse populations: Cultural implications for health care professionals.* Pittsburgh: Oncology Nursing Society.

Markowitz, S., & Bertagnolli, M. (2009). Molecular origins of cancer: Molecular basis of colorectal cancer. *New England Journal of Medicine, 361*(25), 2449-2460.

McCance, K., Huether, S., Brashers, V., & Rote, N. (2010). *Pathophysiology: The biologic basis for disease in adults and children* (6th ed.). St. Louis: Mosby.

Pesquera, M., Yoder, L., & Lynk, M. (2008). Improving cross-cultural awareness and skills to reduce health disparities in cancer. *MEDSURG Nursing, 17*(2), 114-120.

Touhy, T., & Jett, K. (2010). *Ebersole and Hess' gerontological nursing & healthy aging* (3rd ed.). St. Louis: Mosby.

U.S. Department of Health and Human Services, Public Health Service, National Toxicology Program. (2011). *Report on carcinogens* (12th ed.). Retrieved July 2011 from http://ntp.niehs.nih.gov/go/roc12.

Wells, S. (2008). Cervical cancer: An overview with suggested practice and policy goals. *MEDSURG Nursing, 17*(1), 43-50.

Chapter 24

Abarado, C., & Mahon, S. (2010). Androgen-deprivation bone loss in patients with prostate cancer. *Clinical Journal of Oncology Nursing, 14*(2), 191-198.

American Cancer Society. (2011). *Cancer facts and figures—2011.* Report No. 00-300M–No. 5008.11. Atlanta: Author.

Bieck, T., Phillips, S., & Steele-Moses, S. (2010). Appraising the evidence for avoiding lotions or topical agents prior to radiation therapy. *Clinical Journal of Oncology Nursing, 14*(1), 103-105.

Binner, M., Ross, D., & Browner, I. (2011). Chemotherapy-induced peripheral neuropathy: Assessment of oncology nurses' knowledge and practice. *Oncology Nursing Forum, 38*(4), 448-454.

Borsellino, M., & Young, M. (2011). Anticipatory coping: Taking control of hair loss. *Clinical Journal of Oncology Nursing, 15*(3), 311-315.

Breem, S., & Kumar, N. (2011). Management of treatment-related symptoms in patients with breast cancer: Current strategies and future directions. *Clinical Journal of Oncology Nursing, 15*(1), 63-71.

Brown, C. (Ed.). (2010). *A guide to oncology symptom management.* Pittsburgh: Oncology Nursing Society.

Byar, K., & Workman, M. (2012). Targeted therapies to treat cancer. In J. Kee, E. Hayes, & L. McCuistion (Eds.), *Pharmacology: A nursing process approach* (7th ed., pp. 543-567). St. Louis: Saunders.

Camporeale, J. (2008). Basics of radiation therapy. *Clinical Journal of Oncology Nursing, 12*(2), 193-195.

Canadian Cancer Society's Steering Committee. (2010). *Canadian cancer statistics, 2010.* Toronto: Canadian Cancer Society.

Collins, A., & Garner, M. (2007). Caring for lung cancer patients receiving photodynamic therapy. *Critical Care Nurse, 27*(2), 53-60.

*Cope, D., & Reb, A. (Eds.). (2006). *An evidence-based approach to the treatment and care of the older adult with cancer.* Pittsburgh: ONS Publishing.

Donovan, D. (2009). Management of peripheral neuropathy caused by microtubule inhibitors. *Clinical Journal of Oncology Nursing, 13*(6), 686-694.

Dunsford, J. (2008). Nursing management of epidermal growth factor receptor inhibitor-induced toxicities. *Clinical Journal of Oncology Nursing, 12*(3), 405-407.

Eaby, B. (2008). Managing skin reactions to targeted cancer therapy. *American Nurse Today, 3*(7), 20-21.

Evens, K., & Eschiti, V. (2009). Cognitive effects of cancer treatment: "Chemo brain" explained. *Clinical Journal of Oncology Nursing, 13*(6), 661-666.

Fitch, M., Maxwell, C., Ryan, C., Löthman, H., Drudge-Coates, L., & Costa, L. (2009). Bone metastases from advanced cancers: Clinical implications and treatment options. *Clinical Journal of Oncology Nursing, 13*(6), 701-710.

Flores, I., & Ershler, W. (2010). Managing neutropenia in older patients with cancer receiving chemotherapy in a community setting. *Clinical Journal of Oncology Nursing, 14*(1), 81-86.

Frankel, C. (2010). Trastuzumab cardio-oncology: Lessons learned. *Clinical Journal of Oncology Nursing, 14*(5), 630-640.

Gosselin, T., Gilliard, L., & Tinnen, R. (2008). Assessing the need for a dietitian in radiation oncology. *Clinical Journal of Oncology Nursing, 12*(5), 781-787.

Gosselin, T., Schneider, S., Plambeck, M., & Rowe, K. (2010). A prospective randomized, placebo-controlled skin care study in women diagnosed with breast cancer undergoing radiation therapy. *Oncology Nursing Forum, 37*(5), 619-626.

Granda-Cameron, C., DeMille, D., Lynch, M. P., Huntzinger, C., Alcorn, T., Levicoff, J., et al. (2010). An interdisciplinary approach to manage cancer cachexia. *Clinical Journal of Oncology Nursing, 14*(1), 72-80.

Hadaway, L. (2009). Preventing and managing peripheral extravasation. *Nursing2009, 39*(10), 26-27.

Harris, D. J., Eilers, J., Harriman, A., Cashavelly, B. J., & Maxwell, C. (2008). Putting evidence into practice: Evidence-based interventions for the management of oral mucositis. *Clinical Journal of Oncology Nursing, 12*(1), 141-152.

Hawkins, R., & Grunberg, S. (2009). Chemotherapy-induced nausea and vomiting: Challenges and opportunities for improved patient outcomes. *Clinical Journal of Oncology Nursing, 13*(1), 54-64.

Huang, R. S., & Ratain, M. (2009). Pharmacogenetics and pharmacogenomics of anticancer agents. *CA: A Cancer Journal for Clinicians, 59*(1), 42-55.

Karius, D. (2010). Intraperitoneal chemotherapy: Improving the odds for ovarian cancer patients. *American Nurse Today, 5*(5), 12-15.

King, J. (2008). What is tumor lysis syndrome? *Nursing2008, 38*(5), 18.

Kuchinski, A., Reading, M., & Lash, A. (2009). Treatment-related fatigue and exercise in patients with cancer: A systematic review. *MEDSURG Nursing, 18*(3), 174-180.

McGraw, B. (2008). At an increased risk: Tumor lysis syndrome. *Clinical Journal of Oncology Nursing, 12*(4), 563-565.

Miller, S. (2010). Anemia. In C. Brown (Ed.), *A guide to oncology symptom management* (pp. 29-47). Pittsburgh: Oncology Nursing Society.

Moody, M., & Jackowski, J. (2010). Are patients on oral chemotherapy in your practice setting safe? *Clinical Journal of Oncology Nursing, 14*(3), 339-346.

Moore, S. (2010). Nonadherence in patients with breast cancer receiving oral therapies. *Clinical Journal of Oncology Nursing, 14*(1), 41-47.

Myers, J., Pierce, J., & Pazdernik, T. (2008). Neurotoxicity of chemotherapy in relation to cytokine release, the blood-brain barrier, and cognitive impairment. *Oncology Nursing Forum, 35*(6), 916-920.

O'Leary, C. (2010). Neutropenia and infection. In C. Brown (Ed.), *A guide to oncology symptom management* (pp. 347-362). Pittsburgh: Oncology Nursing Society.

Poirier, P. (2011). The impact of fatigue on role functioning during radiation therapy. *Oncology Nursing Forum, 38*(4), 457-465.

Polovich, M., Whitford, J., & Olsen, M. (Eds.). (2009). *Chemotherapy and biotherapy guidelines and recommendations for practice* (3rd ed.). Pittsburgh: Oncology Nursing Society.

Quirion, E. (2009). Filgrastim and pegfilgrastim use in patients with neutropenia. *Clinical Journal of Oncology Nursing, 13*(6), 324-328.

Running, A., & Turnbeaugh, E. (2011). Oncology pain and complementary therapy: A review of the literature. *Clinical Journal of Oncology Nursing, 15*(4), 374-379.

Ruppert, R. (2011). Radiation therapy 101: What you need to know to help cancer patients understand their treatment and cope with side effects. *American Nurse Today, 6*(1), 24-29.

Simchowitz, B., Shiman, L., Spencer, J., Brouillard, D., Gross, A., Connor, M., et al. (2010). Perceptions and experiences of patients receiving oral chemotherapy. *Clinical Journal of Oncology Nursing, 14*(4), 447-453.

Simmons, C. (2010). Oral chemotherapy drugs: Handle with care. *Nursing2010, 40*(7), 45-47.

Smink, K., & Schneider, S. (2008). Overview of stereotactic body radiotherapy and the nursing role. *Clinical Journal of Oncology Nursing, 12*(6), 889-893.

Thompson, N. (2009). Keeping neutropenic patients safe. *American Nurse Today, 4*(3), 29-31.

Thompson, N. (2010). When cancer spreads to the bone. *American Nurse Today, 5*(9), 8-10.

Tofthagen, C. (2010). Patient perceptions associated with chemotherapy-induced peripheral neuropathy. *Clinical Journal of Oncology Nursing, 14*(3), E22-E28.

Tofthagen, C., McAllister, D., & McMillan, S. (2011). Peripheral neuropathy in patients with colorectal cancer receiving oxaliplatin. *Clinical Journal of Oncology Nursing, 15*(2), 182-188.

Visovsky, C., Meyer, R., Roller, J., & Poppas, M. (2008). Evaluation and management of peripheral neuropathy in diabetic patients with cancer. *Clinical Journal of Oncology Nursing, 12*(2), 243-247.

Wanchai, A., Armer, J., & Stewart, B. (2011). Nonpharmacologic supportive strategies to promote quality of life in patients experiencing cancer-related fatigue: A systematic review. *Clinical Journal of Oncology Nursing, 15*(2), 203-214.

Waring, J., & Gosselin, T. (2010). Developing a high-dose rate prostate brachytherapy program. *Clinical Journal of Oncology Nursing, 14*(2), 199-203.

Weaver, C. (2009). Caring for a patient after mastectomy. *Nursing2009, 39*(5), 44-48.

Winkeljohn, D. (2010). Adherence to oral cancer therapies: Nursing interventions. *Clinical Journal of Oncology Nursing, 14*(4), 461-466.

Chapter 25

Backman, C., Zoutman, D. E., & Marck, P. B. (2008). An integrative review of the current evidence on the relationship between hand hygiene interventions and the incidence of health care–associated infections. *American Journal of Infection Control, 36*(5), 333-348.

Barnes, B. E., & Sampson, D. A. (2011). A literature review on community-acquired methicillin-resistant *Staphylococcus aureus* in the United States: Clinical information for primary care nurse practitioners. *Journal of the Academy of Nurse Practitioners, 23*(1), 23-32.

*Centers for Disease Control and Prevention (CDC). (2002). Guideline for hand hygiene in health-care settings: Recommendations of the Healthcare Infection Control Practices Advisory Committee and the HICPAC/SHEA/APIC/IDSA Hand Hygiene Task Force. *Morbidity and Mortality Weekly Report, 51*(RR-16), 1-44.

*Cheek, D. J., McGehee-Smith, H., Cunneen, J., & Cartwright, M. (2005). Sepsis: Taking a deeper look. *Nursing2005, 35*(1), 38-42.

Childs, S. G. (2008). Biofilm: The pathogenesis of slime glycocalyx. *Orthopedic Nursing, 27*(6), 361-368.

*Cunha, B. A. (2006). New uses for older antibiotics: Nitrofurantoin, amikacin, colistin, polymyxin B, doxycycline, and minocycline revisited. *Medical Clinics of North America, 90*, 1089-1107.

Grossman, S., & Mager, D. (2010). *Clostridium difficile*: Implications for nursing. *MEDSURG Nursing, 19*(3), 155-158.

Hurlow, J., & Bowler, P. G. (2009). Clinical experience with wound biofilm and management: A case series. *Ostomy and Wound Management, 55*(4), 38-49.

*Korniewicz, D., & Masri, M. E. (2007). Effect of aloe-vera impregnated gloves on hand hygiene attitudes of health care workers. *MEDSURG Nursing, 16*(4), 247-252.

*Lashley, F. R. (2006). Emerging infectious diseases at the beginning of the 21st century. *Online Journal of Issues in Nursing, 11*(1), 1-20.

Lo, S. F., Hayter, M., Change, C. J., Wu, W. Y., & Lee, L. L. (2008). A systematic review of silver-releasing dressings in the management of infected chronic wounds. *Journal of Clinical Nursing, 17*(15), 1973-1985.

*Metlay, J. P., Powers, J. H., Dudley, M. N., Christiansen, K., & Finch, R. G. (2006). Antimicrobial drug resistance, regulation, and research. *Emerging Infectious Diseases, 12*(2), 183-190.

Palese, A., Buchini, S., Deroma, L., & Bartone, F. (2010). The effectiveness of the ultrasound bladder scanner in reducing urinary tract infections: A meta-analysis. *Journal of Clinical Nursing, 19*(21-22), 2970-2979.

Parker, D., Callan, L., Harwood, J., Thompson, D. L., Wilde, M., & Gray, M. (2009). Nursing interventions to reduce the risk of catheter-associated urinary tract infection, Part 1: Catheter selection. *Journal of Wound, Ostomy, Continence Nursing, 36*(1), 23-34.

Ramage, G., Culshaw, S., Jones, B., & Williams, C. (2010). Are we any closer to beating the biofilm: Novel methods of biofilm control. *Current Opinion in Infectious Disease, 23*(6), 560-566.

Richmond, I., Bernstein, A., Creen, C., Cunningham, C., & Rudy, M. (2007). Reducing harm from MRSA. *Nursing Management, 38*(8), 22-27.

*Romero, D. V. (2006). Hand-to-hand combat: Preventing MRSA. *The Nurse Practitioner, 31*(3), 16-23.

Sheff, B. (2005). Avian influenza: Are you ready for a pandemic? *Nursing2005, 35*(9), 26-27.

*Siegel, J. D., Rhinehart, E., Jackson, M., Chiarello, L., the Healthcare Infection Control Practices Advisory Committee. (2007). *Guidelines for isolation precautions: Preventing transmission of infectious agents in healthcare settings 2007.* Atlanta: CDC.

Solseng, T., Vinson, H., Gibbs, P., & Greenwald, B. (2009). Biofilm growth on the Lopez enteral feeding valve cultured in enteral nutrition: Potential implications for medical-surgical patients, nursing care, and research. *MEDSURG Nursing, 18*(4), 225-227, 233.

Stickler, D. J., & Feneley, R. C. (2010). The encrustation and blockage of long-term indwelling catheters: A way forward in prevention and control. *Spinal Cord, 48*(11), 784-790.

Stone, P. W., Pogorzelska, M., Kunches, L., & Hirshhom, L. R. (2008). Hospital staffing and health-care associated infections: A systematic review of the literature. *Current Opinion in Infectious Diseases, 47*(7), 937-944.

*Todd, B. (2006a). Beyond MRSA: VISA and VRSA. *AJN, 106*(4), 28-30.

*Todd, B. (2006b). *Clostridium difficile:* Familiar pathogen, changing epidemiology. *AJN, 106*(5), 33-36.

Chapter 26

American Cancer Society. (2011). *Cancer facts and figures—2011.* Report No. 00-300M–No. 5008.11. Atlanta: Author.

Anderson, J., Langemo, D., Hanson, D., Thompson, P., & Hunter, S. (2007). What you can learn from a comprehensive skin assessment. *Nursing2007, 37*(4), 65-66.

Bianchi, J., & Cameron, J. (2009). Assessment of skin integrity in the elderly 1. Wound care, *British Journal of Community Nursing, 14*, S26-S32.

Bradford, P. (2009). Skin cancer in skin of color. *Dermatology Nursing, 21*(4), 170-178.

*Gaskin, F. C. (1986). Detection of cyanosis in the person with dark skin. *Journal of the National Black Nurses Association, 1*(1), 52-60.

Helfrich, Y., Sachs, D., & Voorhees, J. (2008). Overview of skin aging and photoaging. *Dermatology Nursing, 20*(3), 177-183.

Jarvis, C. (2012). *Physical examination and health assessment* (6th ed.). Philadelphia: Saunders.

LeBlanc, K., & Christensen, D. (2011). Demystifying skin tears, Part 2. *Nursing2011, 41*(7), 16-17.

*Marks, J., & Miller, J. (2006). *Lookingbill and Marks' principles of dermatology* (4th ed.). Philadelphia: Saunders.

McCance, K., Huether, S., Brashers, V., & Rote, N. (2010). *Pathophysiology: The biologic basis for disease in adults and children* (6th ed.). St. Louis: Mosby.

McEnroe-Petitte, D. (2011). Melanoma. *Nursing2011, 41*(5), 45.

Nussbaum, R., McInnes, R., & Willard, H. (2007). *Thompson & Thompson: Genetics in medicine* (7th ed.). Philadelphia: Saunders.

Pagana, K., & Pagana, T. (2010). *Mosby's manual of diagnostic and laboratory tests* (4th ed.). St. Louis: Mosby.

Pullen, R. (2007). Assessing skin lesions. *Nursing2007, 37*(8), 44-45.

Smith, M. (2008). Healthier aging: Taking a closer look for skin cancer. *Nursing2008, 38*(10), 58-60.

*Stanley, W. (2003). Nailing a key assessment. *Nursing2003, 33*(8), 50-51.

The Skin Cancer Foundation. (2010). Understanding melanoma—Warning signs: The ABCDEs of melanoma. Retrieved May 2010, from www.skincancer.org.

Thompson, P., Langemo, D., Hanson, D., Anderson, J., & Hunter, S. (2008). Assessing skin rashes. *Nursing2008, 38*(4), 59.

Touhy, T., & Jett, K. (2010). *Ebersole and Hess' gerontological nursing & healthy aging* (3rd ed.). St. Louis: Mosby.

Wheeler, T. (2008). The role of skin assessment in older people. *British Journal of Community Nursing, 14*(9), 380-384.

Chapter 27

Ackerman, C. (2011). "Not on my watch": Treating and preventing pressure ulcers. *MEDSURG Nursing, 20*(2), 86-93.

Alderden, J., Whitney, J., Taylor, S., & Zaratkiewicz, S. (2011). Risk profile characteristics associated with outcomes of hospital-acquired pressure ulcers: A retrospective review. *Critical Care Nurse, 31*(4), 30-42.

Alexis, A., & Lamb, A. (2009). Concomitant therapy for acne in patients with skin of color: A case-based approach. *Dermatology Nursing, 29*(1), 33-36.

American Cancer Society. (2011). *Cancer facts and figures 2011.* Report No. 00-300M–No. 5008.11. Atlanta: Author.

Aschenbrenner, D. (2011). New drug treats metastatic melanoma. *American Journal of Nursing, 111*(7), 25-26.

Baron, E., Kirkland, E., & Domingo, D. (2008). Advances in photoprotection. *Dermatology Nursing, 20*(4), 265-270, 282-283.

Bianchi, J., & Cameron, J. (2008). Management of skin conditions in the older population 2. *Wound Care, 13*(9), S6-S14.

Bianchi, J., & Cameron, J. (2009). Assessment of skin integrity in the elderly 1. *Wound Care, 14*, S26-S32.

Blaney, W. (2010). Taking steps to prevent pressure ulcers. *Nursing2010, 110*(3), 44-47.

Borlitz, J. (2009). Commonly missed dermatologic conditions. *The Nurse Practitioner, 34*(10), 35-45.

Bradford, P. (2009). Skin cancer in skin of color. *Dermatology Nursing, 21*(4), 170-177, 206.

Broderick, N. (2009). Understanding chronic wound healing. *The Nurse Practitioner, 34*(10), 16-22.

Christopher, G., & Meires, J. (2008). Treating acute onset psoriasis. *The Nurse Practitioner, 33*(7), 8-10.

*Cuzzell, J. (2002a). Wound assessment and evaluation of wound dressings: Confusion or choice? *Dermatology Nursing, 14*(3), 187-188, 191.

*Cuzzell, J. (2002b). Wound assessment and evaluation: Wound documentation guidelines. *Dermatology Nursing, 14*(4), 265-266.

*Cuzzell, J. (2002c). Wound healing: Translating theory into clinical practice. *Dermatology Nursing, 14*(4), 257-261.

Czerkasij V. (2010). Dermal fillers: Help patients put their best face forward. *The Nurse Practitioner, 35*(10), 43-47.

Day, C., & Boynton, P. (2008). Implementation of wound management in a rural setting, *The Nurse Practitioner, 33*(9), 35-39.

DiAgostino, A. (2009). Skin failure in the acute care setting. *MEDSURG Nursing, 18*(2), 125-126.

Dorner, B., Posthauer. M.E., & Thomas, D. (2009). The role of nutrition in pressure ulcer prevention and treatment: National Pressure Ulcer Advisory Panel white paper. *Advances in Skin & Wound Care, 22*(5), 212-221.

Dunleavy, K. (2008). Putting a dent in pressure ulcer rates. *Nursing2008, 38*(1), 20-21.

Frankel, A.J., & Goldenburg, G. (2010). Insights into treating palmoplantar psoriasis. *Skin & Aging, 18*(8). Retrieved October 2010, from www.skinandaging.com/content/insights-treating-palmoplantar-psoriasis.

Gordon, R. (2009). Skin cancer more than skin deep. *The Nurse Practitioner, 34*(4), 20-27.

Gottlieb, A., Kardos, M., & Yee, M. (2009). Current biologic treatments for psoriasis. *Dermatology Nursing, 21*(5), 259-272.

Hanson, D., Langemo, D., Anderson, J., Hunter, S., & Thompson, P. (2007). Measuring wounds. *Nursing2007, 37*(2), 18-21.

Hanson, D., Langemo, D., Anderson, J., & Thompson, P. (2009). Wound and skin care: Can pressure mapping prevent ulcers? *Nursing2009, 39*(6), 50-51.

Hanson, D., Thompson, P., Langemo, D., Hunter, S., & Anderson, J. (2007). Pressure mapping: A new path to pressure-ulcer prevention. *American Nurse Today, 2*(11), 10-12.

Helfrich, Y., Sachs, D., & Voorhees, J. (2008). Overview of skin aging and photoaging. *Dermatology Nursing, 20*(3), 177-183.

Hess, C. (2009). Wound bed preparation. *Nursing2009, 39*(8), 57.

Hill, M. (2008a). Fungal infections. *Dermatology Nursing, 20*(2), 137-138.

Hill, M. (2008b). Viral infections. *Dermatology Nursing, 20*(1), 57-58.

Hinton, D. (2009). Helping patients with psoriasis. *Dermatology Nursing, 21*(4), 214-215.

Holcomb, S. (2007). Dodging the bullae: Stevens-Johnson syndrome. *Nursing2007, 37*(6), 64cc1-64cc3.

Holcomb, S. (2008). MRSA infections. *Nursing2008, 38*(6), 33.

Jackson, M., McKenney, T., Drumm, J., Merrick, B., LeMaster, T., & VanGilder, C. (2011). Pressure ulcer prevention in high-risk postoperative cardiovascular patients. *Critical Care Nurse, 31*(4), 44-53.

Kayser-Jones, J., Beard, R., & Sharpp, T. (2009). Dying with a stage IV pressure ulcer. *AJN, 109*(1), 40-48.

Kumar, P. (2008). Classification of skin substitutes. *Burns, 34*(1), 148-149.

*Langemo, D., Anderson, J., Hanson, D., Hunter, S., Thompson, P., & Posthauer, M.E. (2006). Nutritional considerations in wound care. *Advances in Skin & Wound Care, 19*(6), 297-303.

Laustsen, G., & Neilson, T. (2007). Prevent shingles with Zostavax. *The Nurse Practitioner, 32*(6), 6-7.

Ledezma, B. (2009). Ipilimumab for advanced melanoma: A nursing perspective. *Oncology Nursing Forum, 36*(1), 97-104.

Lee, M., & Kalb, R. (2008). Systemic therapy for psoriasis. *Dermatology Nursing, 20*(2), 105-111.

Leung-Chen, P. (2008). Everybody's crying MRSA. *AJN, 108*(8), 29-31.

*Marks, J.G., Jr., & Miller, J. (2006). *Lookingbill & Mark's principles of dermatology* (4th ed.). Philadelphia: Saunders.

McCance, K., Huether, S., Brashers, V., & Rote, N. (2010). *Pathophysiology: The biologic basis for disease in adults and children* (6th ed.). St. Louis: Mosby.

McEnroe-Petitte, D. (2011). Melanoma. *Nursing2011, 41*(5), 45.

Meadows-Oliver, M. (2009). Tinea capitis: Diagnostic criteria and treatment options. *Dermatology Nursing, 21*(5), 281-286.

Meehan, M. (2009). Pressure ulcers: The stakes just got higher. *Nursing2009, 39*(10), 45-47.

Mendyk, M. (2008). Community-associated MRSA: Coming to a patient near you? *The Nurse Practitioner, 33*(3), 26-32.

Munn, Z. (2008). Interventions for treating scabies. *Journal of Advanced Nursing, 63*(2), 144-145.

National Pressure Ulcer Advisory Panel (NPUAP). (2010, January). Updated staging system. Retrieved October 2010, from www.npuap.org.

Novatnack, E., & Schweon, S. (2007). Shingles: What you should know. *RN, 70*(6), 27-31.

Nursing2009. (2009a). Head lice. *Nursing2009, 39*(5), 31.

Nursing2009. (2009b). Photosensitivity. *Nursing2009, 39*(9), 32.

Nussbaum, R., McInnes, R., & Willard, H. (2007). *Thompson & Thompson: Genetics in medicine* (7th ed.). Philadelphia: Saunders.

Okan, D., Woo, K., Ayello, E.A., & Sibbald, G. (2007). The role of moisture in wound healing. *Advances in Skin & Wound Care, 20*(1), 39-53.

Pritchard, M. J., & Hwang, S. W. (2009). Cases: Severe anemia from bedbugs. *Canadian Medical Association Journal, 181*(5), 287-288.

Rock, R. (2011). Get positive results with negative-pressure wound therapy. *American Nurse Today, 6*(1), 49-51.

Rubin, K. (2009). Management of metastatic melanoma: Nursing challenges today and tomorrow. *Clinical Journal of Oncology Nursing, 13*(1), 81-89.

Rushing, J. (2008). Assessing a patient for lice infestation. *Nursing2008, 38*(7), 20.

Skin Cancer Foundation. (2010). Understanding melanoma. *The ABCDEs of melanoma.* Retrieved May 2010, from www.skincancer.org/the-abcdes-of-melanoma.html.

Slachta, P. (2008). Caring for chronic wounds: A knowledge update. *American Nurse Today, 3*(7), 27-31.

Smith, L. (2007). Toxic epidermal necrolysis. *Clinical Journal of Oncology Nursing, 11*(3), 333-336.

Smith, M. (2008). Taking a closer look for skin cancer. *Nursing2008, 38*(10), 58-60.

Snow, M. (2007). The truth about scabies. *Nursing2007, 37*(2), 28-30.

Snyder, L. (2008). Wound basics: Type, treatment, and care. *RN, 71*(8), 32-36.

Stranger, C. (2009). Actinic keratosis: Do the numbers add up? *The Nurse Practitioner, 34*(2), 36-39.

Sutton, D., & Thomas, D. (2008). Don't let the bedbugs bite! Identifying and managing infestations. *The Nurse Practitioner, 33*(8), 28-33.

Thackman, J., McElwain, D., & Long, R. (2008). The use of hyperbaric oxygen therapy to treat chronic wounds: A review. *Wound Repair and Regeneration, 16*(3), 321-330.

Thomas, R. (2009). Dishing the dirt on MRSA. *RN, 72*(6), 16-23.

Thomas, S. (2008). Hydrocolloid dressings in the management of acute wounds: A review of the literature. *International Wound Journal, 5*(5), 602-613.

Torrens, R., & Swan, B. (2009). Promoting prevention and early recognition of malignant melanoma. *Dermatology Nursing, 21*(3), 115-122.

Touhy, T., & Jett, K. (2010). *Ebersole and Hess' gerontological nursing & healthy aging* (3rd ed.). St. Louis: Mosby.

United States Food and Drug Administration (FDA). (2011). Approvals. Retrieved April 2011 from www.fda.gov/Drugs/NewsEvents/Newsroom/PressAnnouncements/ucm248390.htm.

van der Veen, V. C., van der Wal, M. B., van Leeuwen, M. C., Ulrich, M. M., & Middelkoop, E. (2010). Biological background of dermal substitutes. *Burns, 36*(3), 305-321.

Van Rijswijk, L. (2009). Wound wise: Pressure ulcer prevention updates. *AJN, 109*(8), 56.

Wallis, L. (2010). FDA warning about negative pressure wound therapy. *AJN, 110*(3), 16.

Wheeler, T. (2008). The role of skin assessment in older people. *British Journal of Community Nursing, 14*(9), 380-384.

Wielowski, I. (2009). Shingles and the vaccine to prevent it. *AJN, 109*(6), 63-65.

Willson, K. (2011). They only come out at night: Bed bugs and their alarming resurgence. *Nursing2011, 41*(1), 54-58.

Woo, K., Ayello, E. A., & Sibbald, R. G. (2007). The edge effect: Current therapeutic options to advance the wound edge. *Advances in Skin & Wound Care, 20*(2), 99-117.

World Health Organization. (2010). Leprosy. Retrieved November 2010, from www.who.int/topics/leprosy/en/.

Yantis, M., O'Toole, K., & Ring, P. (2009). Leech therapy. *AJN, 109*(4), 36-42.

Zulkowski, K., & Gray-Leach, K. (2009). Staging pressure ulcers: What's the buzz in wound care? *AJN, 109*(1), 27-30.

Chapter 28

Alvarado, R., Chung, K., Cancio, L., & Wolf, S. (2009). Burn resuscitation. *Burns, 35*(1), 4-14.

American Burn Association. (2010). National Burn Repository: Summary of the findings 2000-2009. Website: www.ameriburn.org.

Arnoldo, B., Klein, M., & Gibran, B. S. (2006). Practice guidelines for electrical burns. *Journal of Burn Care & Research, 27*(4), 439-447.

Arnstein, P. (2010). What's the best way to cool my patient's burn pain? *Nursing2010, 40*(3), 61-62.

Benner, J. (2008). Online support for burn victims. *Nursing2008, 38*(4), 23.

Blakeney, P., Rosenberg, L., Rosenberg, M., & Faber, A. W. (2008). Psychosocial care of persons with severe burns. *Burns, 34*(4), 433-440.

Brown-Guttovz, H. (2011). Burn injury. *Nursing2011, 41*(5), 72.

Cancio, L. C., Batchinsky, A. I., Dubick, M. A., Park, M. S., Black, I. H., Gomez, R., et al. (2007). Inhalation injury: Pathophysiology and clinical care proceedings of a symposium conducted at the Trauma Institute of San Antonio. *Burns, 33*(6), 681-692.

Carrougher, G., Hoffman, H., Nakamura, D., Lezotte, D., Soltani, M., Leahy, L., et al. (2009). The effect of virtual reality on pain and range of motion in adults with burn injuries. *Journal of Burn Care & Research, 30*(5), 785-791.

Connor-Ballard, P. (2009a). Understanding and managing burn pain: Part 1. *AJN, 109*(4), 48-56.

Connor-Ballard, P. (2009b). Understanding and managing burn pain: Part 2. *AJN, 109*(5), 54-62.

Edelman, D., Maleyko-Jacobs, S., White, M. T., Lucas, C. E., & Ledgerwood, A. M. (2008). Smoking and home oxygen: A preventable public health hazard. *Journal of Burn Care & Research, 29*(1), 119-122.

Harrison, C., & MacNeil, S. (2008). The mechanism of skin graft contracture: An update on current research and potential future therapies. *Burns, 34*(2), 153-163.

Herndon, D. (2007). *Total burn care* (3rd ed.). Philadelphia: Saunders.

Jeffery, S. (2009). Current burn wound management. *Trauma, 11*(4), 241-248.

Klein, J., & Hoffman, C. (2010). Relaxation and visual imagery techniques: Do they work? Can they really help burn patients? *MEDSURG Nursing, 19*(3), 169-175.

Kumar, P. (2008). Classification of skin substitutes. *Burns, 34*(1), 148-149.

Laing, C. (2010). Acute carbon monoxide toxicity. *Nursing2010, 40*(11), 38-43.

Macrino, S., Slater, H., Aballay, A., Goldfarb, I. W., & Caushaj, P. F. (2008). A three decade review of thermal injuries among the elderly at a regional burn centre. *Burns, 34*(4), 509-511.

McCance, K., Huether, S., Brashers, V., & Rote, N. (2010). *Pathophysiology: The biologic basis for disease in adults and children* (6th ed.). St. Louis: Mosby.

Mlcak, R., Suman, O., & Herndon, D. (2007). Respiratory management of inhalation injury. *Burns, 33*(1), 2-13.

Moss, L. (2010). Treatment of the burn patient in primary care. *Nurse Practitioner, 35*(8), 24-31.

Pagana, K., & Pagana, T. (2010). *Mosby's manual of diagnostic and laboratory tests* (4th ed.). St. Louis: Mosby.

Patient education series: Severe sunburn. (2009). *Nursing2009, 39*(7), 31.

Pham, T. N., Cancio, L. C., & Gibran, N. S. (2008). American Burn Association Practice Guidelines: Burn shock resuscitation. *Journal of Burn Care & Research, 29*(1), 257-266.

Prelack, K., Dylewski, M., & Sheridan, R. (2007). Practical guidelines for nutritional management of burn injury and recovery. *Burns, 33*(1), 14-24.

Schnell, H., & Zaspel, J. (2008). Cooling extensive burns: Sprayed coolants can improve initial cooling management. *Burns, 34*(4), 503-508.

Tan, X., Yowler, C., Super, D., & Fratianne, R. (2010). The efficacy of music therapy protocols for decreasing pain, anxiety, and muscle tension levels during burn dressing changes: A prospective randomized crossover trial. *Journal of Burn Care & Research, 31*(4), 590-597.

Thomas, S. (2008). Hydrocolloid dressings in the management of acute wounds: A review of the literature. *International Wound Journal, 5*(5), 602-613.

Touhy, T., & Jett, K. (2010). *Ebersole and Hess' gerontological nursing & healthy aging* (3rd ed.). St. Louis: Mosby.

Van der Veen, V. C., van der Wal, M. B., Van Leeuwen, M. C., Ulrich, M. M., & Middelkoop, E. (2010). Biological background of dermal substitutes. *Burns, 36*(3), 305-321.

Windel, E. M. (2008). Nutrition support in major burn injury: Case analysis of dietetic activity, resource use and cost. *Journal of Human Nutrition and Dietetics, 21*(2), 165-173.

Chapter 29

Benzocaine spray and methemoglobinemia. (2009). *Alberta RN, 7*(2), 28.

Booker, R. (2009). Interpretation and evaluation of pulmonary function tests. *Nursing Standard, 23*(39), 46-56.

Bradley, R. (2007). Improving respiratory assessment skills. *The Journal for Nurse Practitioners, 3*(4), 276-277.

Curran, R. (2009). Vital signs, part 3: Respiratory rate, temperature, and beyond. *EMS Magazine, 38*(5), 38-45.

DeMeulenaere, S. (2007). Pulse oximetry: Uses and limitations. *The Journal for Nurse Practitioners, 3*(5), 312-317.

Evans, T., Lworato, L., & Lord, J. (2008). Capnography: The seventh vital sign. *RT: The Journal for Respiratory Care Practitioners, 21*(1), 30-32.

Fernadez, M., Burns, K., Calhoun, B., George, S., Martin, B., & Weaver, C. (2007). Evaluation of a new pulse oximeter sensor. *American Journal of Critical Care, 16*(2), 146-151.

Gordon, M. (2011). *Manual of nursing diagnosis* (12th ed.). Boston: Jones & Bartlett.

Jarvis, C. (2012). *Physical examination and health assessment* (6th ed.). Philadelphia: Saunders.

McCance, K., Huether, S., Brashers, V., & Rote, N. (2010). *Pathophysiology: The biologic basis for disease in adults and children* (6th ed.). St. Louis: Mosby.

Minini, N., Marino, M., Kohler, W., & Stephan, M. (2009). Pulse oximetry: An essential tool for the busy med-surg nurse. *American Nurse Today, 4*(9), 31-36.

Monitoring your adult patient with bedside pulse oximetry. (2008). *Nursing2008, 38*(9), 42-44.

Murgu, S., Pecson, J., & Colt, H. (2011). Flexible bronchoscopy assisted by noninvasive positive pressure ventilation. *Critical Care Nurse, 31*(3), 70-76.

Nussbaum, R., McInnes, R., & Willard, H. (2007). *Thompson & Thompson: Genetics in medicine* (7th ed.). Philadelphia: Saunders.

Pagana, K., & Pagana, T. (2010). *Mosby's manual of diagnostic and laboratory tests* (4th ed.). St. Louis: Mosby.

Pruitt, B. (2010). Interpreting ABGs: An inside look at your patient's status. *Nursing2010, 40*(7), 31-35.

Pullen, R. (2010). Assessing the paranasal sinuses. *Nursing2010, 40*(5), 49-50.

Ramirez, R., Pickar, T., Frens, S., Cappon, J., & Cleary, J. (2009). Capnography: A better way? *RT: The Journal for Respiratory Care Practitioners, 22*(1), 30-33.

Roberts, M. (2010). Clinical utility and adverse effects of amiodarone therapy. *AACN Advanced Critical Care, 21*(4), 333-338.

*Rushing, J. (2006). Assisting with thoracentesis. *Nursing2006, 36*(12), 18.

Sarna, L., & Bialous, S. (2010). Using evidence-based guidelines to help patients stop smoking. *American Nurse Today, 5*(1), 44-47.

Schwartz, A., & Powell, S. (2009). Brush up on oral assessment and care. *Nursing2009, 39*(3), 30-32.

The Joint Commission. (2010). National Patient Safety Goals. Retrieved November 15, 2010, from www.jointcommission.org/patientsafety/nationalpatientsafetygoals/.

Touhy, T., & Jett, K. (2010). *Ebersole and Hess' gerontological nursing & healthy aging* (3rd ed.). St. Louis: Mosby.

Valdez-Lowe, C., Ghareeb, S., & Artinian, N. (2009). Pulse oximetry in adults. *AJN, 109*(6), 52-59.

*Wesley, C. (2006). Responding to methemoglobinemia after bronchoscopy. *Nursing2006, 36*(12), 64cc1-64cc2.

Workman, M. L., & Winkelman, C. (2008). Genetic influences in common respiratory disorders. *Critical Care Clinics of North America, 20*(2), 171-189.

Chapter 30

Davis, M., & Johnston, J. (2008). Maintaining supplemental oxygen during transport. *AJN, 108*(1), 35-36.

*Dixon, B., & Tasota, F. (2003). Action stat: Inadvertant tracheal decannulation. *Nursing2003, 33*(1), 96.

Edelman, D., Maleyko-Jacobs, S., White, M., et al. (2008). Smoking and home oxygen therapy: A preventable public health hazard. *Journal of Burn Research, 29*(1), 119-122.

Fieder, L., Mitchell, P., & Bridges, E. (2010). Oral care practices for orally intubated critically ill adults. *American Journal of Critical Care, 19*(3), 175-183.

Fischer, R. (2007). Prevent fires when using oxygen cylinder regulators. *Nursing2007, 37*(1), 20.

Fortney, S., & Powers, J. (2008). Dodging a trach tragedy. *American Nurse Today, 3*(10), 42.

Fournier, M. (2010). Derailing disaster after pulmonary aspiration. *American Nurse Today, 5*(7), 41.

Frace, M. (2010). Tracheostomy care on the medical-surgical unit. *MEDSURG Nursing, 19*(1), 58-61.

Grams, L., & Spremulli, M. (2008). Assessing a patient for dysphagia. *Nursing2008, 38*(8), 15.

Halm, M., & Krisko-Hagel, K. (2008). Instilling normal saline with suctioning: Beneficial technique or potentially harmful sacred cow? *American Journal of Critical Care, 17*(5), 469-472.

*Happ, M. B., Tate, J., & Garrett, K. (2006). Nonspeaking older adults in the ICU. *AJN, 106*(5), 29.

*Mahler, D., Fierro-Carrion, G., & Baird, J. (2003). Evaluation of dyspnea in the elderly. *Clinics in Geriatric Medicine, 19*(1), 19-33.

McCance, K., Huether, S., Brashers, V., & Rote, N. (2010). *Pathophysiology: The biologic basis for disease in adults and children* (6th ed.). St. Louis: Mosby.

Pagana, K., & Pagana, T. (2010). *Mosby's manual of diagnostic and laboratory tests* (4th ed.). St. Louis: Mosby.

Pullen, R. (2007). Communicating with a patient on mechanical ventilation. *Nursing2007, 37*(4), 22.

Reed, C., Reineck, C., & Fonseca, I. (2011). Communicating with intubated patients: A new approach. *American Nurse Today, 6*(7), 34-35.

Regan, E., & Dallachiesa, L. (2009). How to care for a patient with a tracheostomy. *Nursing2009, 39*(8), 34-39.

Siela, D. (2010). Evaluation standards for management of artificial airways. *Critical Care Nurse, 30*(4), 76-78.

Sole, M. L., Penoyer, D. A., Su, X., et al. (2009). Assessment of endotracheal cuff pressure by continuous monitoring: A pilot study. *American Journal of Critical Care, 18*(2), 133-143.

Sole, M. L., Su, X., Talbert, S., et al. (2011). Evaluation of an intervention to maintain endotracheal tube cuff pressure within therapeutic range. *American Journal of Critical Care, 20*(2), 109-118.

Stich, J., & Cassella, D. (2009). Getting inspired about oxygen delivery devices. *Nursing2009, 39*(9), 51-54.

Touhy, T., & Jett, K. (2010). *Ebersole and Hess' gerontological nursing & healthy aging* (3rd ed.). St. Louis: Mosby.

Turnbull, D., Furlonger, A., & Andrzejowski, J. (2008). The influence of changes in end-tidal carbon dioxide upon the bispectral index. *Anesthesia, 63*(5), 458-462.

Chapter 31

American Cancer Society (ACS). (2011). *Cancer facts and figures, 2011.* 01-300M–No. 5008.11. Atlanta: Author.

Berry, D. (2008). Case study: Obstructive sleep apnea. *MEDSURG Nursing, 17*(1), 11-16.

Bieck, T., Phillips, S., & Steele-Moses, S. (2010). Appraising the evidence for avoiding lotions or topical agents prior to radiation therapy. *Clinical Journal of Oncology Nursing, 14*(1), 103-105.

Callaway, C. (2011). Rethinking the head and neck cancer population: The human papillomavirus association. *Clinical Journal of Oncology Nursing, 15*(2), 165-170.

Canadian Cancer Society's Steering Committee. (2010). *Canadian cancer statistics, 2010.* Toronto: Canadian Cancer Society.

Duffy, S. A., Scheumann, A. L., Fowler, K. E., Darling-Fisher, C., & Terrell, J. E. (2010). Perceived difficulty quitting predicts enrollment in a smoking-cessation program for patients with head and neck cancer. *Oncology Nursing Forum, 37*(3), 349-356.

Happ, M. B., Sereika, S., Garrett, K., et al. (2011). Nurse-patient communication interactions in the intensive care unit. *American Journal of Critical Care, 20*(2), e28-e40.

Jang, Y., & Kwon, M. (2010). Modified extracorporeal septoplasty technique in rhinoplasty for severely deviated noses. *Annals of Otology, Rhinology, & Laryngology, 119*(5), 331-335.

Lambertz, C. K., Gruell, J., Robenstein, V., Mueller-Funaiole, V., Cummings, K., & Knapp, V. (2010). NO SToPS: Reducing treatment breaks during chemoradiation for head and neck cancer. *Clinical Journal of Oncology Nursing, 14*(5), 585-593.

McCance, K., Huether, S., Brashers, V., & Rote, N. (2010). *Pathophysiology: The biologic basis for disease in adults and children* (6th ed.). St. Louis: Mosby.

Nance-Floyd, B. (2011). Tracheostomy care: An evidence-based guide to suctioning and dressing changes. *American Nurse Today, 6*(7), 14-17.

National Comprehensive Cancer Network. (2010). *Practice guidelines in oncology: Head and neck cancers (version 2.2010).* Fort Washington, PA: Author.

Noonan, B., & Hegarty, J. (2010). The impact of total laryngectomy: The patient's perspective. *Oncology Nursing Forum, 37*(3), 293-301.

Prahlow, J., Prahlow, T., Rakow, R., & Prahlow, N. (2009). Asphyxia caused by inspissated oral and nasopharyngeal secretions. *AJN, 109*(6), 38-50.

Robinson, S., Chia, M., Carney, A. S., Chawla, S., Harris, P., & Esterman, A. (2009). Upper airway reconstructive surgery long-term quality-of-life outcomes compared with CPAP for adult obstructive sleep apnea. *Otolaryngology—Head and Neck Surgery, 141*(2), 257-263.

Rodriguez, C., & Rowe, M. (2010). Use of a speech-generating device for hospitalized postoperative patients with head and neck cancer experiencing speechlessness. *Oncology Nursing Forum, 37*(2), 199-205.

Rushing, J. (2009). Managing epistaxis. *Nursing2009, 39*(6), 12.

Schaller, J. (2008). Myths & facts … about obstructive sleep apnea. *Nursing2008, 38*(1), 27.

Sleep apnea. (2009). *Nursing2009, 39*(6), 48.

Tocco, S. (2008). Preventing airway obstruction. *American Nurse Today, 3*(1), 34.

Touhy, T., & Jett, K. (2010). *Ebersole and Hess' gerontological nursing & healthy aging* (3rd ed.). St. Louis: Mosby.

Townsend-Roccichelli, J., Sanford, J., & VanderWaa, E. (2010). Managing sleep disorders in the elderly. *Nurse Practitioner Journal, 35*(5), 30-37.

Chapter 32

American Cancer Society. (2011). *Cancer facts and figures—2011.* No. 01-300M–No. 5008.11. Atlanta: Author.

Aschenbrenner, D. (2010). Drug watch: New safety requirements for asthma drug. *AJN, 110*(6), 26-27.

Avgeri, S., Matthaiou, D., Dimopoulos, G., Grammatikos, A. P., & Falagas, M. E. (2008). Therapeutic options for *Burkholderia cepacia* infections beyond co-trimoxazole: A systematic review of the clinical evidence. *International Journal of Antimicrobial Agents, 33,* 394-404.

Bauldoff, G. (2009). When breathing is a burden: How to help patients with COPD. *American Nurse Today, 4*(12), 17-21.

Bauman, M., & Handley, C. (2011). Chest-tube care: The more you know, the easier it gets. *American Nurse Today, 6*(9), 27-31.

Bieck, T., & Phillips, S. (2010). Appraising the evidence for avoiding lotions or topical agents prior to radiation therapy. *Clinical Journal of Oncology Nursing, 14*(1), 103-105.

Booker, R. (2009). Interpretation and evaluation of pulmonary function tests. *Nursing Standard, 23*(39), 46-56.

Centers for Disease Control and Prevention (CDC). (2010). FastStats. *National Center for Health Statistics.* Retrieved January 2011, from www.cdc.gov/nchs/fastats/.

Cheng, A. G., Johnston, P. R., Luz, J., Uluer, A., Fligor, B., Licameli, G. R., et al. (2009). Sensorineural hearing loss in patients with cystic fibrosis. *Otolaryngology—Head and Neck Surgery, 141*(1), 86-90.

Chronic bronchitis and emphysema. (2009). *Nursing2009, 39*(4), 29.

Collins, A., & Garner, M. (2007). Care for lung cancer patients receiving photodynamic therapy. *Critical Care Nurse, 27*(2), 53-60.

Corbridge, S., & Corbridge, T. (2010). Asthma in adolescents and adults. *AJN, 110*(5), 28-38.

Crawford, A., & Harris, H. (2008). COPD: Help your patients breathe easier. *RN, 71*(1), 21-26.

Cystic Fibrosis Foundation. (2009). About cystic fibrosis. Retrieved January 2011, from www.cff.org/AboutCF/.

Daly, M. (2009). Stopping a COPD flare-up. *American Nurse Today, 4*(8), 40.

Donahue, D. (2010). Managing pulmonary arterial hypertension. *Nursing2010, 40*(1), 52-54.

Durai, R., Hoque, H., & Davies, T. (2010). Managing a chest tube and drainage system. *AORN Journal, 91*(2), 275-280.

Ellis, K. (2008). Keeping asthma at bay. *American Nurse Today, 3*(2), 20-25.

Gaguski, M. E., Brandsema, M., Gernalin, L., & Martinez, E. (2010). Assessing dyspnea in patients with non–small cell lung cancer in the acute care setting. *Clinical Journal of Oncology Nursing, 14*(4), 509-513.

Global Initiative for Asthma (GINA). (2010). Global strategy for asthma management and prevention. Retrieved June 2011 from: http://www.ginasthma.org/Guidelines/guidelines-resources.html.

Global Initiative for Chronic Obstructive Lung Disease (GOLD). (2009). Global strategy for the diagnosis, management, and prevention of chronic obstructive pulmonary disease. Medical Communications Resources, Inc. Retrieved January 2011, from www.goldcopd.com/guidelineitem.

Halm, M. (2007). To strip or not to strip: Physiological effects of chest tube manipulation. *American Journal of Critical Care, 16*(6), 609-612.

Hansen, F., & Sawatzky, J. (2008). Stress in patients with lung cancer: A human response to illness. *Oncology Nursing Forum, 35*(2), 217-223.

Holcomb, S. (2008). New asthma guidelines: Encourage more activity and a better night's sleep. *Nurse Practitioner Journal, 33*(3), 9-11.

John, L. (2010). Self-care strategies used by patients with lung cancer to promote quality of life. *Oncology Nursing Forum, 37*(3), 339-347.

Kumar, V., Abbas, A., Fausto, N., & Aster, J. (2010). *Robbins and Cotran: Pathologic basis of disease* (8th ed.). Philadelphia: Saunders.

LaRue, L. (2009). Sarcoidosis: A granular view. *Nurse Practitioner Journal, 34*(9), 28-33.

Lawes, R. (2009). Putting the squeeze on asthma. *Nursing2009, 39*(3), 56hn1-56hn4.

Lomas, P., & Fowler, S. (2010). Parents and children with cystic fibrosis: A family affair. *AJN, 110*(8), 30-37.

McCance, K., Huether, S., Brashers, V., & Rote, N. (2010). *Pathophysiology: The biologic basis for disease in adults and children* (6th ed.). St. Louis: Mosby.

McClelland, M. (2010). Paraneoplastic syndromes related to lung cancer. *Clinical Journal of Oncology Nursing, 14*(3), 357-364.

Merton, S., Sawatzky, J., & Diehl-Jones, L. (2009). Getting to the heart of pleural effusion: A case study. *Journal of the American Academy of Nurse Practitioners, 21*(9), 506-512.

Moreland, S. (2010). Nutritional screening and counseling in adults with lung cancer: A systematic review of the evidence. *Clinical Journal of Oncology Nursing, 14*(5), 609-614.

Newton, T. (2009). Respiratory care of the hospitalized patient with cystic fibrosis. *Respiratory Care, 54*(6), 769-776.

Nussbaum, R., McInnes, R., & Willard, H. (2007). *Thompson & Thompson: Genetics in medicine* (7th ed.). Philadelphia: Saunders.

Online Mendelian Inheritance in Man (OMIM). (2010). Asthma, susceptibility to. Retrieved December 2010, from www.ncbi.nlm.nih.gov/omim.

Pagana, K., & Pagana, T. (2010). *Mosby's manual of diagnostic and laboratory tests* (4th ed.). St. Louis: Mosby.

Pruitt, B. (2008). Loosening the bonds of restrictive lung disease. *Nursing2008, 38*(8), 34-39.

Pruitt, B. (2011). Assessing and managing asthma: A global initiative for asthma update. *Nursing2011, 41*(5), 46-52.

Roberts, M. (2010). Clinical utility and adverse effects of amiodarone therapy. *AACN Advanced Critical Care, 21*(4), 333-338.

Rosenblatt, R. (2009). Lung transplantation in cystic fibrosis. *Respiratory Care, 54*(6), 777-787.

Rushing, J. (2007). Managing a water-seal chest drainage unit. *Nursing2007, 37*(12), 12.

Saucier, S., Motyka, C., & Killu, K. (2010). Ultrasonography versus chest radiography after chest tube removal for the detection of pneumothorax. *AACN Advanced Critical Care, 21*(1), 34-38.

Shah, A., & D'Amico, T. (2009). Lung volume reduction surgery for the management of refractory dyspnea in chronic obstructive pulmonary disease. *Current Opinion in Supportive and Palliative Care, 3*(2), 107-111.

Sherry, V., Patton, N., & Stricker, C. (2010). Diagnosis and management of postpneumonectomy empyema with an Eloesser flap. *Clinical Journal of Oncology Nursing, 14*(5), 553-556.

Shutske, K., Baker, D., Zustiak, T., Carlson, A., & Van Riper, K. (2009). Teachable moments: Asthma education in the ED. *American Nurse Today, 4*(8), 24-27.

Smith, B., & Tasota, F. (2011). Smoking out the dangers of COPD. *Nursing2011, 41*(4), 32-39.

Song, M. K., De Vito Dabbs, A., Studer, S. M., & Zangle, S. (2008). Course of illness after the onset of chronic rejection in lung transplant recipients. *American Journal of Critical Care, 17*(3), 246-253.

Thomas, L. (2009). Effective dyspnea management strategies identified by elders with end-stage chronic obstructive pulmonary disease. *Applied Nursing Research, 22*(2), 79-85.

Thompson, N. (2010). When cancer spreads to the bone. *American Nurse Today, 5*(9), 8-10.

Touhy, T., & Jett, K. (2010). *Ebersole and Hess' gerontological nursing & healthy aging* (3rd ed.). St. Louis: Mosby.

Vacca, V. (2009). On the alert for pulmonary arterial hypertension. *Nursing2009, 39*(12), 36-40.

Walker, S. (2008). Updates in non–small-cell lung cancer. *Clinical Journal of Oncology Nursing, 12*(4), 587-596.

Walker, S., & Bryden, G. (2010). Managing pleural effusions: Nursing care of patients with a Tenckhoff catheter. *Clinical Journal of Oncology Nursing, 14*(1), 59-64.

Walz, D. (2010). Cancer-related anorexia-cachexia syndrome. *Clinical Journal of Oncology Nursing, 14*(3), 283-287.

Weber, C., Silver, M., Cromer, D., Kaminski, S., Wirick, T., & Vallejo, J. (2011). Under pressure: Pulmonary arterial hypertension. *Critical Care Nurse, 31*(4), 87-94.

Weiss, S., Raby, B., & Rogers, A. (2009). Asthma genetics and genomics 2009. *Current Opinion in Genetics and Development, 19*(3), 279-282.

Wells, M., Sarna, L., Cooley, M. E., Brown, J. K., Chernecky, C., Williams, R. D., et al. (2007). Use of complementary and alternative medicine therapies to control symptoms in women living with lung cancer. *Cancer Nursing, 30*(1), 45-55.

White, K., & Ruth-Sahd, L. (2007). Bronchiolitis obliterans organizing pneumonia. *Critical Care Nurse, 27*(3), 53-66.

Widlitz, A., McDevitt, S., Ward, G. R., & Krichman, A. (2007). Practical aspects of continuous intravenous treprostinil therapy. *Critical Care Nurse, 27*(2), 41-50.

Wise, R., & Tashkin, D. (2007). Optimizing treatment of chronic obstructive pulmonary disease: An assessment of current therapies. *American Journal of Medicine, 120*(8 Suppl. A), S4-S13.

Workman, M. L., & Winkelman, C. (2008). Genetic influences in common respiratory disorders. *Critical Care Nursing Clinics of North America, 20*(2), 171-189.

Chapter 33

American Association of Critical-Care Nurses (AACN). (2008). Ventilator-associated pneumonia. *Critical Care Nurse, 28*(3), 83-85.

American Lung Association (ALA). (2010a). Trends in pneumonia and influenza morbidity and mortality. Retrieved January 2010, from www.lungusa.org/finding-cures/our-research/trend-reports/pi-trend-report.pdf.

American Lung Association (ALA). (2010b). Trends in tuberculosis morbidity and mortality. Retrieved January 2010, from www.lungusa.org/finding-cures/our-research/trend-reports/TB-Trend-Report.pdf.

Ames, N. (2011). Evidence to support tooth brushing in critically ill patients. *American Journal of Critical Care, 20*(3), 242-250.

Centers for Disease Control and Prevention (CDC). (2010a). Cover your cough. Retrieved January 2011, from www.cdc.gov/flu/protect/covercough.htm.

Centers for Disease Control and Prevention (CDC). (2010b). 2009 H1N1: Overview of a pandemic. Retrieved January 2011, from www.cdc.gov/h1n1flu/yearinreveiw/yir5.htm.

Centers for Disease Control and Prevention (CDC). (2010c). Prevention & control of influenza with vaccines: Recommendations of the Advisory Committee on Immunization Practices (ACIP). *Morbidity and Mortality Weekly Report, 59*, 1-62.

Curtin, L. (2011). Preventing ventilator-associated pneumonia: A nursing-intervention bundle. *American Nurse Today, 6*(3), 9-11.

Dobbin, K. (2009). Understanding empyema. *Nursing2009, 39*(6), 56cc1-56cc3.

Dobbin, K., & Howard, V. (2011). Listen closely to detect healthcare-associated pneumonia. *Nursing2011, 41*(7), 59-62.

Eisenstadt, E. (2010). Dysphagia and aspiration pneumonia in older adults. *Journal of the American Academy of Nurse Practitioners, 22*(1), 17-22.

Ferguson, L., & Rhoads, J. (2009). Multidrug-resistant and extensively drug-resistant tuberculosis: The new face of an old disease. *Journal of the American Academy of Nurse Practitioners, 21*(11), 603-609.

Fowler, S. (2008). Community-acquired pneumonia: Follow the guidelines to better outcomes. *American Nurse Today, 3*(9), 26-30.

Garcia, R., Jendresky, L., Colbert, L., Bailey, A., Zaman, M., & Majumder, M. (2009). Reducing ventilator-associated pneumonia through advanced oral-dental care: A 48-month study. *American Journal of Critical Care, 18*(6), 523-534.

Gribble, E., & Williams, A. (2010). Break through multidrug-resistant TB. *The Nurse Practitioner, 35*(3), 14-22.

Hoyle, C. (2009). Make your strep diagnosis spot on. *The Nurse Practitioner, 34*(10), 46-52.

Kapustin, J. (2008). The 2008-09 influenza season: Are you ready? *The Nurse Practitioner, 33*(10), 12-19.

Knechel, N. (2009). Tuberculosis: Pathophysiology, clinical features, and diagnosis. *Critical Care Nurse, 29*(2), 34-43.

Kung, Y. (2010). A close-up view of flu. *The Nurse Practitioner, 35*(4), 47-52.

Lessons learned from the 2009 H1N1 pandemic flu. (2010). *AJN, 110*(10), 22-23.

Luttenberger, K. (2010). Battling VAP from a new angle. *Nursing2010, 40*(2), 52-55.

McCance, K., Huether, S., Brashers, V., & Rote, N. (2010). *Pathophysiology: The biologic basis for disease in adults and children* (6th ed.). St. Louis: Mosby.

Nelson, R. (2010). Drug-resistant tuberculosis. *AJN, 110*(10), 55-57.

Regan, E. (2009). Diagnosis rhinitis: Viral and allergic characteristics. *The Nurse Practitioner, 33*(9), 20-26.

Rushing, J. (2007). Obtaining a throat culture. *Nursing2007, 37*(3), 20.

Schappert, S., & Rechsteiner, E. (2008). Ambulatory medical care utilization estimates for 2006. *National Health Statistics Report, 8*. Retrieved January 2011, from www.cdc.gov/nchs/data/nhsr/nhsr008.pdf.

Schweon, S. (2010). Double jeopardy: Pneumococcal pneumonia following seasonal influenza. *Nursing2010, 40*(12), 60-61.

The war on tuberculosis. (2010). *AJN, 110*(7), 20-22.

Todd, B. (2010). Sepsis and pneumonia take their toll. *AJN, 110*(8), 60-61.

Touhy, T., & Jett, K. (2010). *Ebersole and Hess' gerontological nursing & healthy aging* (3rd ed.). St. Louis: Mosby.

Trossman, S. (2008). New interest in an old health threat. *American Nurse Today, 3*(1), 37-38.

Tucker, S., Poland, G., & Jacobson, R. (2008). Requiring influenza vaccination for health care workers. *AJN, 108*(2), 32-34.

World Health Organization (WHO). (2010). Global tuberculosis control 2010. Retrieved January 2011, from www.who.int/tb/publications/global_report/2010/en/index.html.

Chapter 34

Andrews, P., & Habashi, N. (2010). Detecting, managing, and preventing pulmonary embolism. *American Nurse Today, 5*(9), 21-25.

ARDS Foundation. (2010). Facts About ARDS. Retrieved June 2010, from www.ardsil.com/facts.htm.

Badet, M., Bayle, F., Richard, J. C., & Guérin, C. (2009). Comparison of optimal positive end-expiratory pressure and recruitment maneuvers during lung-protective mechanical ventilation in patients with acute lung injury/acute respiratory distress syndrome. *Respiratory Care, 54*(7), 847-854.

Bahloul, M., Chaari, A., Kallel, H., Abid, L., Hamida, C. B., Dammak, H., et al. (2010). Pulmonary embolism in intensive care unit: Predictive factors, clinical manifestations and outcomes. *Annals of Thoracic Medicine, 5*(2), 97-103.

Balk, R. (2009). Strategies to improve oxygenation in ALI and ARDS. *Journal of Respiratory Therapy, 22*(11), 10-14.

Briggs, D. (2010). Nursing care and management of patients with intrapleural drains. *Nursing Standard, 24*(21), 47-55.

Briggs, S., Goettler, C. E., Schenarts, P. J., et al. (2009). High-frequency oscillatory ventilation as a rescue therapy for adult trauma patients. *American Journal of Critical Care, 18*(2), 144-148.

Chan, L. Y., Jones, A. Y., Chung, R. C., & Hung, K. N. (2010). Peak flow rate during induced coughing: A predictor of successful decannulation of a tracheotomy tube in neurosurgical patients. *American Journal of Critical Care, 19*(3), 278-284.

Colonel, P., Houzé, M. H., Vert, H., et al. (2008). Swallowing disorders as a predictor of unsuccessful extubation: A clinical evaluation. *American Journal of Critical Care, 17*(6), 504-510.

Curry, K., Cobb, S., Kutash, M., & Diggs, C. (2008). Characteristics associated with unplanned extubations in a surgical intensive care unit. *American Journal of Critical Care, 17*(1), 45-52.

Davis, M., & Johnston, J. (2008). Maintaining supplemental oxygen during transport. *American Journal of Nursing, 108*(1), 35-36.

Day, M. (2011). On alert for iatrogenic pneumothorax. *Nursing2011, 41*(6), 66-67.

Documenting pneumothorax. (2008). *Nursing2008, 38*(9), 19.

Dunn, J., & Baker, M. (2011). Daily sedation breaks and breathing trials help wean patients from ventilators safely. *American Nurse Today, 6*(3), 12-14.

El-Khatib, M., Zeineldine, S., Ayoub, C., Husari, A., & Bou-Khalil, P. K. (2010). Critical care clinicians' knowledge of evidence-based guidelines for preventing ventilator-associated pneumonia. *American Journal of Critical Care, 19*(3), 272-277.

Farley, A., McLafferty, E., & Hendry, C. (2009). Pulmonary embolism: Identification, clinical features and management. *Nursing Standard, 23*(28), 49-56.

Feider, L., Mitchell, P., & Bridges, E. (2010). Oral care practices for orally intubated critically ill adults. *American Journal of Critical Care, 19*(2), 175-183.

Frace, M. (2010). Tracheostomy care on the medical-surgical unit. *MEDSURG Nursing, 19*(1), 58-61.

Gallagher, J. (2009). Taking aim at ARDS. *Nursing2009, 39*(10), 49-54.

Gay, S. (2010). An inside view of venous thromboembolism. *The Nurse Practitioner, 35*(9), 32-39.

Grap, M. (2009). Not-so-trivial pursuit: Mechanical ventilation risk reduction. *American Journal of Critical Care, 18*(4), 299-309.

Grossbach, I., Chlan, L., & Tracy, M. (2011). Overview of mechanical ventilatory support and management of patient- and ventilator-related responses. *Critical Care Nurse, 31*(3), 30-44.

Grossbach, I., Stranberg, S., & Chlan, L. (2011). Promoting effective communication for patients receiving mechanical ventilation. *Critical Care Nurse, 31*(3), 46-60.

Halm M., & Armola, R. (2009). Effect of oral care on bacterial colonization and ventilator-associated pneumonia. *American Journal of Critical Care, 18*(3), 275-278.

Kallus, C. (2009). Building a solid understanding of mechanical ventilation. *Nursing2009, 39*(6), 22-28.

Khalid, I., Doshi, P., & DiGiovine, B. (2010). Early enteral nutrition and outcomes of critically ill patients treated with vasopressors and mechanical ventilation. *American Journal of Critical Care, 19*(3), 261-268.

Kjonegaard, R., Fileds, W., & King, M. (2010). Current practice in airway management: A descriptive evaluation. *American Journal of Critical Care, 19*(2), 168-174.

Kleinman, S., Gajic, O., & Nunes, E. (2007). Promoting recognition of transfusion-related acute lung injury. *Critical Care Nurse, 27*(4), 49-53.

Konstantinides, S. (2008). Acute pulmonary embolism. *New England Journal of Medicine, 359*(26), 2804-2813.

Le, R., & Dewan, N. (2009). Pulmonary embolectomy: Should it be offered earlier rather than later? *Respiratory Care, 54*(3), 390-392.

Lyerla, F., LeRouge, C., Cooke, D. A., (2010). A nursing clinical decision support system and potential predictors of head-of-bed position for patients receiving mechanical ventilation. *American Journal of Critical Care, 19*(1), 39-47.

McAdams-Jones, D. (2009). What's causing this respiratory distress? How to recognize and reverse transfusion-related acute lung injury. *American Nurse Today, 4*(5), 28.

McCance, K., Huether, S., Brashers, V., & Rote, N. (2010). *Pathophysiology: The biologic basis for disease in adults and children* (6th ed.). St. Louis: Mosby.

Mellott, K. G., Grap, M. J., Munro, C. L., (2009). Patient-ventilator dyssynchrony: Clinical significance and implications for practice. *Critical Care Nurse, 29*(6), 41-55.

Morrell, N. (2010). Prone positioning in patients with acute respiratory distress syndrome. *Nursing Standard, 24*(21), 42-45.

Powers, J. (2007). The five P's spell positive outcomes for ARDS patients. *American Nurse Today, 2*(3), 34-38.

Powers, K., & Talbot, L. (2011). Fat embolism syndrome after femur fracture with intramedullary nailing: Case report. *American Journal of Critical Care, 20*(3), 264-265, 267.

Qasim, Z., & Gwinnutt, C. (2009). Flail chest: Pathophysiology and management. *Trauma, 11*, 63-70.

Racco, M. (2009). Nutrition in the ICU: Nutritional support for the mechanically ventilated patient in the ICU. *RN, 72*(1), 26-30.

Regan, E., & Dallachiesa, L. (2009). How to care for a patient with a tracheostomy. *Nursing2009, 39*(8), 34-39.

Rodriguez, C., & Rowe, M. (2010). Use of a speech-generating device for hospitalized postoperative patients with head and neck cancer experiencing speechlessness. *Oncology Nursing Forum, 37*(2), 199-205.

Roman, M. (2010). Pneumothorax. *MEDSURG Nursing, 19*(3), 183-184.

Rose, L. (2008). High-frequency oscillatory ventilation in adults. *AACN Advanced Critical Care, 19*(4), 412-420.

Ruiz, C. (2011). Thwarting a pneumothorax. *American Nurse Today, 6*(5), 32.

Schwartz, A., & Powell, S. (2009). Brush up on oral assessment and care. *Nursing2009, 39*(3), 30-32.

Stuban, S. (2010). Home mechanical ventilation. *AJN, 110*(5), 63-67.

Tracy, M., & Chlan, L. (2011). Nonpharmacologic interventions to manage common symptoms in patients receiving mechanical ventilation. *Critical Care Nurse, 31*(3), 19-28.

Winkelman, C. (2008). Inflammation and genomics in the critical care unit. *Critical Care Nursing Clinics of North America, 20*(2), 213-221.

Winkelman, C. (2009). Bed rest in health and critical illness: A body systems approach. *AACN Advanced Critical Care, 20*(3), 254-266.

Winkelman, C., & Chiang, L. (2010). Manual turns in patients receiving mechanical ventilation. *Critical Care Nurse, 30*(4), 36-43.

Workman, M. L., & Winkelman, C. (2008). Genetic influences in common respiratory disorders. *Critical Care Nursing Clinics of North America, 20*(2), 171-189.

Chapter 35

American Heart Association (AHA). (2010a). *Dietary and lifestyle recommendations* (updated: May 21, 2010). Retrieved August 29, 2010, from www.heart.org/HEARTORG/GettingHealthy/Diet-and-Lifestyle-Recommendations_UCM_305855_Article.jsp.

American Heart Association (AHA). (2010b). Heart disease and stroke statistics 2010 update. Retrieved July 23, 2010, from www.americanheart.org.

Cheek, D., & Tester, J. (2008). Women and heart disease: What's new? *Nursing2008, 38*(1), 37-42.

*DeVon, H. A., & Zerwic, J. J. (2003). The symptoms of unstable angina: Do women and men differ? *Nursing Research, 52*(2), 108-118.

*Giuliano, K. K., Scott, S. S., Brown, V., & Olson, M. (2003). Backrest angle and cardiac output measurement in critically ill patients. *Nursing Research, 52*(4), 242-248.

*Gordon, M. (2011). *Manual of nursing diagnosis* (12th ed.). Boston: Jones & Bartlett.

*Greenland, P., Bonow, R. O., Brundage, B. H., Budoff, M. J., Eisenberg, M. J., Grundy, S. M., et al. (2007). ACCF/AHA clinical expert consensus document on coronary artery calcium scoring by computed tomography in global cardiovascular risk assessment and in evaluation of patients with chest pain. *Circulation, 115*(3), 402-426.

Howie-Esquivel, J., & White, M. (2008). Biomarkers in acute cardiovascular disease. *Journal of Cardiovascular Nursing, 23*(2), 124-131.

Jarvis, C. (2012). *Physical examination and health assessment* (6th ed.). St. Louis: Mosby.

Landgraf, J., Wishner, S. H., & Kloner, R. A. (2010). Comparison of automatic oscillometric versus auscultatory blood pressure measurement. *American Journal of Cardiology, 106*(3), 386-388.

Lloyd-Jones, D., Adams, R., Carnethon, M., Simone, G., Ferguson, T. B., Flegal, K., et al. (2009). Heart disease and stroke statistics—2009 update: A report from the American Heart Association Statistics Committee and Stroke Statistics Subcommittee. *Circulation, 119*, e21-e181.

*Mehta, M. (2003). Assessing cardiovascular status. *Nursing2003, 33*(1), 56-57.

Metcalf, P. A., Scragg, R. K., Schaaf, L. D., Dyall, L., Black, P. N., et al. (2008). Comparison of different markers of socioeconomic status with cardiovascular disease and diabetes risk factors in the Diabetes, Heart and Health survey. *Journal of the New Zealand Medical Association, 121*(1269). Retrieved August, 1, 2010, from www.nzma.org.nz/journal/121-1269/2929/.

*National Cholesterol Education Program. (2002). *Third report of the Expert Panel on Detection, Evaluation, and Treatment of High Blood Cholesterol in Adults (Adult Treatment Panel III)*. NIH Publication No. 02-5215. Bethesda: National Heart, Lung, and Blood Institute.

*National High Blood Pressure Education Program. (2003). *The seventh report of the Joint National Committee on Prevention, Detection, Evaluation, and Treatment of High Blood Pressure*. NIH Publication No. 03-5233. Bethesda: National Heart, Lung, and Blood Institute.

Ott, L. K. (2008). Assessing blood flow with CT angiography. *Nursing2008, 38*(1), 26.

Pagana, K. D., & Pagana, T. J. (2010). *Mosby's diagnostic and laboratory tests* (4th ed.). St. Louis: Mosby.

Pearson, T. L. (2010). Ankle brachial index as a prognostic tool for women with coronary artery disease. *Journal of Cardiovascular Nursing, 25*(1), 20-24.

Ridker, P. M., Paynter, N. P., Rifai, N., Gaziano, M., & Cook, N. R. (2008). C-reactive protein and parental history improve global cardiovascular risk prediction. *Circulation, 118*(22), 2243-2251.

Sanborn, T. A., Ebrahimi, R., Manoukian, S. V., McLaurin, B. T., Cox, D. A., Feit, F., et al. (2010). Impact of femoral vascular closure devices and antithrombotic therapy on access site bleeding in acute coronary syndromes. *Circulation: Cardiovascular Interventions, 3*(1), 57-62.

Sulzbach-Hoke, L. M., Ratcliffe, S. J., Kimmel, S. E., Kolansky, D. M., & Polomano, R. (2010). Predictors of complications following sheath removal with percutaneous coronary intervention. *Journal of Cardiovascular Nursing, 25*(3), e1-e8.

*The New York Heart Association. (1964). *Diseases of the heart and blood vessels: Nomenclature and criteria for diagnosis* (6th ed.). Boston: Little, Brown.

Wright, J. D., Hirsch, R., & Wang, C.-Y. (2009). One-third of U.S. adults embraced most heart healthy behaviors in 1999-2002. *National Center for Health Statistics data brief, (17)*. Hyattsville, MD: National Center for Health Statistics. Retrieved July 28, 2010, from www.cdc.gov/nchs/data/databriefs/db17.htm.

Chapter 36

American Heart Association (AHA). (2010). Highlights of the 2010 American Heart Association Guidelines for CPR and ECC. Retrieved September 18, 2011, from http://www.heart.org/idc/groups/heart-public/@wcm/@ecc/documents/downloadable/ucm_317350.pdf.

Atwood, S., Stanton, C., & Davenport, J. S. (2009). *Introduction to basic cardiac dysrhythmias* (4th ed.). St. Louis: Mosby/JEMS.

Bardy, G. H., Lee, K. L., Mark, D. B., Poole, J. E., Toff, W. D., Tonkin, A. M., et al. (2008). Home use of automated external defibrillators for sudden cardiac arrest. *New England Journal of Medicine, 358*(7), 1793-1804.

Batista, L., Lima, F., Januzzi, J., Donahue, V., Snydeman, C., & Greer, D. (2010). Feasibility and safety of combined percutaneous coronary intervention and therapeutic hypothermia following cardiac arrest. *Resuscitation, 81*(4), 398-403.

Brady, A., Malone, A., & Fleming, S. (2009). A literature review of the individual and systems factors that contribute to medication errors in nursing practice. *Journal of Nursing Management, 17*(6), 679-697.

Chalupka, A. N. (2010). Radiofrequency catheter ablation for atrial fibrillation. *American Association of Occupational Health Nurses, 58*(5), 220.

Cheng, J. M. (2010). New and emerging antiarrhythmic and anticoagulant agents for atrial fibrillation. *American Journal of Health-System Pharmacy, 67*(9), S26-S34.

Chilukuri, K., Dalal, D., Gadrey, S., Marine, J. E., MacPherson, E., Henrikson, C. A., et al. (2010). A prospective study evaluating the role of obesity and obstructive sleep apnea for outcomes after catheter ablation of atrial fibrillation. *Journal of Cardiovascular Electrophysiology, 21*(5), 521-525.

Craig, K. J., & Day, M. P. (2011). Are you up to date on the latest BLS and ACLS guidelines? *Nursing2011, 41*(5), 40-44.

Crandall, M., Bradley, D., Packer, D., & Asirvatham, S. (2009). Contemporary management of atrial fibrillation: Update on anticoagulation and invasive management strategies. *Mayo Clinic Proceedings, 87*(7), 643-662.

Crossley, G. H., Chen, J., Choucair, W., Cohen, T. J., Gohn, D. C., Johnson, W. B., et al. (2009). Clinical benefits of remote versus transtelephonic monitoring of implanted pacemakers. *Journal of the American College of Cardiology, 54*(22), 2012-2019.

Dagres, N., & Anastasiou-Nana, M. (2010). Atrial fibrillation and obesity: An association of increasing importance. *Journal of the American College of Cardiology, 55*(21), 2328-2329.

Davies, A. (2009). Permanent pacemakers: An overview. *British Journal of Cardiac Nursing, 4*(6), 262-269.

DeVon, H. A., Hogan, N., Ochs, A. L., & Shapiro, M. (2010). Time to treatment for acute coronary syndromes: The cost of indecision. *Journal of Cardiovascular Nursing, 25*(2), 106-114.

Dobromir, D., & Nattel, S. (2010). New antiarrhythmic drugs for treatment of atrial fibrillation. *The Lancet, 375*(9721), 1212-1223.

Epstein, A. E., DiMarco, J. P., Ellenbogen, K. A., Estes, N., Freedman, R. A., Gettes, L. S., et al. (2008). ACC/AHA/HRS 2008 guidelines for device-based therapy of cardiac rhythm abnormalities: Executive summary. *Circulation, 117*, 2820-2840.

Franklin, D., & Bono, M. (2008). Guide to antiarrhythmic therapies. *Emergency Medicine, 40*(1), 36-39.

Garlitski, A. C., & Estes, N. A. III. (2010). Emerging therapies for atrial fibrillation: Is the paradigm shifting? *Journal of Interventional Cardiac Electrophysiology, 28*(1), 1-4.

Goodrich, C. (2009). Cardiopulmonary resuscitation: Where are we now? *AACN Advanced Critical Care, 20*(4), 373-383.

Green, J. M., & Chiaramida, A. J. (2010). *12 lead EKG confidence: A step-by-step guide.* New York: Springer.

Grigoriyan, A., Vazquez, R., Palvinskaya, T., Bindelglass, G., Rishi, A., Amoateng-Adjepong, Y., et al. (2009). Outcomes of cardiopulmonary resuscitation for patients on vasopressors or inotropes: A pilot study. *Journal of Critical Care, 24*(3), 415-418.

Grmec, S., & Mally, S. (2009). Timeliness of administration of vasopressors in CPR. *Critical Care, 13*(1), 401.

Hallas, C., Burke, J., White, D., & Connelly, D. (2010). A prospective 1-year study of changes in neuropsychological functioning after implantable cardioverter-defibrillator surgery. *Circulation: Arrhythmia and Electrophysiology, 3,* 170-177.

Harden, J. (2011). Taking a cool look at therapeutic hypothermia. *Nursing2011, 41*(9), 46-52.

Hardin, S. R., & Steele, J. R. (2008). Atrial fibrillation among older adults: Pathophysiology, symptoms, and treatment. *Journal of Gerontological Nursing, 34*(7), 26-32.

Holding, S., Tyndall, K., Russell, C., & Cowan, C. (2009). The impact of a nurse-led rapid-access atrial fibrillation clinic. *British Journal of Cardiac Nursing, 4*(6), 276-281.

Hunt, E. A., Mancini, M. E., Smyth, M., & Truitt, T. L. (2009). Using the American Heart Association's national registry of cardiopulmonary resuscitation for performance improvement. *Joint Commission Journal on Quality & Patient Safety, 35*(1), 13-20.

Jost, D., Degrange, H., Verret, C., Hersan, O., Banville, I. L., Chapman, F. W., et al. (2010). A randomized controlled trial of the effect of automated external defibrillator cardiopulmonary resuscitation protocol on outcome from out-of-hospital cardiac arrest. *Circulation, 121,* 1614-1622.

Kalahasty, G., & Ellenbogen, K. (2009). The role of pacemakers in the management of patients with atrial fibrillation. *Cardiology Clinics, 27*(1), 137-150.

Keseg, D. P. (2010). Reducing interruptions: Continuous compression CPR & minimally interrupted CPR result in improved survival. *Journal of Emergency Medical Services, 35*(1), 14-17.

Lloyd-Jones, D., Adams, R., Carnethon, M., De Simone, G., Ferguson, R. B., Flegal, K., et al. (2009). Heart disease and stroke statistics—2009 update: A report from the American Heart Association Statistics Committee and Stroke Statistics Subcommittee. *Circulation, 119*(3), 480-486.

Marcus, G. M., Olgin, J. E., Whooley, M., Vittinghoff, E., Stone, K. L., Mehra, R., et al. (2010). Racial differences in atrial fibrillation prevalence and left atrial size. *American Journal of Medicine, 123*(4), 375.e1-7.

McDonough, M. (2009). Mission control: Managing atrial fibrillation. *Nursing2009, 39*(11), 58-63.

Michaels, A. D., Spinler, S. A., Leeper, B., Ohman, E. M., Alexander, K. P., Newby, L. K., et al. (2010). Medication errors in acute cardiovascular and stroke patients: A scientific statement from the American Heart Association. *Circulation, 121,* 1664-1682.

Mitka, M. (2009). Researchers seek MRI-safe pacemakers. *Journal of the American Medical Association, 301*(5), 476.

Morrison, D., & Smith, J. (2009). Taking a vested interest in a wearable cardioverter defibrillator. *Nursing2009, 39*(6), 29-32.

New 80-lead EKG is easy to interpret. (2008). *ED Nursing, 8,* 112-113.

Onalan, O., Cumurcu, G., & Bekar, L. (2008). Complete atrioventricular block associated with concomitant use of

metoprolol and paroxetine. *Mayo Clinic Proceedings, 83*(5), 595-599.

Pagana, K. D., & Pagana, T. J. (2010). *Mosby's manual of diagnostic and laboratory tests* (4th ed.). St. Louis: Mosby.

Palatnik, A. (2009). Too fast, too slow, too ugly: Dysrhythmias that every nurse should recognize. *Nursing2009, 39*(9), 38-46.

Pelter, M. (2010). Time to treatment for acute coronary syndromes: The cost of indecision. *Journal of Cardiovascular Nursing, 25*(2), 115-116.

Quirino, G., Giammaria, M., Corbucci, G., Pistelli, P., Turri, E., Mazza, A., et al. (2009). Diagnosis of paroxysmal atrial fibrillation in patients with implanted pacemakers: Relationship to symptoms and other variables. *Pacing & Clinical Electrophysiology, 32*(1), 91-98.

Ristagno, G., Tang, W., Huang, L., Fymat, A., Chang, Y. T., Sun, S., et al. (2009). Epinephrine reduces cerebral perfusion during cardiopulmonary resuscitation. *Critical Care Medicine, 37*(4), 1408-1415.

Roguin, A. (2009). Magnetic resonance imaging in patients with implantable cardioverter-defibrillators and pacemakers. *Journal of the American College of Cardiology, 54*(6), 556-557.

Rose, E., Chinitz, L. A., Holmes, D. S., & Aizer, A. (2010). A novel mechanism of failure to detect atrial arrhythmias by pacemakers and implantable cardioverter defibrillators. *Journal of Cardiovascular Electrophysiology, 21*(3), 325-328.

Ruiter, J. H., Mulder, E., Schuchert, A., Burri, H., Stuhlinger, M. C., Hartikainen, J., et al. (2010). The feasibility of fully automated pacemaker advise in treating atrial tachyarrhythmias. *Pacing & Clinical Electrophysiology, 33*(5), 605-614.

Sayre, M. R., Berg, R. A., Cave, D. M., Page, R. L., Potts, J., White, R. D., et al. (2008). Hands-only (compression-only) cardiopulmonary resuscitation: A call to action for bystander response to adults who experience out-of-hospital sudden cardiac arrest. *Circulation, 117*(16), 2162-2167.

Sellers, M. B., & Newby, L. K. (2011). Atrial fibrillation, anticoagulants, fall risk, and outcomes in elderly patients. *American Heart Journal, 161*(2), 241-246.

Sherrard, H. (2008). An automated external defibrillator in the home did not reduce all-cause mortality in patients at risk of cardiac arrest. *Evidence-Based Nursing, 11*(4), 113.

Sheu, S., Wei, I., Chen, C., Yu, S., & Tang, F. (2009). Using snowball sampling method with nurses to understand medication administration errors. *Journal of Clinical Nursing, 18*(4), 559-569.

Skidmore-Roth, L. (2011). *Mosby's 2011 nursing drug reference* (24th ed.). St. Louis: Mosby.

Tedrow, U. B., Conen, D., Ridker, P. M., Cook, N. R., Koplan, B. A., Manson, J. E., et al. (2010). The long- and short-term impact of elevated body mass index on the risk of new atrial fibrillation: The WHS (Women's Health Study). *Journal of the American College of Cardiology, 55*(21), 2319-2327.

Wilber, D. J., Pappone, C., Neuzil, P., De Paola, A., Marchlinski, F., Natale, A., et al. (2010). Comparison of antiarrhythmic drug therapy and radiofrequency catheter ablation in patients with paroxysmal atrial fibrillation. *Journal of the American Medical Association, 303*(4), 333-340.

Wokhlu, A., Monahan, K. H., Hodge, D. O., Asirvatham, S. J., Friedman, P. A., Munger, T. M., et al. (2010). Long-term quality of life after ablation of atrial fibrillation: The impact of recurrence, symptom relief, and placebo effect. *Journal of the American College of Cardiology, 55*(21), 2308-2316.

Worth, T. (2009). CPR and PCI. *AJN, 109*(10), 22.

Wung, S., & Kozik, T. (2008). Electrocardiographic evaluation of cardiovascular status. *Journal of Cardiovascular Nursing, 23*(2), 169-174.

Yeung, J., & Perkins, G. D. (2010). Timing of drug administration during CPR and the role of simulation. *Resuscitation, 81*(3), 265-266.

Chapter 37

Albert, N., Trochelman, K., Li, J., & Lin, S. (2009). Signs and symptoms of heart failure: Are you asking the right questions? *American Journal of Critical Care, 19*(5), 443-452.

Andrews, T. (2009). Restarting the clock … again: Ethical considerations in retransplantation. *Dimensions of Critical Care Nursing, 28*(5), 209-213.

*Carelock, J., & Clark, A. P. (2003). Heart failure: Pathophysiologic mechanisms. *AJN, 101*(12), 26-35.

Chapa, D., Lee, H., Kaoe, C., Friedmann, E., Thomas, S., Anderson, J., et al. (2008). Reducing mortality with device therapy in heart failure patients without ventricular arrhythmias. *American Journal of Critical Care, 17*, 443-452.

Chen, W., Tran, K., & Maisel, A. (2010). Biomarkers in heart failure. *Heart, 96*, 314-320.

Christensen, D. (2008). Extreme heart makeover: Understanding mechanical circulatory support. *Nursing2008, 38*(5), 48-53.

Dakin, C. L. (2008). New approaches to heart failure in the ED. *AJN, 108*(3), 68-71.

DiSalvo, T., Acker, M., Dec, W., & Byrne, J. (2010). Mitral valve surgery in advanced heart failure. *Journal of the American College of Cardiology, 55*(4), 271-282.

Donlan, S., Quattromani, E., Pang, P., & Gheorghiade, M. (2009). Therapy for acute heart failure syndromes. *Current Cardiology Reports, 11*, 192-201.

Duffy, J., Hoskins, L., & Dudley-Brown, S. (2009). Improving outcomes for older adults with heart failure: A randomized trial using a theory-guided nursing intervention. *Journal of Nursing Care Quality, 25*(1), 56-64.

Dworakowski, R., Prendergast, B., Wendler, O., & MacCarthy, P. (2010). Treatment of acquired valvular heart disease: Percutaneous alternatives. *Clinical Medicine, 10*(2), 181-187.

Eisen, H., & Ross, H. (2010). Prevention and treatment of cardiac transplant vasculopathy. *UpToDate*. Retrieved June 26, 2010, from www.uptodate.com/patients/content/topic.do?topicKey=~rZWWnH5TdOdTou.

Hill, C. (2009). Acute heart failure: Too sick for discharge teaching? *Critical Care Nursing Quarterly, 32*(2), 106-111.

*Hoercher, K. J., Vacha, C. J., & McCarthy, P. M. (2002). Left ventricular splints and wraps for end-stage heart failure: A new approach in the new millennium. *Journal of Cardiovascular Nursing, 16*(3), 82-86.

Jessup, M., Abraham, W. T., Casey, D. E., Feldman, A. M., Francis, G. S., Ganiats, T. G., et al., writing on behalf of the 2005 guideline update for the diagnosis and management of chronic heart failure in the adult writing committee. (2009). 2009 Focused update: ACCF/AHA guidelines for the diagnosis and management of heart failure in adults: a report of the American College of Cardiology Foundation/American Heart Association Task Force on practice guidelines. *Circulation, 119*(14), 1977-2016.

Joseph, S., Cedars, A., Ewald, G., Geltman, E., & Mann, D., (2009). Acute decompensated heart failure contemporary medical management. *Texas Heart Institute Journal, 36*(6), 510-520.

Kale, P., & Fang, J. (2008). Devices in acute heart failure. *Critical Care Medicine, 31*(Suppl. 1), S121-S128.

Lea, P. (2009). The effects of depression in heart failure. *Dimensions of Critical Care Nursing, 28*(4), 164-168.

Lindgren, T. G., Fukuoka, Y., Rankin, S. H., Cooper, B. A., Carroll, D., & Munn, Y. L. (2008). Cluster analysis of elderly cardiac patients' prehospital symptomatology. *Nursing Research, 57*(1), 14-23.

McCalmont, V., & Ohler, L. (2008). Cardiac transplantation candidate identification, evaluation and management. *Critical Care Nursing Quarterly, 31*(3), 216-229.

McCance, K. L., Huether, S. E., Brashers, V. L., & Rote, N. S. (2010). *Pathophysiology: The biologic basis for disease in adults and children* (6th ed.). St. Louis: Mosby.

Moertl, D., Berger, R., Hammer, A., Huelsmann, M., Hutuleac, R., & Pacher, R. (2009). B-type natriuretic peptide predicts benefit from a home-based nurse care in chronic heart failure. *Journal of Cardiac Failure, 15*(3), 233-240.

Noveanu, M., Breidthardt, T., Cayir, S., Potocki, M., Laule, K., & Mueller, C. (2009). B-type natriuretic peptide-guided management and outcome in patients with obesity and dyspnea: Results from the BASEL study. *American Heart Journal, 158*(3), 488-495.

Osaki, S., Edwards, N., Velez, M., Johnson, M., Murray, M., Hoffman, J., et al. (2008). Improved survival in patients with ventricular assist device therapy: The University of Wisconsin experience. *European Journal of Cardio-Thoracic Surgery, 34*(2), 281-288.

Ramani, G., Uber, P., & Mehra, M. (2010). Chronic heart failure: Contemporary diagnosis and management. *Mayo Clinic Proceedings, 85*(2), 180-195.

Ray, S. (2010). Changing epidemiology and natural history of valvular heart disease. *Clinical Medicine, 10*(2), 168-171.

Rogers, J., Aaronson, K., Boyle, A., Russell, S., Milano, C., Pagani, F., et al. (2010). Continuous flow left ventricular assist device improves functional capacity and quality of life of advanced heart failure patients. *Journal of the American College of Cardiology, 55*(17), 1826-1834.

Saunders, M. (2010). A comparison of employed and unemployed caregivers of older heart failure patients. *Holistic Nursing Practice, 24*(1), 16-22.

Seward, J., & Casaclang-Verzosa, G. (2010). Infiltrative cardiovascular diseases. *Journal of the American College of Cardiology, 55*(17), 1769-1779.

Seyfarth, M., Sibbing, D., Baurer, I., Frohlich, G., Bott-Flugel, L., Byrne, R., et al. (2008). A randomized clinical trial to evaluate the safety and efficacy of a percutaneous left ventricular assist device versus intra-aortic balloon pumping for treatment of cardiogenic shock caused by myocardial infarction. *Journal of the American College of Cardiology, 52*(19), 1584-1588.

Sherrod, M., Graulty, R., Crawford, M., & Cheek, D. (2009). Intravenous heart failure medications. *Home Healthcare Nurse, 27*(10), 610-619.

Thomas, S. A., Chapa, D. V., Friedman, E., Durden, C., Ross, A., Lee, M. C. Y., et al. (2008). Depression in patients with heart failure: Prevalence, pathophysiological mechanisms, and treatment. *Critical Care Nurse, 28*(2), 40-55.

Thompson, B. (2009). Sudden cardiac death and heart failure. *AACN Advanced Critical Care, 20*(4), 356-365.

Wexler, R., Elton, T., Pleister, A., & Feldman, D. (2009). Cardiomyopathy: An overview. *American Academy of Family Physicians, 79*(9), 778-784.

Wingate, S., & Wiegland, D. L. M. (2008). End-of-life care in the critical care unit for patients with heart failure. *Critical Care Nurse, 28*(2), 84-94.

Chapter 38

*ALLHAT Officers and Coordinators for the ALLHAT Collaborative Research Group. (2002a). Major outcomes in high-risk hypertensive patients randomized to angiotensin-converting enzyme inhibitor or calcium channel blocker vs diuretic. The Antihypertensive and Lipid-Lowering Treatment to Prevent Heart Attack Trial (ALLHAT). *Journal of the American Medical Association, 288*(23), 2981-2997.

*ALLHAT Officers and Coordinators for the ALLHAT Collaborative Research Group. (2002b). Major outcomes in moderately hypercholesterolemic, hypertensive patients randomized to pravastatin vs usual care. The Antihypertensive and Lipid-Lowering Treatment to Prevent Heart Attack Trial (ALLHAT-LLT). *Journal of the American Medical Association, 288*(23), 2998-3007.

American Heart Association (AHA). (2010). *Heart disease and stroke statistics—2010 update.* Dallas: Author.

Anderson, D. J., Anderson, M. A., & Hill, P. D. (2010). Location of blood pressure measurement. *MEDSURG Nursing, 19*(5), 287-294.

Braverman, A. C. (2010). Acute aortic dissection. *Circulation, 122*(2), 184.

*Bussard, M. E. (2002). Reteplase: Nursing implications for catheter-directed thrombolytic therapy for peripheral vascular occlusions. *Critical Care Nurse, 22*(3), 57-63.

Cranwell-Bruce, L. A. (2008). Antihypertensives. *MEDSURG Nursing, 17*(5), 337-342.

*Day, M. W. (2003). Recognizing and managing deep vein thrombosis. *Nursing2003, 33*(5), 36-42.

*Douglas, J. G., Bakris, G. L., Epstein, M., Ferdinand, K. C., Ferrario, C., Flack, J. M., et al. (2003). Consensus statement of the Hypertension in African Americans Working Group of the International Society on Hypertension in Blacks: Management of high blood pressure in African Americans. *Archives of Internal Medicine, 163*(5), 525-541.

*Eichinger, S., Minar, E., Bialonczyk, C., Hirschl, M., Quehenberger, P., Schneider, B., et al. (2003). D-dimer levels and risk of recurrent venous thromboembolism. *Journal of the American Medical Association, 290*(8), 1071-1074.

Forsdahl, S. H., Singh, K., Solberg, S., & Jacobsen, B. K. (2009). Risk factors for abdominal aortic aneurysms. *Circulation, 119*(16), 2202-2208.

Gay, V., Hamilton, R., Heiskell, S., & Sparks, A. M. (2009). Influence of bedrest or ambulation in the clinical treatment of acute deep vein thrombosis on patient outcomes: A review and synthesis of the literature. *MEDSURG Nursing, 18*(5), 293-299.

Harris, W. S., Miller, M., Tighe, A. P., Davidson, M. H., & Schaefer, E. J. (2008). Omega-3 fatty acids and coronary heart disease: Clinical and mechanistic perspectives. *Atherosclerosis, 197*(1), 12-24.

Hermida, R. C., Ayala, D. E., Mojon, A., & Fernandez, J. R. (2009). Ambulatory blood pressure control with bedtime administration in subjects with prehypertension. *American Journal of Hypertension, 22*, 896-903.

*Hess, C. T. (2003). Managing your patient's arterial ulcer. *Nursing2003, 33*(5), 17.

Hiratzka, L. F., Bakris, G. L., Beckman, J. A., Bersin, R. M., Carr, V. F., Casey, D. E., et al. (2010). *Guidelines for the diagnosis and management of patients with thoracic aortic disease.* Philadelphia: Lippincott Williams & Wilkins.

Horne, E. M., & Gordon, P. M. (2009). Taking aim at hypertensive crisis. *Nursing2009, 39*(3), 48-53.

Husten, C. G. (2008). Tobacco use: Ending the epidemic. *MEDSURG Nursing, 17*(5), 345-354.

Jarvis, C. (2012). *Physical examination and health assessment* (6th ed.). St. Louis: Mosby.

*Joint National Committee. (2003). *The Seventh Report of the Joint National Committee on Prevention, Detection, Evaluation, and Treatment of High Blood Pressure. NIH Publication No. 03-5233.* Bethesda, MD: National Heart, Lung, and Blood Institute.

Levi, M. (2008). Self-management of anticoagulation. *Expert Review of Cardiovascular Therapy, 6*(7), 979-985.

*Lichtenstein, A. H., Appel, L. J., Brands, M., Carnethon, M., Daniels, S., Franch, H. A., et al. (2006). Diet and lifestyle recommendations revision 2006: A scientific statement from the American Heart Association Nutrition Committee. *Circulation, 2006*(114), 82-96. Retrieved October 4, 2010, from circ.ahajournals.org.

Lloyd-Jones, D., Adams, R. J., Brown, T. M., Carnethon, M., Dai, S., De Simone, G., et al. (2010). Heart disease and stroke statistics 2010 updated: A report from the American Heart Association. *Circulation, 121*(7), e46-e215.

*Malacaria, B., & Feloney, C. D. H. (2003). Going with the flow of anticoagulant therapy. *Nursing2003, 33*(3), 36-42.

McCance, K. L., Huether, S. E., Brashers, V. L., & Rote, N. S. (2010). *Pathophysiology: The biologic basis for disease in adults and children* (6th ed.). St. Louis: Mosby.

National Center for Complementary and Alternative Medicine. (2010). Herbs at a glance: Garlic. Retrieved June 11, 2010 from http://nccam.nih.gov/health/garlic/ataglance.htm.

*National Cholesterol Education Program. (2002). *Third Report of the Expert Panel on Detection, Evaluation, and Treatment of High Blood Cholesterol in Adults (Adult Treatment Panel III). NIH Publication No. 02-5215.* Bethesda, MD: National Heart, Lung, and Blood Institute.

Pagana, K. D., & Pagana, T. J. (2010). *Mosby's manual of diagnostic and laboratory tests* (4th ed.). St. Louis: Mosby.

Safar, M. E., Priollet, P., Luizy, F., Mourad, J. J., Cacoub, P., Levesque, H., et al. (2009). Peripheral arterial disease and isolated systolic hypertension: The ATTEST study. *Journal of Human Hypertension, 2009*(23), 182-187.

Schmid, A., Damush, T., Plue, L., Submanian, U., Bakas, T., & Williams, L. (2009). Current blood pressure self-management: A qualitative study. *Rehabilitation Nursing, 34*(6), 223-229.

Sieggreen, M. (2008). Understanding critical limb ischemia. *Nursing2008, 38*(10), 50-56.

Van Tongeren, R., Bastiaansen, A., Van Wissen, R., Le Cessie, S., Hamming, J., & Van Bockel, J. (2010). A comparison of the Doppler-derived maximal systolic acceleration versus the ankle-brachial pressure index or detecting and quantifying peripheral arterial occlusive disease in diabetic patients. *Journal of Cardiovascular Surgery, 51*(3), 391-398.

Verdecchia, P., Angeli, F., Mazzotta, G., Gentile, G., & Reboldi, G. (2009). Home blood pressure measurements will not replace 24-hour ambulatory blood pressure monitoring. *Hypertension, 2009*(54), 188-195.

Winslow, E. H., & Brosz, D. L. (2008). Graduated compression stockings in hospitalized postoperative patients: Correctness of usage and size. *AJN, 108*(9), 40-50.

Chapter 39

Abbas, A., Lichtman, A., & Pillai, S. (2010). *Cellular and molecular immunology* (updated 6th ed.). Philadelphia: Saunders.

*Angus, D., Linde-Zwirble, W., Lidicker, J., Clermanit, G., Carcillo, J., & Pinsky, M. (2001). Epidemiology of severe sepsis in the United States: Analysis of incidence, outcome, and associated costs of care. *Critical Care Medicine, 29*(7), 1303-1310.

Centers for Disease Control and Prevention. (2010). FastStats. *National Center for Health Statistics.* Retrieved January 2011, from www.cdc.gov/nchs/fastats/.

Cooper, B. (2008). Review and update on inotropes and vasopressors. *AACN Advanced Critical Care, 19*(1), 5-15.

Dellacroce, H. (2009). Surviving sepsis: The role of the nurse. *RN, 72*(7), 16-21.

Dellinger, R. P., Levy, M. M., Carlet, J. M., Bion, J., Parker, M. M., Jaeschke, R., et al. (2008). Surviving Sepsis Campaign—International guidelines for management of severe sepsis and septic shock: 2008. *Intensive Care Medicine, 34*(1), 17-60.

Dodge, M. (2010). SIRS: A systematic approach for medical-surgical nurses to stop the progression to sepsis. *MEDSURG Nursing, 19*(1), 11-15.

Ecklund, M., & Ecklund, C. (2007). How to recognize and respond to hypovolemic shock. *American Nurse Today, 2*(4), 28-31.

El Solh, A. A., Akinnusi, M. E., Alsawalha, L. N., & Pineda, L. A. (2008). Outcome of septic shock in older adults after implementation of the sepsis "bundle." *Journal of the American Geriatrics Society, 56*(2), 272-278.

Giuliano, K., Lecardo, M., & Staul, L. (2011). Impact of protocol watch on compliance with the surviving sepsis campaign. *American Journal of Critical Care, 20*(4), 313-321.

Gobel, B., & Peterson, G. (2010). Sepsis and septic shock. *Clinical Journal of Oncology Nursing, 14*(6), 793-797.

Hatler, C., Hebden, J., Kaler, W., & Zack, J. (2010). Walk the walk to reduce catheter-related bloodstream infections. *American Nurse Today, 5*(1), 26-30.

Held, M., & Sturtz, M. (2009). Managing acute decompensated heart failure. *American Nurse Today, 4*(2), 18-22.

King, K., & Olson, D. (2007). What you should know about neurogenic shock. *American Nurse Today, 2*(2), 36-39.

Landis, R. C. (2009). Redefining the systemic inflammatory response. *Seminars in Cardiothoracic and Vascular Anesthesia, 13*(2), 87-94.

Mattiace, R. (2008). Preventing hypovolemic shock. *American Nurse Today, 3*(3), 28.

McCance, K., Huether, S., Brashers, V., & Rote, N. (2010). *Pathophysiology: The biologic basis for disease in adults and children* (6th ed.). St. Louis: Mosby.

Miller, J. (2007). Keeping your patient hemodynamically stable. *Nursing2007, 37*(5), 36-41.

Moureau, N. (2009). Reducing the cost of catheter-related bloodstream infections. *Nursing2009, 39*(7), 14-15.

Nelson, D. P., Lemaster, T. H., Plost, G. N., & Zahner, M. L. (2009). Recognizing sepsis in the adult patient. *AJN, 109*(3), 40-45.

Pagana, K. (2009). What does the absolute neutrophil count tell you? *American Nurse Today, 4*(2), 12-13.

Pagana, K., & Pagana, T. (2010). *Mosby's manual of diagnostic and laboratory tests* (4th ed.). St. Louis: Mosby.

Powers, K., & Burchell, P. (2010). Sepsis alert: Avoiding the shock. *Nursing2010, 40*(4), 34-38.

Schuetz, P., Christ-Crain, M., & Müller, B. (2008). Procalcitonin and other biomarkers for the assessment of disease severity and guidance of treatment in bacterial infections. *Advances in Sepsis, 6*(3), 82-89.

Stricker, J. (2010). Traumatic hypovolemic shock: Halt the downward spiral. *Nursing2010, 40*(10), 34-39.

Thierry, R., & Thierry, C. (2010). Interleukin-33 safeguards neutrophils in sepsis. *Nature Medicine, 16*(6), 638-639.

Touhy, T., & Jett, K. (2010). *Ebersole and Hess' gerontological nursing & healthy aging* (3rd ed.). St. Louis: Mosby.

Toussaint, S., & Gerlach, H. (2009). Activated protein C for sepsis. *New England Journal of Medicine, 361*(27), 2646-2652.

Zimmermann, P. (2009). Stemming a lethal immunologic response. *American Nurse Today, 4*(9), 58.

Chapter 40

Albert, N. M., & Lewis, C. (2008). Recognizing and managing left ventricular dysfunction: After myocardial infarction. *Critical Care Nurse, 28*(2), 20-37.

Allen, J., & Dennison, C. (2010). Randomized trials of nursing interventions for secondary prevention in patients with coronary artery disease and heart failure. *Journal of Cardiovascular Nursing, 25*(3), 207-220.

American Heart Association (AHA). (2010). *Heart disease and stroke statistics—2010 update.* Dallas, TX: Author. Retrieved June 16, 2011, from http://circ.ahajournals.org/cgi/reprint/CIRCULATIONAHA.109.192667.

*Anderson, J. L. (2007). ACC/AHA 2007 guidelines for the management of patients with unstable angina/non ST-elevation myocardial infarction. Executive summary: A report of the American College of Cardiology/American Heart Association Task Force on Practical Guidelines (Writing Committee to revise the 2002 guidelines for the management of patients with unstable angina/non-ST elevation myocardial infarction). *Journal of the American College of Cardiology, 50*(7), 652-726.

*Bellasi, A., Raggi, P., Merz, C., & Shaw, L. (2007). New insights into ischemic heart disease in women. *Cleveland Clinic Journal of Medicine, 74*(8), 585-594.

Dolansky, M. A., Xu, F., Zullio, M., Shishehbor, B., Moore, S. M., & Rimm, A. A. (2010). Post–acute care services received by older adults following a cardiac event: A population-based analysis. *Journal of Cardiovascular Nursing, 25*(4), 342-349.

Dressler, D. (2009). Death by clot: Acute coronary syndromes, ischemic stroke, pulmonary embolism, and disseminated intravascular coagulation. *AACN Advanced Critical Care, 20*(2), 166-176.

Ebbing, M., Bleive, Ø., Ueland, P., Nordrehaug, J., Nilsen, D., Vollset, S., et al. (2008). Mortality and cardiovascular events in patients treated with homocysteine-lowering B vitamins after coronary angiography: A randomized controlled trial. *Journal of the American Medical Association, 300*(7), 795-804.

Flicker, L. (2010). Cardiovascular risk factors, cerebrovascular disease burden and healthy brain aging. *Clinics in Geriatric Medicine, 26*(1), 17-27.

*Grundy, S. M., Cleeman, J. I., Daniels, S. R., Donato, K. A., Eckel, R. H., Franklin, B. A., et al. (2005). Diagnosis and management of the metabolic syndrome: An American Heart Association/National Heart, Lung, and Blood Institute Scientific Statement. *Circulation, 112*(17), 2735-2752.

Harris, W. S., Mozaffarian, D., Rimm, E., Kris-Etherton, P., Rudel, L. L., Appel, L. J., et al. (2009). Omega-6 fatty acids and risk for cardiovascular disease: A science advisory from the American Heart Association Nutrition Subcommittee of the Council on Nutrition, Physical Activity and Metabolism; Council on

Cardiovascular Nursing; and Council on Epidemiology and Prevention. *Circulation, 119*(6), 902-907.

Hayman, L. L., & Hughes, S. (2008). Progress in prevention: Preventing heart disease—a global challenge and a call to action. *Journal of Cardiovascular Nursing, 23*(1), 65-66.

*Kip, K. E., Marroquin, O. C., Kelley, D. E., Johnson, B. D., Kelsey, S. F., Shaw, L. J., et al. (2004). Clinical importance of obesity versus metabolic syndrome I cardiovascular risk in women: A report from the Women's Ischemia Syndrome Evaluation (WISE) study. *Circulation, 109*(6), 706-713.

*Knox, J., & Gaster, B. (2007). Dietary supplements for the prevention and treatment of coronary artery disease. *Journal of Alternative and Complementary Medicine, 13*(1), 83-95.

*Kushner, F. G., Hand, M., Smith, S. C., Jr., King, S. B., 3rd., Anderson, J. L., Antaman, E. M., et al. (2009). 2009 focused updates: ACC/AHA guidelines for the management of patients with ST-elevation myocardial infarction (Updating the 2004 guideline and 2007 focused update) and the ACC/AHA/SCAI guidelines on percutaneous coronary intervention (Updating the 2005 guideline and 2007 focused update): A report of the American College of Cardiology Foundation/American Heart Association task force on practice guidelines. *Journal of the American College of Cardiology, 54*(27), 2228-2241.

McCance, K., Huether, S., Brashers, V. L., & Rote, N. S. (2010). *Pathophysiology: The biologic basis for disease in adults and children* (6th ed.). St. Louis: Mosby.

McSweeney, J. C., O'Sullivan, P., Cleves, M. A., Lefler, L. L., Cody, M., Moser, D. K., et al. (2010). Racial differences in women's prodromal and acute symptoms of myocardial infarction. *American Journal of Critical Care, 19*(1), 63-73.

Mente, A., deKoning, L., Shannon, H. S., & Anand, S. S. (2009). A systematic review of the evidence supporting a causal link between dietary factors and coronary heart disease. *Archives of Internal Medicine, 169*(7), 659-669.

Moser, D. K., & Riegel, B. (2008). *Cardiac nursing: A companion to Braunwald's heart disease.* St. Louis: Mosby.

Mullen-Fortino, M., & O'Brien, N. (2008). Caring for a patient after coronary artery bypass graft surgery. *Nursing2008, 38*(3), 46-52.

O'Keefe, J. H., Carter, M. D., & Lavie, C. J. (2009). Primary and secondary prevention of cardiovascular diseases: A practical evidence-based approach. *Mayo Clinic Procedures, 84*(8), 741-757.

Overbaugh, K. (2009). Acute coronary syndrome, *AJN, 109*(5), 42-52.

Pagana, K. D., & Pagana, T. J. (2010). *Mosby's manual of diagnostic and laboratory tests* (4th ed.). St. Louis: Mosby.

Sanz, J., Moreno, P. R., & Fuster, V. (2010). The year in atherothrombosis. *Journal of the American College of Cardiology, 55*(14), 1487-1498.

Scirica, B. (2010). Acute coronary syndrome: Emerging tools for diagnosis and risk assessment. *Journal of the American College of Cardiology, 55*(14), 1403-1415.

Shaw, L. J., Bugiardini, R., & Merz, C. N. (2009). Women and ischemic heart disease: Evolving knowledge. *Journal of the American College of Cardiology, 54*(17), 1561-1575.

Shoulders-Odom, B. (2008). Management of patients after percutaneous coronary interventions. *Critical Care Nurse, 28*(5), 26-41.

*Siniorakis, E., Arvanitakis, S., Voyatzopoulos, G., Hatziandreou, P., Plataris, G., et al. (2000). Hemodynamic classification in acute myocardial infarction: Has anything changed in the last 3 decades? *Chest, 117,* 1286-1290.

Stangl, V., Witzel, V., Baumann, G., & Stangl, K. (2008). Current diagnostic concepts to detect coronary artery disease in women. *European Heart Journal, 29,* 707-717.

Summers, K., Martin, K., & Watson, K. (2010). Impact and clinical management of depression in patients with coronary artery disease. *Pharmacotherapy, 30*(3), 304-322.

Surette, M. (2008). The science behind dietary omega-3 fatty acids. *Canadian Medical Association Journal, 178*(2), 177-180.

Suzuki, K., Elkind, M. S., Boden-Albala, B., Jin, Z., Berry, G., DiTullio, M. R., et al. (2009). Moderate alcohol consumption is associated with better endothelial function: A cross sectional study. *BMC Cardiovascular Disorders, 9,* 8.

Weustink, A. C., Mollet, N. R., Neefjes, L. A., Meijboom, W. B., Galema, T. W., van Mieghem, C. A., et al. (2010). Diagnostic accuracy and clinical utility of noninvasive testing for coronary artery disease. *Annals of Internal Medicine, 152*(10), 630-639.

Wiviott, S. D., Braunwald, E., McCabe, C. H., Montalescot, G., Ruzyllo, W., Gottlieb, S., et al. (2007). Prasugrel verses clopidogrel in patients with acute coronary syndromes. *New England Journal of Medicine, 357*(20), 2001-2015.

Chapter 41

Beattie, S. (2007). Bone marrow aspiration and biopsy. *RN, 70*(2), 41-43.

Bucciarelli, P. & Mannucci, P. (2009). The hemostatic system through aging and menopause. *Climacteric, 12*(Suppl. I), 47-51.

Gordon, M. (2011). *Manual of nursing diagnosis* (12th ed.). New York: Jones & Bartlett.

Jarvis, C. (2012). *Physical examination and health assessment* (6th ed.). Philadelphia: Saunders.

Matthews, J., & Newton, S. (2010). The Coombs test. *Clinical Journal of Oncology Nursing, 14*(2), 143-145.

McCance, K., Huether, S., Brashers, V., & Rote, N. (2010). *Pathophysiology: The biologic basis for disease in adults and children* (6th ed.). St. Louis: Mosby.

Miller, J., & Starks, B. (2010). Deciphering clues in the CBC count. *Nursing2010, 40*(7), 52-55.

Nussbaum, R., McInnes, R., & Willard, H. (2007). *Thompson & Thompson: Genetics in medicine* (7th ed.). Philadelphia: Saunders.

Pagana, K., & Pagana, T. (2010). *Mosby's manual of diagnostic and laboratory tests* (4th ed.). St. Louis: Mosby.

Ruegg, T., Curran, C., & Lamb, T. (2009). Use of buffered lidocaine in bone marrow biopsies: A randomized, controlled trial. *Oncology Nursing Forum, 36*(1), 52-60.

Touhy, T. & Jett, K. (2010). *Ebersole and Hess' gerontological nursing & healthy aging* (3rd ed.). St. Louis: Mosby.

Weyland, P. (2009). Warfarin therapy management: Tap in to new ways to slow the clot. *Nurse Practitioner Journal, 34*(3), 22-28.

*Woodrow, P. (2003). Assessing blood results in older people: Haematology and liver function tests. *Nursing Older People, 15*(3), 29-31.

Chapter 42

Afable, M., & Lyon, D. (2008). Severe fatigue: Could it be aplastic anemia? *Clinical Journal of Oncology Nursing, 12*(4), 569-573.

Allen-Bard, S. (2009). Suboptimal responses to imatinib in chronic myelogenous leukemia: What are they and how do they affect treatment? *Clinical Journal of Oncology Nursing, 13*(5), 537-542.

American Cancer Society. (2011). *Cancer facts and figures 2011.* Report No. 01-300M–No. 5008.11. Atlanta: Author.

Ault, P., & Jones, K. (2009). Understanding iron overload: Screening, monitoring, and caring for patients with transfusion-dependent anemia. *Clinical Journal of Oncology Nursing, 13*(1), 511-517.

Baker, M. (2010). Graft-versus-host disease following autologous transplantation. *Oncology Nursing Forum, 37*(3), 269-272.

Bauer, S., & Romvari, E. (2009). Treatment of chronic myeloid leukemia following imatinib resistance: A nursing guide to second-line treatment options. *Clinical Journal of Oncology Nursing, 13*(5), 523-534.

Belavic, J. (2010). Drug approvals. *The Nurse Practitioner, 35*(2), 12-23.

Bertolotti, P., Bilotti, E., Colson, K., Curran, K., Doss, D., Faiman, B., et al. (2008). Management of side effects of novel therapies for multiple myeloma: Consensus statements developed by the IMF Nurse Leadership Board. *Clinical Journal of Oncology Nursing, 12*(Suppl. 3), 9-12.

Bevans, M., Tierney, D. K., Bruch, C., Burgunder, M., Castro, K., Ford, R., et al. (2009). Hematopoietic stem cell transplantation nursing: A practice variation study. *Oncology Nursing Forum, 36*(6), E317-E325.

Bielefeldt, S., & DeWitt, J. (2009). The rules of blood transfusion: Best practices for blood product administration. *American Nurse Today, 4*(2), 27-28.

Brown, C. (Ed.). (2010). *A guide to oncology symptom management.* Pittsburgh: Oncology Nursing Society.

Byar, K., & Workman, M. (2012). Targeted therapies to treat cancer. In J. Kee, E. Hayes, & L. McCuistion (Eds.), *Pharmacology: A nursing process approach* (7th ed.). St. Louis: Saunders.

Collins, T. (2011). Packed red blood cell transfusions in critically ill patients. *Critical Care Nurse, 31*(1), 25-33.

Cook, L. (2009). Learning about blood component therapy. *Nursing2009, 39*(4), 30-33.

Coyer, S., & Lash, A. (2008). Pathophysiology of anemia and nursing care implications. *MEDSURG Nursing, 17*(2), 77-83, 91.

Devine, H., Tierney, K., Schmit-Pokorny, K., & McDermott, K. (2010). Mobilization of hematopoietic stem cells for use in autologous transplantation. *Clinical Journal of Oncology Nursing, 14*(2), 212-222.

Dohnalek, L. (2007). Blood transfusions: How technology can improve patient safety. *American Nurse Today, 2*(5), 46-47.

Elphee, E. (2008). Caring for patients with chronic lymphocytic leukemia. *Clinical Journal of Oncology Nursing, 12*(3), 417-423.

Glass, M., & Spitrey, J. (2009). Heparin-induced thrombocytopenia: Your questions answered. *AACN Advanced Critical Care, 20*(1), 5-9.

Goy, A. (2009). Diffuse large B-cell lymphoma: An evolving paradigm of care. *The Oncology Nurse, 1*(Suppl. 4), 4-11.

Granados, R., & Jacob, E. (2009). Pain experience in hospitalized adults with sickle cell disease. *MEDSURG Nursing, 18*(3), 161-167.

Hernandez, S., & Patterson, G. E. (2009). What you need to know about acute chest syndrome. *Nursing2009, 39*(6), 42-45.

Hunt, C. (2010). Immune thrombocytopenia purpura. *MEDSURG Nursing, 19*(4), 237-239.

Huntley, A. (2009). Transfusion reaction. *Nursing2009, 39*(1), 72.

Katz, E. (2009). Blood transfusion: Friend or foe. *AACN Advanced Critical Care, 20*(2), 155-163.

Keisner, S., & Shah, S. (2009). Advances in the treatment of multiple myeloma. *The Oncology Nurse, 2*(Suppl. 8), 14-15.

Kurtin, S., & Demakos, E. (2010). An update on the treatment of myelodysplastic syndrome. *Clinical Journal of Oncology Nursing, 14*(3), E295.

Kuman, V., Abbas, A., Fausto, N., & Aster, J. (2010). *Robbins and Cotran: Pathologic basis of disease* (8th ed.). Philadelphia: Saunders.

Kyle, R., & Rajkumar, S. V. (2009). Treatment of multiple myeloma: A comprehensive review. *Clinical Lymphoma & Myeloma, 9*(4), 278-288.

Lambing, A. (2007). Bleeding disorders: Patient history key to diagnosis. *The Nurse Practitioner, 32*(12), 16-24.

Leighton, S. (2008). The spin on apheresis. *Nursing2008, 38*(4), 29-31.

Mann-Jiles, V., & Morris, D. (2009). Quality of life of adult patients with sickle cell disease. *Journal of the American Academy of Nurse Practitioners, 21*(6), 340-349.

McCance, K., Huether, S., Brashers, V., & Rote, N. (2010). *Pathophysiology: The biologic basis for disease in adults and children* (6th ed.). St. Louis: Mosby.

McNally, G. (2011). B-cell lymphoma, unclassifiable: A review of the literature. *Clinical Journal of Oncology Nursing, 15*(2), 189-193.

MD Consult. http://www.mdconsult.com.

Miceli, T., Colson, K., Faiman, B., Miller, K., Tariman, J.; IMF Nurse Leadership Board. (2011). Maintaining bone health in patients with multiple myeloma: Survivorship care plan of the International Myeloma Foundation Nurse Leadership Board. *Clinical Journal of Oncology Nursing, 15*(4), 9-23.

Miceli, T., Colson, K., Gavino, M., Lilleby, K., IMF Nurse Leadership Board. (2008). Myelosuppression associated with novel therapies in patients with multiple myeloma: Consensus statement of the IMF Nurse Leadership Board. *Clinical Journal of Oncology Nursing, 12*(Suppl. 3), 13-19.

Miller, K., Musial, L., Whitworth, A., & Chanan-Kahn, A. (2010). Management of patients with chronic lymphocytic leukemia treated with lenalidomide. *Clinical Journal of Oncology Nursing, 14*(4), 491-499.

Mullen, E., & Mendez, N. (2008). Hyperviscosity syndrome in patients with multiple myeloma. *Oncology Nursing Forum, 35*(3), 350-352.

Munro, N. (2009). Hematologic complications of critical illness: Anemia, neutropenia, thrombocytopenia, and more. *AACN Advanced Critical Care, 20*(2), 145-154.

Myers, F., & Reyes, C. (2011). Blood cultures: 5 steps to doing it right. *Nursing2011, 41*(3), 62-63.

National Hemophilia Foundation. (2010). MASAC recommendations concerning products licensed for the treatment of hemophilia and other bleeding disorders. Retrieved December 2010, from http://hemophilia.org.

Nettina, S. (2009). A new look at vitamin B_{12} deficiency. *The Nurse Practitioner, 34*(11), 18-24.

Nussbaum, R., McInnes, R., & Willard, H. (2007). *Thompson & Thompson: Genetics in medicine* (7th ed.). Philadelphia: Saunders.

Pack-Mabien, A., & Haynes, J. (2009). A primary care provider's guide to preventive and acute care management of adults and children with sickle cell disease. *Journal of the American Academy of Nurse Practitioners, 21*(5), 250-257.

Pagana, K. (2009). What does the absolute neutrophil count tell you? *American Nurse Today, 4*(2), 12-13.

Pagana, K., & Pagana, T. (2010). *Mosby's manual of diagnostic and laboratory tests* (4th ed.). St. Louis: Mosby.

Rome, S., Doss, D., Miller, K., Westphal, J.; IMF Nurse Leadership Board. (2008). Thromboembolic events associated with novel therapies in patients with multiple myeloma: Consensus statement of the IMF Nurse Leadership Board. *Clinical Journal of Oncology Nursing, 12*(Suppl. 3), 21-27.

Sickle Cell Information Center. (2010). Frequently asked questions. Emory University. Atlanta, GA. Website: www.scinfo.org/faq/

Simmons, S. (2010). Anemia. *Nursing2010, 40*(6), 34.

Smart, M. (2010). Pharmacy corner: Ofatumumab used to treat chronic lymphocytic leukemia. *Oncology Nursing Forum, 37*(2), 223.

Smith, L., Bertolotti, P., Curran, K., Jenkins, B.; IMF Nurse Leadership Board. (2008). Gastrointestinal side effects associated with novel therapies in patients with multiple myeloma: Consensus statement of the IMF Nurse Leadership Board. *Clinical Journal of Oncology Nursing, 12*(Suppl. 3), 37-51.

Sparks, M. (2009). Argatroban therapy in heparin-induced thrombocytopenia. *AACN Advanced Critical Care, 20*(1), 37-43.

Tariman, J., Love, G., McCullagh, E., Sandifer, S.; IMF Nurse Leadership Board. (2008). Peripheral neuropathy associated with novel therapies in patients with multiple myeloma: Consensus statement of the IMF Nurse Leadership Board. *Clinical Journal of Oncology Nursing, 12*(Suppl. 3), 29-35.

The Joint Commission (TJC). (2010). National Patient Safety Goals. Retrieved October 2010, from www.jointcommission.org/patientsafety/nationalpatientsafetygoals/.

United States National Library of Medicine (2011). Genetics home reference: Sickle cell disease. Retrieved June 2011 from http://ghr.nlm.nih.gov/condition/sickle-cell-disease.

Walker, D., & Held-Warmkessel, J. (2010). Acute promyelocytic leukemia: An overview with implications for oncology nurses. *Clinical Journal of Oncology Nursing, 14*(6), 747-759.

Whelton, S. (2007). Radioimmunotherapy in the treatment of non-Hodgkin's lymphoma. *The Nurse Practitioner, 32*(12), 35-38.

Winkeljohn, D. (2010). Idiopathic thrombocytic purpura. *Clinical Journal of Oncology Nursing, 14*(4), 411-413.

Zimmermann, P. (2010). Revisiting IM injections. *AJN, 110*(2), 60-61.

Chapter 43

Agrawal, Y., Carey, J. P., Della Santina, C. C., Schubert, M. C., & Minor, L. B. (2009). Disorders of balance and vestibular function in U.S. adults. *Archives of Internal Medicine, 169*(10), 938-944.

Gordon, M. (2011). *Manual of nursing diagnosis* (12th ed.). New York: Jones & Bartlett.

Hickey, J. V. (2008). *The clinical practice of neurological and neurosurgical nursing* (6th ed.). Philadelphia: Lippincott Williams & Wilkins.

Jarvis, C. (2012). *Physical examination and health assessment* (6th ed.). Philadelphia: Saunders.

*Lower, J. (2003). Using pain to assess neurologic response. *Nursing2003, 33*(60), 56-57.

*Milisen, K., Braes, T., Fick, D. M., & Foreman, M. D. (2006). Cognitive assessment and differentiating the 3 D's (dementia, depression, delirium). *Nursing Clinics of North America, 41*(1), 1-21.

Pagana, K. D., & Pagana, T. J. (2010). *Mosby's manual of diagnostic and laboratory tests* (4th ed.). St. Louis: Mosby.

Palmieri, R. L. (2009). Wrapping your head around cranial nerves. *Nursing2009, 39*(9), 24-30.

*Photo Guide. (2006). Assessing the cranial nerves. *Nursing2006, 36*(11), 47-49.

*Rushing, J. (2007). Assisting with lumbar puncture. *Nursing2007, 37*(1), 23.

Solomon, E. P. (2009). *Introduction to human anatomy and physiology* (3rd ed.). Philadelphia: Saunders.

*Thompson, H. J. (2006). *Neurological assessment of the older adult: A guide for nurses*. Chicago: American Association of Neuroscience Nurses.

Vance, D. E. (2009). Speed of processing in older adults: A cognitive review for nursing. *Journal of Neuroscience Nursing, 41*(6), 290-297.

Chapter 44

*Backer, J. H. (2006). The symptom experience of patients with Parkinson's disease. *Journal of Neuroscience Nursing, 38*(1), 51-57.

Bradway, C., & Hirschman, K. B. (2008). Working with families of hospitalized older adults with dementia. *AJN, 108*(10), 52-60.

Chadwick, C. (2008). Steady your sights on Parkinson's disease. *Nursing2008, 38*(12), 56hn1-56hn4.

Cotter, V. T., & Evans, L. K. (2008). Try this: Avoiding restraints in older adults with dementia. *AJN, 108*(3), 45-46.

Cranwell-Bruce, L. A. (2010). Drugs for Parkinson's disease. *MEDSURG Nursing, 19*(6), 347-350.

Ellison, D., Williams, M. L., Moodt, G., & Farrar, F. C. (2010). Electrodiagnostic studies. *Critical Care Clinics of North America, 22*(1), 7-18.

Feinberg, L. F. (2008). Caregiver assessment: Understanding the issues. *AJN, 108*(Suppl. 9), 38-39.

Fincher, L., Ward, C., Dawkins, V., Magee, V., & Willson, P. (2009). Using telehealth to educate Parkinson's disease patients about complicated medication regimens. *Journal of Gerontological Nursing, 35*(2), 16-24.

Haahr, A., Kirkevold, M., Hall, E. O., & Ostergaard, K. (2011). Living with advanced Parkinson's disease: A constant struggle with unpredictability. *Journal of Advanced Nursing, 67*(2), 408-417.

Heavey, E. (2010). An update on meningococcal meningitis. *Nursing2010, 40*(10), 61-62.

*Howland, R. H. (2007). What is vagal nerve stimulation? *Journal of Psychosocial Nursing and Mental Health Services, 44*(8), 11-14.

Huntington's Disease Society of America (HDSA). (2010). *Fast facts about HD*. New York City: Author.

Klager, J., Duckett, A., Sandler, S., & Moskowitz, C. (2008). Huntington's disease: A caring approach to end of life. *Journal of Care Management, 9*(2), 75-81.

Lilley, L. L., Collins, S. R., Harrington, S., & Snyder, J. S. (2011). *Pharmacology and the nursing process*. St. Louis: Mosby.

*Matthews, C., Miller, L., & Mott, M. (2007). Getting ahead of meningitis and encephalitis. *Nursing2007, 107*(11), 37-42.

McCance, K. L., Huether, S. E., Brashers, V. L., & Rote, N. R. (2010). *Pathophysiology: The biologic basis for disease in adults and children* (6th ed.). St. Louis: Mosby.

Miller, C. A. (2008). Communication difficulties in hospitalized older adults with dementia. *AJN, 108*(3), 58-66.

Moloney, M. F., & Cranwell-Bruce, L.A. (2010). Pharmacologic management of migraine headaches. *Nurse Practitioner, 35*(9), 16-22.

*Nussbaum, R. L., McInnes, R. R., & Willard, H. F. (2007). *Thompson & Thompson genetics in medicine* (7th ed.). Philadelphia: Saunders.

Pagana, K. D., & Pagana, T. J. (2010). *Manual of diagnostic and laboratory tests* (4th ed.). St. Louis: Mosby.

Rank, W. (2008). Interrupting status epilepticus. *Nursing2008*, *38*(10), 56cc1-56cc3.

Roberts, B. R. (2010). Caring for patients with Parkinson's disease. *Nursing2010*, *40*(7), 58-64.

Rowe, M. (2008). Wandering in hospitalized older patients. *AJN*, *108*(10), 62-70.

*Sanchez-del-Rio, M., Reuter, U., & Moskowitz, M. (2006). New insights into migraine pathophysiology. *Current Opinion in Neurology*, *19*(3), 294-298.

Schulz, R., & Sherwood, P. R. (2008). Physical and mental health effects of family caregiving. *AJN*, *108*(Suppl. 9), 23-27.

*Schutte, D. L. (2006). Alzheimer disease and genetics: Anticipating the questions. *AJN*, *106*(12), 40-46.

Sharer, J. (2008). Tackling sundowning in a patient with Alzheimer's disease. *MEDSURG Nursing*, *17*(1), 27-30.

Stockdell, R., & Amella, E. (2008). The Edinburgh Feeding Evaluation in Dementia Scale. *AJN*, *108*(8), 46-54.

*Tan, H. J., Suganthi, C., Dhachayani, S., Rizal, A. M., & Raymond, A. A. (2007). The coexistence of anxiety and depressive personality traits in migraine. *Singapore Medical Journal*, *48*(4), 307-310.

*Vacca, V. M., & Olson, A. (2007). Epilepsy in the elderly. *Advance for Nurses MD/DC/VA*, *2*, 39-40.

Walker, E. R., Wexler, B., Dilorio, C., Escoffery, C., McCarty, F., & Yeager, K. A. (2009). Content and characteristics of goals created during a self-management intervention for people with epilepsy. *Journal of Neuroscience Nursing*, *41*(6), 312-321.

Welsh, M. (2008). Treatment challenges in Parkinson's disease. *The Nurse Practitioner*, *33*(7), 32-38.

*Yaari, R., & Correy-Bloom, J. (2007). Alzheimer's disease. *Seminars in Neurology*, *27*(1), 32-41.

Zarit, S., & Femia, E. (2008). Behavioral and psychological interventions for family caregivers. *AJN*, *108*(9), 47-53.

Chapter 45

*Amato, M. P., Portaccio, E., & Zipoli, V. (2006). Are there protective treatments for cognitive decline in MS? *Journal of Neurological Science*, *245*(1-2), 183-186.

*American Association of Neuroscience Nurses. (2007). *Cervical spine surgery: A guide to preoperative and postoperative patient care*. Chicago: Author.

*Copeland, B. (2007). Surgical versus nonsurgical treatment for back pain. *New England Journal of Medicine*, *357*(12), 1255.

DeSanto-Madeya, S. (2009). Adaptation to spinal cord injury for families post-injury. *Nursing Science Quarterly*, *22*(1), 57-66.

Duddy, M., Haghikia, A., Cocco, E., Eggers, C., Drulovic, J., Carmona, O., et al. (2011). Managing MS in a changing treatment landscape. *Journal of Neurology, Mar25* (Epub ahead of print). Retrieved March 26, 2011, from www.ncbi.nlm.nih.gov/pubmed/21437661.

Esmonde, L., & Long, A. F. (2008). Complementary therapy use by persons with multiple sclerosis: Benefits and research priorities. *Complementary Therapies in Clinical Practice*, *14*(3), 176-184.

Fraser, C., Mahoney, J., & McGurl, J. (2008). Correlates of sexual dysfunction in men and women with multiple sclerosis. *Journal of Neuroscience Nursing*, *40*(5), 312-317.

*International Multiple Sclerosis Genetics Consortium; Hafler, D. A., Compston, A., Sawcer, S., Lander E. S., Daly, M. J., De Jager, P. L., et al. (2007). Risk alleles for multiple sclerosis identified by a genomewide study. *New England Journal of Medicine*, *357*(9), 851-862.

Liedstrom, E., Isaksson, A. K., & Ahlstrom, G. (2010). Quality of life in spite of an unpredictable future: The next of kin of patients with multiple sclerosis. *Journal of Neuroscience Nursing*, *42*(6), 331-341.

Lohne, V. (2009). Back to life again—Patients' experiences of hope three to four years after a spinal cord injury: A longitudinal study. *Canadian Journal of Neuroscience Nursing*, *31*(2), 20-25.

McCance, K. L., Huether, S. E., Brashers, V. L., & Rote, N. S. (2010). *Pathophysiology: The biologic basis for diseases in adults and children* (6th ed.). St. Louis: Mosby.

*Murphy, J., Henry, R., & Lomen-Hoerth, C. (2007). Establishing subtypes of the continuum of frontal lobe impairment in amyotrophic lateral sclerosis. *Archives of Neurology*, *64*(3), 330-334.

National Spinal Cord Injury Statistical Center. (2010). Spinal cord injury facts and figures at a glance 2010. Retrieved July 19, 2011, from www.fscip.org/facts.htm.

Nayduch, D. A. (2010). Back to basics: Identifying and managing acute spinal cord injury. *Nursing2010*, *40*(9), 24-32.

Newland, P. K., Riley, M. A., Fearing, A. D., Neath, A., & Gibson, D. (2010). Pain in women with relapsing-remitting multiple sclerosis and healthy women: Relationship to demographic variables. *MEDSURG Nursing*, *19*(3), 177-184.

Newman, S. D., & SCI Photovoice Participants. (2010). Evidence-based advocacy: Using Photovoice to identify barriers and facilitators to community participation after spinal cord injury. *Rehabilitation Nursing*, *35*(2), 47-59.

Norton, C., & Chelvanayagam, S. (2010). Bowel problems and coping strategies in people with multiple sclerosis. *British Journal of Nursing*, *19*(4), 220-226.

Palmieri, R. L. (2008). Caring for a medical/surgical patient with MS. *Nursing2008*, *38*(10), 34-40.

*Ridley, B. (2006). Intrathecal baclofen therapy: Challenges in patients with multiple sclerosis. *Rehabilitation Nursing*, *31*(4), 158-164.

Rubinstein, S. M., van Middelkoop, M., Kuijpers, T., Ostelo, R., Verhagen, A. P., de Boer, M. R., et al. (2010). European Spine Journal, *19*(8), 1213-1228.

Ryan, M. (2009). Drug therapies for the treatment of multiple sclerosis. *Journal of Infusion Nursing*, *32*(3), 137-144.

*Sabin, K. L., & Penckofer, S. M. (2007). Patient expectations of quality of life following lumbar spinal surgery. *Journal of Neuroscience Nursing*, *39*(3), 180-189.

Song, H. Y., & Nam, K. A. (2010). Coping strategies, physical function, and social adjustment in people with spinal cord injury. *Rehabilitation Nursing*, *35*(1), 8-15.

van Middelkoop, M., Rubinstein, S. M., Kuijpers, T., Verhagen, A. P., Ostelo, R., Koes, B. W., et al. (2011). A systematic review on the effectiveness of physical rehabilitation interventions for chronic non-specific low back pain. *European Spine Journal*, *20*(1), 19-39.

Chapter 46

*Alexander, D. M. (2007). Facing the pain of trigeminal neuralgia. *Nursing2007*, *37*(7), 18-20.

American Academy of Neurology (AAN). (2011). AAN guideline summary for patients and their families: Treatment for Guillian-Barré syndrome. Retrieved July 20, 2011, from aan.com/professional/practice/pdfs/gbs_guide_pat_care.pdf.

*Atkinson, S. B., Carr, R., Maybee, P., & Haynes, D. (2006). The challenges of managing and treating Guillain-Barré syndrome during the acute phase. *Dimensions of Critical Care Nursing, 25*(6), 256-263.

Bershad, E. M., Feen, E. S., & Suarez, J. I. (2008). Myasthenia gravis crisis. *Southern Medical Journal, 101*(1), 63-69.

*Carlson, D. S., & Pfadt, E. (2005). When your patient has acute facial paralysis. *Nursing2005, 35*(4), 54-55.

Dhar, R. (2008). The morbidity and outcome of patients with Guillain-Barré syndrome admitted to the intensive care unit. *Journal of the Neurological Sciences, 264*(1-2), 121-128.

*Feasby, T. (2007). Guidelines on the use of intravenous immune globulin for neurologic conditions. *Transfusion Medicine Reviews, 21*(Suppl. 1), S57-S107.

Haldeman, D., & Zulkosky, K. (2008). The ascension of Guillain-Barré syndrome. *Critical Care Insider, Spring,* 2-6.

*Hampton, T. (2007). Novel therapies target myasthenia gravis. *Journal of the American Medical Association, 298*(2), 163-164.

Kernich, C. A. (2008). Myasthenia gravis: Maximizing function. *The Neurologist, 14*(1), 75-76.

Lemos, L., Fontes, R., Flores, S., Oliverira, P., & Almeida, A. (2010). Effectiveness of the association between carbamazepine and peripheral analgesic block with ropivacaine for the treatment of trigeminal neuralgia. *Journal of Pain Research, 3,* 201-212.

Leung, N. (2008). Guillain-Barré syndrome in elderly people. *Journal of the American Geriatrics Society, 56*(2), 1381-1382.

Lui, H., Li, H., Xu, M., Chung, K.F., & Zhang, B. P. (2010). A systematic review on acupuncture for trigeminal neuralgia. *Alternative Therapies in Health and Medicine, 16*(3), 30-35.

Maat, A. P. (2008). Inclusion of the transcervical approach in the video-assisted thoracoscopic-extended thymectomy (VATET) for myasthenia gravis: A prospective trial. *Surgical Endoscopy, 22*(1), 265.

National Institute of Neurological Disorders and Stroke. (2011a). Restless legs syndrome fact sheet. Retrieved February 2011, from www.ninds.nih.gov.

National Institute of Neurological Disorders and Stroke. (2011b). Trigeminal neuralgia fact sheet. Retrieved February 2011, from www.ninds.nih.gov.

Simmons, S. (2010). Guillain-Barré syndrome. *Nursing2010, 40*(1), 24-29.

*Slack, C.B., & Landis, C. A. (2006). Improving outcomes for restless legs syndrome. *The Nurse Practitioner, 31*(5), 27-37.

Weigel, G., & Casey, K. F. (2011). Striking back: The trigeminal neuralgia and face pain handbook. Gainsville, FL: TNA Facial Pain Association.

Chapter 47

*Adams, H. P., Jr., del Zoppo, G., Alberts, M. J., Bhatt, D. L., Brass, L., Furlan, A., et al. (2007). Guidelines for the early management of adults with ischemic stroke: A guideline from the American Heart Association/American Stroke Association Stroke Council, Clinical Cardiology Council, Cardiovascular Radiology and Intervention Council, and the Atherosclerotic Peripheral Vascular Disease and Quality of Care Outcomes in Research Interdisciplinary Work Groups. *Stroke, 38*(5), 1655-1711.

Beal, C. (2010). Gender and stroke symptoms: A review of the current literature. *Journal of Neuroscience Nursing, 42*(2), 80-87.

Bederson, J. B., Connolly, E. S., Jr., Batjer, H. H., Dacey, R. G., Dion, J. E., Diringer, M. N., et al. (2009). Guidelines for the management of aneurysmal subarachnoid hemorrhage: A statement for healthcare professionals from a special writing group of the Stroke Council, American Heart Association. *Stroke, 40*(3), 994-1025.

Cahill, J. E., & Armstrong, T. S. (2011). Caring for an adult with a malignant primary brain tumor. *Nursing2011, 41*(6), 28-33.

Centers for Disease Control and Prevention (CDC). (2011). Cerebrovascular disease or stroke. Retrieved July 27, 2011, from www.cdc.gov/nchs/fastats/stroke.htm.

Custer, N. R. (2009). What nurses should know about carotid stents. *MEDSURG Nursing, 18*(5), 277-282.

*Fox, S. W., Mitchell, S. A., & Booth-Jones, M. (2006). Cognitive impairments in patients with brain tumors: Assessment and intervention in the clinic setting. *Clinical Journal of Oncology Nursing, 10*(2), 169-176.

Gramitto, M., & Galitz, D. (2008). Update on stroke: The latest guidelines. *The Nurse Practitioner, 33*(1), 39-47.

Hills, T. E. (2010). Determining brain death: A review of evidence-based guidelines. *Nursing2010, 40*(12), 35-41.

*Hinkle, J. L. (2007). Acute ischemic stroke review. *Journal of Neuroscience Nursing, 39*(5), 285-293, 310.

*Jeong, S., & Kim, M. T. (2007). Effects of a theory-driven music and movement program for stroke survivors in a community setting. *Applied Nursing Research, 20*(3), 125-131.

Kozub, E. (2010). Community stroke prevention programs: An overview. *Journal of Neuroscience Nursing, 42*(3), 143-149.

McNett, M., & Gianakis, A. (2010). Nursing interventions for critically ill traumatic brain injury patients. *Journal of Neuroscience Nursing, 42*(2), 71-77.

Miller, J., & Mink, J. (2009). Acute ischemic stroke: Not a moment to lose. *Nursing2009, 39*(5), 37-42.

Mink, J., & Miller, J. (2011a). Opening the window of opportunity for treating acute ischemic stroke. *Nursing2011, 41*(1), 24-32.

Mink, J., & Miller, J. (2011b). Respond aggressively to hemorrhagic stroke. *Nursing2011, 41*(3), 36-43.

Morrison, K. (2007). Improving the care of stroke patients. *American Nurse Today, 2*(4), 38-44.

Oran, N., & Oran, I. (2010). Carotid angioplasty and stenting in carotid artery stenosis: Neuroscience nursing implications. *Journal of Neuroscience Nursing, 42*(1), 3-11.

*Palmieri, R. L. (2006). Carotid artery stenosis paves the way for a stroke. *Nursing2006, 36*(6), 36-42.

*Palmieri, R. L. (2007). Responding to primary brain tumor. *Nursing2007, 37*(1), 36-43.

Simpson, J. R., Zahuranec, D. B., Lisabeth, L. D., Sanchez, B. N., Skolarus, L. E., Mendizabal, J. E., et al. (2010). Mexican Americans with atrial fibrillation have more recurrent strokes than do non-Hispanic whites. *Stroke, 41*(10), 2132-2136.

Summers, D., Leonard, A., Wentworth, D., Saver, J. L., Simpson, J., Spilker, J. A., Hock, N., et al. (2009). Comprehensive overview of nursing and interdisciplinary care of the acute ischemic stroke patient: A scientific statement from the American Heart Association. *Stroke, 40*(8), 2911-2944.

Wijdicks, E. F. M., Varelas, P. N., Gronseth, G. S., et al. (2010). Evidence-based guideline update: Determining brain death in adults: Report of the Quality Standards Subcommittee of the American Academy of Neurology. *Neurology, 74*(23), 1911-1918.

Chapter 48

Cannon, J. (2010). Assessing visual acuity. *Nursing2010, 40*(8), 65.

Gordon, M. (2011). *Manual of nursing diagnosis* (12th ed.). New York: Jones & Bartlett.

Jarvis, C. (2012). *Physical examination and health assessment* (6th ed.). Philadelphia: Saunders.

Keeping an eye on abnormalities. (2008). *Nursing2008, 38*(1), 48-49.

McCance, K., Huether, S., Brashers, V., & Rote, N. (2010). *Pathophysiology: The biologic basis for disease in adults and children* (6th ed.). St. Louis: Mosby.

Nussbaum, R., McInnes, R., & Willard, H. (2007). *Thompson & Thompson: Genetics in medicine* (7th ed.). Philadelphia: Saunders.

Rushing, J. (2007). Administering eyedrops. *Nursing2007, 37*(5), 18.

*Sackett, C., & Schenning, S. (2003). Eye safety in the workplace. *Insight (American Society of Ophthalmic Registered Nurses), 27*(4), 101-102.

Touhy, T., & Jett, K. (2010). *Ebersole and Hess' gerontological nursing & healthy aging* (3rd ed.). St. Louis: Mosby.

*Vaughan, D., Asbury, T., & Riordan-Eva, P. (Eds.). (2004). *General ophthalmology* (16th ed.). New York: McGraw-Hill.

Chapter 49

American Cancer Society. (2011). *Cancer facts and figures 2011.* Report No. 00-300M–No. 5008.11. Atlanta: Author.

Ayers, D. (2010). Take a closer look at LASIK surgery. *Nursing2010, 40*(48), 48-51.

Foundation Fighting Blindness. (2010). Retrieved February 2011, from www.blindness.org.

Jarvis, C. (2012). *Physical examination and health assessment* (6th ed.). Philadelphia: Saunders.

Kaufman, S. (2009). Developments in age-related macular degeneration: Diagnosis and treatment. *Geriatrics, 64*(3), 16-19.

Kock, J., & Sikes, K. (2009). Getting the red out: Primary angle-closure glaucoma. *The Nurse Practitioner, 34*(5), 6-9.

Lockey, J. (2009). The provision of information for patients prior to cataract surgery. *British Journal of Nursing, 18*(19), 1207-1211.

McCance, K., Huether, S., Brashers, V., & Rote, N. (2010). *Pathophysiology: The biologic basis for disease in adults and children* (6th ed.). St. Louis: Mosby.

National Eye Institute of the National Institutes of Health. (2010). Prevalence of cataract and pseudophakia/aphakia among adults in the United States. Retrieved February 2011, from www.nei.nih.gov/eyedata/pbd6.asp.

Noble, J., & Chaudhary, V. (2010). Five things to know about age-related macular degeneration. *Canadian Medical Association Journal, 182*(16), 1759.

Nussbaum, R., McInnes, R., & Willard, H. (2007). *Thompson & Thompson: Genetics in medicine* (7th ed.). Philadelphia: Saunders.

Pullen, R., & Hall, D. (2010). Sjögren syndrome: More than dry eyes. *Nursing2010, 40*(8), 37-41.

Saligan, L., & Yeh, S. (2008). Seeing red: Guiding the management of ocular hyperemia. *The Nurse Practitioner, 33*(6), 14-20.

Sharts-Hopko, N., & Glynn-Milley, C. (2009). Primary open-angle glaucoma: Catching and treating the "sneak thief of sight." *AJN, 109*(2), 40-47.

Simar, K. (2009). The fundamentals of uveal melanoma. *Clinical Journal of Oncology Nursing, 13*(5), 483-485.

Statistics Canada. (2010). Retrieved February 2011, from www.statcan.gc.ca.

Tao, Y., Libondi, T., & Jonas, J. (2010). Long-term follow-up after multiple intravitreal bevacizumab injections for exudative age-related macular degeneration. *Journal of Ocular Pharmacology and Therapeutics, 26*(1), 79-83.

Touhy, T., & Jett, K. (2010). *Ebersole and Hess' gerontological nursing & healthy aging* (3rd ed.). St. Louis: Mosby.

Watkinson, S. (2009). Visual impairment in older people. *Nursing Older People, 21*(8), 30-36.

Watkinson, S. (2010). Management of older people with dry and wet age-related macular degeneration. *Nursing Older People, 22*(5), 21-26.

Chapter 50

Bess, F. H., & Humes, L. E. (2007). *Audiology: The fundamentals* (4th ed.). Baltimore: Lippincott Williams & Wilkins.

Boys Town National Research Hospital. (2010). Hearing loss. Retrieved August 2010, from www.boystownhospital.org/.

Centers for Disease Control and Prevention. (2010). Hearing loss. Retrieved December 2010, from www.cdc.gov/ncbddd/hearingloss/index.html.

Diagnostic tests for vestibular disorders. (2011). Retrieved January 2011, from www.vestibular.org/vestibular-disorders/diagnostic-tests.php.

Gordon, M. (2011). *Manual of nursing diagnosis* (12th ed.). New York: Jones & Bartlett.

Holcomb, S. (2009). Get an earful of the new cerumen impaction guidelines. *The Nurse Practitioner Journal, 34*(4), 14-19.

Jarvis, C. (2012). *Physical examination and health assessment* (6th ed.). Philadelphia: Saunders.

Kutten, J., & Reedy, S. (2009). Are you tuned in to your deaf patients? *The Nurse Practitioner, 34*(8), 44-49.

Laubach, G. (2010). Speaking up for older patients with hearing loss. *Nursing2010, 40*(1), 60-62.

Lieu, C., Sadler, G., Fullerton, J., & Stohlmann, P. (2007). Communication strategies for nurses interacting with deaf patients. *MEDSURG Nursing, 16*(4), 239-245.

*Lusk, S. L. (1997). Noise exposures: Effects of hearing and prevention of noise induced hearing loss. *AAOHN Journal, 45*(8), 397-405, 409-410.

McCance, K., Huether, S., Brashers, V., & Rote, N. (2010). *Pathophysiology: The biologic basis for disease in adults and children* (6th ed.). St. Louis: Mosby.

Nussbaum, R., McInnes, R., & Willard, H. (2007). *Thompson & Thompson: Genetics in medicine* (7th ed.). Philadelphia: Saunders.

Pagana, K., & Pagana, T. (2010). *Mosby's manual of diagnostic and laboratory tests* (4th ed.). St. Louis: Mosby.

Stach, B., Hornsby, B., Rosenfeld, M., & DeChicchis, A. (2009). The complexity of auditory aging. *Seminars in Hearing, 30*(2), 94-111.

Stephenson, M. (2009). Hearing protection in the 21st century: They're not your father's earplugs anymore. *Seminars in Hearing, 30*(1), 56-64.

Touhy, T., & Jett, K. (2010). *Ebersole and Hess' gerontological nursing & healthy aging* (3rd ed.). St. Louis: Mosby.

Chapter 51

Bassim, M., & Fayad, J. (2010). Implantable middle ear hearing devices: A review. *Seminars in Hearing, 31*(1), 28-36.

Bauer, C., & Brozoski, T. (2008). Tinnitus assessment and treatment: Integrating clinical experience with the basic science of tinnitus. *Seminars in Hearing, 29*(4), 371-385.

Holcomb, S. (2009). Get an earful of the new cerumen impaction guidelines. *The Nurse Practitioner, 34*(4), 14-19.

Humes, L., Ahistrom, J., Bratt, G., & Peek, B. (2009). Studies of hearing-aid outcome measures in older adults: A comparison of technologies and an examination of individual differences. *Seminars in Hearing, 30*(2), 112-128.

Ko, J. (2010). Presbycusis and its management. *British Journal of Nursing, 19*(3), 160-165.

Kutten, J., & Reedy, S. (2009). Are you tuned in to your deaf patients? *The Nurse Practitioner, 34*(8), 44-49.

Laubach, G. (2010). Speaking up for older patients with hearing loss. *Nursing2010, 40*(1), 60-62.

Lee, L., & Pensak, M. (2008). Contemporary role of endolymphatic mastoid shunt surgery in the era of transtympanic perfusion strategies. *Annals of Otology, Rhinology, & Laryngology, 117*(12), 871-875.

Lee, M. R., Pawlowski, K. S., Luong, A., Furze, A. D., & Roland, P. S. (2009). Biofilm presence in humans with chronic suppurative otitis media. *Otolaryngology—Head & Neck Surgery, 141*(5), 567-571.

Lieu, C. C. (2007). Communication strategies for nurses interacting with deaf patients. *MEDSURG Nursing, 16*(4), 239-245.

*McAleer, M. (2006). Communicating effectively with deaf patients. *Nursing Standard, 20*(19), 51-54.

McCance, K., Huether, S., Brashers, V., & Rote, N. (2010). *Pathophysiology: The biologic basis for disease in adults and children* (6th ed.). St. Louis: Mosby.

Newman, C., Sandridge, S., Meit, S., & Cherian, N. (2008). Strategies for managing patients with tinnitus: A clinical pathway model. *Seminars in Hearing, 29*(3), 300-309.

Nussbaum, R., McInnes, R., & Willard, H. (2007). *Thompson & Thompson: Genetics in medicine* (7th ed.). Philadelphia: Saunders.

Online Mendelian Inheritance in Man, OMIM™. (2010). McKusick-Nathans Institute for Genetic Medicine, Johns Hopkins University (Baltimore, MD) and National Center for Biotechnology Information, National Library of Medicine (Bethesda, MD). Retrieved July 2011 from www.ncbi.nlm.nih.gov/omim/.

Pagana, K., & Pagana, T. (2010). *Mosby's manual of diagnostic and laboratory tests* (4th ed.). St. Louis: Mosby.

Peate, I. (2009). Ménière's disease: Helping and understanding. *British Journal of Healthcare Assistants, 3*(12), 578-581.

Pratt, S. R., Kuller, L., Talbott, E. O., McHugh-Pemu, K., Buhari, A. M., & Xu, X. (2009). Prevalence of hearing loss in black and white elders: Results of the cardiovascular health study. *Journal of Speech, Language, and Hearing Research, 52*(4), 973-989.

Scheier, D. (2009). Barriers to health care for people with hearing loss: A review of the literature. *Journal of the New York State Nurses Association, 40*(1), 4-10.

Stach, B., Hornsby, B., Rosenfeld, M., & DeChicchis, A. (2009). The complexity of auditory aging. *Seminars in Hearing, 30*(2), 94-111.

Stephenson, M. (2009). Hearing protection in the 21st century: They're not your father's earplugs anymore. *Seminars in Hearing, 30*(1), 56-64.

Touhy, T., & Jett, K. (2010). *Ebersole and Hess' gerontological nursing & healthy aging* (3rd ed.). St. Louis: Mosby.

U.S. Food and Drug Administration. (2010). Medical devices—Recently approved devices. Retrieved January 2011, from www.fda.gov/MedicalDevices/ProductsandMedicalProcedures/.

Warren, E. (2008). ENT in primary care: Vertigo. *Practice Nurse, 35*(10), 39-41.

Chapter 52

Bigony, L. (2008). Arthroscopic surgery: A historical perspective. *Orthopaedic Nursing, 27*(6), 349-354.

Collyott, C. L., & Brooke, M. V. (2008). Evaluation and management of joint pain. *Orthopaedic Nursing, 27*(4), 246-250.

Gordon, M. (2011). *Manual of nursing diagnosis* (12th ed.). New York: Jones & Bartlett.

Jarvis, C. (2012). *Physical examination and health assessment* (6th ed.). St. Louis: Mosby.

Kress, T., Krueger, D., & Ziccardi, S. (2008). Creatine kinase: An assay with muscle. *Nursing2008, 38*(10), 62.

*Maher, A. B. (2002). Assessment of the musculoskeletal system. In A. B. Maher, S. W. Salmond, & T. A. Pellino (Eds.), *Orthopaedic nursing* (3rd ed.). Philadelphia: Saunders.

Mosher, C. M. (2010). *An introduction to orthopaedic nursing.* (4th ed.). Chicago, IL: National Association of Orthopaedic Nurses.

*Nussbaum, R. L., McInnes, R. R., & Willard, H. F. (2007). *Thompson & Thompson genetics in medicine* (7th ed.). Philadelphia: Saunders.

Pagana, K. D., & Pagana, T. J. (2010). *Mosby's diagnostic and laboratory test reference* (4th ed.). St. Louis: Mosby.

Pullen, R. L. (2008). Preparing a patient for magnetic resonance imaging. *Nursing2008, 38*(10), 22.

*Taggart, H. M. (2007). *Core curriculum for orthopaedic nursing* (6th ed.). Boston: Pearson.

Chapter 53

Chang, S. F., Yang, R. S., Chung, U. L., Chen, C. M., & Cheng, M. H. (2010). Perception of risk factors and DXA T-score among at-risk females of osteoporosis. *Journal of Clinical Nursing, 19*(13-14), 1795-1802.

Cohen, H. V. (2010). Bisphosphonate-associated osteonecrosis of the jaw—Patient care considerations: Overview for the orthopaedic nursing healthcare professional. *Orthopaedic Nursing, 29*(3), 176-180.

Doheny, M. O., Sedlak, C. A., Zeller, R., & Estok, P. J. (2010). Validation of the Osteoporosis Smoking Health Belief instrument. *Orthopaedic Nursing, 29*(1), 11-16.

*Estok, P. J., Sedlak, C. A., Doheny, M. O., & Hall, R. (2007). Structural model for osteoporosis preventing behavior in postmenopausal women. *Nursing Research, 56*(7), 148-158.

Gloth, F. M., 3rd, & Simonson, W. (2008). Osteoporosis is underdiagnosed in skilled nursing facilities: A large-scale heel BMD screening study. *Journal of the American Medical Directors Association, 9*(3), 190-193.

Greene, D., & Dell, R. M. (2010). Outcomes of an osteoporosis disease-management program managed by nurse practitioners. *Journal of the American Academy of Nurse Practitioners, 22*(6), 326-329.

*Iacono, M. V. (2007). Osteoporosis: A national public health priority. *Journal of Perianesthesia Nursing, 22*(3), 175-193.

Institute for Safe Medication Practices. (2008). ISMPs list of high-alert medications. Retrieved February 2011, from www.ismp.org/Tools/highalertmedications.pdf.

Johnson, M. A., Davery, A., Park, S., Hausman, D. B., & Poon, L. W. (2008). Age, race and season predict vitamin D status in African American and white octogenarians and centenarians. *Journal of Nutrition and Healthy Aging, 12*(10), 690-695.

Lee, J. (2009). Complication related to bisphosphonate therapy: Osteonecrosis of the jaw. *Journal of Infusion Nursing, 32*(6), 330-335.

Lilley, L. L., Rainforth Collins, S., Harrington, S., & Snyder, J. S. (2011). *Pharmacology and the nursing process* (6th ed.). St. Louis: Mosby.

Matzo, M. (2008). Agents for preventing fractures in osteoporosis. *AJN*, *108*(8), 73.

McCance, K. L., Huether, S. E., Brashers, V. L., and Rote, N. R. (2010). *Pathophysiology: The biologic basis for disease in adults and children* (6th ed.). St. Louis: Mosby.

Najat, D., Garner, T., Hagen, T., Shaw, B., Sheppard, P. W., Falchetti, A., et al. (2009). Characterization of a non-UBA domain missense mutation of sequestosome (SQSTM1) in Paget's disease of bone. *Journal of Bone and Mineral Research*, *24*(4), 632-642.

National Institute of Arthritis and Musculoskeletal and Skin Diseases. (2010). Information for patients about Paget's disease of bone. Retrieved February 2011, from www.niams.nih.gov/ Health_Info/Bone/pagets/patient_info.asp.

National Osteoporosis Foundation. (2010). *Clinician's guide to prevention and treatment of osteoporosis*. Washington, DC: Author.

*Nussbaum, R., McInnes, R., & Willard, H. (2007). *Thompson & Thompson: Genetics in medicine* (7th ed.). Philadelphia: Saunders.

Pagana, K. D., & Pagana, T. J. (2010). *Mosby's manual of diagnostic and laboratory tests* (4th ed.). St. Louis: Mosby.

Parikh, S., Avorn, J., & Solomon, D. H. (2009). Pharmacological management of osteoporosis in nursing home populations: A systematic review. *Journal of the American Geriatric Society*, *57*(2), 327-334.

Przybelski, R., Agrawal, S., Krueger, D., Engelke, J. A., Walbrun, F., & Binkley, N. (2008). Rapid correction of low vitamin D status in nursing home residents. *Osteoporosis International*, *19*(11), 1621-1628.

*Sadler, C., & Huff, M. (2007). African-American women: Health beliefs, lifestyle, and osteoporosis. *Orthopaedic Nursing*, *26*(2), 96-101.

Sambrook, P. N., Cameron, I. D., Chen, J. S., March, L. M., Simpson, J. M., Cumming, R. G., et al. (2010). Oral bisphosphonates are associated with reduced mortality in frail older people: A prospective five-year study. *Osteoporosis International*, *21*(10), Epub ahead of print.

Seton, M., Moses, A. M., Bode, R. K., & Schwartz, C. (2011). Paget's disease of bone: The skeletal distribution, complications, and quality of life as perceived by patients. *Bone*, *48*(2), 281-285.

Swislocki, A., Green, J. A., Heinrich, G., Barnett, C. A., Meadows, I. D., Harmon, E. B., et al. (2010). Prevalence of osteoporosis in men in a VA rehabilitation center. *American Journal of Managed Care*, *16*(6), 427-433.

Voda, S. C. (2009a). Dangerous curves: Treating adult idiopathic scoliosis. *Nursing2009*, *39*(12), 42-46.

Voda, S. C. (2009b). Help older men bone up on osteoporosis. *Nursing2009*, *39*(12), 66-67.

*Woman's Health Initiative. (2005). Findings from the WHI postmenopausal hormone therapy trials. Retrieved April 18, 2007, from www.nhlbi.nih.gov/whi/index.html.

Chapter 54

Al-Shaer, D., Hill, P. D., & Anderson, M. A. (2011). Nurses' knowledge and attitudes regarding pain assessment and intervention. *MEDSURG Nursing*, *20*(1), 7-12.

Altizer, L. L. (2008). Colles' fracture. *Orthopaedic Nursing*, *27*(2), 140-145.

Barry, M. (2010). Bringing Achilles tendinopathy to heel. *Nursing2010*, *40*(10), 30-33.

Chang, H. J., Burke, A. E., & Glass, R. M. (2010). Achilles tendinopathy. *Journal of the American Medical Association*, *303*(2), 188.

Day, M. W. (2008). Fracture in the field. *Nursing2008*, *38*(6), 72.

*Folden, S., & Tappen, R. (2007). Factors influencing function and recovery following hip repair surgery. *Orthopaedic Nursing*, *26*(4), 234-241.

Herr, K., & Titler, M. (2009). Acute pain assessment and pharmacological management practices for the older adult with a hip fracture: Review of ED trends. *Journal of Emergency Nursing*, *35*(4), 312-320.

*Holmes, S. B., & Brown, S. J. (2005). Skeletal pin site care: National Association of Orthopaedic Nurses guidelines for orthopaedic nursing. *Orthopaedic Nursing*, *24*(2), 99-107.

Hsu, E. (2009). Practical management of complex regional pain syndrome. *American Journal of Therapeutics*, *16*(2), 147-154.

Huisstede, B. M., Randsdorp, M. S., Coert, J. H., Glerum, S., van Middlekoop, M., & Koes, B. W. (2010). Carpal tunnel syndrome. Part II—Effectiveness of surgical treatments: A systematic review. *Archives of Physical Medicine and Rehabilitation*, *91*(7), 1005-1024.

Ketz, A. K. (2008). Pain management in the traumatic amputee. *Critical Care Nursing Clinics of North America*, *20*(1), 51-57.

*Laskowski-Jones, L. (2006). First aid for amputation. *Nursing2006*, *36*(4), 50-52.

Lowe, J., & Tariman, J. D. (2008). Lower extremity amputations: Black men with diabetes overburdened. *Advance for Nurse Practitioners*, *16*(11), 28.

Montana, C., & Kautz, D. D. (2011). Turning the nightmare of complex regional pain syndrome into a time of healing, renewal, and hope. *MEDSURG Nursing*, *20*(3), 139-142.

Nahm, E. S., Resnick, B., Orwig, D., Magaziner, J., & Degrezia, M. (2010). Exploration of informal caregiving following hip fractures. *Geriatric Nursing*, *31*(4), 254-262.

National Institute of Neurological Disorders and Stroke. (2011). Complex regional pain syndrome fact sheet. Retrieved March 4, 2011, from www.ninds.nih.gov/disorders/reflex_ sympathetic_dystrophy/detail.htm.

*Olsson, L. E., Karlsson, J., & Ekman, I. (2007). Effects of nursing interventions within an integrated care pathway for patients with hip fracture. *Journal of Advanced Nursing*, *58*(2), 116-125.

Pagana, K. D., & Pagana, T. J. (2010). *Mosby's manual of diagnostic and laboratory tests* (4th ed.). St. Louis: Mosby.

Pullen, R. L. (2010). Caring for a patient after amputation. *Nursing2010*, *40*(1), 15.

Satryb, S. A., Wilson, T. J., & Patterson, M. M. (2011). Casting: All wrapped up. *Orthopedic Nursing*, *30*(1), 37-41.

Schoen, D. C. (2008). Preventing hip fractures. *Orthopaedic Nursing*, *27*(2), 148-152.

Schoen, D. C. (2009). The hand. *Orthopaedic Nursing*, *28*(4), 194-198.

Small, K. (2009). Ankle sprains and fractures in adults. *Orthopaedic Nursing*, *28*(6), 314-320.

Smith, M. A., & Smith, W. T. (2010). Rotator cuff tears: An overview. *Orthopaedic Nursing*, *29*(5), 319-322.

Uchiyama, S., Itsubo, T., Nakamura, K., Kato, H., Yasutomi, T., & Momose, T. (2010). Current concepts of carpal tunnel syndrome: Pathophysiology, treatment, and evaluation. *Journal of Orthopaedic Science*, *15*(1), 1-13.

Voda, S. C. (2011). Bad breaks—A nurse's guide to distal radius fractures. *Nursing2011*, *41*(8), 34-40.

Chapter 55

American Cancer Society. (2010). American Cancer Society Guidelines for the early detection of cancer. Retrieved August 5, 2011, from www.cancer.org/Healthy/FindCancerEarly/CancerScreeningGuidelines.

Bruesehoff, M. P. (2010). ERCP—Much ado about blockages: Update your knowledge about the diagnostic and therapeutic uses for endoscopic retrograde cholangiopancreatography. *Nursing2010, 40*(9), 46-50.

Ellett, M. L. (2010). A literature review of the safety and efficacy of using propofol for sedation in endoscopy. *Gastroenterology Nursing, 33*(2), 113-117.

Gordon, M. (2011). *Manual of nursing diagnosis* (12th ed.). New York: Jones & Bartlett.

*Greenwald, B. (2006). A pilot study evaluating two alternate methods of stool collection for the fecal occult blood test. *MEDSURG Nursing, 15*(2), 89-94.

*Heseltine, P. (2007, January). Fecal immunochemical test. *Clinical Laboratory News*. Retrieved March 24, 2008, from www.aacc.org.

Hulse, R. S., Stuart-Shor, E. M., & Russo, J. (2010). Endoscopic procedure with a modified Reiki intervention: A pilot study. *Gastroenterology Nursing, 33*(1), 20-26.

Jarvis, C. (2012). *Physical examination and health assessment* (6th ed.). Philadelphia: Saunders.

Keske, L. A., & Letizia, M. (2010). *Clostridium difficile* infection: Essential information for nurses. *MEDSURG Nursing, 19*(6), 329-333.

*Madsen, D., Sebolt, T., Cullen, L., Folkedahl, B., Mueller, T., Richardson, C., et al. (2005). Listening to bowel sounds: An evidence-based practice project. *AJN, 105*(12), 40-48.

McCance, K. L., Huether, S. E., Brashers, V. L., & Rote, N. R. (Eds.). (2010). *Pathophysiology: The biologic basis for disease in adults & children* (6th ed.). St. Louis: Mosby.

Pagana, K. D., & Pagana, T. J. (2010). *Mosby's manual of diagnostic and laboratory tests* (4th ed.). St. Louis: Mosby.

Society of Gastroenterology Nurses and Associates. (2008). *Gastroenterology nursing: A core curriculum* (4th ed.). Chicago: Author.

*Yu, M. (2002). M2A Capsule Endoscopy: A breakthrough diagnostic tool for small intestine imaging. *Gastroenterology Nursing, 25*(1), 24-27.

Chapter 56

*American Dietetic Association. (2007). Position of the American Dietetic Association: Oral health and nutrition. Retrieved July 23, 2011, from www.eatright.org.

*Berry, A. M., Davidson, P. M., Masters, J., & Rolls, K. (2007). Systematic literature review of oral hygiene practices for intensive care patients receiving mechanical ventilation. *American Journal of Critical Care, 16*(6), 552-562.

Cancer Research UK. (2010). Types of mouth and oropharyngeal cancer. Retrieved June 16, 2011, from www.cancerhelp.org.uk.

*Chia-Hui Chen, C. (2003). The Geriatric Oral Health Assessment Index (GOHAI). *Try this: Best practices in nursing for older adults, 14*(6), 5-6.

Duffin, C. (2008). Brushing up on oral hygiene. *Nursing Older People, 20*(2), 14-16.

Feider, L., Mitchell, P., & Bridges, E. (2010). Oral care practices for orally intubated critically ill adults. *American Journal of Critical Care, 19*(2), 175-183.

Finlayson, T., Williams, D., Siefert, K., Jackson, J., & Ruth, N. (2010). Oral health disparities and psychosocial correlates of self-rated oral health in the National Survey of American Life. *American Journal of Public Health, 100*(Suppl. 1), S246-S255.

Jarvis, C. (2012). *Physical examination and health assessment* (6th ed.). Philadelphia: Saunders.

*McCance, K. L., Huether, S. E., Brashers, V. L., & Rote, N. R. (2010). *Pathophysiology: The biologic basis for disease in adults & children* (6th ed.). St. Louis: Mosby.

National Institute of Dental and Craniofacial Research. (2008). Bringing the promise of molecular medicine to oral cancer screening. Retrieved December 2010, from www.nidcr.nih.gov.

Oral Cancer Foundation. (2010). Oral cancer facts. Retrieved December 15, 2010, from www.oralcancerfoundation.org.

Oral CDx. (2008). The Oral CDx Brush Test. Retrieved December 15, 2010, from www.sopreventable.com.

Purandare, N., Woods, E., Butler, S., & Julie, M. (2010). Dental health of community-living older people attending secondary healthcare: A cross-sectional comparison between those with and without diagnosed mental illness. *International Psychogeriatrics, 22*(3), 417-423.

Winkeljohn, D. (2010). Adherence to oral cancer therapies: Nursing interventions. *Clinical Journal of Oncology Nursing, 14*(4), 461-466.

Chapter 57

A new horizon: Recommendations and treatment guidelines for Barrett's esophagus. (2009). *Gastroenterology Nursing, 32*(3), 211-212.

American Cancer Society. (2010). Cancer facts and figures 2010. Retrieved February 12, 2011, from www.cancer.org.

Bresalier, R. S. (2009). Barrett's esophagus and esophageal adenocarcinoma. *Annual Review of Medicine, 60*, 221-231.

Bulsiewicz, W. J., & Shaheen, N. J. (2011). The role of radiofrequency ablation in the management of Barrett's esophagus. *Gastroenterological Endoscopy Clinics of North America, 21*(1), 95-109.

Chait, M. M. (2010). Gastroesophageal reflux disease: Important considerations for older patients. *World Journal of Gastrointestinal Endoscopy, 2*(12), 388-396.

Edmondson, D., & Schiech, L. (2008). Esophageal cancer: A tough pill to swallow. *Nursing2008, 38*(4), 44-51.

Hard to swallow: Understanding dysphagia. (2008). *Nursing2008, 38*(3), 44-45.

*Jacobson, B. C., Somers, S. C., Fuchs, C. S., Kelly, C. P., & Camargo, C. A., Jr. (2006). Body-mass index and symptoms of gastrointestinal reflux in women. *New England Journal of Medicine, 354*(22), 2340-2348.

Jaromahum, J., & Fowlers, S. (2010). Lived experiences of eating after esophagectomy: A phenomenological study. *MEDSURG Nursing, 19*(2), 96-100.

Ji, F., Wang, Z., Wu, J., Gao, X., & Chen, X. (2010). The Stretta procedure eliminated arrhythmia due to gastroesophageal reflux disease. *Gastroenterology Nursing, 33*(5), 344-346.

*Lawrence, B. L., & Taylor, D. (2007). Esophageal pH monitoring goes wireless. *Nursing2007, 37*(10), 26-27.

McCance, K. L., Huether, S. E., Brashers, V. L., & Rote, N. R. (2010). *Pathophysiology: The biologic basis for disease in adults and children* (6th ed.). St. Louis: Mosby.

*McCormick, D. G. (2004). Stretta procedure for the treatment of gastroesophageal reflux disease. *Gastroenterology Nursing, 27*(1), 22-28.

*Nussbaum, R. L., McInnes, R. R., & Willard, H. F. (2007). *Thompson and Thompson's genetics in medicine*. Philadelphia: Saunders.

Sweed, M. R., Edmondson, D., & Cohen, S. J. (2009). Tumors of the esophagus, gastroesophageal junction, and stomach. *Seminars in Oncology Nursing, 25*(1), 61-75.

*Tawk, M., Goodrich, S., Kinasewitz, G., & Orr, W. (2006). The effect of 1 week of continuous positive airway pressure treatment in obstructive sleep apnea patients with concomitant gastroesophageal reflux. *Chest, 130*(4), 1003-1008.

Tomizawa, Y., & Wang, K. K. (2009). Changes in screening, prognosis and therapy for esophageal adenocarcinoma in Barrett's disease. *Current Opinion in Gastroenterology, 25*(4), 358-368.

Chapter 58

*Cope, D. G., & Reb, A. M. (2006). *An evidence-based approach to the treatment and care of the older adult with cancer*. Pittsburgh, PA: Oncology Nursing Society.

Fromm, A. (2009). Care of older adult populations diagnosed with *Helicobacter pylori*: A review of current literature. *Gastroenterology Nursing, 32*(6), 393-398.

Halpin, A., Huckabay, L. M., Kozuki, J. L., & Forsythe, D. (2010). Weigh the benefits of using a 0-to-5 nausea scale. *Nursing2010, 40*(11), 18-20.

Kwok, C. S., Yeong, J. K., & Loke, Y. K. (2010). Meta-analysis: Risk of fractures with acid-suppressing medication. *Bone, 48*(4), 768-776.

Loffroy, R., & Guiu, B. (2009). Role of transcatheter arterial embolization for massive bleeding from gastroduodenal ulcers. *World Journal of Gastroenterology, 15*(47), 5889-5897.

McCance, K. L., Huether, S. E., Brashers, V. L., & Rote, N. S. (2010). *Pathophysiology: The biologic basis for disease in adults and children* (6th ed.). St. Louis: Mosby.

National Cancer Institute. (2010). SEER stat fact sheets: Stomach. Retrieved March 22, 2011, from www.seer.cancer.gov/statfacts/html/stomach.html.

National Digestive Disease Information Clearinghouse. (2011). H. pylori and peptic ulcer. National Institute of Diabetes and Digestive and Kidney Diseases home page. Retrieved August 6, 2011, from www.niddk.nih.gov./health/digest/pubs/hpylori/hypylori.htm.

Olsson, U., Bosaeus, I., & Bergbom, I. (2010). Patients' experiences of the recovery period 12 months after upper gastrointestinal surgery. *Gastroenterology Nursing, 33*(6), 422-431.

Pagana, K. D., & Pagana, T. J. (2010). *Mosby's manual of diagnostic and laboratory tests* (4th ed.). St. Louis: Mosby.

*Ramakrishnan, K., & Salina, R. C. (2007). Peptic ulcer disease. *American Family Physician, 76*(7), 1005-1012.

Saif, W. W., Makrilia, N., Zalonis, A., Merikas, M., & Syrigos, K. (2010). Gastric cancer in the elderly: An overview. *European Journal of Oncology, 36*(8), 709-717.

*Schmidt, E. (2005). Nebulised lidocaine before nasogastric tube insertion reduced patient discomfort but increased risk of nasal bleeding. *Evidence-Based Nursing, 8*(2), 16.

Schrauwen, R. W., Janssen, M. J., & de Boer, W. A. (2009). Seven-day PPI-triple therapy with levofloxacin is very effective for *Helicobacter pylori* eradication. *Netherlands Journal of Medicine, 67*(3), 96-101.

*Schuler, A. (2007). Risks versus benefits of long-term proton pump inhibitor therapy in the elderly. *Geriatric Nursing, 28*(4), 225-229.

Chapter 59

American Cancer Society (ACS). (2010). *Cancer facts and figures 2010*. Atlanta: Author.

Anastasi, J. K., McMahon, D. J., & Kim, G. H. (2009). Symptom management for irritable bowel syndrome: A pilot randomized controlled trial of acupuncture/moxibustion. *Gastroenterology Nursing, 32*(4), 243-255.

Barkhordari, E., Rezaei, N., Ansaripour, B., Larki, P., Alighardashi, M., Ahmad-Ashtiani, H. R., et al. (2010). Proinflammatory cytokine gene polymorphisms in irritable bowel syndrome. *Journal of Clinical Immunology, 30*(1), 74-79.

Bengtsson, M., Ulander, K., Borgdal, E. B., & Ohlsson, B. (2010). A holistic approach for planning care of patients with irritable bowel syndrome. *Gastroenterology Nursing, 33*(2), 98-108.

Berger, A. M., Grem, J. L., Visovsky, C., Marunda, H. A., & Yurkovich, J. M. (2010). Fatigue and other variables during adjuvant chemotherapy for colon and rectal cancer. *Oncology Nursing Forum, 37*(1), 59-69.

*Brush, K. A. (2007). Measuring intra-abdominal pressure. *Nursing2007, 37*(7), 42-43.

Carlsson, E., Berndtsson, I., Hallen, A. M., Lindholm, E., & Persson, E. (2010). Concerns and quality of life before surgery and during the recovery period in patients with rectal cancer and an ostomy. *Journal of Wound, Ostomy, and Continence Nursing, 37*(6), 654-661.

*Freeman, L. C. (2007). Responding to small-bowel obstruction. *Nursing2007, 37*(5), 56hn1-56hn6.

Good, K., Niziolek, J., Yoshida, C., & Rowlands, A. (2010). Insights into barriers that prevent African Americans from seeking colorectal screenings: A qualitative study. *Gastroenterology Nursing, 33*(3), 204-208.

Gwee, K. A., Bak, Y. T., Ghoshal, U. C., Gonlachanvit, S., Lee, O. Y., Fock, K. M., et al. (2010). Asian consensus on irritable bowel syndrome. *Journal of Gastroenterology and Hepatology, 25*(7), 1189-1205.

Hamlyn, S. (2008). Reducing the incidence of colorectal cancer in African Americans. *Gastroenterology Nursing, 31*(1), 39-42.

Herman, J., Pokkunuri, V., Braham, L., & Pimentel, M. (2010). Gender distribution in irritable bowel syndrome is proportional to the severity of constipation relative to diarrhea. *Gender Medicine: The Journal for the Study of Sex & Gender Differences, 7*(3), 240-246.

Kerckhoffs, A. P., Ben-Amor, K., Samsom, M., van der Rest, M. E., de Vogel, J., Knol, J., et al. (2011). Molecular analysis of faecal and duodenal samples reveals significantly higher prevalence and numbers of *Pseudomonas aeruginosa* in irritable bowel syndrome. *Journal of Medical Microbiology, 60*, 236-245.

Lindberg, D. A. (2009). Hydrogen breath testing in adults: What is it and why is it performed? *Gastroenterology Nursing, 32*(1), 19-24.

Lyra, A., Krogius-Kurikka, L., Nikkila, J., Malinen, E., Kajander, K., Kurikka, K., et al. (2010). Effect of a multispecies probiotic supplement on quantity of irritable bowel syndrome-related intestinal microbial phylotypes. *BMC Gastroenterology, 10*, 110.

Malinen, E., Krogius-Kurikka, L., Lyra, A., Nikkila, J., Jaaskelainen, A., Rinttila, T., et al. (2010). Association of symptoms with gastrointestinal microbiota in irritable bowel syndrome. *World Journal of Gastroenterology, 16*(36), 4532-4540.

McCance, K. L., Huether, S. E., Brashers, V. L., & Rote, N. R. (2010). *Pathophysiology: The biologic basis for disease in adults and children* (6th ed.). St. Louis: Mosby.

National Comprehensive Cancer Network. (2008). Clinical practice guidelines in oncology: Colorectal cancer screening. Retrieved March 27, 2011, from http://nccn.org/professionals/physician_gls/PDF/colorectal_screening.pdf.

Nicholl, B. I., Halder, S. L., Macfarlane, G. L., Thompson, D. G., O'Brien, S., Musleh, M., et al. (2008). Psychosocial risk markers for new onset irritable bowel syndrome: Results of a large prospective population-based study. *Pain, 137*(1), 147-155.

*Norton, C. K., Linenfelser, P. I., Cyron, K. E., & Casey, K. A. (2006). Trauma and intraabdominal hypertension. *AJN, 106*(7), 51-55.

*Nussbaum, R. L., McInnes, R. R., & Willard, H. F. (2007). *Thompson and Thompson's genetics in medicine*. Philadelphia: Saunders.

Pagana, K. D., & Pagana, T. J. (2010). *Mosby's manual of diagnostic and laboratory tests* (4th ed.). St. Louis: Mosby.

Pimental, M., Lembo, A., Chey, W. D., Zakko, S., Ringel, Y., Yu, J., et al. (2011). Rifaximin therapy for patients with irritable bowel syndrome without constipation. *New England Journal of Medicine, 364*(1), 22-32.

Pirotta, M. (2009). Irritable bowel syndrome: The role of complementary medicines in treatment. *Australian Family Physician, 38*(12), 966-968.

*Pontieri-Lewis, V. (2006). Basics of ostomy care. *MEDSURG Nursing, 15*(4), 199-202.

*Pullen, R. L. (2006). Teaching your patient to irrigate a colostomy. *Nursing2006, 36*(4), 22.

Stubenrauch, J. M. (2010). Rectal cancer rates rising in patients under 40. *AJN, 110*(11), 15.

Symms, M. R., Rawl, S. M., Grant, M., Wendel, C. S., Coons, S. J., Hickey, S., et al. (2008). Sexual health and quality of life among male veterans with intestinal ostomies. *Clinical Nurse Specialist, 22*(1), 30-40.

Weingarten, M. A., Zalmanovici, A., & Yaphe, J. (2008). Dietary calcium supplementation for preventing colorectal cancer and adenomatous polyps. *Cochrane Database of Systematic Reviews, 23*(1), CD003548.

Wood, G. A., & Sauder, B. L. (2009). Sexual side effects in women with anal carcinoma. *Oncology Nursing Forum, 36*(3), 275-278.

Chapter 60

Cooper, J. M., Collier, J., James, V., & Hawkey, C. J. (2010). Beliefs about personal control and self-management in 30-40 year olds living with inflammatory bowel disease: A qualitative study. *International Journal of Nursing Studies, 47*(12), 1500-1509.

Crohn's and Colitis Foundation of America. (2008). *About ulcerative colitis and proctitis*. New York: Author.

Cronin, E. (2010). Prednisolone in the management of patients with Crohn's disease. *British Journal of Nursing, 19*(21), 1333-1336.

Crumbock, S. C., Loeb, S. J., & Fick, D. M. (2009). Physical activity, stress, disease activity, and quality of life in adults with Crohn disease. *Gastroenterology Nursing, 32*(3), 188-195.

Dolejs, S., Kennedy, G., & Heise, C. P. (2011). Small bowel obstruction following restorative proctocolectomy: Affected by a laparoscopic approach? *Journal of Surgical Research*, March 29 (Epub ahead of print). Retrieved April 10, 2011, from www.ncbi.nlm.nih.gov/pubmed/21474147.

Dudley-Brown, S., Nag, A., Cullinan, C., Ayers, M., Hass, S., & Panjabi, S. (2009). Health-related quality-of-life evaluation of Crohn disease patients after receiving natalizumab therapy. *Gastroenterology Nursing, 32*(5), 327-339.

Fajardo, A. D., Dharmarajan, S., George, V., Hunt, S. R., Birnbaum, E. H., Fleshman, J. W., et al. (2010). Laparoscopic versus open 2-stage ileal pouch: Laparoscopic approach allows for faster restoration of intestinal continuity. *Journal of the American College of Surgeons, 211*(3), 377-383.

*Heuer, O. E., Hammerum, A. M., Collignon, P., & Wegener, H. C. (2006). Human health hazard from antimicrobial-resistant enterococci in animals and food. *Clinical Infectious Diseases, 43*(7), 911-916.

Howard, D. D., White, C. Q., Harden, T. R., & Ellis, C. N. (2009). Incidence of surgical site infections postcolorectal resections without preoperative mechanical or antibiotic bowel preparation. *American Journal of Surgery, 75*(8), 659-663.

Kessler, H., Mudter, J., & Hohenberger, W. (2011). Recent results of laparoscopic surgery in inflammatory bowel disease. *World Journal of Gastroenterology, 17*(9), 1116-1125.

*Lichtenstein, G., Abreu, M., Cohen, R., & Tremaine, W. (2006). American Gastroenterological Association Institute medical position statement on corticosteroids, immunomodulators, and infliximab in inflammatory bowel disease. *Gastroenterology, 130*(3), 935-939.

McCance, K. L., Huether, S. E., Brashers, V. L., & Rote, N. R. (2010). *Pathophysiology: The biologic basis for disease in adults and children* (6th ed.). St. Louis: Mosby.

*Nussbaum, R. L., McInnes, R. R., & Willard, H. F. (2007). *Thompson & Thompson genetics in medicine* (7th ed.). Philadelphia: Saunders.

Pagana, K. D., & Pagana, T. J. (2010). *Mosby's manual of diagnostic and laboratory tests* (4th ed.). St. Louis: Mosby.

Pihl-Lesnovska, K., Hjortswang, H., Ek, A. C., & Frisman, G. H. (2010). Patients' perspective of factors influencing quality of life while living with Crohn disease. *Gastroenterology Nursing, 33*(1), 37-44.

*Present, D. H. (2006). *Current and investigational approaches in the management of ulcerative colitis*. Secaucus, NJ: Thomson Professional Postgraduate Services/Shire Pharmaceuticals, Inc. December, 1-17.

*Rocca, J. D. (2007). Minimizing the perils of appendicitis. *Nursing2007, 37*(1), 64hn1-64hn3.

*Sands, B. E. (2006). Clinical pearls from ACG 2006: Advances in diagnosis, staging and treatment of Crohn's disease. *Therapeutic Window, LLC CME Certified Newsletter*, November, 1-11.

Savard, J., & Woodgate, R. (2009). Young peoples' experience of living with ulcerative colitis and an ostomy. *Gastroenterology Nursing, 32*(1), 33-41.

*Snow, M. (2006). Preventing *Salmonella* infection. *Nursing2006, 36*(9), 17.

Spencer, C. (2010). Ulcerative colitis. *Nursing Standard, 24*(52), 59.

*Willcutts, K., Scarano, K., & Eddins, C. W. (2005). Ostomies and fistulas: A collaborative approach. *Practical Gastroenterology, 29*(11), 63-79.

Chapter 61

American Liver Foundation. (2010). *Hepatitis B*. New York: Author.

American Liver Foundation. (2011). *Position statement on hepatitis A and vaccination*. New York: Author.

Augustin, S., Gonzalez, A., & Genesca, J. (2010). Acute esophageal variceal bleeding: Current strategies and new perspectives. *World Journal of Hepatology, 2*(7), 261-274.

*Garcia-Tsao, G., Sanyal, A. J., Grace, N. D., & Carey, W.; Practice Guidelines Committee of the American Association for the Study of Liver Diseases; Practice Parameters Committee of the American College of Gastroenterology. (2007). Prevention and management of gastroesophageal varices and variceal hemorrhage in cirrhosis. *Hepatology, 46*(3), 922-938.

Kelso, L. A. (2008). Cirrhosis: Caring for patients with end-stage liver failure. *The Nurse Practitioner, 33*(7), 24-30.

Kinder, M. (2009). The lived experience of treatment for hepatitis C. *Gastroenterology Nursing, 32*(6), 401-408.

Lee, H., Park, W., Yang, J. H., & You, K. S. (2010). Management of hepatitis B virus infection. *Gastroenterology Nursing, 33*(2), 120-126.

Lindor, K. D., Gershwin, M. E., Poupon, R., Kaplan, M., Bergasa, N. V., & Heathcote, E. J.; American Association for the Study of Liver Diseases. (2009). AASLD practice guidelines: Primary biliary cirrhosis. *Hepatology, 50*(1), 291-308.

Lok, A. S. F., & McMahon, B. J. (2009). AASLD: Chronic hepatitis B: Update 2009. *Hepatology, 50*(3), 661-662.

McCance, K. L., Huether, S. E., Brashers, V. L., & Rote, N. S. (2010). *Pathophysiology: The biologic basis for disease in adults and children* (6th ed.). St. Louis: Mosby.

Minano, C., & Garcia-Tsao, G. (2010). Clinical pharmacology of portal hypertension. *Gastroenterology Clinics of North America, 39*(3), 681-695.

*Moore, S. (2007). Management of hepatic colorectal metastases: A shifting paradigm. *Colorectal Cancer Nursing, 1*(2), 4-7.

Pagana, K., & Pagana, T. (2010). *Mosby's manual of diagnostic and laboratory tests* (4th ed.). St. Louis: Mosby.

Pozza, R. (2008). Clinical management of HIV/hepatitis C virus coinfection. *Journal of the American Academy of Nurse Practitioners, 20*(10), 496-505.

Rossi, L., Zoratto, F., Papa, A., Iodice, F., Minozzi, M., Frati, L., et al. (2010). Current approach in the treatment of hepatocellular carcinoma. *World Journal of Gastroenterology Oncology, 2*(9), 348-359.

Sgorbini, M., O'Brien, L., & Jackson, D. (2009). Living with hepatitis C and treatment: The personal experience of patients. *Journal of Clinical Nursing, 18*(16), 2282-2291.

Chapter 62

American Cancer Society (ACS). (2010). *Cancer facts and figures—2010.* Atlanta: Author.

*Amerine, E. (2007). Get optimum outcomes for acute pancreatitis patients. *The Nurse Practitioner, 32*(6), 44-48.

Attasaranya, S., Fogel, E. L., & Lehman, G. A. (2008). Choledocholithiasis, ascending cholangitis, and gallstone pancreatitis. *Medical Clinics of North America, 92*(4), 925-960.

Bharwani, N., Patel, S., Prabhusesal, S., Fortheringham, T., & Power, N. (2011). Acute pancreatitis: The role of imaging in diagnosis and management. *Clinical Radiology, 66*(2), 164-175.

Binenbaum, S. J., Teixeira, J. A., Forrester, G. L., Harvey, E. J., Afthinos, J., Kim, G. J., et al. (2009). Single-incision laparoscopic cholecystectomy using a flexible endoscope. *Archives of Surgery, 144*(8), 734-738.

Comstock, D. (2008). Dealing with postcholecystectomy syndrome. *Nursing2008, 38*(4), 17-19.

Daniak, C. N., Peretz, D., Fine, J. M., Wang, Y., Meinke, A. K., & Hale, W. B. (2008). Factors associated with time to laparoscopic cholecystectomy for acute cholecystitis. *World Journal of Gastroenterology, 14*(7), 1084-1090.

Fusaroli, P., Spada, A., Mancino, M. G., & Caletti, G. (2010). Contrast harmonic echo-endoscopic ultrasound improves accuracy in diagnosis of solid pancreatic masses. *Journal of Gastroenterology and Hepatology, 8*(7), 629-634.

*Halls, B. S., & Ward-Smith, P. (2007). Identifying early symptoms of pancreatic cancer. *Clinical Journal of Oncology Nursing, 11*(2), 245-248.

*Holcomb, S. S. (2007). Stopping the destruction of acute pancreatitis. *Nursing2007, 37*(6), 43-48.

Hubb, H. A., & Saunders, M. (2011). The yellow bird of jaundice: Recognizing biliary obstruction. *Nursing2011, 41*(10), 28-36.

McCance, K. L., Huether, S. E., Brashers, V. L., & Rote, N. R. (2010). *Pathophysiology: The biologic basis for disease in adults and children* (6th ed.). St. Louis: Mosby.

Midha, S., Khajuria, R., Shastri, S., Kabra, M., & Garg, P. K. (2010). Idiopathic chronic pancreatitis in India: Phenotypic characterization and strong genetic susceptibility due to SPINK1 and CFTR gene mutations. *Gut, 59*(6), 800-807.

Navarra, G., La Malfa, G., Lazzara, S., Ullo, G., & Curro, G. (2010). SILS and NOTES cholecystectomy: A tailored approach. *Journal of Laparoscopic and Advanced Surgical Technologies, 20*(6), 511-514.

Novotny, I., Dite, P., Lata, J., Nechutova, H., & Klanicka, B. (2010). Autoimmune pancreatitis: Recent advances. *Digestive Diseases, 28*(2), 334-338.

Pagana, K. D., & Pagana, T. J. (2010). *Mosby's manual of diagnostic and laboratory tests* (4th ed.). St. Louis: Mosby.

*Riehl, M. (2007). Help your patient cope with pancreatic cancer. *Nursing2007, 37*(4), 54-57.

Simmons, S. (2010). Gallstones. *Nursing2010, 37*(11), 37.

Targarona, E. M., Maldonado, M., Marzol, J. A., & Marinello, F. (2010). Natural orifice transluminal endoscopic surgery: The transvaginal route moving forward from cholecystectomy. *World Journal of Gastroenterology Surgery, 2*(6), 179-186.

Van Laethem, J. L., & Marechal, R. (2007). Emerging drugs for the treatment of pancreatic cancer. *Expert Opinion on Emerging Drugs, 12*(2), 301-311.

Chapter 63

American Heart Association. (2010). Knowing your fats. Retrieved March 30, 2011, from www.heart.org.

Bankhead, R., Boullata, J., Brantley, S., Corkins, M., Guenter, P., Krenitsky, J., et al. (2009). Enteral nutrition administration. In A.S.P.E.N. enteral nutrition practice recommendations. *Journal of Parenteral Enteral Nutrition, 33*(2), 149-158.

*Barth, M. M., & Jenson, C. E. (2006). Postoperative nursing care of gastric bypass patients. *American Journal of Critical Care, 15*(4), 378-388.

*Bender, S., Pusateri, M., Cook, A., Ferguson, M., & Hall, J. C. (2000). Malnutrition: Role of the TwoCal® HN Med Pass Program. *MEDSURG Nursing, 9*(6), 284-296.

Camden, S. G. (2009). Obesity: An emerging concern for patients and nurses. *OJIN: The Online Journal of Issues in Nursing, 14*(1). Retrieved March 30, 2011, from http://nursingworld.org/MainMenuCategories/ANAMarketplace/ANAPeriodicals/OJIN/TableofContents/Vol142009/No1Jan09.

Centers for Disease Control and Prevention (CDC). (2009). About BMI for adults. Retrieved March 30, 2011, from www.cdc.gov/healthyweight/assessing/bmi/adult_bmi/index.html.

Clancy, C. (2010). Focus on obesity. Retrieved March 30, 2011, from www.ahrq.gov.

Clutts, B. (2009). Recognition and management of complications following Roux-en-Y gastric bypass: A guide for health care workers in non-bariatric hospitals. *MEDSURG Nursing, 18*(6), 335-341.

Conte, C., Cascino, A., Bartali, B., Donini, L., Rossi-Fanelli, F., & Vaiano, A. (2009). Anorexia of aging. *Current Nutrition & Food Science, 5,* 9-12.

*DiMaria-Ghalili, R. A., & Amella, E. (2005). Nutrition in older adults. *AJN, 105*(3), 40-50.

DiMaria-Ghalili, R. A., & Guenter, P. (2008). The Mini Nutritional Assessment. *AJN, 108*(2), 48-49.

*Elpern, E. H., Killeen, K., Talla, E., Perez, G., & Gurka, D. (2007). Capnometry and air insufflation for assessing initial placement of gastric tubes. *American Journal of Critical Care, 16*(6), 544-550.

*Grindel, M. E., & Grindel, C. G. (2006). Nursing care of the person having bariatric surgery. *MEDSURG Nursing, 15*(3), 129-144.

* Harrington, L. (2006). Postoperative care of patients undergoing bariatric surgery. *MEDSURG Journal, 15*(6), 357-363.

*Health Canada. (2007). Eating well with Canada's Food Guide: First Nations, Inuit, and Métis. Retrieved on August 19, 2011 from www.hc-sc.gc.ca/fn-an/food-guide-aliment/index_e.html.

Jarvis, C. (2012). *Physical examination and health assessment* (6th ed.). Philadelphia: Saunders.

Kaser, N. J., & Kukla, A. (2009). Weight loss surgery. *OJIN: The Online Journal of Issues in Nursing, 14*(1). Retrieved March 30, 2011, from http://nursingworld.org/MainMenuCategories/ANAMarketplace/ANAPeriodicals/OJIN/TableofContents/Vol142009/No1Jan09.

Kulie, T., Slattengren, A., Redmer, J., Counts, H., Eglash, A., & Schranger, S. (2011). Obesity and women's health: An evidence-based review. *Journal of the American Board of Family Medicine, 24*(1), 75-78.

Lee, J., Visser, M., Tylavsky, F., Kritchevsky, S., Schwartz, A., Sahyoun, N., et al. (2010). Weight loss and regain and effects on body composition: The health, aging, and body composition study. *The Journals of Gerontology, Series A, 65*(1), 78-83.

McCance, K. L., Huether, S. E., Brashers, V. L., & Rote, N. R. (2010). *Pathophysiology: The biologic basis for disease in adults and children* (6th ed.). St. Louis: Mosby.

Mehanna, H. M., Moledina, J., & Travis, J. (2008). Refeeding syndrome: What it is, and how to prevent and treat it. *BMJ, 336,* 1495-1498.

Muir, M., & Archer-Heese, G. (2009). Essentials of a bariatric patient handling program. *OJIN: The Online Journal of Issues in Nursing, 14*(1). Retrieved March 30, 2011, from http://nursingworld.org/MainMenuCategories/ANAMarketplace/ANAPeriodicals/OJIN/TableofContents/Vol142009/No1Jan09.

National Agriculture Library. (2008). Vegetarian nutrition resource list. Retrieved March 30, 2011, from www.nal.usda.gov.

National Heart, Lung, and Blood Institute. (2011). Calculating your body mass index. Retrieved March 30, 2011, from www.nhlbisupport.com/bmi/.

National Institute of Diabetes and Digestive and Kidney Diseases. (2008). Weight and waist measurement: Tools for adults. Retrieved March 30, 2011, from www.win.niddk.nih.gov.

Pagana, K. D., & Pagana, T. J. (2010). *Mosby's manual of diagnostic and laboratory tests* (4th ed.). St. Louis: Mosby.

Palmer, J. L., & Metheney, N. A. (2008). Preventing aspiration in older adults with dysphagia. *AJN, 108*(2), 40-47.

Pettit, E. (2009). Treating morbid obesity: Surgery is often a last resort, but can be a life-saving choice that improves self-esteem and overall quality of life. *RN, 72*(2), 30-35.

*Sudakin, T. (2006). T.E.N. or T.P.N. *Nursing2006, 36*(12), 52-55.

Tufts University. (2011). Modified MyPyramid for older adults. Retrieved March 30, 2011, from nutrition.tufts.edu.

U.S. Department of Agriculture (USDA). (2010). Dietary guidelines for Americans, 2010. Retrieved August 19, 2011, from www.cnpp.usda.gov/DGAs2010-DGACReport.htm.

Yantis, M. A., & Verlander, R. (2011). Untangling enteral nutrition guidelines. *Nursing2011, 41*(9), 33-39.

Yoon, M. N., Lowe, M., Budgell, M., & Steele, C. M. (2011) An exploratory investigation using appreciative inquiry to promote nursing oral care. *Geriatric Nursing, 32*(5), 326-340.

Chapter 64

Davis, G. (2007). Hormonal control and the endocrine system: Achieving homeostasis. *Nurse Prescribing, 4*(11), 446-453.

Gordon, M. (2011). *Manual of nursing diagnosis* (12th ed.). New York: Jones & Bartlett.

Jarvis, C. (2012). *Physical examination and health assessment* (6th ed.). Philadelphia: Saunders.

Klee, G. (2008). Laboratory techniques for recognition of endocrine disorders. In H. Kronenberg, S. Melmed, K. Polonsky, & P. R. Larsen (Eds.), *Williams' textbook of endocrinology* (11th ed.). Philadelphia: Saunders.

Kronenberg, H., Melmed, S., Polonsky, K., & Larsen, P. R. (Eds.). (2008). *Williams' textbook of endocrinology* (11th ed.). Philadelphia: Saunders.

Lamberts, S. (2008). Endocrinology and aging. In H. Kronenberg, S. Melmed, K. Polonsky, & P. R. Larsen (Eds.), *Williams' textbook of endocrinology* (11th ed.). Philadelphia: Saunders.

McCance, K., Huether, S., Brashers, V., & Rote, N. (2010). *Pathophysiology: The biologic basis for disease in adults and children* (6th ed.). St. Louis: Mosby.

Nussbaum, R., McInnes, R., & Willard, H. (2007). *Thompson & Thompson: Genetics in medicine* (7th ed.). Philadelphia: Saunders.

Pagana, K., & Pagana, T. (2010). *Mosby's manual of diagnostic and laboratory tests* (4th ed.). St. Louis: Mosby.

Touhy, T., & Jett, K. (2010). *Ebersole and Hess' gerontological nursing & healthy aging* (3rd ed.). St. Louis: Mosby.

Chapter 65

Belavic, J. (2010). Drug approvals. *The Nurse Practitioner, 35*(2), 12-23.

Collins, M., & Claros, E. (2011). Recognizing the face of dehydration. *Nursing2011, 41*(8), 26-31.

Cook, L. (2009). Pheochromocytoma. *AJN, 109*(2), 50-53.

Crawford, A., & Harris, H. (2011). Balancing act: Na+ and K+. *Nursing2011, 41*(7), 44-50.

Daub, K. (2008). Pheochromocytoma: An elusive diagnosis. *Nursing2008, 38*(1), 56hn1-56hn2.

Fitzgerald, M. (2008). Hyponatremia associated with SSRI use in a 65-year-old woman. *The Nurse Practitioner, 33*(2), 11-12.

Fraser, L., & Van Uum, S. (2010). Work-up for Cushing syndrome. *Canadian Medical Association Journal, 182*(6), 584-587.

Graham, S. M., Iseli, T. A., Karnell, L. H., Clinger, J. D., Hitchon, P. W., & Greenlee, J. D. (2009). Endoscopic approach for pituitary surgery improves rhinologic outcomes. *Annals of Otology, Rhinology & Laryngology, 118*(9), 630-635.

McCance, K., Huether, S., Brashers, V., & Rote, N. (2010). *Pathophysiology: The biologic basis for disease in adults and children* (6th ed.). St. Louis: Mosby.

Melmed, S., & Kleinberg, D. (2008). Anterior pituitary. In H. Kronenberg, S. Melmed, K. Polonsky, & P. R. Larsen (Eds.), *Williams' textbook of endocrinology* (11th ed., pp. 155-261). Philadelphia: Saunders.

Pagana, K., & Pagana, T. (2010). *Mosby's manual of diagnostic and laboratory tests* (4th ed.). St. Louis: Mosby.

Radovich, P. (2010). Primary adrenal insufficiency: Elusive and potentially life-threatening. *American Nurse Today, 5*(3), 37-39.

Robinson, A., & Verbalis, J. (2008). Posterior pituitary. In H. Kronenberg, S. Melmed, K. Polonsky, & P. R. Larsen (Eds.), *Williams' textbook of endocrinology* (11th ed., pp. 263-295). Philadelphia: Saunders.

Rottmann, C. (2007). SSRIs and the syndrome of inappropriate antidiuretic hormone secretion. *AJN, 107*(1), 51-58.

Simmons, S. (2010). Flushing out the truth about diabetes insipidus. *Nursing2010, 40*(1), 55-59.

Stewart, P. (2008). The adrenal cortex. In H. Kronenberg, S. Melmed, K. Polonsky, & P. R. Larsen (Eds.), *Williams' textbook of endocrinology* (11th ed., pp. 445-503). Philadelphia: Saunders.

Touhy, T., & Jett., K. (2010). *Ebersole and Hess' gerontological nursing & healthy aging* (3rd ed.). St. Louis: Mosby.

Tsegay, E., Anyango, G., Van Sell, S., & Miller-Anderson, M. (2008). Pheochromocytoma: A rare tumor in adults and children. *RN, 71*(6), 31-34.

Young, W. (2008). Endocrine hypertension. In H. Kronenberg, S. Melmed, K. Polonsky, & P. R. Larsen (Eds.), *Williams' textbook of endocrinology* (11th ed., pp. 505-537). Philadelphia: Saunders.

Chapter 66

Al-Shakhrah, I. (2008). Radioprotection using iodine-131 for thyroid cancer and hyperthyroidism: A review. *Clinical Journal of Oncology Nursing, 12*(6), 905-912.

American Cancer Society. (2011). *Cancer facts and figures 2011.* Report No. 00-300M—No. 5008.11. Atlanta: Author.

Aschenbrenner, D. (2009). Treatment for Graves' disease poses risk of liver failure. *AJN, 109*(10), 33.

Brent, G., Larsen, P. R., & Davies, T. (2008). Hypothyroidism and thyroiditis. In H. Kronenberg, S. Melmed, K. Polonsky, & P. R. Larsen (Eds.), *Williams' textbook of endocrinology* (11th ed., pp. 377-409). Philadelphia: Saunders.

Burton, J. (2011). Hyperthyroidism. *MEDSURG Nursing, 20*(3), 152-153.

Crawford, A., & Harris, H. (2011). Balancing act: Hypomagnesemia and hypermagnesemia. *Nursing2011, 41*(10), 52-55.

Davies, T., & Larsen, P. R. (2008). Thyrotoxicosis. In H. Kronenberg, S. Melmed, K. Polonsky, & P. R. Larsen (Eds.), *Williams' textbook of endocrinology* (11th ed., pp. 333-375). Philadelphia: Saunders.

Devdhar, M., Ousman, Y., & Burman, K. (2007). Hypothyroidism. *Endocrinology and Metabolism Clinics of North America, 36*(4), 595-615.

Kasputin, J. (2010). Hypothyroidism: An evidence-based approach to a complex disorder. *The Nurse Practitioner, 35*(8), 44-53.

Kessenich, C., & Higgs, D. (2010). Understanding amiodarone-induced hypothyroidism. *The Nurse Practitioner, 35*(6), 14-15.

Kronenberg, H., Melmed, S., Polonsky, K., & Larsen, P. R. (Eds.). (2008). *Williams' textbook of endocrinology* (11th ed.). Philadelphia: Saunders.

Leung, M.-K., Platt, M., & Metson, R. (2009). Revision endoscopic orbital decompression in the management of Graves' orbitopathy. *Otolaryngology-Head and Neck Surgery, 141*(1), 46-51.

McAdams-Jones, D. (2008). Calming a thyroid storm. *American Nurse Today, 3*(12), 31.

McCance, K., Huether, S., Brashers, V., & Rote, N. (2010). *Pathophysiology: The biologic basis for disease in adults and children* (6th ed.). St. Louis: Mosby.

Nussbaum, R., McInnes, R., & Willard, H. (2007). *Thompson & Thompson: Genetics in medicine* (7th ed.). Philadelphia: Saunders.

Pagana, K., & Pagana, T. (2010). *Mosby's manual of diagnostic and laboratory tests* (4th ed.). St. Louis: Mosby.

Simmons, S. (2010). A delicate balance: Detecting thyroid disease. *Nursing2010, 40*(7), 29.

Snissarenko, E. P., Kim, G. H., Simental, A. A., Jr., Zwart, J. E., Ransbarger, D. M., & Kim, P. D. (2009). Minimally invasive video-assisted thyroidectomy: A retrospective study over two years of experience. *Otolaryngology-Head and Neck Surgery, 141*(1), 29-33.

Touhy, T., & Jett, K. (2010). *Ebersole and Hess' gerontological nursing & healthy aging* (3rd ed.). St. Louis: Mosby.

Chapter 67

Acee, A. (2010). Detecting and managing depression in type II diabetes: PHQ-9 is the answer! *MEDSURG Nursing, 19*(1), 32-37.

American Association of Diabetes Educators (AADE). (2008). Position statement: Diabetes and exercise. *The Diabetes Educator, 34*(1), 37-40.

American Association of Diabetes Educators (AADE). (2009a). Position statement: Diabetic kidney disease. *The Diabetes Educator, 35*(Suppl. 3), 53-56.

American Association of Diabetes Educators (AADE). (2009b). Position statement: Primary prevention of type 2 diabetes. *The Diabetes Educator, 35*(Suppl. 3), 57-59.

American Diabetes Association (ADA). (2008). Position statement: Nutritional recommendations and interventions for diabetes. *Diabetes Care, 31*(Suppl. 1), 61-78.

American Diabetes Association (ADA). (2009). ADA Workgroup report: International expert committee report on the role of the A_{1c} assay in the diagnosis of diabetes. *Diabetes Care, 32*(7), 1327-1334.

American Diabetes Association (ADA). (2010a). Position statement: Diagnosis and classification of diabetes mellitus. *Diabetes Care, 33*(Suppl. 1), 14.

American Diabetes Association (ADA). (2010b). Position statement: Standards of medical care in diabetes—2010. *Diabetes Care, 33*(Suppl. 1), 11-61.

American Diabetes Association (ADA). (2010c). Executive summary: Standards of medical care in diabetes—2010. *Diabetes Care, 33*(Suppl. 1), 4-10.

American Diabetes Association (ADA). (2011). National diabetes fact sheet. Retrieved September 2011 from www.diabetes.org/diabetes-basics/diabetes-statistics/.

Appel, S. (2011). Tapping incretin-based therapy for type 2 diabetes. *Nursing2011, 41*(3), 49-51.

Appel, S., Wright, M., Hill, A., & Ovalle, F. (2008). Uncovering imperative interventions in prediabetes & type 2 diabetes. *The Nurse Practitioner, 33*(8), 20-26.

Bedlack, R. (2009). The management of diabetic neuropathy and glycemic control in long-term care facilities. *Clinical Geriatrics, 17*(4), 4-9.

Belavic, J. (2010). A new treatment option for type 2 diabetes. *The Nurse Practitioner, 35*(1), 51-52.

Cranwell-Bruce, L. (2009). Update in diabetes management. *MEDSURG Nursing, 18*(1), 51-53.

Deatcher, J. (2008). Prediabetes. *AJN, 108*(7), 77-79.

Fleury-Milfort, E. (2009). Optimizing outcomes with incretin-based therapies: Practical information for nurse practitioners to share with patients. *Journal of the American Academy of Nurse Practitioners, 21*(Suppl. 1), 642-650.

Flood, L. (2009). Nurse-patient interactions related to diabetes foot care. *MEDSURG Nursing, 18*(6), 361-368.

Foot care for people with diabetes. (2010). *Nursing2010, 40*(1), 33.

Fowler, M. (2009). Hyperglycemic crisis in adults: Pathophysiology, presentation pitfalls, and prevention. *Clinical Diabetes, 27*(1), 19-23.

Hill, A., & Appel, S. (2009). Signs of improvement: Diabetes update 2009. *The Nurse Practitioner, 34*(6), 12-22.

Longo, R. (2010). Understanding oral antidiabetic agents: How to make sense of this vast armamentarium. *AJN, 110*(2), 49-52.

Martin, C. (2010). DPP-4 inhibitors: A new option for diabetes management. *American Nurse Today, 35*(11), 29-31.

McCance, K. L., Huether, S. E., Brashers, V., & Rote, N. (Eds.). (2010). Pathophysiology: The biologic basis for disease in adults & children (6th ed.). St. Louis: Mosby.

Meneily, G. (2010). Pathophysiology of diabetes in the elderly. *Clinical Geriatrics, 18*(4), 25-28.

Moghissi, E. S., Korytkowski, M. T., DiNardo, M., Einhorn, D., Hellman, R., Hirsch, I. B., et al. (2009). American Association of Clinical Endocrinologists and American Diabetes Association consensus statement on inpatient glycemic control. *Diabetes Care, 32*(6), 1119-1131.

Mozaffarian, D., Kamineni, A., Carnethon, M., Djoussé, L., Mukamal, K. J., & Siscovik, D. (2009). Lifestyle risk factors and new onset diabetes mellitus in older adults: The cardiovascular health study. *Archives of Internal Medicine, 169*(8), 798-807.

National Institute of Diabetes and Digestive and Kidney Diseases (NIDDK) of the National Institutes of Health. (2011). National Diabetes Information Clearing House: National diabetes statistics, 2011. Retrieved March, 2011, from www.diabetes.niddk.nih.gov/dm/pubs/statistics/.

Nussbaum, R., McInnes, R., & Willard, H. (2007). *Thompson & Thompson: Genetics in medicine* (7th ed.). Philadelphia: Saunders.

Peyrot, M., Rubin, R., Kruger, D., & Travis, L. (2010). Correlates of insulin injection omission. *Diabetes Care, 33*(2), 240-245.

Roberts, R. O., Geda, Y. E., Knopman, D. S., Christianson, T. J., Pankratz, V. S., Boeve, B. F., et al. (2008). Association of duration and severity of diabetes mellitus with mild cognitive impairment. *Archives of Neurology, 65*(8), 1066-1073.

Robertson, C. (2009). New developments in incretin-based therapies: The current state of the field. *Journal of the American Academy of Nurse Practitioners, 21*(Suppl. 1), 631-641.

Roelker, E. (2008). Screening for coronary artery disease in patients with diabetes. *Diabetes Spectrum, 21*(3), 166-171.

Voda, S. (2008). Improving diabetes education for minority groups. *Nursing2008, 38*(7), 12-13.

Wick, A., & Newlin, K. (2009). Incretin-based therapies: Therapeutic rationale and pharmacological promise for type 2 diabetes. *Journal of the American Academy of Nurse Practitioners, 21*(Suppl. 1), 623-630.

Young, J. (2011). Educating staff nurses on diabetes: Knowledge enhancement. *MEDSURG Nursing, 20*(3), 143-146, 150.

Chapter 68

Bixby, M., & Giuliano, K. (2008). Bladder pressure monitoring. *AACN Advanced Critical Care, 19*(4), 349-353.

Brenner, B. M. (Ed.). (2008). *Brenner & Rector's the kidney* (8th ed.). Philadelphia: Saunders.

Counts, C. (Ed.). (2008). *Core curriculum for nephrology nursing* (5th ed.). Pitman, NJ: American Nephrology Nurses Association.

Daniel, K., & Cason, C. (2007). Estimating glomerular filtration rate in the elderly. *Journal for Nurse Practitioners, 3*(4), 242-244.

Dong, K., & Quan, D. (2010). Appropriately assessing renal function for drug dosing. *Nephrology Nursing Journal, 37*(3), 304-308.

Fields, W., Tedeschi, C., Foltz, J., Myers, T., Heaney, K., Bosak, K., et al. (2008). Reducing preventable safety events by recognizing renal risk. *Clinical Nurse Specialist, 22*(2), 73-78.

Gordon, M. (2011). *Manual of nursing diagnosis* (12th ed.). New York: Jones & Bartlett.

Gray-Vickery, P. (2010). Gathering "pearls" of knowledge for assessing older adults. *Nursing2010, 40*(3), 34-42.

Harris, T. A. (2010). Changing practice to reduce the use of urinary catheters. *Nursing2010, 40*(2), 18-20.

Jarvis, C. (2012). *Physical examination and health assessment* (6th ed.). Philadelphia: Saunders.

Kohtz, C., & Thompson, M. (2007). Preventing contrast medium–induced nephropathy. *AJN, 107*(9), 40-49.

Matteucci, R. (2009). *Urinary catheter use and prevention of infection. Evidence-Based Care Sheet*, Glendale, CA: CINAHL Information Systems.

McCance, K., Huether, S., Brashers, V., & Rote, N. (2010). *Pathophysiology: The biologic basis for disease in adults and children* (6th ed.). St. Louis: Mosby.

Morrell, G. (2010). False reading of retained urine from a bladder scan. *Urologic Nursing, 30*(2), 147-148.

Newman, D. (2009). Talking to patients about bladder control problems. *The Nurse Practitioner, 34*(12), 33-45.

Nussbaum, R., McInnes, R., & Willard, H. (2007). *Thompson & Thompson: Genetics in medicine* (7th ed.). Philadelphia: Saunders.

Pagana, K. D., & Pagana, T. J. (2010). *Mosby's manual of diagnostic and laboratory tests* (4th ed.). St. Louis: Mosby.

Potter, P., Perry, A., Stockert, P., & Hall, A. (2011). *Basic nursing* (7th ed.). St. Louis: Mosby.

Touhy, T., & Jett, K. (2010). *Ebersole and Hess' gerontological nursing & healthy aging* (3rd ed.). St. Louis: Mosby.

U.S. Renal Data Systems. (2010). *USRDS 2009 annual data report.* Bethesda, MD: The National Kidney and Urologic Diseases Information Clearinghouse (NKUDIC). National Institutes of Health.

Voss, A. (2009). Incidence and duration of urinary catheters in hospitalized older adults before and after implementing a geriatric protocol. *Journal of Gerontological Nursing, 35*(6), 35-41.

Wein, A. J., Kavoussi, L. R., Novick, A. C., Partin, A. W., & Peters, C. A. (2007). *Campbell-Walsh urology* (9th ed.). Philadelphia: Saunders.

Woodward, S. (2010). The need for best practice in catheterization. *British Journal of Nursing, 19*(12), 740.

Chapter 69

*Agency for Health Care Policy and Research (AHCPR). (1996). (Revised 2001a). *Urinary incontinence in adults: Acute and chronic management. Clinical practice guideline.* AHCPR Publication No. 96-0682. Rockville, MD: Agency for Health Care Policy and Research, Public Health Service, U.S. Department of Health and Human Services.

*Agency for Health Care Policy and Research (AHCPR). (1996). (Revised 2001b). *Urinary incontinence in adults: Helping people with incontinence. Clinical practice guideline.* AHCPR Publication No. 96-0683. Rockville, MD: Agency for Health Care Policy and Research, Public Health Service, U.S. Department of Health and Human Services.

American Cancer Society (ACS). (2011). *Cancer facts and figures 2011.* Report No. 01-300M–5008.11. Atlanta: Author.

Belavic, J. (2009). Fesoterodine for the treatment of overactive bladder. *The Nurse Practitioner, 34*(8), 14-15.

Bixby, M., & Giuliano, K. (2008). Bladder pressure monitoring. *AACN Advanced Critical Care, 19*(4), 349-353.

Bowen, A., & Hellstrom, W. J. G. (2007). Urinary tract infections: A primer for clinicians. Retrieved June 15, 2007, from www.Medscape.com.

Bradway, C., & Rodgers, J. (2009). Evaluation and management of genitourinary emergencies. *The Nurse Practitioner, 34*(5), 36-43.

Bray, B., Van Sell, S., & Miller-Anderson, M. (2007). Stress incontinence: It's no laughing matter. *RN, 70*(4), 25-29.

Brenner, B. (2008). *Brenner & Rector's the kidney* (8th ed.). Philadelphia: Saunders.

Carpenter, D., & Visovsky, C. (2010). Stress urinary incontinence: A review of treatment options. *AORN Journal, 91*(4), 471-480.

Centers for Disease Control and Prevention (CDC). (2009). Guideline for prevention of catheter-associated urinary tract infections, 2009. Retrieved October 15, 2010, from www.cdc.gov/hicpac/cauti/001_cauti.html.

Crestodina, L. (2007). Assessment and management of urinary incontinence in the elderly male. *The Nurse Practitioner, 32*(9), 26-34.

Dowling-Castronovo, A., & Specht, J. (2009). Assessment of transient urinary incontinence in older adults. *AJN, 109*(2), 62-71.

Ellsworth, P., & Kirshenbaum, E. (2010). Update on the pharmacologic management of overactive bladder: The present and the future. *Urologic Nursing, 30*(1), 29-38, 53.

Elpern, E. H., Killeen, K., Ketchem, A., Wiley, A., Patel, G., & Lateef, O. (2009). Reducing use of indwelling urinary catheters and associated urinary tract infections. *American Journal of Critical Care, 18*(6), 535-541.

Evans, R. J., & Sant, G. R. (2007). Current diagnosis of interstitial cystitis: An evolving paradigm. *Urology, 69*(Suppl. 4), S64-S72.

Forrest, J. B., & Dell, J. R. (2007). Successful management of interstitial cystitis in clinical practice. *Urology, 69*(Suppl. 4), S82-S86.

Gemmill, R., Ferrell, B., Krouse, R., & Grant, M. (2010). Going with the flow: Quality-of-life outcomes of cancer survivors with urinary diversion. *Journal of the Wound, Ostomy and Continence Nurses, 37*(1), 65-72.

Gray, M. (2010). Reducing catheter-associated urinary tract infections in the critical care unit. *AACN Advanced Critical Care, 21*(3), 247-257.

Harris, T. (2010). Changing practice to reduce the use of urinary catheters. *Nursing2010, 40*(2), 18-20.

Kannankeril, A., Lam, H., Reyes, E., & McCartney, J. (2011). Urinary tract infection rates associated with re-use of catheters in clean intermittent catheterization of male veterans. *Urologic Nursing, 31*(1), 41-48.

Katz, A. (2009). When worlds collide: Urinary incontinence and female sexuality. *AJN, 109*(3), 59-63.

Kessenich, C. (2010). Urosepsis in the elderly. *The Nurse Practitioner, 35*(11), 10-11.

McCance, K., Huether, S., Brashers, V., & Rote, N. (2010). *Pathophysiology: The biologic basis for disease in adults and children* (6th ed.). St. Louis: Mosby.

McDermott, P. (2009). Painful bladder syndrome/interstitial cystitis (history, epidemiology, symptoms, diagnosis and treatments). *International Journal of Urological Nursing, 3*(1), 16-23.

Newman, D. (2009). Talking to patients about bladder control problems. *The Nurse Practitioner, 34*(12), 33-45.

Newman, D., & Willson, M. (2011). Review of intermittent catheterization and current best practices. *Urologic Nursing, 31*(1), 12-29, 48.

Nussbaum, R., McInnes, R., & Willard, H. (2007). *Thompson & Thompson: Genetics in medicine* (7th ed.). Philadelphia: Saunders.

Pagana, K., & Pagana, T. (2010). *Mosby's manual of diagnostic and laboratory tests* (4th ed.). St. Louis: Mosby.

Pelter, M., & Stephens, K. (2008). Evaluation of a device to facilitate female catheterization. *MEDSURG Nursing, 17*(1), 19-25.

Pelvic Pain and Urgency Frequency symptom scale: PUF questionnaire. (2005). Retrieved June 17, 2007, from www.orthoelmiron.com/orthoelmiron/hcptools_puf.html?host=www.orthoelmiron.com.

Saldano, D. (2008). Urinary tract infection: Finding an answer when conventional testing is not helpful. *Urologic Nursing, 28*(4), 267-268.

Siegel, J., Sand, P., & Sasso, K. (2008). Vulvodynia and pelvic pain? Think interstitial cystitis. *The Nurse Practitioner, 33*(10), 40-45.

Touhy, T., & Jett, K. (2010). *Ebersole and Hess' gerontological nursing & healthy aging* (3rd ed.). St. Louis: Mosby.

U.S. Renal Data Systems. (2010). *USRDS 2009 annual data report.* Bethesda, MD: The National Kidney and Urologic Diseases Information Clearinghouse (NKUDIC). National Institutes of Health.

Washburn, D. (2007). Intravesicular antineoplastic therapy following transurethral resection of bladder tumors: Nursing implications from the operating room to discharge. *Clinical Journal of Oncology Nursing, 11*(4), 553-559.

Zurakowski, T., Taylor, M., & Bradway, C. (2006). Effective teaching strategies for the older adult with urologic concerns. *Urologic Nursing, 26*(5), 355-360.

Chapter 70

American Cancer Society. (2011). *Cancer facts and figures 2011.* Report No. 00-300M–No. 5008.11. Atlanta: Author.

Bilous, R. (2010). Diabetic nephropathy: Diagnosis, screening and management. *Diabetes & Primary Care, 12*(2), 105-114.

Brenner, B. (Ed.). (2008). *Brenner & Rector's the kidney* (8th ed.). Philadelphia: Saunders.

Byar, K., & Workman, M. (2012). Targeted therapies to treat cancer. In J. Kee, E. Hayes, & L. McCuistion (Eds.), *Pharmacology: A nursing process approach* (7th ed.). St. Louis: Saunders.

*Cope, D, & Reb, A. (Eds.). (2006). *An evidence-based approach to the treatment and care of the older adult with cancer.* Pittsburgh: Oncology Nursing Society.

Creel, P. (2009). Management of mTOR inhibitor side effects. *Clinical Journal of Oncology Nursing, 13*(6), 19-23.

De Zeeuw, D. (2007). Albuminuria: A target for treatment of type 2 diabetic nephropathy. *Seminars in Nephrology, 27*(2), 172-181.

Dong, K., & Quan, D. (2010). Appropriately assessing renal function for drug dosing. *Nephrology Nursing Journal, 37*(3), 304-308.

Garcia, J. A., & Rini, B. I. (2007). Recent progress in the management of advanced renal cell carcinoma. *CA: A Cancer Journal for Clinicians, 57*(2), 112-125.

Gomez, N. (Ed.). (2008). *Core curriculum for nephrology nursing* (5th ed.). Pitman, NJ: American Association of Nephrology Nurses.

Jemal, A., Siegel, R., Ward, E., Murray, T., Xu, J., & Thun, M. J. (2007). Cancer statistics, 2007. *CA: A Cancer Journal for Clinicians, 57*(1), 43-67.

Joseph, J., & Chowdhury, P. (2009). Percutaneous renal biopsy. *British Journal of Hospital Medicine, 70*(4), M59-M61.

Kidney Cancer Association. (2010). About kidney cancer. Retrieved September 2011, from www.kidneycancer.org/.

Kodner, C. (2009). Nephrotic syndrome in adults: Diagnosis and management. *American Family Physician, 80*(10), 1129-1134, 1136.

LeHir, M., & Kriz, W. (2007). New insights into structural patterns encountered in glomerulosclerosis. *Current Opinions in Nephrology and Hypertension, 16*(3), 184-191.

Malizzia, L., & Hsu, A. (2008). Temsirolimus, an mTOR inhibitor for treatment of patients with advanced renal cell carcinoma. *Clinical Journal of Oncology Nursing, 12*(4), 639-646.

McCance, K., Huether, S., Brashers, V., & Rote, N. (2010). *Pathophysiology: The biologic basis for disease in adults and children* (6th ed.). St. Louis: Mosby.

Moldawer, N., & Figlin, R. (2008). Renal cell carcinoma: The translation of molecular biology into new treatments, new patient outcomes, and nursing implications. *Oncology Nursing Forum, 35*(4), 699-708.

National Institute for Health and Clinical Excellence (NICE). (2008). *Chronic kidney disease: Early identification and management of chronic kidney disease in adults in primary and secondary care* (Clinical guideline; No. 73). Retrieved October 20, 2010, from www.guideline.gov/content.aspxid=14330.

Nussbaum, R., McInnes, R., & Willard, H. (2007). *Thompson & Thompson: Genetics in medicine* (7th ed.). Philadelphia: Saunders.

Pagana, K., & Pagana, T. (2010). *Mosby's manual of diagnostic and laboratory tests* (4th ed.). St. Louis: Mosby.

Polycystic Kidney Disease Foundation. (2010). 10 things every nephrologists should know about PKD. Retrieved September 2011 from www.pkdcure.org/home.html.

Russell, S. (2008). Responding to threats to the kidney. *Nursing2008, 38*(2), 36-40.

Shoham, D. A., Vupputuri, S., Diez Roux, A. V., Kaufman, J. S., Coresh, J., Kshirsagar, A. V., et al. (2007). Kidney disease in life-course socioeconomic context: The Atherosclerosis Risk in Communities (ARIC) Study. *American Journal of Kidney Disease, 49*(2), 217-226.

Thompson, J. (2009). Metastatic renal cell carcinoma: Current standards of care. *Clinical Journal of Oncology Nursing, 13*(6), 8-12.

Touhy, T., & Jett, K. (2010). *Ebersole and Hess' gerontological nursing & healthy aging* (3rd ed.). St. Louis: Mosby.

U.S. Renal Data Systems. (2010). *USRDS 2009 annual data report.* Bethesda, MD: The National Kidney and Urologic Diseases Information Clearinghouse (NKUDIC). National Institutes of Health.

Walker, P. (2009). The renal biopsy. *Archives of Pathological and Laboratory Medicine, 133*(2), 181-188.

Wood, L. (2007). Sorafenib: A promising new targeted therapy for renal cell carcinoma. *Clinical Journal of Oncology Nursing, 11*(5), 649-656.

Wood, L. (2009a). Management of vascular endothelial growth factors and multikinase inhibitor side effects. *Clinical Journal of Oncology Nursing, 13*(6), 13-18.

Wood, L. (2009b). Renal cell carcinoma: Screening, diagnosis, and prognosis. *Clinical Journal of Oncology Nursing, 13*(6), 3-7.

Wood, L. (2010). New therapeutic strategies for renal cell carcinoma. *Urologic Nursing, 30*(1), 40-53.

Chapter 71

Alcaraz, M., Brzostowicz, M., & Moran, J. (2008). Decreasing peritonitis infection rates. *Nephrology Nursing Journal, 35*(4), 421-423.

Ali, B., & Gray-Vickrey, P. (2011). Limiting the damage from acute kidney injury. *Nursing2011, 41*(3), 22-31.

Ali, T., Khan, I., Simpson, W., Prescott, G., Townend, J., Smith, W., et al. (2007). Incidence and outcomes in acute kidney injury: A comprehensive population-based study. *Journal of the American Society of Nephrology, 18*(4), 1282-1298.

Bagshaw, S. M. (2008). Short- and long-term survival after acute kidney injury. *Nephrology Dialysis Transplant, 23*(7), 2126-2128.

*Barone, C., Martin-Watson, A., & Barone, G. (2004). The postoperative care of the adult renal transplant recipient. *MEDSURG Nursing, 13*(5), 296-302.

Basile, C. (2008). The long-term prognosis of acute kidney injury: Acute renal failure as a cause of chronic kidney disease. *Journal of Nephrology, 21*(5), 657-662.

Bednarski, D., Castner, D., & Douglas, C. (2009). Interventions for acute tubular necrosis. *The Nurse Practitioner, 34*(8), 7-10.

Beto, J., & Nicholas, M. (2009). So just what can I eat? Nutritional care in patients with diabetes mellitus and chronic kidney disease. *Nephrology Nursing Journal, 36*(5), 497-505.

Boyle, M., & Baldwin, I. (2010). Understanding the continuous replacement therapy circuit for acute renal failure support. *AACN Advanced Critical Care, 21*(4), 367-375.

Brites, F. D., Fernandez, K. M., Verona, J., Malusardi, M. C., Ischoff, P., Beresan, H., et al. (2007). Chronic renal failure in diabetic patients increases lipid risk factors for atherosclerosis. *Diabetes Research and Clinical Practice, 75*(1), 35-41.

Broden, C. (2009). Acute renal failure and mechanical ventilation: Reality or myth? *Critical Care Nurse, 29*(2), 62-75.

Brown, L. J., Clark, P. C., Armstrong, K. A., Liping, Z., & Dunbar, S. B. (2010). Identification of modifiable chronic kidney disease risk factors by gender in an African-American cohort. *Nephrology Nursing Journal, 37*(2), 133-142.

Cano, N. (2007). Nutritional supplementation in adult patients on hemodialysis. *Journal of Renal Nutrition, 17*(1), 103-105.

Castner, D. (2008). Kidney dialysis. *Nursing2008, 38*(9), 45.

Castner, D. (2010). Understanding the stages of chronic kidney disease. *Nursing2010, 40*(5), 25-31.

Castro, M. (2009). Kidney transplant. *Nursing2009, 39*(3), 33.

Catizone, R., Malacarne, F., Bortot, A., Annaloro, M., Russo, G., Barilla, A., et al. (2010). Renal replacement therapy in elderly patients: Peritoneal dialysis. *Journal of Nephrology, 23*(Suppl. 15), S90-S97.

Chen, S., Chang, J., Chou, M., Lin, M., Chen, J., Sun, J., et al. (2008). Slowing renal function decline in chronic kidney disease patients after nephrology referral. *Nephrology, 13*(8), 730-736.

Chow, S., & Wong, F. (2010). Health-related quality of life in patients undergoing peritoneal dialysis: Effects of a nurse-led case management program. *Journal of Advanced Nursing*, 66(8), 1780-1792.

Coorey, G. M., Paykin, C., Singleton-Driscoll, L. C., & Gaston, R. S. (2009). Barriers to preemptive kidney transplantation. *AJN*, 109(11), 28-37.

Crowley, S. T., & Peixoto, A. J. (2009). Acute kidney injury in the intensive care unit. *Clinical Chest Medicine*, 30(1), 28-43.

Denhaerynck, K., Manhaeve, D., Dobbles, F., Garzoni, D., Nolte, C., & De Geest, S. (2007). Prevalence and consequences of nonadherence to hemodialysis regimens. *American Journal of Critical Care*, 16(3), 222-235.

Dinwiddie, L. (2008). A new long-term vascular access device for catheter dependent patients. *Nephrology Nursing*, 35(2), 170.

Dirkes, S. (2011). Acute kidney injury: Not just acute renal failure anymore? *Critical Care Nurse*, 31(1), 37-49.

Dirkes, S., & Hodge, K. (2007). Continuous renal replacement therapy in the adult intensive care unit: History and current trends. *Critical Care Nurse*, 27(2), 61-80.

Doss, S., Schiller, B., & Moran, J. (2008). Buttonhole cannulation: An unexpected outcome. *Nephrology Nursing Journal*, 35(4), 417-419.

Eskridge, M. (2010). Hypertension and chronic kidney disease: The role of lifestyle modification and medication management. *Nephrology Nursing Journal*, 37(1), 55-60, 99.

Gevirtz, C. (2009). Controlling pain: Managing post-transplantation pain syndromes. *Nursing2009*, 39(2), 60-61.

Jepson, R. (2009). Protect your patient from dialysis hypotension. *Nursing2009*, 39(11), 55-56.

Jepson, R., & Alonso, E. (2009). Overheated dialysate: A case report and review. *Nephrology Nursing Journal*, 36(5), 551-553.

Kohtz, C., & Thompson, M. (2007). Preventing contrast medium–induced nephropathy. *AJN*, 107(9), 40-49.

Kopyt, N. (2007). Management and treatment of chronic kidney disease. *The Nurse Practitioner*, 32(11), 14-23.

Kuchta, K., VanBuskirk, S., & Houglum, M. (2007). Helping patients with end-stage renal disease. *AJN*, 107(5), 35-36.

Landreneau, K., Lee, K., & Landreneau, M. (2010). Quality of life in patients undergoing hemodialysis and renal transplantation: A meta-analytic review. *Nephrology Nursing Journal*, 37(1), 37-45.

LaRocco, S. (2011). Treatment options for patients with kidney failure. *AJN*, 111(10), 57-62.

Lopez, C. (2008). Cultural diversity and the renal diet: The Hispanic population. *Nephrology Nursing Journal*, 35(1), 69-72.

Lowell, J., Go, A., Chertow, G., McCulloch, C., Fan, D., Ordonez, J., et al. (2009). Dialysis-requiring acute renal failure increases the risk of progressive chronic kidney failure. *Kidney International*, 76(8), 893-899.

Mahoney, C. (2007). Should patients eat during dialysis? *Nursing2007*, 37(10), 57-58.

Martchev, D. (2008). Improving quality of life for patients with kidney failure. *RN*, 71(4), 31-36.

Martin, R. (2010). Acute kidney injury: Advances in definition, pathophysiology, and diagnosis. *AACN Advanced Critical Care*, 21(4), 350-356.

McCance, K., Huether, S., Brashers, V., & Rote, N. (2010). *Pathophysiology: The biologic basis for disease in adults and children* (6th ed.). St. Louis: Mosby.

Mehrotra, R. (2009). Long-term outcomes in automated peritoneal dialysis: Similar or better than continuous ambulatory peritoneal dialysis? *Peritoneal Dialysis International*, 29(Suppl. 2), S111-S114.

Merhaut, S., & Trupp, R. (2010). Cardiorenal dysfunction. *AACN Advanced Critical Care*, 21(4), 357-364.

Myers, L. (2008). Novel therapies to reduce rejection in kidney transplant recipients. *Nephrology Nursing Journal*, 35(6), 591-593.

National Kidney and Urologic Diseases Information Clearinghouse (NKUDIC). (2010a). *Treatment methods for kidney failure: Hemodialysis, peritoneal dialysis, kidney transplantation.* Retrieved September 2011 from http://kidney.niddk.nih.gov/kudiseases/pubs/.

National Kidney & Urologic Diseases Information Clearinghouse (NKUDIC) (2010b). *Vascular access for hemodialysis.* Retrieved September 2011 fromhttp://kidney.niddk.nih.gov/kudiseases/pubs/vascularaccess/index.htm.

Nussbaum, R., McInnes, R., & Willard, H. (2007). *Thompson & Thompson: Genetics in medicine* (7th ed.). Philadelphia: Saunders.

Okusa, M. D., Chertow, G. M., Portilla, D.; Acute Kidney Injury Advisory Group of the American Society of Nephrology. (2009). The nexus of acute kidney injury, chronic kidney disease and World Kidney Day 2009. *Clinical Journal of the American Society of Nephrology*, 4(3), 520-522.

Pagana, K., & Pagana, T. (2010). *Mosby's manual of diagnostic and laboratory tests* (4th ed.). St. Louis: Mosby.

Pathophysiology review. (2010). *Nursing2010*, 40(4), 46-47.

Peacock, P., & Sinert, R. (2010). *Acute renal failure.* Retrieved February 2011, from www.emedicine.medscape.com/article/243492-overview.

Pearce, J. (2007). Documenting peritoneal dialysis. *Nursing2007*, 37(10), 28.

Pradeep, A., & Verrelli, M. (2010). *Chronic renal failure.* Retrieved February 2011, from www.emedicine.medscape.com/article/238798-overview.

Sahjian, M., & Frakes, M. (2007). Crush injuries: Pathophysiology and current treatment. *The Nurse Practitioner*, 32(9), 13-18.

Salinitri, F., Berlie, H., & Desai, N. (2009). Pharmacotherapeutic blood pressure management in a chronic kidney disease patient. *AACN Advanced Critical Care*, 20(3), 205-213.

Smith, K., & Smelt, S. (2009). Consequences of chronic kidney disease—mineral and bone disorder: A progressive disease. *Nephrology Nursing Journal*, 36(1), 49-55.

Solomon, D. (2010). *Patient information: Nonsteroidal anti-inflammatory drugs (NSAIDs).* Retrieved February 2011, from www.update.com/contents/patient-information-nonsteroidal-antiinflammatory-drugs-nsaids.

Stall, S. (2008). Protein recommendations for individuals with CKD stages 1-4. *Nephrology Nursing Journal*, 35(3), 279-282.

Szromba, C. (2010). Heparin-induced thrombocytopenia (HIT) in patients on hemodialysis: An update. *Nephrology Nursing Journal*, 37(2), 185-187.

Tseke, P., Androulaki, M., & Andrikos, E. (2010). Peritoneal dialysis versus hemodialysis: Comparing the comparable. *International Journal of Artificial Organs*, 33(6), 408-409.

United Network for Organ Sharing (UNOS) online. (2011). Living donation types. Retrieved September 2011 from www.unos.org.

U.S. Renal Data Systems (USRDS). (2010). *USRDS 2009 annual data report.* Bethesda, MD: The National Kidney and Urologic Diseases Information Clearinghouse (NKUDIC). National Institutes of Health.

Venkataraman, R., & Kellum, J. (2007). Prevention of acute renal failure. *Chest, 131*(1), 300-308.

Warise, L. (2010). Update: Diuretic therapy in acute renal failure: A clinical case study. *MEDSURG Nursing, 19*(3), 149-152.

Zeigler, S. (2007). Prevent dangerous hemodialysis catheter disconnection. *Nursing2007, 37*(3), 70.

Chapter 72

American Cancer Society (ACS). (2010). *Cancer facts and figures 2010.* Atlanta: Author.

American Cancer Society (ACS). (2011). *Guidelines for the early detection of cancer.* Atlanta: Author.

Dean, R. A. K. (2010). Cultural competence: Nursing in a multicultural society. *Nursing for Women's Health, 14*(1), 50-59.

Gordon, M. (2011). *Manual of nursing diagnosis* (12th ed.). New York: Jones & Bartlett.

Jarvis, C. (2012). *Physical examination and health assessment* (6th ed.). St. Louis: Saunders.

Lowdermilk, D. L., & Perry, S. E. (2011). *Maternity and women's health care* (10th ed.). St. Louis: Mosby.

Pagana, K., & Pagana, T. (2010). *Mosby's manual of diagnostic and laboratory tests* (4th ed.). St. Louis: Mosby.

Ruhl, C. (2010). Sleep is a vital sign: Why assessing sleep is an important part of women's health. *Nursing for Women's Health, 14*(3), 243-247.

Wallace, M. A. (2008). Assessment of sexual health in older adults: Using the PLISSIT model to talk about sex. *AJN, 108*(7), 52-60.

Chapter 73

Aitaoto, N., Tsark, J., Tomiyasu, D., Yamashita, B., & Braun, K. (2009). Strategies to increase breast and cervical cancer screening among Hawaiian, Pacific Islander, and Filipina women in Hawai'i. *Hawaii Medical Journal, 68*(9), 215-222.

American Cancer Society (ACS). (2010a). *Breast cancer facts & figures 2009-2010.* Atlanta: Author.

American Cancer Society (ACS). (2010b). *Breast cancer detailed guide.* Atlanta: Author.

American Cancer Society (ACS). (2010c). *Breast cancer facts & figures for African Americans 2009-2010.* Atlanta: Author.

American Cancer Society (ACS). (2010d). *Breast cancer facts & figures for Hispanics/Latinos 2009-2011.* Atlanta: Author.

American College of Obstetricians and Gynecologists (ACOG). (2011). Annual mammogram should start at age 40 years. *Contemporary OB/GYN, 56*(9), 20.

Association of Women's Health, Obstetric, and Neonatal Nursing (AWHONN). (2010). Breast cancer screening: A AWHONN position statement. *Journal of Obstetric, Gynecologic, & Neonatal Nursing, 39*(5), 608-610.

Bluming, A. Z., & Tavris, C. (2009). Hormone replacement therapy: Real concerns and false alarms. *Cancer Journal, 15*(2), 93-104.

Burstein, H. (2010). Avastin, ODAC, and the FDA: Are we drafting the right players? *Journal of the National Comprehensive Cancer Network, 8*(8), 833-834.

Camp-Sorrell, D. (2009). Cancer and its treatment effect on young breast cancer survivors. *Seminars in Oncology Nursing, 25*(4), 251-258.

Cangiarella, J., Guth, A., Axelrod, D., Darvishian, F., Singh, B., Simsir, A., et al. (2008). Is surgical excision necessary for the management of atypical lobular hyperplasia and lobular carcinoma in situ diagnosed on core needle biopsy? A report of 38 cases and review of the literature. *Archives of Pathology & Laboratory Medicine, 132*(6), 979-983.

Cunningham, J., Montero, A., Garrett-Mayer, E., Berkel, H., & Ely, B. (2010). Racial differences in the incidence of breast cancer subtypes defined by combined histologic grade and hormone receptor status. *Cancer Causes & Control, 21*(3), 399-409.

Dizon, D. (2009). Quality of life after breast cancer: Survivorship and sexuality. *The Breast Journal, 15*(5), 500-504.

Enderlin, C., Coleman, E., Stewart, C., & Hakkak, R. (2009). Dietary soy intake and breast cancer risk. *Oncology Nursing Forum, 36*(5), 531-539.

English, K., Fairbanks, J., Finster, C., Rafelito, A., Luna, J., & Kennedy, M. (2008). A socioecological approach to improving mammography rates in a tribal community. *Health Education & Behavior, 35*(3), 396-409.

Food and Drug Administration (FDA). (2010). *Summary minutes of the Oncologic Drugs Advisory Committee, July 10, 2010.* Washington, D.C.: Author. Retrieved October 30, 2010, from www.fda.gov.

Fu, M., Axelrod, D., & Haber, J. (2008). Breast-cancer-related lymphedema: Information, symptoms, and risk-reduction behaviors. *Journal of Nursing Scholarship, 40*(4), 341-348.

Han, H-R., Lee, J-E., Kim, J., Hedlin, H. K., Song, H., & Kim, M. T. (2009). A meta-analysis of interventions to promote mammography among ethnic minority women. *Nursing Research, 58*(4), 246-254.

Hines, L., Risendal, B., Slattery, M., Baumgartner, K., Giuliano, A., Sweeney, C., et al. (2010). Comparative analysis of breast cancer risk factors among Hispanic and non-Hispanic white women. *Cancer, 116*(13), 3215-3223.

Jemal, A., Siegel, R., Xu, J., & Ward, E. (2010). Cancer statistics, 2010. *CA: A Cancer Journal for Clinicians, 60*(5), 277-300.

Lally, R. (2010). Acclimating to breast cancer: A process of maintaining self-integrity in the pretreatment period. *Cancer Nursing, 33*(4), 268-279.

Lee, E. (2009). Evidence-based management of benign breast diseases. *American Journal for Nurse Practitioners, 13*(7-8), 22-29.

Liu, M., Huang, W., Wang, A., Huang, C., Huang, C., Chang, T., et al. (2010). Prediction of outcome of patients with metastatic breast cancer: Evaluation with prognostic factors and Nottingham prognostic index. *Supportive Care in Cancer, 18*(12), 1553-1564.

Mattarella, A. (2010). Breast cancer in men. *Radiologic Technology, 81*(4), 361M-378M.

Maughan, K., Lutterbie, M., & Ham, P. (2010). Treatment of breast cancer. *American Family Physician, 81*(11), 1339-1346.

McLachlan, K. (2009). Information and support needs of young women with breast cancer. *Cancer Nursing Practice, 8*(8), 21-24.

Morris, L. (2010). Targeting the red-hot danger of inflammatory breast cancer. *Nursing2010, 40*(9), 58-62.

Muggerud, A., Hallett, M., Johnsen, H., Kleivi, K., Zhou, W., Tahmasebpoor, S., et al. (2010). Molecular diversity in ductal carcinoma in situ (DCIS) and early invasive breast cancer. *Molecular Oncology, 4*(4), 357-368.

Nothacker, M., Duda, V., Hahn, M., Warm, M., Degenhardt, F., Madjar, H., et al. (2009). Early detection of breast cancer: Benefits and risks of supplemental breast ultrasound in asymptomatic women with mammographically dense breast tissue. A systematic review. *BMC Cancer, 9*, 335.

Owns, B., Jackson, M., & Berndt, A. (2009). Pilot study of a structured aerobic exercise program for Hispanic women during treatment for early-stage breast cancer. *MEDSURG Nursing, 18*(1), 23-30.

Pollán, M. (2010). Epidemiology of breast cancer in young women. *Breast Cancer Research and Treatment, 123*(Suppl. 1), 3-6.

Skaane, P. (2009). Studies comparing screen-film mammography and full-field digital mammography in breast cancer screening: Updated review. *Acta Radiologica, 50*(1), 3-14.

Smith, B., Arthur, D., Buchholz, T., Haffty, B., Hahn, C., Hardenbergh, P., et al. (2009). Accelerated partial breast irradiation consensus statement from the American Society for Radiation Oncology (ASTRO). *International Journal of Radiation Oncology, Biology, Physics, 74*(4), 987-1001.

Sotiriou, C., & Pusztai, L. (2009). Gene-expression signatures in breast cancer. *The New England Journal of Medicine, 360*(8), 790-800.

U.S. Preventive Services Task Force (USPSTF). (2009). Screening for breast cancer: U.S. Preventive Services Task Force recommendations statement. *Annals of Internal Medicine, 151,* 716-726.

Wanchai, A., Armer, J. M., & Stewart, B. R. (2010). Complementary and alternative medicine use among women with breast cancer: A systematic review. *Clinical Journal of Oncology Nursing, 14*(4), 45-55.

Weaver, C. (2009). Caring for a patient after mastectomy. *Nursing2009, 39*(5), 44-48.

Weigelt, B., Geyer, F., & Reis-Filho, J. (2010). Histological types of breast cancer: How special are they? *Molecular Oncology, 4*(3), 192-208.

Wingo, P., King, J., Swan, J., Coughlin, S., Kaur, J., Erb-Alvarez, J., et al. (2008). Breast cancer incidence among American Indian and Alaska Native women: US, 1999-2004. *Cancer, 113*(Suppl. 5), 1191-1202.

Wyatt, G., Sikorskii, A., Wills, C., & Su, H. (2010). Complementary and alternative medicine use, spending, and quality of life in early stage breast cancer. *Nursing Research, 59*(1), 58-66.

Xie, L., Brisson, J., Holowaty, E., Villeneuve, P., & Mao, Y. (2010). The influence of cosmetic breast augmentation on the stage distribution and prognosis of women subsequently diagnosed with breast cancer. *International Journal of Cancer, 126*(9), 2182-2190.

Zakhireh, J., Fowble, B., & Esserman, L. (2010). Application of screening principles to the reconstructed breast. *Journal of Clinical Oncology, 28*(1), 173-180.

Chapter 74

American Cancer Society (ACS). (2010). *Cancer facts and figures 2010.* Atlanta: Author.

Ayers, D. M., & Montgomery, M. (2009). Putting a stop to dysfunctional uterine bleeding. *Nursing2009, 39*(1), 44-50.

Blewitt, K. (2010). Ovarian cancer: Listen for the disease that whispers. *Nursing2010, 40*(11), 24-32.

*Bohnenkamp, S., LeBaron, V., & Yoder, L. H. (2007a). The medical-surgical nurse's guide to ovarian cancer: Part I. *MEDSURG Nursing, 16*(4), 259-266.

*Bohnenkamp, S., LeBaron, V., & Yoder, L. H. (2007b). The medical-surgical nurse's guide to ovarian cancer: Part II. *MEDSURG Nursing, 16*(5), 323-330.

*Cayir, G., Beji, N. K., & Yalcin, O. (2007). Effectiveness of nursing care after surgery for stress incontinence. *Urological Nursing, 27*(1), 25-33.

Everett, T. R., & Crawford, R. A. (2010). Laparoscopic assisted vaginal hysterectomy and bilateral salpingo-oophorectomy as a day surgery procedure: A promising option. *Journal of Obstetrics and Gynaecology, 30*(7), 697-700.

Fanning, J., Hojat, R., Johnson, J., & Fenton, B. (2010). Laparoscopic cytoreduction for primary advanced ovarian cancer. *Journal of the Society of Laparoscopic Surgeons, 14*(1), 80-82.

Fanning, J., & Hossler, C. (2010). Laparoscopic conversion rate for uterine cancer surgical staging. *Obstetrics and Gynecology, 116*(6), 1354-1357.

*Kelley, C. (2007). Estrogen and its effect on vaginal atrophy in post-menopausal women. *Urologic Nursing, 27*(1), 40-45.

Lowdermilk, D. L., & Perry, S. E. (2011). *Maternity and women's health care* (10th ed.). St. Louis: Mosby.

*MacDonald, D. J., Sarna, L., Ulman, G. C., Grant, M., & Weitzel, J. (2006). Cancer screening and risk-reducing behaviors of women seeking genetic cancer risk assessment for breast and ovarian cancers. *Oncology Nursing Forum, 33*(2), 27-35.

*Martin, V. R. (2007). Ovarian cancer: An overview of treatment options. *Clinical Journal of Oncology Nursing, 11*(2), 201-207.

Matthews, C. A., Reid, N., Ramakrishnan, V., Hull, K., & Cohen, S. (2010). Evaluation of the introduction of robotic technology on route of hysterectomy and complications in the first year of use. *American Journal of Obstetrics and Gynecology, 203*(5), 499. e1-5.

McCance, K. L., Huether, S. E., Brashers, V. L., & Rote, N. R. (2010). *Pathophysiology: The biological basis for disease in adults and children* (6th ed.). St. Louis: Mosby.

Mirsaidi, N. (2009). Looking into problems with transvaginal mesh. *Nursing2009, 39*(7), 54.

*Nussbaum, R. L., McInnes, R. R., & Willard, H. F. (2007). *Thompson & Thompson genetics in medicine* (7th ed.). Philadelphia: Saunders.

Pagana, K., & Pagana, T. (2010). *Mosby's manual of diagnostic and laboratory tests* (4th ed.). St. Louis: Mosby.

Schiech, L. (2010). HPV-related cancer. *Nursing2010, 40*(10), 22-28.

Stone, P., Burnett, A., Burton, B., & Roman, J. (2010). Overcoming extreme obesity with robotic surgery. *International Journal of Medical Robotics, 6*(4), 382-385.

Wells, S. F. (2008). Cervical cancer: An overview with suggested practice and policy goals. *MEDSURG Nursing, 17*(1), 43-51.

Chapter 75

Agbabiaka, T. B., Pittler, M. H., Wider, B., & Ernst, E. (2009). *Serenoa repens* (saw palmetto): A systematic review of adverse events. *Drug Safety, 32*(8), 637-647.

American Cancer Society (ACS). (2011). *Testicular cancer.* Retrieved April 19, 2011, from www.cancer.org/cancer/testicularcancer/detailedguide/testicular-cancer-key-statistics.

Bohenkamp, S., & Yoder, L. H. (2009). The medical-surgical nurse's guide to testicular cancer. *MEDSURG Nursing, 18*(2), 116-124.

Eltabey, M. A., Sherif, H., & Hussein, A. A. (2010). Holmium laser enucleation versus transurethral resection of the prostate. *Canadian Journal of Urology, 17*(6), 5447-5452.

Hamilton-Reeves, J. M., Rebello, S. A., Thomas, W., Kurzer, M. S., & Slaton, J. W. (2008). Effects of soy protein isolate consumption on prostate cancer biomarkers in men with HGPIN, ASAP, and low-grade prostate cancer. *Nutrition and Cancer, 60*(1), 7-13.

Held-Warmkessel, J. (2008). Caring for a patient with metastatic prostate cancer. *Nursing2008, 38*(6), 52-56.

Hemminki, K., Sundquist, J., & Bermejo, J. L. (2008). Familial risks for cancer as the basis for evidence-based clinical referral and counseling. *The Oncologist, 13*(3), 239-247.

Johnson, T. V., Abbasi, A., Ehrlich, S. S., Kleris, R. S., Chirumamilla, S. L., Schoenberg, E. D., et al. (2010). Major depression drives severity of American Urological Association Symptom Index. *Urology, 76*(6), 1317-1320.

*Leman, E. S., Cannon, G. W., Trock, B. J., Sokoll, L. J., Chan, D. W., Mangold, R., et al. (2007). EPCA-2: A highly specific serum marker for prostate cancer. *Urology, 69*(4), 714-720.

*Matthews, P. A. (2007). Hormone ablation therapy: Lightening the load for today's prostate cancer patient. *Urology Nursing, 27*(Suppl.), 3-11.

McCance, K., Huether, S., Brashers, V. L., & Rote, N. R. (2010). *Pathophysiology: The biologic basis for disease in adults and children* (6th ed.). St. Louis: Mosby.

*National Comprehensive Cancer Network (NCCN). (2007). NCCN Clinical Practice Guidelines in Oncology. *Prostate cancer early detection.* Retrieved April 18, 2011, from www. nccn.org/professionals.

Pagana, K. D., & Pagana, T. J. (2010). *Mosby's manual of diagnostic and laboratory tests* (4th ed.). St. Louis: Mosby.

Pesquera, M., Yoder, L., & Lynk, M. (2008). Improving cross-cultural awareness and skills to reduce health disparities in cancer. *MEDSURG Nursing, 17*(2), 114-121.

Roehrborn, C. G. (2011). Male lower urinary tract symptoms (LUTS) and benign prostatic hyperplasia (BPH). *Medical Clinics of North America, 95*(1), 87-100.

Slovin, S. F. (2008). Pitfalls or promise in prostate cancer immunotherapy: Which is winning? *Cancer Journal, 14*(1), 26-34.

Strief, D. M. (2008). An overview of prostate cancer: Diagnosis and treatment. *MEDSURG Nursing, 17*(4), 258-264.

Tackland, J., MacDonald, R., Rutks, I., & Wilt, T. J. (2009). *Serenoa repens* for benign prostatic hyperplasia. *Cochrane Database Systematic Reviews,* April 15(2), CD001423. Retrieved April 15, 2011, from www.ncbi.nlm.nih.gov/pubmed/19370565.

*Wallace, M., & Storms, S. (2007). The needs of men with prostate cancer: Results of a focus group study. *Applied Nursing Research, 20*(4), 181-187.

Wang, C. J., Lin, Y. N., Huang, S. W., & Chang, C. H. (2011). Low dose oral desmopressin for nocturnal polyuria in patients with benign prostatic hyperplasia: A double-blind, placebo controlled, randomized study. *Journal of Urology, 185*(1), 219-223.

Zarowitz, B. J. (2010). Opportunity to optimize management of benign prostatic hyperplasia. *Geriatric Nursing, 31*(6), 441-445.

Chapter 76

Bavis, M. P., Smith, D. Y., & Siomos, M. Z. (2009). Genital herpes: Diagnosis, treatment, and counseling in the adolescent patient. *Journal for Nurse Practitioners, 5*(6), 415-420.

*Centers for Disease Control and Prevention (CDC). (2006). *Expedited partner therapy in the management of sexually transmitted diseases.* Atlanta: U.S. Department of Health and Human Services. Retrieved September 27, 2010, from www.cdc. gov/std/treatment/EPTFinalReport2006.pdf.

*Centers for Disease Control and Prevention (CDC). (2007a). Update to CDC's sexually transmitted diseases treatment guidelines, 2006: Fluoroquinolones no longer recommended

for treatment of gonococcal infections. *Morbidity and Mortality Weekly Report, 56*(14), 332-336.

*Centers for Disease Control and Prevention (CDC). (2007b). Quadrivalent human papilloma virus vaccine: Recommendations of the Advisory Committee on Immunization Practices (ACIP). *Morbidity and Mortality Weekly Report, 56*(RR-2), 1-24.

Centers for Disease Control and Prevention (CDC). (2008). Summary of notifiable diseases—United States, 2006. *Morbidity and Mortality Weekly Report, 55*(53), 1-94. Retrieved December 11, 2010, from www.cdc.gov/mmwr/preview/mmwrhtml/ mm5553a1.htm.

Centers for Disease Control and Prevention (CDC). (2009). *Sexually transmitted disease surveillance, 2008.* Atlanta: U.S. Department of Health and Human Services. Retrieved January 14, 2011, from www.cdc.gov/std/stats08/default.htm.

Centers for Disease Control and Prevention (CDC). (2010a). Sexually transmitted diseases treatment guidelines, 2010. *Morbidity and Mortality Weekly Report, 59*(RR-12), 1-110.

Centers for Disease Control and Prevention (CDC). (2010b). Seroprevalence of herpes simplex virus type 2 among persons aged 14-49 years—United States, 2005-2008. *Morbidity and Mortality Weekly Report, 59*(15), 456-459.

Centers for Disease Control and Prevention (CDC). (2010c). *Basic information about antibiotic-resistant gonorrhea (ARG).* Retrieved January 14, 2011, from www.cdc.gov/std/gonorrhea/ arg/basic.htm.

Centers for Disease Control and Prevention (CDC). (2010d). *Pelvic inflammatory disease: CDC fact sheet.* Retrieved December 12, 2010, from www.cdc.gov/std/PID/STDFact-PID.htm.

Centers for Disease Control and Prevention (CDC). (2010e). *Legal status of expedited partner therapy (EPT).* Retrieved December 12, 2010, from www.cdc.gov/std/ept/legal/default.htm.

Centers for Disease Control and Prevention (CDC). (2010f). Youth risk behavior surveillance—United States, 2009: Surveillance summaries, June 4, 2010. *Morbidity and Mortality Weekly Report, 59*(SS-5), 1-148.

Chaturvedi, A. K., Engels, E. A., Anderson, W. F., & Gillison, M. L. (2008). Incidence trends for human papillomavirus–related and –unrelated oral squamous cell carcinomas in the United States. *Journal of Clinical Oncology, 26*(4), 612-619.

*Datta, S. D., Sternberg, M., Johnson, R. E., Berman, S., Papp, J. R., McQuillan, G., et al. (2007). Gonorrhea and chlamydia in the United States among persons 14 to 39 years of age, 1999 to 2002. *Annals of Internal Medicine, 147*(2), 89-96.

Drugge, J. M., & Allen, P. J. (2008). A nurse practitioner's guide to the management of herpes simplex virus-1 in children. *Dermatology Nursing, 20*(6), 455-466.

*Dunne, E. F., Unger, E. R., Sternberg, M., McQuillan, G., Swan, D., Patel, S. S., et al. (2007). Prevalence of HPV infection among females in the United States. *Journal of the American Medical Association, 297*(8), 813-819.

Fortuna, R. F., Robbins, B. R., & Halterman, J. S. (2009). Ambulatory care among young adults in the United States. *Annals of Internal Medicine, 151*(6), 379-385.

Holmes, K. K., Sparling, P. F., Stamm, W. E., Wasserheit, J. N., Corey, L., et al. (Eds.), (2008). *Sexually transmitted diseases* (4th ed.). New York: McGraw-Hill.

Johns Hopkins Point of Care-IT Center. (2010). *Antibiotic guide.* Retrieved November 15, 2010, from http://hopkins-abxguide. org/.

Kim, J. J. (2010). Targeted human papillomavirus vaccination of men who have sex with men in the USA: A cost-effectiveness modeling analysis. *The Lancet Infectious Diseases, 10*(12), 845-852.

*Lajiness, M. J. (2007). The new vaccine to prevent HPV. *Urologic Nursing, 27*(2), 153-154.

Muñoz, N., Kjaer, S. K., Sigurdsson, K., Iversen, O. E., Hernandez-Avila, M., Wheeler, C. M., et al. (2010). Impact of human papillomavirus (HPV)–6/11/16/18 vaccine on all HPV-associated genital diseases in young women. *Journal of the National Cancer Institute, 102*(5), 325-329.

Owusu-Edusei, K., Jr., Gift, T. L., & Chesson, H. W. (2010). Treatment cost of acute gonococcal infections: Estimates from employer-sponsored private insurance claims data in the United States, 2003-2007. *Sexually Transmitted Diseases, 37*(5), 316-318.

Pagana, K., & Pagana, T. (2010). *Mosby's manual of diagnostic and laboratory tests* (4th ed.). St. Louis: Mosby.

Pultorak, E., Wong, W., Rabins, C., & Mehta, S. D. (2009). Economic burden of sexually transmitted infections: Incidence and direct medical cost of chlamydia, gonorrhea, and syphilis among Illinois adolescents and young adults, 2005-2006. *Sexually Transmitted Diseases, 36*(10), 629-636.

Spinola, S. M. (2008). Chancroid and *Haemophilus ducreyi*. In K. K. Holmes, P. F. Sparling, W. E. Stamm, J. N. Wasserheit, L. Corey, et al. (Eds.), *Sexually transmitted diseases* (4th ed., pp. 689-699). New York: McGraw-Hill.

Stamm, W. E. (2008a). Chlamydia trachomatis infections of the adult. In K. K. Holmes, P. F. Sparling, W. E. Stamm, J. N. Wasserheit, L. Corey, et al. (Eds.), *Sexually transmitted diseases* (4th ed., pp. 575-593). New York: McGraw-Hill.

Stamm, W. E. (2008b). Lymphogranuloma venereum. In K. K. Holmes, P. F. Sparling, W. E. Stamm, J. N. Wasserheit, L. Corey, et al. (Eds.), *Sexually transmitted diseases* (4th ed., pp. 595-605). New York: McGraw-Hill.

*Trelle, S., Shang, A., Nartey, L., Cassell, J. A., & Low, N. (2007). Improved effectiveness of partner notification for patients with sexually transmitted infections: Systematic review. *BMJ, 334*(7589), 354.

U.S. Department of Health and Human Services (USDHHS), Office of Disease Prevention and Health Promotion. (2010). *Healthy People 2020*. Retrieved September 27, 2011, from www.healthypeople.gov/hp2020/.

U.S. Preventive Service Task Force (USPSTF), Agency for Healthcare Research and Quality. (2010). *Guide to clinical preventive services, 2010-2011*. Retrieved September 27, 2011, from www.ahrq.gov/clinic/pocketgd.htm.

Winer, R. L., & Koutsky, L. A. (2008). Genital human papillomavirus infection. In K. K. Holmes, P. F. Sparling, W. E. Stamm, J. N. Wasserheit, L. Corey, et al. (Eds.), *Sexually transmitted diseases* (4th ed., pp. 489-508). New York: McGraw-Hill.

Do-Not-Use Abbreviations and Symbols

Symbol or Abbreviation	Intended Meaning	Potential Problem	Preferred Term
μg	Microgram	Mistaken as "mg" (milligram)	Use "mcg"
ʒ	Dram	Symbol for dram mistaken as "3"	Use the metric system
℔	Minim	Symbol for minim mistaken as "mL" (milliliter)	Use the metric system
@	At	Mistaken as "2"	Use "at"
&	And	Mistaken as "2"	Use "and"
+	Plus or and	Mistaken as "4"	Use "and"
°	Hour	Mistaken as a zero (e.g., q2° seen as "q20")	Use "hr," "h," or "hour"
Ø	Zero, null sign	Mistaken as the numerals 4, 6, or 9	Use the number "0" or the word "zero"
ī/d	One daily	Mistaken as "tid" (three times daily)	Use "1 daily"
/ (slash mark)	Separates two doses or indicates "per"	Mistaken as the number 1 (e.g., "25 units/10 units" misread as "25 units and "110 units")	Use "per" rather than a slash mark to separate doses
> and <	Greater than and less than	Mistaken as opposite of intended; mistakenly use incorrect symbol; "<10" mistaken as "40"	Use "greater than" or "less than"
AD, AS, AU	Right ear, left ear, each ear	Mistaken as OD, OS, OU (right eye, left eye, each eye)	Use "right ear," "left ear," or "each ear"
ARA A	vidarabine	Mistaken as cytarabine (ARA C)	Use complete drug name
AZT	zidovudine (Retrovir)	Mistaken as azathioprine or aztreonam	Use complete drug name
BT	Bedtime	Mistaken as "BID" (twice daily)	Use "bedtime"
cc	Cubic centimeter	Mistaken as "u" (unit)	Use "mL" (milliliter)
CPZ	Compazine (prochlorperazine)	Mistaken as chlorpromazine	Use complete drug name
D/C	Discharge or discontinue	Premature discontinuation of medications if D/C (intended to mean "discharge") has been misinterpreted as "discontinued" when followed by a list of discharge medications	Use "discharge" and "discontinue"
DPT	Demerol-Phenergan-Thorazine	Mistaken as diphtheria-pertussis-tetanus (vaccine)	Use complete drug name
DTO	Diluted tincture of opium, or deodorized tincture of opium (Paregoric)	Mistaken as tincture of opium	Use complete drug name
HCl	hydrochloric acid or hydrochloride	Mistaken as potassium chloride (the "H" is misinterpreted as "K")	Use complete drug name unless expressed as a salt of a drug
HCT	hydrocortisone	Mistaken as hydrochlorothiazide	Use complete drug name

Symbol or Abbreviation	Intended Meaning	Potential Problem	Preferred Term
HCTZ	hydrochlorothiazide	Mistaken as hydrocortisone (seen as HCT250 mg)	Use complete drug name
HS	Half-strength	Mistaken as bedtime	Use "half-strength" or "bedtime"
hs	At bedtime, hours of sleep	Mistaken as half-strength	Use "half-strength" or "bedtime"
IJ	Injection	Mistaken as "IV" or "intrajugular"	Use "injection"
IN	Intranasal	Mistaken as "IM" or "IV"	Use "intranasal" or "NAS"
IU	International unit	Mistaken as IV (intravenous) or 10 (ten)	Use "unit"
"IV Vanc"	Intravenous vancomycin	Mistaken as Invanz	Use complete drug name
MgSO$_4$	Magnesium sulfate	Mistaken as morphine sulfate	Use complete drug name
MS, MSO$_4$	Morphine sulfate	Mistaken as magnesium sulfate	Use complete drug name
MTX	methotrexate	Mistaken as mitoxantrone	Use complete drug name
"Nitro" drip	nitroglycerin infusion	Mistaken as sodium nitroprusside infusion	Use complete drug name
"Norflox"	norfloxacin	Mistaken as Norflex	Use complete drug name
OD, OS, OU	Right eye, left eye, each eye	Mistaken as AD, AS, AU (right ear, left ear, each ear)	Use "right eye," "left eye," or "each eye"
o.d. or OD	Once daily	Mistaken as "right eye" (OD—oculus dexter), leading to oral liquid medications administered in the eye	Use "daily"
OJ	Orange juice	Mistaken as OD or OS (right or left eye); drugs meant to be diluted in orange juice may be given in the eye	Use "orange juice"
PCA	procainamide	Mistaken as patient-controlled analgesia	Use complete drug name
Per os	By mouth, orally	The "os" can be mistaken as "left eye" (OS—oculus sinister)	Use "PO," "by mouth," or "orally"
PTU	propylthiouracil	Mistaken as mercaptopurine	Use complete drug name
q.d. or QD	Every day	Mistaken as q.i.d., especially if the period after the "q" or the tail of the "q" is misunderstood as an "i"	Use "daily"
qhs	Nightly at bedtime	Mistaken as "qhr" or every hour	Use "nightly"
qn	Nightly or at bedtime	Mistaken as "qh" (every hour)	Use "nightly" or "at bedtime"
q.o.d. or QOD	Every other day	Mistaken as "q.d." (daily) or "q.i.d." (four times daily) if the "o" is poorly written	Use "every other day"
q1d	Daily	Mistaken as q.i.d. (four times daily)	Use "daily"
q6PM, etc.	Every evening at 6 PM	Mistaken as every 6 hours	Use "daily at 6 PM" or "6 PM daily"
SC, SQ, sub q	Subcutaneous	SC mistaken as SL (sublingual); SQ mistaken as "5 every"; the "q" in "sub q" has been mistaken as "every" (e.g., a heparin dose ordered "sub q 2 hours before surgery" misunderstood as every 2 hours before surgery)	Use "subcut" or "subcutaneously"
ss	Sliding scale (insulin) or ½ (apothecary)	Mistaken as "55"	Spell out "sliding scale"; use "one-half" or "½"
SSRI	Sliding scale regular insulin	Mistaken as selective-serotonin reuptake inhibitor	Spell out "sliding scale (insulin)"
SSI	Sliding scale insulin	Mistaken as Strong Solution of Iodine (Lugol's)	Spell out "sliding scale (insulin)"

Symbol or Abbreviation	Intended Meaning	Potential Problem	Preferred Term
T3	Tylenol with codeine No. 3	Mistaken as liothyronine	Use complete drug name
TAC	triamcinolone	Mistaken as tetracaine, Adrenalin, cocaine	Use complete drug name
TNK	TNKase	Mistaken as "TPA"	Use complete drug name
TIW or tiw	3 times a week	Mistaken as "3 times a day" or "twice in a week"	Use "3 times weekly"
U or u	Unit	Mistaken as the number 0 or 4, causing a tenfold overdose or greater (e.g., 4U seen as "40" or 4u seen as "44"); mistaken as "cc" so dose given in volume instead of units (e.g., 4u seen as "4cc")	Use "unit"
×3d	For 3 days	Mistaken as "3 doses"	Use "for 3 days"
ZnSO$_4$	zinc sulfate	Mistaken as morphine sulfate	Use complete drug name
Trailing zero after decimal point (e.g., 1.0 mg)	1 mg	Mistaken as 10 mg if the decimal point is missed	Do not use trailing zeroes for doses expressed in whole numbers
No leading zero before a decimal dose (e.g., .5 mg)	0.5 mg	Mistaken as 5 mg if the decimal point is not seen	Use zero before a decimal point when the dose is less than a whole unit
Drug name and dose run together (especially problematic for drug names that end in "l," such as Inderal40 mg; Tegretol300 mg)	Inderal 40 mg Tegretol 300 mg	Mistaken as Inderal 140 mg Mistaken as Tegretol 1300 mg	Place adequate space between the drug name, dose, and unit of measure
Numerical dose and unit of measure run together (e.g., 10mg, 100mL)	10 mg 100 mL	The "m" is sometimes mistaken as a zero or two zeros, risking a 10- to 100-fold overdose	Place adequate space between the dose and unit of measure
Abbreviations such as mg. or mL. with a period after the abbreviation	mg mL	The period is unnecessary and could be mistaken as the number 1 if written poorly	Use mg, mL, etc. without a terminal period
Large doses without properly placed commas (e.g., 100000 units; 1000000 units)	100,000 units 1,000,000 units	100000 has been mistaken as "10,000" or "1,000,000"; 1000000 has been mistaken as "100,000"	Use commas for dosing units at or above 1,000, or use words such as 100 "thousand" or 1 "million" to improve readability

Data from Institute for Safe Medication Practices (www.ismp.org): *ISMP's list of error-prone abbreviations, symbols, and dose designations, 2010*; and The Joint Commission (www.jointcommission.org): *The official "do not use" list, 2005*.

Communication Quick Reference for Spanish-Speaking Patients

The Body—El Cuerpo (ehl koo-EHR-poh)

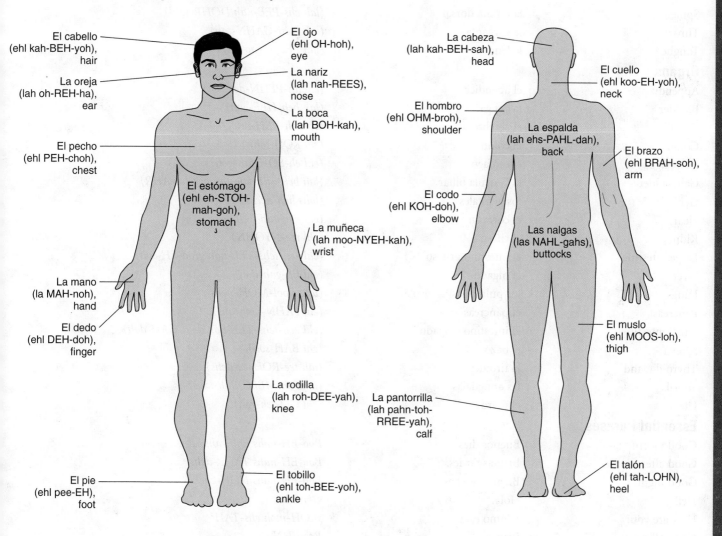

El cabello
(ehl kah-BEH-yoh),
hair

La oreja
(lah oh-REH-ha),
ear

El pecho
(ehl PEH-choh),
chest

El estómago
(ehl eh-STOH-
mah-goh),
stomach

La mano
(la MAH-noh),
hand

El dedo
(ehl DEH-doh),
finger

El pie
(ehl pee-EH),
foot

El ojo
(ehl OH-hoh),
eye

La nariz
(lah nah-REES),
nose

La boca
(lah BOH-kah),
mouth

La muñeca
(lah moo-NYEH-kah),
wrist

La rodilla
(lah roh-DEE-yah),
knee

El tobillo
(ehl toh-BEE-yoh),
ankle

La cabeza
(lah kah-BEH-sah),
head

El cuello
(ehl koo-EH-yoh),
neck

El hombro
(ehl OHM-broh),
shoulder

La espalda
(lah ehs-PAHL-dah),
back

El brazo
(ehl BRAH-soh),
arm

El codo
(ehl KOH-doh),
elbow

Las nalgas
(las NAHL-gahs),
buttocks

El muslo
(ehl MOOS-loh),
thigh

La pantorrilla
(lah pahn-toh-
RREE-yah),
calf

El talón
(ehl tah-LOHN),
heel

Common Instructions to Be Used with the Body Parts

Move the	Mueva	*(mooh-EH-bah)*
Touch the	Toque	*(TOH-keh)*
Point to the	Señale	*(seh-NYAH-leh)*

More Parts of the Body

English	Spanish	Pronunciation
Armpit	la axila	(lah ahk-SEE-lah)
Breasts	los senos	(lohs SEH-nohs)
Collarbone	la clavícula	(lah klah-BEE-koo-lah)
Diaphragm	el diafragma	(ehl dee-ah-FRAHG-mah)
Forearm	el antebrazo	(ehl ahn-teh-BRAH-soh)
Groin	la ingle	(lah EEN-gleh)
Hip	la cadera	(lah kah-DEH-rah)
Kneecap	la rótula	(lah ROH-too-lah)
Nail	la uña	(lah OO-nyah)
Pelvis	la pelvis	(lah PEHL-bees)
Rectum	el recto	(ehl REHK-toh)
Rib	la costilla	(lah kohs-TEE-yah)
Spine	la espina dorsal	(lah ehs-PEE-nah DOHR-sahl)
Throat	la garganta	(lah gahr-GAHN-tah)
Tongue	le lengua	(lah LEHN-goo-ah)

Organs

English	Spanish	Pronunciation
Appendix	el apéndice	(ehl ah-PEHN-dee-seh)
Bladder	la vejiga	(lah beh-HEE-gah)
Brain	el cerebro	(ehl seh-REH-broh)
Colon	el colon	(ehl KOH-lohn)
Esophagus	el esófago	(ehl eh-SOH-fah-goh)
Gallbladder	la vesícula biliar	(lah beh-SEE-koo-lah bee-lee-AHR)
Genitals	los genitales	(lohs heh-nee-TAH-lehs)
Heart	el corazón	(ehl koh-rah-SOHN)
Kidney	el riñón	(ehl ree-NYOHN)
Large intestine	el intestino grueso	(ehl een-tehs-TEE-noh groo-EH-soh)
Liver	el hígado	(ehl EE-gah-doh)
Lungs	los pulmones	(lohs pool-MOH-nehs)
Pancreas	el páncreas	(ehl PAHN-kreh-ahs)
Small intestine	el intestino delgado	(ehl een-tehs-TEE-noh dehl-GAH-doh)
Spleen	el bazo	(ehl BAH-soh)
Thyroid gland	la tiroides	(lah tee-ROH-ee-dehs)
Tonsils	las amígdalas	(lahs ah-MEEG-dah-lahs)
Uterus	el útero	(ehl OO-teh-roh)

Essential Phrases

English	Spanish	Pronunciation
Good morning.	Buenos días.	Boo-EH-nohs DEE-ahs.
Good afternoon.	Buenas tardes.	Boo-EH-nahs TAHR-dehs.
Good night.	Buenas noches.	Boo-EH-nahs NOH-chehs.
Hello.	Hola.	OH-lah.
How are you?	¿Cómo está?	¿KOH-moh ehs-TAH?
Good (Fine).	Bien.	Bee-EHN.
Bad, Better, Worse.	Mal, Mejor, Peor.	Mahl, Meh-OHR, Peh-OHR.
The same.	Igual.	Ee-GOO-ahl.
Do you speak English?	¿Habla Inglés?	¿AH-blah een-GLEHS?
I don't understand.	No comprendo.	Noh kom-PREHN-doh.
Excuse me.	Discúlpeme.	Dees-KOOL-peh-meh.
Please speak slowly.	Por favor, hable más lento.	Pohr fah-VOHR, AH-bleh mahs LEHN-toh.
Are you in pain?	¿Está adolorido(a)?	¿Ehs-TAH ah-doh-loh-REE-doh(dah)?

Essential Phrases—cont'd

Yes, No.	Sí, No.	See, Noh.
Tell me where it hurts.	Dígame donde le duele.	DEE-gah-meh DOHN-deh leh doo-EH-leh.
Here, There.	Aquí, Ahi.	Ah-KEE, Ah-EE.

Description of Pain

Is your pain ...	Tiene un dolor ...	Tee-EH-neh oon doh-LOHR ...
burning?	¿que arde?	¿keh AHR-deh?
constant?	¿constante?	¿kohns-TAHN-teh?
dull?	¿amortiguado?	¿ah-MOHR-tee-goo-AH-doh?
intermittent?	¿intermitente?	¿een-tehr-mee-TEHN-teh?
mild?	¿moderado?	¿moh-deh-RAH-doh?
severe?	¿muy fuerte?	¿MOO-ee foo-EHR-teh?
sharp?	¿agudo?	¿ah-GOO-doh?
throbbing?	¿pulsante?	¿pool-SAHN-teh?
worse?	¿peor?	¿peh-OHR?
Are you allergic to any medication?	¿Es usted alérgico(a) a algun medicamento?	¿Ehs oos-TEHD ah-LEHR-hee-koh(kah) ah ahl-GOON meh-dee-kah-MEHN-toh?
I'm here to help you.	Estoy aquí para ayudarle.	Ehs-TOH-ee ah-KEE pah-rah ah-yoo-DAHR-leh.
Calm down.	Cálmese.	KAHL-meh-seh.
Please.	Por favor.	Pohr fah-VOHR.
Thank you.	Gracias.	GRAH-see-ahs.
You're welcome.	De nada.	Deh NAH-dah.
May I?	¿Puedo?	¿Poo-EH-doh?
Who, What, When, Where?	¿Quién, Qué, Cuándo, Dónde?	¿Kee-EHN, Keh, Koo-AHN-doh, DOHN-deh?
Zero, One, Two, Three, Four	Cero, Uno, Dos, Tres, Cuatro	SEH-roh, OO-noh, dohs, trehs, koo-AH-troh
Five, Six, Seven, Eight, Nine, Ten	Cinco, Seis, Siete, Ocho, Nueve, Diez	SEEN-koh, SEH-ees, see-EH-teh, OH-choh, noo-EH-beh, dee-EHS

Preliminary Examination

My name is __, and I am your nurse.	Me llamo __, y soy su enfermera(o).	Meh YAH-moh ___, ee SOH-ee soo ehn-fehr-MEH-rah(roh).
I'm going to ...	Le voy a ...	Leh VOH-ee ah ...
take your vital signs.	tomar los signos vitales.	toh-MAHR lohs SEEG-nohs vee-TAH-lehs.
weigh you.	pesar.	peh-SAHR.
take your blood pressure.	tomar la presión.	toh-MAHR lah preh-see-OHN.
Extend your arm and relax.	Extienda su brazo y descánselo.	Ehks-tee-EHN-dah soo BRAH-soh ee dehs-KAHN-seh-loh.
I'm going to take your ...	Le voy a tomar ...	Leh voy ah toh-MAHR ...
pulse.	el pulso.	ehl POOL-soh.
temperature.	su temperatura.	soo tehm-peh-rah-TOO-rah.
I'm going to count your respirations.	Voy a contar sus respiraciones.	VOH-ee ah kohn-TAHR soos rehs-pee-rah-see-OH-nehs.

Obtaining a Blood Sample

I need to draw a blood sample.	Necesito tomar una muestra de la sangre.	Neh-seh-SEE-toh toh-MAHR OO-nah moo-EHS-trah deh lah SAHN-greh.
Please give me your arm.	Por favor, déme el brazo.	Pohr fah-VOHR, DEH-meh ehl BRAH-soh.
It may cause a little discomfort.	Le puede causar alguna molestia.	Leh poo-EH-deh kah-OO-sahr ahl-GOO-nah moh-LEHS-tee-ah.
I am going to put a tourniquet around your arm.	Le voy a poner una liga alrededor del brazo.	Leh VOH-ee ah poh-NEHR OO-nah LEE-gah ahl-reh-deh-DOHR dehl BRAH-soh.
I am going to draw blood from this vein.	Voy a sacar la sangre de esta vena.	VOH-ee ah sah-KAHR lah SAHN-greh deh EHS-tah VEH-nah.

Obtaining Blood from a Finger Stick

I need to take a few drops of blood from your finger.	Necesito sacar unas gotas de sangre de uno de sus dedos.	*Neh-seh-SEE-toh sah-KAHR OO-nahs GOH-tahs deh SAHN-greh deh OO-noh deh soos DEH-dohs.*

Obtaining a Urine Sample

We also need a urine sample.	También necesitamos una muestra de la orina.	*Tahm-bee-EHN neh-seh-see-TAH-mohs OO-nah moo-EHS-trah deh lah oh-REE-nah.*
It has to be from the middle of the stream.	Tiene que ser de la mitad del chorro.	*Tee-EH-neh keh sehr deh lah mee-TAHD dehl CHOH-rroh.*
Put the urine in this cup.	Ponga la orina en esta tasa.	*POHN-gah lah oh-REE-nah ehn EHS-tah TAH-sah.*

Obtaining a Stool Specimen

I need a sample of your stool.	Necesito una muestra de su excremento.	*Neh-seh-SEE-toh OO-nah moo-EHS-trah deh soo ehks-kreh-MEN-toh.*
Please put a small amount in this cup.	Por favor ponga un poco en esta tasa.	*Pohr fa-VOHR POHN-gah oon POH-koh ehn EHS-tah TAH-sah.*

Obtaining a Sputum Specimen

I need a sample of your sputum.	Necesito una muestra de su esputo.	*Neh-seh-SEE-toh OO-nah MWEHS-trah deh soo ehs-POO-toh.*
Please spit in this cup.	Por favor, escupa en este vaso.	*Pohr fah-VOHR, ehs-KOO-pah ehn EHS-teh VAH-soh.*

Orders

You need…	Necesita …	*Neh-seh-SEE-tah…*
a bandage.	un vendaje.	*oon behn-DAH-heh.*
a blood transfusion.	una transfusión de sangre.	*OO-nah trahns-foo-see-OHN deh SAHN-greh.*
a cast.	un molde de yeso.	*oon MOHL-deh deh YEH-soh.*
gauze.	la gasa.	*lah GAH-sah.*
intensive care.	cuidado intensivo.	*koo-ee-DAH-doh een-tehn-SEE-boh.*
intravenous fluids.	líquidos intravenosos.	*LEE-kee-dohs een-trah-beh-NOH-sohs.*
an operation.	una operación.	*OO-nah oh-peh-rah-see-OHN.*
physical therapy.	terapia física.	*teh-RAH-pee-ah FEE-see-kah.*
a shot.	una inyección.	*OO-nah een-yehk-see-OHN.*
x-rays.	rayos equis.	*RAH-yohs EH-kees.*
We're going to …	Vamos a …	*VAH-mohs ah …*
change the bandage.	cambiarle el vendaje.	*kahm-bee-AHR-leh ehl behn-DAH-heh.*
give you a bath.	darle un baño.	*DAHR-leh oon BAH-nyoh.*
take out the I.V.	sacarle el tubo intravenoso.	*sah-KAHR-leh ehl TOO-boh een-trah-beh-NOH-soh.*

Description of Tubes

The tube in your …	El tubo en su …	*Ehl TOO-boh ehn soo …*
arm is for I.V. fluids.	brazo es para líquidos intravenosos.	*BRAH-soh ehs PAH-rah LEE-kee-dohs een-trah-beh-NOH-sohs.*
bladder is for urinating.	vejiga es para orinar.	*beh-HEE-gah ehs PAH-rah oh-ree-NAHR.*
stomach is for the food.	estómago es para los alimentos.	*ehs-TOH-mah-goh ehs PAH-rah lohs ah-lee-MEN-tohs.*
throat is for breathing.	garganta es para respirar.	*gahr-GAHN-tah ehs PAH-rah rehs-pee-RAHR.*

A

A delta fiber Myelinated fiber found primarily in the skin and muscle; carries rapid, sharp, pricking, or piercing sensations that can generally be localized to a well-defined area; also called "mechanical nociceptor."

abdominoperineal (AP) resection The surgical removal of the sigmoid colon, rectum, and anus through combined abdominal and perineal incisions. This resection is performed when rectal tumors are present.

ablation The process or act of removing.

abscess A localized collection of pus caused by an inflammatory response to bacteria in tissues or organs.

absence seizure A type of generalized seizure consisting of brief periods of loss of consciousness and blank staring, as if daydreaming. The patient returns to baseline immediately after the seizure. This type is more common in children and tends to run in families. Left untreated, seizures may occur frequently throughout the day, interfering with daily life.

absolute neutrophil count (ANC) The percentage and actual number of mature circulating neutrophils; used to measure a patient's risk for infection. The higher the numbers, the greater the resistance to infection.

absorbable suture A type of suture digested over time by body enzymes.

absorption The uptake from the intestinal lumen of nutrients produced by digestion.

abstinence syndrome Symptoms that occur when a patient who is physically dependent on opioids abruptly ceases using them. Slowly tapering (weaning) the drug dosage lessens or alleviates the physical withdrawal symptoms in a patient who is opioid dependent.

acalculia Difficulty with math calculations; caused by brain injury or disease.

acalculous cholecystitis Inflammation of the gallbladder occurring in the absence of gallstones; typically associated with biliary stasis caused by any condition that affects the regular filling or emptying of the gallbladder.

acceleration-deceleration Forces involved in high-speed crashes or falls from a great height; produce injury by tearing, shearing, and compressing anatomic structures.

acclimatization The process of adapting to a high altitude; involves physiologic changes that help the body compensate for less available oxygen in the atmosphere.

accommodation The process of maintaining a clear visual image when the gaze is shifted from a distant object to a near object. The eye adjusts its focus by changing the curvature of the lens.

achalasia An esophageal motility disorder believed to result from esophageal denervation; involves a failure to relax the smooth muscle fibers of the gastrointestinal tract and

characterized by chronic and progressive dysphagia. The term is typically used to refer to failure of the lower esophageal sphincter to relax properly with swallowing and to the replacement of normal peristalsis of the esophagus with abnormal contractions.

achlorhydria The absence of hydrochloric acid from gastric secretions.

acid A substance that releases hydrogen ions when dissolved in water. The strength of an acid is measured by how easily it releases hydrogen ions in solution.

acidosis An acid-base imbalance in which blood pH is below normal.

acinus The structural unit of the lower respiratory tract consisting of a respiratory bronchiole, an alveolar duct, and an alveolar sac.

Acorn cardiac support device A polyester mesh jacket that is placed over the ventricles to provide support and avoid overstretching the myocardial muscle in the patient with heart failure; reduces heart muscle hypertrophy and assists with improvement of ejection fraction.

acoustic neuroma A benign tumor of cranial nerve VIII; symptoms include damage to hearing, facial movements, and sensation. The tumor can enlarge into the brain, damaging structures in the cerebellum.

activated protein C An enzyme that helps prevent inappropriate clot formation. It is activated when it binds to healthy endothelial cells of the blood vessels; reduced levels are an indicator of sepsis and septic shock.

active euthanasia Purposeful action that directly causes death; not supported by most professional organizations, including the American Nurses Association.

active immunity Resistance to infection that occurs when the body responds to an invading antigen by making specific antibodies against the antigen. Immunity lasts for years and is natural by infection or artificial by stimulation (e.g., vaccine) of the body's immune defenses.

activities of daily living (ADLs) The activities performed in the course of a normal day, such as bathing, dressing, feeding, and ambulating.

activity therapist A member of the rehabilitation health care team who works to help patients continue or develop hobbies or interests; also called "recreational therapist."

acupoint One of the specific areas for acupressure and acupuncture located on meridians throughout the body.

acupressure A traditional Chinese medicine therapy in which the fingers are used to press certain points on the body to increase the flow of energy and promote the body's self-healing ability.

acupuncture A traditional Chinese medicine therapy in which tiny needles are inserted into the skin and subcutaneous tissues at certain

areas of the body to deliver manual vibration or electrical stimulation.

acute Having relatively greater intensity; marked by a sudden onset and short duration.

acute adrenal insufficiency A life-threatening event in which the need for cortisol and aldosterone is greater than the available supply; also called "Addisonian crisis."

acute arterial occlusion The sudden blockage of an artery, typically in the lower extremity, in the patient with chronic peripheral arterial disease.

acute compartment syndrome (ACS) A complication of a fracture characterized by increased pressure within one or more compartments and causing massive compromise of circulation to the area. Compartments are sheaths of inelastic fascia that support and partition muscles, blood vessels, and nerves in the body.

acute coronary syndrome (ACS) A disorder, including unstable angina and myocardial infarction, that results from obstruction of the coronary artery by ruptured atherosclerotic plaque and leads to platelet aggregation, thrombus formation, and vasoconstriction.

acute gastritis Inflammation of the gastric mucosa or submucosa after exposure to local irritants. Various degrees of mucosal necrosis and inflammatory reaction occur in acute disease. Complete regeneration and healing usually occur within a few days.

acute hematogenous infection An infection resulting from bacteremia, disease, or nonpenetrating trauma that is disseminated by the blood through the circulation.

acute ischemic stroke (AIS) A stroke caused by the occlusion (blockage) of a cerebral artery by either a thrombus or an embolus.

acute kidney failure A rapid decrease in kidney function that leads to the accumulation of metabolic wastes in the body. It is caused by inadequate kidney perfusion; damage to the glomeruli, interstitial tissue, or tubules; or obstructed urine flow. It can progress to end-stage kidney disease in patients with chronic renal insufficiency.

acute kidney injury A rapid decrease in kidney function, leading to the collection of metabolic wastes in the body; formerly called "acute renal failure (ARF)."

acute pain The unpleasant sensory and emotional experience associated with tissue damage that results from acute injury, disease, or surgery.

acute pancreatitis A serious inflammation of the pancreas characterized by a sudden onset of abdominal pain, nausea, and vomiting. It is caused by premature activation of pancreatic enzymes that destroy ductal tissue and pancreatic cells and results in autodigestion and fibrosis of the pancreas.

acute paronychia Inflammation of the skin around the nail, which usually occurs with a torn cuticle or an ingrown toenail.

acute pericarditis An inflammation or alteration of the pericardium, the membranous sac that encloses the heart; may be fibrous, serous, hemorrhagic, purulent, or neoplastic.

acute pyelonephritis Active bacterial infection in the kidney.

acute respiratory distress syndrome (ARDS) Respiratory failure marked by hypoxemia that persists even when 100% oxygen is given, as well as decreased pulmonary compliance, dyspnea, noncardiac-associated bilateral pulmonary edema, and dense pulmonary infiltrates on x-ray.

acute sialadenitis Inflammation of a salivary gland; can be caused by infectious agents, irradiation, or immunologic disorders.

adaptive immunity The immunity that a person's body makes (or can receive) as an adaptive response to invasion by organisms or foreign proteins; occurs either naturally or artificially through lymphocyte responses and can be either active or passive.

adaptive mechanism The means of producing compensation; also called "compensatory mechanism."

addiction A primary, chronic neurobiologic disease characterized by impaired control over drug use, compulsive use, continued use despite harm, and craving.

addisonian crisis Acute adrenal insufficiency; a life-threatening event in which the need for cortisol and aldosterone is greater than the available supply.

additive In pharmacology, a drug that adds an effect, either harmful or beneficial, when given with another drug.

adenocarcinoma Tumor that arises from the glandular epithelial tissue.

adenohypophysis The anterior lobe of the pituitary gland, which makes up about 70% of the gland.

adiponectin An anti-inflammatory and insulin sensitizing hormone.

adipose Fatty.

adjuvant A substance that aids another substance, such as a cancer treatment that uses chemotherapy in addition to surgery.

adjuvant drug Drug used to relieve pain either alone or in combination with an analgesic to enhance the effectiveness of the analgesic.

adjuvant therapy Chemotherapy that is used along with surgery or radiation.

adrenal crisis Acute adrenocortical insufficiency, which can be life threatening.

adrenal Cushing's disease An excess of glucocorticoids caused by a problem in the adrenal cortex, usually a benign tumor (adrenal adenoma). This usually occurs in only one adrenal gland.

adrenal steroid Any of the hormones produced and secreted by the adrenal cortex; also called "corticosteroid."

advance directive A written document prepared by a competent person to specify what,

if any, extraordinary actions he or she would want when no longer able to make decisions about personal health care.

adverse drug event (ADE) An unintended harmful reaction to an administered drug.

aerophagia The excessive swallowing of air.

aerosolization Transmission via fine airborne droplets.

aesthetic plastic surgery Plastic surgery that is cosmetic and aims to alter a person's physical appearance.

afferent arteriole The smallest, most distal portion of the renal arterial system that supplies blood to the nephron. From the afferent arteriole, blood flows into the glomerulus, a series of specialized capillary loops.

afferent loop syndrome Chronic partial obstruction of the duodenal loop after partial gastrectomy and gastrojejunostomy, resulting in abdominal bloating and pain after eating; often followed by nausea and vomiting.

after-drop A continued decrease in core body temperature after a victim is removed from a cold environment; results from equilibration of core and peripheral blood temperature and counter-current cooling of the blood perfusing cold tissue.

afterload The pressure or resistance that the ventricles must overcome to eject blood through the semilunar valves and into the peripheral blood vessels; the amount of resistance is directly related to arterial blood pressure and blood vessel diameter.

agglutination A clumping action that results during the antibody-binding process when antibodies link antigens together to form large and small immune complexes.

aggregation Clumping together.

agnosia A general term for a loss of sensory comprehension; may include an inability to write, comprehend reading material, or use an object correctly.

agraphia Loss of the ability to write; caused by brain injury or disease.

Airborne Precautions Infection control guidelines from the Centers for Disease Control and Prevention; used for patients with infections spread by the airborne transmission route, such as tuberculosis. Negative airflow rooms are required to prevent the airborne spread of microbes.

akinesia Slow or no movement, as seen in a patient with Parkinson disease; also called "bradykinesia."

alanine aminotransferase (ALT) An enzyme found in the liver. Levels of this enzyme are elevated in patients with liver disease, infectious mononucleosis, and other disorders.

albuminuria The presence of albumin in the urine.

alcohol abuse A condition in which a person has problems related to alcohol use but does not have a strong craving for alcohol, loss of control, or physical dependence.

alcoholic hepatitis Liver inflammation caused by the toxic effect of alcohol on hepatocytes. The liver becomes enlarged, with cellular

degeneration and infiltration by fat, leukocytes, and lymphocytes.

alcoholism A disease in which a person has a strong need or compulsion to consume alcohol, is unable to quit once he or she begins drinking, experiences a physical dependence, and needs to increase the amount of alcohol to get "high."

aldosterone The chief mineralocorticoid produced by the adrenal cortex. Aldosterone increases kidney reabsorption of sodium and water, thus restoring blood pressure, blood volume, and blood sodium levels. Aldosterone secretion is regulated by the renin-angiotensin system, serum potassium ion concentration, and adrenocorticotropic hormone.

alert Awake and responsive to stimulation.

alexia Problems understanding written language; caused by brain injury or disease.

alkaline reflux gastropathy A complication of gastric surgery in which the pylorus is bypassed or removed. Endoscopic examination reveals regurgitated bile in the stomach and mucosal hyperemia. Symptoms include early satiety, abdominal discomfort, and vomiting; also called "bile reflux gastropathy."

alkalosis An acid-base imbalance in which blood pH is above normal.

allele An alternate form (or variation) of a gene.

allergen A foreign protein that is capable of causing a hypersensitivity response, or allergy, that ranges from uncomfortable (itchy, watery eyes or sneezing) to life threatening (allergic asthma, anaphylaxis, bronchoconstriction, or circulatory collapse); causes a release of natural chemicals, such as histamine, in the body.

allergy An increased or excessive response to the presence of a foreign protein or allergen (antigen) to which the patient has been previously exposed.

allogenic Having cell types that are antigenically distinct; for example, bone marrow transplantation in which the patient receives bone marrow or peripheral blood taken from a healthy donor. Compare with autologous bone marrow transplantation, in which patients receive their own cells, which were collected earlier.

allogenic bone marrow transplantation The transplantation of bone marrow from a sibling.

allogenic transplant Type of bone marrow transplant in which a closely HLA-matched sibling or an unrelated but matched donor provides the stem cells.

allograft A graft of tissue or bone between individuals of the same species but a different genotype; the donor may be a cadaver or a living person, either related or unrelated; also called "homograft."

alopecia Hair loss.

alveolitis Inflammation of the alveoli.

Alzheimer's disease (AD) A chronic, progressive, degenerative disease that accounts for 60% of the dementias occurring in people older than 65 years; characterized by loss of memory, judgment, and visuospatial perception and by a change in personality. Over time, the patient becomes increasingly cognitively impaired. Severe physical deterioration takes place, and death occurs as a result of complications of immobility; also called "dementia, Alzheimer type."

amaurosis fugax A transient, brief episode of blindness in one eye.

ambulatory A term that refers to a patient who goes to the hospital or physician's office and returns home on the same day.

ambulatory aid Assistive device such as a cane or a walker.

ambulatory pump Infusion therapy pump generally used with a home care patient to allow a return to his or her usual activities while receiving infusion therapy.

amebic hepatic abscess A liver abscess caused by the protozoan *Entamoeba histolytica;* may occur after amebic dysentery and usually occurs as a single abscess in the right hepatic lobe.

amenorrhea The absence of menstrual periods in women.

amnesia Loss of memory.

amputation The removal of a limb or other appendage of the body.

amyotrophic lateral sclerosis (ALS) A progressive and degenerative disease of the motor system that is characterized by atrophy of the hands, forearms, and legs and results in paralysis and death. There is no known cause, no cure, no specific treatment, no standard pattern of progression, and no method of prevention; also called "Lou Gehrig's disease."

anabolic hormone A hormone that stimulates growth.

anabolic steroids Synthetic substances that mimic the actions of testosterone. Prescribed for people with hormonal difficulties such as delayed puberty or impotence and misused by athletes to increase strength and performance.

anaerobic Lacking adequate oxygen.

anaerobic cellular metabolism Metabolism without oxygen.

anal fissure A painful ulcer at the margin of the anus.

analgesia Pain relief or pain suppression.

analgesia team Team typically consisting of one or more nurses, pharmacists, case managers, and physicians who consult with staff and prescribers on how best to control the patient's pain; also called "multidisciplinary pain team."

anaphylaxis The widespread reaction that occurs in response to contact with a substance to which the person has a severe allergy (antigen); characterized by blood vessel and bronchiolar smooth muscle involvement causing widespread blood vessel dilation, decreased cardiac output, and bronchoconstriction; results in cell damage and the release of large amounts of histamine, severe hypovolemia, vascular collapse, decreased cardiac contraction, and dysrhythmias and causes extreme whole-body hypoxia.

anasarca Generalized edema.

anastomosis Surgical reattachment; also a general term meaning a connection.

anatomic dead space Places in which air flows but the structures are too thick for gas exchange.

androgen Any substance, such as testosterone, that promotes masculinization; male hormones.

anemia A clinical sign of some abnormal condition related to a reduction in one of the following: number of red blood cells, amount of hemoglobin, or hematocrit (percentage of packed red blood cells per deciliter of blood).

anergy The inability to mount an immune response to an antigen.

anesthesia An induced state of partial or total loss of sensation with or without loss of consciousness.

anesthetic Agent that produces loss of sensation.

aneuploid An abnormal karyotype with more or fewer than 23 pairs of chromosomes.

aneurysm A permanent localized dilation of an artery (to at least two times its normal diameter) that forms when the middle layer (media) of the artery is weakened, stretching the inner (intima) and outer (adventitia) layers. As the artery widens, tension in the wall increases and further widening occurs, thus enlarging the aneurysm.

aneurysmectomy A surgical procedure performed to excise an aneurysm.

angina pectoris Literally, "strangling of the chest"; a temporary imbalance between the ability of the coronary arteries to supply oxygen and the demand for oxygen by the cardiac muscle. As a result, the patient experiences chest discomfort.

angioedema Diffuse swelling resulting from a vascular reaction in the deep tissues; can occur in a patient having an anaphylactic reaction.

anion Ion that has a negative charge.

anisocoria A difference in the size of the pupils.

ankle-brachial index (ABI) A ratio derived by dividing the ankle blood pressure by the brachial blood pressure; this calculation is used to assess the vascular status of the lower extremities. To obtain the ABI, a blood pressure cuff is applied to the lower extremities just above the malleoli. The systolic pressure is measured by Doppler ultrasound at both the dorsalis pedis and posterior tibial pulses. The higher of these two pressures is then divided by the higher of the two brachial pulses.

ankylosing spondylitis A form of rheumatoid arthritis that affects the vertebral column and causes spinal deformities.

anomia Inability to find words.

anorectal abscess A localized induration and fluctuance that is caused by inflammation of the soft tissue near the rectum or anus and is most often the result of obstruction of the ducts of glands in the anorectal region by feces, foreign bodies, or trauma.

anorectic drugs Drugs that suppress appetite, which reduces food intake and, over time, may result in weight loss; may be prescribed for

obese patients in a comprehensive weight reduction program.

anorexia The loss of appetite for food.

anorexia nervosa An eating disorder of self-induced starvation resulting from a fear of fatness, even though the patient is underweight.

anorexin Neuropeptide that decreases appetite.

anoxic Completely lacking oxygen.

antalgic gait A term that refers to an abnormality in the stance phase of gait. When part of one leg is painful, the person shortens the stance phase on the affected side.

anterior colporrhaphy Surgery for severe symptoms of cystocele in which the pelvic muscles are tightened for better bladder support.

anterior cord syndrome A condition caused by cervical injuries; results from damage to the anterior portion of both the gray and white matter of the spinal cord, usually as a result of decreased blood supply. Motor function and pain and temperature sensation are lost below the level of injury, but the sensations of touch, position, and vibration remain intact.

anterior nares The nostrils or external openings into the nasal cavities.

antibody-mediated immune system The defense response that produces antibodies directed against certain pathogens. The antibodies inactivate the pathogens and protect against future infection from that microorganism.

anticoagulant Something that limits blood clot formation.

antidepressants A group of drugs that help manage clinical depression.

antiepileptic drugs (AEDs) A class of drugs used to control seizures; also called "anticonvulsants."

antigen A foreign protein or allergen that is capable of causing an immune response; protein on the surface of a cell.

antiplatelet agents Drugs that destroy blood platelets.

anuria Complete lack of urine output; usually defined as less than 100 mL/24 hr.

anuric Characterized by anuria (complete lack of urine output).

aortic regurgitation The flow of blood from the aorta back into the left ventricle during diastole; occurs when the aortic valve leaflets do not close properly during diastole and the annulus (the valve ring that attaches to the leaflets) is dilated or deformed.

aortic stenosis Narrowing of the aortic valve orifice and obstruction of left ventricular outflow during systole.

aortic valve The semilunar valve of the heart that separates the left ventricle from the aorta.

aphasia Inability to use or comprehend spoken or written language due to brain injury or disease.

aphonia Inability to produce sound; complete but temporary loss of the voice.

aphthous stomatitis Noninfectious stomatitis.

apical impulse The pulse located at the left fifth intercostal space in the midclavicular line in the mitral area (the apex of the heart); also called the "point of maximal impulse."

aplastic anemia A deficiency of circulating red blood cells because of failure of the bone marrow to produce these cells; usually occurs with leukopenia and thrombocytopenia.

apolipoprotein E One of several regulators of lipoprotein metabolism.

apoptosis Programmed cell death that occurs when deoxyribonucleic acid in the telomere is gone and the chromosomes unravel.

appendectomy Surgical removal of the inflamed appendix.

appendicitis Acute inflammation of the vermiform appendix, which is the blind pouch attached to the cecum of the colon, which is usually located in the right iliac region just below the ileocecal valve.

approximated In a clean laceration or a surgical incision to be closed with sutures or staples, the act of bringing together the wound edges with the skin layers lined up in correct anatomic position so they can be held in place until healing is complete.

apraxia The loss of the ability to carry out a purposeful motor activity.

aqueous humor The clear, watery fluid that is continually produced by the ciliary processes and fills the anterior and posterior chambers of the eye. This fluid drains through the canal of Schlemm into the blood to maintain balanced intraocular pressure (pressure within the eye).

arcus senilis An opaque ring within the outer edge of the cornea caused by fat deposits. Its presence does not affect vision.

areflexic bladder Urinary retention and overflow (dribbling) caused by injuries to the lower motor neuron at the spinal cord level of S2 to S4 (e.g., multiple sclerosis and spinal cord injury below T12). Bladder emptying may be achieved by performing a Valsalva maneuver or tightening the abdominal muscles. The effectiveness of these maneuvers should be ascertained by catheterizing the patient for residual urine after voiding. Also called "flaccid bladder."

aromatherapy A complementary therapy that uses essential oils obtained from plants to enhance psychological and physical well-being; may be applied in compresses, used in baths, or applied topically to the skin.

arrhythmogenic right ventricular cardiomyopathy (dysplasia) A form of cardiomyopathy that results from the replacement of myocardial tissue with fibrous and fatty tissue.

arterial revascularization The surgical procedure most commonly used to increase arterial blood flow in the affected limb of a patient with peripheral arterial disease.

arterial ulcers A painful complication in the patient with peripheral arterial disease. Typically, the ulcer is small and round, with a "punched out" appearance and well-defined borders. Ulcers develop on the toes (often the great toe), between the toes, or on the upper aspect of the foot. With prolonged occlusion, the toes can become gangrenous.

arteriography Angiography of the arterial vessels; this invasive diagnostic procedure involves fluoroscopy and the use of a contrast medium and is performed when an arterial obstruction, narrowing, or aneurysm is suspected.

arteriosclerosis A thickening, or hardening, of the arterial wall.

arteriotomy A surgical opening into an artery.

arteriovenous malformation (AVM) An abnormality that occurs during embryonic development, resulting in a tangled mass of malformed, thin-walled, dilated vessels. The congenital absence of a capillary network in these vessels forms an abnormal communication between the arterial and venous systems and increases the risk that the vessels may rupture, causing bleeding into the subarachnoid space or into the intracerebral tissue. In the absence of the capillary network, the thin-walled veins are subjected to arterial pressure.

arteritis Inflammation of arterial walls.

arthralgia Pain in a joint.

arthritis Inflammation of one or more joints.

arthrodesis The surgical fusion of a joint.

arthrogram An x-ray study of a joint after contrast medium (air or solution) has been injected to enhance its visualization.

arthroscopy Examination of the interior of a joint with an arthroscope (a fiberoptic tube).

articulations Joint surfaces.

artifact In the electrocardiogram, interference that is seen on the monitor or rhythm strip and may look like a wandering or fuzzy baseline; can be caused by patient movement, loose or defective electrodes, improper grounding, or faulty equipment.

ascending paralysis Paralysis that begins in the legs and spreads to the arms and upper body.

ascending tracts Groups of nerves that originate in the spinal cord and end in the brain.

ascites The accumulation of free fluid within the peritoneal cavity. Increased hydrostatic pressure from portal hypertension causes this fluid to leak into the peritoneal cavity.

aseptic meningitis A type of meningitis that often occurs after viral illnesses such as measles, herpes simplex, coxsackievirus, and echovirus and is marked by inflammation over the cerebral cortex, white matter, and meninges. The formation of exudate (common in bacterial meningitis) does not occur, and no organisms are obtained from the cerebrospinal fluid. Also called "viral meningitis."

aseptic necrosis See *avascular necrosis (AVN)*.

ASKED Model of Cultural Competence created by Dr. Josie Campinha-Bacote that provides a beginning self-assessment tool for cultural competence.

aspartate aminotransferase (AST) An enzyme found in the liver. Levels of this enzyme are elevated in patients with liver disorders and are highest in conditions that cause necrosis, such as severe viral hepatitis.

assistive/adaptive device Any item that enables the patient to perform all or part of an activity independently.

asterixis A coarse tremor characterized by rapid, nonrhythmic extensions and flexions in the wrists and fingers; a motor disturbance seen in portal-systemic encephalopathy; also called a "liver flap" or "flapping tremor."

astigmatism A refractive error caused by unevenly curved surfaces on or in the eye (especially of the cornea) that distort vision.

asynchronous (fixed-rate) pacing mode The mode of temporary cardiac pacing in which the pulse generator does not sense any intrinsic beats of the patient but fires at a fixed rate, regardless of the intrinsic rhythm. Used when the patient is asystolic or profoundly bradycardic, as may occur after open-heart surgery.

ataxia Gait disturbance or loss of balance.

atelectasis Collapse of alveoli.

atherectomy An invasive nonsurgical technique in which a high-speed, rotating metal burr uses fine abrasive bits to scrape plaque from inside an artery while minimizing damage to the vessel surface.

atherosclerosis A type of arteriosclerosis that involves the formation of plaque within the arterial wall; the leading contributor to coronary artery and cerebrovascular disease.

atonic (akinetic) seizure A type of generalized seizure characterized by a sudden loss of muscle tone that lasts for seconds and is followed by postictal confusion. These seizures usually cause the patient to fall, which may result in injury.

atresia Congenital absence of a normal body orifice or tubular organ, such as the ear canal.

atrial fibrillation (AF) A cardiac dysrhythmia in which multiple rapid impulses from many atrial foci, at a rate of 350 to 600 times per minute, depolarize the atria in a totally disorganized manner, with no P waves, no atrial contractions, a loss of the atrial kick, and an irregular ventricular response.

atrial flutter A cardiac dysrhythmia that involves rapid atrial depolarization and occurs at a rate of 250 to 350 times per minute.

atrial gallop An abnormal fourth heart sound that occurs as blood enters the ventricles during the active filling phase at the end of ventricular diastole; may be heard in patients with hypertension, anemia, ventricular hypertrophy, myocardial infarction, aortic or pulmonic stenosis, and pulmonary emboli.

atrial overdrive pacing A type of pacing that may be used to terminate symptomatic tachydysrhythmias such as atrial flutter or atrial fibrillation. Overdrive pacing is accomplished by rapidly pacing the atrium to capture the heart and control depolarization and is followed by no pacing in the hope that the sinus node will regain control of the heart.

atrioventricular (AV) block The delay or blockage of supraventricular impulses in the atrioventricular node or intraventricular conduction system; usually classified as first-, second-, or third-degree block. Conduction may be transiently or permanently abnormal.

atrioventricular (AV) junction In the cardiac conduction system, the area consisting of a transitional cell zone, the atrioventricular (AV) node itself, and the bundle of His. The AV node lies just beneath the right atrial endocardium, between the tricuspid valve and the ostium of the coronary sinus.

at-risk drinking Drinking behavior in which five or more alcoholic beverages for men (four or more for women) are consumed.

atrophic gastritis A type of chronic gastritis that is seen most often in older adults. It can occur after exposure to toxic substances in the workplace (e.g., benzene, lead, and nickel) or *Helicobacter pylori* infection, or it can be related to autoimmune factors.

attenuated The quality of making a substance weaker; for example, antigens that are used to make vaccines are specially processed to make them less likely to grow in the body.

atypical angina Angina that manifests itself as indigestion, pain between the shoulders, an aching jaw, or a choking sensation that occurs with exertion. Many women experience atypical angina.

atypical migraine The least common of the three types of migraine headaches, after migraines with aura and migraines without aura; the atypical category includes menstrual and cluster migraines.

audiogram The graphic record of the results of pure-tone audiometry.

audiometer An electronic device that produces pure tones at various frequencies; used in determining hearing acuity.

aura A sensation that signals the onset of a headache or seizure; the patient may experience visual changes, flashing lights, or double vision.

autoamputation of the distal digits A condition in which the tips of the digits fall off spontaneously; can occur in severe cases of Raynaud's phenomenon.

autoantibodies Antibodies directed against self tissues of cells.

autocontamination The occurrence of infection in which the patient's own normal flora overgrows and penetrates the internal environment.

autodigestion Self-digestion. Specifically, the process of the stomach digesting itself if there is a break in its protective mucosal barrier.

autoimmune pancreatitis A chronic inflammatory form of pancreatitis that can also affect the bile ducts, kidneys, and other major connective tissues.

autologous blood transfusion Reinfusing the patient's own blood during surgery.

autologous donation The donation of a patient's own blood before scheduled surgery for use, if needed, during the surgery to eliminate transfusion reactions and reduce the risk of bloodborne disease.

autologous transplant A type of bone marrow transplant in which patients receive their own stem cells, which were collected before high-dose therapy.

autolysis The spontaneous disintegration of tissue by the action of the patient's own cellular enzymes.

automaticity The ability of a cell to initiate an impulse spontaneously and repetitively; in cardiac electrophysiology, the ability of primary pacemaker cells (SA node, AV junction) to generate an electrical impulse.

automatism Behavior of which the patient is not aware and which is not under the patient's control, such as lip smacking or picking at clothes; occurs in some types of seizure disorders.

autonomic dysreflexia A syndrome that affects the patient with an upper spinal cord injury; characterized by severe hypertension and headache, bradycardia, nasal stuffiness, and flushing; caused by a noxious stimulus, usually a distended bladder or constipation. This is a neurologic emergency and must be promptly treated to prevent a hypertensive brain attack.

autonomic nervous system (ANS) The part of the nervous system that is not under conscious control; consists of the sympathetic nervous system and the parasympathetic nervous system.

autoregulation The tendency of an organ or system to maintain blood flow at a fairly constant rate by dilating or constricting arteries in response to changes in blood pressure, carbon dioxide tension, and oxygen tension.

autosome Any of the 22 pairs of human chromosomes containing genes that code for all the structures and regulatory proteins needed for normal function but do not code for the sexual differentiation of a person.

avascular Lacking a blood supply.

avascular necrosis (AVN) The death of bone tissue, usually because the blood supply to the bone is disrupted. It is usually a complication of a hip fracture or any fracture in which there is displacement of bone; also called "osteonecrosis."

axial loading A mechanism of injury that involves vertical compression. An example is a diving accident, in which the blow to the top of the head causes the vertebrae to shatter and pieces of bone enter the spinal canal and damage the cord.

azoospermia The absence of living sperm in the semen.

azotemia An excess of nitrogenous wastes (urea) in the blood.

B

B-type natriuretic peptide (BNP) A peptide produced and released by the ventricles when the patient has fluid overload as a result of heart failure (HF).

Babinski's sign Dorsiflexion of the great toe and fanning of the other toes, which is an abnormal reflex in response to testing the plantar reflex with a pointed (but not sharp) object; indicates the presence of central nervous system disease. The normal response is plantar flexion of all toes.

bacteremia The presence of bacteria in the bloodstream.

bacteriuria Bacteria in the urine.

bad death A death embodied by pain, not having one's wishes followed at the end of one's life, isolation, abandonment, and constant agonizing about losses associated with death.

Baker's cyst Enlarged popliteal bursa.

balanced analgesia See *multimodal analgesia.*

balanitis circinata Ringlike inflammation of the glans penis.

Ballance's sign During percussion, resonance over the right flank with the patient lying on the left side; this is an abnormal sign associated with abdominal trauma and is found with a ruptured spleen.

ballottement A maneuver to detect fluid in the knee by grasping the medial and lateral aspect of the knee between the thumb and third finger and pushing down on the top surface of the patella with the forefinger. If fluid is present, the patella can be pressed down a distance and rises back up when the forefinger is removed.

banding See *endoscopic variceal ligation.*

barbiturate coma The use of drugs such as pentobarbital sodium or sodium thiopental at dosages to maintain complete unresponsiveness; used for patients whose increased intracranial pressure cannot be controlled by other means. These drugs decrease the metabolic demands of the brain and cerebral blood flow, stabilize cell membranes, decrease the formation of vasogenic edema, and produce a more uniform blood supply. The patient in a barbiturate coma requires mechanical ventilation, sophisticated hemodynamic monitoring, and intracranial pressure monitoring.

bariatrics Branch of medicine that manages obesity and its related diseases.

barium enema See *lower GI series.*

baroreceptors Sensory receptors in the arch of the aorta and at the origin of the internal carotid arteries that are stimulated when the arterial walls are stretched by an increased blood pressure.

barotrauma An injury caused by rapid changes of pressure; usually refers to injury to the eardrum caused by an increase in pressure within the middle ear or to lung damage from excessive pressure.

Barrett's epithelium Columnar epithelium (instead of the normal squamous cell epithelium) that develops in the lower esophagus during the process of healing from gastroesophageal reflux disease. It is considered premalignant and is associated with an increased risk of cancer in patients with prolonged disease.

Barrett's esophagus Ulceration of the lower esophagus caused by exposure to acid and pepsin, leading to the replacement of normal distal squamous mucosa with columnar epithelium as a response to tissue injury.

basal insulin secretion The low levels of insulin that are secreted during fasting.

basal rate A type of regimen for continuous infusion of patient-controlled analgesia that provides more consistent analgesia.

base A substance that binds (reduces) free hydrogen ions in solution. Strong bases bind hydrogen ions easily; weak bases bind less readily.

Bell's palsy Acute paralysis of cranial nerve VII; characterized by a drawing sensation and paralysis of all facial muscles on the affected side. The patient cannot close the eye, wrinkle the forehead, smile, whistle, or grimace. The face appears masklike and sags; also called "facial paralysis."

beneficence The ethical principle of preventing harm and ensuring the patient's well-being.

benign Altered cell growth that is harmless and does not require intervention.

benign prostatic hyperplasia (BPH) Age-associated enlargement of the prostate gland in men, which may cause bladder compression and can obstruct urinary flow.

benign tumor cells Normal cells growing in the wrong place or at the wrong time.

bereavement Grief and mourning experienced by the survivor before and after a death.

bicaval technique Surgical technique in heart transplantation in which the intact right atrium of the donor heart is preserved by anastomoses at the recipient's superior and inferior vena cavae.

bifurcation The point of division of a single structure into two branches.

bigeminy A type of premature complex that exists when normal complexes and premature complexes occur alternately in a repetitive two-beat pattern, with a pause occurring after each premature complex so that complexes occur in pairs.

bilateral orchiectomy The surgical removal of both testes, typically performed as palliative surgery in patients with prostate cancer. It is not intended to cure the prostate cancer but to arrest its spread by removing testosterone.

bilateral salpingo-oophorectomy (BSO) Surgical removal of both fallopian tubes and both ovaries.

biliary colic Intense pain due to obstruction of the cystic duct of the gallbladder from a stone moving through or lodged within the duct. Tissue spasm occurs in an effort to mobilize the stone through the small duct.

biliary stent A plastic or metal device that is placed percutaneously to keep a duct of the biliary system open in patients experiencing biliary obstruction.

biofilm A complex group of microorganisms that functions within a "slimy" gel coating on medical devices.

biological response modifiers (BRMs) A class of immunomodulating drugs that attempt to modify the course of disease.

biologically based therapies Therapies that use natural substances for healing, including herbs, foods, vitamins, and minerals.

bivalve To cut a cast lengthwise into two equal pieces.

black box warning A governmental designation indicating that a drug has at least one serious side effect and must be used with caution.

bladder ultrasound Less invasive test to determine postvoiding residual urine volumes for the patient with a reflex (upper motor neuron) or uninhibited bladder; often used to measure residual urine in the bladder of patients with spinal cord injury.

blanch To whiten.

blast effect Injury resulting from impact forces such as that of an exploding bomb.

blast phase cell Immature cell that divides.

blepharitis An inflammation of the eyelid edges.

bloodborne metastasis The release of tumor cells into the blood; the most common cause of cancer spread.

blood pressure (BP) The force of blood exerted against the vessel walls.

Blumberg's sign Pain felt on abrupt release of steady pressure (rebound tenderness) over the site of abdominal pain.

blunt trauma Injury resulting from impact forces such as those sustained in a motor vehicle crash or a fall.

body mass index (BMI) A measure of nutritional status that does not depend on frame size; indirectly estimates total fat stores within the body by the relationship of weight to height.

bolus feeding A method of tube feeding that involves intermittent feeding of a specified amount of enteral product at specified times during a 24-hour period, typically every 4 hours.

bone mineral density (BMD) The quality of bone that determines bone strength. It peaks between 30 and 35 years of age, when both bone resorption activity and bone-building activity occur at a constant rate. When bone resorption activity exceeds bone-building activity, bone density decreases.

bone remodeling The process of bone tissue constantly undergoing change.

bone resorption Loss of bone density due to demineralization resulting from the release of calcium from storage areas in bones.

bone scan A radionuclide test in which radioactive material is injected for visualization of the entire skeleton; used to detect tumors, arthritis, osteomyelitis, osteoporosis, vertebral compression fractures, and unexplained bone pain.

bony ossicle Small bone; in the ear, the malleus, the incus, and the stapes, which are found in the epitympanum.

borborygmus (borborygmi) Bowel sounds, especially loud gurgling sounds, resulting from hypermotility of the bowel.

boring In pain, the type of intense pain that feels like it is going through the body.

botulism A paralytic disease resulting from ingestion of a toxin in food contaminated with *Clostridium botulinum*. Botulism is associated with home-canned foods, commercially prepared products, and products not adequately heated to destroy toxins. Initial symptoms include diplopia, dysphagia, and dysarthria. Illness may be mild or severe, with paralysis, respiratory failure, and death.

Bouchard's nodes Swelling at the proximal interphalangeal joints in osteoarthritis involving the hands.

bowel training A program for patients with neurologic problems that is designed to include a combination of suppository use and a consistent toileting schedule.

boxer's ear See *cauliflower ear*.

bradycardia Slowness of the heart rate; characterized as a pulse rate less than 50 to 60 beats/min.

bradydysrhythmia An abnormal heart rhythm characterized by a heart rate less than 60 beats/min.

bradykinesia Slow or no movement, as seen in a patient with Parkinson disease; also called "akinesia."

brain abscess A collection of pus that forms in the extradural, subdural, or intracerebral area of the brain as a result of a purulent infection, usually due to bacteria invading the brain directly or indirectly.

brain attack Stroke; disruption in the normal blood supply to the brain, either as an interruption in blood flow (ischemic stroke) or as bleeding within or around the brain (hemorrhagic stroke). A medical emergency that occurs suddenly, a stroke should be treated immediately to prevent neurologic deficit and permanent disability. Formerly called "cerebrovascular accident," the National Stroke Association now uses the term "brain attack" to describe stroke.

brain herniation syndrome In the patient with untreated increased intracranial pressure, protrusion (herniation) of the brain downward toward the brainstem or laterally from a unilateral lesion within one cerebral hemisphere, causing irreversible brain damage and possibly death.

breast One of a pair of mammary glands that develop in response to secretions from the hypothalamus, pituitary gland, and ovaries. Breasts are an accessory of the reproductive system meant to nourish the infant after birth. They also are organs for sexual arousal in the mature adult.

breast augmentation Cosmetic surgical procedure to enhance the size, shape, or symmetry of the breasts.

breast-conserving surgery Surgical method for breast cancer that removes the bulk of the tumor rather than the entire breast.

Broca's aphasia See *expressive aphasia*.

Broca's area An important speech area of the cerebrum. It is located in the frontal lobe and is composed of neurons responsible for the formation of words, or speech.

bronchoscopy Insertion of a tube in the airway, usually as far as the secondary bronchi, for the purpose of visualizing airway structures and obtaining tissue samples for biopsy or culture.

Brown-Séquard syndrome A condition caused by cervical injuries; generally results from penetrating injuries that cause hemisection of the spinal cord or injuries that affect half of the spinal cord. Motor function, proprioception, vibration, and deep touch sensations are lost on the same side of the body as the lesion (ipsilateral). On the opposite side of the body (contralateral), the sensations of pain, temperature, and light touch are affected.

bruit Swishing sound in the larger arteries (carotid, aortic, femoral, and popliteal) that can be heard with a stethoscope or Doppler probe; may indicate narrowing of the artery and is usually associated with atherosclerotic disease.

bulbar Pertaining to the muscles involved in facial expression, chewing, and speech.

bulimia nervosa An eating disorder that is characterized by episodes of binge eating in which the patient ingests a large amount of food in a short time, followed by purging behavior such as self-induced vomiting or excessive use of laxatives and diuretics.

bunion Hallux valgus deformity of the foot in which lateral deviation of the great toe causes the first metatarsal head to become enlarged.

bunionectomy Surgical removal of the hallux valgus deformity (bunion) of the foot.

bursae The small sacs lined with synovial membrane that are located at joints and bony prominences to prevent friction between bone and structures adjacent to bone.

butterfly rash A dry, scaly, raised rash on the face; the major skin manifestation of systemic lupus erythematosus.

C

C fiber Unmyelinated or poorly myelinated fiber found in muscle, periosteum, and viscera; conducts thermal, chemical, and strong mechanical impulses that produce diffuse, persistent, and dull, burning, or achy sensations.

cachexia Extreme body wasting and malnutrition that develop from an imbalance between food intake and energy use.

calculi An abnormal formation of a mass of mineral salts that can occur in the body; forms in the kidney when excess calcium precipitates out of solution; also called "stones."

calculous cholecystitis Inflammation of the gallbladder usually following and created by obstruction of the cystic duct by a stone (calculus).

callus The loose, fibrous, vascular tissue that forms at the site of a fracture as the first phase of healing and is normally replaced by hard bone as healing continues.

calyx The anatomic term for a cuplike structure.

Canadian Triage Acuity Scale (CTAS) A standardized model for triage in which lists of descriptors are used to establish the triage level.

cancellous The softer tissue inside bones that contains large spaces, or trabeculae, that are filled with red and yellow marrow.

cancer control See *cytoreductive surgery.*

candidiasis An infection caused by the fungus *Candida albicans.*

canthus The place where the upper and lower eyelids meet at the corner of either side of the eye.

capillary closing pressure The amount of pressure needed to occlude skin capillary blood flow.

capillary leak syndrome The response of capillaries to the presence of biologic chemicals (mediators) that change blood vessel integrity and allow fluid to shift from the blood in the vascular space into the interstitial tissues.

Caplan's syndrome The presence of pneumoconiosis and rheumatoid nodules in the lungs; noted primarily in coal miners and asbestos workers.

capsule The layer of fibrous tissue on the outer surface of the kidney, which provides protection and support. The renal capsule itself is surrounded by layers of fat and connective tissue.

carboxyhemoglobin Carbon monoxide on oxygen-binding sites of the hemoglobin molecule.

carcinoembryonic antigen (CEA) An oncofetal antigen that may be elevated in 70% of people with colorectal cancer. CEA is not specifically associated with the colorectal cancer and may be elevated in the presence of other benign or malignant diseases and in smokers. CEA is often used to monitor the effectiveness of treatment and to identify disease recurrence.

carcinogen Any substance that changes the activity of the genes in a cell so that the cell becomes a cancer cell.

carcinogenesis Cancer development.

cardiac axis In electrocardiography (ECG), the direction of electrical current flow in the heart. The relationship between the cardiac axis and the lead axis is responsible for the deflections seen on the ECG pattern.

cardiac catheterization The most definitive but most invasive test in the diagnosis of heart disease; involves passing a small catheter into the heart and injecting contrast medium.

cardiac index A calculation of cardiac output requirements to account for differences in body size; determined by dividing the cardiac output by the body surface area.

cardiac output (CO) The volume of blood ejected by the heart each minute; normal range in adults is 4 to 7 L/min.

cardiac rehabilitation The process of actively assisting the patient with cardiac disease to achieve and maintain a productive life while remaining within the limits of the heart's ability to respond to increases in activity and stress. *Phase 1* begins with the acute illness and ends with discharge from the hospital. *Phase 2* begins after discharge and continues through convalescence at home. *Phase 3* refers to long-term conditioning.

cardiac resynchronization therapy (CRT) In patients with some types of heart failure, the use of a permanent pacemaker alone or in combination with an implantable cardioverter-defibrillator to provide biventricular pacing.

cardiac tamponade Compression of the myocardium by fluid that has accumulated around the heart; this compresses the atria and ventricles, prevents them from filling adequately, and reduces cardiac output.

cardiogenic shock Post–myocardial infarction heart failure in which necrosis of more than 40% of the left ventricle has occurred; also called "class IV heart failure."

cardiomegaly Enlarged heart.

cardiomyopathy A subacute or chronic disease of cardiac muscle; classified into four categories based on abnormalities in structure and function: dilated, hypertrophic, restrictive, and arrhythmogenic.

cardiopulmonary bypass (CPB) Diversion of the blood from the heart to a bypass machine, where it is heparinized, oxygenated, and returned to the circulation through a cannula placed in the ascending aortic arch or femoral artery to provide oxygenation, circulation, and hypothermia during induced cardiac arrest for coronary artery bypass surgery. This process ensures a motionless operative field and prevents myocardial ischemia.

cardiopulmonary resuscitation (CPR) A procedure that involves ventilating the patient who has stopped breathing, as well as giving chest compressions in the absence of a carotid pulse.

cardioversion A synchronized countershock that may be performed in emergencies for hemodynamically unstable ventricular or supraventricular tachydysrhythmias or electively for stable tachydysrhythmias that are resistant to medical therapies. The shock depolarizes a critical mass of myocardium simultaneously during intrinsic depolarization and is intended to stop the re-entry circuit and allow the sinus node to regain control of the heart.

carina The point at which the trachea branches into the right and left mainstem bronchi.

caring A process, set of actions, and attitude that show genuine physical and emotional concern for others.

carotid endarterectomy Removal of atherosclerotic plaque from the inner lining of the carotid artery to open the artery enough to re-establish blood flow and decrease risk for brain attack. This surgical procedure prevents progression of brain attack in symptomatic patients with recurrent transient ischemic attacks or carotid stenosis.

carotid sinus massage A method of vagal stimulation of the cardiac conduction system in which the physician massages over one carotid artery for a few seconds and observes for a change in cardiac rhythm. Massaging the carotid sinus causes vagal stimulation, thus slowing sinoatrial and atrioventricular nodal conduction.

carpal tunnel syndrome (CTS) A common condition in which the median nerve in the wrist becomes compressed, causing pain and numbness.

carrier (1) A person who harbors an infectious agent without symptoms of active disease; (2) in genetics, a person who has one mutated allele for a recessive genetic disorder. A carrier does not usually have any manifestations of the disorder but can pass the mutated allele to his or her children.

case management The process of assessment, planning, implementation, evaluation, and interaction for patients who have complex health problems and incur a high cost to the health care system. Goals include promoting quality of life, decreasing fragmentation and duplication of care across health care settings, and maintaining cost-effectiveness.

caseation necrosis A type of necrosis in which tissue is turned into a granular mass.

cast A rigid device that immobilizes the affected body part while allowing other body parts to move. It is most commonly used for fractures but may also be applied to correct deformities (e.g., clubfoot) or to prevent deformities (e.g., those seen in some patients with rheumatoid arthritis).

catabolism Any destructive metabolic process by which organisms convert substances into excreted compounds.

cataract A lens opacity that distorts the image projected onto the retina.

catechol *O*-methyltransferase (COMT) inhibitors Enzymes that inactivate dopamine, thereby blocking dopamine activity and increasing the effectiveness of levodopa; a class of drugs prescribed for patients with Parkinson disease.

catecholamines Hormones (dopamine, epinephrine, and norepinephrine) released by the adrenal medulla in response to stimulation of the sympathetic nervous system.

cation Ion that has a positive charge.

cauliflower ear A deformed and hardened auricle caused by trauma and resulting in a hematoma that hardens unless the blood is removed by needle aspiration; also called "boxer's ear."

cell-mediated immunity Microbial resistance that is mediated by the action of specifically sensitized T-lymphocytes.

cellulitis An acute, spreading, edematous inflammation of the deep subcutaneous tissues; usually caused by infection of a wound or burn.

central cord syndrome A condition caused by cervical injuries that involve lesions of the central portion of the spinal cord. Loss of motor function is more pronounced in the upper extremities than in the lower extremities; varying degrees and patterns of sensation remain intact.

central IV therapy IV therapy in which a vascular access device (VAD) is placed in a central blood vessel, such as the superior vena cava.

cerebral angiography (arteriography) Visualization of the cerebral circulation (carotid and vertebral arteries) after injecting a contrast medium into an artery (usually the femoral).

cerebral blood flow (CBF) Useful in evaluating cerebral vasospasm; can be measured in many areas of the brain with the use of radioactive substances.

cerebral perfusion pressure (CPP) The pressure gradient over which the brain is perfused. It is influenced by oxygenation, cerebral blood volume, blood pressure, cerebral edema, and intracranial pressure (ICP) and is determined by subtracting the mean ICP from the mean arterial pressure. A cerebral perfusion pressure above 70 mm Hg is generally accepted as an appropriate goal of therapy.

cerebral salt-wasting (CSW) The primary cause of hyponatremia in the neurosurgical population; characterized by hyponatremia, decreased serum osmolality, and decreased blood volume. It is thought to result from the extrarenal influence of atrial natriuretic factor.

cerumen The wax produced by glands within the external ear canal; helps protect and lubricate the ear canal.

cervical polyp Tumor that arises from the mucosa and extends to the opening of the cervical os. Polyps result from hyperplasia of the endocervical epithelium, inflammation, or an abnormal local response to hormonal stimulation or localized vascular congestion of the cervical blood vessels. Polyps are the most common benign growth of the cervix.

cervix The lower, narrowed portion of the uterus that extends into the vagina. It is the passage site for sperm to enter the uterus and the passage site for menstrual flow to exit the uterus.

chalazion An inflammation of a sebaceous gland in the eyelid.

chancre The ulcer that is the first sign of syphilis. It develops at the site of entry (inoculation) of the organism, usually 3 weeks after exposure. The lesion may be found on any area of the skin or mucous membranes but occurs most often on the genitalia, lips, nipples, and hands and in the oral cavity, anus, and rectum.

chancroid A sexually transmitted disease characterized by painful genital ulcerations and caused by infection with *Haemophilus ducreyi*. Infection develops as a result of sexual exposure or self-contamination from a lesion elsewhere on the body. Incubation period varies from 3 to 10 days. A tender papule appears at the site of inoculation and rapidly breaks down to form an irregularly shaped, deep ulcer that has a purulent discharge and bleeds easily.

chelation A general term referring to a drug or substance that binds or attaches to another substance.

chemoreceptor Specialized sensory receptor in the bifurcation of the carotid arteries and in the aortic arch; sensitive to hypoxemia. When stimulated, the carotid chemoreceptors send impulses along Hering's nerves and the aortic chemoreceptors send impulses along the vagus nerves to activate a vasoconstrictor response.

chemotaxin Substance secreted by damaged tissues and blood vessels that attracts neutrophils and macrophages so that phagocytosis can occur; also called "leukotaxin."

chemotherapy The treatment of cancer with chemical agents that have systemic effects; used to cure and to increase survival time.

chemotherapy-induced peripheral neuropathy (CIPN) The loss of sensory or motor function of peripheral nerves associated with exposure to certain anticancer drugs.

chest tube A drain placed in the pleural space to allow closed–chest drainage, which restores intrapleural pressure and allows re-expansion of the lung after surgery in patients who have undergone thoracotomy (incision of the chest wall).

Cheyne-Stokes respirations Common sign of nearing death in which apnea alternates with periods of rapid breathing.

choked disc See *papilledema*.

cholecystectomy The surgical removal of the gallbladder.

cholecystitis Inflammation of the gallbladder.

cholecystokinin A hormone that stimulates digestive juices and may work with leptin to increase or decrease appetite.

choledochojejunostomy Surgical anastomosis of the common bile duct with the jejunum.

cholelithiasis The presence of gallstones.

cholesteatoma A benign overgrowth of squamous cell epithelium.

cholinergic crisis Overmedication with cholinesterase inhibitors.

cholinesterase inhibitors Drugs that improve cholinergic neurotransmission in the central nervous system by delaying the destruction of acetylcholine by acetylcholinesterase, thus delaying the onset of cognitive decline. These are approved for symptomatic treatment of Alzheimer's disease but do not affect the course of the disease.

chondrogenic Originating from cartilage.

chondroitin A supplement that may play a role in strengthening cartilage.

choreiform movement Rapid, jerky movement.

chorioretinitis Inflammation of both the choroid and the retina.

chronic Having a slow onset and symptoms that persist for an extended period.

chronic calcifying pancreatitis (CCP) Alcohol-induced chronic pancreatitis that is characterized by protein precipitates that plug the ducts and lead to ductal obstruction, atrophy, and dilation. The epithelium of the ducts undergoes histologic changes, resulting in metaplasia (cell replacement) and ulceration. This inflammatory process causes fibrosis of the pancreatic tissue.

chronic cancer pain Persistent or recurrent pain that results from cancer or another progressive disease or life-threatening condition.

chronic constrictive pericarditis A fibrous thickening of the pericardium that prevents adequate filling of the ventricles and eventually results in cardiac failure; caused by chronic pericardial inflammation due to tuberculosis, radiation therapy, trauma, kidney failure, or metastatic cancer.

chronic fatigue syndrome (CFS) A chronic illness characterized by severe fatigue for 6 months or longer, usually following flu-like symptoms. At least four of the following criteria are required for diagnosis: sore throat; substantial impairment in short-term memory or concentration; tender lymph nodes; muscle pain; multiple joint pain with redness or swelling; headaches of a new type, pattern, or severity; unrefreshing sleep; and postexertional malaise lasting more than 24 hours.

chronic gastritis A patchy, diffuse inflammation of the mucosal lining of the stomach. Chronic gastritis usually heals without scarring but can progress to hemorrhage and ulcer formation.

chronic health problem A condition that has existed for at least 3 months.

chronic hepatitis Chronic liver inflammation that usually occurs as a result of hepatitis B or C. Superimposed infection with hepatitis D (HDV) in patients with chronic HBV may also result in chronic hepatitis. Can lead to cirrhosis and liver cancer.

chronic non-cancer pain Persistent or recurrent pain associated with a tissue injury that has healed or is not associated with cancer, such as arthritis.

chronic obstructive pancreatitis Pancreatitis that develops from inflammation, spasm, and obstruction of the sphincter of Oddi. Inflammatory and sclerotic lesions occur in the head of the pancreas and around the ducts, causing obstruction and backflow of pancreatic secretions.

chronic obstructive pulmonary disease (COPD) Any lung disease characterized by bronchospasm and dyspnea, such as emphysema and chronic bronchitis.

chronic osteomyelitis Bone infection that persists over a long time due to misdiagnosis or inadequate treatment; also called "subchronic osteomyelitis."

chronic pain Pain that persists or recurs for indefinite periods (usually more than 3 months), often involves deep body structures, is poorly localized, and is difficult to describe. Also called "persistent pain."

chronic pancreatitis A progressive, destructive disease of the pancreas characterized by remissions and exacerbations. Inflammation and fibrosis of the tissue contribute to pancreatic insufficiency and diminished function of the organ.

chronic paronychia Inflammation of the skin around the nail that persists for months. People at risk for chronic paronychia are those with frequent exposure to water, such as homemakers, bartenders, and laundry workers.

chronic pyelonephritis A kidney disorder that results from repeated or continued upper urinary tract infections or the effects of such infections.

chronic stable angina (CSA) Type of angina characterized by chest discomfort that occurs with moderate to prolonged exertion and in a pattern that is familiar to the patient.

chyme The liquid formed when food is transformed during the digestion process in the gastrointestinal tract.

cilia Hairlike projections from epithelial cells; also, the eyelids or eyelashes.

circle of Willis At the base of the brain, the ring formed by the anterior, middle, and posterior cerebral arteries where they are joined together by small communicating arteries.

circumcision The surgical removal of the prepuce or foreskin of the penis.

circumferential Referring to something that completely surrounds an extremity or the thorax.

cirrhosis Liver disease that is characterized by extensive scarring of the liver and is usually caused by a chronic irreversible reaction to hepatic inflammation and necrosis; disease typically develops insidiously and has a prolonged, destructive course.

classic heat stroke A form of heat stroke in which the body's ability to dissipate heat is significantly impaired; occurs over time as a result of long-term exposure to a hot, humid environment such as a home without air-conditioning in the high heat of the summer.

claudication Pain in the muscles resulting from an inadequate blood supply.

climacteric The phase of a woman's life from the initial decline in the amount of estrogen produced by the ovaries to the end of symptoms. The lay term for this phase is "the change of life."

clinical practice guideline An "official recommendation" based on evidence to diagnose and/or manage a health problem (e.g., pain management).

clinically competent The condition of being legally competent and having decisional capacity.

clitoris A small, cylindric organ of the external female genitalia that is composed of erectile tissue with a high concentration of sensory nerve endings.

clonic Pertaining to a state of alternating muscle stiffness followed by rhythmic jerking motions, as in a tonic-clonic seizure.

clonic seizure A type of generalized seizure lasting several minutes and characterized by muscle contraction and relaxation.

clonus The sudden, brief, jerking contraction of a muscle or muscle group often seen in seizures.

closed fracture A fracture that does not extend through the skin and therefore has no visible wound; also called "simple fracture."

closed head injury A type of traumatic primary brain injury that occurs as the result of blunt trauma; the integrity of the skull is not violated, and damage to brain tissue depends on the degree and mechanisms of injury.

closed reduction A nonsurgical method for managing a simple fracture. While applying a manual pull, or traction, on the bone, the health care provider manipulates the bone ends so they realign.

clubbing Changes in the tissue beds of the fingers and toes, with the base of the nail becoming spongy; results from chronic oxygen deprivation in the tissue beds.

cluster headache A type of oculotemporal or oculofrontal headache marked by unilateral, excruciating, nonthrobbing pain that is felt deep in and around the eye and may radiate to the forehead, temple, cheek, ear, occiput, or neck. Average duration is 10 to 45 minutes. Headaches occur every 8 to 12 hours and up to 24 hours daily at the same time for about 6 to 8 weeks (hence the term "cluster"), followed by remission for 9 months to a year. Cause and mechanism are unknown but have been attributed to vasoreactivity and oxyhemoglobin desaturation.

CO₂ narcosis Loss of sensitivity to high levels of $Paco_2$. For these patients, the stimulus to breathe is a decreased arterial oxygen level.

coagulopathy Clotting abnormalities.

cochlea The spiral organ of hearing within the inner ear.

cognition The ability of the brain to process, store, retrieve, and manipulate information.

cognitive therapist A member of the rehabilitative health care team, usually a neuropsychologist, who works primarily with patients who have experienced head injuries and have cognitive impairments.

cohorting The practice of grouping patients who are colonized or infected with the same pathogen.

coitus Sexual intercourse.

cold antibody anemia A form of immunohemolytic anemia (in which the immune system attacks a person's own red blood cells for unknown reasons) that occurs with complement protein fixation on immunoglobulin M (IgM). In this condition, the arteries in the hands and feet constrict profoundly in response to cold temperatures or stress.

cold phase A phase after peripheral nerve trauma resulting in complete denervation in which the skin appears cyanotic, mottled, or reddish blue and feels cool compared with the contralateral, unaffected extremity. The cold phase follows the warm phase, which lasts 2 to 3 weeks after injury.

colectomy Surgical removal of part or all of the colon.

collaboration The planning, implementing, and evaluation of patient care using an interdisciplinary (ID) plan of care.

collaborative nursing function Activity that is mutually determined by the nurse and the physician or other health care team member or that is directed or prescribed by the health care provider but requires nursing judgment to perform.

collateral circulation Circulation that provides blood to an area with altered tissue perfusion through smaller vessels that develop and compensate for the occluded vessels.

colon interposition A surgical procedure that may be performed in patients with an esophageal tumor when the tumor involves the stomach or the stomach is otherwise unsuitable for anastomosis. In colon interposition, a section of right or left colon is removed and brought up into the thorax to substitute for the esophagus.

colon resection Surgery performed for colorectal cancer in which the tumor and regional lymph nodes are removed.

colonization The presence of microorganisms in the tissues of the host without causing symptomatic disease.

colonoscopy The endoscopic examination of the entire large bowel.

colostomy The surgical creation of an opening between the colon and the surface of the abdomen.

colposcopy Examination of the cervix and vagina using a colposcope, which allows three-dimensional magnification and intense illumination of epithelium with suspected disease. This procedure can locate the exact site of precancerous and malignant lesions for biopsy.

comatose A state of being unconscious and unarousable.

comedones Plural form of "comedo." Blackheads and whiteheads, the noninflammatory lesions of acne.

command center See *emergency operations center.*

commando (co-mandible) procedure (COMbined neck dissection, MANDibulectomy, and Oropharyngeal resection) A procedure in which the surgeon removes a segment of the mandible with the oral lesion and performs a radical neck dissection.

comminuted fracture A type of fracture that involves fragmentation of the bone.

commitment Occurrence in which early embryonic cells start changing into differentiated cells.

communicable The ability of an infection, such as influenza, to be transmitted from person to person.

comorbidity Pre-existing disease state that must be included in patient assessment in regard to how the condition might adversely affect a seemingly unrelated health problem.

compartment syndrome A condition in which increased tissue pressure in a confined anatomic space causes decreased blood flow to the area, leading to hypoxia and pain.

compensated cirrhosis A form of cirrhosis in which the liver has significant scarring but is still able to perform essential functions without causing significant symptoms.

compensatory mechanism The means of producing compensation; also called "adaptive mechanism."

complement activation and fixation Actions triggered by some classes of antibodies that can remove or destroy antigen.

complementary and alternative medicine The broad range of healing philosophies, approaches, and therapies that mainstream Western medicine does not commonly use.

complete spinal cord injury An injury in which the spinal cord has been severed or damaged in a way that eliminates all innervation below the level of the injury.

complex partial seizure A type of partial seizure that occurs in patients with epilepsy, causing loss of consciousness for 1 to 3 minutes. Characteristic behaviors known as "automatisms" may occur, such as lip smacking or picking at clothes. The patient may experience amnesia after the seizure. Because the area of the brain most often involved is the temporal lobe, complex partial seizures are often called "psychomotor seizures" or "temporal lobe seizures."

complex regional pain syndrome (CRPS) A complex disorder that includes debilitating pain, atrophy, autonomic dysfunction (excessive sweating, vascular changes), and motor impairment (most notably muscle paresis), probably caused by an abnormally hyperactive sympathetic nervous system. This syndrome most often results from traumatic injury and commonly occurs in the feet and hands; formerly called "reflex sympathetic dystrophy (RSD)."

compliance In respiratory physiology, a measure of elasticity within the lung. Also, a patient's fulfillment of a caregiver's prescribed course of treatment.

compound fracture See *open fracture.*

compression fracture A fracture that is produced by a loading force applied to the long axis of cancellous bone. These fractures commonly occur in the vertebrae of patients with osteoporosis.

computed tomography coronary angiography (CTCA) 64-slice diagnostic scan used to diagnose coronary artery disease in symptomatic patients.

computed tomography (CT) scanning Use of a computer to take pictures at many horizontal levels, or slices, of the area being studied. The cross-sectional slices build up three-dimensional pictures; a contrast medium may be used to enhance the image.

concentration gradient Movement across a membrane from an area of higher concentration to an area of lower concentration.

concussion A type of closed head injury that is caused by blunt trauma (e.g., a blow to the head) and is characterized by a brief loss of consciousness.

conductive hearing loss Hearing loss that results from any physical obstruction of sound wave transmission (e.g., a foreign body in the external canal, a retracted or bulging tympanic membrane, or fused bony ossicles).

conductivity The ability of a cell to transmit an electrical stimulus from cell membrane to cell membrane.

congestive heart failure (CHF) Former term for "left-sided heart failure." Categorized as either systolic heart failure or diastolic heart failure that may be acute or chronic and mild to severe.

conization The removal of a cone-shaped sample of tissue from the cervix for cytologic study.

conjunctivae The mucous membranes of the eye that line the undersurface of the eyelids (palpebral conjunctiva) and cover the sclera (bulbar conjunctiva).

connective tissue disease (CTD) A group of diseases that are the major focus of rheumatology (the study of rheumatic diseases); most are musculoskeletal disorders.

consensual response In assessing pupillary reaction to light, a slight constriction of the pupil of the eye not being tested when a penlight is brought in from the side of the patient's head and shined into the eye being tested as soon as the patient opens his or her eyes.

consolidation Solidification; lack of air spaces in the lung, such as occurs in pneumonia.

contact laser prostatectomy (CLP) Procedure for treating benign prostatic hyperplasia that uses laser energy to coagulate excess tissue. Also called "interstitial laser coagulation (ILC)."

Contact Precautions Infection control guidelines from the Centers for Disease Control and Prevention; used for patients with infections spread by direct contact or contact with items in the patient's environment, such as pediculosis.

contiguous Something in direct contact with, or adjacent to, another area or structure.

continence The ability to voluntarily control emptying the bladder and colon. Continence is a learned behavior whereby a person can suppress the urge to urinate until a socially appropriate location is available.

continuous feeding A method of tube feeding in which small amounts of enteral product are continuously infused (by gravity drip or by a pump or controller device) over a specified time.

continuous positive airway pressure (CPAP) A respiratory treatment that improves obstructive sleep apnea in patients with heart failure.

contractility The ability of a cell to contract in response to an impulse. In cardiac electrophysiology, the ability of atrial and ventricular muscle cells to shorten their fiber length in response to electrical stimulation, generating sufficient pressure to propel blood forward. Contractility is the mechanical activity of the heart.

contraction The closure of a wound as new collagen replaces damaged tissue, pulling the wound edges inward along the path of least resistance.

contralateral Pertaining to the opposite side.

contrecoup injury Bruising of the brain tissue, with damage occurring on the side opposite the site of impact.

controller A stationary, pole-mounted electronic device that uses a sensor to monitor fluid flow during infusion therapy and to detect flow interruption.

contusion A bruise; when referring to closed head injury, a bruising of brain tissue usually found at the site of impact (coup injury). Compare with *contrecoup injury.*

cor pulmonale Right-sided heart failure caused by pulmonary disease.

cordectomy Excision of a vocal cord in surgery for laryngeal cancer.

cordotomy Surgical technique in which the surgeon cuts the pain pathways at the midline portion of the spinal cord, before nerve impulses ascend to the spinothalamic tract. Used to relieve intractable pain in patients with metastatic cancer by interrupting the transmission of pain.

cornea The clear layer that forms the external coat on the front of the eye.

corneal abrasion Scrape or scratch of the cornea that disrupts its integrity.

corneal ulceration Deep disruption of the corneal epithelium that extends into the stromal layer and is caused by bacteria, protozoa, or fungi.

coronary artery bypass graft A surgical procedure in which occluded coronary arteries are bypassed with the patient's own venous or arterial blood vessels or synthetic grafts.

coronary artery calcium (CAC) score A measure of the amount of coronary artery calcification present.

coronary artery disease (CAD) Disease affecting the arteries that provide blood, oxygen, and nutrients to the myocardium; partial or complete blockage of the blood flow through the coronary arteries, causing ischemia and infarction of the myocardium, angina pectoris, and acute coronary syndromes.

coronary artery vasculopathy (CAV) A form of coronary artery disease that presents as diffuse plaque in the arteries of the donor heart in patients who have received a heart transplant.

cortex The outer layer of an organ or body structure.

cortical A term referring to compact bone of the shaft of a bone.

corticosteroids The hormones produced and secreted by the adrenal cortex; also called "adrenal steroids."

cortisol The main glucocorticoid produced by the adrenal cortex.

coryza The common cold, or acute viral rhinitis.

cough assist A technique for assisting the tetraplegic patient to cough. Place his or her hands on either side of the rib cage or upper abdomen below the diaphragm; then, as the patient exhales, push upward to help expand the lungs and cough.

craniotomy Surgical incision into the cranium.

creatine kinase (CK) An enzyme specific to cells of the brain, myocardium, and skeletal muscle. Its appearance in the blood indicates tissue necrosis or injury, with levels following a predictable rise and fall during a specified period.

Credé maneuver A technique used to assist in urination in which a patient places his or her hand in a cupped position directly over the bladder area and pushes inward and downward gently as if massaging the bladder to empty.

cremasteric reflex Stimulation of the skin on the front and inner side of the thigh retracts the testicle and scrotum on the same side. An intact reflex indicates integrity of the first lumbar nerve segment of the spinal cord.

crepitus (crepitation) A continuous grating sensation caused when irregular cartilage or bone fragments rub together and which may be felt or heard as a joint is put through passive range of motion; also, a crackling sensation that can be felt on a patient's chest, indicating that air is trapped within the tissues.

CREST syndrome In patients with systemic sclerosis, the combination of **c**alcinosis (calcium deposits), **R**aynaud's phenomenon, **e**sophageal dysmotility, **s**clerodactyly (scleroderma of the digits), and **t**elangiectasia (spider-like hemangiomas).

cricothyroidotomy Surgical procedure in which an opening is made between the thyroid cartilage and cricoid cartilage ring and results in a tracheostomy; also called "cricothyrotomy." The procedure is used in an emergency for access to the lower airways.

crises In the patient with sickle cell disease, periodic episodes of extensive cellular sickling that have a sudden onset and can occur as often as weekly or as seldom as once a year.

critical access hospital A small rural facility of 15 or fewer inpatient beds that provides around-the-clock emergency care services 7 days per week. Considered a necessary provider of health care to community residents who are not close to other hospitals in a given region.

critical thinking Purposeful, outcome-directed thinking that is used to make clinical judgments based on scientific evidence rather than on tradition or conjecture (guesswork).

cross-contamination A type of contamination in which organisms from another person or from the environment are transmitted to the patient.

cryoanalgesia The use of cold to achieve permanent ablation of nerve roots.

cryoprecipitate A highly concentrated blood product that is derived from plasma and includes clotting factors VIII and XIII, von Willebrand's factor, and fibrinogen.

cryosurgery Destruction of tissue by applying extreme cold; may reduce pain and tumor size in patients with metastatic cancer.

cryotherapy (1) A way of decreasing muscle pain by "cooling down" the area with a local, short-acting gel or cream, such as after physical therapy; (2) in ophthalmologic surgery, use of a freezing probe to repair retinal detachment.

cryptorchidism Failure of the testes to descend into the scrotum.

Cullen's sign The presence of a bluish discoloration around the umbilicus, which is an indication of intra-abdominal bleeding.

cultural competence The ability of health care provider or organization to understand and respond effectively to the cultural and linguistic needs that patients bring to the health care setting.

cultural diversity The differences among people, which may or may not be visible.

cultural sensitivity The way that one responds to cultural differences.

culture (1) A procedure for identifying a microorganism by cultivating and isolating it in tissue cultures or artificial media; (2) an integrated pattern of human behavior that is learned and transmitted to succeeding generations and includes thought, speech, action, and artifacts.

curandero A folk healer in the Mexican-American medicine system who considers health and health care from a holistic, spiritual perspective rather than the traditional scientific viewpoint.

curative surgery Surgery done to remove all cancer tissue.

Curling's ulcer Acute ulcerative gastroduodenal disease, which may develop within 24 hours of a severe burn injury because of reduced gastrointestinal blood flow and mucosal damage.

Cushing's disease (Cushing's syndrome) Hypercortisolism caused by oversecretion of hormones by the adrenal cortex.

Cushing's triad A classic yet late sign of increased intracranial pressure (ICP) manifested by severe hypertension with a widened pulse pressure and bradycardia. As ICP increases, the pulse becomes thready, irregular, and rapid. Cerebral blood flow increases in response to hypertension.

Cushing's ulcer Acute ulcerative gastroduodenal disease that may develop as a result of increased intracranial pressure.

cutaneous reflexes Superficial reflexes. Usually the plantar and abdominal reflexes are tested.

cuticle A layer of keratin at the nail fold, which attaches the nail plate to the soft tissue of the nail fold.

cyanosis Bluish or darkened discoloration of the skin and mucous membranes; results from an increased amount of deoxygenated hemoglobin.

cyclic feeding A method of tube feeding similar to continuous feeding (see definition of *continuous feeding*) except the infusion is stopped for a specified time in each 24-hour period ("down time"); the down time typically occurs in the morning to allow bathing, treatments, and other activities.

cyst Firm, flesh-colored nodule that contains liquid or semisolid material.

cystectomy (1) Removal of a cyst; (2) surgical removal of the bladder and surrounding tissue.

cystitis Inflammation of the bladder.

cystocele Herniation of the bladder into the vagina.

cytokines Small protein hormones produced by white blood cells.

cytopenia Low blood count.

cytoprotectant Drug that protects specific healthy cells; given to patients to decrease the impact of chemotherapy on normal tissues.

cytoreductive surgery Surgery done to remove part of a tumor while leaving a known amount of gross tumor behind; also called "cancer control."

cytotoxic Having cell-damaging effects.

D

dandruff An accumulation of patchy or diffuse white or gray scales on the surface of the scalp.

dawn phenomenon In the patient with diabetes, a condition of fasting hyperglycemia resulting from a nighttime release of growth hormone that causes blood glucose elevations at about 5 to 6 AM. Providing more insulin for the overnight period helps avoid this condition.

death When illness or trauma overwhelms the compensatory mechanisms of the body and the lungs and heart cease to function.

death rattle Loud, wet respirations caused by secretions in the respiratory tract and oral cavity of a patient who is near death.

débridement The removal of infected tissue from a healing wound.

debriefing After a mass casualty incident or disaster, (1) the provision of sessions for small groups of staff in which teams are brought in to discuss effective coping strategies (critical incident stress debriefing), and (2) the administrative review of staff and system performance during the event to determine opportunities for improvement in the emergency management plan.

debris Dead cells and tissues in a wound.

decerebrate posturing Abnormal posturing and rigidity characterized by extension of the arms and legs, pronation of the arms, plantar flexion, and opisthotonos; usually associated with dysfunction in the brainstem area. Also called "decerebration."

decerebration See *decerebrate posturing*.

decompensated cirrhosis A form of cirrhosis in which liver function is significantly impaired with obvious manifestations of liver failure.

decompressive laminectomy Removal of one or more laminae in the patient with spinal cord injury and compression; allows for cord expansion from edema if more conventional measures fail to prevent neurologic deterioration.

decorticate posturing Abnormal posturing seen in the patient with lesions that interrupt the corticospinal pathways. The arms, wrists, and fingers are flexed with internal rotation and plantar flexion of the legs. Also called "decortication."

decortication See *decorticate posturing*.

deep tendon reflexes Tested as part of the neurologic assessment. An intact reflex arc is indicated when the muscle contracts in response to the tendon being struck with a hammer.

deep vein thrombophlebitis Presence of a thrombus associated with inflammation in the deep veins, usually in the legs. Compared with superficial thrombophlebitis, it presents a greater risk for pulmonary embolism; also called "deep vein thrombosis."

deep vein thrombosis (DVT) Common term for deep vein thrombophlebitis.

defibrillation An asynchronous countershock that depolarizes a critical mass of myocardium simultaneously to stop the re-entry circuit, allowing the sinus node to regain control of the heart.

degradation The process of breaking down.

dehiscence A partial or complete separation of the outer layers of a wound, sometimes described as a "splitting open" of the wound.

dehydration Fluid intake less than what is needed to meet the body's fluid needs.

delayed union Term describing a fracture that has not healed within 6 months of injury.

delegation The process of transferring to a competent person the authority to perform a selected nursing task or activity in a selected patient care situation.

delirium An acute state of confusion, usually short-term and reversible within 3 weeks. Often seen among older adults in a hospital or other unfamiliar setting.

delirium tremens (DTs) Tremors of the entire body; a symptom of alcohol withdrawal.

demand dose An amount of drug specified by the health care provider that is programmed into a patient-controlled analgesia infusion pump.

dementia A syndrome of slowly progressive cognitive decline with global impairment of intellectual function. The most common type is Alzheimer's disease.

demyelination Destruction of myelin between the nodes of Ranvier; a major pathologic finding in Guillain-Barré syndrome.

demyelinization Occurrence of multiple sclerosis in which the myelin sheath is damaged and its thickness is reduced.

deoxyribonucleic acid (DNA) The basic genetic material required for cell division and growth.

dependence A condition that causes a habitual, compulsive, and uncontrollable urge to use a substance; without the substance, the body experiences severe physiologic, psychological, and emotional disturbances.

depolarization The ability of a cell to respond to a stimulus by initiating an impulse; also called "excitability."

depressant A drug that reduces the activity of the central nervous system, such as a benzodiazepine or barbiturate.

depressed fracture A type of skull fracture in which the bone is pressed inward into brain tissue.

depression A response to multiple life stresses, a single situation, a primary disorder, or a problem associated with dementia; this response can range from mild, transient feelings of sadness to a severe sense of helplessness and hopelessness.

dermal appendages Collectively, the sweat and oil glands and the hair follicles. The depth of dermal appendages varies from one body area to another.

dermal papillae Fingerlike projections of dermal tissue that anchor the epidermis to the dermis.

dermatomes Specific areas of the skin that receive sensory input from spinal nerves.

dermatomyositis Polymyositis that is accompanied by a rash.

descending tracts Groups of nerves that begin in the brain and end in the spinal cord.

desquamation The shedding or peeling of skin.

diagnostic peritoneal lavage (DPL) Test that determines the presence of internal bleeding following abdominal trauma.

diagnostic surgery Surgery done to remove all or part of a suspected lesion for examination and testing; also called "biopsy."

dialysate The solution used in dialysis. It is composed of water, glucose, sodium chloride, potassium, magnesium, calcium, and bicarbonate; dialysate composition may be altered according to the patient's needs for treatment of electrolyte imbalances.

dialyzer The apparatus used to perform hemodialysis. Also known as the "artificial kidney," it has four parts: a blood compartment, a dialysate compartment, a semipermeable membrane, and an enclosed structure to support the membrane.

diaphoresis Abnormally profuse sweating.

diaphysis The shaft, or elongated cylindric portion, between the ends of a long bone.

diastole The phase of the cardiac cycle that consists of relaxation and filling of the atria and ventricles; normally about two thirds of the cardiac cycle.

diastolic blood pressure The amount of pressure/force against the arterial walls during the relaxation phase of the heart.

diastolic heart failure Heart failure that occurs when the left ventricle is unable to relax adequately during diastole, which prevents the ventricle from filling with sufficient blood to ensure adequate cardiac output.

diathermy The use of a high-frequency current to heat body tissues.

Dietary Guidelines for Americans Recommendations made by the USDA and U.S. Department of Health and Human Services to help people maintain nutritional health; updated every 5 years.

dietitian A member of the health care team who ensures patients meet their nutritional needs. Also called "nutritionist."

diffuse axonal injury (DAI) A type of closed head injury that is usually related to high-speed acceleration/deceleration, as with motor vehicle crashes. There is significant damage to axons in the white matter, and there are lesions in the corpus callosum, midbrain, cerebellum, and upper brainstem. Patients with severe injury may present with immediate coma, and most survivors require long-term care.

diffuse light reflex A description of a light reflex that is spotty or multiple because of a changed eardrum shape from either retraction or bulging.

diffuse scleroderma Skin thickening on the trunk, face, and proximal and distal extremities in patients with systemic sclerosis.

diffusion The spontaneous, free movement of particles (solute) across a permeable membrane down a concentration gradient; that is, from an area of higher concentration to an area of lower concentration.

digestion The mechanical and chemical process in which complex foodstuffs are broken down into simpler forms that can be used by the body.

digitalis toxicity A reaction to therapy with digitalis derivatives (digoxin) that is identified by monitoring serum digoxin and potassium levels (hypokalemia potentiates digitalis toxicity). Signs of toxicity are nonspecific (anorexia, fatigue, changes in mental status). Toxicity may cause dysrhythmia, most commonly premature ventricular contractions.

dilated cardiomyopathy (DCM) A type of cardiomyopathy that involves extensive damage to the myofibrils and interference with myocardial metabolism. There is normal ventricular wall thickness but dilation of both ventricles and impairment of systolic function.

dilation Increase in the diameter of blood vessels.

diplopia Double vision.

direct contact A mode of infection transmission in which microorganisms are transferred directly by physical contact from one person to another.

direct current stimulation (DCS) The placement of an implantable device to promote bone fusion; used as an adjunct for patients for whom spinal fusion may be difficult.

direct inguinal hernia A sac formed from the peritoneum that contains a portion of the intestine and passes through a weak point in the abdominal wall.

direct response Pupil constriction in response to bringing a penlight in from the side of the patient's head and shining the light in the eye being tested as soon as the patient opens his or her eyes.

directly observed therapy (DOT) A technique in which a health care professional watches the patient swallow prescribed drugs.

disabling health problem Any physical or mental health problem that can cause disability.

disaster A mass casualty incident in which the number of casualties exceeds the resource capabilities of a particular community or hospital facility.

disaster triage tag system A system that categorizes triage priority by colored and numbered tags.

discoid lesion Round lesion in patients who have discoid lupus erythematosus; evident when exposed to sunlight or ultraviolet light.

disease-modifying antirheumatic drugs (DMARDs) Drugs prescribed to slow the progression of mild rheumatoid disease before it worsens, such as hydroxychloroquine, sulfasalazine, or minocycline.

disequilibrium A condition in which the hydrostatic pressure is not the same in the two fluid spaces on either side of a permeable membrane.

disinfection A method of infection control in which the level of disease-causing organisms is reduced but the organisms are not killed; adequate when an item is entering a body area that has resident bacteria or normal flora, such as the respiratory tract.

diskitis Disk inflammation.

dislocation of a joint Occurrence of the articulating surfaces of two or more bones moving away from each other.

dissociate The act of separating and releasing ions.

distal protection device A device that is placed beyond (distal to) the stenosis during an angioplasty/stenting procedure for the purpose of catching debris that breaks off during the procedure.

divalent cation An ion having two positive charges.

diverticula Sacs resulting from the herniation of the mucosa and submucosa of a tubular organ into surrounding tissue.

diverticulitis The inflammation of one or more diverticula.

diverticulosis The presence of many abnormal pouchlike herniations (diverticula) in the wall of the intestine.

dizziness A disturbed sense of a person's relationship to space.

DNA replication The process of making a new copy of an entire strand of DNA.

dopamine agonist A class of drugs that mimic dopamine. Dopamine agonists stimulate dopamine receptors and are typically the most effective during the first 3 to 5 years of use. Prescribed for the patient with Parkinson disease to reduce dyskinesias (problems with movement).

dose (1) In radiation therapy, the amount of radiation absorbed by recipient tissue during radiation therapy as determined by intensity of exposure, duration of exposure, and closeness of the radiation source to the cells; (2) the amount of drug or other substance to be administered at one time.

dose-dense chemotherapy Chemotherapy that uses higher doses more often for aggressive cancer treatment, especially breast cancer.

double-barrel stoma The least common type of colostomy, which is created by dividing the bowel and bringing both the proximal and distal portions to the abdominal surface to create two stomas.

doubling time The amount of time it takes for a tumor to double in size.

Dressler's syndrome Pericarditis, fever, and pericardial and pleural effusions occurring together from 1 to 12 weeks after myocardial infarction.

droplet The small particles produced when a person coughs or sneezes; may be involved in indirect transmission of infection.

Droplet Precautions Infection control guidelines from the Centers for Disease Control and Prevention; used for patients with infections spread by the droplet transmission route, such as influenza.

drug holiday Period of time lasting up to 10 days in which the patient with Parkinson disease receives no drug therapy.

dual x-ray absorptiometry (DXA) A type of radiographic scan that measures bone mineral density in the hip, wrist, or vertebral column; used as a screening and diagnostic tool for diagnosis and for follow-up evaluation of treatment of osteoporosis.

ductal carcinoma in situ (DCIS) An early, noninvasive form of breast cancer in which cancer cells are located within the duct and have not invaded the surrounding fatty breast tissue.

ductal ectasia A benign breast disease caused by dilation and thickening of the collecting ducts in the subareolar area. The ducts become distended and filled with cellular debris, which activates an inflammatory response. It is usually seen in women approaching menopause.

dull A term that describes the medium-pitched, soft, thudlike sound over a solid organ (e.g., liver) that is obtained upon percussion of the abdomen.

dumping syndrome A constellation of vasomotor symptoms that typically occur within 30 minutes after eating; believed to occur as a result of the rapid emptying of gastric contents into the small intestine, which shifts fluid into the gut and causes abdominal distention. Early manifestations include vertigo, tachycardia, syncope, sweating, pallor, and palpitations.

Dupuytren's contracture A slowly progressive contracture of the palmar fascia that results in flexion of the fourth or fifth digit of the hand and occasionally affects the third digit. Although a fairly common problem, the cause is unknown. It usually occurs in older men, tends to occur in families, and can be bilateral.

durable power of attorney (DPOA) for health care A legal document in which a person appoints someone else to make health care decisions in the event he or she becomes incapable of making decisions.

dysarthria Slurred speech.

dysfunctional uterine bleeding (DUB) A nonspecific term to describe bleeding that is excessive or abnormal in amount or frequency without predisposing anatomic or systemic conditions. Such bleeding occurs most often at either end of the span of a woman's reproductive years, when ovulation is becoming established or when it is becoming irregular at menopause.

dyskinesia Difficulty with movement.

dysmenorrhea Painful menstruation.

dysmetria The inability to direct or limit movement.

dyspareunia Painful sexual intercourse.

dyspepsia Indigestion or heartburn following meals.

dysphagia Difficulty in swallowing.

dyspnea Difficulty in breathing or breathlessness.

dyspnea on exertion (DOE) Dyspnea that is associated with activity, such as climbing stairs.

dysrhythmia A disorder of the heartbeat involving a disturbance in cardiac rhythm; irregular heartbeat.

dystrophic Pertaining to or characterized by dystrophy; abnormal.

dystrophin A muscle protein that maintains muscle integrity by sending signals to coordinate smooth, synchronous muscle fiber contraction. Faulty action of this protein causes muscular dystrophy.

dysuria Painful urination.

E

early-onset seizure Seizure that occurs within 7 days of a head injury.

Eaton-Lambert syndrome A form of myasthenia gravis that affects the muscles of the trunk and the pelvic and shoulder girdles; often observed in combination with small cell carcinoma of the lung. Although weakness increases after exertion, there may be a temporary increase in muscle strength during the first few contractions, followed by a rapid decline.

ecchymoses Large purple, blue, or yellow bruises of the skin resulting from small hemorrhages; these bruises are larger than petechiae.

ecchymotic Pertaining to a bruise.

ECG caliper A measurement tool used in analysis of an electrocardiographic (ECG) rhythm strip.

echocardiography In cardiovascular assessment, the use of ultrasound waves to assess cardiac structure and mobility, particularly of the valves; a noninvasive, risk-free test that is easily performed at the bedside or on an ambulatory care basis.

echolalia Automatic repetition of what another person says.

ectopic Out of place.

ectopic beats Heartbeats generated outside the normal conduction system in the ventricles; a cardiac manifestation of hyperkalemia.

ectropion A turning outward and sagging of the eyelid, which is caused by relaxation of the orbicular muscle.

edema Tissue swelling as a result of the accumulation of excessive fluid in the interstitial spaces.

edentulous Without teeth.

efferent arterioles The extremely small blood vessels that carry the remaining blood out of the glomerulus (once the glomerulus has filtered the blood to make urine) and into one of two additional capillary systems (the peritubular capillaries or the vasa recta).

effluent Drainage.

effusion An accumulation of fluid, such as in a joint (where it may limit movement).

ejection fraction The percentage of blood ejected from the heart during systole.

elastin The major component of the elastic fibers that are scattered among the collagen fibers. Elasticity of the skin depends on both the amount and quality of the elastic fibers.

electrical bone stimulation The use of an electronic device (e.g., magnetic coils applied on the skin or over a cast to deliver a pulsed magnetic field) to promote bone union after a fracture. The exact mechanism of action is unknown, but this procedure is based on research showing that bone has inherent electrical properties that are used in healing.

electrocardiogram (ECG) A graphic recording of the electrical current generated by the heart. The ECG provides information about cardiac dysrhythmias, myocardial ischemia, site and extent of myocardial infarction, cardiac hypertrophy, electrolyte imbalances, and effectiveness of cardiac drugs. It is a routine part of cardiovascular evaluation and is a valuable diagnostic test.

electroencephalography (EEG) A recording of the electrical activity of the cerebral hemispheres; it represents the voltage changes in various areas of the brain as determined by recording the difference between two electrodes.

electrolyte A substance in body fluids that carries an electrical charge; also called an "ion."

electromyography (EMG) A recording of the electrical activity of peripheral nerves by testing muscle activity.

electrophysiologic study (EPS) In cardiovascular assessment, an invasive procedure performed in a catheterization laboratory during which programmed electrical stimulation of the heart is used to induce and evaluate lethal dysrhythmias and conduction abnormalities to permit accurate diagnosis and effective treatment. The study is used in patients who have survived cardiac arrest, have recurrent tachydysrhythmias, or experience unexplained syncopal episodes.

electrovaporization of the prostate (EVAP) Procedure for treating benign prostatic hyperplasia with high-frequency electrical current to cut and vaporize excess tissue.

emboli (1) Tumor pieces that spread to distant body areas; (2) small blood clots that can enter circulation.

embolic protection device (EPD) A device that is placed beyond the stenosis during an angioplasty/stenting procedure to catch debris that breaks off during the procedure.

embolus The occurrence of inflammation and thickening of the vein wall around a clot (thrombus).

emergence Recovery from anesthesia.

emergency medical technician (EMT) Prehospital care provider who supplies basic life-support interventions such as oxygen, basic wound care, splinting, spinal immobilization, and monitoring of vital signs.

emergency medicine physician A member of the emergency health care team with education and training in the specialty of emergency patient management.

emergency operations center (EOC) A designated location in the Hospital Incident Command System (HICS) with accessible communication technology; also called the "command center."

emergency preparedness A goal or plan to meet the extraordinary need for hospital beds, staff, drugs, personal protective equipment, supplies, and medical devices such as mechanical ventilators.

Emergency Severity Index (ESI) A standardized model for triage that categorizes both patient acuity and resource utilization into five levels, from most urgent to least urgent.

emergent triage In a three-tiered triage scheme, the category that includes any condition or injury that poses an immediate threat to life or limb, such as crushing chest pain or active hemorrhage.

emetogenic A substance that induces nausea and vomiting.

emission The first stage of the male orgasm in which the prostate gland secretes its fluid at the same time as the vas deferens.

emmetropia The state of perfect refraction of the eye; with the lens at rest, light rays from a distant source are focused into a sharp image on the retina.

emotional abuse The intentional use of threats, humiliation, intimidation, and isolation to another person.

emotional lability Having uncontrollable emotions; for example, the patient laughs and then cries unexpectedly for no apparent reason.

empyema A collection of pus in the pleural space.

encephalitis An inflammation of the brain parenchyma (brain tissue) and meninges that affects the cerebrum, brainstem, and cerebellum; usually caused by a virus.

endogenous Originating inside the body.

endometrial ablation Procedure for dysfunctional uterine bleeding that removes a built-up uterine lining using a laser, roller ball, or balloon.

endometrial cancer Cancer of the inner uterine lining.

endometriosis The abnormal occurrence of endometrial tissue outside the uterine cavity.

endometritis An infection of the endometrium.

endorphins Morphine-like substances in the body that are released when the large-diameter nerve fibers are stimulated. They close the gate and decrease pain transmission.

endoscope A tube that allows viewing and manipulation of internal body areas.

endoscopic retrograde cholangiopancreatography (ERCP) The visual and radiographic examination of the liver, gallbladder, bile ducts, and pancreas by means of an endoscope and the injection of radiopaque dye to identify the cause and location of obstruction.

endoscopic variceal ligation (EVL) The application of small "O" bands around the base of the esophageal varices to cut off their blood supply; also called "banding."

endoscopy The direct visualization of the gastrointestinal tract by means of a flexible fiberoptic endoscope.

endothelin A secretion produced by the endothelial cells when they are stretched.

endotoxin Any toxic substance that is produced in the cell walls of certain bacteria and released only with cell lysis. Typhoid and meningococcal diseases are caused by endotoxins.

endovascular stent graft The repair of an abdominal aortic aneurysm using a stent made of flexible material; the stent is inserted through a skin incision into the femoral artery by way of a catheter-based system.

endoventricular circular patch cardioplasty In the patient with heart failure, a procedure in which the surgeon removes portions of the cardiac septum and left ventricular wall and grafts a circular patch (synthetic or autologous) into the opening. This procedure provides a more normal shape to the left ventricle to improve hemodynamics.

end-stage kidney disease (ESKD) Acute renal failure combined with chronic renal insufficiency, resulting in the inability of the kidney to excrete waste products normally. The patient may need hemodialysis or a kidney transplant.

energy conservation Strategies to reduce the fatigue associated with chronic and disabling conditions, such as allowing rest periods and setting priorities.

engraftment The successful transplantation of cells in the patient's bone marrow.

enophthalmos Backward displacement of the eyeball into the orbit so that the eye appears sunken.

enteroscopy Visualization of the small intestine.

enterostomal feeding tube A tube used for patients who need long-term enteral feeding; the physician directly accesses the gastrointestinal tract using surgical, endoscopic, and laparoscopic techniques.

entropion The turning inward of the eyelid, causing the eyelashes to rub against the eye.

enucleation The surgical removal of the entire eyeball.

envenomation Venom injection from a snake bite.

epididymectomy Surgical excision of the epididymis from the testicle.

epididymis The cordlike structure along the posterior border of the testis; it is the first portion of a ductal system that transports sperm from the testes to the urethra.

epididymitis Inflammation of the epididymis.

epidural Term for the space between the dura mater and vertebrae; it consists of fat, connective tissue, and blood vessels.

epidural analgesia The instillation of a pain-blocking agent into the epidural space (between the dura mater and the vertebral column).

epidural catheter A transducer or sensor that is placed between the skull and the dura (leaving the dura intact) to monitor intracranial pressure.

epidural hematoma An accumulation of clotted blood resulting from arterial bleeding into the space between the dura and the skull; a neurosurgical emergency.

epidural hemorrhage Arterial bleeding into the space between the dura and the skull.

epiglottis A leaf-shaped, elastic structure that is attached along one edge to the top of the larynx; it closes over the glottis during swallowing to prevent food from entering the trachea and opens during breathing and coughing.

epilepsy A chronic disorder characterized by recurrent, unprovoked seizure activity; may be caused by an abnormality in electrical neuronal activity, an imbalance of neurotransmitters, or a combination of both.

epiphyses The two knoblike ends of a long bone.

epistaxis Nosebleed.

epitympanum The upper portion of the tympanic cavity; a compartment containing the three bony ossicles.

equianalgesic Refers to the dose and route of administration of one drug that produces approximately the same degree of analgesia as the given dose and route of another drug.

equilibrium (1) A state of balance; (2) a condition in which there is no hydrostatic pressure difference between the two fluid spaces on either side of a permeable membrane.

erectile dysfunction (ED) The inability to achieve or maintain a penile erection sufficient for sexual intercourse.

ergonomics An applied science in which the workplace is designed to increase worker comfort (thus reducing injury) while increasing efficiency and productivity.

erosion Ulceration.

eructation The act of belching.

erythema Redness of the skin.

erythema migrans A round or oval flat or slightly raised rash.

erythrocyte A red blood cell. Red blood cells are the major cells in the blood and are responsible for tissue oxygenation.

erythroplakia A velvety red mucosal lesion, most often occurring in the oral cavity.

erythroplasia Red, velvety patches on a mucous membrane.

erythropoiesis The selective maturation of stem cells into mature erythrocytes.

eschar The crust of dead tissue that forms from coagulated particles of destroyed dermis in a patient with a full-thickness burn injury.

escharotomy Incision made through tight eschar to relieve pressure and allow normal blood flow and breathing.

esophageal stricture Narrowing of the esophageal opening.

esophageal varices The distention of fragile, thin-walled esophageal veins due to increased pressure; the increased pressure is a result of portal hypertension, in which the blood backs up from the liver and enters the esophageal and gastric vessels that carry it into the systemic circulation.

esophagectomy The surgical removal of all or part of the esophagus.

esophagitis Inflammation of the esophagus.

esophagogastroduodenoscopy (EGD) The visual examination of the esophagus, stomach, and duodenum by means of a fiberoptic endoscope.

esophagogastrostomy The surgical creation of a communication between the stomach and the esophagus; it involves the removal of part of the esophagus and proximal stomach.

esophagomyotomy A surgical procedure in which the lower esophageal sphincter is incised to facilitate the passage of food for patients with achalasia.

essential hypertension Elevated blood pressure that is not caused by a specific disease. The major risk factor is a family history of hypertension; also called "primary hypertension."

ethnopharmacology The study of how ethnicity affects how drugs work in the body, including drug absorption, distribution, metabolism, and excretion.

euploid Having the correct number of chromosome pairs for the species.

euploidy The normal diploid number for a cell.

eustachian tube Tube that connects the nasopharynx with the middle ear and opens during swallowing to equalize pressure within the middle ear.

euthyroid Having normal thyroid function.

evidence-based practice Care that nurses provide that is based on research and identified standards and considers the patient's preferences and values and the nurse's clinical expertise.

evisceration The total separation of all layers of a wound and the protrusion of internal organs through the open wound.

evoked potentials Tests to measure the electrical signals to the brain generated by hearing, touch, or sight; also called "evoked response."

exacerbate To increase in severity of disease or its symptoms.

exacerbation An increase in severity of a disease; also called "flare-up."

excision Removal of a lesion and local surrounding tissue.

excitability The ability of a cell to respond to a stimulus by initiating an impulse; also called "depolarization." In cardiac electrophysiology, it is the ability of non-pacemaker myocardial cells to respond to an electrical impulse generated from pacemaker cells and to depolarize.

exercise electrocardiography In cardiovascular assessment, a test that assesses cardiovascular response to an increased workload; also called "exercise tolerance" or a "stress test." Exercise electrocardiography helps determine the functional capacity of the heart, screens for coronary artery disease, and identifies dysrhythmias that develop during exercise. It also aids in evaluating the effectiveness of anti-dysrhythmic drugs.

exertional dyspnea Breathlessness or difficulty breathing that develops during activity or exertion.

exertional heat stroke A form of heat stroke with a sudden onset, typically due to strenuous physical activity in hot, humid conditions. Lack of acclimatization to hot weather and wearing clothing too heavy for the environment are common contributing factors.

exogenous Originating outside the body.

exogenous hyperthyroidism Hyperthyroidism caused by excessive use of thyroid replacement hormones.

exophthalmos Abnormal protrusion of the eyeball (proptosis).

exotoxin Any toxic substance that is produced and released by certain bacteria into the surrounding environment. Botulism, tetanus, and diphtheria are attributed to exotoxins.

expedited partner therapy (EPT) Therapy used to treat chlamydia in which patients are given a drug or prescription with specific instructions for administration to their partners without direct evaluation by a health care provider; also called "patient-delivered partner therapy."

exploratory laparotomy A surgical opening of the abdominal cavity to investigate the cause of an obstruction or peritonitis.

exposure (1) The final component of the primary survey that allows for thorough assessment of the trauma patient; (2) in radiation therapy, the amount of radiation that is delivered to a tissue.

expressed gene When a particular gene has been "turned on."

expression (gene) The selective activation of a particular gene in a specific cell type.

expressive aphasia A type of aphasia resulting from damage in Broca's area of the frontal lobe of the brain. A motor speech problem in which the patient understands what is said but is unable to communicate verbally and has difficulty writing; rote speech and automatic speech, such as responses to a greeting, are often intact. The patient is aware of the deficit and may become frustrated and angry. Also called "Broca's aphasia" or "motor aphasia."

expressivity In genetics, the degree of expression a person has when a specific autosomal dominant gene is present. The gene is always expressed, but some people have more severe results.

external catheter An epidural catheter, a portion of which exits the skin.

external fixation A system in which pins or wires are passed through skin and bone and connected to a rigid external frame to immobilize a fracture during healing.

external hemorrhoid A hemorrhoid that lies below the anal sphincter and can be seen on inspection of the anal region.

external otitis A painful irritation or infection of the skin of the external ear, with resulting allergic response or inflammation. When it occurs in patients who participate in water sports, external otitis is called "swimmer's ear."

external urethral sphincter The sphincter composed of the skeletal muscle that surrounds the urethra.

extracapsular Located outside the joint capsule.

extracellular fluid (ECF) The portion of total body water (about one third) that is in the space outside the cells. This space also includes interstitial fluid, blood, lymph, bone, and connective tissue water, and the transcellular fluids.

extracranial-intracranial bypass A surgical procedure in which the surgeon performs a craniotomy and bypasses the blocked artery by making a graft (bypass) from the first artery to the second artery to establish blood flow around the blocked artery and re-establish blood flow to the involved areas.

extramedullary tumor A tumor found within the spinal dura but outside the cord.

extrapulmonary Involving nonpulmonary tissues.

extravasation Escape of fluids or drugs into the subcutaneous tissue; a complication of intravenous infusion.

extrinsic factor In hematology, an event (e.g., trauma) that occurs outside the blood to cause platelet plugs to form.

extubation The removal of an endotracheal tube.

exudate Pus.

F

facial paralysis See *Bell's palsy*.

facilitated diffusion Diffusion across a cell membrane that requires the assistance of a transport system or membrane-altering system; also called "facilitated transport."

facilitated transport See *facilitated diffusion*.

failed back surgery syndrome (FBSS) A combination of organic, psychological, and socioeconomic factors in patients for whom back surgery is not successful. Discouraged by repeated surgical procedures, these patients must continue long-term nonsurgical management of pain, including nerve blocks.

fall An unintentional change in body position that results in the patient's body coming to rest on the floor or ground.

fallophobia In some older adults, the fear of falling and sustaining a serious injury.

fallopian tubes The tubes that insert into the fundus of the uterus, extending laterally close to the ovaries, and provide a duct between the ovaries and uterus for the passage of ova and sperm; also called "uterine tubes."

far point of vision The farthest point at which the eye can see an object.

fascia An inelastic tissue that surrounds groups of muscles, blood vessels, and nerves in the body.

fasciculation Abnormal, involuntary twitching of a muscle.

fasciotomy A surgical procedure in which an incision is made through the skin and subcutaneous tissues into the fascia of the affected compartment to relieve the pressure in and restore circulation to the affected area in the patient with acute compartment syndrome.

fat embolism syndrome (FES) A serious complication, usually resulting from a fracture, in which fat globules are released from the yellow bone marrow into the bloodstream. This syndrome usually occurs within 48 hours of the fracture and can result in respiratory failure or death, often from pulmonary edema.

fatigue (stress) fracture A fracture that results from excessive or repeated strain and stress on a bone.

fatty liver (steatosis) Caused by the accumulation of fats in and around the hepatic cells. It may be caused by alcohol abuse or other factors.

fecal occult blood test (FOBT) A diagnostic test that measures the presence of blood in the stool from gastrointestinal bleeding; this is a common finding associated with colorectal cancer.

Felty's syndrome The combination of rheumatoid arthritis, hepatosplenomegaly (enlarged liver and spleen), and leukopenia.

femoral hernia A hernia that protrudes through the femoral ring.

fetor hepaticus The distinctive fruity or musty breath odor of chronic liver disease and portal-systemic encephalopathy.

fibrinolysis The breakdown of a clot.

fibrinolytic Drug that targets the fibrin component of the coronary thrombosis; used to dissolve thrombi in the coronary arteries and restore myocardial blood flow; examples include tissue plasminogen activator, anisoylated plasminogen-streptokinase activator complex, and reteplase.

fibroadenoma A solid, slowly enlarging, benign mass of connective tissue that is unattached to the surrounding breast tissue and is typically discovered by the patient herself. The mass is usually round, firm, easily movable, nontender, and clearly delineated from the surrounding tissue.

fibrocystic breast condition (FBC) Physiologic nodularity of the breast that is thought to be caused by an imbalance in the normal estrogen-to-progesterone ratio. It is the most common breast problem of women between 20 and 30 years of age.

fibrogenic Originating from fibrous tissue.

fibroids See *leiomyomas*.

fibromyalgia syndrome (FMS) A chronic pain syndrome characterized by pain and tenderness at specific sites in the back of the neck, upper chest, trunk, low back, and extremities along with fatigue, sleep disturbances, and headache.

fibrosis Replacement of normal cells with connective tissue and collagen (scar tissue).

filter The movement of fluid from the space with higher hydrostatic pressure through the membrane into the space with lower hydrostatic pressure.

filtration The movement of fluid through a cell or blood vessel membrane because of hydrostatic pressure differences on both sides of the membrane.

financial abuse Mismanagement or misuse of the patient's property or resources.

first intention healing Healing in which the wound can be easily closed and dead space eliminated without granulation, which thus shortens the phases of tissue repair. Inflammation resolves quickly, and connective tissue repair is minimal, resulting in a thin scar.

fistula An abnormal opening between two adjacent organs or structures.

five cardinal manifestations of inflammation Warmth, redness, swelling, pain, and decreased function.

fixed occlusion Wiring the jaws together in the mouth closed position.

flaccid bladder See *areflexic bladder.*

flaccid paralysis Paralysis of a part of the body that is characterized by loss of muscle tone due to hypotonia; may be seen in the patient who has experienced a brain attack.

flail chest Inward movement of the thorax during inspiration, with outward movement during expiration; results from multiple rib fractures caused by blunt chest trauma that leaves a segment of the chest wall loose.

flatulence The presence of an excessive amount of gas in the stomach or intestines.

fluid overload An excess of body fluid. Also called "overhydration."

folliculitis A superficial bacterial infection involving only the upper portion of the hair follicle.

forced expiratory volume in the first second (FEV$_1$) Volume of air blown out as hard and fast as possible during the first second of the most forceful exhalation after the greatest full inhalation.

forced vital capacity (FVC) Volume of air exhaled from full inhalation to full exhalation.

forensic nurse examiner Emergency department specialist who is trained to recognize evidence of abuse and to intervene on the patient's behalf and who obtains patient histories, collects forensic evidence, and offers counseling and follow-up care for victims of rape, child abuse, and domestic violence.

fracture A break or disruption in the continuity of a bone.

frameshift mutation A mutation that occurs as a result of adding or deleting a single base or a group of bases.

fremitus Vibration.

frequency (1) The highness or lowness of tones (expressed in hertz). The greater the number of vibrations per second, the higher the frequency (pitch) of the sound; the fewer the number of vibrations per second, the lower the pitch; (2) an urge to urinate frequently in small amounts.

fresh frozen plasma (FFP) Plasma that is frozen immediately after donation so that the clotting factors are preserved.

friable Easily crumbled or damaged.

frostbite A cold injury characterized by the degree of tissue freezing and the resultant damage it produces. Frostbite injuries can be superficial, partial, or full thickness.

frostnip A form of superficial frostbite (typically on the face, fingers, or toes) that produces pain, numbness, and pallor but is easily remedied with the application of warmth and does not induce tissue injury.

full agonist Morphine-like opioid analgesic that binds to mu receptors and blocks the release of substance P, preventing the transmission of pain; the most potent of all analgesics.

Fulmer SPICES A framework that identifies six serious "marker conditions" that can lead to longer hospital stays for patients, higher medical costs, and deaths.

fulminant hepatitis A severe acute and often fatal form of hepatitis caused by failure of the liver cells to regenerate, with progression to necrosis.

fundoplication A procedure in which the fundus of the stomach is wrapped around the lower end of the esophagus to anchor it and reinforce the lower esophageal sphincter; the most common surgical technique for hiatal hernia repair. A laparoscopic Nissen fundoplication is one variation of this type of procedure; a traditional, open surgical approach (using a large abdominal incision) is another variation.

furuncle A localized inflammation of the skin caused by bacterial infection, usually *Staphylococcus*, of a hair follicle; also called "a boil."

G

G$_1$ phase Phase of cell division in which the cell gets ready for division by taking on extra nutrients, making more energy, growing extra membrane, and increasing the amount of cytoplasm.

G$_2$ phase Phase of cell division in which the cell makes proteins that will be used in actual cell division and in normal physiologic function after cell division is complete.

gallium scan A test that is similar to the bone scan but uses the radioisotope *gallium citrate* and is more specific and sensitive in detecting bone problems. This substance also migrates to brain, liver, and breast tissue and therefore is used to examine these structures when disease is suspected.

gamma globulin See *immunoglobulin.*

ganglion A round, cystlike lesion, often overlying a wrist joint or tendon.

gas bloat syndrome A common, usually temporary, complication of fundoplication surgery. In this syndrome, patients are unable to voluntarily eructate (belch).

gastrectomy The surgical removal of part or all of the stomach.

gastric bypass (Roux-en-Y gastric bypass) A type of gastric restriction surgery in which gastric resection is combined with malabsorption surgery. The patient's stomach, duodenum, and part of the jejunum are bypassed so that fewer calories can be absorbed.

gastric lavage Procedure of irrigating the stomach in which a large-bore nasogastric tube is inserted into the stomach and room-temperature solution is instilled in volumes of 200 to 300 mL. The solution and blood are repeatedly withdrawn manually until returns are clear or light pink and without clots.

gastrinoma A non–beta cell islet tumor of the pancreas; the usual cause of Zollinger-Ellison syndrome.

gastritis An inflammation of the gastric mucosa (stomach lining).

gastroenteritis An increase in the frequency and water content of stools or vomiting as a result of inflammation of the mucous membranes of the stomach and intestinal tract. It affects primarily the small bowel and can be of either viral or bacterial origin.

gastroesophageal reflux disease (GERD) An upper gastrointestinal disease caused by the backward flow (reflux) of gastrointestinal contents into the esophagus.

gastrojejunostomy Surgical anastomosis of the stomach to the jejunum.

gastroparesis Delay in gastric emptying.

gastrostomy A stoma created from the abdominal wall into the stomach.

gate control theory A theory to explain the observed relationship between pain and emotion; a gating mechanism occurs in the spinal cord. Nerve fibers (A delta and C fibers) transmit pain impulses from the periphery of the body. The impulses travel to the dorsal horns of the spinal cord, specifically to the *substantia gelatinosa*. The cells of the substantia gelatinosa can inhibit or facilitate the pain impulses transmitted to the trigger cells (T-cells). When T-cell activity is inhibited, the gate is closed and impulses are less likely to be transmitted to the brain. When the gate is opened, pain impulses ascend to the brain.

gel phenomenon In patients with rheumatoid arthritis, morning stiffness that lasts between 45 minutes and several hours after awakening.

gene The deoxyribonucleic acid (DNA) in the form of chromosomes within the nucleus of each cell that contains the instructions for making all the different proteins any organism makes. Every human cell with a nucleus contains the entire set of human genes.

general anesthesia A reversible loss of consciousness induced by inhibiting neuronal impulses in the central nervous system.

generalized seizure One of the three broad categories of seizure disorders along with partial seizures and unclassified seizures. There are six types: tonic-clonic, tonic, clonic, absence, myoclonic, and atonic (akinetic).

generation time The time it takes one cell to divide into two cells.

genetics The science concerned with the general mechanisms of heredity and the variation of inherited traits.

genital herpes (GH) An acute, recurring, incurable viral disease of the genitalia caused by the herpes simplex virus and transmitted through contact with an infected person. An outbreak typically is preceded by a tingling sensation of the skin followed by the appearance of vesicles (blisters) on the penis, scrotum, vulva, perineum, vagina, cervix, or perianal region. The blisters rupture spontaneously, leaving painful erosions. After the lesions heal, the virus remains dormant, periodically reactivating with a recurrence of symptoms.

genome The complete set of human genes. Each human cell with a nucleus contains the entire set of human genes. The human genome contains about 35,000 individual genes.

genomics The science focusing on the function of all of the human DNA, including genes and noncoding DNA regions.

genomic health care The application of known genetic variation to enhance health care to individuals and their families.

genotype The actual alleles for a genetic trait, not just what can be observed.

genu valgum A deformity in which the knees are abnormally close together and the space between the ankles is increased; also called "knock-knee."

genu varum A deformity in which the knees are abnormally separated and the lower extremities are bowed inward; also called "bowleg."

Geriatric Depression Scale—Short Form A valid and reliable screening tool to help determine if an older patient has clinical depression.

geriatric failure to thrive (GFTT) A complex syndrome including under-nutrition, impaired physical functioning, depression, and cognitive impairment.

Ghon tubercle A mass of necrotic lung tissue, visible on x-ray, that is the primary lesion of tuberculosis.

ghrelin The "hunger hormone" that is secreted in the stomach; increases in a fasting state and decreases after a meal.

Glasgow Coma Scale An objective and widely accepted tool for neurologic assessment and documentation of level of consciousness. It establishes baseline data for eye opening, motor response, and verbal response. The patient is assessed and assigned a numerical score for each of these areas. A score of 15 represents normal neurologic functioning, and a score of 3 represents a deep coma state.

glaucoma A group of ocular diseases resulting in increased intraocular pressure, causing reduced blood flow to the optic nerve and retina and followed by tissue damage.

glomerulus A series of specialized capillary loops that receive blood from the afferent arteriole and then filter water and small particles from the blood to make urine. The remaining blood leaves the glomerulus via the efferent arteriole.

glossectomy The partial or total surgical removal of the tongue.

glossitis A smooth, beefy red tongue.

glottis The opening between the true vocal cords inside the larynx.

glucagon A hormone secreted by the pancreas that increases blood glucose levels. It is a "counterregulatory" hormone that has actions opposite those of insulin. It causes the release of glucose from cell storage sites whenever blood glucose levels are low.

gluconeogenesis The conversion of proteins and amino acids to glucose in the body.

glucosamine A supplement that may decrease inflammation.

glycemic A term referring to blood glucose.

glycogenesis The production of glycogen in the body.

glycogenolysis The breakdown of glycogen into glucose.

glycoprotein IIa/IIIb inhibitors Drugs that target the platelet component of the thrombus. They are administered intravenously to prevent fibrinogen from attaching to activated platelets at the site of a thrombus and are given to patients with acute coronary syndromes (especially unstable angina and non–Q-wave myocardial infarction). Examples include abciximab, eptifibatide, and tirofiban.

"go bag" See *personal readiness supplies.*

goiter Enlargement of the thyroid gland.

gonadotropins Hormones that stimulate the ovaries and testes to produce sex hormones.

gonads The male and female reproductive endocrine glands. Male gonads are the testes, and female gonads are the ovaries.

goniometer An instrument for measuring angles; also refers to a tool used to measure joint range of motion.

good death A death that is free from avoidable distress and suffering for patients, families, and caregivers; in agreement with patients' and families' wishes; and consistent with clinical practice standards.

gout A systemic disease in which urate crystals deposit in the joints and other body tissues, causing inflammation.

gradient A graded difference of hydrostatic pressure in a state of disequilibrium; that is, one fluid space has a higher hydrostatic pressure than the other.

grading System of classifying cellular aspects of a cancer tumor.

granulation The formation of scar tissue for wound healing to occur.

granulocyte Neutrophil that contains a large number of granules.

granuloma Growth that develops in the lungs of patients with sarcoidosis and contains lymphocytes, macrophages, epithelioid cells, and giant cells; scar tissue.

granuloma inguinale An ulcerative disease of the genital area that appears as a painless nodule.

Graves' disease Toxic diffuse goiter characterized by hyperthyroidism, enlargement of the thyroid gland, abnormal protrusion of the eyes, and dry, waxy swelling of the front surfaces of the lower legs.

gray (gy) Unit of measurement for an absorbed radiation dose.

gray matter In the spinal cord, neuron cell bodies.

grief The emotional feeling related to the perception of loss.

grommet A polyethylene tube that is surgically placed through the tympanic membrane to allow continuous drainage of middle-ear fluids in the patient with otitis media.

ground substance A lubricant composed of protein and sugar groups that surrounds the dermal cells and fibers and contributes to the skin's normal suppleness and turgor.

guardian A person appointed to make health care decisions for a patient who is determined to not be legally competent.

guided imagery An alternative therapy technique in which the patient is provided with images or prompts by a nurse, family member, or friend or via a tape.

Guillain-Barré syndrome (GBS) An acute autoimmune disorder characterized by varying degrees of motor weakness and paralysis. It may be referred to by a variety of other names, such as "acute idiopathic polyneuritis" and "polyradiculoneuropathy."

gynecomastia Abnormal enlargement of the breasts in men.

H

H_2-receptor antagonists A group of drugs that inhibit gastric acid secretion by blocking the effects of histamine on parietal cell receptors in the stomach.

halitosis A foul odor of the mouth.

hallucinogens Chemical substances that possess mind-altering or perception-altering properties, such as lysergic acid (LSD), phencyclidine (PCP), and marijuana.

hallux valgus A common deformity of the foot that occurs when the great toe deviates laterally at the metatarsophalangeal joint; sometimes referred to as a "bunion."

halo fixator A static traction device used for immobilization of the cervical spine. Four pins or screws are inserted into the skull, and a metal halo ring is attached to a plastic vest or cast when the spine is stable, allowing increased patient mobility.

hammertoe The dorsiflexion of any metatarsophalangeal joint with plantar flexion of the adjacent proximal interphalangeal joint. The second toe is most often affected.

hand hygiene Infection control protocol that refers to both handwashing and alcohol-based hand rubs.

handwashing The process of wetting, soaping, lathering, applying friction under running water for at least 15 seconds, rinsing, and drying the hands; an important part of infection control.

health care–acquired infections (HAIs) Infections that are associated with the provision of health care; for example, microorganisms can enter the body through the genitourinary tract in patients with indwelling urinary catheters.

Healthy People 2020 A program created by the U.S. Department of Health and Human Services with the goal of eliminating differences in health status among racial and ethnic minorities while continually improving the overall health of all Americans through research, preventive programs, and inclusion of members of minority groups.

heart failure A general term for the inadequacy of the heart to pump blood throughout the body, causing insufficient perfusion of body tissues with vital nutrients and oxygen; also called "pump failure."

heart rate (HR) Term referring to the number of times the ventricles contract each minute.

heart reduction surgery Partial left ventriculectomy; in the patient with heart failure, a surgical procedure to remove a triangle-shaped section of the weakened heart in the left lateral ventricle to reduce the ventricle's diameter and decrease wall tension.

heart transplantation A surgical procedure in which a heart from a donor with a comparable body weight and ABO compatibility is transplanted into a recipient less than 6 hours after procurement. It is the treatment of choice for patients with severe dilated cardiomyopathy and may be considered for patients with restrictive cardiomyopathy.

heat exhaustion A syndrome primarily caused by dehydration from heavy perspiration and inadequate fluid and electrolyte consumption during heat exposure over hours to days; if left untreated, can be a precursor to heat stroke.

heat stroke A true medical emergency in which the victim's heat regulatory mechanisms fail and are unable to compensate for a critical elevation in body temperature; if uncorrected, organ dysfunction and death will ensue.

Heberden's nodes Swelling at the distal interphalangeal joints in osteoarthritis that involves the hands.

helminths Parasitic worms that are capable of causing infectious disease with gastrointestinal symptoms in humans. The three general categories are roundworms (nematodes), flukes (trematodes), and tapeworms (cestodes).

hematemesis The vomiting of blood.

hematochezia The passage of red blood via the rectum.

hematocrit The percentage of packed red blood cells per deciliter of blood.

hematogenous Disseminated by the blood through the circulation.

hematogenous tuberculosis A form of tuberculosis that spreads throughout the body when a large number of organisms enter the blood. Also called "miliary tuberculosis."

hematopoiesis The production of blood cells, which occurs in the red marrow of bones.

hematuria Blood in the urine.

hemianopsia Blindness in half of the visual field of one or both eyes; also called "hemianopia."

hemiarthroplasty Surgical replacement of part of the shoulder joint, typically the humeral component, as an alternative to total shoulder arthroplasty.

hemiparesis Weakness on one side of the body.

hemiplegia Paralysis on one side of the body.

hemoconcentration Elevated plasma levels of hemoglobin, hematocrit, serum osmolarity, glucose, protein, blood urea nitrogen, and electrolytes that occur when only the water is lost and other substances remain.

hemodilution Excessive water in the vascular space.

hemodynamic monitoring An invasive system that directly measures pressures in the heart and great vessels; used in critical care areas to provide quantitative information about vascular capacity, blood volume, pump effectiveness, and tissue perfusion.

hemoglobin A (HbA) Normal adult hemoglobin. The molecule has two alpha chains and two beta chains of amino acids.

hemolytic The characteristic of destroying red blood cells.

hemoptysis Coughing up blood or blood-stained sputum.

hemorrhoid Unnaturally swollen or distended vein in the anorectal region.

hemorrhoidectomy The excision of a hemorrhoid.

hemostasis The multi-step process of controlled blood clotting.

heparin-induced thrombocytopenia and thrombosis (HIT) The aggregation of platelets into "white clots" that can cause thrombosis, usually in the form of an acute arterial occlusion; occurs with heparin administration; also called "white clot syndrome."

hepatic coma See *portal-systemic encephalopathy.*

hepatic encephalopathy See *portal-systemic encephalopathy.*

hepatitis The widespread inflammation of liver cells.

hepatitis A Hepatitis that is caused by the hepatitis A virus (HAV) and is characterized by a mild course similar to that of a typical viral syndrome and often goes unrecognized. It is spread via the fecal-oral route by oral ingestion of fecal contaminants. Sources of infection include contaminated water, shellfish caught in contaminated water, and food contaminated by infected food handlers. The virus may also be spread by oral-anal sexual activity. The incubation period is usually 15 to 50 days. The disease is usually not life threatening but may be more severe in people older than 40 years. It can also complicate pre-existing liver disease.

hepatitis B A form of hepatitis that is caused by the hepatitis B virus, which is shed in the body fluids of infected people and asymptomatic carriers. It is spread through unprotected sexual intercourse with an infected partner, needle sharing, blood transfusions, and other modes. Symptoms usually occur within 25 to 180 days of exposure and include nausea, fever, fatigue, joint pain, and jaundice. Most adults who get hepatitis B recover, clear the virus from their body, and develop immunity; however, up to 10% of patients with the disease do not develop immunity and become carriers.

hepatitis C Hepatitis that is caused by the hepatitis C virus. Transmission is blood to blood, most commonly by needle sharing or needle stick injury with contaminated blood. The rate of sexual transmission is very low; it is not spread by casual contact and is rarely transmitted from mother to fetus. The average incubation period is 7 weeks. Most people are asymptomatic and are not diagnosed until long after the initial exposure when an abnormality is detected during a routine laboratory evaluation or when symptoms of liver impairment appear. Hepatitis C causes chronic inflammation in the liver that eventually causes the hepatocytes to scar and may progress to cirrhosis.

hepatitis carrier Person who has had hepatitis B but has not developed immunity. Hepatitis carriers can infect others even though they are not sick and demonstrate no obvious signs of disease. Chronic carriers are at high risk for cirrhosis and liver cancer.

hepatitis D The hepatitis D virus (HDV) co-infects with hepatitis B virus (HBV) and needs the presence of HBV for viral replication. HDV can co-infect a patient with HBV or can occur as a superinfection in a patient with chronic HBV. Superinfection usually develops into chronic HDV infection. The incubation period is 14 to 56 days. As with HBV, the disease is transmitted primarily by parenteral routes.

hepatitis E Hepatitis E virus (HEV) was originally identified by its association with water-borne epidemics of hepatitis in the Indian subcontinent. Since then, it has occurred in epidemics in Asia, Africa, the Middle East, Mexico, and Central and South America, typically after heavy rains and flooding. In the United States, hepatitis E has been found only in travelers returning from endemic areas. The virus is transmitted via the fecal-oral route, and the clinical course resembles that of hepatitis A. HEV has an incubation period of 15 to 64 days. There is no evidence at this time of a chronic form of hepatitis E.

hepatocyte Liver cell.

hepatomegaly Enlargement of the liver.

hepatorenal syndrome (HRS) A state of progressive oliguric renal failure associated with hepatic failure, resulting in functional impairment of kidneys with normal anatomic and morphologic features. It indicates a poor prognosis for the patient with hepatic failure and is often the cause of death in patients with cirrhosis.

herbal preparation Plant used for medicinal purposes.

hereditary chronic pancreatitis Pancreatitis that may be associated with *SPINK1* and *CFTR* gene mutations.

heritability The risk that a disorder can be transmitted to one's children in a recognizable pattern.

hernia A weakness in the abdominal muscle wall through which a segment of the bowel or other abdominal structure protrudes.

herniated nucleus pulposus (HNP) The protrusion (herniation) of the pulpy material from the center of a vertebral disk; herniated disks occur most often between the fourth and fifth lumbar vertebrae (L4-5) but may occur at other levels. A herniation in the lumbosacral area can press on the adjacent spinal nerve (usually the sciatic nerve), causing severe burning or stabbing pain into the leg or foot, or it may press on the spinal cord itself, causing leg weakness and bowel and bladder dysfunction. The specific area of pain depends on the level of herniation.

hernioplasty Surgical repair of a hernia in which the surgeon reinforces the weakened outside muscle wall with a mesh patch.

herniorrhaphy The surgical repair of a hernia.

heterotopic ossification Abnormal bony overgrowth, often into muscle; seen as a complication of prolonged immobility in patients with spinal cord injury.

hiatal hernia Protrusion of the stomach through the esophageal hiatus of the diaphragm and into the thorax; also called "diaphragmatic hernia."

high altitude Elevations above 5000 feet, which can produce a range of physiologic consequences in the body.

high altitude disease (HAD) Pathophysiologic responses in the body caused by exposure to low partial pressure of oxygen at high elevations.

high altitude pulmonary edema (HAPE) A form of acute mountain sickness often seen with high altitude cerebral edema. Clinical indicators include persistent dry cough, cyanosis of the lips and nail beds, tachycardia and tachypnea at rest, and rales auscultated in one or both lungs. Pink, frothy sputum is a late sign.

highly sensitive C-reactive protein (hsCRP) A serum marker of inflammation and a common and critical component to the development of atherothrombosis.

high-output heart failure Heart failure that occurs when cardiac output remains normal or above normal. It is usually caused by increased metabolic needs or hyperkinetic conditions such as septicemia (fever), anemia, and hyperthyroidism. This type of heart failure is different from left- and right-sided heart failure, which are typically low-output states, and is not as common as other types.

hilum The area of the kidney in which the renal artery and nerve plexus enter and the renal vein and ureter exit. This area is not covered by the renal capsule.

hirsutism Abnormal growth of body hair, especially on the face, chest, and the linea alba of the abdomen of women.

holistic care The connection and integration of the mind, body, and spirit.

homeopaths Care providers who plan individualized care by prescribing small doses of specially prepared plant and animal extracts and minerals to promote healing.

homeopathic medicine Practice of medicine that uses small doses of specially prepared plant extracts and minerals to promote healing.

homeostasis The narrow range of normal conditions (e.g., body temperature, blood electrolyte values, blood pH, blood volume) in the human body; the tendency to maintain a constant balance in normal body states.

homeostatic mechanism A safeguard or control mechanism within the human body that prevents dangerous changes.

homocysteine An essential sulfur-containing amino acid that is produced when dietary protein breaks down; elevated values (greater than 15 mmol/L) may be a risk factor for the development of cardiovascular disease.

homonymous hemianopsia Condition in which there is blindness in the same side of both eyes.

hordeolum An infection of the sweat glands in the eyelid.

hormone Chemical produced in the body that exerts its effects on specific tissues known as "target tissues."

hospice care An interdisciplinary approach to facilitate quality of life and a "good" death for patients near the end of their lives, with care provided in a variety of settings.

Hospital Incident Command System (HICS) An organizational model for disaster management in which roles are formally structured under the hospital or long-term care facility incident commander, with clear lines of authority and accountability for specific resources.

hospital incident commander As defined in a hospital's emergency response plan, the person (either an emergency physician or administrator) who assumes overall leadership for implementing the institutional plan at the onset of a mass casualty incident. The hospital incident commander has a global view of the entire situation, facilitates patient movement through the system, and brings in resources to meet patient needs.

hospitalist Family practitioner or internist employed by a hospital.

Huber needle A noncoring port access needle used in central IV therapy.

human leukocyte antigen (HLA) Antigen that is present on the surfaces of nearly all body cells as a normal part of the person and acts as an antigen only if it enters another person's body.

human papilloma virus (HPV) test A test that can identify many high-risk types of HPV associated with the development of cervical cancer.

humoral immunity A type of immunity provided by antibodies circulating in body fluids.

Huntington disease (HD) A hereditary disorder transmitted as an autosomal dominant trait at the time of conception (formerly called "Huntington chorea"). Men and women between 35 and 50 years of age are affected; clinical onset is gradual. The two main symptoms are progressive mental status changes (leading to dementia) and choreiform movements (rapid, jerky movements) in the limbs, trunk, and facial muscles.

hydrocephalus The abnormal accumulation of cerebrospinal fluid within the skull.

hydronephrosis Abnormal enlargement of the kidney caused by a blockage of urine lower in the tract and filling of the kidney with urine.

hydrophilic Tending to absorb water readily.

hydrophobic Not readily absorbing water; waterproof.

hydrostatic pressure The force of the weight of water molecules pressing against the confining walls of a space.

hydrotherapy The application of water for treatment of injury or disease.

hydroureter Abnormal distention of the ureters.

hyperacusis An intolerance for sound levels that do not bother other people.

hyperaldosteronism Excessive mineralocorticoid production.

hypercalcemia A total serum calcium level above 10.5 mg/dL or 2.75 mmol/L, which can cause fatigue, anorexia, nausea and vomiting, constipation, polyuria, and serious damage to the urinary system.

hypercapnia Increased arterial carbon dioxide levels.

hypercarbia Increased partial pressure of arterial carbon dioxide ($Paco_2$) levels.

hypercellularity An abnormal number of cells.

hyperemia Increased blood flow to an area.

hyperesthesia Abnormally increased sensation.

hyperextension A mechanism of injury that occurs when a part of the body is suddenly accelerated and then decelerated, causing extreme extension.

hyperflexion A mechanism of injury that occurs when a part of the body is suddenly and forcefully accelerated forward, causing extreme flexion.

hyperglycemia Abnormally high levels of blood glucose.

hyperglycemic-hyperosmolar state (HHS) State of increased blood osmolarity caused by hyperglycemia.

hyperinsulinemia Chronic high blood insulin levels.

hyperkalemia An elevated level of potassium in the blood.

hyperlipidemia An elevation of serum lipid (fat) levels in the blood.

hypermagnesemia A serum magnesium level above 2.1 mEq/L.

hypernatremia An excessive amount of sodium in the blood.

hyperopia An error of refraction that occurs when the eye does not refract light enough, causing images to fall (converge) behind the retina and resulting in poor near vision; also called "farsightedness."

hyperosmotic Describes fluids with osmolarities (solute concentrations) greater than 300 mOsm/L; hyperosmotic fluids have a greater osmotic pressure than do isosmotic fluids and tend to pull water from the isosmotic fluid space into the hyperosmotic fluid space until an osmotic balance occurs. Also called "hypertonic."

hyperphosphatemia A serum phosphorus level above 4.5 mg/dL.

hyperpituitarism Hormone oversecretion that occurs with pituitary tumors or hyperplasia.

hyperplasia Growth that causes tissue to increase in size by increasing the number of cells; abnormal overgrowth of tissue.

hyperpnea An abnormal increase in the depth of respiratory movements.

hypersensitivity An overreaction to a foreign substance.

hypertension A cardiovascular condition pertaining to people who have a systolic blood pressure of 140 mm Hg or higher or a diastolic blood pressure of 90 mm Hg or higher or who take medication to control blood pressure; approximately 1 of every 5 Americans has hypertension.

hyperthermia Elevated body temperature; fever.

hyperthyroidism A condition caused by excessive production of thyroid hormone.

hypertonia A condition of excessive muscle tone, which tends to cause fixed positions or contractures of the involved extremities and restricted range of motion of the joints.

hypertonic See *hyperosmotic.*

hypertriglyceridemia Elevated levels (150 mg/dL or above) of triglyceride in the blood.

hypertrophic cardiomyopathy (HCM) A type of cardiomyopathy that involves disarray of the myocardial fibers and asymmetric ventricular hypertrophy; leads to a stiff left ventricle that results in diastolic filling abnormalities.

hypertrophy The enlargement or overgrowth of an organ; tissue increases in size by the enlargement of each cell.

hyperuricemia An excess of uric acid in the blood.

hyperventilation A state of increased rate and depth of breathing.

hyperviscosity Excessively thick or concentrated, as of the blood.

hyperviscous The quality of being thicker than normal.

hypervolemia Increased plasma volume; or fluid excess.

hyphema A hemorrhage in the anterior chamber of the eye that occurs when a force is applied to the eye and breaks the blood vessels.

hypnosis An altered state of consciousness in which a person enters a trance and loses an overall sense of reality.

hypocalcemia A total serum calcium level below 9.0 mg/dL or 2.25 mmol/L.

hypocapnia Decreased arterial carbon dioxide levels.

hypodermoclysis The slow infusion of isotonic fluids into subcutaneous tissue.

hypoesthesia Abnormally decreased sensation.

hypoglycemia Abnormally low levels of glucose in the blood.

hypokalemia A decreased serum potassium level; a common electrolyte imbalance.

hypomagnesemia Decreased serum magnesium levels.

hyponatremia A serum sodium level below 136 mEq/L (mmol/L).

hypo-osmotic Describes fluids with osmolarities of less than 270 mOsm/L. Hypo-osmolar fluids have a lower osmotic pressure than isosmotic fluids, and water tends to be pulled from the hypo-osmotic fluid space into the isosmotic fluid space until an osmotic balance occurs. Also called "hypotonic."

hypoperfusion Decreased blood flow through an organ.

hypophonia Soft voice.

hypophosphatemia Inadequate levels of phosphate in the blood (below 3.0 mg/dL).

hypophysectomy Surgical removal of the pituitary gland.

hypoplasia Reduced production of cells.

hypoproteinemia A decrease in serum proteins.

hyporeflexia A decreased response to deep tendon reflex stimulation.

hyposthenuria The inability to form urine of high specific gravity; loss of urine-concentrating ability.

hypothalamic-hypophysial portal system The small, closed circulatory system that the hypothalamus shares with the anterior pituitary gland, which allows hormones produced in the hypothalamus to travel directly to the anterior pituitary gland.

hypothalamus A structure within the brain; an integral part of autonomic nervous system control (controlling temperature and other functions) that is essential in intellectual function.

hypothermia A core body temperature less than 95° F (35° C).

hypotonia An abnormal condition of inadequate muscle tone, with an inability to maintain balance.

hypotonic See *hypo-osmotic.*

hypoventilation A state in which gas exchange at the alveolar-capillary membrane is inadequate so that too little oxygen reaches the blood and carbon dioxide is retained.

hypovolemia Abnormally decreased volume of circulating fluid in the body; fluid deficit.

hypoxemia (hypoxemic) Decreased blood oxygen levels; hypoxia.

hypoxia (hypoxic) A reduction of oxygen supply to the tissues.

hysterosalpingogram An x-ray of the cervix, uterus, and fallopian tubes that is performed after injection of a contrast medium. This test is used in infertility workups to evaluate tubal anatomy and patency and uterine problems such as fibroids, tumors, and fistulas.

hysteroscopy Examination of the interior of the uterus and cervical canal using an endoscope.

I

icterus Yellow discoloration of the sclerae.

idiopathic chronic pancreatitis Pancreatitis that may be associated with *SPINK1* and *CFTR* gene mutations.

idiopathic epilepsy See *primary epilepsy.*

idiopathic seizure See *unclassified seizure.*

idioventricular rhythm A heart rhythm in which the ventricular nodal cells pace the ventricles at a rate that is usually less than 40 beats/min; also called "ventricular escape rhythm."

ileostomy The surgical creation of an opening into the ileum, usually by bringing the end of the terminal ileum through the abdominal wall and forming a stoma, or ostomy.

imagery In complementary medicine, a mind-body therapy or form of distraction in which the patient is encouraged to visualize or think about some pleasant or desirable feeling, sensation, or event.

immediate memory Short-term or new memory. Test by asking the patient to repeat two or three unrelated words to make sure they were heard; after about 5 minutes, while continuing the examination, ask the patient to repeat the words.

immunity Resistance to infection; usually associated with the presence of antibodies or cells that act on specific microorganisms.

immunocompetence Full immunity, which requires the interaction of the processes of inflammation, antibody-mediated immunity (humoral immunity), and cell-mediated immunity.

immunocompetent Having proper functioning of the body's ability to maintain itself and defend against disease.

immunoglobulin Antibody; also called "gamma globulin."

impedance The pressure that the heart must overcome to open the aortic valve. The amount of impedance depends on aortic compliance and total systemic vascular resistance, a combination of blood viscosity and arteriolar constriction.

impedance cardiography (ICG) A noninvasive monitoring system that measures the total impedance (resistance) to the flow of electricity in the heart and provides measures of thoracic fluid, left ventricular function (cardiac output and cardiac index), preload, afterload, and contractility of the heart.

impermeable Not porous.

implanted port A device used for long-term or frequent infusion therapy; consists of a portal body, a dense septum over a reservoir, and a catheter that is surgically implanted on the upper chest or upper extremity.

inactivation The process of binding an antibody to an antigen to cover the antigen's active site and to make the antigen harmless without destroying it; also called "neutralization."

incisional hernia Protrusion of the intestine at the site of a previous surgical incision resulting from inadequate healing. Most often caused by postoperative wound infections, inadequate nutrition, and obesity.

incomplete spinal cord injury An injury in which the spinal cord has been damaged in a way that allows some function or movement below the level of the injury.

incontinence   Involuntary loss of urine or stool severe enough to cause social or hygienic problems.

incus   One of the three bony ossicles of the ear; also called the "anvil."

independent living skills   See *instrumental activities of daily living (IADLs)*.

independent nursing function   A nursing function initiated and carried out by the nurse without direction from the health care provider.

indirect contact   A mode of infection transmission in which microorganisms are transferred passively from a contaminated inanimate object to a susceptible person.

indirect inguinal hernia   A sac formed from the peritoneum that contains a portion of the intestine or omentum. The hernia pushes downward at an angle into the inguinal canal. In males, indirect inguinal hernias can become large and often descend into the scrotum.

indolent   Slow-growing.

induration   Hardening.

infarction   Necrosis, or cell death.

infective endocarditis   A microbial infection (e.g., viruses, bacteria, fungi) involving the endocardium; previously called "bacterial endocarditis."

inferior vena cava filtration   Surgical procedure in which the surgeon inserts a filter device percutaneously into the inferior vena cava of a patient with recurrent deep vein thrombosis (to prevent pulmonary emboli) or pulmonary emboli that do not respond to medical treatment. The device is meant to trap emboli in the inferior vena cava before they progress to the lungs. Holes in the device allow blood to pass through, thus not significantly interfering with the return of blood to the heart.

inferior wall myocardial infarction   A type of myocardial infarction that occurs in patients with obstruction of the right coronary artery, causing significant damage to the right ventricle.

infertility   Difficulty becoming pregnant.

infiltrating ductal carcinoma   The most common type of breast cancer; it originates in the mammary ducts and grows in the epithelial cells lining these ducts.

infiltration   The leakage of IV solution into the tissues around the vein.

inflammatory breast cancer   A rare but highly aggressive form of invasive breast cancer. Symptoms include swelling, skin redness, and pain in the breasts.

inflammatory cytokines   Proteins produced primarily by white blood cells that assist in the inflammatory and immune responses of the body (e.g., tumor necrosis factor, interleukins).

inflow disease   Chronic peripheral arterial disease with obstruction at or above the common iliac artery, abdominal aorta, or profunda femoris artery. The patient experiences discomfort in the lower back, buttocks, or thighs after walking a certain distance. The pain usually subsides with rest.

informatics   A specialized computer science that involves using information and technology to communicate, manage knowledge, mitigate error, and support decision making.

infrapatellar notch   The area directly below the knee.

infratentorial   Located below the tentorium of the cerebellum.

infusate   A solution that is infused into the body.

infusion therapy   The delivery of parenteral medications and fluids through a variety of catheter types and locations using multiple techniques and procedures, such as intravenous and intra-arterial therapy to deliver solutions into the vascular system.

inhalants   Breathable chemical vapors that produce psychoactive effects.

initial   First or, in phases of shock, early.

initiation   In oncology, the first step in carcinogenesis; caused by damage to the genes.

innate-native immunity   Also called "natural immunity"; a type of immunity that cannot be developed or transferred from one person to another and is not an adaptive response to exposure or invasion by foreign proteins.

inpatient   A patient who is admitted to a hospital.

insensible water loss   Water loss from the skin, lungs, and stool that cannot be controlled.

instrumental activities of daily living (IADLs)   Special activities performed in the course of a day such as using the telephone, shopping, preparing food, and housekeeping. Also called "independent living skills."

insufflation   The practice of injecting gas or air into a cavity before surgery to separate organs and improve visualization.

insulin resistance   A reduced ability of most cells to respond to insulin. It is associated with type 2 diabetes.

insulinoma   A usually benign tumor of the islets of Langerhans that causes excessive insulin secretion and subsequent hypoglycemia (low serum glucose); the most common type of neuroendocrine pancreatic tumor, even though it is rare.

integrative medicine   Practice of medicine that combines therapies from traditional Western medicine and complementary and alternative medicine (CAM).

intensity   A quality of sound that is expressed in decibels; generally, having a high degree of energy or activity.

intensivist   A physician who specializes in critical care.

intention tremor   A tremor that occurs when performing an activity.

interbody cage fusion   Cagelike spinal device that is implanted into the space where a disk was removed. Bone graft tissue grows into and around the cage and creates a stable spine at that level.

intercostally   Located between the ribs.

interdisciplinary pain team   Team typically consisting of one or more nurses, pharmacists, case managers, and physicians who consult with staff and prescribers on how best to control the patient's pain; also called "analgesia team."

intermittent claudication   A characteristic leg pain experienced by patients with chronic peripheral arterial disease. Typically, patients can walk only a certain distance before a cramping muscle pain forces them to stop. As the disease progresses, the patient can walk only shorter and shorter distances before pain recurs. Ultimately, pain may occur even at rest.

internal derangement   A broad term for disturbances of an injured knee joint.

internal fixation   The use of metal pins, screws, rods, plates, or prostheses to immobilize a fracture during healing. The surgeon makes an incision (open reduction) to gain access to the broken bone and implants one or more devices.

internal hemorrhoid   A hemorrhoid that is located above the anal sphincter and cannot be seen on inspection of the perineal area.

internal urethral sphincter   The smooth detrusor muscle that lines the interior of the bladder neck.

interstitial cystitis   A bladder inflammation of unknown etiology that occurs predominantly in women and is characterized by urinary frequency and pain on bladder filling.

interstitial fluid   A portion of the extracellular fluid that is between cells, sometimes called the "third space."

interstitial laser coagulation (ILC)   Procedure for treating benign prostatic hyperplasia that uses laser energy to coagulate excess tissue. Also called "contact laser prostatectomy (CLP)."

intra-abdominal hypertension (IAH)   Condition of sustained or repeated intra-abdominal pressure of 12 mm Hg or higher.

intra-abdominal pressure   Pressure contained within the abdominal cavity.

intra-aortic balloon pump (IABP)   An intra-aortic counterpulsation device. It may be used as an invasive intervention to improve myocardial perfusion during an acute myocardial infarction, reduce preload and afterload, and facilitate left ventricular ejection. It is also used when patients do not respond to drug therapy with improved tissue perfusion, decreased workload of the heart, and increased cardiac contractility.

intra-arterial thrombolysis   Therapy for brain attack that delivers the thrombolic agent directly into the thrombus within 6 hours of the attack's onset.

intracapsular   Located within the joint capsule.

intracellular fluid (ICF)   The portion of total body water (about two thirds) that is found inside the cells.

intracerebral hemorrhage   Bleeding within the brain tissue caused by the tearing of small arteries and veins in the subcortical white matter.

intracorporeal   Situated or occurring inside the body.

intractable pain   Chronic pain that cannot be managed using standard therapies.

intramedullary tumor Tumor originating within the spinal cord in the central gray matter and anterior commissure. It is often malignant.

intraocular pressure (IOP) Pressure of the fluid within the eye; may be measured by methods that involve direct contact with the eye or by noncontact techniques.

intraoperative During surgery.

intraosseous (IO) therapy Infusion therapy that is delivered to the vascular network in the long bones.

intraperitoneal (IP) therapy The administration of antineoplastic agents into the peritoneal cavity.

intrapulmonary Within the respiratory tract.

intrarenal/intrinsic renal failure Decreased renal function resulting from damage to the glomeruli, interstitial tissue, or tubules. It can contribute to acute renal failure.

intrathecal Referring to the spine.

intrathecal (subarachnoid) analgesia The introduction of a pain-blocking agent into the space between the arachnoid mater and pia mater of the spinal cord (where the cerebrospinal fluid is located).

intravascular ultrasonography (IVUS) In cardiac catheterization, the use of a flexible catheter with a miniature transducer that emits sound waves. Sound waves are reflected off the plaque and the arterial wall, creating an image of the blood vessel; used as an alternative to injecting a contrast medium into the coronary arteries.

intravenous (systemic) fibrinolytic therapy The intravenous administration of thrombolytic agents to dissolve a thrombus.

intraventricular catheter (IVC) A small tube that is inserted into the anterior horn of the lateral ventricle of the nondominant cerebral hemisphere to monitor intracranial pressure; can also be used to drain cerebrospinal fluid to decrease pressure and obtain specimens for laboratory analysis.

intravesical Situated inside the bladder.

intrinsic factor A substance normally secreted by the gastric mucosa and needed for intestinal absorption of vitamin B_{12}. A deficiency of intrinsic factor and the resulting failure to absorb vitamin B_{12} leads to pernicious anemia.

intussusception The telescoping of a segment of the intestine within itself.

invasive Pertaining to the ability to penetrate nearby tissue; said of cancers.

invasive temporary pacemaker A cardiac pacing system consisting of an external battery-operated pulse generator and pacing electrodes, or lead wires, that attach to the generator on one end and are in contact with the heart on the other end. Electrical pulses are emitted from the negative terminal of the generator, flow through a lead wire, and stimulate the cardiac cells to depolarize. The current seeks ground by returning through the other lead wire to the positive terminal of the generator, thus completing a circuitous route.

ion A substance found in body fluids that carries an electrical charge; also called "electrolyte."

iontophoresis A treatment for lower back pain in which a small electrical current and dexamethasone are typically used.

ipsilateral Occurring on the same side.

iris The colored portion of the external eye; its center opening is the pupil. Muscles of the iris contract and relax to control pupil size and the amount of light entering the eye.

iritis Inflammation of the iris.

irreducible hernia A hernia that cannot be reduced or placed back into the abdominal cavity; requires immediate surgical evaluation.

irreversible stage The former name for the refractory stage of shock. See *refractory stage*.

irritability An overresponse to stimuli.

irritable bowel syndrome (IBS) A chronic gastrointestinal disorder characterized by chronic or recurrent diarrhea, constipation, and/or abdominal pain and bloating; also called "spastic colon," "mucous colon," or "nervous colon."

ischemia Blockage of blood flow through a blood vessel. Prolonged severe ischemia can cause irreversible damage to tissue.

ischemic Cell dysfunction or death from a lack of oxygen resulting from decreased blood flow in a body part.

ischemic stroke A type of brain attack caused by occlusion of a cerebral artery by either a thrombus or an embolus. About 80% of all brain attacks are ischemic.

Ishihara chart The most commonly used tool for testing color vision. The chart shows numbers composed of dots of one color within a circle of dots of a different color. Each eye is tested separately by asking the patient what numbers he or she sees on the chart; reading the numbers correctly indicates normal color vision.

isoelectric Having equal electric potentials, such as in the heart.

isosmotic Having the same osmotic pressures; also called "isotonic" or "normotonic."

isosthenuria Excretion of urine with the same osmolality as that of plasma; occurs in patients with declining renal function due to chronic renal failure.

isotonic See *isosmotic*.

isotope A different form of a specific element; has a slightly different atomic weight and number of neutrons.

"itch-scratch-itch" cycle A pattern seen in patients with pruritus who try to relieve the itching sensation by scratching the skin, further stimulating the itch receptors and causing the itching sensation to continue.

J

jaundice A syndrome characterized by excessive circulating bilirubin levels. Liver cells cannot effectively excrete bilirubin, and skin and mucous membranes become characterized by a yellow coloration.

jejunostomy The surgical creation of an opening between the jejunum and the surface of the abdominal wall.

joint The place at which two or more bones come together; also referred to as "articulation" of the joint. The primary function is to provide movement and flexibility in the body.

journaling A mind-body therapy in which the patient records the process of life and reflects on it to express feelings, gain new perspectives, and pay attention to what is in the unconscious.

jugular venous distention (JVD) Enlargement of the jugular vein of the neck; caused by an increase in jugular venous pressure.

justice The ethical principle that refers to patient equality.

juxtaglomerular complex Specialized cells that produce and store renin in the afferent arteriole, efferent arteriole, and distal collecting tubule; taken together, the juxtaglomerular cells and the macula densa.

K

karyotype Technique used to make an organized arrangement of all the chromosomes within one cell during the metaphase section of mitosis.

Kehr's sign Pain in the left shoulder resulting from diaphragmatic irritation; may be present in splenic injury.

keratin The protein produced by keratinocytes; makes the outermost skin layer waterproof.

keratoconjunctivitis sicca A condition of the eyes that results from changes in tear composition, lacrimal gland malfunction, or altered tear distribution; also called "dry eye syndrome."

keratoconus The degeneration of the corneal tissue resulting in abnormal corneal shape.

keratoplasty Corneal transplant. The surgical removal of diseased corneal tissue and replacement with tissue from a human donor cornea.

ketogenesis The conversion of fats to acids in the body.

ketone bodies Substances, including acetone, that are produced as by-products of the incomplete metabolism of fatty acids. When insulin is not available (as in uncontrolled diabetes mellitus), they accumulate in the blood and cause metabolic acidosis; also called "ketones."

ketorolac (Toradol) Popular nonsteroidal anti-inflammatory drug prescribed for short-term use in acute pain because it can be given orally, intramuscularly, or by IV push.

knee height caliper Device that uses the distance between the patella and heel to estimate height.

Kupffer cells Phagocytic cells that are part of the body's reticuloendothelial system and are involved in the protective function of the liver. Kupffer cells engulf harmful bacteria and anemic red blood cells.

Kussmaul respiration A type of breathing that occurs when excess acids caused by the absence of insulin increase hydrogen ion and carbon dioxide levels in the blood. This state triggers an increase in the rate and depth of respiration in an attempt to excrete more carbon dioxide and acid.

kwashiorkor Lack of protein quantity and quality in the presence of adequate calories. Body weight is somewhat normal, and serum proteins are low.

kyphoplasty A minimally invasive surgery for managing vertebral fractures in patients with osteoporosis. Bone cement is injected into the fracture site to provide pain relief, and an inflated balloon is used to restore height to the vertebra.

L

labia majora Two vertical folds of adipose tissue that extend posteriorly from the mons pubis to the perineum.

labia minora Two thinner, vertical folds of reddish epithelium that are surrounded by the labia majora.

labyrinthectomy Surgical removal of the labyrinth; used as a radical treatment of Ménière's disease when medical therapy is ineffective and the patient already has significant hearing loss.

labyrinthitis An infection of the labyrinth of the ear; may occur as a complication of acute or chronic otitis media.

laceration A type of wound characterized by tearing or mangling and usually caused by sharp objects and projectiles.

lacrimal gland A small gland that produces tears; located in the upper outer part of each ocular orbit.

lacto-ovo-vegetarian A vegetarian diet pattern in which milk, cheese, eggs, and dairy foods are eaten but meat, fish, and poultry are avoided.

lactose intolerance The inability to convert lactose (found in milk and dairy products) to glucose and galactose in the body.

lacto-vegetarian A vegetarian diet pattern in which milk, cheese, and dairy foods are eaten but meat, fish, poultry, and eggs are avoided.

lacunae Small, deep cavities within the brain that result from occlusion of a small vessel; this leads to infarct and necrosis of the area of the brain supplied by the affected vessel.

laparoscopy A minimally invasive procedure in which the surgeon makes several small incisions near the umbilicus through which a small endoscope is placed to examine the abdomen; direct examination of the pelvic cavity through an endoscope.

laparotomy An open surgical approach in which a large abdominal incision is made.

laryngitis Inflammation of the mucous membranes lining the larynx.

laryngectomee A person who has had a laryngectomy.

laryngopharynx The area behind the larynx that extends from the base of the tongue to the esophagus. It is the critical dividing point at which solid foods and fluids are separated from air.

larynx The "voice box"; it is composed of several cartilages and is located above the trachea and just below the throat at the base of the tongue; part of the upper respiratory tract.

laser An acronym for light amplification by stimulated emission of radiation. As a surgical tool, a laser emits a high-powered beam of light that cuts tissue more cleanly than do scalpel blades. A laser creates intense heat, rapidly clots blood vessels or tissue, and turns target tissue (e.g., a tumor) into vapor.

laser-assisted angioplasty A procedure using heat from a laser probe that is advanced through a cannula to vaporize arteriosclerotic plaque and open the occluded or stenosed artery.

latency period The time between the initiation of a cell and the development of an overt tumor.

late-onset seizure Seizure that occurs initially more than 7 days after a head injury.

latex allergy Reactions to exposure to latex in gloves and other medical products; reactions include rashes, nasal or eye symptoms, and asthma.

latrodectism A syndrome caused by the venom of a black widow spider bite in which neurotransmitter releases from nerve terminals to cause severe abdominal pain, muscle rigidity and spasm, hypertension, and nausea and vomiting.

lead In an ECG, the provider of one view of the heart's electrical activity.

lead axis In electrocardiography, the imaginary line that joins the positive and negative poles of the lead systems.

left shift An increase in the band cells (immature neutrophils) in the white blood cell differential count; an early indication of infection.

left-sided heart (ventricular) failure Inadequacy of the left ventricle of the heart to pump adequately; results in decreased tissue perfusion from poor cardiac output and pulmonary congestion from increased pressure in the pulmonary vessels; typical causes include hypertensive, coronary artery, or valvular disease involving the mitral or aortic valve. Most heart failure begins with failure of the left ventricle and progresses to failure of both ventricles.

legally competent A person 18 years of age or older, a pregnant or a married minor, a legally emancipated (free) minor who is self-supporting, or a person not declared incompetent by a court of law.

leiomyomas Benign, slow-growing solid tumors of the uterine myometrium (muscle layer). These are the most commonly occurring pelvic tumors; also called "myomas" and "fibroids."

lens The circular, convex structure of the eye that lies behind the iris and in front of the vitreous body. Normally transparent, the lens bends the rays of light entering through the pupil so they focus on the retina. The curve of the lens changes to focus on near or distant objects.

leprosy (Hansen's disease) A chronic, contagious, systemic mycobacterial infection of the peripheral nervous system with skin involvement. The clinical course is either progressive or self-limiting depending on the immunologic status of the host. Although the exact mechanism of infection remains unknown, studies suggest transmission via the airborne route, by insects, or through direct contact with skin lesions.

leptin A hormone that is released by fat cells and possibly by gastric cells; it also acts on the hypothalamus to control appetite.

lethargic A state of drowsiness or sleepiness.

leukemia A type of cancer with uncontrolled production of immature white blood cells in the bone marrow; the bone marrow becomes overcrowded with immature, nonfunctional cells, and the production of normal blood cells is greatly decreased.

leukocyte White blood cell (WBC); this immune system cell protects the body from the effects of invasion by organisms.

leukocytosis An elevated white blood cell count.

leukopenia A reduction in the number of white blood cells.

leukoplakia White, patchy lesions on a mucous membrane.

level I trauma center According to the American College of Surgeons, a regional resource facility that is capable of "providing leadership and total care for every aspect of injury, from prevention through rehabilitation."

level II trauma center A community facility that is capable of providing care to the vast majority of injured patients but may not be able to meet the resource needs of patients who require very complex injury management.

level III trauma center A critical link to higher-capability trauma centers in communities that do not have ready access to level I or level II centers; the primary focus is injury stabilization and patient transfer.

level IV trauma center A facility that offers advanced life support care in rural or remote settings that do not have ready access to a higher-level trauma center, such as a ski area.

LGBT Acronym for "lesbian, gay, bisexual, and transgender" culture.

libido Sexual desire.

lichenification An abnormal thickening of the skin to a leathery appearance; can occur in patients with chronic dermatitis because of their continual rubbing of the area to relieve itching.

Lichtenberg figures Branching or ferning marks that appear on the skin as a result of a lightning strike; also called "keraunographic markings" or "erythematous arborization."

life review A structured process of reflecting on one's life that is often facilitated by an interviewer.

ligament One of many bands of tissue that attach bones to other bones at joints and serve to support joints.

light reflex The reflection of the otoscope's light off the eardrum in the form of a clearly demarcated triangle of light in the normal ear.

limited scleroderma Thick skin that is limited to sites distal to the elbow and knee but also involves the face and neck.

linear fracture   A type of bone fracture involving a simple, clean break in which the impacted area of bone bends inward and the area around it bends outward.

lipid   Fat, including cholesterol and triglycerides, that can be measured in the blood.

lipoatrophy   The loss or atrophy of subcutaneous fat; in patients with diabetes, the loss of fat tissue in areas of repeated insulin injection.

lipohypertrophy   The enlargement or hypertrophy of subcutaneous fat; in patients with diabetes, an increased swelling of fat that occurs at the site of repeated insulin injections.

lipolysis   The decomposition or splitting up of fat to provide fuel for energy when liver glucose is unavailable.

liposuction   A cosmetic procedure to reduce the amount of adipose tissue in selected areas of the body.

lithotripsy   The use of sound, laser, or dry shock wave energy to break a kidney stone into small fragments; also called "extracorporeal shock wave lithotripsy."

living will   A legal document that instructs physicians and family members about what life-sustaining treatment is wanted (or not wanted) if the patient becomes unable to make decisions.

lobectomy   Surgical removal of an entire lung lobe.

lobular carcinoma in situ (LCIS)   A noninvasive form of breast cancer that does not show up as a calcified cluster on a mammogram and is therefore most often diagnosed incidentally during a biopsy for another problem.

local anesthesia   Anesthesia that is delivered by applying it to the skin or mucous membranes of the area to be anesthetized or by injecting it directly into the tissue around an incision, wound, or lesion.

localized pain   Confined to the site of origin.

lockout interval   A specific interval between doses programmed into a patient-controlled analgesia infusion pump. No drug is administered if the patient attempts to access the drug before the interval has elapsed.

locus   The specific chromosome location for a gene.

log rolling   Turning technique in which the patient turns all at once while his or her back is kept as straight as possible.

long-term nonprogressor (LTNP)   A person who has been infected with the human immune deficiency virus for at least 10 years and has remained asymptomatic with CD4+ cell counts within a normal range. About 1% of those infected are long-term nonprogressors.

loop electrosurgical excision procedure (LEEP)   Diagnostic procedure/treatment in which a thin loop-wire electrode that transmits a painless electrical current is used to cut away affected cervical cancer tissue.

lordosis   The anterior concavity in the curvature of the lumbar and cervical spine when viewed from the side; a common finding in pregnancy and abdominal obesity.

Lou Gehrig's disease   See *amyotrophic lateral sclerosis (ALS)*.

low back pain (LBP)   Pain in the lumbosacral region of the back caused by muscle strain or spasm, ligament sprain, disk degeneration, or herniation of the nucleus pulposus from the center of the disk. Herniated disks occur most often between the fourth and fifth lumbar vertebrae (L4-5) but may occur at other levels.

lower esophageal sphincter (LES)   The portion of the esophagus proximal to the gastroesophageal junction; when at rest, the sphincter is closed to prevent reflux of gastric contents into the esophagus.

lower GI series   Radiographic visualization of the large intestine; usually ordered for a patient with a complaint of blood or mucus in the stool or a change in bowel pattern, such as diarrhea or constipation; also called a "barium enema."

lower motor neurons   Neurons that carry motor impulses to skeletal muscles. Patients with spinal cord injuries involving lower motor neuron lesions experience muscle wasting due to long-term flaccid paralysis.

lower urinary tract symptom (LUTS)   Any of a collection of symptoms seen in benign prostatic hyperplasia, including hesitancy, intermittency, reduced force and size of the urinary stream, a sensation of incomplete bladder emptying, and postvoid dribbling.

low-intensity pulsed ultrasound   A method using ultrasonic waves to promote bone union in slow-healing fractures or for new fractures as an alternative to surgery.

low-profile gastrostomy device (LPGD)   A gastrostomy device that uses a firm or balloon-style internal bumper or retention disk; an antireflux valve keeps gastric contents from leaking onto the skin.

loxoscelism   Systemic effects from the injected toxin of a spider bite.

lumbar puncture   The insertion of a spinal needle into the subarachnoid space between the third and fourth (sometimes the fourth and fifth) lumbar vertebrae to withdraw spinal fluid for analysis; also called a "spinal tap."

lumen   The inside cavity of a tube or tubular organ, such as a blood vessel or airway.

lung compliance   The quality of elasticity of the lungs.

lunula   The white crescent-shaped portion of the nail at the lower end of the nail plate.

lurch   An abnormality in the swing phase of gait; occurs when the muscles in the buttocks or legs are too weak to allow the person to change weight from one foot to the other.

luteal   Pertaining to the post-ovulation phase of the menstrual cycle.

Lyme disease   A systemic infectious disease that is caused by the spirochete *Borrelia burgdorferi* and results from the bite of an infected deer tick. Signs and symptoms include a large "bull's-eye" circular rash, malaise, fever, headache, and muscle or joint aches.

lymph   Fluid that has moved out of the capillaries and is returned to the systemic circulation.

lymphadenopathy   Persistently enlarged lymph nodes.

lymphedema   Abnormal accumulation of protein fluid in the subcutaneous tissue of the affected limb after a mastectomy.

lymphoblastic   Pertaining to abnormal leukemic cells that come from the lymphoid pathways and develop into lymphocytes.

lymphocytic   Pertaining to abnormal leukemic cells that come from the lymphoid pathways.

lymphokine   Cytokine produced by T-cells.

lysergic acid (LSD)   The prototype major hallucinogenic drug that is odorless and colorless with a slightly bitter taste; also called "acid."

lysis   Breakage, for example, of a cell membrane.

lysozyme   A component that is present in large quantities in many body secretions and dissolves the cell walls of some bacteria.

M

M phase   The phase of cell division in which a single cell splits into two cells (actual mitosis).

macrocytic anemia   A form of vitamin B_{12} deficiency anemia characterized by abnormally large precursor cells.

macrovascular   Referring to large blood vessels.

macular   A term referring to a macula, a discolored spot on the skin that is not raised above the surface.

macular degeneration   The deterioration of the macula, the area of central vision.

magnesium (Mg^{2+})   A mineral that forms a cation when dissolved in water.

magnetoencephalography (MEG)   A noninvasive imaging technique that measures the magnetic fields produced by electrical activity in the brain via extremely sensitive devices such as superconducting quantum interference devices (SQUIDs).

malabsorption   A syndrome associated with a variety of disorders and intestinal surgical procedures and characterized by impaired intestinal absorption of nutrients.

malignant   Referring to cancer.

malignant cell growth   Altered cell growth that is serious and, without intervention, leads to death; cancer.

malignant hypertension   A severe type of elevated blood pressure that rapidly progresses, with systolic blood pressure greater than 200 mm Hg and diastolic blood pressure greater than 150 mm Hg (greater than 130 mm Hg when there are pre-existing complications).

malignant transformation   The process of changing a normal cell into a cancer cell.

malleus   The outermost bony ossicle of the ear; also called the "hammer."

malpighian layers   The stratified layers of the epithelium that are formed when older keratinocytes are pushed upward.

mammography   An x-ray of the soft tissue of the breast.

mandibulectomy   Surgical removal of the jaw.

Manning criteria   A collective term for the characteristic symptoms of irritable bowel syndrome: abdominal pain relieved by defecation or associated with changes in stool frequency or consistency, abdominal distention, the sensation of incomplete evacuation of stool, and the presence of mucus with stool passage.

marasmic-kwashiorkor A combined protein and energy malnutrition that often presents clinically when metabolic stress is imposed on a chronically starved patient.

marasmus A calorie malnutrition in which body fat and protein are wasted but serum proteins are often preserved.

marsupialization Surgical formation of a pouch that is a new duct opening.

masklike facies Facial expression characterized by wide-open, fixed, staring eyes caused by rigidity of the facial muscles; often seen in patients with Parkinson disease.

mass casualty event A situation affecting the public health that is defined based on the resource availability of a particular community or hospital facility. When the number of casualties exceeds the resource capabilities, a disaster situation is recognized to exist.

massage The use of various strokes and pressure to manipulate soft tissues for therapeutic purposes.

mastication The process of chewing.

mastoid process The bony ridge located over the temporal bone behind the pinna; part of the external ear.

mastoiditis An acute or chronic infection of the mastoid air cells caused by untreated or inadequately treated otitis media.

matrix In referring to bone, the substance of bone consisting chiefly of collagen, mucopolysaccharides, and lipids. Deposits of inorganic calcium salts (carbonate and phosphate) in the matrix provide the hardness of bone.

maze procedure An open chest surgical technique often performed with coronary artery bypass grafting for patients in atrial fibrillation with decompensation.

McMurray test A common diagnostic technique for the patient with a torn meniscus. The examiner flexes and rotates the knee and then presses on the medial aspect while slowly extending the leg. The test result is positive if clicking is palpated or heard; however, a negative finding does not rule out a tear.

mean arterial pressure (MAP) The arterial blood pressure (between 60 and 70 mm Hg) necessary to maintain perfusion of major body organs, such as the kidneys and brain.

mechanical débridement Method of débriding a wound by mechanical entrapment and detachment of dead tissue.

mechanical obstruction The physical obstruction of the bowel by disorders outside the intestine (e.g., adhesions or hernias) or by blockages in the lumen of the intestine (e.g., tumors, inflammation, strictures, or fecal impactions).

mechanical patient lift Electrically operated device used to lift, transfer, move, and reposition patients.

mechanism of injury (MOI) The manner in which a patient's traumatic event occurred, such as a high-speed motor vehicle crash or gunshot wound.

mediastinal shift A shift of central thoracic structures toward one side; seen on chest x-ray.

mediastinitis Infection of the mediastinum.

medical command physician As defined in a hospital's emergency response plan, the person responsible for determining the number, acuity, and medical resource needs of victims arriving from the incident scene and for organizing the emergency health care team response to injured or ill patients.

medical harm Physician incidents and all errors caused by members of the health care team or system that lead to patient injury or death.

medical nutritional supplements (MNSs) Enteral products taken by patients who cannot consume enough nutrients in their usual diet (e.g., Ensure, Boost).

medication overuse headache See *rebound headache.*

meditation A mind-body therapy using self-directed practices to relax the body and calm the mind.

medulla A general term for the most interior portion of an organ or structure.

melena Blood in the stool, with the appearance of black tarry stools.

memory cell A type of B-lymphocyte that remains sensitized but does not start to produce antibodies until the next exposure to the same antigen.

menarche A female's first menstruation, which is one sign of puberty.

Ménière's disease Tinnitus, one-sided sensorineural hearing loss, and vertigo that is related to overproduction or decreased reabsorption of endolymphatic fluid and causes a distortion of the entire inner canal system.

meninges The immediate protective covering of the brain and the spinal cord.

meningioma A type of benign brain tumor that arises from the coverings of the brain (the meninges) and causes compression and displacement of adjacent brain tissue.

meningitis Inflammation, usually bacterial or viral, of the arachnoid and pia mater of the brain and spinal cord and the cerebrospinal fluid. May be caused by bacteria or viruses; symptoms are the same regardless of the causative organism.

meniscectomy Surgical excision of a meniscus, as in a knee joint.

menopause The end of menstruation and the biologic end of reproductive ability. The term applies only to the last menstrual period. The actual date of menopause cannot be determined until at least 1 year has passed without menses.

menses The monthly flow of blood from the genital tract of women.

menstruation The cyclic shedding of the endometrial lining of the uterus.

metabolic syndrome A collection of related health problems with insulin resistance as a main feature. Other features include obesity, low levels of physical activity, hypertension, high blood levels of cholesterol, and elevated triglyceride levels. Metabolic syndrome increases the risk for coronary heart disease. Also called "syndrome X."

metastasis The growth and spread of cancer.

metastasize To spread cancer from the main tumor site to many other body sites.

metastatic Referring to disease, such as cancer, that transfers from one organ to another organ or part not directly connected; pertains to additional tumors that form after cancer cells move from the primary location by breaking off from the original group and establishing remote colonies.

methemoglobinemia The conversion of normal hemoglobin to methemoglobin.

microalbuminuria The presence of very small amounts of albumin in the urine that are not measurable by a urine dipstick or usual urinalysis procedures. Specialized assays are used to analyze a freshly voided urine specimen for microscopic levels of albumin.

microcytic Abnormally small in size, such as an abnormally small red blood cell.

microvascular Referring to small blood vessels.

microvascular decompression A surgical procedure to relieve the pain of trigeminal neuralgia by relocating a small artery that compresses the trigeminal nerve as it enters the pons. The surgeon carefully lifts the loop of the artery off the nerve and places a small silicone sponge between the vessel and the nerve.

midline catheter A type of catheter that is 6 to 8 inches long and inserted through the veins of the antecubital fossa; used in therapies lasting from 1 to 4 weeks.

migraine headache An episodic familial disorder manifested by a unilateral, frontotemporal, throbbing pain that is often worse behind one eye or ear. It is often accompanied by a sensitive scalp, anorexia, photophobia, and nausea with or without vomiting. Three categories of migraine headache are migraines with aura, migraines without aura, and atypical migraines.

migratory arthritis In the early stage of rheumatoid arthritis, symptoms that are migrating or involve more joints.

miliary tuberculosis See *hematogenous tuberculosis.*

mineralocorticoids Corticosteroids produced in the zona glomerulosa of the adrenal gland to help control the body's sodium and potassium content.

minimally invasive direct coronary artery bypass (MIDCAB) Surgical procedure that does not require cardiopulmonary bypass and may be used for patients with a lesion of the left anterior descending artery.

minimally invasive esophagectomy (MIE) A laparoscopic surgical procedure to remove part of the esophagus; may be performed in patients with early-stage cancer.

minimally invasive inguinal hernia repair (MIIHR) Surgical repair of an inguinal hernia through a laparoscope, which is the treatment of choice.

minimally invasive surgery (MIS) A general term for any surgery performed using laparoscopic technique.

miosis Constriction of the pupil of the eye.

mitochondria Within the cytoplasm of cells, the sites of production of adenosine triphosphate.

mitosis Cell division.

mitotic index The percentage of actively dividing cells within a tumor.

mitral (bicuspid) valve The atrioventricular valve that separates the left atrium of the heart from the left ventricle.

mitral regurgitation Inability of the mitral valve to close completely during systole, which allows the backflow of blood into the left atrium when the left ventricle contracts; usually due to fibrosis and calcification caused by rheumatic disease. Also called "mitral insufficiency."

mitral stenosis Thickening of the mitral valve due to fibrosis and calcification and usually caused by rheumatic fever. The valve leaflets fuse and become stiff, the chordae tendineae contract, and the valve opening narrows, preventing normal blood flow from the left atrium to the left ventricle. As a result, left atrial pressure rises, the left atrium dilates, pulmonary artery pressures increase, and the right ventricle hypertrophies.

mitral valve prolapse (MVP) Dysfunction of the mitral valve that occurs because the valvular leaflets enlarge and prolapse into the left atrium during systole; usually benign but may progress to pronounced mitral regurgitation.

mixed conductive-sensorineural hearing loss A profound hearing loss that results from a combination of both conductive and sensorineural types of hearing loss.

modifiable risk factor A factor in disease development that can be altered or controlled by the patient. Examples include elevated serum cholesterol levels, cigarette smoking, hypertension, impaired glucose tolerance, obesity, physical inactivity, and stress.

modified radical mastectomy Surgical procedure for breast cancer in which the affected breast is completely removed.

monokine Cytokine made by macrophages, neutrophils, eosinophils, and monocytes.

monosyllabic One-syllable words, such as *day, toe,* and *ran,* used in speech discrimination testing to determine the patient's ability to discriminate among similar sounds or among words that contain similar sounds.

mons pubis The fat pad that covers the symphysis pubis and protects it during sexual intercourse; it becomes prominent and covered with hair during puberty.

morbid obesity A weight that has a severely negative effect on health; usually more than 100% above ideal body weight or a body mass index greater than 40.

morbidity An illness or an abnormal condition or quality.

mortality Death.

Morton's neuroma Plantar digital neuritis, a condition in which a small tumor grows in a digital nerve of the foot. The patient usually describes the pain as an acute, burning sensation in the web space that involves the entire surface of the third and fourth toes.

motor Facilitating movement.

motor aphasia See *expressive aphasia.*

motor cortex Area in the frontal lobe of the brain that controls voluntary movement.

motor end plate The junction of a peripheral motor nerve and the muscle cells that it supplies.

mourning The outward social expression of loss.

mu opioids Drugs that cause side effects that include constipation, nausea and vomiting, urinary retention, pruritus (itching), sedation, and respiratory depression because of their action on the mu receptor, the most important type of opioid receptor.

mucosa The innermost layer of the gastrointestinal tract; consists of a thin layer of smooth muscle and specialized exocrine gland cells.

mucositis Open sores on mucous membranes.

multi-casualty event A disaster event in which a limited number of victims or casualties are involved and can be managed by a hospital using local resources.

multifocal Having multiple points of origin.

multigated blood pool scanning In nuclear cardiology, cardiac blood pool imaging is a noninvasive test to evaluate cardiac motion and calculate ejection fraction by using a computer to synchronize the patient's electrocardiogram with pictures obtained by a gamma-scintillation camera. In multigated blood pool scanning, the computer breaks the time between R waves into fractions of a second, called "gates." The camera records blood flow through the heart during each gate. By analyzing information from multiple gates, the computer can evaluate ventricular wall motion and calculate ejection fraction (percentage of the left ventricular volume that is ejected with each contraction) and ejection velocity.

multimodal analgesia The use of a combination of opioids, non-opioids, and local anesthetics for postoperative pain; also called "balanced analgesia."

multiple organ dysfunction syndrome (MODS) The sequence of inadequate blood flow to body tissues, which deprives cells of oxygen and leads to anaerobic metabolism with acidosis, hyperkalemia, and tissue ischemia; this is followed by dramatic changes in vital organs and leads to the release of toxic metabolites and destructive enzymes.

multiple sclerosis (MS) A chronic autoimmune disease that affects the myelin sheath and conduction pathway of the central nervous system. It is one of the leading causes of neurologic disability in persons 20 to 40 years of age.

murmur Abnormal heart sound that reflects turbulent blood flow through normal or abnormal valves; murmurs are classified according to their timing in the cardiac cycle (systolic or diastolic) and their intensity depending on their level of loudness.

Murphy's sign A sign of gallbladder disease consisting of pain that increases with deep inspiration with right subcostal palpation.

muscle biopsy The extraction of a muscle specimen for the diagnosis of atrophy (as in muscular dystrophy) and inflammation (as in polymyositis).

muscular dystrophy (MD) A group of degenerative myopathies characterized by weakness and atrophy of muscle without nervous system involvement. At least nine types have been clinically identified and can be broadly categorized as slowly progressive or rapidly progressive.

mutation A change in deoxyribonucleic acid (DNA) that is passed from one generation to another.

myalgia Muscle aches/muscle pain.

myasthenia gravis (MG) A chronic autoimmune disease of the neuromuscular junction. It is characterized by remissions and exacerbations, with fatigue and weakness primarily in the muscles innervated by the cranial nerves and in the skeletal and respiratory muscles. It ranges from mild disturbances of the ocular muscles to a rapidly developing, generalized weakness that may lead to death from respiratory failure.

myasthenic crisis Undermedication with cholinesterase inhibitors.

mydriasis Dilation of the pupil of the eye.

myelin sheath A white, lipid covering of the axon.

myelocytic Pertaining to leukemias in which the abnormal cells come from the myeloid pathways.

myelogenous Pertaining to leukemias in which the abnormal cells come from the myeloid pathways.

myelography Radiography of the spine after injection of contrast medium into the subarachnoid space of the spine; used to visualize the vertebral column, intervertebral disks, spinal nerve roots, and blood vessels.

myelosuppression Suppression of bone marrow activity that causes decreased numbers of blood cells (pancytopenia).

myocardial contractility The force of cardiac contraction independent of preload.

myocardial hypertrophy Enlargement of the myocardium.

myocardial infarction (MI) Injury and necrosis of myocardial tissue that occurs when the tissue is abruptly and severely deprived of oxygen; usually caused by atherosclerosis of a coronary artery, rupture of the plaque, subsequent thrombosis, and occlusion of blood flow.

myocardial nuclear perfusion imaging (MNPI) The use of radionuclide techniques in which radioactive tracer substances are used to view, record, and evaluate cardiovascular abnormalities; useful for detecting myocardial infarction and decreased myocardial blood flow and for evaluating left ventricular ejection.

myocardium The heart muscle.

myoclonic seizure A type of generalized seizure characterized by a brief jerking or stiffening of the extremities. The contractions last for just a few seconds and may be symmetric or asymmetric.

myofibril sarcomere The basic contractile unit of the myocardial cell.

myoglobin A low–molecular-weight heme protein found in cardiac and skeletal muscle; an early marker of myocardial infarction.

myoglobinuria The release of muscle myoglobulin into the urine.

myoglobinuric renal failure Renal failure that is caused by the release of myoglobulin (muscle protein) from injured muscle tissues into the circulation. Myoglobulin, which is believed to have a direct toxic effect on the kidney, can occlude the distal convoluted tubule and precipitate acute renal failure.

myomectomy The surgical removal of leiomyomas with preservation of the uterus.

myometrium The thick, middle, muscular layer of the body of the uterus. Contraction of these muscle fibers can expel the products of conception and can constrict the blood vessels to control bleeding after childbirth.

myopathy A problem in muscle tissue.

myopia An error of refraction that occurs when the eye over-refracts or over-bends the light and focuses images in front of the retina; this results in normal near vision but poor distance vision; also called "nearsightedness."

myositis Inflammation of a muscle.

myosplint Electrical stimulation of tension splints in the heart to help the ventricle change to a more normal shape in the patient with heart failure; under investigation in Europe and the United States.

myringoplasty Surgical reconstruction of the eardrum.

myringotomy The surgical creation of a hole in the eardrum; performed to drain middle-ear fluids and relieve pain in the patient with otitis media (middle-ear infection).

myxedema Dry, waxy swelling of the skin that is accompanied by nonpitting edema (especially around the eyes, in the hands and feet, and between the shoulder blades) and is associated with primary hypothyroidism.

myxedema coma A rare, serious complication of untreated or poorly treated hypothyroidism in which decreased metabolism causes the heart muscle to become flabby and the chamber size to increase, resulting in decreased cardiac output and decreased perfusion to the brain and other vital organs.

N

nadir In chemotherapy, the period of greatest bone marrow suppression, when the patient's platelet count may be very low.

nasoduodenal tube (NDT) A tube that is inserted through a nostril and into the small intestine.

nasoenteric tube (NET) Any feeding tube that is inserted nasally and then advanced into the gastrointestinal tract.

nasogastric (NG) tube A tube that is inserted through a nostril and into the stomach for liquid feeding or for withdrawing gastric contents.

nasotracheal The route for inserting a tube into the trachea via the nose.

National Patient Safety Goals Goals published by The Joint Commission that require health care organizations to focus on specific priority safety practices.

natural chemical débridement Method of débriding a wound by creating an environment that promotes self-digestion of dead tissues by bacterial enzymes.

naturopath Holistic care provider who uses a combination of physical therapies, herbal preparations, homeopathic remedies, acupuncture, and lifestyle changes to improve health.

naturopathic medicine The practice of medicine that incorporates herbs and nutrition into its health care practice.

near point of vision The closest distance at which the eye can see an object clearly.

near-drowning Recovery after submersion in a liquid medium (usually water); this term is no longer used because language that describes drowning incidents has been standardized.

near-euglycemic A term that refers to near-normal blood glucose levels.

near-syncope Dizziness with an inability to remain in an upright position.

necrosis Cell death, or infarction.

necrotic arachnidism A necrotic wound resulting from a spider bite.

necrotizing hemorrhagic pancreatitis (NHP) Inflammation of the pancreas that is characterized by diffusely bleeding pancreatic tissue with fibrosis and tissue death. This form affects about 20% of patients with pancreatitis.

necrotizing vasculitis A group of diseases whose primary manifestation is inflammation of arterial walls, which causes ischemia in the tissues usually supplied by the involved vessels.

needle thoracostomy A quick, temporary method of chest decompression in which a large-bore needle is used to vent trapped air pending chest tube insertion.

negative deflection In electrocardiography, the flow of electrical current in the heart (cardiac axis) away from the positive pole and toward the negative pole.

negative feedback control mechanism The condition of maintaining a constant output of a system by exerting an inhibitory control on a key step by a product of that system. Used in a series of reactions that control hormone secretion and cellular activity based on responses to correct any movement away from normal function. An example of a simple negative feedback hormone response is the control of insulin secretion in which the action of insulin (decreasing blood glucose levels) is the opposite of the condition that stimulated insulin secretion (elevated blood glucose levels).

negative nitrogen balance A net loss of protein that occurs when the breakdown (degradation) of protein exceeds buildup (synthesis).

neglect In nursing, failure to provide for a patient's basic needs.

neoadjuvant therapy Treatment of a cancerous tumor with chemotherapy to shrink the tumor before it is surgically removed.

neoplasia Any new or continued cell growth not needed for normal development or replacement of dead and damaged tissues.

nephrectomy The surgical removal of the kidney.

nephrolithiasis The formation of stones in the kidney.

nephron The "working" unit of the kidney where urine is formed from blood. Each kidney consists of about 1 million nephrons, and each nephron separately makes urine. There are two types of nephrons: cortical and juxtamedullary.

nephropathy Pathologic change in the kidney that reduces kidney function and leads to renal failure.

nephrosclerosis Thickening in the nephron blood vessels that results in narrowing of the vessel lumen, with decreased renal blood flow and chronically hypoxic kidney tissue.

nephrostomy The surgical creation of an opening directly into the kidney; performed to divert urine externally and prevent further damage to the kidney when a stricture is causing hydronephrosis and cannot be corrected with urologic procedures.

nephrotic syndrome (NS) A condition of increased glomerular permeability that allows larger molecules to pass through the membrane into the urine and be removed from the blood. This process causes massive loss of protein into the urine, edema formation, and decreased plasma albumin levels.

nephrotoxicity (nephrotoxic) The disruption of kidney function.

neuritic plaques Degenerating nerve terminals found particularly in the hippocampus, an important part of the limbic system, and marked by increased amounts of an abnormal protein called "beta amyloid"; a characteristic change of the brain found in patients with Alzheimer's disease.

neuroaxial Referring to the epidural or spinal area.

neuroendocrine regulation The regulation of overall body function by the combined actions of the endocrine system and the nervous system.

neurofibrillary tangles Tangled masses of fibrous elements throughout the neurons; a classic finding at autopsy in the brains of patients with Alzheimer's disease.

neurogenic shock Hypotension and bradycardia associated with cervical spinal injuries and caused by a loss of autonomic function. The patient is at greatest risk in the first 24 hours after injury.

neuroglial cells Cells of varying size and shape that provide protection, structure, and nutrition for the neurons.

neurohypophysis The posterior lobe of the pituitary gland that stores hormones produced in the hypothalamus.

neurolysis Permanent nerve destruction.

neuroma A sensitive tumor consisting of nerve cells and nerve fibers.

neuropathic pain A type of chronic noncancer pain that results from a nerve injury. Examples of causes include diabetic neuropathy, postherpetic neuralgia, radiculopathy (spinal nerve damage), and trigeminal neuralgia. Neuropathic pain is described as burning, shooting, stabbing, and the sensation of "pins and needles."

neuropathy A progressive deterioration of nerves that results in loss of nerve function. A common complication of diabetes, it often involves all parts of the body.

neurotransmitter Regulatory chemical that exerts inhibitory (slowing down) or excitatory (speeding up) activity at postsynaptic nerve cell membranes. Acetylcholine, norepinephrine, epinephrine, dopamine, and serotonin are neurotransmitters.

neurovascular assessment Assessment of the neuromuscular system that includes inspection of skin color, temperature, and capillary refill distal to an injury, surgical procedure, or cast. Palpation of pulses in the extremities below level of injury and assessment of sensation, movement, and pain in the injured part give a complete assessment.

neutralization See *inactivation*.

neutropenia Decreased numbers of leukocytes, especially neutrophils, which causes immunosuppression.

neutrophilia Increased number of circulating neutrophils.

nevus A mole; a benign skin growth of the pigment-forming cells.

new-onset angina Cardiac chest pain that occurs for the first time.

nitroglycerin (NTG) A drug prescribed for patients with angina. It increases collateral blood flow, redistributes blood flow toward the subendocardium, and causes dilation of the coronary arteries.

nits Lice eggs.

NMDA (*N*-methyl-D-aspartate) receptor antagonist A group of drugs that block excess amounts of glutamate, which damages nerve cells in the brain; used to treat Alzheimer's disease.

nociceptive pain Pain related to the skin, musculoskeletal structures, or body organs.

nocturia The need to urinate excessively at night. Also called "nocturnal polyuria."

nocturnal polyuria See *nocturia*.

nodule A small node. In the vocal cords, enlarged fibrous tissue caused by infectious processes or overuse of the voice.

nonabsorbable suture Suture that becomes encapsulated in the tissue during the healing process and remains in the tissue unless removed; made of silk, cotton, steel, nylon, polyester, or other synthetic material.

nonadherence In health care, accidental failure by a patient to take medication.

noncompliance In health care, deliberate failure by a patient to take medication.

non-exertional heat stroke See *classic heat stroke*.

noninvasive temporary pacing (NTP) Cardiac pacing that is accomplished through the application of two large external electrodes attached to an external pulse generator; used as an emergency measure to provide demand ventricular pacing in a profoundly bradycardic or asystolic patient until invasive pacing can be instituted or the patient's intrinsic rate returns to normal.

nonmechanical obstruction Intestinal obstruction that does not involve a physical obstruction in or outside the intestine. Instead, decreased or absent peristalsis results in a slowing of the movement or a backup of intestinal contents. This is also known as "paralytic ileus" or "adynamic ileus" because it is a result of neuromuscular disturbance.

nonmodifiable risk factor Factor in disease development that cannot be altered or controlled by the patient. Examples include age, gender, family history, and ethnic background.

nonprogressive (compensatory) stage of shock The stage of shock that occurs when kidney and hormonal mechanisms are activated because cardiovascular compensation alone is not enough to maintain mean arterial pressure and supply needed oxygen to the vital organs.

nonsteroidal anti-inflammatory drugs (NSAIDs) Potent anti-inflammatory agents that inhibit the synthesis of prostaglandins, thus decreasing pain and inflammation.

nonsustained ventricular tachycardia (NSVT) Occurrence of three or more successive premature ventricular complexes.

nontunneled percutaneous central catheter A type of catheter, usually 15 to 20 cm long and with dual or triple lumens, that is inserted through the subclavian vein in the upper chest or through the jugular veins in the neck using sterile technique.

nonurgent In a three-tiered triage scheme, the category that includes patients who can generally tolerate waiting several hours for health care services without a significant risk of clinical deterioration, such as those with sprains, strains, or simple fractures.

"normal" adult blood pressure According to 2003 guidelines, blood pressure less than 120 mm Hg systolic *and* less than 80 mm Hg diastolic in adults.

normal flora The microorganisms living in or on the human host without causing disease; the bacteria that are characteristic of each body location. Normal flora often compete with and prevent infection from unfamiliar microorganisms attempting to invade a body site.

normal sinus rhythm (NSR) The rhythm originating from the sinoatrial node (dominant pacemaker), with atrial and ventricular rates of 60 to 100 beats/min and regular atrial and ventricular rhythms.

normotonic See *isosmotic*.

North American pit vipers The Crotalidae, one of two families of indigenous poisonous snakes in North America; named for the characteristic depression between each eye and nostril. They include rattlesnakes, copperheads, and water moccasins and account for most poisonous snakebites in the United States.

nosocomial infection Acquired in an inpatient health care setting; for example, infections that were not present at hospital admission; also called "hospital-acquired infections" and "health care–associated infections."

nothing by mouth (NPO) No eating, drinking (including water), or smoking.

nuchal rigidity Stiff neck, which can be a sign of cerebrospinal fluid leak; nuchal rigidity is not checked until a spinal cord injury is ruled out.

nucleoside What the four bases in deoxyribonucleic acid (DNA) (adenine, guanine, cytosine, thymine) become when a five-sided sugar (deoxyribose sugar) attaches to them.

nucleotide The final form of a base that actually gets put into the strand of deoxyribonucleic acid. A nucleoside becomes a complete nucleotide by the attachment of phosphate groups.

nulliparity The condition of never having given birth.

nurse technician See *nursing assistant*.

nursing assistant A member of the rehabilitative health care team who assists the registered nurse in the care of patients.

nutritional screening A screening by the health care provider that includes visual inspection, measured height and weight, weight history, usual eating habits, ability to chew and swallow, and any recent changes in appetite or food intake. The screening is a way to determine which patients need more extensive nutritional assessment.

nutritional status Reflects the balance between nutrient requirements and intake.

nutritionist A member of the health care team who ensures patients meet their nutritional needs. Also called "dietitian."

nystagmus Involuntary, rapid eye movements.

O

obesity An increase in body weight at least 20% above the upper limit of the normal range for ideal body weight, with an excess amount of body fat; in an adult, a body mass index greater than 30.

obligatory urine output The minimum amount of urine per day needed to dissolve and excrete toxic waste products.

obstipation The inability to pass stool; intractable constipation.

obstruction Blockage.

obstructive jaundice Jaundice caused by an impediment to the flow of bile from the liver to the duodenum; may be caused by edema of the ducts or gallstones.

occlusion Blockage.

occlusive stroke A type of brain attack caused by ischemia (interruption in blood flow) in the brain tissue supplied by the affected artery.

Occupational Safety and Health Administration (OSHA) A federal agency that protects workers from injury or illness at their place of employment.

occupational therapist (OT, OTR) A member of the rehabilitation health care team who works to develop the patient's fine motor skills used for activities of daily living and the skills related to coordination and cognitive retraining.

odynophagia Pain on swallowing.

oligomenorrhea Scant or infrequent menses.

oligospermia Low sperm count.

oliguria Decreased excretion of urine in relation to amount of fluid intake; usually defined as urine output less than 400 mL/day.

omentectomy Surgical removal of the connective tissues covering the pelvic organs.

oncogene Proto-oncogene that has been "turned on" and can cause cells to change from normal cells to cancer cells.

oncogenesis Cancer development.

oncogenic osteomalacia Osteomalacia that is caused by malignant tumors of the bone; also called "tumor-induced osteomalacia."

oncovirus Virus that causes cancer.

oophorectomy Surgical removal of the ovary.

open fracture A fracture in which the skin surface over the broken bone is disrupted, causing an external wound; also called "compound fracture."

open head injury A type of traumatic primary brain injury that occurs with a skull fracture or when the skull is pierced by a penetrating object. The integrity of the brain and the dura is violated and there is exposure to outside contaminants, with damage to the underlying vessels, dural sinus, brain, and cranial nerves.

open reduction The reduction of a fracture after surgical incision into the site to allow direct visualization of the fracture. See *internal fixation*.

ophthalmoplegia Paralysis or weakness of the eye muscles.

opioids Any of a group of drugs made from the Asian poppy or produced as a synthetic drug that produces the same effects of the opium plant. The street term for opioids is "narcotics" or "narcs."

opportunistic infection Infection caused by organisms that are present as part of the normal environment and would be kept in check by normal immune function.

optic disc The point at the inside back of the eye where the optic nerve enters the eyeball. It appears as a creamy pink to white depressed area in the retina and contains only nerve fibers and no photoreceptor cells.

optic fundus The area at the inside back of the eye that can be seen with an ophthalmoscope.

optic nerve The nerve of sight; connects the optic disc to the brain.

orbit The bony socket of the skull that surrounds and protects the eye along with the attached muscles, nerves, vessels, and tear-producing glands.

orchiectomy The surgical removal of one or both testes.

orchitis An acute testicular inflammation resulting from trauma or infection.

orexin Neuropeptide that is an appetite stimulant.

organ of Corti The receptor end-organ of hearing located on the basilar membrane of the cochlea; contains hair cells that detect vibration from sound and stimulate the eighth cranial nerve.

orotracheal The route for inserting a tube into the trachea via the mouth.

orthopnea Shortness of breath that occurs when lying down but is relieved by sitting up.

orthostatic Pertaining to or caused by standing erect.

orthostatic hypotension A decrease in blood pressure (20 mm Hg systolic and/or 10 mm Hg diastolic) that occurs during the first few seconds to minutes after changing from a sitting or lying position to a standing position; also called "postural hypotension."

orthotopic transplantation The most common type of transplantation procedure in which a diseased organ is removed and a donor organ is grafted in its place. For example, during heart transplantation, the surgeon removes the diseased heart and leaves the posterior walls of the patient's atria, which serve as the anchor for the donor heart; anastomoses are made between the recipient and donor atria, aorta, and pulmonary arteries.

osmolality The number of milliosmoles in a kilogram of solution.

osmolarity The number of milliosmoles in a liter of solution.

osmosis The movement of a solvent across a semipermeable membrane (a membrane that allows the solvent, but not the solute, to pass through) from a lesser to a greater concentration.

osteitis deformans A metabolic disorder of bone remodeling, or turnover, in which increased resorption or loss results in bone deposits that are weak, enlarged, and disorganized; also called "Paget's disease."

osteoarthritis Noninflammatory form of arthritis characterized by the progressive deterioration and loss of cartilage in one or more joints; most common form of arthritis.

osteoblast Cell associated with formation of bone.

osteoblastic Referring to bone production activity.

osteoclast Cell associated with destruction or resorption of bone.

osteoclastic Referring to bone destruction.

osteocyte Bone cell.

osteogenic Originating from bone.

osteomalacia Abnormal softening of the bone tissue characterized by inadequate mineralization of osteoid. It is the adult equivalent of rickets (vitamin D deficiency) in children.

osteomyelitis An inflammation of bone tissue caused by pathogenic microorganisms; produces an increased vascularity and edema often involving the surrounding soft tissues.

osteonecrosis See *avascular necrosis*.

osteopenia A condition of low bone mass that occurs when there is a disruption in the bone remodeling process.

osteophyte Bone spur.

osteoporosis A metabolic disease in which bone demineralization results in decreased density and subsequent fractures.

osteotomy Surgical resection of bone.

ostomate A patient with an ostomy.

ostomy The surgical creation of an opening, usually referring to an opening in the abdominal wall; stoma.

otorrhea Ear discharge.

otosclerosis Irregular bone growth around the ossicles.

otoscope An instrument used to examine the ear; consists of a light, a handle, a magnifying lens, and a pneumatic bulb for injecting air into the external canal to test mobility of the eardrum.

ototoxic Having a toxic effect on the inner ear structures.

ototoxicity Disruption of hearing and/or balance.

outflow disease Chronic peripheral arterial disease with obstruction at or below the superficial femoral or popliteal artery. The patient experiences burning or cramping in the calves, ankles, feet, and toes after walking a certain distance; the pain usually subsides with rest.

outpatient A patient who goes to the hospital for treatment and returns home on the same day.

ovaries A pair of almond-shaped organs that are located near the lateral walls of the upper pelvic cavity. They develop and release ova and produce the sex steroid hormones (estrogen, progesterone, androgen, and relaxin).

overflow (urinary) incontinence The involuntary loss of urine when the bladder is overdistended.

overhydration See *fluid overload*.

overweight An increase in body weight for height compared with a reference standard (e.g., the Metropolitan Life height and weight tables) or 10% greater than ideal body weight. However, this weight may not reflect excess body fat, which in an adult is a body mass index of 25 to 30.

ovoid pupil In evaluating pupils for size and reaction to light, the midstage between a normal-size pupil and a dilated pupil; indicates the development of increased intracranial pressure.

ovulation The cyclic maturation of a dominant follicle (the graafian follicle) in the ovary and the subsequent release of the ovum.

oxygen concentrator A machine that removes nitrogen, water vapor, and hydrocarbons from room air.

oxygen dissociation The transfer of oxygen from hemoglobin to tissues.

P

P wave In the electrocardiogram, the deflection representing atrial depolarization.

pacemaker In the cardiac conduction system, the sinus node.

pack-years The number of packs of cigarettes per day multiplied by the number of years the patient has smoked; used in recording the patient's smoking history.

Paget's disease An alternative name for "osteitis deformans," a metabolic disorder of bone remodeling, or turnover, in which increased resorption or loss results in bone deposits that are weak, enlarged, and disorganized.

pain An unpleasant sensory and emotional experience associated with actual or potential tissue damage; the most reliable indication of pain is the patient's self-report.

palliation Relieving symptoms.

palliative care A compassionate and supportive approach to patients and families who are living with life-threatening illnesses; involves a holistic approach that provides relief of symptoms experienced by the dying patient.

palliative sedation A care management approach involving the administration of drugs such as benzodiazepines for the purpose of lowering of patient consciousness.

palliative surgery Surgery done to make the patient more comfortable.

palpitations A feeling of fluttering in the chest, an unpleasant awareness of the heartbeat, and an irregular heartbeat; may result from a change in heart rate or rhythm or from an increase in the force of heart contractions.

pancreatic abscess A collection of purulent material that results from extensive inflammatory necrosis of the pancreas after infection by organisms such as *Escherichia coli;* the most serious complication of pancreatitis. It is fatal if left untreated.

pancreatic pseudocyst A false cyst, so named because, unlike a true cyst, it does not have an epithelial lining. It is an encapsulated saclike structure that forms on or surrounds the pancreas and develops as a complication of acute or chronic pancreatitis. It may contain up to several liters of straw-colored or dark-brown viscous fluid, the enzymatic exudate of the pancreas.

pancreaticojejunostomy Surgical anastomosis of the pancreatic duct with the jejunum.

pancytopenia A deficiency of all three cell types (red blood cells, white blood cells, and platelets) of the blood.

pandemic A general epidemic spread over a wide geographic area and affecting a large proportion of the population.

panhypopituitarism The decreased production of all anterior pituitary hormones; an extremely rare condition.

panniculectomy The surgical removal of any panniculus, most often the abdominal apron; usually done as a follow-up to bariatric surgery in an obese patient.

panniculitis Infection of the panniculus.

panniculus A layer of membrane; also used to refer to skinfold areas in the obese patient.

pannus Vascular granulation tissue composed of inflammatory cells that forms in a joint space; erodes articular cartilage and eventually destroys bone.

Papanicolaou test (Pap smear) A cytologic study that is effective in detecting precancerous and cancerous cells obtained from the cervix.

papilla The anatomic term for a small, nipple-shaped projection or structure.

papilledema Edema and hyperemia of the optic disc; a sign of increased intracranial pressure found on ophthalmoscopic examination; also called a "choked disc."

papilloma A pedunculated outgrowth of tissue.

papillotomy An incision of a papilla, a small nipple-shaped projection or structure.

papular Referring to a papule, a small, solid elevation of the skin.

paracentesis A procedure in which the physician inserts a trocar catheter into the abdomen to remove and drain ascitic fluid from the peritoneal cavity.

paradoxical blood pressure (paradoxical pulse) An exaggerated decrease in systolic pressure by more than 10 mm Hg during the inspiratory phase of the respiratory cycle (normal is 3 to 10 mm Hg); clinical conditions that may produce a paradoxical blood pressure include pericardial tamponade, constrictive pericarditis, and pulmonary hypertension.

paradoxical chest movement The "sucking inward" of the loose chest area during inspiration and a "puffing out" of the same area during expiration in a patient with a flail chest.

paradoxical splitting Abnormal splitting of the S_2 heart sound heard in patients with severe myocardial depression; causes early closure of the pulmonic valve or a delay in aortic valve closure.

paralysis Absence of movement.

paralytic ileus Absence of peristalsis.

paramedic Prehospital care provider for patients who require care that exceeds basic life support resources. Advanced life support (ALS) may include cardiac monitoring, advanced airway management and intubation, establishing IV access, and administering drugs en route to the emergency department.

paranasal sinuses The air-filled cavities within the bones that surround the nasal passages. Lined with ciliated membrane, the sinuses provide resonance during speech and decrease the weight of the skull.

paraparesis Weakness that involves only the lower extremities, as seen in lower thoracic and lumbosacral injuries or lesions.

paraplegia Paralysis that involves only the lower extremities, as seen in lower thoracic and lumbosacral injuries or lesions.

parathyroid hormone (PTH) A hormone released from the parathyroid glands in response to decreased serum calcium levels.

parenchyma A general term for the functional elements of an organ as differentiated from its framework (stroma).

paresis Weakness.

paresthesia Abnormal or unusual nerve sensations of touch, such as tingling and burning.

parietal cells Cells lining the wall of the stomach that secrete hydrochloric acid and produce intrinsic factor.

Parkinson disease (PD) A debilitating neurologic disease that affects motor ability and is characterized by four cardinal symptoms: tremor, rigidity, akinesia (slow movement), and postural instability. It is the third most common neurologic disorder of older adults; also called "paralysis agitans."

parotidectomy The surgical removal of the parotid glands.

paroxysmal nocturnal dyspnea (PND) In the patient with heart disease, difficulty breathing that develops after lying down for several hours and causes the patient to awaken abruptly with a feeling of suffocation and panic. Occurs because the heart is unable to compensate for the increased volume when blood from the lower extremities is redistributed to the venous system, which increases venous return to the heart. A diseased heart is ineffective in pumping the additional fluid into the circulatory system, and pulmonary congestion results.

paroxysmal supraventricular tachycardia (PSVT) A form of supraventricular tachycardia that occurs when the rhythm is intermittent, initiated suddenly by a premature complex such as a premature atrial complex, and terminated suddenly with or without intervention.

partial seizure One of the three broad categories of seizure disorders along with generalized seizure and unclassified seizure. Partial seizures are of two types: complex and simple. Partial seizures begin in a part of one cerebral hemisphere; some can evolve into generalized tonic-clonic, tonic, or clonic seizures. They are most often seen in adults and in general are less responsive to medical treatment; also called "focal seizures" or "local seizures."

passive euthanasia See *withdrawing or withholding life-sustaining therapy.*

passive immunity Resistance to infection that is of short duration (days or months) and either natural by transplacental transfer from the mother or artificial by injection of antibodies (e.g., immunoglobulin).

passive smoking The exposure to secondhand smoke produced by a person smoking cigarettes.

pathogen Any microorganism capable of producing disease.

pathogenicity The ability to cause disease.

pathologic (spontaneous) fracture A fracture that occurs after minimal trauma to a bone that has been weakened by a disease such as bone cancer or osteoporosis.

patient-centered care Care that recognizes the patient or designee as the source of control and full partner in providing compassionate and coordinated care based on respect for the patient's preferences, values, and needs.

patient-controlled analgesia A method that allows the patient to control the dosage of opioid analgesia received by using an infusion pump to deliver the desired amount of medication through a conventional IV route.

patients Recipients of care in mutually trusting relationships with nurses and other members of the health care team.

PDSA Acronym for plan, do, study, analysis.

peak expiratory flow (PEF) The fastest airflow rate reached at any time during exhalation.

peau d'orange A dimpled appearance of the skin, resembling an orange peel.

pedal Pertaining to the feet.

pediculosis An infestation by human lice.

pedigree A graph of a family history for a specific trait or health problem over several generations.

pelvic inflammatory disease (PID) Any infection of the pelvis involving the upper genital tract beyond the cervix in women. It occurs when organisms from the lower genital tract migrate from the endocervix upward through the uterine cavity into the fallopian tubes.

pemphigus vulgaris A rare, chronic blistering disease that can occur anywhere on the skin and is associated with high morbidity and mortality rates. It is caused by an autoimmune disorder that occurs most often during middle and old age.

penectomy Surgical removal of the penis.

penetrance In genetics, how often or how well a gene is expressed when it is present within a population.

penetrating injury See *penetrating trauma.*

penetrating trauma Injuries caused by piercing; classified by the velocity of the vehicle (e.g., knife or bullet) causing the injury. Low-velocity injuries from knife wounds cause damage directly at the site; high-velocity injuries from gunshot wounds cause both direct and indirect damage; also called "penetrating injury."

penis An organ for urination and intercourse. It consists of the body or shaft and the glans penis (the distal end of the penis).

peptic ulcer A mucosal lesion of the stomach or duodenum.

peptic ulcer disease (PUD) The impairment of gastric mucosal defenses so they no longer protect the epithelium from the effects of acid and pepsin.

percussion notes The sounds heard upon striking a part of the body with short, sharp blows; aids diagnosis through a systematic assessment of changes in the sound quality obtained.

percutaneous Performed through the skin.

percutaneous alcohol septal ablation Surgical procedure for hypertrophic cardiomyopathy (HCM) in which alcohol is injected into a target septal branch of the left anterior descending coronary artery to produce a small

septal infarction. This procedure also widens the left ventricular outflow tract.

percutaneous electrical nerve stimulation (PENS) See *transcutaneous electrical nerve stimulation (TENS).*

percutaneous endoscopic gastrostomy (PEG) A stoma created from the abdominal wall into the stomach for insertion of a short feeding tube.

percutaneous stereotactic rhizotomy (PSR) Procedure performed under general anesthesia to treat trigeminal neuralgia; a hollow needle is passed through the inside of the patient's cheek into the trigeminal nerve fibers, and a heating current (radiofrequency thermocoagulation) goes through the needle to destroy some of the fibers.

percutaneous transhepatic cholangiography (PTC) The radiographic study of the biliary duct system using an iodinated dye instilled via a percutaneous needle inserted through the liver into the intrahepatic ducts. It may be performed when a patient has jaundice or persistent upper abdominal pain, even after cholecystectomy, but it is rarely performed as a diagnostic procedure.

percutaneous transluminal angioplasty (PTA) A nonsurgical method of improving arterial flow by opening the vessel lumen and creating a smooth inner vessel surface. One or more arteries are dilated with a balloon catheter advanced through a cannula, which is inserted into or above an occluded or stenosed artery.

percutaneously Performed through the skin and other tissues.

perforate To break open or pierce through a part.

pericardial effusion Complication of pericarditis that occurs when the space between the parietal and visceral layers of the pericardium fills with fluid.

pericardial friction rub An abnormal sound that originates from the pericardial sac and occurs with the movements of the heart during the cardiac cycle; usually transient and a sign of inflammation, infection, or infiltration; may be heard in patients with pericarditis resulting from myocardial infarction, cardiac tamponade, or post-thoracotomy.

pericardiectomy Surgical excision of the pericardium (the sac around the heart).

pericardiocentesis Withdrawal of pericardial fluid through a catheter inserted into the pericardial space to relieve the pressure on the heart.

perichondrium A tough, fibrous tissue layer that surrounds the ear cartilage and gives shape to the pinna.

perimenopause Menopause transition; changes in spontaneous ovarian function that precede the last menstrual period and occur gradually. Common features are a change in the woman's usual menstrual periods and the beginning of vasomotor symptoms, such as hot flushes and night sweats.

perineum The area between the vaginal opening and the anus. The skin of the

perineum covers the muscles, fascia, and ligaments that support the pelvic structures.

periodontal disease Gum disease in which mandibular bone loss has occurred.

perioperative The operative experience consisting of the preoperative, intraoperative, and postoperative time periods.

peripheral blood stem cells (PBSCs) Stem cells that are collected from peripheral blood for transplantation into the patient.

peripheral chemoreceptors Several 1- to 2-mm collections of tissue identified in the carotid arteries and along the aortic arch.

peripheral IV therapy IV therapy in which a vascular access device (VAD) is placed in a peripheral vein, usually in the arm.

peripheral neuropathy (PN) A general term for inflammation of peripheral nerves; also called "polyneuritis" and "polyneuropathy."

peripheral vascular disease (PVD) Any disorder that alters the natural flow of blood through the arteries and veins of the peripheral circulation.

peripherally inserted central catheter (PICC) A long catheter inserted through a vein of the antecubital fossa (inner aspect of the bend of the arm) or the middle of the upper arm.

peritonitis Acute inflammation of the visceral/parietal peritoneum and endothelial lining of the abdominal cavity, or peritoneum.

peritonsillar abscess (PTA) A complication of acute tonsillitis. The infection spreads from the tonsil to the surrounding tissue, which forms an abscess.

periungual lesion Skin lesion around the nail bed.

permeable The quality of being porous.

pernicious anemia A form of megaloblastic anemia caused by failure to absorb vitamin B_{12} because of a deficiency of intrinsic factor (normally secreted by the gastric mucosa) needed for intestinal absorption of vitamin B_{12}.

PERRLA An acronym that stands for the phrase "Pupils should be equal in size, round and regular in shape, and react to light and accommodation."

persistent pain See *chronic pain.*

personal emergency preparedness plan An individual plan that outlines specific arrangements in the event of disaster, such as childcare, pet care, and older adult care.

personal protective equipment (PPE) Infection control protocol that refers to the use of gloves, isolation gowns, face protection, and respirators with N95 or higher filtration.

personal readiness supplies A preassembled disaster supply kit for the home and/or automobile that contains clothing and basic survival supplies; also called a "go bag."

petechiae Pinpoint red spots on the mucous membranes, palate, conjunctivae, or skin.

pH A measure of the free hydrogen ion level in body fluid.

phagocytosis The process of engulfing, ingesting, killing, and disposing of an invading organism by neutrophils and macrophages; a key process of inflammation.

Phalen's maneuver (or Phalen's wrist test) Test to determine the presence of carpal tunnel syndrome (CTS); a positive test for CTS cause paresthesia in the medial nerve distribution of the palm of the hand in 60 seconds.

phantom limb pain (PLP) A frequent complication of amputation in which the patient perceives sensation in the absent (amputated) foot or hand. This sensation usually diminishes over time.

pharmacologic stress echocardiogram A form of echocardiography in which either dobutamine (increases heart's contractility) or adenosine (dilates coronary arteries) is given to the patient; usually used when patients cannot tolerate exercise.

pharynx The throat, which extends from the soft palate to the esophagus and is lined with mucous membrane; part of the upper respiratory tract.

phenotype Any genetic characteristic that can actually be observed or, in some cases, determined by laboratory test.

pheochromocytoma A tumor of the adrenal medulla, which can cause excessive secretion of catecholamines.

pheresis A procedure in which whole blood is withdrawn from the patient, a blood component (such as stem cells) is filtered out, and the plasma is returned to the patient.

phimosis A tight foreskin of the penis, which cannot be retracted.

phlebitis Inflammation of a vein, which can predispose patients to thrombosis.

phlebothrombosis Presence of a thrombus in a vein without inflammation.

phlebotomy Drawing of blood from a vein.

phonation Normal speech.

phonophobia Abnormal sensitivity to sound.

phonophoresis Treatment for back pain in which a topical drug (e.g., lidocaine, hydrocortisone) is applied followed by continuous ultrasound for 10 minutes.

photocoagulation Use of a laser, such as in treatment of retinal detachment.

photophobia Abnormal sensitivity to light.

photopsia The appearance of bright flashes of light due to the onset of retinal detachment.

physiatrist A physician who specializes in rehabilitative medicine.

physical abuse The use of a physical force, such as hitting, burning, pushing, and molesting the patient, that results in bodily injury.

physical dependence The adaptation manifested by a drug class–specific withdrawal syndrome. Manifestations can be produced by abrupt cessation, rapid dose reduction, decreasing blood level of the drug, or administration of an antagonist.

physical therapist (PT, RPT) A member of the rehabilitation health care team who helps the patient achieve mobility and who teaches techniques for performing certain activities of daily living.

piggyback set See *secondary administration set.*

pilonidal cyst A lesion of the sacral area that often has a sinus track extending into deeper tissue structures.

pinna The external ear, which is composed of cartilage covered by skin.

pitting Indentation of the skin; often occurs with edema.

pituitary Cushing's disease Oversecretion of ACTH by the anterior pituitary gland, which causes hyperplasia of the adrenal cortex in both adrenal glands and an excess of most hormones secreted by the adrenal cortex.

placebo Substance or action that produces an effect regardless of its known intrinsic value or specific physical or chemical properties.

placebo effect A patient's favorable response to a placebo.

plantar fasciitis An inflammation of the plantar fascia, which is located in the area of the arch of the foot. It is often seen in athletes, especially runners.

plasma cell A short-lived B-lymphocyte that begins functioning immediately to produce antibodies against sensitizing antigens.

plasmapheresis The separation of plasma from whole blood, after which the blood cells are returned to the patient without the plasma to eliminate antibodies.

pleiotropic Having widespread or numerous effects.

plethoric A flushed appearance of the skin.

pleura The continuous smooth membrane composed of two surfaces that totally enclose the lungs.

pleural effusion Fluid in the pleural space.

pleuritic chest pain A stabbing pain on taking a deep breath.

pleurodesis An inflammation created by instilling a sclerosing agent through a chest tube into the pleural space, which causes the pleura to stick to the chest wall and prevent formation of effusion fluid.

plexus Cluster of nerves.

ploidy The number and appearance of chromosomes; used to describe cancer cells.

pluripotency The unlimited potential of early embryonic cells to mature into any body cell; also called "multipotency" or "totipotency."

pluripotent stem cell The precursor cell involved in the production of red blood cells.

pneumonectomy Removal of an entire lung, including all blood vessels.

pneumothorax Air in the pleural (chest) cavity.

podagra Inflammation of the metatarsophalangeal joint of the great toe.

point of maximal impulse (PMI) See *apical impulse.*

point mutation The substitution of one base for another.

polyarthralgia Aching around multiple joints.

polycystic kidney disease (PKD) An inherited disorder in which fluid-filled cysts develop in the kidneys.

polycythemia An excess of red blood cells.

polycythemia vera (PV) A disease that involves massive production of red blood cells, leukocytes, and platelets.

polydipsia Excessive intake of water.

polymedicine The use of many drugs to treat multiple health problems for older adults.

polymorphism A variation in form.

polymyalgia rheumatica (PMR) A clinical syndrome characterized by stiffness, weakness, aching of the proximal musculature (the shoulder and pelvic girdles), and systemic manifestations such as low-grade fever, arthralgias and stiffness, fatigue, and weight loss.

polymyositis A diffuse inflammatory disease of skeletal (striated) muscle that causes symmetric weakness and atrophy.

polyp An abnormal outgrowth from a mucous membrane.

polypectomy Surgical removal of a polyp, such as a nasal polyp.

polyphagia Excessive eating.

polypharmacy The use of many drugs to treat multiple health problems for older adults.

polyuria Frequent and excessive urination.

pores Openings or spaces.

portal hypertension An abnormal persistent increase in pressure within the portal vein; a major complication of cirrhosis.

portal hypertensive gastropathy A complication that can occur in patients with portal hypertension, with or without esophageal varices. Slow gastric mucosal bleeding may result in chronic slow blood loss, occult positive stools, and anemia.

portal-systemic encephalopathy (PSE) A clinical disorder seen in hepatic failure and cirrhosis; it is manifested by neurologic symptoms and is characterized by an altered level of consciousness, impaired thinking processes, and neuromuscular disturbances; also called "hepatic encephalopathy" and "hepatic coma."

positive deflection In electrocardiography, the flow of electrical current in the heart (cardiac axis) toward the positive pole.

positive inotropic agents Drugs that increase myocardial contractility and are prescribed to improve cardiac output.

positron emission tomography (PET) A diagnostic tool that provides information about the function of the brain, specifically glucose and oxygen metabolism and cerebral blood flow. The patient is injected with the molecule *deoxyglucose,* which is tagged to an isotope. The isotope emits activity in the form of positrons, which are scanned and converted into a color image by a computer.

postanesthesia care unit (PACU) Recovery room.

postcholecystectomy syndrome (PCS) The occurrence of the clinical manifestations of biliary tract disease following cholecystectomy; caused by residual or recurring calculi, inflammation, or stricture of the common bile duct.

post-concussion syndrome A group of clinical manifestations following a concussion that consist of personality changes, irritability, headaches, dizziness, restlessness, nervousness, insomnia, memory loss, and depression.

The prolonged pattern is classified as post-trauma syndrome.

posterior colporrhaphy The surgical procedure to repair a rectocele by strengthening pelvic supports and reducing the bulging.

posterior cord lesion A condition caused by cervical injuries; results from damage to the posterior gray and white matter of the spinal cord. Motor function remains intact, but the patient experiences a loss of vibratory sense, crude touch, and position sensation; this is the opposite of anterior cord syndrome.

posteroanterior Back to front; position for standard chest x-rays.

postherpetic neuralgia Pain that persists after herpes zoster lesions have resolved.

postictal stage Referring to the time immediately after a seizure.

postoperative After surgery.

postpericardiotomy syndrome Symptoms, including pericardial and pleural pain, pericarditis, friction rub, elevated temperature and white blood cell count, and dysrhythmias, that occur in patients after cardiac surgery; may occur days to weeks after surgery and seems to be associated with blood that remains in the pericardial sac.

postrenal failure Decrease in renal function related to an obstruction in the flow of urine. It can progress to acute renal failure.

postural (orthostatic) hypotension A decrease of more than 20 mm Hg of systolic pressure or more than 10 mm Hg of diastolic pressure, with a 10% to 20% increase in heart rate; patients may report dizziness or lightheadedness when they move from a lying to a sitting or standing position.

post-void residual (PVR) The amount of urine remaining in the bladder within 20 minutes after voiding.

potency The ability to have and sustain an erection.

PQRST A mnemonic (memory device) that may help in the current problem assessment of patients with gastrointestinal tract disorders. The letters represent the following areas <u>P</u>, precipitating or palliative (What brings it on? What makes it better or worse?); <u>Q</u>, quality or quantity (How does it look, feel, or sound?); <u>R</u>, region or radiation (Where is it? Does it spread anywhere?); <u>S</u>, severity scale (How bad is it [on a scale of 1 to 10]? Is it getting better, worse, or staying the same?); <u>T</u>, timing (Onset, duration, and frequency?).

PR interval In the electrocardiogram, the interval measured from the beginning of the P wave to the end of the PR segment; represents the time required for atrial depolarization as well as impulse delay in the atrioventricular node and travel time to the Purkinje fibers.

PR segment In the electrocardiogram, the isoelectric line from the end of the P wave to the beginning of the QRS complex, when the electrical impulse is traveling through the atrioventricular node, where it is delayed.

prandial insulin secretion The increased levels of insulin that are secreted after eating.

Within 10 minutes of eating, an early burst of insulin secretion occurs, which is followed by an increasing insulin release that lasts as long as hyperglycemia is present.

prealbumin (PAB) A protein secreted by the liver that binds thyroxine.

precipitation The formation of large, insoluble antigen-antibody complexes during the antibody-binding process.

prediabetes An impaired fasting glucose (IFG) or impaired glucose tolerance (IGT).

pre-emptive analgesia A technique to decrease postoperative pain and the requirements for analgesia, improve morbidity, and decrease hospital stay by administering local anesthetics, opioids, and nonsteroidal anti-inflammatory drugs in the preoperative, intraoperative, or postoperative period.

prehospital care provider Typically, any of the first caregivers encountered by the patient if he or she is transported to the emergency department by an ambulance or helicopter.

prehypertension A blood pressure category that includes blood pressure readings of 120 to 139 mm Hg systolic or 80 to 89 mm Hg diastolic. Prehypertensive patients are at a higher risk for the development of hypertension.

preictal phase Referring to events that a patient experiences before a seizure, such as the presence of an aura.

preinfarction angina Chest pain that occurs in the days or weeks before a myocardial infarction.

preload The degree of myocardial fiber stretch at the end of diastole and just before contraction; determined by the amount of blood returning to the heart from both the venous system (right heart) and the pulmonary system (left heart).

premature atrial complex (PAC) In the electrocardiogram, an early complex that occurs when atrial tissue becomes irritable. This ectopic focus fires an impulse before the next sinus impulse is due, thus usurping the sinus pacemaker. The premature P wave from the atrial focus is early and has a shape different from that of the P wave generated from the sinus node.

premature complex In the electrocardiogram, an early complex that occurs when a cardiac cell or cell group other than the sinoatrial node becomes irritable and fires an impulse before the next sinus impulse is generated. After the premature complex, there is a pause before the next normal complex, which creates an irregularity in the rhythm.

premature ventricular complex (PVC) In the electrocardiogram, an early ventricular complex is followed by a pause that results from increased irritability of ventricular cells. The QRS complexes may be unifocal or uniform (of the same shape), or multifocal or multiform (of different shapes).

premenstrual dysphoric disorder (PMDD) A more disabling and severe form of premenstrual syndrome.

premenstrual syndrome (PMS) A collection of symptoms that occur in the 2 weeks before menstruation and are followed by relief with menses and a symptom-free phase. Symptoms may include emotional, physical, and cognitive manifestations such as irritability, breast tenderness, and short-term memory problems.

preoperative Before surgery.

prepuce The foreskin of the penis.

prerenal failure Condition that causes inadequate kidney perfusion; can progress to acute renal failure.

presbycusis The loss of hearing, especially for high-pitched sounds; occurs as a result of aging.

presbyopia An age-related impairment of vision characterized by a loss of lens elasticity and the ability of the eye to accommodate. The near point of vision increases, and near objects must be placed farther from the eye to be seen clearly.

presence A type of communication that consists of listening and acknowledging the legitimacy of the patient's and/or family's pain.

pressure ulcer Tissue damage caused when the skin and underlying soft tissue are compressed between a bony prominence and an external surface for an extended period; commonly occurs over the sacrum, hips, and ankles.

pretibial Pertaining to the front of the leg below the knee.

pretibial myxedema Dry, waxy swelling of the front surfaces of the lower legs.

preventive therapy drugs For asthma, drugs that are used every day regardless of symptoms to change airway responsiveness and prevent asthma attacks from occurring.

priapism An abnormal, long-maintained erection without sexual desire, which causes the penis to become large, hard, and painful. It can occur from neural, vascular, or pharmacologic causes.

primary angle-closure glaucoma A form of glaucoma characterized by a narrowed angle and forward displacement of the iris so that movement of the iris against the cornea narrows or closes the chamber angle, obstructing the outflow of aqueous humor. It can have a sudden onset and is an emergency; also called "closed-angle glaucoma," "narrow-angle glaucoma," or "acute glaucoma."

primary arthroplasty A total joint arthroplasty procedure that has been performed for the first time.

primary epilepsy Epilepsy that is not associated with any identifiable brain lesion or other specific cause; however, genetic factors most likely play a role in its development.

primary gout The most common type of gout; results from one of several inborn errors of purine metabolism.

primary lesions In describing skin disease, the initial reaction to a problem that alters one of the structural components of the skin.

primary open-angle glaucoma (POAG) The most common form of primary glaucoma;

characterized by reduced outflow of aqueous humor through the chamber angle. Because the fluid cannot leave the eye at the same rate it is produced, intraocular pressure gradually increases.

primary prevention Strategies used to avoid or delay the actual occurrence of a specific disease.

primary progressive multiple sclerosis A type of multiple sclerosis (MS) that involves a steady and gradual neurologic deterioration without remission of symptoms. Patients with this type of MS are usually between 40 and 60 years of age at onset of the disease and experience progressive disability with no acute attacks.

primary survey Priorities of care addressed in order of immediate threats to life as part of the initial assessment in the emergency department. Survey is based on an "ABC" mnemonic with "D" and "E" added for trauma patients: airway/cervical spine (A), breathing (B), circulation (C), disability (D), and exposure (E).

primary tumor The original tumor, usually identified by the tissue from which it arose (parent tissue), such as in breast cancer or lung cancer.

progressive multifocal leukoencephalopathy (PML) Rare disease affecting the white matter of the brain caused by a virus that attacks the cells that make myelin; occurs most often in patients who are immunosuppressed.

progressive stage of shock The stage of shock that occurs with a sustained decrease in mean arterial pressure, when compensatory mechanisms are functioning but are no longer delivering sufficient oxygen, even to vital organs.

progressive-relapsing multiple sclerosis A type of multiple sclerosis (MS) that occurs in only 5% of patients with MS. It is characterized by the absence of periods of remission, and the patient's condition does not return to baseline. Progressive cumulative symptoms and deterioration occur over several years.

proinsulin A precursor of insulin that includes the alpha and beta chains of the insulin molecule.

projected pain Pain that occurs along a specific nerve or nerves.

proliferative diabetic retinopathy (PDR) A form of retinopathy associated with diabetes mellitus in which a network of fragile new blood vessels develops, leaking blood and protein into surrounding tissue. The new blood vessels are stimulated by retinal hypoxia that results from poor capillary perfusion of the retinal tissues. New blood vessels grow in the retina, onto the iris, and into the back of the vitreous. The vitreous contracts and pulls away from the retina, causing blood vessels to break and bleed into the vitreous.

promoter In oncology, a substance that promotes or enhances growth of the initiated cancer cell; may be a hormone, drug, or chemical.

pronator drift Occurs in a patient with muscle weakness due to cerebral or brainstem reasons. The arm on the weak side tends to fall, or "drift," with the palm pronating (turning inward) after the patient has closed his or her eyes and held the arms perpendicular to the body with the palms up for 15 to 30 seconds; part of the neurologic assessment.

prophylactic mastectomy Highly controversial practice of surgically removing the breast in order to reduce the risk of breast cancer.

prophylactic surgery Surgery done to remove "at-risk" tissue to prevent cancer development.

proportional pulse pressure A measurement of cardiac output that is calculated from blood pressure measurements, as follows: subtract diastolic from systolic blood pressure, and divide the result by systolic blood pressure. A proportional pulse pressure less than 25% indicates severely compromised cardiac output.

proprioception Position sense.

proprioceptive Awareness of body position.

prosopagnosia The inability to recognize oneself and other familiar faces; occurs in patients in the later stages of Alzheimer's disease.

prostaglandins Chemicals that are produced in the cells and cause inflammation and swelling.

prostate gland A large accessory gland of the male reproductive system. It secretes a milky alkaline fluid that adds bulk to the semen, enhances sperm motility, and neutralizes acidic vaginal secretions.

prostatectomy Surgical removal of the prostate.

prostate-specific antigen (PSA) A glycoprotein produced solely by the prostate. The normal blood level of PSA is less than 4 ng/mL; levels are higher in patients with increased prostatic tissue as a result of benign prostatic hyperplasia, prostatic infarction, prostatitis, and prostate cancer. Levels associated with prostate cancer are usually much higher than those occurring with other prostate tissue enlargement.

prostatitis Inflammation of the prostate.

prostatodynia Pain in the prostate with manifestations of prostatitis but no inflammation of the prostate and a negative urine culture.

prostration Extreme exhaustion.

protein-calorie malnutrition (PCM) A disorder of nutrition that may present in three forms: marasmus, kwashiorkor, and marasmic-kwashiorkor; also called "protein-energy malnutrition."

protein-energy malnutrition (PEM) See *protein-calorie malnutrition.*

protein synthesis The process by which genes are used to make the proteins needed for physiologic function.

proteinuria The presence of protein in the urine.

proteolysis The breakdown of proteins to provide fuel for energy when liver glucose is unavailable.

proton-pump inhibitor (PPI) A group of drugs that inhibit the proton pump in the stomach to decrease gastric acid production.

pruritus An unpleasant itching sensation.

pseudoaddiction An iatrogenic syndrome created by the undertreatment of pain and characterized by patient behaviors such as anger and escalating demands for more or different medications; results in suspicion and avoidance by staff. Pseudoaddiction can be distinguished from true addiction because the behaviors resolve when pain is effectively treated.

pseudogout A disease that mimics the clinical manifestations of gout; however, the crystals deposited in the joints are calcium pyrophosphate, not sodium urate.

psoriatic arthritis (PsA) A syndrome of inflammatory arthritis associated with psoriasis, the skin condition characterized by a scaly, itchy rash.

psychiatric crisis nurse team An emergency department specialty team whose nurses interact with patients and families in crisis.

psychotropic drugs Antipsychotic and neuroleptic drugs. These are appropriately given to patients with emotional and behavioral health problems (e.g., hallucinations and delusions) that accompany dementia but are sometimes inappropriately used for agitation, combativeness, or restlessness. They are considered chemical restraints because they decrease mobility and patients' ability to care for themselves.

ptosis Drooping of the eyelid.

pulmonary artery occlusive pressure (PAOP) See *pulmonary artery wedge pressure.*

pulmonary artery wedge pressure (PAWP) Measurement of pressure in the left atrium using a balloon-tipped catheter introduced into the pulmonary artery. When the balloon at the catheter tip is inflated, the catheter advances and wedges in a branch of the pulmonary artery. The tip of the catheter is able to sense pressures transmitted from the left atrium, which reflect left ventricular end-diastolic pressure; also called "pulmonary artery occlusive pressure."

pulmonary autograph The relocation of the patient's own pulmonary valve to the aortic position for aortic valve replacement (Ross procedure).

pulmonary embolism (PE) A collection of particulate matter, most commonly a blood clot, that enters venous circulation and lodges in the pulmonary vessels, obstructing pulmonary blood flow and leading to decreased systemic oxygenation, pulmonary tissue hypoxia, and potential death.

pulmonic valve The semilunar valve of the heart that separates the right ventricle from the pulmonary artery.

pulse deficit The difference between the apical and peripheral pulses.

pulse pressure The difference between the systolic and diastolic pressures.

pulse therapy Any therapy given at a high dose for a short duration.

pulsus alternans A type of pulse in which a weak pulse alternates with a strong pulse despite a regular heart rhythm; seen in patients with severely depressed cardiac function.

pump A pole-mounted or portable device that pumps medication or fluid under pressure during infusion therapy.

pump failure See *heart failure*.

punctum The opening through which tears drain; located at the nasal side of the eyelid edges.

pupil The opening through which light enters the eye; located in the center of the iris of the eye.

pure tones Tones generated by an audiometer to determine hearing acuity.

Purkinje cells In the cardiac conduction system, the cells that make up the bundle of His, bundle branches, and terminal Purkinje fibers. These cells are responsible for the rapid conduction of electrical impulses throughout the ventricles, leading to ventricular depolarization and subsequent ventricular muscle contraction.

purpura Purple patches on the skin that may be caused by blood disorders, vascular abnormalities, or trauma.

pyelolithotomy The surgical removal of a stone from the kidney.

pyelonephritis A bacterial infection in the kidney and renal pelvis (the upper urinary tract).

pyloromyotomy An incision through the serosa and muscularis of the pylorus, down to the mucosa; created to prevent gastric motility disturbances in patients who have undergone esophagectomy.

pyogenic liver abscess A liver abscess resulting from bacterial infection by *Escherichia coli* and *Klebsiella, Enterobacter, Salmonella, Staphylococcus,* and *Enterococcus* species. A pyogenic abscess is generally solitary and is confined to the right lobe, but occasionally abscesses are multiple.

pyramid The fan-shaped structures that constitute the medulla of the kidney. Each kidney has 12 to 18 pyramids.

pyuria The presence of white blood cells (pus) in the urine.

Q

QRS complex In the electrocardiogram, the portion consisting of the Q, R, and S waves, representing ventricular depolarization.

QRS duration In the electrocardiogram, the time required for depolarization of both ventricles; measured from the beginning of the QRS complex to the J point (the junction where the QRS complex ends and the ST segment begins).

QT interval In the electrocardiogram, the time from the beginning of the QRS complex to the end of the T wave. It represents the total time required for ventricular depolarization and repolarization.

quadriceps-setting exercise Postoperative leg exercise performed by straightening the legs and pushing the back of the knees into the bed.

quadrigeminy A type of premature complex consisting of a repetitive four-beat pattern; usually occurs as three sequential normal complexes followed by a premature complex and a pause, with the same pattern repeating itself in a four-beat pattern.

quadriparesis Weakness that involves all four extremities; seen with cervical spinal cord injury.

qualitative question A clinical question that focuses on the meanings and interpretations of human phenomena or experience of people and usually analyzes the content of what a person says during an interview or what a researcher observes.

quality improvement A competency that nurses can achieve by using data to monitor the outcomes of care processes and using improvement methods to design and test changes to continuously improve the quality and safety of health care systems.

quantitative question A clinical question that asks about the relationship between or among defined, measurable phenomena and includes statistical analysis of information that is collected to answer a question.

R

Rad Older acronym for "radiation absorbed dose."

radiating pain Diffuse, unlocalized pain around the site of origin.

radiation dose The amount of radiation absorbed by the tissue.

radiation exposure The amount of radiation delivered to a tissue during radiation therapy.

radiation proctitis Rectal mucosa inflammation that results from external beam radiation therapy.

radical cystectomy Removal of the bladder and surrounding tissue with urinary diversion.

radical vulvectomy The surgical removal of the entire vulva skin, labia, clitoris, subcutaneous tissues, and possibly inguinal and femoral node dissection.

radicular Referring to a nerve root.

radiculopathy Referring to radicular pain; spinal nerve root involvement.

radiofrequency ablation The use of heat to achieve permanent ablation of nerve roots.

radiofrequency catheter ablation An invasive procedure that uses radiofrequency waves to abolish an irritable focus that is causing a supraventricular or ventricular tachydysrhythmia.

Rapid Response Team Team of critical care experts that save lives and decrease the risk for harm by providing care to patients before a respiratory or cardiac arrest occurs. Also called "Medical Emergency Team."

rebound headache Headache that occurs as a side effect of a drug that has relieved an initial migraine headache; also called "medication overuse headache."

recall memory Recent memory, which can be tested during the history taking by asking about items such as the dates of clinic or physician appointments.

receptive aphasia A type of aphasia caused by injury to Wernicke's area in the temporo-parietal area of the brain and characterized by an inability to understand the spoken and written word; both reading and writing ability are equally affected. Although the patient can talk, the language is often meaningless and neologisms (made-up words) are common parts of speech. Also called "Wernicke's aphasia" or "sensory aphasia."

reconstructive plastic surgery Type of plastic surgery that corrects or improves functional defects that have occurred as a result of congenital problems, trauma and scarring, or other types of therapy.

reconstructive surgery Surgery done to increase function, enhance appearance, or both; also called "rehabilitative surgery."

recreational exercise A type of exercise that includes hobbies and sports, with no planned purpose other than relaxation.

recreational therapist A member of the health care team who works to help patients continue or develop hobbies or interests; also called "activity therapist."

rectocele A protrusion of the rectum through a weakened vaginal wall.

red reflex A reflection of light on the retina seen as a red glare during ophthalmoscopic examination. An absent red reflex may indicate a lens opacity or cloudiness of the vitreous.

redirection An intervention to help with communication problems in patients with dementia; consists of attracting the patient's attention before conversing, keeping the environment as free of distractions as possible, and speaking directly to the patient in a distinct manner using clear and short sentences.

reducible hernia A hernia that can be placed back into the abdominal cavity by gentle pressure.

reduction mammoplasty Breast reduction surgery in which the surgeon removes excess breast tissue and then repositions the nipple and remaining skin flaps to produce an optimal cosmetic effect.

Reed-Sternberg cell A specific cancer cell type, found in lymph nodes, that is a marker for Hodgkin's lymphoma.

re-epithelialization In partial-thickness (superficial) wounds involving damage to the epidermis and upper layers of the dermis, a form of healing by means of the production of new skin cells by undamaged epidermal cells in the basal layer of the dermis.

refeeding syndrome Life-threatening metabolic complication that can occur when nutrition is restarted for a patient who is in a starvation state.

referred pain Perceived pain in an area distant from the site of painful stimuli.

reflex arc A closed circuit of spinal and peripheral nerves that requires no control by the brain.

reflex bladder Incontinence characterized by sudden, gushing voids, usually without completely emptying the bladder; caused by neurologic problems affecting the upper motor neuron, such as with spinal cord injuries above the twelfth thoracic vertebra; also called "spastic bladder."

reflex sympathetic dystrophy (RSD) See *complex regional pain syndrome*.

reflux Reverse or backward flow.

reflux esophagitis Damage to the esophageal mucosa, often with erosion and ulceration, in patients with gastroesophageal reflux disease.

refract To cause to bend.

refraction The bending of light rays.

refractory stage The stage of shock that occurs when too much cell death and tissue damage result from too little oxygen reaching the tissues; the vital organs have overwhelming damage, and the body is unable to respond effectively to interventions. Formerly called the "irreversible stage."

regional anesthesia A type of local anesthesia that blocks multiple peripheral nerves in a specific body region.

regurgitation Flowing in the opposite direction from normal, as the occurrence of warm fluid traveling up the throat, unaccompanied by nausea, in the patient with gastroesophageal reflux disease.

rehabilitation The process of learning to live with chronic and disabling conditions by returning the patient to the fullest possible physical, mental, social, vocational, and economic capacity.

rehabilitation case manager Nurse or other health care professional who coordinates health care for patients undergoing rehabilitation in home or acute care settings.

rehabilitation nurse Nurse who coordinates the efforts of health care team members for patients undergoing rehabilitation in the inpatient setting; may be designated as the patient's case manager.

rehabilitative surgery See *reconstructive surgery*.

relapsing-remitting multiple sclerosis A type of multiple sclerosis that occurs in 85% of cases and is characterized by a mild or moderate course, depending on the degree of disability. Relapses develop over 1 to 2 weeks and resolve over 4 to 8 months, after which the patient returns to baseline.

religion The formal expression of spirituality.

relocation stress syndrome Physiologic or psychosocial distress following transfer from one environment to another, such as after admission to a hospital or nursing home; also called "relocation trauma."

reminiscence The process of randomly reflecting on memories of events in one's life.

remote memory Long-term memory of events; can be tested by asking patients about their birth date, schools attended, city of birth, or anything from the past that can be verified.

renal calculi Kidney stones.

renal colic Severe pain associated with distention or spasm of the ureter, such as with an obstruction or the passing of a stone; the pain radiates into the perineal area, groin, scrotum, or labia. Pain may be intermittent or continuous and may be accompanied by pallor, diaphoresis, and hypotension.

renal columns Cortical tissue that dips into the interior of the kidney and separates the pyramids in the medulla; also called "columns of Bertin."

renal cortex The outermost layer of functional kidney tissue lying beneath the renal capsule.

renal osteodystrophy The problems in bone metabolism and structure caused by renal failure–induced hypocalcemia and hyperphosphatemia.

renal pelvis The expansion from the upper end of the ureter into which the calices of the kidney open.

renal threshold The limit to the amount of glucose that the kidney can reabsorb as glucose is filtered from the blood; also called the "transport maximum."

renin A hormone that is produced in the juxtaglomerular complex of the kidney and helps regulate blood flow, glomerular filtration rate, and blood pressure. Renin is secreted when sensing cells (macula densa) in the distal convoluted tubule sense changes in blood volume and pressure.

repetitive stress injury (RSI) Injury caused by repeated movements of the same part of the body (e.g., carpal tunnel syndrome).

replication The reproduction of DNA that occurs each time a cell divides.

repolarization A return to baseline after depolarization.

rescue drugs For asthma, drugs that are used to actually stop an asthma attack once it has started.

reservoir In health care, a source of infectious agents. Animate reservoirs include people, animals, and insects. Inanimate reservoirs include environmental sources and medical equipment. Community reservoirs include sewage, contaminated water, and improperly handled foods.

resistin A hormone produced by fat cells that creates resistance to insulin activity.

resorption In referring to bone, the loss of bone minerals and density; the release of free calcium from bone storage sites directly into the extracellular fluid.

restorative aid A member of the health care team, often with the nursing department, who assists the therapists, especially in the long-term care setting.

restraint Any device (physical restraint) or drug (chemical restraint) that prevents the patient from moving freely.

restrictive cardiomyopathy A form of cardiomyopathy that restricts the filling of the ventricles; a type of lung disease that prevents good expansion and recoil of the gas exchange unit.

restrictive disorders Disorders that prevent good expansion and recoil of the gas exchange unit.

restrictive lung disorder Any lung disorder that prevents good expansion and recoil of the gas exchange unit.

resurfacing Regrowth of new skin cells across the open area of a wound as it heals.

resuscitation phase The first phase of a burn injury, beginning at the onset of injury and continuing to about 48 hours.

rete pegs The fingers of epidermal tissue that project into the dermis.

reticular activating system (RAS) Special cells throughout the brainstem that constitute the system that controls awareness and alertness.

retina The innermost layer of the eye, made up of sensory receptors that transmit impulses to the optic nerve. It contains blood vessels and two types of photoreceptors called "rods" and "cones." Rods work at low light levels and provide peripheral vision; cones are active at bright light levels and provide color and central vision.

retinal detachment Separation of the retina from the epithelium.

retinal hole A break in the retina; can be caused by trauma or can occur with aging.

retinal tear Jagged and irregularly shaped break in the retina resulting from traction on the retina.

retinitis Inflammation of the retina.

retinopathy Inflammation of the retina; also used as a general term for vision problems.

retrograde Going against the normal direction of flow.

retrograde ejaculation Condition in which semen flows backwards into the bladder so that only a small amount is ejaculated from the penis.

retroviruses The family of viruses that includes the human immune deficiency virus.

reversible ischemic neurologic deficit (RIND) A type of transient focal neurologic dysfunction resulting from a brief interruption in cerebral blood flow; symptoms last longer than 24 hours but less than a week.

revision arthroplasty Surgical replacement of a prosthesis that has loosened and is causing pain.

rhabdomyolysis The breakdown or disintegration of muscle tissue; associated with excretion of myoglobin in the urine.

rheumatic carditis Inflammatory lesions in the heart due to a sensitivity response that develops after an upper respiratory tract infection with group A beta-hemolytic streptococci, which occurs in about 40% of patients with rheumatic fever. Inflammation results in impaired contractile function of the myocardium, thickening of the pericardium, and valvular damage.

rheumatic disease Any disease or condition involving the musculoskeletal system.

rheumatoid arthritis (RA) A chronic, progressive, systemic, inflammatory autoimmune disease process that primarily affects the synovial joints; one of the most common connective tissue diseases and the most destructive to the joints.

rhinitis   An inflammation of the nasal mucosa.

rhinitis medicamentosa   Nasal congestion from overuse of nose drops or sprays.

rhinoplasty   A surgical reconstruction of the nose done for cosmetic purposes and improvement of airflow.

rhinorrhea   Watery drainage from the nose; a "runny" nose.

rhizotomy   Surgical technique in which sensory nerve roots are destroyed where they enter the spinal cord; used to interrupt the transmission of pain.

rhytidectomy   Plastic surgery to eliminate wrinkles from the facial skin; commonly known as a "face lift."

rickets   Vitamin D deficiency in children.

right-sided heart (ventricular) failure   The inability of the right ventricle to empty completely, resulting in increased volume and pressure in the systemic veins and systemic venous congestion with peripheral edema.

rigidity   Abnormal resistance to passive movement of the extremities, an early sign of Parkinson disease.

rigors   Severe chills.

Romberg sign   Swaying or falling when the patient is standing with arms at the sides, feet and knees close together, and eyes closed; a test of equilibrium in neurologic assessment.

rotation   A mechanism of injury in which the head is turned excessively beyond the normal range.

rubor   Dusky red discoloration of the skin.

rugae   Folds, as of a mucous membrane.

S

S phase   The phase of cell division in which the cell doubles its deoxyribonucleic acid (DNA) content by separating the double strands of DNA and building a new strand complementary to the original strand (DNA synthesis).

S₃ gallop   The third heart sound; an early diastolic filling sound that indicates an increase in left ventricular pressure and may be heard on auscultation in patients with heart failure.

salpingitis   Infection of the fallopian tube.

sanguineous   Having a bloody appearance.

sarcoidosis   A granulomatous disorder of unknown cause that can affect any organ but most often involves the lung.

SBAR   Acronym for a formal method of communication between two or more members of the health care team. It is used most often when there is an unmet patient need or problem but can also be used to communicate continuing care issues when a patient is discharged from one agency to another. It consists of four steps Situation, Background, Assessment, Recommendation.

scabies   A contagious skin disease caused by mite infestations.

sclera   The external white layer of the eye.

scleroderma   See *systemic sclerosis.*

sclerosing agent   An irritant that causes inflammation; often used to relieve pleural effusion.

sclerotherapy   The injection of a sclerosing agent via a catheter, usually in an endoscopic procedure, to stop variceal bleeding.

sclerotic   Hard, or hardening.

scoliosis   An abnormal lateral curve in the spine, which normally should be a straight vertical line.

scotoma   Blind spot in the visual field.

scrotum   A thin-walled, fibromuscular pouch that lies behind the penis and is suspended below the pubic bone. This pouch protects the testes, epididymis, and vas deferens in a space that is slightly cooler than inside the abdominal cavity.

seborrhea   Excessive secretion of sebum, resulting in greasy, itchy scaling.

sebum   A mildly bacteriostatic, fat-containing substance produced by the sebaceous glands. Sebum lubricates the skin and reduces water loss from the skin surface.

second intention healing   Healing of deep tissue injuries or wounds with tissue loss in which a cavity-like defect requires gradual filling of the dead space with connective tissue, which prolongs the repair process.

secondary administration set   A short conduit that is attached to the primary administration set at a Y-injection site and is used to deliver intermittent medications; also called a "piggyback set."

secondary gout   Gout involving hyperuricemia.

secondary hypertension   Elevated blood pressure that is related to a specific disease (e.g., kidney disease) or medication (e.g., estrogen).

secondary lesion   Describing skin disease in terms of changes in the appearance of the primary lesion. These changes occur with progression of an underlying disease or in response to a topical or systemic therapeutic intervention.

secondary prevention   Early detection of a disease or condition, sometimes before signs and symptoms are evident, to prevent or limit permanent disability or death.

secondary progressive multiple sclerosis   A type of multiple sclerosis that begins with a relapsing-remitting course and later becomes steadily progressive. Attacks and partial recoveries may continue to occur.

secondary seizure   Non-epileptic seizure that results from an underlying brain lesion, most commonly a tumor or trauma.

secondary survey   In the emergency department, a more comprehensive head-to-toe assessment performed to identify other injuries or medical issues that need to be managed or that might impact the course of treatment.

secondary tumor   Additional tumor that is established when cancer cells move from the primary location to another area in the body; also called "metastatic tumor."

second-look surgery   Surgery done to assess the disease status in patients who have been

treated and have no symptoms of remaining cancer tumor.

segmentectomy   A lung resection (segmental resection) that includes the bronchus, pulmonary artery and vein, and tissue of the involved lung segment or segments, which are divisions of lobes.

seizure   An abnormal, sudden, excessive, uncontrolled electrical discharge of neurons within the brain that may result in an alteration in consciousness, motor or sensory ability, and/or behavior. A single seizure may occur for no known reason; however, seizures may be due to a pathologic condition of the brain, such as a tumor.

self-determination   An individual sense of autonomy; capable of making informed decisions about care. Also called "self-management."

self-management   See *self-determination.*

self-tolerance   In immunology, the ability to recognize self cells versus non-self cells, which is necessary to prevent healthy body cells from being destroyed along with invading cells.

semicircular canals   Within the inner ear, tubes made of cartilage that contain fluid and hair cells and are connected to the sensory nerve fibers of the vestibular portion of the eighth cranial nerve. The fluid and hair cells within the canals help maintain the sense of balance.

sensitivity   The likelihood that infecting bacterial organisms will be killed or stopped by a particular antibiotic drug. Sensitivity is determined by testing different antibiotics against the organisms. Organisms are "sensitive" if the antibiotic is effective in stopping their growth; organisms are "resistant" if the antibiotic is not effective.

sensorineural hearing loss   Hearing loss that results from a defect in the cochlea, the eighth cranial nerve, or the brain itself. Exposure to loud noises and music may cause this type of hearing loss as a result of damage to the cochlear hair cells.

sensory   Facilitating sensation.

sensory aphasia   See *receptive aphasia.*

sepsis   Systemic infection.

septic shock   The type of shock that occurs when large amounts of toxins and endotoxins produced by bacteria are released into the blood, causing a whole-body inflammatory reaction.

septicemia   Systemic disease associated with sepsis; the presence of pathogens in the blood.

sequestrum   A piece of necrotic bone that has separated from surrounding bone tissue; a common complication of osteomyelitis.

serologic testing   Laboratory testing that is performed to identify pathogens by detecting antibodies to the organism.

serositis   Inflammation of a serous membrane, such as the pleura or peritoneum.

serous   Having a serum-like appearance, or yellow color.

serum sickness   A type III hypersensitivity reaction that develops first as a skin rash and occurs within 3 to 21 days of the administration of antivenin (Crotalidae) polyvalent. This allergic response is often accompanied by other manifestations such as fever, arthralgias (joint pains), and pruritus (itching).

severe acute respiratory syndrome (SARS) An easily spread respiratory infection first identified in China in November 2002. At first appearing as an atypical pneumonia, it is caused by a new, more virulent form of coronavirus, and there is no known effective treatment.

severe sepsis The progression of sepsis with an amplified inflammatory response.

sex chromosomes The pair of chromosomes containing the genes for sexual differentiation in humans. In males, the sex chromosomes are an X and a Y; in females, the sex chromosomes are two Xs.

sexually transmitted diseases (STDs) Any of a group of diseases caused by infectious organisms that have been passed from one person to another through intimate contact. Some organisms that cause these diseases are transmitted only through sexual contact. Other organisms are transmitted by parenteral exposure to infected blood, fecal-oral transmission, intrauterine transmission to the fetus, and perinatal transmission from mother to neonate.

SHARE Acronym standing for *S*tandardize critical content, *H*ardwire within your system, *A*llow opportunity to ask questions, *R*einforce quality and measurement, *E*ducate and coach.

shift to the left An increased number of immature neutrophils found on a differential count in patients with infections; can be characterized by changes in percentages of different types of leukocytes.

shock The whole-body response to poor tissue oxygenation. Any problem that impairs oxygen delivery to tissues and organs can start the syndrome of shock and lead to a life-threatening emergency.

short peripheral catheter A catheter that consists of a plastic cannula built around a sharp stylet for venipuncture, which extends slightly beyond the cannula and is advanced into the vein.

sialagogue An agent that stimulates the flow of saliva.

simple fracture See *closed fracture.*

simple partial seizure A type of partial seizure in which the patient remains conscious, often reporting an aura (e.g., perception of an offensive smell) before the seizure occurs. Characterized by unilateral movement of an extremity, unusual sensations, and autonomic or psychic symptoms. Autonomic changes include a change in heart rate, skin flushing, and epigastric discomfort.

single-photon emission computed tomography (SPECT) A diagnostic tool using a radiopharmaceutical (agent that enables radioisotopes to cross the blood-brain barrier) that is administered by IV injection, after which the patient is scanned.

sinoatrial (SA) node In the cardiac conduction system, the primary pacemaker of the heart; located close to the epicardial surface of the right atrium near its junction with the superior vena cava. It can spontaneously and rhythmically generate electrical impulses at a rate of 60 to 100 beats/min; also called the "sinus node."

sinus arrhythmia A variant of normal sinus rhythm that results from changes in intrathoracic pressure during breathing; heart rate increases slightly during inspiration and decreases slightly during exhalation. Atrial and ventricular rates are between 60 and 100 beats/min, and atrial and ventricular rhythms are irregular.

sinus bradycardia A cardiac dysrhythmia caused by a decreased rate of sinus node discharge, with a heart rate that is less than 60 beats/min.

sinusitis An inflammation of the mucous membranes of the sinuses.

Sjögren's syndrome In patients with advanced rheumatoid arthritis, the triad of dry eyes, dry mouth, and dry vagina caused by the obstruction of secretory ducts and glands by inflammatory cells and immune complexes.

skin fold measurement Measurement that estimates body fat.

skinning vulvectomy The surgical removal of superficial vulvar skin (without removal of the clitoris) and the replacement of removed skin with split-thickness grafts.

sleep apnea A breathing disruption during sleep that lasts at least 10 seconds and occurs a minimum of 5 times in an hour.

sliding board Alternative transfer technique for a patient who cannot bear weight but who has balance skills.

smart pump An infusion pump with dosage calculation software.

smegma A white, cheesy secretion from the sebaceous glands in the glans; may accumulate under the foreskin of the penis. This secretion is not present in the circumcised male.

social worker Member of the health care team who helps patients identify support services and resources and who coordinates transfers to or discharges from the rehabilitation setting.

sodium (Na⁺) A mineral that is the major cation in the extracellular fluid and maintains extracellular fluid (ECF) osmolarity.

solubility The degree to which a solute dissolves in water.

solute A particle dissolved or suspended in the water portion (solvent) of body fluids; a solution consists of a solute and a solvent.

solvent The water portion of fluids.

Somogyi's phenomenon In the patient with diabetes, morning hyperglycemia from the effective counterregulatory response to nighttime hypoglycemia. Treat by ensuring adequate dietary intake at bedtime and by evaluating the insulin dose and exercise programs to prevent conditions that lead to hypoglycemia.

spastic bladder See *reflex bladder.*

spastic paralysis Paralysis of a part of the body that is characterized by spasticity of muscles due to hypertonia; may be seen in the patient who has experienced a brain attack.

specialized nutritional support (SNS) Total nutritional intake orally or intravenously with commercially prepared products (either total enteral nutrition or total parenteral nutrition).

speech-language pathologist (SLP) A member of the rehabilitation health care team who evaluates and retrains patients with speech, language, or swallowing problems.

spermatogenesis Normal sperm production and maturation.

sphincter of Oddi The sheath of muscle fibers surrounding the papillary opening of the duodenum.

sphincterotomy A procedure for opening a sphincter.

spica cast A type of cast that encases a portion of the trunk and one or two extremities; contrasted with a body cast, which encircles the trunk of the body.

spider angiomas Vascular lesions with a red center and radiating branches; also called "telangiectasias," "spider nevi," or "vascular spiders."

spinal fusion (arthrodesis) A surgical procedure to stabilize the spine after repeated laminectomies have been unsuccessful. Chips of bone are removed (typically from the iliac crest) or are obtained from donor bone; the chips are grafted between the vertebrae for support and to strengthen the back.

spinal shock See *spinal shock syndrome.*

spinal shock syndrome Loss of reflex activity below the level of a spinal lesion; occurs immediately after injury as a result of disruption in the communication pathways between the upper motor neurons and the lower motor neurons; also called "spinal shock."

spinal stenosis Narrowing of the spinal canal; typically seen in people older than 60 years.

spirituality The connection to self, others, the environment, and a "higher power."

spiritual counselor Counselor who specializes in spiritual assessments and care, usually a member of the clergy.

splenectomy Surgical removal of the spleen.

splenomegaly Enlargement of the spleen.

splint Any object or device that extends to the joints above and below a fracture to immobilize it.

splinter hemorrhage Black longitudinal line or small red streak on the distal third of the nail bed; seen in patients with infective endocarditis.

spondee Two-syllable words in which there is generally equal stress on each syllable, such as *airplane, railroad,* and *cowboy;* used in testing speech reception threshold.

spondylolisthesis Condition in which one vertebra slips forward on the one below it, often as a result of spondylolysis. This problem causes pressure on the nerve roots, leading to pain in the lower back and into the buttocks.

spondylolysis A defect in one of the vertebrae; usually found in the lumbar spine.

spontaneous bacterial peritonitis (SBP) Bacterial infection of the abdominal peritoneum caused by ascites; often seen in patients with cirrhosis of the liver.

spore An encapsulated, inactive organism.

sprain Excessive stretching of a ligament.

ST segment In the electrocardiogram, the line (normally isoelectric) representing early ventricular repolarization. It occurs from the J point to the beginning of the T wave.

staging System of classifying clinical aspects of a cancer tumor.

Standard Precautions Infection control guidelines from the Centers for Disease Control and Prevention stating that all body excretions, secretions, and moist membranes and tissues are potentially infectious; combines protective measures from Universal Precautions and Body Substance Isolation.

stapes One of the three bony ossicles of the ear; also called the "stirrup."

stasis dermatitis In patients with venous insufficiency, discoloration of the skin along the ankles, which extends up to the calf.

stasis ulcer In patients with long-term venous insufficiency, ulcer formed as a result of edema or minor injury to the limb; typically occurs over the malleolus.

status epilepticus Prolonged seizures lasting more than 5 minutes or repeated seizures over the course of 30 minutes; a potential complication of all types of seizures.

steatorrhea An excessive amount of fat in the stool.

stem cell An immature, undifferentiated cell produced by the bone marrow.

stent A small tube that is placed in a tubular structure to dilate it; a wirelike device that may be used along with percutaneous transluminal angioplasty to help keep the vessel open.

stereotactic pallidotomy A surgical treatment for the patient with Parkinson disease when drugs are ineffective in symptom management. An electrode is used to create a lesion in a targeted area within the pallidum, with the goal of reducing tremor and rigidity.

stereotyping Assuming that all people in a particular culture have the group's values and beliefs or practice the group's customs.

sterilization A method of infection control in which all living organisms and bacterial spores are destroyed; used on items that invade human tissue where bacteria are not commonly found.

stimulant Any of a group of drugs that excite the cerebral cortex of the brain, producing a variety of behavioral responses and causing an increase in body activity, such as caffeine, nicotine, amphetamines, and methamphetamines.

stimulation test A type of test for pituitary function that involves injecting agents known to stimulate secretion of specific pituitary hormones and then measuring the response.

stoma The surgical creation of an opening; usually refers to an opening in the abdominal wall.

stomatitis Inflammation of the oral mucosa; characterized by painful single or multiple ulcerations that impair the protective lining of the mouth. The ulcerations are commonly referred to as "canker sores."

strain Excessive stretching of a muscle or tendon when it is weak or unstable; sometimes referred to as "muscle pulls."

strangulated hernia A tightly constricted hernia that compromises the blood supply to the herniated segment of the bowel as a result of pressure from the hernial ring (the band of muscle around the hernia); leads to ischemia and obstruction of the bowel loop, with necrosis of the bowel and possibly bowel perforation.

strangulated obstruction Intestinal obstruction with compromised blood flow.

stratum corneum The outermost layer of the skin.

stress test See *exercise electrocardiography.*

stress ulcers Multiple shallow erosions of the proximal stomach and occasionally the duodenum.

stress urinary incontinence Loss of urine during activities that increase intra-abdominal pressure, such as laughing, coughing, sneezing, or lifting heavy objects.

striae Reddish purple streaks on the skin, also called "stretch marks."

stricture Narrowing.

stridor A high-pitched crowing sound caused by laryngospasm or edema above or below the glottis; heard during respiration.

stroke Former name for "brain attack"; see *brain attack.*

stroke volume The amount of blood ejected by the left ventricle during each heartbeat.

stuporous A state of being arousable only with vigorous or painful stimulation.

subarachnoid See *subarachnoid space.*

subarachnoid screw or bolt A hollow device placed into the subarachnoid space for direct measurement of intracranial pressure. It does not allow drainage of cerebrospinal fluid to treat increased pressure, but it is less invasive, which lowers the risk of infection. Compare with "intraventricular catheter."

subarachnoid space Term for the space between the arachnoid mater and pia mater of the spinal cord; also called "subarachnoid."

subcutaneous emphysema The presence of bubbles under the skin because of air trapping; an uncommon late complication of fracture.

subcutaneous nodule Characteristic round, movable, nontender swelling under the skin of the arm or fingers in patients with severe rheumatoid arthritis.

subcutaneous therapy Infusion therapy that is delivered under the skin when patients cannot tolerate oral medications, when intramuscular injections are too painful, or when vascular access is not available.

subdural hematoma (SDH) The collection of clotted blood that typically results from venous bleeding into the space beneath the dura and above the arachnoid.

subdural hemorrhage Venous bleeding into the space beneath the dura and above the arachnoid.

subdural space Term for the space between the dura mater and the middle layer (arachnoid).

subendocardial myocardial infarction An infarction that involves only the subendocardium, the inner layer of the cardiac muscle.

subluxation Partial joint dislocation.

submucous resection (SMR) Surgical procedure to straighten a deviated septum when chronic symptoms or discomfort occur; also called "nasoseptoplasty."

substance abuse The overindulgence of a chemical substance and the resulting dependence that interferes with life's activities.

substance misuse The taking of chemicals for reasons other than their intended action.

substance use The taking of chemicals for pleasure without dependence.

substernally Located below the ribs.

subtotal thyroidectomy The surgical removal of part of the thyroid tissue.

sundowning In patients with Alzheimer's disease, increased confusion at night or when excessively fatigued.

superinfection Reinfection or a second infection of the same type.

supervision Guidance or direction, evaluation, and follow-up by the nurse to ensure that the task or activity is performed appropriately.

suppressed gene A particular gene that has been "turned off."

suprapatellar area The area directly above the knee.

supratentorial Located within the cerebral hemispheres, in the area above the tentorium of the cerebellum; the tentlike fold of dura that surrounds the cerebellar hemisphere and supports the occipital lobe.

supraventricular tachycardia (SVT) A form of tachycardia that involves the rapid stimulation of atrial tissue at a rate of 100 to 280 beats/min. It is most often due to a re-entry mechanism in which one impulse circulates repeatedly throughout the atrial pathway, re-stimulating the atrial tissue at a rapid rate.

surfactant A fatty protein secreted by type II pneumocytes to reduce surface tension in the alveoli.

surgical débridement Method of débriding a wound by removing thick, adherent wound crust using a scalpel or scissors.

surveillance Term used to describe the tracking of infections by health care agencies.

susceptibility The risk of the host to infection; may be increased by the breakdown of host defenses against pathogens.

swimmer's ear See *external otitis.*

sympathectomy Surgical cutting of the sympathetic nerve branches via endoscopy through a small axillary incision.

sympathetic tone A state of partial blood vessel constriction caused when nerves from the sympathetic division of the autonomic nervous system continuously stimulate vascular smooth muscle.

synapse The area through which impulses are transmitted to their eventual destination.

synchronous (demand) pacing mode The mode of temporary cardiac pacing in which the pacemaker's sensitivity is set to sense the patient's own beats. When the patient's intrinsic rate is above the rate set on the pulse generator, the pacemaker is inhibited from firing. When the patient's rate is below that set on the generator, the pacemaker fires electrical impulses to stimulate depolarization.

syncope Transient loss of consciousness (blackouts), most commonly caused by decreased perfusion to the brain.

syndrome of inappropriate antidiuretic hormone (SIADH) Persistent hyponatremia, hypovolemia, and inappropriately elevated urine osmolality that occurs when vasopressin (antidiuretic hormone) is secreted even when plasma osmolarity is low or normal.

syndrome X See *metabolic syndrome.*

syngeneic transplant Bone marrow transplant in which stem cells are taken from the patient's own identical sibling.

synovectomy The surgical removal of synovium.

synovial joint Type of joint lined with synovium, a membrane that secretes synovial fluid for lubrication and shock absorption.

synovitis Inflammation of synovial membrane.

synthesis The process of building up.

syphilis A complex sexually transmitted disease that can become systemic and cause serious complications and even death. It is caused by the spirochete *Treponema pallidum,* which is found in the mouth, intestinal tract, and genital areas of people and animals. The infection is usually transmitted by sexual contact, but transmission can occur through close body contact and kissing.

syringe pump Pump for infusion therapy that uses a battery-powered piston to push the plunger continuously at a selected mL/hr rate; limited to small-volume continuous or intermittent infusions.

systemic Affecting the body system as a whole.

systemic lupus erythematosus (SLE) A chronic, progressive, inflammatory connective tissue disorder that can cause major body organs and systems to fail; characterized by spontaneous remissions and exacerbations.

systemic sclerosis (SSc) A chronic connective tissue disease characterized by inflammation, fibrosis, and sclerosis of the skin and vital organs; also called "scleroderma" and formerly called "progressive systemic sclerosis."

systemic vascular resistance The resistance to the flow of blood through the body's blood vessels; it increases when vessels constrict and decreases when vessels dilate.

systole The phase of the cardiac cycle that consists of the contraction and emptying of the atria and ventricles.

systolic blood pressure The amount of pressure/force generated by the left ventricle to distribute blood into the aorta with each contraction of the heart.

systolic heart failure (systolic ventricular dysfunction) Heart failure that results when the heart is unable to contract forcefully enough during systole to eject adequate amounts of blood into the circulation.

T

T wave In the electrocardiogram, the deflection that follows the ST segment and represents ventricular repolarization.

tachycardia An excessively fast heart rate; characterized as a pulse rate greater than 100 beats/min.

tachydysrhythmia An abnormal heart rhythm with a rate greater than 100 beats/min.

tachypnea An increased rate of breathing.

tactile (vocal) fremitus A vibration of the chest wall produced when the patient speaks; can be palpated on the chest wall.

tai chi A holistic movement therapy derived from a traditional Chinese martial art; has been adapted as a mind-body exercise that integrates body movements, mental concentration, muscle relaxation, and breathing to promote the flow of *qi,* or energy, in the body.

target tissues The tissues that respond specifically to a given hormone.

taut Tightly stretched.

telemetry In electrocardiography (ECG), the use of a battery-powered transmitter system for monitoring an ambulatory patient; allows freedom of movement within a certain radius without losing transmission of the ECG.

telesurgery The use of robotics to perform surgical procedures over long distances.

telomeres The "tips" of the chromosomes.

temporal field blindness A decrease in lateral peripheral vision.

temporary pacing A nonsurgical intervention for cardiac dysrhythmia that provides a timed electrical stimulus to the heart when either the impulse initiation or the intrinsic conduction system of the heart is defective.

tendon Any one of many bands of tough, fibrous tissue that attach muscles to bones.

tendon transplant Removal of a tendon from one part of the body and transplantation into the affected area to replace a ruptured tendon that cannot be repaired surgically.

tenesmus Straining, especially painful straining to defecate.

tension headache A type of headache characterized by neck and shoulder muscle tenderness and bilateral pain at the base of the skull and in the forehead; usually treated with non-opioid analgesics such as acetaminophen, aspirin, and nonsteroidal anti-inflammatory drugs.

teratogenic Tending to produce birth defects.

tetany Continuous contractions of muscle groups; hyperexcitability of nerves and muscles.

tetraplegia Another term for quadriplegia (paralysis that involves all four extremities).

thalamotomy An alternative to stereotactic pallidotomy as a surgical treatment for the patient with Parkinson disease; uses thermocoagulation of brain cells to reduce tremor. Usually only unilateral surgery is performed to benefit the side of the body most affected by the disease.

thalamus A structure within the brain; functions as the "central switchboard" for the central nervous system.

thallium scan A test that is similar to the bone scan but uses the radioisotope *thallium* and is more sensitive in diagnosing the extent of disease in patients with osteosarcoma.

The Joint Commission An organization that offers peer evaluation for accreditation every 3 years for all types of health care agencies that meet their standards. Formerly known as the "Joint Commission for Accreditation of Healthcare Organizations (JCAHO)."

therapeutic exercise A type of exercise that includes carefully planned activities designed to improve muscle strength, muscle tone, and joint range of motion and to reduce pain and improve the patient's psychological health.

thermotherapy Technique for treating benign prostatic hyperplasia that uses a variety of heat methods to destroy excess prostate tissue.

third intention healing Delayed primary closure of a wound with a high risk for infection. The wound is intentionally left open for several days until inflammation has subsided and is then closed by first intention.

thoracentesis The aspiration of pleural fluid or air from the pleural space.

threshold In evaluating hearing, the lowest level of intensity at which pure tones and speech are heard by a patient; in general, the lowest level at which a stimulus is perceived.

thrombectomy Removal of a clot (thrombus) from a blood vessel.

thrombocytopenia A reduction in the number of blood platelets below the level needed for normal coagulation, resulting in an increased tendency to bleed.

thrombophlebitis The presence of a thrombus associated with inflammation; usually occurs in the deep veins of the lower extremities.

thrombosis The formation of a blood clot (thrombus) within a blood vessel.

thrombus A blood clot believed to result from an endothelial injury, venous stasis, or hypercoagulability.

thymectomy Removal of the thymus gland.

thymoma An encapsulated tumor of the thymus gland.

thyrocalcitonin (TCT) A hormone produced and secreted by the parafollicular cells of the thyroid gland to help regulate serum calcium levels; secreted in response to excess plasma calcium.

thyroid storm (thyroid crisis) A life-threatening event that occurs in patients with uncontrolled hyperthyroidism and is usually caused by Graves' disease. Key manifestations include fever, tachycardia, and systolic hypertension.

thyrotoxicosis The condition caused by excessive amounts of thyroid hormones.

thyroxine (T_4) A hormone that is produced by the follicular cells of the thyroid gland and increases metabolism.

Tinel's sign Test that confirms a diagnosis of carpal tunnel syndrome; a positive test causes palmar paresthesias when the area of the median nerve is tapped lightly.

tinnitus A continuous ringing or noise perception in the ears.

titration Adjustment of IV fluid rate on the basis of the patient's urine output plus serum electrolyte values.

TNM (tumor, node, metastasis) System developed by the American Joint Committee on Cancer to describe the anatomic extent of cancers.

toe brachial pressure index (TBPI) Toe systolic pressure divided by brachial (arm) systolic pressure; may be performed instead of or in addition to ankle-brachial index to determine arterial perfusion in the feet and toes.

tolerance A state of adaptation in which exposure to a drug induces changes that result in a decrease in one or more of the drug's effects over time.

tomography An imaging technique that produces planes, or slices, for focus and blurs the images of other structures; different from standard x-rays, which superimpose one structure on another.

tonic Pertaining to a state of stiffening or rigidity of the muscles, particularly of the arms and legs, and immediate loss of consciousness.

tonic seizure A type of generalized seizure characterized by an abrupt increase in muscle tone, loss of consciousness, and loss of autonomic signs; lasts from 30 seconds to several minutes.

tonic-clonic seizure A type of generalized seizure consisting of a tonic phase (characterized by stiffening or rigidity of the muscles and immediate loss of consciousness); this is followed by clonic or rhythmic jerking of the extremities and lasts 2 to 5 minutes. The patient may bite his or her tongue and may become incontinent of urine or feces. Fatigue, confusion, and lethargy may last up to an hour after the seizure.

tonsillitis An inflammation and infection of the tonsils and lymphatic tissues located on each side of the throat.

tophi A collection of uric acid crystals that form hard, irregular, painless nodules on the ears, arms, and fingers of patients with gout.

torsades de pointes A type of ventricular tachycardia that is related to a prolonged QT interval.

total body surface area (TBSA) The total amount of skin surface for one person.

total hysterectomy Removal of the uterus and cervix; the procedure may be vaginal or abdominal.

total joint arthroplasty (TJA) Surgical creation of a joint, or total joint replacement; commonly performed in patients with osteoarthritis. Also called "total joint replacement (TJR)."

total joint replacement (TJR) See *total joint arthroplasty*.

total parenteral nutrition (TPN) Provision of intensive nutritional support for an extended time; delivered to the patient through access to central veins, usually the subclavian or internal jugular veins.

total thyroidectomy The surgical removal of all of the thyroid tissue.

touch discrimination Part of the neurologic examination. The patient closes his or her eyes while the practitioner touches the patient with a finger and asks that the patient point to the area touched.

toxic and drug-induced hepatitis Liver inflammation resulting from exposure to hepatotoxins (e.g., industrial toxins, alcohol, and medications).

toxic epidermal necrolysis (TEN) A rare acute drug reaction of the skin that results in diffuse erythema and blister formation, with mucous membrane involvement and systemic toxicity.

toxic megacolon Acute enlargement of the colon along with fever, leukocytosis, and tachycardia; usually associated with ulcerative colitis.

toxic multinodular goiter Hyperthyroidism caused by multiple thyroid nodules, which may be enlarged thyroid tissues or adenomas, and a goiter that has been present for several years.

toxic shock syndrome (TSS) A severe illness caused by a toxin produced by certain strains of *Staphylococcus aureus*. It was first recognized in 1980 as related to menstruation and tampon use. It is characterized by abrupt onset of a high fever and headache, sore throat, vomiting, diarrhea, generalized rash, and hypotension. The most common manifestations are skin changes (initially a rash that resembles a severe sunburn and changes to a macular erythema similar to a drug-related rash).

toxin Protein molecule released by bacteria that affects host cell at a distant site. Continued multiplication of a pathogen is sometimes accompanied by toxin production.

trabecular Spongy bone; also called "cancellous bone."

trabeculation An abnormal thickening of the bladder wall caused by urinary retention and obstruction.

tracheostomy The (tracheal) stoma, or opening, that results from a tracheotomy.

tracheotomy The surgical incision into the trachea for the purpose of establishing an airway.

trachoma A chronic conjunctivitis caused by *Chlamydia trachomatis*.

traction The application of a pulling force to a part of the body to provide reduction, alignment, and rest.

transcellular fluid Any of the fluids in special body spaces, including cerebrospinal fluid, synovial fluid, peritoneal fluid, and pleural fluid.

transcultural nursing The area of study and practice that focuses on the care, health, and illness patterns of people with similarities and differences in their cultural beliefs, values, and practices; also, care that considers the cultural aspects of the patient.

transcutaneous electrical nerve stimulation (TENS) The use of a battery-operated device to deliver small electrical currents to the skin and underlying tissues for pain management; also called "percutaneous electrical nerve stimulation (PENS)."

transesophageal echocardiography (TEE) A form of echocardiography performed transesophageally (through the esophagus); an ultrasound transducer is placed immediately behind the heart in the esophagus or stomach to examine cardiac structure and function.

transferrin An iron-transport protein that can be measured directly or calculated as an indirect measurement of total iron-binding capacity.

transient ischemic attack (TIA) A brief attack (lasting a few minutes to less than 24 hours) of focal neurologic dysfunction caused by a brief interruption in cerebral blood flow, possibly resulting from cerebral vasospasm or transient systemic arterial hypertension. Repeated attacks may damage brain tissue; multiple attacks indicate significant increased risk for brain attack.

transmitted In genetics, the passage of a gene for a specific trait from one human generation to the next.

transmural myocardial infarction An infarction that involves all three layers of cardiac muscle.

transmyocardial laser revascularization A new surgical procedure for patients with unstable angina and inoperable coronary artery disease with areas of reversible myocardial ischemia. After a single-lung intubation, a left anterior thoracotomy is performed and the heart is visualized. A laser is used to create 20 to 24 long, narrow channels through the left ventricular muscle to the left ventricle. The channels eventually allow oxygenated blood to flow from the left ventricle during diastole to nourish the muscle.

transport maximum See *renal threshold*.

transurethral microwave therapy (TUMT) Procedure for treating benign prostatic hyperplasia using high temperatures to heat and destroy excess tissue.

transurethral needle ablation (TUNA) Procedure for treating benign prostatic hyperplasia using low radiofrequency energy to shrink the prostate.

transurethral resection of the prostate (TURP) The traditional "closed" surgical procedure for removal of the prostate. In this procedure, the surgeon inserts a resectoscope (an instrument similar to a cystoscope, but with a cutting and cauterizing loop) through the urethra. The enlarged portion of the prostate gland is then resected in small pieces.

trauma Bodily injury.

trauma activation criteria Certain injury mechanisms associated with life-threatening consequences that serve as criteria for summoning the trauma team for a rapid and coordinated resuscitation response.

trauma center Specialty care facility that provides competent and timely trauma services to patients depending on its designated level of capability.

trauma nursing Nursing specialty that encompasses the continuum of care from injury prevention and prehospital services to acute care, rehabilitation and, ultimately, community reintegration.

trauma system An organized and integrated approach to trauma care designed to ensure that all critical elements of trauma care delivery are aligned to meet the injured patient's needs.

triage In the emergency department, sorting or classifying patients into priority levels depending on illness or injury severity, with the highest acuity needs receiving the quickest evaluation and treatment.

triage officer In a hospital's emergency response plan, the person who rapidly evaluates each patient who arrives at the hospital. In a large hospital, this person is generally a physician who is assisted by triage nurses; however, a nurse may assume this role when physician resources are limited.

tricuspid valve The atrioventricular valve of the heart; separates the right atrium from the right ventricle.

tricyclic antidepressants Drugs used to treat depression.

trigeminy A type of premature complex consisting of a repetitive three-beat pattern; usually occurs as two sequential normal complexes followed by a premature complex and a pause, with the same pattern repeating itself in triplets.

trigger points In patients with fibromyalgia syndrome, tender areas that can typically be palpated to elicit pain in a predictable, reproducible pattern.

triiodothyronine (T₃) A hormone produced by the follicular cells of the thyroid gland.

tropic hormones Hormones secreted by the anterior pituitary gland that stimulate other endocrine glands.

tropical sprue A disease caused by an infectious agent that has not been identified but is thought to be bacterial. Tropical sprue results in malabsorption of fat, folic acid, and vitamin B₁₂ in later stages of the disease.

troponin A myocardial muscle protein released into the bloodstream after injury to myocardial muscle. Because it is not found in healthy patients, any rise in values indicates cardiac necrosis or acute myocardial infarction.

truss A device, usually a pad made with firm material, that is held in place over the hernia with a belt to keep the abdominal contents from protruding into the hernial sac.

tube thoracostomy A method of chest decompression performed after needle thoracostomy in which a chest tube is inserted in the fifth intercostal space, just anterior to the midaxillary line, to promote air and fluid drainage.

tuberculosis (TB) A highly communicable disease caused by *Mycobacterium tuberculosis*. It is the most common bacterial infection worldwide.

tumescence The condition of being swollen.

tumor-induced osteomalacia See *oncogenic osteomalacia*.

tunneled central venous catheter A type of catheter used for long-term infusion therapy in which a portion of the catheter lies in a subcutaneous tunnel, separating the points where the catheter enters the vein from where it exits the skin.

turbidity Cloudiness of a solution.

turbinates Three bony projections that protrude into the nasal cavities from the walls of the internal portion of the nose.

turgor The condition of being swollen and congested; indicates the amount of skin elasticity; the normal resiliency of a pinched fold of skin.

Turner's sign Ecchymosis on either flank, which may indicate retroperitoneal bleeding into the abdominal wall.

tympanic A term that describes the high-pitched, loud, musical sound heard over an air-filled intestine; obtained upon percussion of the abdomen.

tympanic membrane The eardrum; a thick, transparent sheet of tissue that provides a barrier between the external ear and the middle ear.

type A gastritis A form of chronic gastritis associated with the presence of antibodies to parietal cells and intrinsic factor. An autoimmune pathogenesis for this type of gastritis has been proposed.

type B gastritis The most common form of chronic gastritis; caused by *Helicobacter pylori* infection; 50% of patients who have gastric ulcers have associated chronic gastritis.

tyrosine kinase inhibitors (TKIs) Drugs with the main action of inhibiting activation of tyrosine kinases. There are many different TKIs. Some are unique to the cell type; others may be present only in cancer cells that express a specific gene mutation. As a result, the different TKI drugs are effective in disrupting the growth of some cancer cell types and not others.

U

U wave In the electrocardiogram, the deflection that follows the T wave and may result from slow repolarization of ventricular Purkinje fibers. When present, it is of the same polarity as the T wave, although generally smaller. Abnormal prominence of the U wave suggests an electrolyte abnormality or other disturbance.

ulcerative colitis (UC) A chronic inflammatory process that affects the mucosal lining of the colon or rectum; one of a group of bowel diseases of unknown etiology characterized by remissions and exacerbations. It can result in loose stools containing blood and mucus, poor absorption of vital nutrients, and thickening of the colon wall.

umbilical hernia Protrusion of the intestine at the umbilicus; can be congenital or acquired. Congenital umbilical hernias appear in infancy. Acquired umbilical hernias directly result from increased intra-abdominal pressure and are most commonly seen in obese people.

unclassified seizure One of the three broad categories of seizure disorders along with partial seizure and generalized seizure. They occur for no known reason, do not fit into the generalized or partial classifications, and account for about half of all seizure activity; also called "idiopathic seizures."

uncus The inner part of the temporal lobe of the brain that can move downward and cause pressure on the brainstem; the vital sign center.

undermining Separation of the skin layers at the wound margins from the underlying granulation tissue.

unilateral body neglect syndrome In the patient who has had a brain attack, an unawareness of the existence of the paralyzed side. For example, the patient may believe he or she is sitting up straight when actually he or she is leaning to one side. Another typical example is the patient who washes or dresses only one side of the body.

uninhibited bladder May occur with a neurologic problem that affects the cortical bladder center of the brain (frontal lobe), such as brain attack or brain injury. The patient has little sensorimotor control and cannot wait until he or she is on the commode or bedpan before voiding.

Unna boot A wound dressing constructed of gauze moistened with zinc oxide; used to promote venous return in the ambulatory patient with a stasis ulcer and to form a sterile environment for the ulcer. The boot is applied to the affected limb, from the toes to the knee, after the ulcer has been cleaned with normal saline solution and covered with an elastic wrap. The dressing hardens like a cast.

unroofing Lifting or puncturing of the outer surface of a skin lesion to obtain specimens for bacterial culture.

unstable angina Chest pain or discomfort that occurs at rest or with exertion and causes marked limitation of activity; characterized by an increase in the number of attacks and an increase in the intensity of pain. Pain may last longer than 15 minutes or may be poorly relieved by rest or nitroglycerin.

upper esophageal sphincter (UES) The ringlike band of muscle fibers at the upper end of the esophagus. When at rest, the sphincter is closed to prevent air from entering into the esophagus during respiration.

upper GI (gastrointestinal) radiographic series The radiographic visualization of the gastrointestinal tract from the oral part of the pharynx to the duodenojejunal junction; used to detect disorders of structure or function of the esophagus (barium swallow), stomach, or duodenum.

upper motor neurons Neurons that carry motor impulses from the cerebral cortex to the cerebral nerves. Patients with spinal cord injuries involving upper motor neuron lesions experience muscle spasticity, which can lead to contractures after spinal shock has resolved.

uremia The accumulation of nitrogenous wastes in the blood (azotemia); a result of renal failure, with clinical symptoms including nausea and vomiting.

uremic frost A layer of urea crystals from evaporated sweat; may appear on the face, eyebrows, axilla, and groin in patients with advanced uremic syndrome.

uremic syndrome The systemic clinical and laboratory manifestations of end-stage kidney disease.

ureterolithiasis Formation of stones in the ureter.

ureteropelvic junction (UPJ) The narrow area in the upper third of the ureter at the point at which the renal pelvis becomes the ureter.

ureteroplasty Surgical repair of the ureter.

ureterovesical junction (UVJ) The point at which each ureter becomes narrow as it enters the bladder.

urethral meatus The opening at the endpoint of the urethra.

urethral stricture An obstruction that occurs low in the urinary tract due to decreased diameter of the urethra, causing bladder distention before hydroureter and hydronephrosis.

urethritis An inflammation of the urethra that causes symptoms similar to urinary tract infection.

urethroplasty Surgical treatment of the urethral stricture to remove the affected area with or without grafting to create a larger opening.

urgency The feeling that urination will occur immediately.

urgent triage In a three-tiered triage scheme, the category that includes patients who should be treated quickly but in whom an immediate threat to life does not currently exist, such as those with abdominal pain or displaced fractures or dislocations.

urinary tract infection (UTI) An infection in the normally sterile urinary system. The unobstructed and complete passage of urine from the renal and urinary systems is critical in maintaining a sterile urinary tract. When any structural abnormality is present, the risk for damage as a result of infection is greatly increased.

urolithiasis The presence of calculi (stones) in the urinary tract.

urosepsis The spread of an infection from the urinary tract to the bloodstream, resulting in systemic infection accompanied by fever, chills, hypotension, and altered mental status.

urticaria A transient vascular reaction of the skin marked by the development of wheals (hives).

uterine artery embolization Treatment for leiomyomas in which a radiologist uses a percutaneous catheter inserted through the femoral artery to inject polyvinyl alcohol pellets into the uterine artery. The resulting blockage starves the tumor of circulation, allowing it (or them) to shrink.

uterine prolapse Downward displacement of the uterus into the vagina.

uvea The middle layer of the eye, which consists of the choroid, ciliary body, and iris. The choroid has many blood vessels that supply nutrients to the retina.

uveitis Inflammation of part or all of the uvea.

V

vagal maneuver Nonsurgical management of cardiac dysrhythmias that is intended to induce vagal stimulation of the cardiac conduction system, specifically the sinoatrial and atrioventricular nodes. Vagal maneuvers may be attempted to terminate supraventricular tachydysrhythmia.

vagina The collapsible hollow tube with thin, muscular walls lined by mucous membrane and many blood vessels; extends from the vestibule to the uterus. It is the channel for the passage of menstrual flow, allows reception of the penis during intercourse, and allows passage of the fetus during a vaginal birth.

vaginectomy Surgical removal of part or all of the vagina.

vagotomy syndrome Diarrhea that develops as a result of the interruption of vagal fibers to the abdominal viscera during esophageal surgery.

validation therapy For the patient with moderate or severe Alzheimer's disease, the process of recognizing and acknowledging the patient's feelings and concerns without reinforcing an erroneous belief (e.g., if the patient is looking for his or her deceased mother).

Valsalva maneuver A form of vagal stimulation of the cardiac conduction system in which the health care provider instructs the patient to bear down as if straining to have a bowel movement.

variant (Prinzmetal's) angina A type of angina caused by coronary vasospasm (vessel spasm); usually associated with elevation of the ST segment on an electrocardiogram obtained during anginal attacks.

varicocelectomy The surgical removal of a varicocele (a cluster of dilated veins behind and above the testis).

varicose veins Distended, protruding veins that appear darkened and tortuous; common in patients older than 30 years whose occupations require prolonged standing. As the vein wall weakens and dilates, venous pressure increases and the valves become incompetent (defective). The incompetent valves enhance the vessel dilation, and the veins become tortuous and distended.

vas deferens A firm, muscular tube that continues from the tail of each epididymis and is a reservoir for sperm and tubular fluids. They merge with ducts from the seminal vesicle to form the ejaculatory ducts at the base of the prostate gland. Sperm from the vas deferens and secretions from the seminal vesicles are transported through the ejaculatory duct to mix with prostatic fluids in the prostatic urethra. Also called "ductus deferens."

vascular access device A catheter; a plastic tube placed in a blood vessel to deliver fluids and medications.

vasculitis Blood vessel inflammation.

vasoconstriction Decrease in diameter of blood vessels.

vaso-occlusive event (VOE) A blood vessel obstruction caused by masses of sickled RBCs.

vasopressin Secretion of the posterior pituitary gland, also known as "antidiuretic hormone" or "ADH."

vasospasm A sudden and transient constriction of a blood vessel.

Vaughn-Williams classification System used to categorize antidysrhythmic agents according to their effects on the action potential of cardiac cells.

vegan A vegetarian diet pattern in which only foods of plant origin are eaten.

venous beading A complication of diabetes; the abnormal appearance of retinal veins in which areas of swelling and constriction along a segment of vein resemble links of sausage. Such bleeding occurs in areas of retinal ischemia and is a predictor of proliferative diabetic retinopathy.

venous duplex ultrasonography A noninvasive test using ultrasonic waves; the preferred diagnostic test for deep vein thrombosis.

venous insufficiency Alteration of venous efficiency by thrombosis or defective valves; caused by prolonged venous hypertension, which stretches the veins and damages the valves, resulting in further venous hypertension, edema and, eventually, venous stasis ulcers, swelling, and cellulitis.

venous thromboembolism (VTE) A term that refers to both deep vein thrombosis and pulmonary embolism; obstruction by a thrombus.

ventilation assistance Process or devices to help the patient breathe easily (e.g., mechanical ventilation assistance).

ventral hernia Protrusion of the intestine at the site of a previous surgical incision resulting from inadequate healing. Most often caused by postoperative wound infections, inadequate nutrition, and obesity.

ventricular asystole The complete absence of any ventricular rhythm. There are no electrical impulses in the ventricles and therefore no ventricular depolarization, no QRS complex, no contraction, no cardiac output, and no pulse, respirations, or blood pressure. The patient is in full cardiac arrest.

ventricular fibrillation (VF) A cardiac dysrhythmia that results from electrical chaos in the ventricles; impulses from many irritable foci fire in a totally disorganized manner so that ventricular contraction cannot occur; there is no cardiac output or pulse and therefore no cerebral, myocardial, or systemic perfusion. This rhythm is rapidly fatal if not successfully terminated within 3 to 5 minutes.

ventricular gallop An abnormal third heart sound that arises from vibrations of the valves and supporting structures and is produced during the rapid passive filling phase of ventricular diastole when blood flows from the atrium to a noncompliant ventricle. In patients older than 35 years, it is an early sign of heart failure or ventricular septal defect.

ventricular remodeling (1) Progressive myocyte (myocardial cell) contractile dysfunction over time; results from activation of the renin-angiotensin system caused by reduced blood flow to the kidneys, a common occurrence in low-output states; (2) after a myocardial infarction, permanent changes in the size and shape of the left ventricle due to scar tissue; such remodeling may decrease left ventricular function, cause heart failure, and increase morbidity and mortality.

ventricular tachycardia (VT) An abnormal heart rhythm that occurs with repetitive firing of an irritable ventricular ectopic focus, usually at a rate of 140 to 180 beats/min or more.

ventriculomyomectomy The surgical excision of a portion of the hypertrophied ventricular septum to create a widened outflow tract in patients with obstructive hypertrophic cardiomyopathy.

ventriculostomy The surgical placement of an intraventricular catheter to drain cerebrospinal fluid in patients with increased intracranial pressure and rapidly deteriorating neurologic function.

vertebroplasty A minimally invasive surgery for managing vertebral fractures in patients with osteoporosis. Bone cement is injected directly into the fracture site to provide immediate pain relief.

vertigo A sense of spinning movement that may result from diseases of the inner ear.

vesicant Chemical that causes tissue damage on direct contact.

vesicant medication A drug that causes tissue damage when extravasated.

vesicle In health care, a small bladder or blister.

vestibule A longitudinal area between the labia minora, the clitoris, and the vagina that contains Bartholin glands and the openings of the urethra, Skene's glands (paraurethral glands), and vagina.

viral hepatitis Inflammation of the liver that results from an infection caused by one of five major categories of viruses (hepatitis A, B, C, D, or E). Viral hepatitis is the most common type and can be either acute or chronic.

viral load testing Test that measures the presence of human immune deficiency virus genetic material (ribonucleic acid) or other viral proteins in the patient's blood.

viral meningitis A type of meningitis that often occurs after viral illnesses such as

measles, herpes simplex, coxsackievirus, and echovirus; it is marked by inflammation over the cerebral cortex, white matter, and meninges. The formation of exudate (common in bacterial meningitis) does not occur, and no organisms are obtained from the cerebrospinal fluid. Also called "aseptic meningitis."

Virchow's triad The occurrence of stasis of blood flow, endothelial injury, or hypercoagulability; often associated with thrombus formation.

viremia The presence of viruses in the blood.

virilization The presence of male secondary sex characteristics.

virtual colonoscopy A noninvasive alternative to the colonoscopy procedure. A scanner is used to view the colon.

virulence A term used to describe the frequency with which a pathogen causes disease (degree of communicability) and its ability to invade and damage a host. Virulence can also indicate the severity of the disease; often used as a synonym for pathogenicity.

visceral proteins Proteins such as albumin that circulate in the bloodstream and may be produced by the liver.

viscous Of thick consistency.

vitiligo An abnormality of the skin characterized by patchy areas of pigment loss with increased pigmentation at the edges. It is seen with primary hypofunction of the adrenal glands and is due to autoimmune destruction of melanocytes in the skin.

vitrectomy The surgical removal of the vitreous.

vitreous body The clear, thick gel that fills the vitreous chamber of the eye (the space between the lens and the retina). This gel transmits light and shapes the eye.

vocational counselor A member of the rehabilitative health care team who assists the patient with job placement, training, or further education.

volutrauma Damage to the lung by excess volume delivered to one lung over the other.

volvulus Obstruction of the bowel caused by twisting of the bowel.

vulva The external female genitalia; extends from the mons pubis to the anal opening.

vulvar self-examination (VSE) A method for self-examination of the external female genitalia for early detection of diseases of the vulva.

vulvectomy Surgical removal of the vulva, labia majora, labia minora, and, possibly, the clitoris.

vulvovaginitis Inflammation of the lower genital tract resulting from a disturbance of the balance of hormones and flora in the vagina and vulva.

W

warm antibody anemia A form of immunohemolytic anemia (in which the immune system attacks a person's own red blood cells for unknown reasons) that occurs with immunoglobulin G antibody excess and may be

triggered by drugs, chemicals, or other autoimmune problems.

warm phase A phase lasting 2 to 3 weeks after peripheral nerve trauma resulting in complete denervation; the extremity is warm, and the skin appears flushed or rosy. The warm phase is gradually superseded by a cold phase.

water brash Reflex salivary hypersecretion that occurs in response to reflux in the patient with gastroesophageal reflux disease.

wean The process of going from ventilatory dependence to spontaneous breathing.

"wearing off" phenomenon Loss of response over time to a medication.

wedge resection Removal of small, localized areas of disease.

Wernicke's aphasia See *receptive aphasia*.

Wernicke's area An important speech area of the cerebrum. It is located in the temporal lobe and plays a significant role in higher-level brain function. It enables the processing of words into coherent thought and recognition of the idea behind written or printed words (language).

Whipple procedure (radical pancreaticoduodenectomy) A surgical treatment for cancer of the head of the pancreas. The procedure entails removal of the proximal head of the pancreas, the duodenum, a portion of the jejunum, the stomach (partial or total gastrectomy), and the gallbladder, with anastomosis of the pancreatic duct (pancreaticojejunostomy), the common bile duct (choledochojejunostomy), and the stomach (gastrojejunostomy) to the jejunum.

white matter In the spinal cord, myelinated axons that surround the gray matter (neuron cell bodies).

Williams position A position in which the patient lies in the semi-Fowler's position and flexes the knees to relax the muscles of the lower back and relieve pressure on the spinal nerve root. This is typically more comfortable and therapeutic for the patient with low back pain.

withdrawal syndrome Symptoms that occur when a patient who is physically dependent on opioids abruptly stops using them. Slowly tapering (weaning) the drug dosage lessens or alleviates the physical withdrawal symptoms in a patient who is opioid dependent. Also called "abstinence syndrome."

withdrawing or withholding life-sustaining therapy (WWLST) The withdrawal or withholding of one or more therapies that might prolong the life of a person who cannot be cured by the therapy; the withdrawal of therapy does not directly cause death. Formerly called "passive euthanasia."

work-related musculoskeletal disorders (MSDs) Disorders caused by heavy lifting and dependent transfers by staff members.

X

xenograft Tissue transplanted (grafted) from another species; for example, a heart valve transplanted from a pig to a human.

xeroradiography A diagnostic x-ray technique in which images are produced electrically rather than chemically, permitting lower exposure times and radiation energies than those of ordinary x-rays. The images exhibit "edge contrast," which is useful for identifying minute calcifications in the breast.

xerosis Abnormally dry skin.

xerostomia Abnormal dryness of the mouth caused by a severe reduction in the flow of saliva.

x-ray Radiation that is generated by machine.

Z

Zollinger-Ellison syndrome (ZES) The occurrence of upper gastrointestinal tract ulceration, increased gastric acid secretion, and the presence of a non–beta cell islet tumor of the pancreas, called a "gastrinoma." Affected people may have more than one gastrinoma.

Chapter 2
p. 10   B
p. 13   A, B, C, D, E

Chapter 3
p. 18   A
p. 22   A

Chapter 4
p. 33   C

Chapter 5
p. 49   D
p. 52   0.25 mL
p. 56   B

Chapter 8
p. 94   B
p. 104   D

Chapter 9
p. 113   B, C, D, E
p. 114   B, C, D, F

Chapter 10
p. 127   B
p. 128   B, C, D, E, A
p. 134   B

Chapter 11
p. 139   C
p. 153   D
p. 148   B, C, D, E
p. 152   A

Chapter 12
p. 158   C
p. 161   B, C

Chapter 13
p. 171   C
p. 180   A
p. 182   C
p. 187   D
p. 190   A

Chapter 14
p. 203   A

Chapter 15
p. 213   D
p. 216   125 mL/hr

Chapter 16
p. 246   B
p. 247   D
p. 248   C
p. 252   C
p. 254   A

Chapter 17
p. 266   C
p. 270   B
p. 275   D

Chapter 18
p. 285   D
p. 289   C
p. 292   A
p. 295   B

Chapter 20
p. 328   B, D, E
p. 331   A
p. 336   B, C, D, E, F
p. 347   C
p. 350   A

Chapter 21
p. 369   A
p. 375   C
p. 375   C
p. 377   B

Chapter 22
p. 386   B
p. 394   B

Chapter 24
p. 410   D
p. 414   C
p. 421   C
p. 422   B
p. 433   C

Chapter 25
p. 440   C
p. 443   A, B, D, E

Chapter 26
p. 454   D
p. 463   A
p. 468   A

Chapter 27
p. 472   B
p. 477   D
p. 488   A
p. 501   C
p. 507   A

Chapter 28
p. 515   D
p. 523   B
p. 523   A
p. 526   B
p. 527   A
p. 528   C
p. 532   D
p. 539   A

Chapter 29
p. 548   B
p. 551   D
p. 555   C
p. 556   A
p. 560   C

Chapter 30
p. 565   A
p. 570   D
p. 574   B
p. 575   C

Chapter 31
p. 583   B
p. 584   D
p. 591   C
p. 595   D

Chapter 32
p. 610   A
p. 617   D
p. 620   C
p. 622   B
p. 631   C
p. 637   A

Chapter 33
p. 645   B
p. 647   D
p. 657   B

Chapter 34
p. 667   D
p. 668   A
p. 675   C
p. 679   C
p. 681   B

Chapter 35
p. 694   C
p. 708   C

Chapter 36
p. 721   B
p. 731   B
p. 732   C
p. 737   C
p. 738   A, D, C, B, E

Chapter 37
p. 749   A, D
p. 752   B
p. 753   B
p. 763   D

Chapter 38
p. 775   C
p. 784   D

p. 789   B
p. 795   B
p. 801   C
p. 803   C
p. 804   A

Chapter 39
p. 812   D
p. 819   A
p. 822   B

Chapter 40
p. 834   B, C, D, F
p. 840   D
p. 849   B

Chapter 41
p. 859   B
p. 863   D
p. 866   A

Chapter 42
p. 873   D
p. 875   A
p. 878   D
p. 881   A
p. 885   B
p. 891   C
p. 896   A
p. 901   A

Chapter 43
p. 919   A
p. 922   B

Chapter 44
p. 931   D
p. 936   B, D, E
p. 951   C
p. 953   A

Chapter 45
p. 965   D
p. 972   B

Chapter 46
p. 990   D
p. 994   A, B, C, E
p. 995   A, C, E, F

Chapter 47
p. 1007 B
p. 1013 D
p. 1017 C
p. 1026 D
p. 1035 C

Chapter 48
p. 1045 D
p. 1048 C

Chapter 49
p. 1056   D
p. 1059   B
p. 1062   C
p. 1067   B
p. 1070   B
p. 1075   C

Chapter 50
p. 1082   D
p. 1086   C

Chapter 51
p. 1090   D
p. 1096   B
p. 1097   A

Chapter 52
p. 1112   B, C
p. 1117   C

Chapter 53
p. 1124   B
p. 1131   D

Chapter 54
p. 1154   B, C, D
p. 1164   C
p. 1169   C, D, E, F

Chapter 55
p. 1184   C, A, B, D
p. 1187   A

Chapter 56
p. 1195   B
p. 1200   A, C, D, E

Chapter 57
p. 1208   D
p. 1212   A, C, D, E

Chapter 58
p. 1225   B, E, F
p. 1228   D
p. 1234   A, C, E

Chapter 59
p. 1245   D
p. 1251   A, C

Chapter 60
p. 1270   B, C, D
p. 1274   B
p. 1278   C
p. 1287   C

Chapter 61
p. 1299   C, D, E
p. 1305   A

Chapter 62
p. 1320   D
p. 1328   B
p. 1333   A, B, E

Chapter 63
p. 1339   49.1
p. 1344   A, C, D, F

Chapter 64
p. 1364   C
p. 1367   B

Chapter 65
p. 1373   C
p. 1378   D
p. 1380   B
p. 1381   B
p. 1388   A

Chapter 66
p. 1396   C
p. 1403   A
p. 1404   A
p. 1405   B

Chapter 67
p. 1413   C
p. 1416   A
p. 1418   D
p. 1430   C
p. 1431   C
p. 1439   B

Chapter 68
p. 1476   B
p. 1482   C
p. 1486   A

Chapter 69
p. 1494   C
p. 1504   B
p. 1507   D
p. 1515   A

Chapter 70
p. 1523   D
p. 1526   C
p. 1532   D

Chapter 71
p. 1543   C
p. 1546   B
p. 1546   B
p. 1548   D
p. 1551   B
p. 1555   A

Chapter 72
p. 1583   C
p. 1586   B

Chapter 73
p. 1594   B
p. 1603   D

Chapter 74
p. 1614   A
p. 1620   A

Chapter 75
p. 1636   D
p. 1645   A

Chapter 76
p. 1656   A
p. 1665   D

Chapter 2

2-1, From Potter, P.A., & Perry, A.G. (2001). *Fundamentals of nursing* (5th ed.). St. Louis: Mosby; **2-2,** from Grodner, M., Roth, S.L., & Walkingshaw, B.C. (2012). *Nutritional foundations and clinical applications: A nursing approach* (5th ed.). St. Louis: Mosby; **2-3, 2-4,** from Potter, P.A., & Perry, A.G. (2009). *Fundamentals of nursing* (7th ed.). St. Louis: Mosby.

Chapter 3

3-3, From the Aging Clinical Research Center (ACRC), a joint project of Stanford University and the VA Palo Alto Health Care System, Palo Alto, CA, funded by the National Institute of Aging and the Department of Veterans Affairs.

Chapter 4

4-1, 4-3, From Harkreader, H., Hogan, M.A., & Thobaben, M. (2007). *Fundamentals of nursing: Caring and clinical judgment* (3rd ed.). Philadelphia: Saunders.

Chapter 5

5-2, From Melzack, R. (1975). The McGill Pain Questionnaire: Major properties and scoring methods. *Pain, 1,* 272-281; **5-3,** Simple Descriptive Pain Distress Scale, 0-10 Numeric Pain Distress Scale, and Visual Analog Scale redrawn from Acute Pain Management Guideline Panel. (1992). *Acute pain management: Operative or medical procedures and trauma. Clinical practice guideline.* AHCPR Pub. No. 92-0032. Rockville, MD: Agency for Health Care Policy and Research, Public Health Service, U.S. Department of Health and Human Services; Pain Relief Visual Analog Scale redrawn from Fishman, B., Pasternak, S., Wallenstein, S.L., Houde, R.W., Holland, J.C., & Foley, K.M. (1987). The Memorial Pain Assessment Card: A valid instrument for the evaluation of cancer pain. *Cancer, 60*(5), 1151-1158; Percent Relief Scale redrawn from the Brief Pain Inventory. Pain Research Group, Department of Neurology, University of Wisconsin—Madison; **5-4,** CADD-PCA is a registered trademark of Pharmacia Deltec, St. Paul, MN; **5-5,** courtesy Medtronic, Inc., Columbia Heights, MN.

Chapter 6

6-2, Modified from Nussbaum, R., McInnes, R., & Willard, H. (2007). *Thompson & Thompson: Genetics in medicine* (7th ed.). Philadelphia: Saunders; **6-7,** modified from Jorde, L., Carey, J., Bamshad, M., & White, R. (2000). *Medical genetics* (2nd ed.). St. Louis: Mosby; **6-10,** modified from Jorde, L., Carey, J., & Bamshad, M. (2010). *Medical genetics* (4th ed.). St. Louis: Mosby.

Chapter 7

7-1, © 2010. Rona F. Levin & Jeffrey M. Keefer; **7-2,** © 2010. R.E. Burke & R.F. Levin; **7-3,** © 2007. Visiting Nurse Service of New York and Rona F. Levin.

Chapter 8

8-4, From Potter, P., & Perry, A. (2009). *Fundamentals of nursing* (7th ed.). St. Louis: Mosby.

Chapter 9

9-1, © 2005. National Hospice and Palliative Care Organization, 2007 Revised. All rights reserved. Reproduction and distribution by an organization or organized group without the written permission of the National Hospice and Palliative Care Organization is expressly forbidden. Visit caringinfo.org for more information.

Chapter 10

10-3, From Henry M., & Stapleton, E. (2010). *EMT prehospital care* (4th ed.). St. Louis: Mosby.

Chapter 11

11-1, From Auerbach, P.S. (2008). *Wilderness medicine* (5th ed.). Philadelphia: Mosby; courtesy Michael Cardwell & Carl Barden Venom Laboratory; **11-2,** from Auerbach, P.S. (2008). *Wilderness medicine* (5th ed.). Philadelphia: Mosby; courtesy Sherman Minton, MD; **11-3,** from Auerbach, P.S. (2008). *Wilderness medicine* (5th ed.). Philadelphia: Mosby; courtesy Michael Cardwell & Jude McNally; **11-4,** from Auerbach, P.S. (2008). *Wilderness medicine* (5th ed.). Philadelphia: Mosby; courtesy Indiana University Medical Center; **11-5,** from Auerbach, P.S. (2008). *Wilderness medicine* (5th ed.). Philadelphia: Mosby; courtesy Paul Auerbach, MD; **11-6,** from Auerbach, P.S. (2008). *Wilderness medicine* (5th ed.) Philadelphia: Mosby; **11-7,** from Auerbach, P.S. (2008). *Wilderness medicine* (5th ed.). Philadelphia: Mosby; courtesy Cameron Bangs, MD.

Chapter 12

12-2, Courtesy Ann Breslin; **12-3,** courtesy Jeanne McConnell, MSN, RN.

Chapter 13

13-2, 13-7, 13-10, ©1992 by M. Linda Workman. All rights reserved.

Chapter 14

14-3, 14-12, ©1992 by M. Linda Workman. All rights reserved.

Chapter 15

15-1, From Perry, A., & Potter, P. (2010). *Clinical nursing skills & techniques* (7th ed.). St. Louis: Mosby; **15-2,** courtesy Becton Dickinson Infusion Therapy Systems, Sandy, UT; **15-3,** courtesy AccuVein, LLC; **15-7,** courtesy Edwards Lifesciences, Irvine, CA; **15-11,** courtesy NowMedical, Chadds Ford, PA; **15-12,** from Potter, P., & Perry, A. (2009). *Fundamentals of nursing* (7th ed.). St. Louis: Mosby; **15-13,** courtesy I-Flow, Inc., Lake Forest, CA; **15-14,** courtesy Venetec International, San Diego, CA; **15-15,** courtesy I.V. House, Hazelwood, MO.

Chapter 16

16-1, From Association of periOperative Registered Nurses: *Comprehensive surgical checklist.* Retrieved October 27, 2010, from www.aorn.org/docs/assets/6014C0F7-B3AB-38C4-C3D370D159B8B068/ComprehenisveSurgicalChecklist.pdf. © 2010. AORN, Inc. Used with permission. **16-2, 16-6,** courtesy Christiana Care Health Services, Newark, DE; **16-4,** from

Perry, A.G., & Potter, P.A. (2010). *Clinical nursing skills and techniques* (7th ed.). St. Louis: Mosby; **16-5, A,** courtesy The Kendall Healthcare Company, Mansfield, MA; **16-5, B,** courtesy Venodyne, Inc., Norwood, MA; **16-5, C,** courtesy Huntleigh Healthcare, Eatontown, NJ.

Chapter 17

17-1, Courtesy Christiana Care Health Services, Newark, DE; **17-5,** redrawn with permission by Intuitive Surgical, Inc., 2007.

Chapter 18

18-1, Courtesy Forrest General Hospital, Hattiesburg, MS; **18-2, 18-5,** from Harkreader, H., Hogan, M.A., & Thobaben, M. (2007). *Fundamentals of nursing: Caring and clinical judgment* (3rd ed.). Philadelphia: Saunders; **18-3, C, D,** courtesy CR Bard, Inc., Covington, GA.

Chapter 19

19-3, Modified from Goldman, L., & Schafer, A. (Eds.). (2012). *Goldman's Cecil medicine* (24th ed.). Philadelphia: Saunders.

Chapter 20

20-2, A, From Jebson, L.R., & Coons, D.D. (1998). Total hip arthroplasty. *Surgical Technologist, 30*(10), 12-21; **B,** from Mercier, L.R. (2000). *Practical orthopaedics* (5th ed.). St. Louis: Mosby; **20-5,** from Damjanov, I. (2006). *Pathophysiology for the health professions* (3rd ed.). Philadelphia: Saunders; **20-8,** from Goldman L., & Ausiello, D. (2007). *Cecil medicine* (23rd ed.). Philadelphia: Saunders.

Chapter 21

21-1, From Kumar, V., Abbas, A., & Fausto, N. (2010). *Robbins & Cotran pathologic basis of disease* (8th ed.). Philadelphia: Saunders; **21-4,** from McCance, K.L., & Huether, S.E. (2002). *Pathophysiology: The biologic basis for disease in adults and children* (4th ed.). St. Louis: Mosby; **21-5,** from The Centers for Disease Control and Prevention. (2011). *HIV surveillance report: Diagnosis of HIV infection and AIDS in the United States and dependent areas,* 2009. Vol. 21, Atlanta: Author; **21-6,** from Marks, J., & Miller, J. (2006). *Lookingbill & Marks' principles of dermatology* (4th ed.). Philadelphia: Saunders; **21-7,** from Leonard, P.C. (2009). *Building a medical vocabulary* (7th ed.). St. Louis: Saunders.

Chapter 22

22-2, Courtesy Dey, Napa, CA; **22-3,** from Auerbach, P. (2008). *Wilderness medicine* (5th ed.). Philadelphia: Mosby; courtesy Sheryl Olson.

Chapter 23

23-6, From American Cancer Society. *Cancer facts and figures 2011.* Atlanta, GA: Author.

Chapter 24

24-3, From Weinzweig, J., & Weinzweig, N. (2005). *The mutilated hand,* St. Louis: Mosby; **24-4,** from Workman, M.L., & LaCharity, L. (2011). *Understanding pharmacology: Essentials for medication safety.* St. Louis: Saunders; **24-5,** from Kee, J., Hayes, E., & McCuistion, L. (2012). *Pharmacology: A nursing process approach,* St. Louis: Saunders; **24-7,** from Forbes, C.D.,

& Jackson, W.F. (2003). *Colour atlas and text of clinical medicine* (3rd ed.). London: Mosby.

Chapter 25

25-1, A, From deWit, S.C. (2009). *Fundamental concepts and skills for nursing* (3rd ed.). Philadelphia: Saunders; **B,** from Elkin, M.C., Perry, A., & Potter, P.A. (2007). *Nursing interventions and clinical skills* (4th ed.). St. Louis: Mosby; courtesy Kimberly-Clark Health Care, Roswell, GA.

Chapter 26

26-14, From Marks, J., & Miller, J. (2007). *Lookingbill and Marks' principles of dermatology* (4th ed.). Philadelphia: Saunders.

Chapter 27

27-2, Modified from Swaim, S.F. (1980). *Surgery of traumatized skin.* Philadelphia: Saunders; **27-4,** from Barbara Braden & Nancy Bergstrom. © 1988. Reprinted with permission; **27-5,** illustrations from the National Pressure Ulcer Advisory Panel and European Pressure Ulcer Advisory Panel. (2009). *Pressure ulcer prevention and treatment: Clinical practice guideline.* Washington, DC: NPUAP. Used with permission; **27-9,** from The Centers for Disease Control and Prevention, Atlanta, GA (www.bt.cdc.gov/agent/anthrax/anthrax-images/); **27-10,** from Marks, J., & Miller, J. (2006). *Lookingbill & Marks' principles of dermatology* (4th ed.). Philadelphia: Saunders; **27-12,** from Lookingbill, D.P., & Marks, J.G. (2000). *Principles of dermatology* (3rd ed.). Philadelphia: Saunders; **27-17,** courtesy Stevens Johnson Syndrome Foundation, Littleton, CO.

Chapter 28

28-1, Modified from Moritz, A.R. (1947). Studies of thermal injuries. II: The relative importance of time and surface temperature in causation of cutaneous burns. *American Journal of Pathology, 23,* 695; **28-14,** from Hanke, C.W., & Sattler, G. (2006). *Procedures in cosmetic dermatology series: Liposuction.* Philadelphia: Saunders.

Chapter 29

29-12, From Young, A.P., & Proctor, D. (2008). *Kinn's the medical assistant: An applied learning approach* (10th ed.). St. Louis: Saunders; **29-13,** from Harkreader, H., Hogan, M.A., & Thobaben, M. (2007). *Fundamentals of nursing: Caring and clinical judgment* (3rd ed.). Philadelphia: Saunders.

Chapter 30

30-3, 30-9, 30-10, From Perry, A.G., & Potter, P.A. (2010). *Clinical nursing skills and techniques* (7th ed.). St. Louis: Mosby; **30-11,** courtesy Chad Therapeutics, Chatsworth, CA; **30-13,** courtesy Mallinckrodt, Inc., Shiley Tracheostomy Products, St. Louis, MO; **30-14,** courtesy J.T. Posey Company, Arcadia, CA; **30-15,** courtesy Dale Medical Products, Inc., Plainville, MA.

Chapter 31

31-1, From Tardy, M.E. (1997). *Rhinoplasty: The art and science.* Philadelphia: Saunders. Used with permission; **31-2, A,** courtesy Invotec International, Jacksonville, FL; **31-5,** courtesy InHealth Technologies, a division of Helix Medical, LLC, Carpinteria, CA.

Chapter 32

32-3, From Jarvis, C. (2012). *Physical examination and health assessment* (6th ed.). Philadelphia: Saunders; **32-4,** from Aehlert, B. (2011). *Paramedic practice today: Above and beyond.* St. Louis: Mosby; **32-11,** modified from Gift, A. (1989). A dyspnea assessment guide. *Critical Care Nurse, 9*(8), 79. Used with permission; **32-12,** from Swartz, M.H. (2009). *Textbook of physical diagnosis: History and examination* (6th ed.). Philadelphia: Saunders; **32-13,** courtesy Axcan Pharma, Mont-Saint-Hilaire, Quebec, Canada; **32-18,** courtesy Atrium Medical Corporation, Hudson, NH.

Chapter 33

33-1, Courtesy Covidien, AG, Switzerland; **33-2,** illustration from Workman, M.L., & LaCharity, L. (2011). *Understanding pharmacology.* St. Louis: Saunders; photo from Kumar, V., Abbas, A., Fausto, N., & Aster, J. (2009). *Robbins and Cotran pathologic basis for disease* (8th ed.). Philadelphia: Saunders; **33-3,** from Zitelli, B.J., & Davis, H.W. (2007). *Atlas of pediatric physical diagnosis* (5th ed.). Philadelphia: Saunders; courtesy Kenneth Schuitt, MD; **33-4,** courtesy Uvex Safety, Smithfield, RI.

Chapter 34

34-2, Modified from Gift, A. (1989). A dyspnea assessment guide. *Critical Care Nurse, 9*(8), 79. Used with permission; **34-3, A,** courtesy Sims Porter, Inc.; **34-4,** © Dräger Medical AG & Co. KG, Lübeck, Germany. All rights reserved. Not to be reproduced without written permission, not to be saved or copied in any electronic format, not to be transmitted electronically or mechanically by way of photocopying or photographing, in any way, shape or form, whether fully or partially; **34-5,** from McCance, K.L. Huether S.E., Brashers, V.L., & Rote, N.S. (2010). *Pathophysiology: The biologic basis for disease in adults and children* (6th ed.). St. Louis: Mosby.

Chapter 36

36-14, 36-16, Courtesy Medtronic, Inc., Minneapolis, MN. Reproduced with permission; **36-15,** courtesy Philips Medical Systems, Andover, MA.

Chapter 37

37-1, From McCance, K.L., & Huether, S.E. (2002). *Pathophysiology: The biologic basis for disease in adults and children* (4th ed.). St. Louis: Mosby; **37-2,** courtesy Abiomed, Inc., Danvers, MA; **37-3, A, B,** courtesy Medtronic, Inc., Minneapolis, MN; **C** courtesy Baxter Healthcare Corporation, Edwards CVS Division, Santa Ana, CA.

Chapter 38

38-4, From Brooks, M., & Jenkins, M.P. (2008). Acute and chronic ischaemia of the limb. *Surgery 26*(1), 17-20; **38-8,** from Rutherford, R. (2005). *Vascular surgery* (6th ed.). Philadelphia: Saunders; **38-9,** from Forbes, C.D., & Jackson, W.F. (2003). *Colour atlas and text of clinical medicine* (3rd ed.). London: Mosby.

Chapter 40

40-1, From Huether S.E., McCance, K.L., Brashers, V.L., & Rote, N.S. (2008). *Understanding pathophysiology* (4th ed.). St. Louis: Mosby.

Chapter 42

42-3, From Feldman, M., Friedman, L., & Brandt, L. (2010). *Sleisenger and Fordtran's gastrointestinal and liver disease* (9th ed.). Philadelphia: Saunders; **42-4,** from Leonard, P.C. (2009). *Building a medical vocabulary: With Spanish translations* (7th ed.). St. Louis: Saunders; **42-7,** from DeWit, S.C. (2009). *Concepts and skills for nursing* (3rd ed.). St. Louis: Saunders.

Chapter 44

44-1, From Salvo, S.G. (2009). *Mosby's pathology for massage therapists* (2nd ed.). St. Louis: Mosby; **44-2, A,** from Mini-Mental State Examination © 1975, 1998, 2001 by MiniMental, LLC. All rights reserved. Published 2001 by Psychological Assessment Resources, Inc. May not be reproduced in whole or in part in any form or by any means without written permission of Psychological Assessment Resources, Inc., 16204 N. Florida Ave., Lutz, FL 33549; (800) 331-8378, www4.parinc.com/. **B,** from Seidel, H.M., Ball, J.W., Dains, J.E., Benedict, G.W. (2003). *Mosby's guide to physical examination* (5th ed.). St. Louis: Mosby.

Chapter 45

45-5, From Harkreader, H. (2007). *Fundamentals of nursing: Caring and clinical judgment* (3rd ed.). Philadelphia: Saunders.

Chapter 47

47-3, From Seidel, H.M., Ball, J.W., Dains, J.E., Flynn, J.A., Solomon, B.S., & Stewart, R.W. (2011). *Mosby's guide to physical examination* (7th ed.). St. Louis: Mosby; **B,** modified from Stein, H.A., Slatt, B.J., & Stein, R.M. (1994). *The ophthalmic assistant* (6th ed.). St. Louis: Mosby. **47-10,** from Flint, P.W., Haughey, B.H., Lund, V.J., Niparko, J.K., Richardson, M.A., Robbins, K.T., et al. (2010). *Cummings otolaryngology: Head & neck surgery* (5th ed.). Philadelphia: Mosby; courtesy Elekta, Inc.

Chapter 48

48-8, Courtesy the National Society to Prevent Blindness; **48-13,** courtesy Medtronic Ophthalmics, Minneapolis, MN.

Chapter 49

49-4, Courtesy John A. Costin, MD; **49-6,** from Patton, K.T., & Thibodeau, G.A. (2010). *Anatomy and physiology* (7th ed.). St. Louis: Mosby; **49-8,** from Workman, M.L., LaCharity, L., & Kruchko, S.C. (2011). *Understanding pharmacology.* St. Louis: Saunders; courtesy Pfizer, Inc., New York; **49-9,** from Workman, M.L., LaCharity, L., & Kruchko, S.C. (2011). *Understanding pharmacology.* St. Louis: Saunders.

Chapter 52

52-4, Modified from Jarvis, C. (2012). *Physical examination and health assessment* (6th ed.). St. Louis: Saunders.

Chapter 54

54-3, 54-4, 54-9, Courtesy Smith & Nephew, Inc., Orthopaedics Divisions, Memphis, TN; **54-5,** from Christensen, B.L.. & Kockrow, E.O. (2011). *Adult health nursing* (6th ed.). St. Louis: Mosby; **54-6,** from McCance, K.L., Huether, S.E., Brashers, V.L., & Rote, N.S. (2010). *Pathophysiology: The biologic basis for disease in adults and children* (6th ed.). St. Louis: Mosby; **54-13,** courtesy Zimmer, Inc., Warsaw, IN.

Chapter 56

56-1, From Friedman-Kien, A.E., & Cockerell, C.J. (1996). *Color atlas of AIDS* (2nd ed.). Philadelphia: Saunders.

Chapter 59

59-3, From Swartz, M. (2009). *Textbook of physical diagnosis: History and examination* (6th ed.). Philadelphia: Saunders; **59-7,** from Evans, S. (2009). *Surgical pitfalls.* Philadelphia: Saunders.

Chapter 60

60-3, B, From Perry, A.G., & Potter, P.A. (2006). *Clinical nursing skills & techniques* (6th ed.). St. Louis: Mosby; courtesy ConvaTec, Princeton, NJ; **60-5,** courtesy ConvaTec, a Bristol-Myers Squibb Company, Princeton, NJ.

Chapter 63

63-1, From U.S. Department of Agriculture, 2011, www.ChooseMyPlate.gov; **63-2,** ® Société des Produits Nestlé S.A., Vevey, Switzerland, Trademark Owners; **63-3, A,** from Lilley, L., Rainforth Collins, S., Harrington, S., & Snyder, J. (2011). *Pharmacology and the nursing process* (6th ed.). St. Louis: Mosby; **B,** from Harkreader, H. (2007). *Fundamentals of nursing* (3rd ed.). St. Louis: Saunders; courtesy C.R. Bard, Inc., Billerica, MA; **C,** from Harkreader, H. (2007). *Fundamentals of nursing* (3rd ed.). St. Louis: Saunders; courtesy Ballard Medical Products, Draper, UT.

Chapter 64

64-4, From Guyton, A., & Hall, J. (2006). *Textbook of medical physiology* (11th ed.). Philadelphia: Saunders.

Chapter 65

65-1, From Mendelhoff, A., & Smith, D.E. (Eds.). (1956). Acromegaly, diabetes, hypermetabolism, proteinuria, and heart failure. Clinical Pathological Conference, *American Journal of Medicine, 20,* 133; **65-2,** from Chabner, D.E. (2011). *The language of medicine* (9th ed.). St. Louis: Saunders; **65-3,** from Wilson J.D., Foster, D., Kronenberg, H., & Larsen, P.R. (1998). *Williams textbook of endocrinology* (9th ed.). Philadelphia: Saunders; courtesy Dr. H. Patrick Higgins; **65-4,** from Wenig B.M., Heffess, C.S., & Adair, C.F. (1997). *Atlas of endocrine pathology.* Philadelphia: Saunders.

Chapter 67

67-6, 67-8, Courtesy MiniMed, Inc., Northridge, CA; **67-7,** courtesy Becton, Dickinson and Company, Franklin Lakes, NJ; **67-9,** from Frykberg, R.G., Zgonis, T., Armstrong, D.G.,

Driver, V.R., Giurini, J.M., Kravitz, S.R., et al. (2006). Diabetic foot disorders: A clinical practice guideline—2006 revision. *The Journal of Foot and Ankle Surgery, 45*(5), S1-S66.

Chapter 68

68-10, Courtesy Verathon Corporation, Bothell, WA.

Chapter 69

69-1, A, Courtesy ConvaTec, A Bristol-Meyers Squibb Company, a Division of E.R. Squibb & Sons, Inc., Princeton, NJ; **69-2,** from Pollack, H.M. (2000). *Clinical urography* (2nd ed.). Philadelphia: Saunders; **69-3,** modified from Singal, R.K., & Denstedt, J.D. (1997). Contemporary management of ureteral stones. *The Urologic Clinics of North America, 24*(1), 59-70.

Chapter 70

70-2, From Kumar, V., Abbas, A., Fausto, N., & Aster, J. (2010). *Robbins and Cotran pathologic basis of disease* (8th ed.). Philadelphia: Saunders.

Chapter 71

71-1, Courtesy Kendall Company, Bothell, WA; **71-5,** courtesy GAMBRO Healthcare, Stockholm, Sweden; **71-10, A,** from Geary, D.F., & Schaefer, F. (2008). *Comprehensive pediatric nephrology.* Philadelphia: Mosby; **71-15,** courtesy Baxter International, Inc., Deerfield, IL.

Chapter 73

73-1, From Swartz, M.H. (2009). *Textbook of physical diagnosis: History and examination* (6th ed.). Philadelphia: Saunders; **73-2,** from Mansel, R., & Bundred, N. (1995). *Color atlas of breast disease.* St. Louis: Mosby; **73-3,** from Gallager, H.S., Leis, H.P. Jr., Snyderman, R.K., & Urban, J.A. (1978). *The breast.* St. Louis: Mosby.

Chapter 75

75-2, From American Urological Association Practice Guidelines Committee. (2003). Guideline on the management of benign prostatic hyperplasia (BPH). *Journal of Urology, 170*(2 Pt 1), 530-547; **75-6,** from Seidel H.M., Ball, J.W., Dains, J.E., Flynn, J.A., Solomon, B.S., & Stewart, R.W. (2011). *Mosby's guide to physical examination* (7th ed.). St. Louis: Mosby.

Chapter 76

76-1, 76-2, From Morse, S., Ballard, R., Holmes, K., & Moreland, A. (2003). *Atlas of sexually transmitted diseases and AIDS* (3rd ed.). Edinburgh: Mosby.

Page numbers followed by "f" indicate
figures, "t" indicate tables, and "b" indicate boxes.